SECOND EDITION

# TEXTBOOK OF PSYCHIATRY

for southern Africa

Edited by
Jonathan Burns • Louw Roos

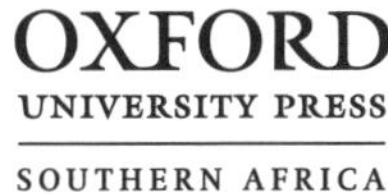

OXFORD
UNIVERSITY PRESS

Oxford University Press is a department of the University of Oxford.
It furthers the University's objective of excellence in research, scholarship,
and education by publishing worldwide. Oxford is a registered trade mark of
Oxford University Press in the UK and in certain other countries

Published in South Africa by
Oxford University Press Southern Africa (Pty) Limited

Vasco Boulevard, Goodwood, N1 City, P O Box 12119, Cape Town,
South Africa



Second edition published in 2016



**Textbook of Psychiatry for southern Africa**

ISBN 978 0 19 904632 4

Typeset in Palatino LT Std 9.5pt on 12pt
Printed on [insert paper quality e.g. acid-free paper]

**Acknowledgements**
Publisher: Lydia Reid
Project managers: Tanya Paulse /Lindsay-Jane Lücks
Copy editor: Hanneke Gagiano
Proof reader: Annette de Villiers and Gail Learmont
Indexer: Jeanne Cope
Designer: Shaun Andrews
Cover designer: Judith Cross
Illustrator: Craig Farham
Typesetter: Orchard Publishing
Printed and bound by: Shumani Mills Communications, Parow, Cape Town

SW60315

# Table of contents

# Contributors

**Prof. Colleen Adnams**
*Department of Psychiatry & Mental Health*
*University of Cape Town*

**Prof. Orlando Alonso Betancourt**
*Head of Department*
*Department of Psychiatry*
*Walter Sisulu University*

**Dr Laila Asmal**
*Department of Psychiatry*
*Stellenbosch University*

**Dr Manfred Böhmer**
*Department of Psychiatry*
*University of Pretoria*

**Dr Belinda Bruwer**
*Department of Psychiatry*
*Stellenbosch University*

**Prof. Jonathan Burns**
*Head of Department*
*Department of Psychiatry*
*University of KwaZulu-Natal*

**Dr Bonginkosi Chiliza**
*Department of Psychiatry*
*Stellenbosch University*

**Dr Franco Colin**
*Department of Psychiatry*
*University of Pretoria*

**Dr Giada del Fabro**
*Hyde Park*
*Johannesburg*

**Prof. Paul de Wet**
*Department of Psychiatry*
*University of Pretoria*

**Dr Ilse du Plessis**
*Department of Psychiatry*
*University of Pretoria*

**Dr Willem Esterhuysen**
*Department of Psychiatry*
*Walter Sisulu University*

**Dr Gerhard Grobler**
*Department of Psychiatry*
*University of Pretoria*

**Prof. Stoffel Grobler**
*Department of Psychiatry*
*Walter Sisulu University*

**Prof. Brian Harvey**
*Department of Pharmacology*
*North-West University*

**Prof. Yasmien Jeenah**
*Department of Psychiatry*
*Faculty of Health Sciences*
*University of Witwatersrand*

**Dr Khatija Jhazbhay**
*Department of Psychiatry*
*University of KwaZulu-Natal*

**Dr Greg Jonsson**
*Department of Psychiatry*
*Faculty of Health Sciences*
*University of Witwatersrand*

**Dr Gerhard Jordaan**
*Department of Psychiatry*
*Stellenbosch University*

**Dr Hester Jordaan**
*Fort England Hospital*
*Grahamstown*

**Prof. John Joska**
*Department of Psychiatry & Mental Health*
*University of Cape Town*

**Dr Enver Karim**
*Department of Psychiatry*
*University of KwaZulu-Natal*

**Dr Nadira Khamker**
*Department of Psychiatry*
*University of Pretoria*

**Dr Howard King**
*Department of Psychiatry*
*University of KwaZulu-Natal*

**Prof. Liezl Koen**
*Department of Psychiatry*
*Stellenbosch University*

**Dr Nastassja Koen**
*Department of Psychiatry & Mental Health*
*University of Cape Town*

**Dr Carla Kotzé**
*Department of Psychiatry*
*University of Pretoria*

**Prof. Christa Krüger**
*Department of Psychiatry*
*University of Pretoria*

**Prof. Angelo Lasich**
*Department of Psychiatry*
*University of KwaZulu-Natal*

**Dr Gian Lippi**
*Department of Psychiatry*
*University of Pretoria*

**Prof. Christine Lochner**
*Department of Psychiatry*
*Stellenbosch University*

**Dr Heidi Loffstadt**
*Department of Psychiatry*
*Walter Sisulu University*

**Dr Kagisho Maaroganye**
*Department of Psychiatry*
*University of Pretoria*

**Dr Thebe Madigoe**
*Department of Psychiatry*
*Faculty of Health Sciences*
*University of Witwatersrand*

**Dr Sibongile Mashaphu**
*Department of Psychiatry*
*University of KwaZulu-Natal*

**Dr Rethabile Mataboge**
*Department of Psychiatry*
*University of Pretoria*

**Prof. Yusuf Moosa**
*Department of Psychiatry*
*Faculty of Health Sciences*
*University of Witwatersrand*

**Dr Mashadi Motlana**
*Department of Psychiatry*
*Faculty of Health Sciences*
*University of Witwatersrand*

**Prof. Mo Nagdee**
*Department of Psychiatry*
*Walter Sisulu University*

**Prof. Richard Nichol**
*Department of Psychiatry*
*University of the Free State*

**Prof. Dana Niehaus**
*Department of Psychiatry*
*Stellenbosch University*

**Dr John Parker**
*Department of Psychiatry & Mental Health*
*University of Cape Town*

**Dr Saeeda Paruk**
*Department of Psychiatry*
*University of KwaZulu-Natal*

**Dr Jacobeth Mosidi Pooe**
*Department of Psychiatry*
*University of Pretoria*

**Dr Felix Potocnik**
*Department of Psychiatry*
*Stellenbosch University*

**Prof. Janus Pretorius**
*Head of Department*
*Department of Psychiatry*
*University of the Free State*

**Dr Suvira Ramlall**
*Department of Psychiatry*
*University of KwaZulu-Natal*

**Prof. Louw Roos**
*Head of Department*
*Department of Psychiatry*
*University of Pretoria*

**Dr Shamima Saloojee**
*Department of Psychiatry*
*University of KwaZulu-Natal*

**Prof. Soraya Seedat**
*Head of Department*
*Department of Psychiatry*
*Stellenbosch University*

**Dr Funeka B Sokudela**
*Department of Psychiatry*
*University of Pretoria*

**Prof. Dan Stein**
*Head of Department*
*Department of Psychiatry & Mental Health*
*University of Cape Town*

**Prof. Ugasvaree Subramaney**
*Department of Psychiatry*
*Faculty of Health Sciences*
*University of Witwatersrand*

**Prof. Christopher Szabo**
*Head of Department*
*Department of Psychiatry*
*Faculty of Health Sciences*
*University of Witwatersrand*

**Prof. Debbie van der Westhuizen**
*Department of Psychiatry*
*University of Pretoria*

**Dr Surita van Heerden**
*Department of Psychiatry & Mental Health*
*University of Cape Town*

**Prof. Werdie van Staden**
*Department of Psychiatry*
*University of Pretoria*

**Dr Naseema Vawda**
*Department of Behavioural Medicine*
*University of KwaZulu-Natal*

**Dr Chris Verster**
*Department of Psychiatry*
*Stellenbosch University*

**Dr Conrad Visser**
*Parktown*
*Johannesburg*

**Prof. James Warwick**
*Department of Medical Imaging and Clinical Oncology*
*Stellenbosch University*

**Prof. Elizabeth Weiss**
*Head of Department*
*Department of Psychiatry*
*University of Limpopo*

**Dr Zukiswa Zingela**
*Department of Psychiatry*
*Walter Sisulu University*

# Preface

Fourteen years have passed since the publication of the 1st edition of the *Textbook of Psychiatry for southern Africa*. We would like to thank the editors of the 1st edition who laid the foundation for this publication: Professors Brian Robertson, Cliff Allwood and Carlo Gagiano.

Research focus, clinical practice and the classification of psychiatric disorders have changed since the 1st edition, resulting in a need for a completely revised and updated textbook which reflects current research evidence in the field, the Mental Health Care Act (2002) as well as the DSM-5 psychiatric classification system. We believe this substantially restructured and expanded 2nd edition, with an additional ten new chapters, will be an indispensable resource within and outside the mental health field in southern Africa.

Textbooks are important repositories of knowledge and guidance. The best textbooks in our view should provide the reader with all of the following attributes: complete and comprehensive coverage of the field, the strongest available evidence, knowledge that is relevant and contextualised, consistency in structure with appropriate emphasis of core topics, clear presentation of the material that is easy to access, and provision of special features (such as case studies) to enhance learning. In this 2nd edition we have attempted to include all these attributes in providing a solid text for any student or practitioner of mental health care within the southern African context.

This project started because we (and others) felt that there was a need for an up-to-date textbook on psychiatry and mental health that is the core reference resource for both the student and health professional studying or working in southern Africa. To achieve this objective, the book needed to be written by local authors representing a range of disciplines and a range of clinical, research and academic experience. Furthermore, we wanted to make this a truly South African book with contributions from all regions of the country. The final product is indeed widely representative of psychiatry and mental health as it is taught, researched and practiced in South Africa today. Sixty-three experts from disciplines such as Psychiatry, Psychology, Radiology and Pharmacology from ten academic institutions and private practice participated in the restructured and expanded 2nd edition. We were fortunate to identify enthusiastic authors to update chapters with the latest scientific findings in the different topics, adding a southern African flavour to the clinical management and approach to the disorders.

This 2nd edition is completely restructured and revised (and in almost all cases rewritten) and has been expanded from the 30 chapters of the 1st edition to its current content of 40 chapters. It is divided into six sections as follows:

- **Section 1** comprises chapters on the background history and evolution of classification systems in psychiatry that provide a basis for conceptualising psychiatric disorders.
- **Section 2** focuses on the causes of psychiatric disorders, presenting detailed chapters on current epidemiological and genetic approaches in the field as well as a comprehensive overview of the neurobiological, psychosocial and cultural aspects of mental health and illness.
- **Section 3** covers the assessment of individuals with mental disorders, including a comprehensive approach to clinical evaluation, the investigation of mental disorders, as well as the very recent move towards a truly person-centered approach to clinical practice.
- **Section 4** consists of 16 chapters, each focused on a major group of psychiatric disorders, providing a complete overview of all conditions affecting adults. Important for the reader to note is the fact that we have not followed the new (life course) approach of DSM-5, where conditions specific to children, adolescents or the elderly are included within the major

disorder chapters. Thus, for example, the childhood anxiety disorder, reactive attachment disorder, is not included in the chapter in this section on adult anxiety disorders (Chapter 14), but is rather included in the next section in a chapter dealing with psychiatry in the young child (Chapter 27). Other differences in approach that we decided to adopt for the sake of coherence and clinical utility are:

- The chapter on cognitive disorders covers issues of classification, clinical approach and management of the major cognitive syndromes of delirium and dementia, but the specific details of individual diseases causing these syndromes (e.g. epilepsy, HIV, Alzheimer's disease) are covered in special topic chapters in the next section (e.g. chapters on neuropsychiatry, HIV and psychogeriatrics).
- Chapter 15 represents what we feel is a logical approach to a range of acute psychiatric disorders/reactions that share the fact that they occur in response to stressful or adverse life events.
- Our handling of the often overlapping conditions and disorders that comprise the OCD-spectrum, somatoform, dissociative and impulse-control disorders is based on the classification contained in DSM-5.
- Problems of substance use and addiction are split between two chapters, the first covering alcohol use and its disorders and the second covering all other substances of use and abuse as well as the addiction syndrome known as gambling disorder.
- Finally, we decided for ease of use to group all conditions and disorders related to sexual dysfunction, preference and identity together in a single chapter. Importantly, this reflects an editorial strategy, not an assumption that these various very different phenomena share anything in common.

▸ **Section 5** comprises ten chapters focused on topics that we feel are of special importance in the study of and practice of psychiatry in the current era. These chapters focus on special populations (e.g. women, children and adolescents, those with intellectual disability, and the elderly), special situations and contexts (e.g. the overlaps between psychiatry and medicine, neuropsychiatry and HIV, as well as the problems of suicide and management of the aggressive patient), and finally special issues (including the legal and ethical aspects of psychiatry).

▸ Finally, **Section 6** covers all the aspects of management of psychiatric disorders, with detailed chapters on pharmacological and other physical treatments (e.g. ECT), psychological treatments, social interventions, the broader approach to public mental health and systems development, and lastly the critically important issue of addressing the stigma that surrounds those living with psychiatric disorders.

The textbook's approach to holistic management for all psychiatric conditions and presentations that is relevant to the southern African context, is based on the best current evidence from both research and clinical practice. It will serve the needs of diverse professional groups working and studying in the field of psychiatry and mental health in southern Africa, including medical students, registrars in Psychiatry, undergraduate and postgraduate students in other mental health disciplines including Nursing, Psychology, Occupational Therapy, Social Work, Pharmacy, Family Medicine, and Public Health, among others.

Our aim with this book is to assist professionals in this field to work competently and deliver quality care to their patients. We believe that this publication will assist in destigmatising psychiatry and promoting the well-being of psychiatric patients who are often neglected in the health-care system.

# PART 1

# Conceptualising psychiatric disorders

CHAPTER

# 1 A brief history of psychiatry

Werdie van Staden

## 1.1 Introduction

This chapter highlights the tendency in history to both oversimplify mental illness and to respond to mental illness (and the study thereof) with **value judgements**. This history may be helpful when we reflect on current and future attitudes, understandings and practices, and thereby guard against oversimplifications that deny the inherent complexities of mental illnesses. It may also be helpful as we scrutinise value judgements and attempt to account for them.

An oversimplification has been to judge mental illness in predominantly naturalistic or moral terms, and to even invoke tensions between these terms. For example, some consider mental illness as merely or predominantly a disease of the brain, while others consider mental illness in the domain of incantations or (bad) choices for which the mentally ill person is to be blamed (Bolton, 2008).

The German historian of psychiatry, Paul Hoff, showed that the worst abuses of psychiatry occur, not through deliberate malpractice, but through psychiatry, in any local context, becoming fixed on and being reduced to what he described as a single-message mythology (Hoff, 2005). In the name of such mythologies, oversimplifications and value judgements have served to stigmatise, patronise or degrade psychiatric patients and psychiatrists. These mythologies may have been underpinned by the emotional responses and/or desperation that psychiatric disorders invoke in some.

In contrast, history has also shown that much sophistication is required to understand the involvement of the brain (one of the most complex organs in the body) in relation to mental illness. Added to this is the values complexity of disease concepts in general and the added values complexity, particularly, entailed in mental illness concepts. It is easy to understand why the term 'madness' has become pejorative in certain contexts, even when used non-pejoratively. 'He got mad at me,' for example, may refer to the other person's anger and not his mental health.

The value-laden concept of 'madness' precedes the term 'psychiatry,' which was coined in 1808 from the Greek words *psyche* (mind) and *iatros* (physician) (Marneros, 2008). The history of psychiatry may be traced back to that of madness, and goes back to ancient times. Ancient history underscores the values complexity contained in considerations of madness and mental illness, and is particularly evident in texts on morals and morality.

## 1.2 Madness in ancient and classical times

The earliest Biblical reference to madness is in Deuteronomy 28:28 (New International Version, 1984) where it is listed as one of the curses of disobedience – clearly expressing a moral aspect. But note also that it is listed in close proximity to tumours, skin conditions and blindness, which may suggest a naturalistic view of madness. Another reference is found in 1 Samuel 21. The young David, not yet king of Israel, had been brought before the Philistine king, Achish, as the expected future king of Israel when David 'changed his behaviour before them, and feigned himself mad in their hands, and made marks on the doors of the gate, and let his spittle fall down upon his beard'. This convinced Achish that David was not fit to be a king and David subsequently escaped. Madness is thus presented as an event that is not unusual, and one that renders a person incapable of carrying responsibility, for example that required of a king.

The view that the incapacitating effects of mental illness may serve as a defence or legitimate excuse is still maintained today (see Chapter 35: Legal and ethical aspects of mental health). The incapacitating effect of mental illness is also seen in secular Greek poetry of about 700 years BC (Robinson, 1996). In Homer's epic poem, the Iliad, King Agamemnon seeks an excuse for his actions that led to the Trojan war: 'It was not that I did it… Zeus and Fate, the erinys that walk in the darkness struck me mad when we were assembled on the day that I took from Achilles the prize that had been awarded him…' (Robinson, 1996). Also, in Book IV of Homer's *Odyssey*, Helen excuses her original abandonment of home as 'the madness that Aphrodite bestowed when she led me there' (Robinson, 1996).

Hippocrates considered madness to be underpinned by physiological abnormalities. When he came across Democritus dissecting animals to find the cause of madness and melancholy, Hippocrates praised Democritus for doing so (Burton, 1881). Hippocrates, like the physicians of his time, subscribed to the theory of the 'harmony of humours' in their understanding of mental disorder. (The humours are blood, phlegm, yellow bile and black bile.) This naturalistic approach contrasts with Plato's moral concept of mental disorder. In *The Republic* he describes a 'harmony of the soul' where reason, appetite and temper are the constituents of the soul (Plato, 2003).

The Roman stoics, like Cicero (106 BC–43 BC) also ascribed to the idea of harmony and balance of the Greeks (Nordenfelt, 1997). This idea has striking similarities with modern-day concepts of 'homeostasis' and 'neurotransmitter imbalances'. Although he ascribed these to naturalistic premises, the core value driving Cicero's classification of mental perturbations was that emotional indifference would be best – emotions should be no more than mild, and are permissible only if conducive to a virtuous life.

## 1.3 The Middle Ages and the Renaissance

During the early Middle Ages the naturalistic view of mental disorder taken by Hippocrates and Galen matched well with similar views in the Arab world (Fulford *et al.*, 2006). Religious value judgements are captured in the Quran's expression of being healthy, for which balance is required among the *ruh* (soul), the *qalb* (connection between the soul and the body), the *aql* (**intellect**) and the *nafs* (**drives** or desires) merging through the *dahmeer* (consciousness). An imbalance results accordingly in physical, mental and/or spiritual illness (Bulbulia and Laher, 2013).

In the European world, madness was predominantly ascribed to being possessed by demons – a version of Hoff's single-message mythology. Being possessed by demons had initially not been considered reason for religious persecution. This changed in the late Middle Ages when the Catholic Church wanted to eradicate heretics and possession was taken as an indication of heresy and witchcraft, leading to many mentally ill people being tried as witches (Fulford *et al.*, 2006).

The late medieval period also saw a revival of Aristotelian naturalistic doctrines. St Thomas Aquinas, for example, distinguished between congenital and non-congenital mental disorder. He considered the insane as lacking in rationality and hence as lacking **capacity** for sin (Fulford *et al.*, 2006). The natural scientists of the time participated in the witch hunts by providing 'expert' evidence whereby a third nipple or pain-insensitive areas would be signs of being a witch. This is also seen in *Malleus Maleficarum* (Kramer and Sprenger, 1996), a widely read textbook that was regarded as a respected authority on witchcraft. The diligence of the authors and their rigorous and meticulous approach, strike even the contemporary reader. The (quasi) scientific evidence to which the Malleus refers, is the inability of a person accused of being a witch to shed tears – a 'most certain' sign of someone being a witch:

> 'If he wishes to find out whether she is endowed with a witch's power of preserving silence, let him take note whether she is able to shed tears when standing in his presence, or when being tortured. For we are taught both by the words of worthy men of old and by our own experience that this is a most certain sign, and it has been found that even if she be urged and exhorted by solemn conjurations to shed tears, if she be a witch she will not be able to weep: although she will assume a tearful aspect and smear her cheeks and eyes with spittle to make it appear that she is weeping; wherefore she must be closely watched by the attendants.'

It is clear from witch hunts that values, in particular a single-message mythology, determined the way signs were interpreted (Fulford *et al.*, 2006). This prompts the question on the values that determine our contemporary interpretations of illness and specifically mental illness, which will be discussed in the last section of this chapter.

The late medieval period also saw the emergence of built institutions for the care for the mentally ill. The first institutions were founded in Baghdad and Cairo early and late in the ninth century respectively (Bulbulia and Laher, 2013). The Maudsley and Bethlem hospitals, as they are known today, were founded in London in 1403. Still in operation today, they have become known internationally for the psychiatric research conducted there (Shorter, 1997).

## 1.4 The great confinement

The emergence of built institutions for specifically the mentally ill gained much momentum from the late medieval period to well into the 20th century. More recently, institutions have been defined more in terms of services and communities rather than a geographical site and built premises. All these changes have been driven by the societal values of the time.

During the early 17th century, religious communities in Europe were charged with the humane care of the mentally ill. They founded boarding houses and many private and public madhouses appeared. These were intended to offer some form of treatment in a caring environment, often with the involvement of a physician or a physician-superintendent. King Louis VIV of France introduced public hospitals for the mentally ill in 1656. In 1713, the Bethel Hospital was opened in Norwich, England, meeting the then requirements for a state-of-the-art asylum. Before 1800, there were only two hospitals for the mentally ill in the USA: the Pennsylvania Hospital (established in 1752) and the New York Hospital that opened in 1791 (Shorter, 1997).

Much of treatment provided involved physical restraint and punitive procedures. One should not assume this treatment was maliciously intended. Overcrowding led to severe neglect and appalling conditions. Some saw a business opportunity and an unscrupulous trade in madness arose in the midst of decreasing resources for a tide of new admissions of allegedly mad people, some of whom were not, in fact, ill (Parry-Jones, 1972).

This evoked a strong reaction by the end of the 18th century, with people calling for a more humanitarian approach. At least in England, this might have been influenced by the **recovery** of King George III from a mental disorder in 1789, by which the public could see mental illness as something that can be treated and cured (Elkes and Thorpe, 1967). A Quaker, William Tuke, established The Retreat in England and offered what was called moral therapy in a more homely environment, which inspired similar institutions across the world. In Paris at the Salpêtrière and Bicêtre Hospitals, Phillipe Pinel and Jean Ettienne Dominique Esquirol had decided to 'throw away the chains' (Shorter, 1997; Fulford, 2006). The next century saw many similar institutions being founded. These asylums, as they were usually called, were often situated in a garden or park-like setting, for the theory was that fresh air, pleasant and beautiful surroundings and useful occupation would aid recovery.

In the Cape of the Good Hope, the Dutch East India Company made provision for settlers and the passing sailors and soldiers who fell mentally ill, and a primitive structure was built adjacent to Van Riebeeck's first fort. It was enlarged in 1674 but owing to growing needs had to be replaced in 1699 by a new hospital adjacent to the Company Gardens. The hospital built in 1772 near the Company Gardens also became overcrowded and patients were transferred to the nearby Slave Lodge. The Somerset Hospital, founded in 1818 by the British colonial government, also provided some beds for those who were called lunatics at the time (Gillis, 2012).

Overcrowding at Somerset Hospital led to the transfer of mentally ill patients to Robben Island in 1836. It had been a convict station but became the place for 'lepers, lunatics and the chronically ill' (Gillis, 2012). The inmates' living conditions were appalling: 'It was quite usual to find them kept in dark insanitary cells, filthy, covered in festering sores and chained to iron rings.' The buildings were 'decrepit, overcrowded and verminous'. This situation changed upon the appointment of Dr JC Minto who improved living conditions and instituted occupations for patients, such as making mats and baskets. He advocated kindness and ordered that mechanical restraint should only be used once seclusion had failed. Bromides were used to settle **agitation**, and in excess might well have induced psychotic symptoms. So-called toxins were evacuated with calomel, which contained mercury and presumably caused serious adverse effects. Psychiatric facilities at Robben Island closed in 1920 (Gillis, 2012).

As was the case in Europe, the USA and many other places in the world, several psychiatric hospitals were built towards the end of the 19th century in South Africa. Under British rule, hospitals conformed more or less to British specifications for asylums. They include Fort England Hospital in Grahamstown (built in 1876), Townhill Hospital in Pietermaritzburg (1882), Oranje Hospital in Bloemfontein (1883), Kowie Hospital in Port Alfred (1889), Valkenberg Hospital in Cape Town (1891), Weskoppies Hospital in Pretoria (1892),and Fort Beaufort in the Eastern Cape (1897) (Gillis, 2012; Sukeri *et al.*, 2014).

All these new facilities, in South Africa and elsewhere, could not provide for a tide of admissions that continued till the middle of the 20th century. By 1950, for example, the Georgia State Sanatorium in the USA had 10 000 beds (Shorter, 1997). Similarly in South Africa, patient populations ranged from 1 000 to 2 000 in some of the above-mentioned hospitals.

As in the 18th century, overcrowding shifted emphasis from treatment to custodial care at these institutions. This changed gradually from the middle of the 20th century onwards, owing to programmes towards de-institutionalisation and developing community care (Shorter, 1997). These contemporary programmes have been value-driven by which the ill effects of institutionalisation and the good and desirable effects of community care had been argued, researched and advocated. Many asylums were closed down – although less so in South Africa – and available dedicated hospital beds have been reduced. In addition to the values driving these changes, the discovery and widespread use of more effective treatments also made further hospitalisation of recovered or partially recovered patients redundant. Some asylums, although now called hospitals, usually situated outside the town, were replaced with smaller, dedicated facilities inside town. Provisions were also made for care inside or next to general hospitals. Progressively, 'psychiatric units' have become and have been referred to as units of psychiatric services and research, more so than being a reference to buildings.

## 1.5 Biological and psychological differentiation

Other than the 'great confinement', the 19th century saw the differentiation of the mental health field into domains of biology and psychology. The term 'psychiatry' was coined in 1808 for designating medically qualified specialists. Many of these specialists advocated for the naturalistic nature of mental disorder, especially with advances in knowledge about brain structures and functions. By the 1860s, for example, Wilhelm Griessinger, professor of psychiatry in Berlin, proffered the aphorism 'Geisteskrankheiten sind Gehirnkrankheiten' (mental illnesses are brain illnesses) (Jaspers, 1946).

This was a time of optimism regarding advances in the study and treatment of mental illnesses and particularly psychoses. Reasons for the optimism stemmed from novel findings in neurology (Fulford *et al.*, 2006). Paul Broca discovered the area in the frontal lobe associated with speech problems in the absence of problems with understanding (referred to today as a motor aphasia). Carl Wernicke found an association between an abnormality in the posterior temporal lobe of the brain and problems of understanding (referred to today as a receptive aphasia). In 1880, Paul Flechsig produced a map of the brain, indicating areas responsible for certain psychological functions. Eduard Halle demonstrated that the brain responds to electric stimulation.

At the same time, psychology emerged as a new discipline, marked by the first textbook of psychology. It was published in 1874 by Wilhelm Wundt, a professor of philosophy at the University of Heidelberg in Germany (Fancher, 1979). In Vienna, Austria, Sigmund Freud resigned as lecturer of neuropathology in 1886 and followed the example of the French neurologist, Charcot, in studying the effects of hypnosis on patients with **conversion** disorder (Gay, 2006). From that, he developed psychoanalysis as a research and a treatment modality and published his findings before the turn of the century.

A build-up of optimism, new discoveries and new knowledge marked the turn of the century. The University of Heidelberg played a pivotal role in the history of psychiatry at the time. In addition to Wilhelm Wundt, Franz Nissl, Emil Kraepelin and Karl Jaspers influenced psychiatry profoundly.

Nissl developed stains by which nerve cells structures could be seen histologically. This made it possible for him and Alois Alzheimer to describe changes in the brain and their distinctive features in respectively Alzheimer's **dementia** and what was called general paralysis of the insane (GPI). This paved the way for Noguchi and Moore to demonstrate, in 1913, the existence of Treponema pallidum in the brain tissue of patients who suffered from GPI. This was an important event: for the first time a clear infective cause was found for psychiatric symptoms (Fulford *et al.*, 2006). There was much optimism for more such discoveries to follow, but the causation of mental disorders proved to be much more complex.

Kraepelin published his *Lehrbuch* (textbook) in 1915. In the midst of a proliferation of diagnostic classifications based on theories of the (potential) causes of mental disorder, he brought order to a situation in which just about every professor of psychiatry had his own classification (Kendell, 1975). Kraepelin first studied histology under Flechsig in Leipzig, but apparently had an eye problem and found it difficult to work with microscopes. Wundt rescued him and was instrumental in his appointment at Heidelberg in 1890, the place where Nissl was at the cutting edge of neuro-histology, and Jaspers was expert on clinically sophisticated and philosophically informed nuances of psychiatric symptomatology. Kraepelin's classification still prevails to some degree in current classifications, for example, the distinction between bipolar disorder and dementia praecox. (Dementia praecox was renamed 'schizophrenia' by Eugen Bleuler in 1912.)

Jaspers joined Nissl's department in 1908 as a young psychiatrist. Nissl commissioned him to write a textbook of psychiatry, which appeared in 1913. This was a seminal and voluminous piece of work, titled *Allgemeine Psychopathologie*, and contained detailed descriptions and examples of psychiatric symptoms and profound considerations of the nature and possibility of knowledge in psychiatry (Jaspers, 1946). Some of his symptomatological distinctions, informed by the philosophy of Immanuel Kant among others, remain in psychiatric use today. For example, the distinction between the form and the content of thoughts and experiences is seen in the mental status examination (see Chapter 7: Clinical assessment in psychiatry).

In an environment with much expectation for the brain sciences to make discoveries, Jaspers was the sceptical gadfly, much like Socrates had been two thousand year before. Jaspers was not killed for this as Socrates had been, but was seemingly sidelined and had to take up a position in the department of philosophy at Heidelberg University. His scepticism was well-founded and turned out spot-on. He said, 'these anatomical constructions, became quite fantastic (e.g., Meynert, Wernicke) and have rightly been called"Brain Mythologies"'(Jaspers, 1946). He warned against the over-simplification of mental disorders by mere causal explanations. He further argued for an account of the meaning of patient experiences in mental disorder. Thus, both *Erklärung* (explanation) and *Verstehen* (understanding) are required. For example, a particular behaviour (e.g. eating) may have both a cause (fasting) and a purpose or reason (to experience delight).

Jasper's scepticism turned out as justified insofar as he had spotted the complexities of mental disorder. The optimism for biological discoveries was not met with much in terms of findings for the next 50 years or so. Instead, for much of the first half of the 20th century, Freud's psychoanalytic theory and the related ideas of his contemporaries and others gained much popularity and informed the dominant treatment modality in psychiatry, especially in the USA and France. It was, in Hoff's terms, the new single-message mythology. Psychoanalysis was offered as a treatment for just about anything distressing, thereby again oversimplifying and reducing the complexities of mental disorders, notwithstanding the worth it has within an appropriately defined scope.

The first half of the 20th century also saw rather desperate treatments of another kind, called physical therapies, and which included barbiturate narcoses, insulin comas, chemically induced convulsions and frontal lobotomies (Shorter, 1997). The use of frontal lobotomies soared: by 1951, no fewer than 18 608 had been performed in the USA since its introduction in 1936. Doing frontal lobotomies was a controversial intervention at the time within psychiatry, mainly for being used indiscriminately by some. Again, one may see the dangers of a single-message mythology to which Hoff alluded. Electroconvulsive treatment (ECT) was also introduced, and, despite its unequivocal **efficacy** for specific disorders, at least some of the negative social sentiments about it arose owing to its use for almost any mental disorder at the time.

The increase in treatment options for mental disorders from the middle of the 20th century onward facilitated the reaction against the inadequacies of psychoanalytic types of **psychotherapy**. Most notably, clinical psychopharmacology made great advances in the 1950s with the discovery of the effects of lithium carbonate on **mania**, chlorpromazine on schizophrenia, and imipramine on depressive illness. Furthermore, the neurotransmitters serotonin and dopamine in the mammalian brain were discovered in the same decade (Shorter, 1997). Several other medications saw the light in subsequent decades.

## 1.6 Growth and role changes in the last three decades

Psychiatry has shown vast growth during the last three decades in many respects: knowledge, research, practice, number of psychiatrists, the establishment of the subspecialties of child and adolescent psychiatry, old-age psychiatry, neuro- and liaison psychiatry, forensic psychiatry, psychiatry of learning and intellectual **disability**, psychotherapy in psychiatry, **addictions** psychiatry, etc. This growth enabled significant shifts in psychiatry's role and its relation with people, its understanding of health and illness complexities, other disciplines and medical specialties.

The recent growth in psychiatry has been propelled, at least in part, by the vast growth and yield from the neurosciences (Van Staden and Fulford, 2007). The complexities have transpired in the form of interacting synaptogenesis, **neurogenesis**, neurotransmitters, neuroreceptors, receptor regulation, cellular messaging across the cell membrane, and **gene expression** as influenced by endocrine, immune, and an array of bodily factors, medications and other substances. The complexities of the genetics of psychiatric disorders called for progress from genealogical inheritance studies to genomic sequencing, linkage studies, world-wide genomic studies, and expansion to include social factors in **epigenetic** studies. Brain imaging has developed into the mapping of brain functions in addition to the structural associations with psychiatric disorders. Research on new compounds for psychiatric disorders has also boomed, with methodologies for establishing their safety as well as efficacy for specific disorders being progressively refined.

A turning point for refinement in clinical psychiatry was brought about by the publication in 1980 of the third edition of the *Diagnostic and Statistical Manual of Mental Disorders* (DSM-III) that contained detailed criteria for the **diagnosis** of the various psychiatric disorders. The DSM-III, its revision in 1987, and the subsequent fourth edition in 1994, brought **reliability** of diagnoses – reliability here means internal consistency of diagnostic criteria and the extent of agreement among psychiatrists that a specific disorder would apply in a given case. More reliability of diagnoses was met concordantly with more specific research and treatment options (American Psychiatric Association, 2013).

The developments in diagnosis, treatment and neurosciences, notwithstanding their successes, rekindled the quest for **biomarkers** for which there had been so much optimism a century ago. The discovery of more biomarkers for mental disorders will certainly open new doors for psychiatry. In the quest for biomarkers (and even in their finding) lurk, in Hoff's terms, a single-message mythology by which the complexity of psychiatric diagnosis would be simple and free of values. However, values in diagnosis are inevitable (Fulford, 1989; Sadler, 2005).

Biomarkers may be valued legitimately in different and even opposing ways. For example, a biomarker may be taken as proof that a mental disorder is not someone's own doing – thus a valid exoneration. Against that, it has been some consolation for many sufferers of mental disorder that they can do something about their disorder: much of psychotherapy and the recovery movement is premised on that (Bracken and Thomas, 2013).

The biomarker single-message mythology, furthermore, had people hoping in the run-up to the publication of the DSM-5 in 2013 that the classification would be based on (genetic) causes. Some even argued that the scientific **validity** of a classification would hinge on it being structured by causes (Kendell and Jablensky, 2003). An example that exposes these expectations as a single-message mythology is that, by that criterion, even the periodic table of the elements in chemistry would fail to be scientifically valid, for it is not causally defined but by the number of protons of each element.

Psychiatric diagnosis is a complex matter – even with biomarkers (Bolton, 2013). For example, delirium, for which there are several biomarkers, is often missed in general hospitals. Causes of psychiatric disorders are often multifactorial, where some are contributory and others necessary. Many factors that appear to be causal may also be the effects of mental disorder. Causation of mental disorders is complex, and in addition there is the role that reasons and purposes play in the emergence of at least some mental disorders, and to which Jaspers alluded a century ago.

Through the history of and the growth in psychiatry, contemporary psychiatry and medicine in general have come to appreciate these complexities (Van Staden, 2010; Van Staden, 2006; Van Staden and Fulford, 2007). Conceptual work done during the last three decades has demonstrated that values not only permeate psychiatry, but also underpin the concepts of illness and disease generally (Fulford, 1989; Sadler, 2005). For example, a blood level of sodium of 105 mmol/ℓ would be of no concern were it not for the fact that it lies outside the values that are compatible with sustained life. Moreover, by generating more choices scientific advances do not resolve value complexity but increase it (Fulford and Van Staden, 2013).

An appreciation of the complexities in psychiatry has led to gradual changes in the role of psychiatry during the last three decades (Fulford and Van Staden, 2013). In relation to patients, a person- and people-centred approach has been developed whereby patients – being the experts by experience – take an active role in psychiatric diagnosis, treatment and research as partners to practitioners who are experts by training (Mezzich *et al.*, 2012; Van Staden, 2013; Bracken and Thomas, 2013). In relation to society, psychiatric patients and psychiatrists have become less stigmatised and psychiatry has seemingly become a more popular speciality (Jury and Del Fabbro, 2014). The complexities in psychiatry have been recognised as such, rather than mistakenly judged as deficiencies (Fulford *et al.*, 2005). Increasingly, psychiatry has espoused a pluralistic view, rather than a single-message mythology, of the multitude of factors that are involved in the diagnosis and treatment of psychiatric disorders. These factors are various: social, societal, personal, interpersonal, psychological, environmental, biological, spiritual, religious, cultural, ethical and professional.

The last three decades have also seen a change of roles in relation to other disciplines. Psychiatry has been increasingly positioned to contribute to other medical disciplines in knowledge and skills (Van Staden, 2012), including:

- sophisticated interpersonal skills (training) for dealing with the increasing complexities in medicine
- **social determinants of health**
- a **person-centred** and people-centred approach
- understanding people in a world of increasing diversity of values
- the complexities of diagnosis and treatment that are usually intensified, rather than resolved, by the discovery of a biomarker, owing to the diagnostic and therapeutic choices afforded by such a discovery
- how humanities may serve as an important resource in dealing with people in their diversity
- practical integration of disparate contributory sciences
- the perils of idealising (or devaluing) either the biological or psychosocial aspects of illness
- socio-political influence (good and bad) in health care
- methodological research rigour (for example, when placebo response rates are high)
- those aspects of medicine that are related more to art than science, which are becoming increasingly challenging, as evident in the surge of health ethics during the last few decades
- complexities of the concepts of health and illness.

## Conclusion

The history of psychiatry reveals the scientific and the values complexities in social and professional responses to the demands brought about by psychiatric disorders. The future of psychiatry will mark how much has been learned in averting alluring oversimplifications and a single-message mythology, and how well will continuous scrutiny and an account of the value judgements that drive pursuits in, and responses to, psychiatry be achieved.

# References


American Psychiatric Association (2013) *Diagnostic and Statistical Manual of Mental Disorders* (5th edition). Arlington, VA: American Psychiatric Association

Bible: New International Version (1984). Grand Rapids: Zondervan

Bolton D (2008) *What is a Mental Disorder? An Essay in Philosophy, Science and Values*. Oxford: Oxford University Press

Bolton D (2013) What is mental illness? In: KWM Fulford, M Davies, RGT Gipps, G Graham, JZ Sadler, G Stanghellini, T Thornton (Eds) *Oxford Handbook of Philosophy and Psychiatry*. Oxford: Oxford University Press

Bracken, P., Thomas P (2013). Challenges to modernist identity of psychiatry: User empowerment and recovery. In Fulford KWM, Davies M, Gipps RGT, Graham G,

Sadler JZ, Stanghellini G, Thornton T (Eds). *Oxford Handbook of Philosophy and Psychiatry*. Oxford: Oxford University Press

Bulbulia T, Laher S (2013) Exploring the role of Islam in perceptions of mental illness in a sample of Muslim psychiatrists based in Johannesburg. *South African Journal of Psychiatry* 19(2): 52–54

Burton R (1881) *The Anatomy of Melancholy*. London: Chatto and Windus

Elkes A, Thorpe JG (1967) *A Summary of Psychiatry*. London: Faber and Faber

Fancher RE (1979) *Pioneers of Psychology*. New York: Norton

Fulford KWM (1989) *Moral Theory and Medical Practice*. Cambridge: Cambridge University Press

Fulford KWM, Broome M, Stanghellini G (2005) Looking with both eyes open: Fact and value in psychiatric diagnosis. *World Psychiatry* 4: 78–86

Fulford KWM, Thornton T, Graham G (2006) *Oxford Textbook of Philosophy and Psychiatry*. Oxford: Oxford University Press

Fulford KWM, Van Staden CW (2013) Values-based practice: Topsy-turvy take-home messages from ordinary language philosophy (and a few next steps). In: Fulford KWM, Davies M, Gipps RGT, Graham G, Sadler JZ, Stanghellini G, Thornton T (Eds). *Oxford Handbook of Philosophy and Psychiatry*. Oxford: Oxford University Press

Gay P (2006) *Freud: a life for our time*. New York: W.W. Norton

Gillis L (2012) The historical development of psychiatry in South Africa since 1652. *South African Journal of Psychiatry* 18(3): 78–82

Hoff P (2005) Die psychopathologische Perspektive. In: M Bormuth, U Wiesing (Eds). *Ethische Aspekte der Forschung in Psychiatrie und Psychotherapie*. Cologne: Deutscher Ärzte-Verlag

Jaspers K (1946) *Allgemeine Psychopathologie*, 4th ed. Berlin: Springer

Jury KL, Del Fabbro G (2014) The attitudes of doctors in South African teaching hospitals towards mental illness and psychiatry (Abstract). *South African Journal of Psychiatry* (3): 101

Kendell R, Jablensky A (2003) Distinguishing between the validity and utility of psychiatric diagnoses. *American Journal of Psychiatry* 160: 4–12

Kendell RE (1975) *The Role of Diagnosis in Psychiatry*. Oxford: Blackwell Scientific Publications

Kramer H, Sprenger J (1996) *Malleus Maleficarum*. London: Bracken Books

Marneros A (2008) Psychiatry's 200th birthday. *The British Journal of Psychiatry* 193: 1–3

Mezzich JE, Miles A, Snaedal J, van Weel C, Botbol M, Salloum I, Van Lerberghe W (2012) The fourth Geneva conference on person-centered medicine: articulating person-centered medicine and people-centered public health. *International Journal of Person-Centered Medicine* 2: 1–5

Nordenfelt L (1997) The stoic conception of mental disorder: The case of Cicero. *Philosophy, Psychiatry and Psychology* 4: 285–291

Parry-Jones W (1972) *The Trade in Lunacy*. London: Routledge and Kegan Paul

Plato (2003) *The Republic*. Harmondsworth, England: Penguin

Robinson D (1996) *Wild Beasts and Idle Humours: The insanity Defense from Antiquity to the Present*. Cambridge, MA: Harvard University Press

Sadler JZ (2005) *Values and Psychiatric Diagnosis*. Oxford: Oxford University Press

Shorter E (1997) *A History of Psychiatry*. New York: John Wiley

Sukeri K, Alonso-Betancourt O, Emsley R (2014) Lessons from the past: Historical perspectives of mental health in the Eastern Cape. *South African Journal of Psychiatry* 20(2): 34–9

Van Staden CW, Fulford KWM (2007) Hypotheses, neuroscience and real persons: The theme of the 10th international conference on philosophy, psychiatry and psychology. *South African Journal of Psychiatry* 13: 68–71

Van Staden CW (2013) Better attitudes and mental health for our future. *South African Journal of Psychiatry* 19(3): 58

Van Staden CW (2012) Building our identity of psychiatry in the past, present and future South Africa. *South African Journal of Psychiatry* 18: 70–71

Van Staden CW (2010) Stuck in the past or heading for flourishing people in diversity. *South African Journal of Psychiatry* 16: 4–6

Van Staden CW (2006) Mind, brain and person: Reviewing psychiatry's constituency. *South African Psychiatry Review* 9: 93–98

# CHAPTER 2 Classification in psychiatry

Manfred Böhmer

'It is real if I choose it to be real.'
*Alice's Adventures in Wonderland,* Lewis Carroll

## 2.1 Introduction

Classification systems are central to science, since such systems help to reduce the complexity of phenomena by arranging them into categories (Zimmerman and Spitzer, 2009). Classifying and establishing classifications are an attempt to help understand the nature of reality. A typical research approach in medicine in developing such systems is first to describe conditions characterised by a particular constellation of symptoms and signs. The initial approach is thus descriptive in nature and these conditions are named syndromes since the underlying aetiology and **pathophysiology** are not known. A condition is called a disease if these underlying factors are elucidated by research (First and Pincus, 2009; First, 2010).

The classification systems used at present in psychiatry are of a descriptive, symptom-based type, since there is still not sufficient understanding of the pathophysiology of mental disorders to justify abandoning this approach in favour of a more aetiologically based alternative (First, 2010). Most psychiatric conditions fall within the definition of a syndrome and are termed a disorder, for example a major depressive disorder (First and Pincus, 2009; First, 2010).

## 2.2 Purposes of classification

According to Zimmerman and Spitzer (2009) and First and Pincus (2009) classification in psychiatry, even though it may not contain information about specific mechanisms or causes for an identified group of symptoms, serves a variety of important purposes, such as:

- facilitating the making of a diagnosis, which is of key importance to the clinician since it is central to the development of a treatment plan and conveys to the patient an understanding of his or her suffering; it gives a name to it
- enabling physicians and researchers to communicate with each other about the disorders or diseases with which they deal
- helping with further research to reach an understanding of underlying causes of disorders.
- being an educational tool.

Diagnoses also serve many functions. Many psychiatric diagnoses are associated with a characteristic course and outcome: knowledge that can be of help to the patient and family. Diagnoses also help to determine the **incidence** and **prevalence** of various diseases throughout the world. A diagnosis can be of importance in litigation and legal matters. Diagnoses are used to make decisions about insurance coverage in many parts of the world. Each time a clinician makes a diagnosis and records it, an awareness of the non-clinical uses to which it may be put should be kept in mind. A careless or hasty diagnosis may have significant legal, financial or other implications for the patient.

In psychiatry there are challenges in making a diagnosis since no objective tests (e.g. blood tests) are available as diagnostic aids. The exceptions here are some of the neurocognitive disorders. Making a diagnosis is still mostly descriptive and based on the history elicited and observations made (First, 2010; Andrews and Peters, 1998; Andrews *et al.*, 1999). The process of making a psychiatric diagnosis is partially simplified by the fact that the American Psychiatric Association (APA) and the World Health Organization (WHO) have formulated manuals that summarise the diagnoses used in psychiatry. These manuals specify the symptoms that must be present to make a particular diagnosis and also organise these diagnoses together into a classification system. Both classification systems have over the years undergone several major revisions.

## 2.3 Definition of a mental disorder

The definition of a mental disorder is of great importance as it distinguishes pathology from what is normal. It can influence estimates of the prevalence of psychiatric disorders and thus allocation of public health funds, influences medical insurance reimbursements and has potential legal implications. Psychiatric diagnoses can also lead to abuse, for example by stigmatising socially undesirable behaviour (Zimmerman and Spitzer, 2009).

Mental disorders, contrary to most medical disorders, are manifested by behaviour, feelings and ways of thinking that differ quantitatively from what is considered to be normal (Zimmerman and Spitzer, 2009). The fifth edition of *The Diagnostic and Statistical Manual of Mental Disorders* (DSM-5) (American Psychiatric Association, 2013) gives the following definition:

- A mental disorder is a syndrome characterized by clinically significant disturbance in an individual's **cognition**, emotion regulation, or behavior that reflects a dysfunction in the psychological, biological, or developmental processes underlying mental functioning.
- Mental disorders are usually associated with significant distress or disability in social, occupational, or other important activities.
- An expectable or culturally approved response to a common stressor or loss, such as the death of a love one, is not a mental disorder.
- Socially deviant behaviour (e.g., political, religious, or sexual) and conflicts that are primarily between the individual and society are not mental disorders unless the deviance or conflict results from a dysfunction in the individual, as described above.

## 2.4 Classification systems

The DSM, published by the APA, is the system most commonly used in South Africa, although there are many controversies around the use of the present edition, *The Diagnostic and Statistical Manual of Mental Disorders*, 5th edition (DSM-5) (see Section 2.5). The official classification system mostly used in Europe and developed by the WHO, is the tenth revision of the *International Classification of Diseases and Related Health Problems* (ICD-10) (Reed *et al.*, 2011; International Advisory Group for the Revision of ICD-10 Mental and Behavioural Disorders, 2011). Both the DSM and ICD follow a descriptive, a-theoretical approach. There are, however, fundamental differences between the two systems. ICD-10 was primarily set up as a classification system, whereas DSM is a diagnostic system (First and Pincus, 2009). While inclusion of a category in the ICD carries with it no implication of diagnostic validity, categories in DSM have been officially sanctioned by the APA as appropriate for clinical and research use (First and Pincus, 2009). Another important difference is that most DSM diagnoses include a 'clinical significance criterion' requiring that the disturbance causes clinical significant distress or **impairment** of functioning. This helps to establish a threshold for making a diagnosis (Zimmerman and Spitzer, 2009; First and Pincus, 2009).

In certain conditions this criterion is unnecessary. In other individuals who have a mental disorder this criterion can create problems, in that they cannot be diagnosed as having the disorder if this criterion is not met. Until the underlying psychological and biological dysfunctions of psychiatric illnesses are identified, the definitions of mental disorders will involve drawing arbitrary lines, such as this clinical significance criterion, to minimise false positive and false negative diagnoses (Zimmerman and Spitzer, 2009).

## 2.4.1 DSM-5

DSM-5 has three sections. Section I is an introductory section, section II lists the diagnostic criteria and codes, while section III has been added to highlight disorders that require further study and are at present not well enough established to be part of the official classification, for example an alternative model for **personality** disorders. This section also includes certain tools and techniques to enhance the decision-making process and to understand the cultural context of mental disorders (American Psychiatric Association, 2013).

The most prominent changes from DSM-IV to DSM-5 are:

- The multi-axial assessment system has been done away with. The five axes included in the DSM-IV classification were:
  - Axis I Clinical disorders
    Other conditions that may be a focus of clinical **attention**
  - Axis II Personality disorders
    Intellectual disability
  - Axis III General medical conditions
  - Axis IV Psychosocial and environmental problems (stressors)
  - Axis V Global assessment of functioning.

  The idea behind the multi-axial system was to promote a comprehensive, bio-psycho-social approach towards clinical assessment and treatment (Zimmerman and Spitzer, 2009).

  In DSM-5, diagnoses previously documented on Axis I to III are listed in a non-axial way. Psychosocial stressors and contextual factors (previously Axis IV) and disability (previously Axis V) are noted separately. This approach implies that there are no fundamental differences in the conceptualisation of Axis I, II or III disorders and that mental disorders as well as general medical conditions are related to physical, biological, behavioural and psychosocial factors or processes.

  In the DSM-IV a patient's overall level of functioning was assessed according to the Global Assessment of Functioning scale. There were, however, concerns about certain aspects of this scale, such as conceptual lack of clarity, since symptoms, suicide risk and behaviour, for example, were included to assess the functioning of the patient. The scale was thus dropped from the DSM-5 and replaced by the World Health Organization Disability Assessment Schedule 2.0 (WHODAS 2.0) in Section III, although it is noted that this needs further study (American Psychiatric Association, 2013).

  The WHODAS 2.0 is self-administered and consists of 36 items to assess disability in adults age 18 years and older. (There is also a proxy-administered version if the patient is unable to complete the form (American Psychiatric Association, 2013).

  The WHODAS 2.0 covers six domains:
  - understanding and communication
  - getting around (standing, moving around, walking)
  - self-care
  - getting along with people
  - life activities at home and at school or work
  - participation in society.
- Autistic disorder, Asperger's disorder and pervasive developmental disorder have been consolidated into autism spectrum disorder.
- The categories of **substance abuse** and **substance dependence** have been eliminated and replaced with an overarching new category of substance use disorders, differentiated in terms of severity.
- Specific types of disorders previously referred to as dementias or organic brain diseases have been described with greater **specificity** as major or mild neurocognitive disorders.
- The subtypes of schizophrenia were eliminated due to their limited diagnostic stability, low reliability and poor validity.
- Obsessive-compulsive disorder has been moved from anxiety disorders and incorporated into a new category of obsessive compulsive and related disorders.

- The classes or groups of conditions have been revised (see Table 2.1).
- The category 'Due to a General Medical Condition' was changed to 'Due to Another Medical Condition' to reflect the fact that psychiatric disorders are regarded as medical conditions themselves.
- The residual category 'Not Otherwise Specified' (NOS) was changed to 'Other Specified Disorders' and 'Unspecified Disorders'. This was done to try to enhance diagnostic specificity. The Other Specified Disorder category allows the clinician to name the specific reason why the criteria of a specific category are not met.

It is important to keep in mind that diagnostic criteria, such as those specified in DSM-5, are guidelines and their use should be informed by clinical judgement (American Psychiatric Association, 2013).

**Table 2.1** Section II: Diagnostic Criteria and Codes

| Section II: Diagnostic Criteria and Codes |
|---|
| Neurodevelopmental Disorders |
| Schizophrenia Spectrum and Other Psychotic Disorders |
| Bipolar and Related Disorders |
| Depressive Disorders |
| Anxiety Disorders |
| Obsessive-Compulsive and Related Disorders |
| Trauma- and Stressor-Related Disorders |
| Dissociative Disorders |
| Somatic Symptom and Related Disorders |
| Feeding and Eating Disorders |
| Elimination Disorders |
| Sleep-Wake Disorders |
| **Sexual Dysfunctions** |
| **Gender Dysphoria** |
| Disruptive, Impulse-Control, and Conduct Disorders |
| Substance-Related and Addictive Disorders |
| Neurocognitive Disorders |
| Personality Disorders |
| **Paraphilic Disorders** |
| Other Mental Disorders |
| Medication-Induced Movement Disorders and Other Adverse Effects of Medication |
| Other Conditions That May Be a Focus of Clinical Attention |

**Source:** Reprinted with permission from the *Diagnostic and Statistical Manual of Mental Disorders*, Fifth Edition, (Copyright 2013). American Psychiatric Association.

If the threshold for a diagnosis is not met, two options in terms of diagnosis are available: other specified disorders and unspecified disorders. The other specified disorder category allows the clinician to state the reasons why the criteria are not met.

### 2.4.1.1 Cultural issues as described in DSM-5

The boundaries between normality and **psychopathology** vary across cultures. The clinician therefore has to consider whether an individual presents with a picture outside of what is considered normal for that culture and society and whether this leads to difficulties in adaptation in his or her culture or social situation.

In DSM-5 (American Psychiatric Association, 2013) the construct of the **culture-bound syndrome** has been replaced by the following three concepts:

- cultural syndrome: a cluster or group of co-occurring symptoms found in a specific cultural group, community or context
- cultural idiom of distress: a way of talking about suffering among individuals of a cultural group referring to shared concepts of pathology and ways of expressing or naming features of distress
- cultural explanation or perceived cause: an explanatory model providing a culturally conceived aetiology or cause for the symptoms or illness.

In Section III of DSM-5 the cultural **formulation** is discussed in detail. A cultural formulation should systematically take into account the patient's cultural background, the role that culture plays in the expression and the evaluation of symptoms and the relationship between the individual and the clinician. This aspect is especially important in southern Africa, where the clinician and patient often not only come from different cultures, but also speak different languages, thereby necessitating the help of an interpreter who sometimes belongs to a third cultural and language group. This is not an ideal situation and especially in the practice of psychiatry clinicians should strive to understand and speak the language of the patients whom they treat, and to learn as much about their cultures as possible.

The DSM-5 suggests that the clinician should try to provide a narrative summary for each of the following categories:

**Cultural identity of the individual**

The individual's cultural or ethnic group should be noted, as well as the degree of involvement with both the culture of origin and the culture of the clinician. Also note language abilities, use and preference. This also applies when treating immigrants and refugees.

**Cultural conceptualisation of distress**

The predominant idioms of distress through which symptoms or the need for social support is communicated should be noted, for example possession by spirits, punishment or instructions given by ancestors and **somatic** complaints. The meaning and perceived severity of the symptoms in relation to the norms of the cultural reference group and the perceived causes or explanations of the illness by the individual and his or her family and extended family should be assessed. Present or past experiences with traditional healers should also be noted.

**Psychosocial stressors and cultural features of vulnerability and resilience**

Key stressors, ways of support as well as the role of religion, family and other social networks should be identified. Levels of functioning, disability and resilience should be assessed within the context of the specific culture.

**Cultural elements of the relationship between the individual and the clinician**

Differences in culture, social status and language must be indicated, especially if these might **affect** diagnosis and treatment.

**Overall cultural assessment**

The implications of the components of the cultural formulation and the implications for diagnosis as well as appropriate treatment and management should be summarised. Further discussion of cultural formulation can be found in Chapter 6: Culture and psychiatry.

## 2.4.2 The International Classification of Diseases system

The ICD-10, of which Chapter V deals with psychiatric disorders, was published in 1992. According to a WPA-WHO global survey, 70% of psychiatrists reported that they mostly use the ICD-10 as classification system in their daily clinical work (Reed *et al.*, 2011).

Based on the WHO's mission and constitution, a classification system must assist in increasing coverage and enhancing mental health care across the world (International Advisory Group for the Revision of ICD-10 Mental and Behavioural Disorders, 2011). Most people with mental disorders in lower and middle-income countries are likely to receive treatment in primary care settings due to local shortages of psychiatrists. It is thus important to have a classification system that is useable and useful in such settings (International Advisory Group for the Revision of ICD-10 Mental and Behavioural Disorders, 2011). For this and other reasons several versions of ICD-10 were developed. The first is designed to be used for statistical purposes. The second version, called the *Clinical Descriptions and Diagnostic Guidelines*, includes definitions of diagnostic terms, categories and sets of criteria and is for use by clinicians. The third version is primarily intended for research and therefore the diagnostic criteria are stricter. The fourth version was produced for use in primary care settings (First and Pincus, 2009) as non-psychiatrists, it is argued, will only use a classification system if it is free of specialist jargon and easy to use (Sartorius, 2009). ICD-10 also follows a phenomenological descriptive approach and uses the term 'disorder' since the pathogenesis of mental disorders is not known and they thus do not qualify for the definition of a disease (Sartorius, 2009).

ICD-10 is multi-axial to allow for different aspects of the patient's health and social situation to be assessed. Axis I includes all the disorders (physical, mental or personality disorders), Axis II deals with the level of functional capacity or disability, and Axis III describes situations that the clinician considers as important in understanding the patient and his or her problem (e.g. 'Problems related to negative events in childhood and adolescence', or 'the circumstances in which the patient lives') (First and Pincus, 2009; Sartorius, 2009). The main features of the patient's condition are thus summarised.

ICD-10 has certain unique characteristics:

- It is based on international consensus among psychiatrists and mental health workers belonging to widely different schools of thought and working in very different conditions (Sartorius, 2009).
- It was produced in several versions for different groups of users and for use in specific situations (Sartorius, 2009).
- Trials in 40 countries were taken into account (Sartorius, 2009).
- ICD-10 was developed in several languages simultaneously. *The Clinical Descriptions and Diagnostic Guidelines* version, for example, is available in 43 languages.
- Additional publications that facilitate its use accompany it, for example research instruments and symptom checklists (Sartorius, 2009).
- The classification relied on a network of collaborating centres of excellence during its development, but also after its publication (Sartorius, 2009).
- The needs of practice with people with mental illness worldwide were taken into account, as well as scientific requirements and public health needs. In line with this, the part dealing with acute and transient psychotic disorders frequently seen in developing countries was expanded and social functioning was avoided as a diagnostic indicator because normal social functioning is so different in various parts of the world (Sartorius, 2009).

### 2.4.3 Differences between ICD and DSM (APA, 2013; International Advisory Group for the Revision of ICD-10 Mental and Behavioural Disorders, 2011; Sartorius, 2009)

- The ICD, once developed, has to be approved by the ICD reference centres and then submitted to the WHO for approval. The 193 countries that are members of the WHO have to accept it (Sartorius, 2009; International Advisory Group for the Revision of ICD-10 Mental and Behavioural Disorders, 2011).
- In its development the views and proposals of all member countries of the WHO were taken into account (Sartorius, 2009).
- Several versions of the ICD have been produced to cater for different needs (Sartorius, 2009).
- The ICD was developed through a process of international consultation and field trials carried out in different parts of the world.
- Functional status and disability do not form part of the ICD definitions and criteria of the diagnostic entities. ICD indicates that mental disorders often interfere with functional impairment, but does not require it in the making of a diagnosis. DSM-5 has also made substantial efforts to separate the concepts of mental disorder and disability; it, however, includes a generic diagnostic criterion requiring distress or disability to establish disorder thresholds. ICD-11 may, however, also refer to specific types of functional impairment as thresholds to separate disorder from non-disorder (International Advisory Group for the Revision of ICD-10 Mental and Behavioural Disorders, 2011; American Psychiatric Association, 2013).

### 2.4.4 ICD-11

ICD-11, expected in 2015, is being developed through an innovative and collaborative process, in which experts and users are for the first time invited to participate in the revision process though a web-based platform. Peer-reviewed comments and input will be added throughout the revision process (World Health Organization, 2015a). Frances (2013a) voices his scepticism about this process. He states that the WHO has limited financial resources for the development of the ICD and that there is less central guidance than with the DSM-5. His concern is that, as with the DSM, this will also lead to diagnostic inflation.

## 2.5 Critique of classification systems in general as well as of DSM-5: Limitations and disadvantages

Before the publication of the DSM-III in 1980, reliability, referring to different psychiatrists coming to the same diagnosis, was poor (Frances, 2013b). The introduction of explicit diagnostic criteria enclosed in a classification system has helped to change this. Agreement, consistency or repeatability between clinicians in terms of diagnostic conclusions has improved (Kendell and Jablensky, 2003). Other important gains achieved through the development and use of classification systems have already been mentioned.

Contemporary classifications have however their problems, inadequacies and failings, such as the following:

- Although in the preface to DSM-5 it is stated that mental disorders do not always fit completely within the boundaries of a single disorder and that scientific evidence places many disorders on a spectrum with closely related disorders, DSM-5 remains mostly a **categorical approach**. Such an approach posits that there are clear boundaries between diagnostic entities, that a disorder is either present or not and thus is, in general, more useful in clinical practice. A dimensional approach states the lack of clear demarcation between normality and illness as well as between different categories (Zimmerman and Spitzer, 2009; First, 2010). Traditionally it has been assumed that most medical diseases are discrete entities, but research strongly suggests that this does not apply to psychiatric disorders (and indeed to some medical disorders such as diabetes which exists as a spectrum of glucose intolerance) (First, 2010; Van Praag, 2010). The hypothesis that DSM-defined syndromes are discrete entities with distinct aetiologies is, for example, undermined by the fact that certain traumas (e.g. sexual abuse) can lead to depression, anxiety, eating disorders or drug abuse; by the high **co-morbidity** rates and the fact that treatments from widely different drug classes are effective for the same diagnosis; and that the same drugs, e.g. SSRIs, can be effective in the treatment of various disorders (First, 2010; Kendell and Jablensky, 2003).

  Another problem with the categorical approach is the question of the threshold for a disorder (Zimmerman and Spitzer, 2009). Too low a threshold will lead to a false positive diagnosis, while too high a threshold results in missed diagnoses or the frequent use of the 'Other Specified' or 'Unspecified categories' (called in previous editions Not Otherwise Specified).

  A categorical approach does not capture the widespread sharing of symptoms and risk factors across many disorders. In future, dimensional approaches that assume that psychopathology lies across a range of dimensions will probably supplement or replace current categorical approaches. In the DSM-5 a dimensional approach augments the categorical approach.
- The validity of the diagnostic concepts cannot be taken for granted (Kendell and Jablensky, 2003). The DSM and ICD are mostly symptom-based classifications without any coherent pathophysiological foundation and thus without fundamental validity (Berk, 2013). Diagnostic categories

are simply concepts, a valuable and useful framework for organising and explaining the complexity of clinical experience. The danger is that such diagnostic concepts, once listed in an official classification system, tend to be reified. People assume that diagnostic categories are clear entities of some kind that can be invoked to explain a patient's symptoms and whose validity need not be questioned (Kendell and Jablensky, 2003). Most psychiatric disorders are not discrete entities, however, and the diagnostic concepts should be seen for what they are: useful tools to practising clinicians and researchers that introduce structure, but are not the final arbitrators. Furthermore, because of the lack of validity, DSM diagnoses are arguably not useful for research (Andreasen, 2007).

- According to Andreasen (2007), the publication of DSM-III in 1980 led to a steady decline in the teaching of careful clinical evaluation, targeted to the individual person's problems and social context, and enriched by a good knowledge of psychopathology. Students are taught to memorise DSM rather than learn more complex psychopathology. DSM criteria were never intended to provide a comprehensive description: they were conceived as the minimum symptoms needed to make a diagnosis and they form only an initial step in a detailed evaluation leading to a formulation and treatment plan.

  Andreasen (2007) also writes that DSM has had a dehumanising impact on the practice of psychiatry. In order to make a DSM diagnosis, clinicians become focused on assessing symptoms and signs - the DSM thus discourages clinicians from getting to know the patient as a person (Frances, 2013a; Andreasen, 2007). The problem might not primarily be the DSM, but rather how it is used. Berk (2013) laments the use of the DSM as a substitute for a comprehensive clinical formulation. Formulations exist in many forms, for example as descriptive, psychodynamic, cognitive-behavioural and systemic formulations and give attention to the unique life history of the patient as person, including the developmental history, **attachment** style, personality structure, conflicts and ability to form relationships (Aveline, 1999; Böhmer, 2011).

- Concern has been voiced about financial considerations playing a role in the development and publication of the DSM. The American Psychiatric Association has made millions of dollars selling the DSM (Zimmerman and Spitzer, 2009). There is also concern about the role of the pharmaceutical industry in present developments, since extending the classification system can be of advantage to the industry (Zimmerman and Spitzer, 2009).
- Many voice the opinion that the DSM-5 is a step backwards. Burns and Alonso-Betancourt (2013) quote criticism levelled at DSM-5, such as concerns about reliability and validity, and argue for the use of the ICD in South African psychiatry. First and Pincus (1999) describe the rigorous way in which the DSM-IV was developed and argue that, especially in the world of research, the DSM (IV) system was the de facto standard. Frances (2013b), chairperson of the taskforce that developed the DSM-IV, writes that psychiatric diagnosis is facing a new crisis of confidence due to diagnostic inflation in the DSM-5. He advises psychiatrists to use the DSM-5 cautiously – if at all. Examples of concern are the loosening of criteria such as for mixed states of bipolar disorder which might contribute to an increase in the diagnosis of bipolar disorder, the lowering of the threshold for various diagnoses and the establishment of new diagnoses (e.g. somatic symptom disorder, binge eating disorder and disruptive mood dysregulation disorder which are all at the fuzzy boundary with normality (Malhi, 2013).

## 2.6 Other developments regarding classification: The NIMH Research Domain Criteria (RDoC) Project

The National Institute of Mental Health (NIMH), a component of the US Department of Health and Human Services, launched a strategic plan in 2008 to, amongst others, '(p)romote discovery in the brain and behavioral sciences to fuel research on the causes of mental disorders'. One of the strategies adopted to reach this goal is to '(d)evelop, for research purposes, new ways of classifying mental disorders based on dimensions of observable behavior and neurobiological measures'. The implementation of this strategy has been named the Research Domain Criteria Project (RDoC) (National Institute of Mental Health, 2008a).

The NIMH states in its strategic plan that currently the diagnosis of mental disorders is based on clinical observation and that the definitions in the present diagnostic system do not incorporate current information from integrative neuroscience research. '(I)n antedating contemporary neuroscience research, the current diagnostic system is not informed by recent breakthroughs in genetics; and molecular, cellular and systems neuroscience' (National Institute of Mental Health, 2008b). Basic biological and behavioural components have to be linked to develop valid, reliable **phenotypes** (measurable **traits** or characteristics) for mental disorders. This will help to elucidate the causes of the disorder and clarify the boundaries and overlap between mental disorders (National Institute of Mental Health, 2008a).

At this stage RDoC is intended as a framework to guide classification of patients for research studies and not as an immediately useful clinical tool. It will follow three guiding principles, all diverging from current diagnostic approaches. According to the guidelines, the RDoC:

- is conceived as a dimensional system spanning the range from normal to abnormal
- is agnostic about current disorder categories – the intent is to generate classifications stemming from basic behavioural neuroscience
- will use several different units of analysis in defining constructs for study, such as imaging, physiological activity, behaviour and self-reporting of symptoms (National Institute of Mental Health, 2008b).

## 2.7 Future research

Psychiatry lacks objective and independent criteria for diagnosing most mental illnesses. Except for certain neurocognitive disorders, no biological or genetic markers have been identified up to now.

Endophenotypes are a relatively new concept in the study of complex neuropsychiatric diseases (Gottesman and Gould, 2003). These are defined as measurable components, unseen by the unaided eye, located between disease and the **genotype** and may be neurophysiological, biochemical, endocrinological, neuro-anatomical, cognitive or neuropsychological. Endophenotypes represent simpler clues to genetic underpinnings than the disease syndrome itself, which may be helpful in genetic analysis. In schizophrenia, eye-tracking dysfunction, working memory and executive cognition can be seen as possible endophenotypes and worthy of further investigation (Gottesman and Gould, 2003).

## 2.8 What is the solution?

The unhappiness with the DSM-5 is probably part of a greater disenchantment with the classification systems as such, since the present approach did not lead to any major new **insights** into aetiology, pathophysiology and treatment. According to Frances (2013b) we will be stuck with **descriptive psychiatry**, such as the ICD and DSM, for the foreseeable future. Such diagnostic concepts do, however, have validity in the sense of being useful concepts that provide useful information (Kendell and Jablensky, 2003). Classification systems are furthermore about learning and understanding. Widiger and Spitzer (1989) write that if a student ignores the caution that DSM represents only an initial step in a comprehensive evaluation, this does not suggest an inadequacy of the manual, but rather a problem in the education of the student by the teacher. Their comment is not totally appropriate, since classification systems do differ in quality, but it does highlight the fact that teachers must be thinkers who are able to keep different points of view in mind. The a-theoretical approach of both classification systems can be a starting point to think about different points of view and to develop a broader perspective of psychopathology as mentioned by Andreasen (2007); it can encourage the consideration of different models of causation and treatment.

Van Praag (2010) reminds us that, although psychiatric disorders are diseases of the brain, they are no less disorders of the soul, of souls in despair. Brain studies have little to offer in understanding the individual soul.

## Conclusion

Classifications systems are an attempt to understand the nature of reality. Neither the DSM nor the ICD classification systems should be reified – they are meant as guides and useful tools in the comprehensive assessment of a patient.

# References


American Psychiatric Association (2013) *Diagnostic and Statistical Manual of Mental Disorders* (5th edition). Arlington, VA: American Psychiatric Association

Andreasen NC (2007) DSM and the death of phenomenology in America: An example of unintended consequences. *Schizophrenia Bulletin* 33(1): 108–12

Andrews G, Peters L (1998) The psychometric properties of the Composite International Diagnostic Interview. *Social Psychiatry and Psychiatric Epidemiology* 33: 80–8

Andrews G, Slade T, Peters L (1999) Classification in psychiatry: ICD-10 versus DSM-IV (editorial). *The British Journal of Psychiatry* 174(1): 3–5

Aveline M (1999) The advantages of formulation over categorical diagnosis in explorative psychotherapy and psychodynamic management. *European Journal of Psychotherapy, Counselling and Health* 2(2): 199–216

Berk M. (2013) The DSM-5: Hyperbole, hope or hypothesis? (editorial) *BMC Medicine* 11: 128–9

Böhmer MW (2011) Dynamic psychiatry and the psychodynamic formulation. *African Journal of Psychiatry* 14(4): 273–7

Burns JK, Alonso-Betancourt O (2013) Are we slaves to DSM? A South African perspective (editorial). *African Journal of Psychiatry* 16: 151–5

Carroll L. (2008) *Alice's Adventures in Wonderland* (Original 1865). Project Gutenberg eBook. Available at: www.gutenberg.org

First MB (2010) Paradigm shifts and the development of the diagnostic and statistical manual of mental disorders: Past experiences and future aspirations. *The Canadian Journal of Psychiatry* 55(11): 692–700

First MB, Pincus HA (2009) Diagnosis and classification. In: Gelder MG, Andreasen NC, López-Ibor Jr JJ, Geddes JR (Eds). *New Oxford Textbook of Psychiatry*. 2nd ed. Oxford: Oxford University Press

First MB, Pincus HA. (1999) Classification in psychiatry: ICD-10 v. DSM-IV: A response (editorial). *The British Journal of Psychiatry* 175(9): 205–9

Frances A (2013a) Interview: The limits and uses of descriptive psychiatry. *Neuropsychiatry* 3(4): 371–5

Frances A (2013b) The new crisis of confidence in psychiatric diagnosis. *Annals of Internal Medicine* 159(3): 221–2

Gottesman II, Gould TD (2003) The endophenotype concept in psychiatry: Etymology and strategic intentions. *The American Journal of Psychiatry* 160: 636–45

International Advisory Group for the Revision of ICD-10 Mental and Behavioural Disorders (2011) A conceptual framework for the revision of the ICD-10 classification of mental and behavioural disorders. *World Psychiatry* 10: 86–92

Kendell R, Jablensky A (2003) Distinguishing between the validity and utility of psychiatric diagnoses. *The American Journal of Psychiatry* 160: 4–12

Malhi GS. (2013) Diagnosis of bipolar disorder: Who is in a mixed state? *The Lancet*, 381(9878): 1599–1600

National Institute of Mental Health (2008a) The National Institute of Mental Health Strategic Plan. Available at: http://www.nimh.nih.gov/about/strategic-planning-reports/index.shtml#strategic-objective1 (Accessed 13 November 2013)

National Institute of Mental Health (2008b) The National Institute of Mental Health Strategic Plan. Available at: http://www.nimh.nih.gov/research-priorities/rdoc/nimh-research-domain-criteria-rdoc.shtml (Accessed 13 November 2013)

Reed GM, Correia JM, Esparza P, Saxena S, Maj M (2011) The WPA-WHO global survey of psychiatrists' attitudes towards mental disorders classification. *World Psychiatry* 10: 118–31

Sartorius N (2009) The classification of mental disorders in the International Classification of Diseases. In: Sadock BJ, Sadock VA, Ruiz P (Eds) *Kaplan & Sadock's Comprehensive Textbook of Psychiatry*, 9th ed. Philadelphia: Lippincott Williams & Wilkins

Van Praag HM (2010) Does psychiatry really know 'solid disease diagnoses'? In: Shorter E, Van Praag HM (Eds). Disease versus dimension in diagnosis. *Canadian Journal of Psychiatry* 55(2): 59–64

Widiger TA, Spitzer RL. (1989) Criticism of DSM-III. *The American Journal of Psychiatry* 146(4): 566–7
World Health Organization (2015a) International Classification of Diseases (ICD) Information Sheet. Available at: http://www.who.int/classifications/icd/factsheet/en/ (Accessed 19 September 2013)
World Health Organization (2015b) *The International Classification of Diseases*, 11th revision is due by 2017. http://www.who.int/classifications/icd/revision/en/ (Accessed 4 April 2015)
Zimmerman M, Spitzer RL (2009) Psychiatric classification. In: Sadock BJ, Sadock VA, Ruiz P (Eds). *Kaplan & Sadock's Comprehensive Textbook of Psychiatry*, 9th ed. Philadelphia: Lippincott Williams & Wilkins

# PART 2

# Causes of psychiatric disorders

CHAPTER

# 3 Psychiatric epidemiology and genetics

Jonathan Burns, Dana Niehaus

## 3.1 Understanding the causes of psychiatric disorders

The history of psychiatry and how society and medicine have understood and responded to mental illness is reviewed in Chapter 1: A brief history of psychiatry of this book. This history is characterised by changes in the understanding of the causes of mental disorders. At different times in both the past and the present, mental disorders have been attributed to:

- supernatural and spiritual forces
- perverse individual choice
- learnt behavior
- **unconscious** psychological processes
- societal forces
- physical disease or degeneration of the brain
- genes.

Each of these **causal attributions** can be linked to beliefs about how mental illness is best treated. Thus we have seen historical and contemporary shifts in popularity and emphasis, between different schools and groups, and different models of illness and associated approaches to treatment. Included in the variety of approaches to treatment are:

- exorcism and other supernatural or spiritual interventions
- forms of punishment or moral treatments
- behavioural and cognitive behavioural approaches
- psychodynamic approaches
- social approaches
- neurobiological interventions.

Against this confusing background of differing (and often conflicting) beliefs, opinions, theories and models, has emerged a recognition that is increasingly supported by scientific evidence, namely that all psychiatric disorders are caused by a complex interaction of multiple factors that are biological, psychological, social, cultural, environmental and even spiritual in nature. According to the bio-psycho-social model of disease, which was based on general systems theory and was constructed to account for the missing dimensions of the biomedical model, each system affects, and is affected by, every other system (Engel, 1980). Therefore no healthy or disordered mental state can be explained on the basis of a single factor, such as a gene.

In the 21st century there is no place for any individual or group that claims to adhere to a scientific world view, to cling to a narrow fundamentalist view that holds up one single factor as the sole cause of mental illness. Individuals are made up of exceedingly complicated molecular entities (established and maintained by the genetic system) that produce and are constantly modified by consciousness, behavior and the environment. The rapid development of the fields of **epigenetics** and **gene-environment interaction** research over the last decade has revealed some of the mechanisms by which genes influence our exposure to environmental factors, how variable genetic makeup modifies individual vulnerability and risk to specific environmental exposures and how environmental exposures alter the expression of inherited genetic information. More recently, **trans-generational** research (Jablonka and Lamb, 2008) provides new evidence for some degree of 'inheritance of acquired characteristics' – a theory first advanced by Jean-Baptiste Lamarck in 1809 in his *Philosophie Zoologique* and rejected for nearly a century. We are appreciating more than ever before that the apparent boundaries between the various genetic, biochemical and environmental factors that contribute to human consciousness are porous and reciprocally connected.

This chapter and several others that follow will review what we know about the causes of psychiatric disorders, including the current evidence for biomedical, psychosocial and cultural factors as they relate to the risk and manifestation of psychopathology. Later in this chapter we will address the issue of genetics and psychiatry and provide an overview of the major genetic approaches and findings in respect of mental disorders.

First, though, we provide a brief overview of a topic that is key to understanding the distribution of and causation of mental disorders: psychiatric epidemiology.

## 3.2 Psychiatric epidemiology

This section will review the key concepts and methods of psychiatric epidemiology, thereby providing a solid foundation for interpreting and understanding the meaning and significance of disorder-specific research findings. The epidemiological findings for psychiatric disorders will be presented in the chapters covering the various disorders.

Psychiatric epidemiology is the study of the distribution of mental disorders in populations and of the risk factors associated with their onset and course (Tohen *et al.*, 2000). Epidemiological methods provide the tools necessary to conduct systematic research into the aetiology and genetics of psychiatric disorders and serve as the basis of outcome studies and clinical trials (Tohen *et al.*, 2000). Epidemiology can be considered one of the scientific foundations of psychiatry (Tohen and Bromet, 1997).

While modern epidemiology has acquired highly sophisticated statistical approaches, its basic theoretical principles, concepts and rules were laid down more than a century ago within the social sciences and medicine (Jablensky, 2002). Thus, the essential elements of any psychiatric epidemiological enquiry still involve the basic notions of determining the frequency and distribution of mental disorders, their associated risk factors and possible interventions to prevent or treat them.

### 3.2.1 Key measures of morbidity and risk

It is important to understand a number of commonly used measures of morbidity and risk. These include prevalence, incidence, morbid risk and measures of effect, each of which is discussed below.

#### 3.2.1.1 Prevalence

Prevalence measures the proportion of individuals who have a particular disease or disorder at a specific point or period in time. The numerator includes both new cases and chronic cases, while the denominator is the total population at risk, including those with the disorder. A distinction is made between point prevalence, which is the number of people affected at a given point in time (e.g. a month or a year), and lifetime prevalence, which includes all people who have had the disorder at any period in their lives. It is important to make this distinction, as lifetime prevalence is usually greater than point prevalence.

#### 3.2.1.2 Incidence

Incidence is the number of people who develop the disorder during a given period of time, divided by the defined population at risk at the beginning of the period. This is the incidence risk and is typically expressed as x per 1 000 (or 10 000) people per annum.

The incidence rate is the number of disease onsets during the period divided by the 'person-years at risk'. In this case, the denominator is defined as the number of people in the population at risk multiplied by the number of years comprising the period under study. It is important to note that the 'population at risk' is the total population, less those who already have the disease and those who fall outside the age range within which onset of the disease normally occurs (Jablensky, 2002). An example of incidence rate would be the following: the incidence rate of first-episode psychosis (FEP) is calculated in a population of 100 000 people over a period of five years. During this period, 150 people develop FEP. The incidence rate is thus 150/500 000 person-years, which could be expressed as 0,3 per 1 000 people.

### 3.2.1.3 Morbid risk (disease expectancy)

Morbid risk (or disease expectancy or lifetime risk) is the probability that a randomly selected member of a defined population will develop a specified disorder if he or she survives to a specified age or over the entire period of risk (Jablensky, 2002).

### 3.2.1.4 Measures of effect

Relative risk, or risk ratio (RR) is the ratio of the occurrence of a given outcome (e.g. disease) in persons exposed to a risk factor compared with the occurrence in the unexposed. In other words, it is a measure of relative difference and equals the incidence risk in the exposed divided by the incidence risk in the unexposed. If incidence rate is used instead of incidence risk, then the ratio is referred to as the rate ratio.

Odds ratio (OR) is similar to relative risk, but is easier to derive. It gives a good approximation of relative risk, especially when rare outcomes are being estimated (Jablensky, 2002). The odds ratio is defined as the ratio of the odds of a given outcome in exposed persons relative to the odds of that outcome among unexposed persons. Both relative risk and odds ratio are quoted together with confidence intervals (CI) that indicate the level of probability of the result. For example, if the RR is 2,3 and the CI is 0,65–4,50, then this is unlikely to be a significant result since the CI

## 3.1 Advanced reading block

**Causality – how do we establish whether a risk factor causes a disease?**

The relationship between a risk factor and a disease outcome is not always a causal relationship. Establishing a causal relationship is difficult and does not simply involve showing an association between a risk factor and a disease outcome. Various epidemiologists have listed criteria for establishing causality. Susser (1991) defined the following criteria for establishing a causal relationship:

1. An association must be shown between risk factor and disease outcome.
2. Temporal priority must be demonstrated, i.e. exposure to the risk factor occurs prior to manifestation of the disease outcome.
3. Direction: changes in the putative cause will actually lead to changes in the outcome; and the association between putative cause and outcome does not derive from a third factor common to both.

Other criteria for causation listed by Hill (1965) include:

1. strength: a dose-response relationship can be demonstrated, i.e. an increase in the magnitude of the risk factor is associated with an increase in the magnitude of the outcome.
2. consistency: the relationship between risk factor and outcome can be demonstrated repeatedly in different experiments.
3. specificity: the risk factor is associated with a specific outcome and not multiple outcomes.
4. plausibility: there must be a plausible biological mechanism linking the exposure (risk factor) and the outcome.

Of the criteria described above, Rothman and Greenland (1998) assert that temporality is the sine qua non for causality.

straddles 1,0 (which is the baseline level of risk in the unexposed group). However, if the RR is again 2,3 and the CI is 1,65–4,20, then this is likely to be a significant result.

Attributable risk (AR, or population attributable risk), is an estimate of the proportion of cases in an exposed population that can be attributed to that exposure and is expressed as a percentage (i.e. AR%). This is useful because it allows one to estimate the net population impact of an exposure (or risk factor) on a particular disease outcome. Attributable risk allows one, for example, to compare the net impact of a common risk factor that is weakly associated (low relative risk) with the outcome, against that of a rare risk factor that is strongly associated (high relative risk) with the same outcome. Attributable risk is useful in public health terms, since it can help to prioritise prevention efforts of various risk factors for disease (Jablensky, 2002).

## 3.2.2 Types of epidemiological study design

The main goal of epidemiological research is to determine associations between exposure and health outcomes. All study designs follow the principles of scientific experiment, but there are a number of factors that determine the choice of design. These include choosing the design that best minimises factors that might **bias** the results, the feasibility of studying a particular population, and the availability of resources. Epidemiological studies can be classified as either descriptive studies, or analytical studies or experimental studies (Jablensky, 2002).

### 3.2.2.1 Descriptive studies

Descriptive studies include cross-sectional studies and prospective surveys of incidence.

Cross-sectional studies involve the collection of data on both exposure(s) and outcome(s) at the same point in time, for example obtaining information about major life events and screening for symptoms of depression. There are two major limitations with this design: firstly, the information provided on exposure (e.g. life events) is retrospective and thus the validity and reliability of this information may be questionable, and secondly, one cannot make any inferences about causality as cause and effect cannot be determined from cross-sectional data. Most of the data we have on the burden of mental disorders worldwide is derived from cross-sectional studies (usually population surveys, which might be either a complete enumeration (census) of an entire population or a statistically representative sample of a population).

Prospective surveys of incidence require continuous monitoring of a defined population in order to detect all new cases emerging during the survey period. This usually requires establishing an active case-finding network that covers all potential gateways where individuals might seek help, throughout the entire catchment area for the period of the study. Alternatively, repeat cross-sectional studies can be conducted periodically in order to detect any new cases that may have emerged between consecutive surveys.

### 3.2.2.2 Analytical studies

Analytical studies include cohort studies, case-control studies and ecological studies.

Cohort studies (or longitudinal studies), collect exposure and outcome data and occur in real time. Data on exposures, for example, can be collected at the time of exposure. Participants are usually selected by a defined characteristic, such as a group who were exposed to a specific experience (e.g. war veterans), or who share a common factor (e.g. born in the same year or during the same period). This allows one to study rare or opportunistic exposures since participants are recruited on the basis of their exposure status (Jablensky, 2002). This group then becomes the cohort. Typically the members of the cohort are re-examined periodically, either at certain points (e.g. after 5 years) or at predetermined milestones (e.g. when a participant reaches a specific age). Cohort studies allow one to make causal inferences based on the temporal relationship between exposures and outcomes. Unlike case-control studies, cohort studies can assess multiple outcomes associated with a single rare or opportunistic exposure (Weich and Prince, 2003). Furthermore, cohort studies minimise information bias (observer bias and recall bias).

The major limitations of cohort studies are:

- cohort attrition (i.e. participants leaving or losing contact with the study)
- studies being restricted to the study of a single exposure and thus generally unsuitable for the study of rare outcomes
- significant time duration
- high cost.

Case-control studies consist of a group of individuals selected because they share a certain disease or risk factor, and are compared with a 'control' group of individuals without the disease or risk factor in terms of factors that may be associated with (or causal of) the outcome of interest (e.g. the disease). Case-control studies are typically cross-sectional in nature or may be prospective where, for example, the effects of a risk factor are followed up over time.

Cases are selected, not to be representative of a population, but rather because of their within-group similarity in terms of the disease or risk factor. For example, if one is studying a group of patients with schizophrenia, it would be important to attempt to include only those individuals with a similar duration of illness or similar treatment history. This within-group homogeneity is aimed at minimising factors that could confound the testing of the study hypothesis (Jablensky, 2002). This means that inclusion and exclusion criteria are critically important (e.g. excluding patients with a relevant comorbid condition such as a diagnosed neurological disorder.)

It is also important for the case group and control group to be as similar as possible across a range of factors such as age, **gender**, ethnicity, socioeconomic status and geographic neighbourhood of residence (i.e. between-group similarity). Thus the control group is matched, either on a one-to-one individual basis (pairwise) or according to the group average or mean for that factor. In selecting control groups it is important not to unnecessarily exclude individuals based on factors that are not directly relevant to the outcome (for example, setting a history of depression as an exclusion factor in a study of schizophrenia), otherwise one may end up with a super-healthy control group, which in turn may exaggerate case-control differences. It is also important to be aware that providing attractive incentives when recruiting control group members may introduce bias through 'control self-selection' (i.e. over-representation of individuals with specific needs or characteristics volunteering as controls).

Ecological studies involve investigating the effects of group level exposures on individual outcomes. Measures of neighbourhood deprivation or **social capital** or population density, for example, may be used as exposure variables or risk factors in looking for associations with mental health outcomes such as depression or substance abuse. Ecological studies have been criticised as suitable only for weak inferences at best because of their vulnerability to what is termed the 'ecological fallacy'. **Ecological fallacy** is the erroneous assumption of association at the individual level based on an observed association at the group level (Jablensky, 2002). The assumption that winter birth is a risk factor for schizophrenia because a large number of people with schizophrenia are born in winter months is an example of an ecological fallacy.

The problem of the ecological fallacy does not, however, reduce the usefulness of ecological studies in generating hypotheses about possible risk factors at the group or societal level. In fact, there is increasing evidence that area-level exposures do indeed play an important role in determining risk for a range of mental disorders (see Chapter 5: Psychosocial determinants of mental disorders). The emergence of the field of social epidemiology over the last decades has seen the emergence of increasingly sophisticated designs aimed at improving ecological research and dealing with a number of methodological problems including ecological fallacy (Berkman and Kawachi, 2000). Multilevel statistical approaches are an important development in this regard and involve the inclusion of both individual and group or area level exposure data in analyses (Blakely and Subramanian,

2006). Thus one may have, for example, data on personal experience of crime gathered from individual participants and also have an independent measure of neighbourhood crime (e.g. police statistics for the area.) This approach is preferable to the traditional approach, which is to derive area level measures from the aggregation of individual measures (e.g. a mean household income measure for the neighbourhood is calculated by adding up all the individual household income figures and dividing the total by the number of households in the neighbourhood).

Ecological studies may be cross-sectional or prospective in nature. Prospective longitudinal ecological studies allow for spatial and temporal analyses: one can look at, not only the possible effects of area-level factors that vary between geographical locations, but also investigate how changes in area-level factors over time impact on changes in outcomes. An example would be to measure levels of sunlight exposure across different geographical locations and at different points in time and then correlate changes in exposure on incidence rate of depression between places and over time.

#### 3.2.2.3 Experimental studies

Experimental studies include intervention studies and clinical trials.

Intervention studies are used to evaluate primary or secondary prevention measures or interventions at the population level (Jablensky, 2002). An example would be to investigate the impact of fluoridation of a region's water supply on the dental health of the population (Tohen *et al.*, 2000). Other examples include studies of prevention interventions for pellagra and its associated psychosis, as well as the prevention of neural tube defects through folate supplementation in pregnancy. As far as psychiatric disorders are concerned, such studies are not yet feasible since almost all psychiatric disorders have multifactorial and often unknown aetiologies.

Clinical trials are essentially epidemiological in design, but are not usually regarded as within the domain of epidemiology (Jablensky, 2002). In clinical trials, patients are exposed to a specific treatment or intervention and outcomes are then measured to determine whether the treatment or intervention has had a positive effect. For a trial to be valid, there must be a comparator group of patients, well matched for demographic and clinical characteristics, who do not receive the specific treatment or intervention. The composition of the intervention and non-intervention groups should be determined through randomisation of patients to each group. Secondly, in order to remove the so-called placebo effect, the comparator group should receive a placebo (or sugar pill), otherwise extraneous factors such as the belief that one is receiving a specific treatment may confound the outcome. In some trials a placebo is not used, for example where one group receives one active treatment (e.g. haloperidol) and the other group receives a different active treatment (e.g. risperidone). Interventions do not always have to comprise physical treatments: for example, one may randomise one group of patients with depression to receive **psycho-education** and **cognitive behavioural therapy**, while the comparator group receives psycho-education only. The final important component of a valid clinical trial is the inclusion of 'blinding'. In a single-blind trial the patient is not aware of the nature of the actual treatment, whereas in a double-blind trial the investigators are also unaware of which treatment the patient is receiving. The reason for single- and double-blind tests is that blinding removes the possibility that knowledge of the nature of a patient's treatment may somehow influence the change in outcome experienced by the patient and/or the evaluation performed by the investigator.

### 3.2.3 Forms of bias in epidemiological research

It is essential to attempt to remove or at least minimise factors that may distort results of epidemiological research thereby leading to incorrect estimates, comparisons and inferences. Such distortions usually relate to forms of bias, which can be considered as errors in the design, conduct or analysis of results of a study. There are three typical forms of bias: selection bias, observation or information bias and **confounding**.

#### 3.2.3.1 Selection bias

Selection bias occurs when the composition of a study group is influenced in such a way that extraneous factors impact on the validity of results. In case-control studies, for example, there may be inappropriate selection of control subjects who are super-healthy (see earlier discussion), or in surveys there may be selection bias if one restricts case recruitment to unrepresentative settings (e.g. hospitals only).

#### 3.2.3.2 Observation bias

Observation bias (or information bias) may occur due to missing data (non-response) that affects part of the sample, such as where participants drop out or do not give information because of a relevant factor more common to this subgroup. Individuals who use cannabis, for example, may be more likely to drop out of the study, thus leaving the impression that cannabis use is somehow reduced as an outcome. Another example is that of recall bias, where one group may tend to recall significant exposures better than a comparison group (e.g. manic patients may recall premorbid life events more readily than normal controls, or mothers of individuals with schizophrenia may over-report pregnancy complications) (Tohen *et al.*, 2000; Jablensky, 2002).

#### 3.2.3.3 Confounding

Confounding occurs where a variable that has an independent effect on the outcome is differentially represented in the groups under comparison (Jablensky, 2002). This means that a variable that is not the risk factor under study is independently associated with both the outcome and the risk factor under study (Tohen *et al.*, 2000). For example, if one is studying the effects of substance abuse on suicide, one must take the presence or absence of depression into account since depression is independently associated with both suicide and substance abuse. In this case, one would have to control, or adjust for, depression in looking at the relationship between substance abuse and suicide.

### 3.2.4 Case definition, identification and measures

The reliable measuring of the prevalence, incidence and associated risk factors of mental disorders or phenomena requires appropriate and accurate definition and identification of cases in a population. This introduces two important concepts: sensitivity and specificity.

Sensitivity refers to the capacity to identify all affected people within a specific population; thus, the measure is sensitive enough to pick up all cases and does not leave out detecting some affected individuals (false negatives).

Specificity refers to the capacity to select true cases that correspond to an established clinical concept: the measure thus predictably and repeatedly detects true cases and does not over-include false positives.

This leads us to a definition of a case. A case, whether one is referring to a person with major depressive disorder or a person who has depressive symptoms above a certain threshold, must be well defined. Measures to detect cases must distinguish between individuals who meet the case definition and those who don't within the population under study. The diagnostic criteria in psychiatry in the form of systems such as DSM-5 and ICD-10 provide definitions for cases of various psychiatric disorders.

Diagnostic instruments have been developed to assist with case identification of psychiatric disorders. These usually consist of structured instruments, such as the Structured Clinical Interview for DSM Disorders (SCID) or Composite International Diagnostic Interview (CIDI) that can be administered and scored by trained lay interviewers or semi-structured interview schedules that require professional clinical judgement, such as the Present State Examination (PSE) or Schedules for Clinical Assessment in Neuropsychiatry (SCAN).

Cases in treatment contact, case registers, case finding in the community, and screening for psychiatric disorders are all approaches to identifying cases.

#### 3.2.4.1 Cases in treatment contact

Recruiting patients from hospitals or clinic settings is relatively easy and economical. However, many factors determine who is able to, or decides to, access these treatment settings. Age-related, gender-related, socioeconomic, geographical and other factors influence whether individuals with health problems enter these clinical populations. There is good evidence that the vast majority of individuals with common mental disorders, such as depression, anxiety and substance use problems, do not access care and treatment. The same is likely to apply for severe mental disorders such as schizophrenia and dementia. Thus clinical populations cannot be considered representative of the actual population of people with these disorders. This form of selection bias means that restricting epidemiological case finding to clinical settings will significantly limit the representativeness of the sample and generalisability of the findings.

#### 3.2.4.2 Case registers

Identifying cases from health records or information systems is a highly cost-effective and feasible form of case identification. In some countries, such as Sweden, the high coverage and quality of clinical records and registers allows for excellent epidemiological research on prevalence, incidence and risk factors for mental disorders. However, in contexts where records may not be consistent in quality and comprehensive in coverage, the reliability of data contained within these records may be questionable. Since such research is generally retrospective, one is further limited by the fact that certain data of interest may not have been recorded, either in full or at all. For example, superficial recording of symptoms and other aspects of clinical assessment within case notes may prevent one from retrospectively feeling confident about diagnosis and thus 'caseness'.

#### 3.2.4.3 Case finding in the community

Where one wishes to find the true prevalence or incidence of a disorder within the general population (rather than the treated or administrative prevalence or incidence), it is necessary to identify cases within the actual community. It is important to ensure inclusion of those individuals not in treatment for whatever reasons. This can be carried out as a population-based survey, which can be of an entire community or of a representative sample of a community. Such surveys include telephonic interviews, self-administered questionnaires and face-to-face interviews. A survey can be conducted as a two-phase study with an initial screening instrument administered first and then a more detailed assessment carried out on those who screen positive. An alternative approach, used in incidence studies, involves monitoring all potential gateways within a defined catchment area for new cases – see earlier discussion of 'Types of epidemiological study design'.

#### 3.2.4.4 Screening for psychiatric disorders

Screening studies are common within populations, whether these are geographical communities or certain patient populations (e.g. screening patients who attend a diabetic clinic for depression). Screening is intended to be a quick and cost-effective method of separating individuals who are likely to have the disorder of interest from those who are likely not to have the disorder. Screening is not diagnostic: it is a method to identify likely cases who can then be assessed for the presence or absence of the disorder using more in-depth assessments. Screening may be conducted using self-administered questionnaires or scales, brief face-to-face or telephonic interviews, or checklists. Examples of screening instruments used commonly in psychiatry are listed in Table 3.1.

Screening instruments should demonstrate both validity and reliability; they also require formal validation when translated into other

**Table 3.1** Screening instruments in common use

| Instrument | Disorders | Application settings |
|---|---|---|
| General Health Questionnaire (GHQ) | anxiety, depression, somatic symptoms, social dysfunction | self-administered; 60, 30 or 12-item versions; community/primary health care, hospitals, |
| Symptom Check List 90 item Revised | symptom dimensions and measures of distress | self-administered; 90 items; community/ primary health care, hospitals |
| Brief Symptom Inventory (BSI) | symptom dimensions and measures of distress | self-administered; 53 items; community/ primary health care, hospitals |
| Kessler Psychological Distress (K10) | global measure of distress; anxiety and depression symptoms | self-administered; 10 items; community/ primary health care, hospitals |
| Hospital Anxiety and Depression Scale (HADS) | anxiety and depression in people with physical health problems | self-administered; 14 items; primary health care, hospitals |
| Hopkins Symptom Checklist (HSCL-25) | anxiety and depression subscales | self-administered; 25 items; community/ PHC and hospitals |
| Zung Self-Rating Anxiety Scale (SAS) | anxiety | self-administered; 20 items; community/ primary health care, hospitals |
| Zung Self-Rating Depression Scale (SDS) | depression | self-administered; 20 items; community/ primary health care, hospitals |
| Centre for Epidemiological Studies Depression Scale (CES-D) | depression | self-administered; 10 or 20-item versions; community/ primary health care, hospitals |
| Beck's Depression Inventory (BDI) | depression | self-administered; 21 items; community/ primary health care, hospitals |
| Patient Health Questionnaire (PHQ-9) | depression | self-administered; 9 items; community/ primary health care, hospitals |
| Edinburgh Postnatal Depression Scale (EPDS) | antenatal or postnatal depression | self-administered; 10 items; community/ primary health care, hospitals |
| Geriatric Depression Scale (GDS) | depression in the elderly | self-administered; 30 items; community/ primary health care, hospitals |
| Trauma Screening Questionnaire (TSQ) | symptoms of post-traumatic stress disorder (PTSD) | self-administered; 10 items; community/ primary health care, hospitals |
| CAGE questionnaire | screening for harmful alcohol use | self-administered; 4 items; community/ primary health care, hospitals |
| Alcohol-Use Disorders Identification Test (AUDIT) | screening for harmful alcohol use | self-administered; 10 items; community/ primary health care, hospitals |
| Brief Psychiatric Rating Scale (BPRS) | screening for psychosis | clinician-rated scale; 18 items |

languages and/or used in different cultural settings.

Validity refers to the extent to which the instrument or measure:

- conforms to agreed concepts about the nature of the object to be measured (content and construct validity)
- concurs with measurements of the same object made with another well-established tool (concurrent validity)
- correctly predicts attributes of the object to be measured (predictive validity).

**Table 3.2** Properties of screening tests

| Screening tool | Actual cases | Non-cases | Total |
|---|---|---|---|
| Positive | a | b | a+b |
| Negative | c | d | c+d |
| Total | a+c | b+d | a+b+c+d |
| | | | |
| Sensitivity (Se) | | Se = a/(a+c) | |
| Proportion false negative: (1-Se) | | (1-Se) = c/(a+c) | |
| Specificity (Sp) | | Sp = d/(b+d) | |
| Proportion false positive (1-Sp) | | (1-Sp) = b/(b+d) | |
| Positive predictive value (PPV) | | PPV = a/(a+b) | |
| Negative predictive value (NPV) | | NPV = d/(c+d) | |

**Source:** Jablensky, 2002; Derogatis *et al.* 1992. Reprinted with permission from Elsevier.

Essentially, validity is the extent to which the tool achieves what it is supposed to measure. Note that sensitivity and specificity (discussed earlier in the chapter) are aspects of validity.

Reliability refers to the extent to which a tool produces consistent results. This includes:

- measures of agreement between independent observers using the tool (inter-rater reliability)
- reproducibility of ratings made by the same observer at different times (test-retest reliability).

The *kappa* coefficient estimates the ratio between actual agreement and the agreement expected to occur by chance. It is a measure of inter-rater agreement and is generally thought to be a more robust measure than simple per cent agreement calculation, since κ takes into account the agreement occurring by chance.

Table 3.2 lists the properties of screening tests with simple explanations of how these properties are statistically determined.

## 3.2.5 Qualitative methods in psychiatric epidemiology

Qualitative methods are an important and indispensable component of psychiatric epidemiology. Where quantitative methods can generate information on frequencies, proportions, rates and associations, qualitative methods allow us to gain an in-depth understanding of the beliefs, attitudes, motivations, and consequences of human behaviours. Qualitative methods can be useful in clarifying important and relevant issues that can then be explored in populations using quantitative approaches. In addition, qualitative methods can be equally useful in gaining further in-depth understanding of findings generated from quantitative approaches.

There are three basic methods of collecting data in qualitative research: in-depth interviews, focus groups and participant observation (Murray, 1998).

#### 3.2.5.1 In-depth interviews

In-depth interviews are conducted on a one-to-one basis and aim to gather detailed narrative information from key informants who have been selected because they are in a prime situation to give insights on the issue under investigation. In-depth interviews are usually semi-structured or may be very loosely guided by a set of topics raised by the interviewer. The latter approach may involve the interviewer posing a very broad question or statement and asking the interviewee to respond freely without any constraints on the response (open-ended interviews).

#### 3.2.5.2 Focus groups

A group of key informants is selected from a population and interview sessions are conducted in a group format (optimally with no more than about ten participants). The investigator performs the role of facilitator and presents the topic for discussion, steering the group discussion so that all the issues are covered.

In both approaches listed above, conversation is recorded using written notes and/or audio-recordings. Recorded material is then transcribed for analysis.

#### 3.2.5.3 Participant observation

Participant observation is carried out in a natural setting with the researcher becoming a temporary member or participant in that setting. The observer aims to understand the social functioning of the setting from the perspectives and behaviours of the people within it. This approach is one of inductive theory building from the bottom up rather than hypothesis testing. The observer may take notes on the behaviour and actions of individuals and may record conversations and informal interviews using written notes and/or audio-recordings for later **transcription** and analysis.

The analysis of transcribed material from qualitative research is known as content or thematic analysis and involves the identification of themes emerging from the material. Statements may be coded or labelled and categorised into common themes presenting a broad range of experiences and views. There are several computer software packages available to facilitate analysis of qualitative data, including ATLAS.ti, NVivo, QSR and ETHNOGRAPH.

There is increasing interest in a so-called mixed-methods approach in epidemiological research. This involves combining both quantitative and qualitative data, methods, methodologies, and/or paradigms in a research study or set of related studies addressing complex problems. Mixed-methods approaches have several advantages.

- Narrow views of the world are often misleading, and approaching a subject from different perspectives or paradigms may help to gain a holistic perspective.
- There are different levels of research (i.e. biological, cognitive, social, etc.), and different methodologies may have particular strengths with respect to these levels. Using more than one method should help to get a clearer picture of the social world and make for more adequate explanations.

## 3.3 Psychiatric genetics

The quest for a clear understanding of the contribution of inherited factors (genetics) to psychiatric disease has been a very frustrating one. The current knowledge base, which comprises data obtained from family, twin and adoption studies, suggests that psychiatric diseases have a genetic or inherited component. The degree of **heritability**, however, varies greatly between disorders, with schizophrenia (>80% heritability), autism spectrum disorder (80% heritability), bipolar disorder (75% heritability) and attention deficit hyperactivity disorder (75% heritability) on the higher end of the spectrum (Sullivan, *et al.*, 2012), while post-traumatic stress disorder, panic disorder and major depressive disorder represent a lower heritability (Goenjian *et al.*, 2008; Sullivan *et al.*, 2012). To understand this, one needs to take a step back and look at some of the basic principles of genetics and how they apply to the study of psychiatry.

## 3.2 Advanced reading block

**Cultural factors in psychiatric epidemiology**

Practising psychiatric epidemiology in diverse social and cultural settings raises a number of important issues including the ways in which we classify psychiatric disorders, measure them, and seek to understand their aetiologies.

The predominant systems of classification and measurement of psychiatric disorders have arisen from Euro-American societies and assume that psychiatric disorders are broadly similar throughout the world and that measurements are universally applicable. This has been termed the **etic approach** and has involved standardisation of what constitutes 'caseness'. Problems with the etic approach include the fact that it ignores observed variations in the epidemiology, **phenomenology** and course and outcome of psychiatric disorders and does not take account of the important role of social, economic and cultural factors in contributing to these variations.

In contrast to the etic approach is the **emic approach** which, influenced heavily by the field of medical anthropology, recognises 'that illness is the result of a 'web of causation' which includes an individual's sociocultural environment' (Heggenhougen and Draper, 1990; Patel, 2003). The emic approach argues that society and culture play such an important role in the presentation of psychiatric disorders that systems of classification and measurement developed in Europe and America cannot be assumed to be universally appropriate (Littlewood, 1990). The emic approach is limited since:

- it cannot provide data that can be compared across cultures
- measurement methods are generally not standardised
- it typically involves small studies that are unable to address questions concerning the long-term course and outcome of disorders (Kirmayer, 1989).

Contemporary epidemiological approaches in cross-cultural settings attempt to integrate etic and emic approaches, establishing a 'culturally sensitive psychiatry' (Kleinman, 1987). This includes efforts to understand

- local explanatory models or causal attributions of illness
- local constructs of psychopathology
- the role of social, economic and cultural factors in determining the risk and course of mental illnesses
- local formal and informal health systems.

Comparisons can be made between diagnoses generated by international measures and local health providers. Measures must be sensitive and valid for the local social and cultural setting, but also be able to generate data that can be compared between different settings. An integrated approach thus should include ethnographic methods within epidemiological approaches and allow ethnography to both guide the epidemiological approach and help to understand the findings derived from the epidemiology.

## 3.3.1 Psychiatric disorders: a complex and multifactorial origin

Although there are a handful of genetic diseases that can be attributed to **mutations** occurring in a single gene, genetic research to date has shown that this does not apply to psychiatric disorders, which, like the majority of other diseases, are multifactoral and complex. Unlike Huntington's disease and cystic fibrosis, whose occurrence can be attributed to mutations occurring in specific genes, namely the Huntington (HTT) and the cystic fibrosis transmembrane conductance regulator (CFTR) genes (Collins 1992; Huntington's Disease Collaborative Research Group, 1993), psychiatric disorders appear to be polygenic (involving many genes) and are brought about by a combination of genetic and environmental factors interacting with one another. It seems likely that these disorders, rather than being caused by the disruption of a single gene, are caused by the disruption of a number of genes possibly occurring in common pathways. By determining which pathways are affected in these disorders we can deepen our understanding of the diseases and in so doing treat them more effectively.

Although psychiatric disorders do involve both gene-gene and gene-environment interactions, in disorders such as schizophrenia, genetics remains the biggest risk factor for developing the disorder. It has been shown that risk factors such as place of birth (urban areas), time of birth (winter), infections, prenatal care and obstetric complications all place individuals at a higher risk for developing schizophrenia. None of these risk factors, however, can more accurately predict the likelihood of developing schizophrenia than family history (Sullivan, 2005).

## 3.3.2 Genetic variants

Even though psychiatric disorders such as schizophrenia, autism spectrum disorder, bipolar disorder and attention deficit hyperactivity disorder are highly heritable, the exact mechanisms that confer this heritability remain elusive. This may in part be attributed to the vast number of variants present in the human genome. Each individual has about 3 million genetic variants in their genome, 20 000 of which are in coding areas and 250-300 of which result in the loss of function of a protein product (1000 Genomes Project Consortium, 2010). It is therefore difficult to filter out the variants that are not involved with disease progression from those that are actually conferring a risk for developing the disorder. Furthermore, there are several different types of genetic variants that have been hypothesised to play a role in placing individuals at an increased risk for developing a psychiatric disorder. These genetic variations include both common and rare genetic variants, in the form of single nucleotide polymorphisms (SNPs), small insertions or deletions of DNA (known as indels), large insertions or deletions of DNA (known as copy number variants (CNVs)) and rearrangements of DNA sequences (Sullivan *et al.*, 2012). In essence, the inherited abnormalities that contribute to psychiatric illness can be due to the interruption of the chromosome structure (such as translocations or inversions of parts of the chromosome) - in a sense a macro abnormality – or can be caused by the interruption of the normal function of a single or multiple genes. The latter can lead to over- or under- production of gene products or changes in the stability or structure of gene products. These variants can alter protein products by:

- changing the amino acid code
- creating or abolishing a start-or-stop codon
- creating or abolishing a splice site
- creating or removing transcription-factor binding sites and, in so doing, changing the amount of protein that is produced.

These 'micro' abnormalities (SNPs and indels), are smaller in size and typically involve one to a few hundred base pairs and are the most common contributing factor to the heritability of psychiatric disorders.

Interruptions of the chromosomal structure are varied in nature and can involve the deletion, translocation or duplication of parts of the chromosome. These defects are usually visible on **karyotypes** and some good examples exist in psychiatry. One of the best examples of the occurrence of 'macro' abnormalities is the deletion of parts of the long arm (q11-13) of chromosome 22 that has been associated with the highest known single-risk factor for schizophrenia. To demonstrate the enormity of this risk, 20-30% of individuals with 22q deletion syndrome develop schizophrenia (Murphy *et al.*, 1999) in comparison to the 1% of individuals in the general population that develop schizophrenia ((http://www.nimh.nih.gov/statistics/prevalence/schziophrenia1SCHIZ.shtml). Another classical example of the effect of interruptions of chromosomes is the translocation of a part of chromosome 1. First discovered in a Scottish family with a high incidence of psychiatric disorders such as schizophrenia, mood disorders and conduct disorder, 70% of the individuals carrying this mutation were shown to have a psychiatric disorder (Porteous *et al.*, 2011).

The translocation point is within a gene that plays an important role in **neurodevelopment** and the disruption of the gene (aptly named Disrupted in Schizophrenia 1 (DISC1) gene) leads to an increase in the risk for psychiatric disease. This translocation was first identified in a survey on juvenile delinquents. When this translocation was examined in other members of this individual's family it was discovered that of the members carrying this mutation, six were diagnosed with schizophrenia or related disorders, five were diagnosed with depression, three were diagnosed with adolescent conduct disorder and two were diagnosed with anxiety disorder (Millar *et al.*, 2000). Although there was much excitement regarding the role that this gene plays in the development of psychiatric disorders, later studies have been unable to consistently replicate these results, as is common with psychiatric genetic research.

### 3.3.3 How do variants and psychiatric disorders link up?

It becomes significantly more complex to link specific 'micro'-abnormalities to psychiatric illness. A look at the literature shows hundreds of different SNPs tested for association with psychiatric illness, either as part of family studies (looking for linkage) or patient-control type of designs. One of the best-curated websites documenting the results obtained from schizophrenia genetic studies has recorded 1 727 studies, which have identified 1 008 genes and 8 788 polymorphisms that are associated with schizophrenia (http://www.szgene.org/). The majority of these findings remain to be replicated. Further complicating psychiatric genetics research, not only are the results obtained inconsistent, but often the same variant is found to be associated with two or three different psychiatric diseases, as was the case with the Scottish family carrying the DISC1 mutation. Besides methodological problems (especially small number of cases), this illustrates the overlap in genetic contribution between some diseases such as bipolar and unipolar depression, obsessive compulsive disorder (OCD) and unipolar depression, as well as bipolar disorder and schizophrenia, to name a few. It has been found that families who are affected by schizophrenia, for instance, also appear to be affected by bipolar disorder, even though these disorders are diagnosed as being distinct from one another. One example of the overlap in genetic findings is the 5-HTTLPR **variable number tandem repeat** polymorphism that occurs in a serotonin transporter gene, SLC6A4, a gene critical to the transport of serotonin. This transporter helps to regulate serotonin availability by moving serotonin from the **synaptic cleft** into the presynaptic neuron (http://www.ncbi.nlm.nih.gov/gene/6532). This particular polymorphism, which has been associated with psychiatric disorders, has two variants, the long allele (L allele) and the short **allele** (S allele). The S allele, which leads to a twofold decrease in the expression of the transporter (Lesch *et al.*, 1996) has been associated with an increased risk for post-traumatic stress syndrome (Xie *et al.*, 2012), anxiety and depression among many other psychiatric diseases (Haddley *et al.*, 2012). Another variant that has been associated with various psychiatric disorders, including OCD and schizophrenia, is the Val158Met polymorphism in the catechol-O-methyltransferase (COMT) gene. This non-synonymous amino-acid change results in a three- to fourfold reduction in the activity of the COMT protein (Lachman *et al.*, 1996), which is responsible for the metabolism of dopamine in the synaptic cleft (http://www.ncbi.nlm.nih.gov/gene/1312). Once again the findings for both COMT and SLC6A4 are inconsistent and the results seem to overlap between different psychiatric disorders. Although psychiatric research often produces highly publicised results that are presented in renowned journals, the results are usually not consistently replicated and as such are hardly ever translated into the clinical setting.

### 3.3.4 The problem of inconsistent findings

There are different approaches to addressing these inconsistent findings. One of the aspects that may need to be considered is the characterisation of patients and controls. Due to the fact that the symptoms of psychiatric disorders are so varied, it may be that the actual phenotypes that are being compared are not the same. Patients and controls may therefore have to be classified into more homogenous groups. One way of doing this is to ensure that the symptoms and outcomes are assessed in a standardised manner and that the patients are at similar stages of disease progression.

Furthermore, instead of looking at the psychiatric disorder as a whole, intermediate traits and measurable biomarkers (known as endophenotypes) can be assessed. Thus, by breaking the disorder up into heritable parts, it may be easier to identify the specific genetic mechanisms involved (Light *et al.*, 2012). One such example is the cortisol awakening response (referring to the difference in cortisol levels between awakening and 20–45 minutes later) that could serve as an endophenotype for major depressive disorder (Goldstein and Klein, 2014). In addition to the characterisation of patients, it is of paramount importance that the controls are well matched to the patients in every aspect (e.g. age, sex, ethnicity) other than the presence of the psychiatric disorder.

Another important consideration with regards to psychiatric genetics is the study design. Initially, genetic studies used linkage mapping, which included affected and unaffected members of a family, to determine which areas of the genome segregate with the disease. As more information became available regarding the function of genes, candidate gene studies became more popular. These studies involve the examination of genetic variants in specific genes. The presence of these variants is then compared between patients and controls to determine if the variants occur at significantly different frequencies between the two groups. The genes chosen for these studies are usually prioritised based on their function and significance for the psychiatric disorder. The dopamine pathway, for example, is thought to be involved in the development of schizophrenia due to the fact that it has been found that changes in the levels of dopamine in certain areas of the brain are related to the different symptoms present in schizophrenia (Keshavan *et al.*, 2008). Based on this hypothesis a candidate gene study would choose genes that are involved in the dopamine pathway, such as the dopamine receptors (e.g. DRD2, DRD3 and DRD4) or the COMT gene that encodes for the enzyme responsible for metabolising dopamine.

The publishing of the first genome-wise association studies (GWAS) (Ozaki *et al.*, 2002; Klein *et al.*, 2005) changed the way that human genetic research was performed. GWAS allows for the simultaneous examination of hundreds of thousands of SNPs throughout the genome. Where candidate gene studies are based on a specific hypothesis, GWAS allows for a hypothesis-free approach, which is particularly useful in psychiatric disorders where little is known regarding the biological mechanisms involved in the development of these disorders. When looking at the catalogue of schizophrenia GWAS published to date, 1 381 results are available (Hindorff *et al.*, 2012). Unfortunately, even though there are a large number of studies that have been performed, they have only played a small role in elucidating the genetic factors involved in psychiatric disorders, which may in part be attributed to sample size. In order to account for the effect of multiple testing due to the vast number of variants that are genotyped, very large cohorts are required in order to obtain genome-wide significance. Thus, multi-collaborative efforts are essential in order to obtain these large cohorts of patients.

The Psychiatric Genomics Consortium is an excellent example of how psychiatric genetic research has done just this. The consortium has recently performed a mega-analysis GWAS for both schizophrenia (9 394 cases and 12 462 controls) and bipolar disorder (7 481 cases and 9 250 controls) (Ripke *et al.*, 2010; Sklar *et al.*, 2011). After replicating the top results in a further 8 000 cases, the schizophrenia study identified 7 loci that appear to be involved in the development of schizophrenia (Ripke *et al.*, 2010). The bipolar disorder study identified two significantly associated loci after replication in an additional 4 500 cases (Sklar *et al.*, 2011). Although both these studies have provided us with new information regarding disease susceptibility for bipolar disorder and schizophrenia, these newly identified variants can only explain a very small portion of the risk for developing the disorders.

## 3.3.5 A look into the future of psychiatric genetics

It is hoped that the rapid advances in sequencing technologies will close the gaps in knowledge that remain. In 2001, the first draft of the human genome was published. This was a huge advancement in genetics and took thirteen years and $3 billion dollars to complete (Wheeler *et al.*, 2008). Today we are able to sequence a genome for about a millionth of this price in a week (Nair, 2011). Furthermore, it is possible to sequence only the coding regions of the genome (1% of the total 3 billion base pairs of DNA) using a technology called exome sequencing, thereby further reducing the associated costs. With this rapid decrease in the cost and time associated with sequencing technology, it has become feasible to use this technology for psychiatric research. One of the big advantages of this is the ability to detect rare variations. This is important as it has been reported that the risk conveyed by genetic variants for psychiatric disorders is inversely proportional to the frequency at which these variants occur in the general population (Kim *et al.*, 2011). In other words, if a variant occurs often in the population, it will increase the risk of developing a psychiatric disorder only slightly; however, if the variant occurs very rarely, the risk that it is likely to confer is bigger. In the past GWAS studies have utilised common SNPs to evaluate genetic disease susceptibility factors; sequencing studies will now allow us to look at rare variants. However, with the analysis of rare variants, even larger samples sizes will be required to detect associations.

It is further hoped that re-sequencing studies will also address the disparities in psychiatric genetics research. In the past, approximately 75% of GWAS have been performed on individuals of European descent (Rosenberg *et al.*, 2010), while very few GWAS and psychiatric genetic studies have been performed on individuals of African descent (Drögemöller *et al.*, 2011; Wright *et al.*, 2011). This can largely be attributed to the fact that the DNA SNP chips used for GWAS were designed according to the genetic variation present in individuals of European descent. Due to the fact that African populations are genetically more diverse than non-African populations, it has been difficult to design chips that are able to capture all the variations present in these populations. Sequencing offers a solution to this by providing the opportunity to look at all the variations in the entire genome. It is hoped that the next phase of psychiatric genetic researchers will include African individuals in their study cohorts.

## 3.3.6 Epigenetics

One last aspect of psychiatric genetics that appears to hold promise for the future is the field of epigenetics. Apart from the genetic variants that have been discussed in this section, there are other genetic mechanisms that may be responsible for contributing to disease susceptibility. This genetic regulation is known as epigenetics. Epigenetics involves the regulation of DNA independent of the DNA sequence. In other words, an external environmental influence will affect how the DNA functions. Examples of this regulation include DNA methylation and histone modification, which involve the DNA becoming less (or more) accessible due to an environmental stimulus. The amount of the gene that is transcribed and eventually translated into a protein is subsequently decreased (or increased). This field is especially promising for psychiatric disorders and other complex diseases due to the fact that it is known that the development of these diseases is brought about by the interaction of genetics and the environment (Labrie *et al.*, 2012). Unfortunately, due to the fact that epigenetic regulation is often tissue specific, the study of this genetic mechanism remains complicated in psychiatric research, as it is usually not possible to obtain brain tissue.

The study of how genetics contributes to the development of psychiatric disorders is very important. Not only do these disorders clearly run in families and show a high heritability, they are also highly stigmatised and treatment is largely ineffective. By identifying genetic factors that contribute to the disease susceptibility, treatment can be improved by targeting the identified genes and pathways involved. Fields such as psychiatric **pharmacogenetics**, which looks at how genetic variants influence treatment efficacy and the occurrence of adverse drug reactions, can be implemented in the clinical setting to replace trial and error based dosing. Additionally, providing a biological basis for the disease should play a role in reducing the **stigma** associated with psychiatric disorders.

## Conclusion

It is not by accident that psychiatric genetics and epidemiology share this chapter. Indeed, these topics share an underlying complexity, with hidden substructures and interactions that still need clarification. A sound knowledge of the basic concepts, as we currently understand them, will allow the student to critically appraise new findings in psychiatric genetics and how these may inform the epidemiological basis of disease and vice versa.

# References


1000 Genomes Project Consortium (2010) A map of human genome variation from population-scale sequencing. *Nature* 467(7319): 1061–73

Berkman LF, Kawachi I (2000) *Social Epidemiology*. Oxford: Oxford University Press

Blakely TA, Subramanian SV (2006) Multilevel studies. In: Oakes JM and Kaufman JS (Eds) *Methods in Social Epidemiology*. San Francisco, CA: Jossey-Bass

Collins FS (1992) Cystic fibrosis: molecular biology and therapeutic implications. *Science* 256(5058): 774–9

Derogatis LR, Dellapietra L, Kilroy V. (1992) Screening for psychiatric disorder in medical populations. In: M Fava, JF Rosenbaum eds. *Research designs and methods in psychiatry*. Amsterdam: Elsevier, 1992, 145–170

Drögemöller BI, Wright GE, Niehaus DJ, Emsley RA, Warnich L (2011) Whole-genome resequencing in pharmacogenomics: moving away from past disparities to globally representative applications. *Pharmacogenomics* 12(12): 1717–28

Engel GL (1980) The clinical application of the biopsychosocial model. *American Journal of Psychiatry* 137: 535–544

Entrez Gene: SLC6A4. Available at http://www.ncbi.nlm.nih.gov/gene/6532. (Accessed 25 July 2012)

Entrez Gene: COMT. Available at http://www.ncbi.nlm.nih.gov/gene/1312. (Accessed 25 July 2012)

Goenjian AK, Noble EP, Walling DP, Goenjian HA, Karayan IS, Ritchie T, Bailey JN. (2008) Heritabilities of symptoms of posttraumatic stress disorder, anxiety, and depression in earthquake exposed Armenian families. *Psychiatric Genetics* 18(6): 261–6

Goldstein BL, Klein DN (2014) A review of selected candidate endophenotypes for depression. *Clinical Psychology Review* 34: 417–427

Haddley K, Bubb VJ, Breen G, Parades-Esquivel UM, Quinn JP (2012) Behavioural Genetics of the Serotonin Transporter. *Current topics in behavioural neurosciences* 12: 503–535

Heggenhougen K, Draper A (1990) *Medical Anthropology and Primary Health Care*. EPC Publication No. 22. London: London School of Hygiene and Tropical Medicine

Hill AB (1965) The environment and disease: Association or causation? *Proceedings of the Royal Society of Medicine* 58: 295–300

Hindorff LA, MacArthur J, Wise A, Junkins HA, Hall PN, Klemm AK, Manolio TA (2012) *A Catalog of Published Genome-Wide Association Studies*. Available at: www.genome.gov/gwastudies. (Accessed 24 July 2012)

Huntington's Disease Collaborative Research Group (1993) A novel gene containing a trinucleotide repeat that is expanded and unstable on Huntington's disease chromosomes. *Cell* 72(6): 971–83

Jablensky A (2002) Research methods in psychiatric epidemiology: An overview. *Australian and New Zealand Journal of Psychiatry* 36: 297–310

Jablonka E, Lamb MJ (2008) Soft inheritance: challenging the modern synthesis. *Genetics and Molecular Biology* 31(2): 389. DOI:10.1590/S1415-47572008000300001

Keshavan MS, Tandon R, Boutros NN, Nasrallah HA (2008) Schizophrenia,"Just the facts": What we know in 2008. Part 3: Neurobiology. *Schizophrenia Research* 106(2-3): 89–107

Kim Y, Zerwas S, Trace SE, Sullivan PF (2011) Schizophrenia genetics: Where next? *Schizophrenia Bulletin* 37(3): 456–63

Kirmayer LJ (1989) Cultural variations in the response to psychiatric disorders and emotional distress. *Social Science and Medicine* 29: 327–339

Klein RJ, Zeiss C, Chew EY, Tsai JY, Sackler RS, Haynes C, Henning AK, SanGiovanni JP, Mane SM, Mayne ST, Bracken MB, Ferris FL, Ott J, Barnstable C, Hoh J (2005) Complement Factor H Polymorphism in Age-Related Macular Degeneration. *Science* 308(5720): 385–9

Kleinman A (1987) Anthropology and psychiatry: the role of culture in cross-cultural research on illness. *British Journal of Psychiatry* 151: 447–454

Labrie V, Pai S, Petronis A (2012) Epigenetics of major psychosis: progress, problems and perspectives. *Trends in Genetics* 28(9): 427–35

Lachman HM, Papolos DF, Saito T, Yu YM, Szumlanski CL, Weinshilboum RM (1996) Human catechol-O-methyltransferasepharmacogenetics: description of a functional polymorphism and its potential application to neuropsychiatric disorders. *Pharmacogenetics* 6(3): 243–50

Lamarck JB (1809, 1914) *Zoological Philosophy* London: MacMillan

Lesch KP, Bengel D, Heils A, Sabol SZ, Greenberg BD, Petri S, Benjamin J, Muller CR, Hamer DH, Murphy DL (1996) Association of anxiety-related traits with a polymorphism in the serotonin transporter gene regulatory region. *Science* 274(5292):1527–31

Light GA, Swerdlow NR, Rissling AJ, Radant A, Sugar CA, Sprock J, Pela M, Geyer MA, Braff DL (2012) Characterization of neurophysiologic and neurocognitive biomarkers for use in genomic and clinical outcome studies of schizophrenia. *PLoS One* 7(7): e39434

Littlewood R (1990) From categories to contexts: A decade of the 'new cross-cultural psychiatry'. *British Journal of Psychiatry* 156: 308–327

Millar JK, Wilson-Annan JC, Anderson S, Christie S, Taylor MS, Semple CA, Devon RS, St Clair DM, Muir WJ, Blackwood DH, Porteous DJ (2000) Disruption of two novel genes by a translocation co-segregating with schizophrenia. *Human Molecular Genetics* 9(9): 1415–23

Murphy KC, Jones LA, Owen MJ (1999) High rates of schizophrenia in adults with velo-cardiofacial syndrome. *Archives of General Psychiatry* 56: 940–5

Murray J (1998) Qualitative Methods. *International Review of Psychiatry* 10: 312–6

Nair P QnAs with Eric S Lander (2011) Proceedings of the National Academy of Science USA 108(28): 11319

Ozaki K, Ohnishi Y, Iida A, Sekine A, Yamada R, Tsunoda T, Sato H, Sato H, Hori M, Nakamura Y, Tanaka T (2002) Functional SNPs in the lymphotoxin-alpha gene that are associated with susceptibility to myocardial infarction. *Nature Genetics* 32(4): 650–4

Patel V (2003) Cultural issues in measurement and research. In: Prince M, Stewart R, Ford T, Hotopf M (Eds) *Practical Psychiatric Epidemiology*. Oxford: Oxford University Press

Porteous DJ, Millar JK, Brandon NJ, Sawa A (2011) DISC1 at 10: connecting psychiatric genetics and neuroscience. *Trends in Molecular Medicine* 17(12): 699–706

Ripke S, Sanders AR, Kendler KS, *et al.* (2011) Genome-wide association study identifies five new schizophrenia loci. *Nature Genetics* 43(10): 969–76

Rosenberg NA, Huang L, Jewett EM, Szpiech ZA, Jankovic I, Boehnke M (2010) Genome-wide association studies in diverse populations. *Nature Reviews Genetics* 11(5): 356–66

Rothman KJ, Greenland S (1998) *Modern Epidemiology*, 2nd ed. Philadelphia, PA: Lippincott-Raven

Sklar P, Ripke S, Scott LJ, *et al.* Large-scale genome-wide association analysis of bipolar disorder identifies a new susceptibility locus near ODZ4. *Nature Genetics* 43(10): 977–83

Sullivan PF (2005) The genetics of schizophrenia. *PLOS Medicine* 2(7): e212

Sullivan PF, Daly MJ, O'Donovan M (2012) Genetic architectures of psychiatric disorders: The emerging picture and its implications. *Nature Reviews Genetics* 13(8): 537–51

Susser M (1991) What is a cause and how do we know one? A grammar for pragmatic epidemiology. *American Journal of Epidemiology* 133: 635–48

SZGene. Available at http://www.szgene.org/ (Accessed 25 July 2012)

Tohen M, Bromet E (1997) Epidemiology in psychiatry. In: Tasman A, Kay J, Lieberman JA, Saunders WB (Eds). *Psychiatry*. New York: Saunders

Tohen M, Bromet E, Murphy JM, Tsuang MT (2000) Psychiatric epidemiology. *Harvard Review of Psychiatry* 8: 111–125

Weich S, Prince M (2003) Cohort studies. In: Prince M, Stewart R, Ford T, Hotopf M (Eds). *Practical Psychiatric Epidemiology*. Oxford: Oxford University Press

Wheeler DA, Srinivasan M, Egholm M, Shen Y, Chen L, McGuire A, He W, Chen YJ, Makhijani V, Roth GT, Gomes X, Tartaro K, Niazi F, Turcotte CL, Irzyk GP, Lupski JR, Chinault C, Song XZ, Liu Y, Yuan Y, Nazareth L, Qin X, Muzny DM, Margulies M, Weinstock GM, Gibbs RA, Rothberg JM (2008) The complete genome of an individual by massively parallel DNA sequencing. *Nature* 452(7189): 872–6

Wright GE, Niehaus DJ, Koen L, Drögemöller BI, Warnich L (2011) Psychiatric genetics in South Africa: cutting a rough diamond. *African Journal of Psychiatry* 14(5): 355–66

Xie P, Kranzler HR, Farrer L, Gelernter J (2012) Serotonin transporter 5-HTTLPR genotype moderates the effects of childhood adversity on posttraumatic stress disorder risk: A replication study. *American Journal of Medical genetics Part B Neuropsychiatric Genetics* DOI: 10.1002/ajmg.b.32068

CHAPTER

# 4 The neurobiology of psychiatric disorders

Brian Harvey, Dana Niehaus

## 4.1 Cellular and molecular principles in psychiatry

Neurons form the hard-wired circuitry of the brain, without which signal transduction and communication would not be possible. In order to better understand the neuropathology of psychiatric illness, as well as response to drug treatment, it is necessary to understand how the brain communicates and how such communication networks go awry to culminate in a given disorder. Although so-called hard-wired circuits that use traditional neurotransmitters are the best-known communication network in the central nervous system (CNS), atypical gaseous neurotransmitters that are synthesised de novo, such as nitric oxide (NO; see Figure 4.1), are analogous to a wi-fi network or wireless connection. Figure 4.1 shows a cartoon of a typical glutamatergic neuron, depicting pre-synaptic release of the typical neurotransmitter, glutamate, and its binding to post-synaptic ionotropic NMDA receptors. Subsequent activation of calcium ($Ca2^{+}$) – dependent nitric oxide synthase (NOS) leads to de novo synthesis of the atypical transmitter nitric oxide (or NO) from the semi-essential amino acid L-arginine and the co-production of *l*-citrulline. *l*-citrulline now acts as a diffusable pre- (retrograde) – and post-synaptic messenger influencing the same and many other neighbouring neurons by activation of the guanylate cyclase-cyclic guanosine monophosphate (GMP) system. cGMP in turn is broken down by cGMP-specific phosphodiesterase (PDE) 5. Due to its high lipid solubility, nitric oxide can diffuse quickly across larger intercellular distances, easily traversing membranes to activate specific subcellular elements (for example guanylyl cyclase) to produce rapid and powerful physiological effects. Nitric oxide

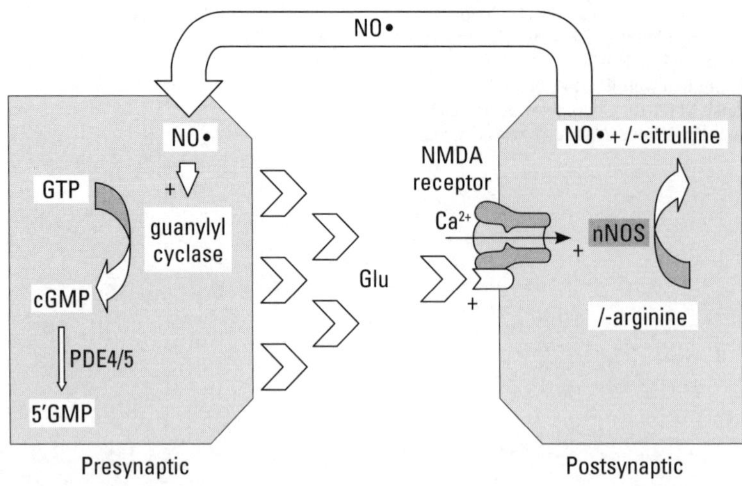


**Figure 4.1** The synthesis and release of the atypical gaseous transmitter, nitric oxide (NO)

has been suggested to be a retrograde messenger central to certain cellular processes such as memory (see Figure 4.1) (Oosthuizen *et al.*, 2005; Harvey, 2006).

A typical neuron (see Figure 4.2) consists of:

- the cell body or soma containing the nucleus and other critical cellular elements
- dendrites that sprout from the cell body making connections with neighbouring neurons and cells
- an axon that projects an extended distance from the cell body (e.g. monoaminergic cell bodies located in the brainstem) to other brain regions (e.g. frontal cortex, striatum, hippocampus)
- axon branches
- axon terminals that sprout from the axon making synaptic connections with the target cells or neurons.

Two types of neurons can be identified: interneurons with short axons that are limited to a single area, such as amino acids, acetylcholine (Ach), and neuropeptides, and neurons with long axons that form specific **projection** pathways to distal regions of the brain. *l*-Norepinephrine (NE) pathways project from the locus coeruleus in the pons to the forebrain, cerebellum and spinal cord. Serotonergic projections start at the raphae nuclei in the mid-brain and pons (raphe) and project to the forebrain, cerebellum and spinal cord. Dopaminergic cell bodies lie predominantly in the midbrain, specifically the ventral tegmental area and the substantia nigra, of which the primary pathways are the nigrostriatal, mesolimbic, mesocortical and tubero-infundibular pathways (see Section 4.5 and Table 4.1). Cholinergic neurons are prominent as interneurons in the striatum, while an important cholinergic pathway projects from the forebrain column, originating in the nucleus basalis of Meynert to innervate the cortex. γ-Amino butyric acid (GABA) and glycine are found diffused in interneurons (supraspinal and spinal), while the nigrostriatal GABA pathway projects from the striatum to the substantia nigra. Histamine enjoys a dense distribution in the central nervous system, especially the hypothalamus. Glutamate is exclusively diffused throughout the brain as relay neurons and interneurons.

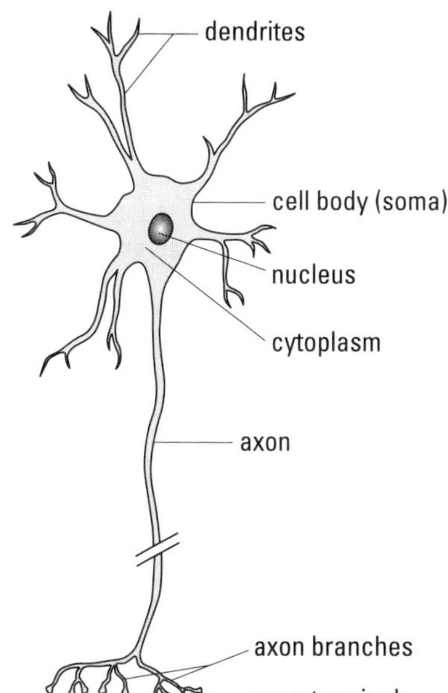


**Figure 4.2** A typical neuron

The overall function of the brain is decentralised to anatomically distinct regions that are dependent on one another, being connected via the myriad of neurotransmitter circuits and networks described above.

Let us now look at the neuroanatomy of the brain.

## 4.2 Functional neuroanatomy of the brain

The brain develops from three embryonic brain vesicles, namely the prosencephalon (combined telencephalon and diencephalon), mesencephalon and rhombencephalon. Both the cerebral cortex and corpus striatum derive from the telencephalon. The thalamus and hypothalamus develop from the diencephalon, the midbrain from the mesencephalon, and the pons, cerebellum and medulla oblongata from the rhombencephalon. Let us consider in more detail the contribution each of these developmental areas makes to our understanding of the functioning of the brain, starting from the outside and moving inwards.

The various regions of the brain are functionally interconnected and thus should not be viewed as independent of each other. The functional arrangement of the nervous system generally involves sensory input, processing and integration, and motor and autonomic output. Sensory organs pick up touch and other sensory inputs which are relayed to the cord or brainstem and transmitted via white matter and intervening neurons to the thalamus and cerebellum, which are the points of convergence of sensory stimuli other than vision and smell. The converged input is then relayed via the thalamus to the cortex via connecting white matter.

Processing takes place first in the primary sensory cortex, then in the unimodal association cortex and finally in the heteromodal association cortex. Cortically processed information (from the unimodal association cortex) is sent to the temporal lobe and hippocampus to be recorded as memory. Memory then flows out via the temporal lobe to the association cortices to be stored as long-term memory. During this process the frontal lobe, with the help of the basal ganglia, acts as an observer and retriever of information and plays an executive role.

Outputs from central processing exert their effects via the motor system and the autonomic (sympathetic and parasympathetic) nervous system. Motor outflow takes place from the primary motor cortex to the cord after processing in the loops of the motor system (primary, premotor and supplementary motor cortex, basal ganglia and cerebellum – where the cerebellum

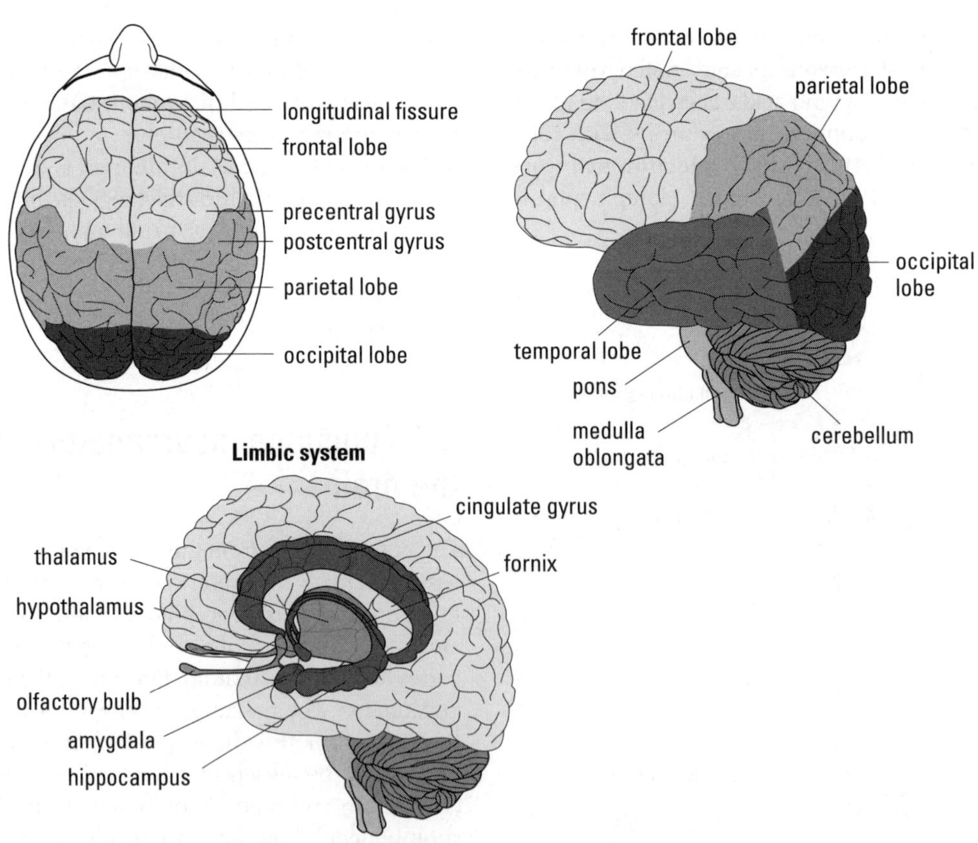


**Figure 4.3** Diagrammatic representation of the brain

facilitates motor learning). Vegetative functions (eating, sleeping, etc.) and autonomic nervous system functions are controlled from the hypothalamus and the reticular activating system. Outflow of the sympathetic and parasympathetic nervous system is crucial for regulating the homeostasis of the body (i.e. fight-or-flight reactions versus maintenance of the body at rest).

## 4.2.1 Cerebral cortex

The outer layer of the brain, the cerebral cortex, is a complex layer divided into a number of lobes.

The cortex is crucial to the execution of higher functions such as reading, writing and understanding our environment on a cognitive or thinking level. The cortex extracts meaning from primary sensory input such as auditory, visual, somatosensory, vestibular and smell (in the primary sensory and unimodal association cortex) and then binds these inputs together to form an integrated experience of the self and the environment (in the heteromodal association cortex).

The cortex extends over the two halves of the brain (right and left hemispheres), which are separated (or rather connected) by the corpus callosum, a massive band of white matter that connects matching areas of the cortex of the two hemispheres. The right and left hemispheres are responsible for different functions (although considerable overlap occurs) in the brain. The hemisphere that contains the speech centres is considered the dominant hemisphere, and not the other way around, which is why left-handed people are still mostly (75%) left hemisphere dominant and the left hemisphere is dominant in right-handed people. The dominant side is associated with language and language-dependent memory, whereas the non-dominant side is responsible for visual and spatial **perception** as well as non-language dependent (visual) memory. The cortex can be divided into five lobes: the frontal, temporal, parietal, occipital, and the limbic lobes. (The limbic lobes are generally referred to as the limbic system.)

It should thus be clear that much of the cortex is devoted to sensory processing and that higher functions (with the exception of the frontal lobe) emerge from junctions (called the heteromodal association cortex) between these areas.

### 4.2.1.1 Frontal lobe

The frontal lobes can be subdivided into the following major areas:

- Motor area (primary motor cortex), which occupies the precentral gyrus (Brodmann area 4). This area is responsible for contralateral voluntary movement.
- Supplementary motor area, which lies anterior to the motor strip. This area co-ordinates and plans motor activity.
- Paracentral lobule, which controls the cortical functions of inhibiting the spinal centre for bladder and bowel voiding until the appropriate time.
- Frontal eye fields, which mediate eye movements in the contralateral direction. This area also plays a role in spatial attention.
- Broca's area (Brodmann areas 44 and 45), usually in the left hemisphere, occupies the inferior prefrontal region. This is the expressive centre for speech.
- Prefrontal cortex proper, which can be subdivided into the dorsolateral prefrontal cortex (DLPFC), the ventromedial prefrontal cortex (VMPFC), and the orbitofrontal cortex (OFC). Pathology in the prefrontal cortex can present as three different prefrontal syndromes. These include the frontal convexity syndrome (predominantly dorsolateral area damage leading to poor abstract thought, indifference and **apathy**), medial frontal syndrome (predominantly ventromedial damage that produces akinesis, incontinence and sparse verbal output) and orbitofrontal syndrome (predominantly orbitofrontal damage which is characterised by **disinhibition**, emotional lability and poor judgement).

It is clear from the variety of critical functions that damage to the frontal lobes can have devastating effects and it is important to note that conditions such as schizophrenia and frontotemporal dementia are linked to dysfunction in the frontal lobes.

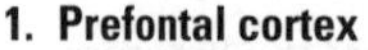

1. **Prefontal cortex**
   – controls personality and behaviour
2. **Premotor cortex**
   – control of movement
3. **Broca's area**
   – controls speech
4. **Primary motor cortex**
   – controls movement
5. **Primary somatosensory cortex**
   – controls sensation
6. **Pareito-occipital sensory association cortex**
   – controls perceptual awareness
7. **Visual cortex**
   – controls vision
8. **Auditory cortex**
   – controls hearing
9. **Temporal sensory association cortex**
   – controls recognition and identification of stimuli (including language)
10. **Cerebellum**
    – controls posture, balance and movement
11. **Brainstem**
    – controls involuntary functions

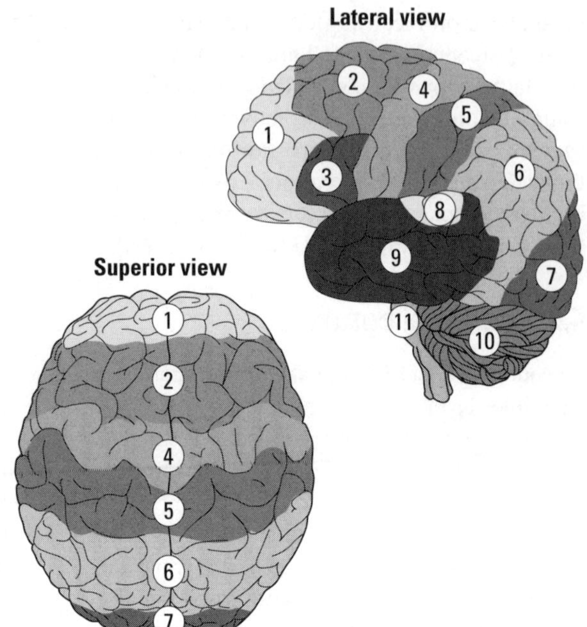


**Figure 4.4** Brain areas and selected functions of each area

### 4.2.1.2 Parietal lobe

The parietal lobe plays a central role in interpreting or making sense of primary somatosensory impulses received from somatosensory receptors across the body. It then integrates these inputs to generate a body map and finally creates a three-dimensional perception of space.

There are two areas in the parietal lobe that play a crucial role in this process:

- the unimodal association cortex receives unprocessed somatosensory input from the periphery, processes the information in areas 1, 2 and 3, and then generates a body map
- the heteromodal association cortex is located in the posterior parietal lobe and binds sensory input from all the modalities as it is received from the respective unimodal cortices – sight, sound, somatosensory, vestibular – and then creates a three-dimensional perception of space (environment).

In addition, the parietal lobes are responsible for higher functions such as calculation, visuospatial function and language function (namely phonological processing in reading).

The most important areas for psychiatry are therefore the postcentral gyrus (where one finds the sensory cortex (Brodmann areas 1, 2 and 3)), the supramarginal gyrus (Brodmann area 40), and the angular gyrus (Brodmann area 39). The latter two form part of Wernicke's language area in the dominant hemisphere. In addition, the fibres of the optic radiation (part of the visual pathway) pass through the depths of the parietal lobe.

The dominant lobe is not only important in terms of language-related functions, but also in the ability to perform calculations, while the non-dominant lobe plays a role in the awareness of one's environment.

Damage to the parietal lobes can cause different clinical signs or symptoms, depending on which hemisphere is affected. Gerstmann's syndrome is a consequence of lesions of the angular gyrus of the dominant hemisphere, the area most associated with writing ability. In Gerstmann's syndrome, the patient shows **dyscalculia,** dysgraphia, right-left disorientation and finger **agnosia** (a deficit in the recognition of body parts). Damage to the non-dominant parietal lobe can lead to anosognosia (lack of awareness of neurological deficit), dressing **apraxia** (difficulty dressing), geographical agnosia (disturbance of geographical memory) and constructional apraxia (inability to copy patterns).

#### 4.2.1.3 Occipital lobe

The occipital lobe is synonymous with the visual pathways. The visual system consists of the following components:

- retinas
- optic tracts that run to the thalamus (lateral geniculate nuclei) and brainstem
- optic radiations that run from the thalamus through the temporal and parietal lobes en route to the occipital cortex, thus connecting the retinas to the brainstem and visual cortex
- cortical areas involved in higher visual functions.

The higher visual functions refer to the process of extracting meaning in the visual cortex. To extract meaning from visual input, two streams of information are needed – a stream of information flowing to the parietal lobe and thus establishing the 'where in space', and a 'what' stream that flows to the temporal lobe and helps with the recognition of objects, colours and faces.

It is important to understand that vision is a crossed sensation. This means that the visual field on the one side of the visual axis registers on the opposite side's visual cortex. Cortical lesions in the occipital lobe can present in different ways depending on the extent of the lesion. Extensive bilateral cortical lesions will result in complete cortical blindness. When the occipital pole is the only area involved, the pathology will involve a central hemianopia (half of the central visual field) defect involving the macula and several different possible combinations of visual impairment. These lesions are relatively rare and it is much more common to see damage to only one occipital lobe, which causes a homonymous hemianopia with central sparing. A very common and useful localising sign is a homonymous hemianopia that follows from a lesion after the optic chiasm.

In addition to vision, the occipital lobe plays an important role in the process of reading. The first step of visual processing involves Brodmann areas 17, 18 and 19 (visual cortex). Two pathways are activated simultaneously: one that passes via the angular gyrus (Brodmann area 39) to Wernicke's area and accesses the temporal lobe memory store for a phonologic representation of every syllable, and a second pathway that accesses the semantic memory store for meaning via the left dorsolateral prefrontal cortex.

#### 4.2.1.4 Temporal lobe

The temporal lobes perform a complex array of functions including hearing, learning and memory. The auditory cortex (Brodmann areas 41 and 42) of the dominant hemisphere is important for the hearing of language, whereas sounds, rhythm and music are functions of the non-dominant hemisphere. Indeed, Wernicke's speech area, which is involved in speech comprehension, is also known as the auditory association cortex (Brodmann area 22). Memory and learning are facilitated by the middle and inferior temporal gyri while visual pathways pass (the 'what' stream) deep in the temporal lobe around the posterior horn of the lateral ventricle to the occipital lobe. One can therefore expect the temporal lobes to play an important role in Alzheimer's dementia.

#### 4.2.1.5 Limbic lobe

The limbic lobes consist of the inferior and medial portions of the temporal lobe, including the hippocampus and parahippocampal gyrus. Two functions important to this lobe are the sensation of olfaction and emotional/affective behaviour. The extended limbic system is sometimes referred to as the circuit of Papez. The extended limbic system is involved in laying down and retrieving episodic memories, again suggesting an important role in cognitive disorders and in the cognitive symptoms of disorders such as depression and post-traumatic stress disorder.

#### 4.2.1.6 White matter

Moving below the cortical grey matter, deeper into the brain, we reach the white matter, which surrounds the deep grey matter islands, or nuclei, of the thalamus, hypothalamus and basal ganglia. An important clinical distinction between cortical and subcortical structures is evident in the anatomy of the dementias, where dementia with white matter changes differs from dementia with predominantly subcortical changes. It is thus important to have a good understanding of these structures.

### 4.2.2 Thalamus and hypothalamus

The thalamus acts as a major relay station and all sensory input (except olfaction) passes through the thalamus before reaching the unimodal association cortex. The ascending reticular activating system (ARAS) is an important component of this connectiveness between senses and the cortex and is able to gate the sensory transmission through the thalamus during sleep.

In a sense the thalamus acts as a radio station, broadcasting news received from its reporters (brainstem, etc.) to a wide audience (the cortex). These structures, and the pathways connecting them, are all involved in attentional processes. The intralaminar nuclei of the thalamus receive inputs from the brainstem nuclei and relay information widely to the cortex. Interestingly, there is also a feedback loop from the cortex to the thalamus that helps to modulate the amount of traffic allowed through the thalamus. The thalamus also forms an important part of the circuit of Papez, which is involved in episodic memory.

The hypothalamus plays a role in functions important for the basic survival of human beings, such as reproduction, growth and metabolism, food and fluid intake, attack and defence, temperature control, the sleep-wake cycle and memory. It also controls the pituitary gland (anterior and posterior lobes) and both divisions of the autonomic nervous system. The sleep-wake cycle is a good example of the key control function of the hypothalamus. The sleep promotor is localised in the ventrolateral pre-optic nucleus (VLPO) of the hypothalamus and is regulated by GABA. The wake promotor is situated within the tuberomammillary nucleus (TMN) of the hypothalamus and is regulated by histamine. Orexin neurons in the lateral hypothalamus stabilise wakefulness, while the suprachiasmatic nucleus acts as the body's internal clock. Since depression is associated with sleep and appetite changes, one can understand why the hypothalamus is implicated in depression and anxiety disorders.

### 4.2.3 Brainstem

The brainstem contains the nuclei of the cranial nerves and is divided into the midbrain (cranial nerve 3 and 4), pons (most of cranial nerve 5-7), medulla (cranial nerve 9-12; with cranial nerve 8 at the pontomedullary junction) and the reticular formation. Most of the medulla is critical to life: it facilitates vegetative functions such as respiration, blood pressure and heart rate control. The reticular formation, which is distributed throughout the brainstem, is important for the initiation of sleep, the production of dreams and the maintenance of alertness by **switching** off the sleep circuits. Large strokes of the brainstem will thus cause coma.

It is important to have a good understanding of the cranial nerves as clinical detection of defects in cranial nerve function help identify the possible location of a lesion:

- The extra-ocular muscle nerve nuclei: the centre for vertical gaze control, the nuclei of the oculomotor nerve (CN III) as well as the trochlear nerve (CN IV) are situated in the midbrain of the brainstem. The abducens nucleus (CN VI) is located in the caudal pons. Together these nuclei are responsible for ocular muscle innervation.
- The lower cranial nerve nuclei (including CN XI): at the bulbar level, the nucleus of the hypoglossal nerve (CNXII), which innervates the tongue, represents the motor somatic column. The dorsal vagal complex consists of the dorsal motor nucleus of the vagus (X) and the solitary nucleus.
- Trigeminal nerve (CN V) nuclei: the general sensory information from the head is conveyed

to nuclei of the trigeminal nerve, which extend along the brainstem as cell columns.

- Vestibulo-cochlear (CN VIII) nuclei and lateral lemniscus: this pathway carries sensory information from the inner ear to the ventral and dorsal cochlear nuclei, located between the medulla and the pons.

Additional structures found in the brainstem include the major descending motor pathways formed by the corticospinal and corticopontine tracts, the pontocerebellar fibre system and the ascending sensory tracts (medial lemniscus and the spinothalamic tract).

### 4.2.4 Cerebellum

Macroscopically, the cerebellum can be subdivided into three different lobes, namely the anterior, posterior and flocculonodular lobes. The anterior lobe receives afferent fibres from the spinal cord and therefore plays an important role in the maintenance of gait. The posterior lobe receives afferent fibres from, and projects efferent fibres to, the motor cortex/vestibular nuclei, pons and basal ganglia. This is important for maintenance of posture and modulation of motor skills. The flocculonodular lobe receives afferent fibres from the vestibular system and helps with the maintenance of balance and control of eye movements.

### 4.2.5 Cerebral spinal fluid and blood supply

In addition to these structures, one cannot neglect to mention that the cerebral spinal fluid system (CSFS) and the cerebral blood supply are critical anatomical aspects of brain function. The cerebral spinal fluid (CSF) is produced by the choroid plexus in the lateral ventricle and then circulates through the ventricular system (lateral, third and fourth ventricles), exits via the foramina, then flows into the subarachnoid space to exit via the arachnoid granulations of the dural venous sinuses and the foramina of Luschka and Magendi to bathe the spinal cord.

The vascular system of the brain is critical to the functioning of the whole brain, interruption of which leads to loss of function (or a 'stroke') in the area supplied by the particular artery. Strokes can affect large areas of the brain or only small localised areas, depending on the size or importance of the arterial blood supply. Although strokes (which are usually caused by either vascular thrombosis or intracranial haemorrhage) are the ambit of neurology, it is nevertheless important to have a good knowledge of the consequences of obstruction of each of the major blood supply components and how this relates to the symptoms and signs described in this chapter.

Having reviewed the most important regions or components of the brain that play a role in psychiatric illness, the next step is to understand how these various brain regions are connected via specific neurocircuitry attended by specific neurotransmitters. We now consider the molecular aspects of neurotransmitter signalling.

## 4.3 Fundamentals of synaptic transmission in psychiatry and psychopharmacology

Having earlier described the neuroanatomy and neurotransmitter circuitry of the brain, let us now focus on the concept of synaptic transmission and how this and the brain neuroanatomy come together to define our understanding of the neurobiology and pharmacology of psychiatric illness (Harvey, 1997; Brink, 2004). Once released into the synaptic cleft, the neurotransmitter can either interact with presynaptic or postsynaptic target receptors (see Figure 4.5), or undergo metabolic breakdown or be taken up into the presynaptic neuron via neurotransmitter transporters (see Figure 4.6). Figure 4.6 provides a diagrammatic representation of pre- and post-synaptic neurons, showing storage of the neurotransmitter (in vesicles), release into the synapse, re-uptake into the pre-synaptic neuron via specific transporters, and metabolism by monoamine oxidase (MAO) and catechol-O-methyl transferase (COMT).

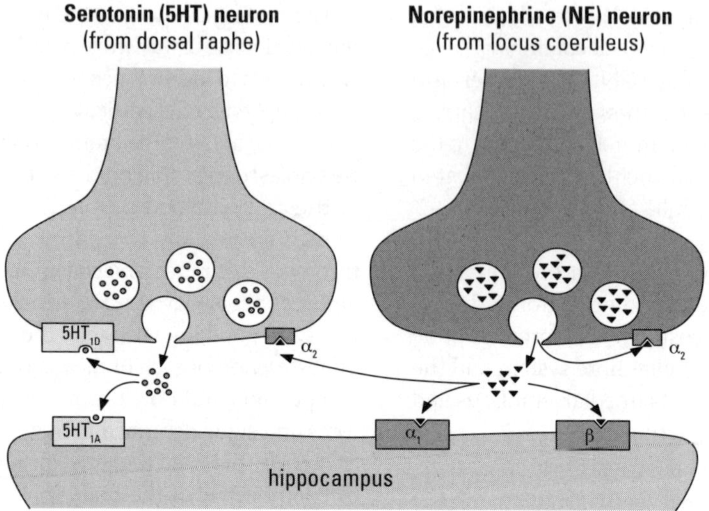


**Figure 4.5** Norepinephrine-serotonin cross-talk in the hippocampus

**Source:** Adapted figure by kind permission of The Lundbeck Institute. http://www.cnsforum.com

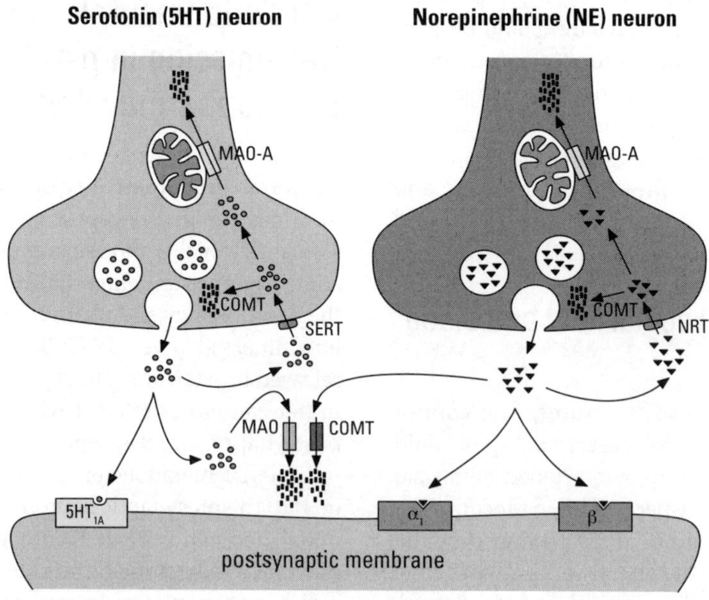


**Figure 4.6** Diagrammatic representation of pre- and postsynaptic neurons showing the molecular targets involved in regulating synaptic neurotransmitter levels

**Source:** Adapted figure by kind permission of The Lundbeck Institute. http://www.cnsforum.com

The figure also indicates post-synaptic binding of the transmitter to its target receptor. Most, if not all, of the pharmacological approaches to treating psychiatric illness are directed at one or more of these receptors, metabolic or reuptake processes, as will be described in subsequent sections (Harvey, 1997). Postsynaptic receptors (e.g. $\alpha_1$-adrenergic, $\beta$ adrenergic, $D_1$, 5-$HT_{2A}$) initiate responses in the target organ or neuron (see Figure 4.5 and Figure 4.6) while these responses are under strict regulation by presynaptic auto-inhibitory receptors, such as $\alpha_2$, $D_2$ and 5-$HT_{1A/D}$ receptors (see Figure 4.5). Carrier molecules (or transporters) located on presynaptic neurons (e.g. 5-HT reuptake transporter (SRT), DA reuptake transporter (DAT) and the NE reuptake transporter (NRT)), regulate synaptic neurotransmitter levels by binding the neurotransmitter and transporting it back into the presynaptic neuron where it is either stored in vesicles or metabolised by monoamine oxidase (MAO) or catechol-O-methyl transferase (COMT; see Figure 4.6). These neurotransmitter reuptake processes are essential components in the brain's ability to self-regulate and to curb excessive release of the neurotransmitter.

While neurotransmitters can regulate their own synthesis and release via actions on presynaptic **autoreceptors** (e.g. $\alpha_2$ receptors on noradrenergic neurons; see Figure 4.5), **heteroreceptors** located on adjacent postsynaptic neurons regulate the function and activity of *other* neuronal networks (e.g. $\alpha_2$ receptors located on serotonergic neurons or 5-$HT_{2A}$ receptors located on dopamine (DA) neurons (not shown). A good clinical example of neuronal cross-talk, where one neurotransmitter can regulate the function of another, relates to the non-specific serotonergic actions of serotonin reuptake inhibitors (SSRI). By inducing an elevation in 5-HT in diverse brain regions, an SSRI can, for example, modulate dopaminergic pathways via a cross-talk mechanism between 5-HT and DA neurons, leading to non-specific side effects such as **dyskinesia** (Harvey, 1997; 1999). Alternatively, targeting such a cross-talk mechanism, by for example blocking $\alpha_2$ receptors, may provide an additional **mode of action** with added therapeutic benefit by disinhibiting NA and S-HT release (e.g. mirtazapine; see Figure 4.5). More often than not a given signal and its associated behavioural response is a cumulative effect of a network of multiple interacting signalling substances.

Finally, the regulation of neurotransmitter anabolism (with precursors such as L-DOPA or L-tyrosine) or the targeting of its metabolism by modulating enzymes such as MAO (e.g. with drugs such as tranylcypromine, moclobemide), COMT (e.g. talcapone) or acetylcholine esterase (e.g. donepezil), are essential mechanisms for controlling neurotransmitter levels and for regulating the availability of precursors for neurotransmitter synthesis (see Figure 4.6). These strategies have therapeutic value in illnesses where there is a relative neurotransmitter deficit (e.g. NE, DA and Ach in depression, Parkinson's disease and Alzheimer's disease, respectively).

Two types of signal transduction systems are evident in the CNS. The opening of ion channels, referred to as ***ionotropic receptors***, mediates the influx or efflux of chloride ($Cl^-$), sodium ($Na^+$) or calcium ($Ca^{2+}$) ions. These receptors provide a rapid response (see Figure 4.7). The second, referred to as **metabotropic receptors**, are **guanosine (G) binding protein**-coupled receptor systems that promote the formation of various **second messenger** molecules, specifically cyclic adenosine monophosphate (cAMP), inositol triphosphate ($IP_3$) and/or diacylglycerol via the enzymatic conversion of specific precursor molecules (e.g. $PIP_2$, ATP; see Figure 4.7) (Brink *et al.*, 2004). Receptor signalling proceeds via either the adenylyl cyclase (AC)-cAMP system or the phospholipase C (PLC)-inositol phosphate system through a process of metabolic conversion of cell membrane precursors or energy-rich phosphates (see Figure 4.7). Sustained response is subsequently mediated by the synthesis of transcription factors. These metabolic processes are time-dependent and hence metabotropic receptor activation is slow, although more long-lasting than ionotropic receptor-mediated events (Harvey and Shahid, 2012).

Once the neurotransmitter (or 'first messenger,' e.g. NE), has activated the postsynaptic

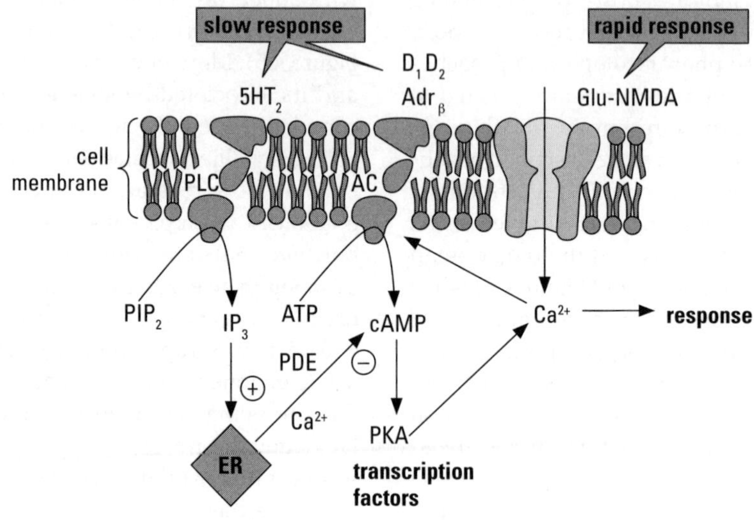


**Figure 4.7** Sub-cellular processes underlying metabotropic and ionotropic receptor signalling

receptor, a cascade of events is initiated within the subcellular domain. This cascade involves activation of various **protein kinase** enzymes (e.g. protein kinase A; PKA) that phosphorylate enzymes, ion channels and other proteins, which in turn culminates in a cellular response (see Figure 4.7) (Brink *et al.*, 2004). While autoreceptor and heteroreceptor directed modulation can control the degree and duration of postsynaptic receptor activation, once the subcellular switch has been turned on it becomes much more difficult and complex to modulate the signal. Nevertheless, an already activated postsynaptic signal can be altered or even reversed by a series of natural homeostatic mechanisms that constantly ensure that neuronal (and by implication brain) function is optimal. Figure 4.7 depicts various neurotransmitters systems (e.g. 5-HT, DA, NE, glutamatergic) impacting on the same postsynaptic membrane. First, because metabotropic signalling takes longer to respond than the rapid signal instated by ionotropic receptors, activation of the ionotropic N-methyl-D-aspartate (NMDA) receptor will evoke a quicker response than metabotropic monoaminergic receptors. However, as illustrated in Figure 4.7, either ionotropic or metabotropic receptor cascade can modulate the events set in place by the other by virtue of an intricate web of interacting and intermodulating neurochemical pathways, such as $Ca^{2+}$-mediated regulation of AC and PKA-mediated regulation of $Ca^{2+}$ signalling, etc. (see Figure 4.7). Thus, as with intra-synaptic receptor cross-talk referred to above, intra-cellular cross-talk between receptor-activated cascades also must be considered, so that receptor selectivity of a particular compound may not necessarily translate into subcellular selectivity (Harvey, 1997; Leonard, 2003).

It is now apparent that 'binding' of a transmitter or drug to a given receptor represents the basis for chemical (or drug)-receptor interactions. Indeed, in the words of one of the fathers of modern pharmacology, Paul Ehrlich, 'agents do not act unless they are bound'.

Let us now consider the physico-chemical aspects of how these substances interact with their receptor, this being fundamental to an understanding of drug action (Brink *et al.*, 2004).

## 4.4 Receptorology in psychiatry and psychopharmacology

The autonomic nervous system's dependence on the secretion of Ach and NE in parasympathetic and sympathetic nerves respectively, provided the first evidence that chemical transmission represents the functional basis for the nervous system. Nerve cells communicate with one another and with adjacent cells by releasing a specific neurotransmitter from the nerve ending into the synaptic cleft. The released neurotransmitter perfuses across this space and binds to a specific surface receptor on the outer side of the presynaptic or postsynaptic cell membrane. These receptors are highly specific for the released neurotransmitter, and in turn mediate various subcellular events that are dependent on that particular neurotransmitter (as discussed in the previous section).

The era of psychopharmacology, beginning in 1949 with the discovery of lithium and the subsequent serendipitous discoveries of chlorpromazine, chlordiaxepoxide and imipramine in the 1950s, emphasised that psychiatric illnesses could be related to imbalances in neurotransmitter signalling that are amenable to modulation by chemicals or drugs. However, the brain can be considered as a mix of neurochemicals and neuronal messengers, all with a distinct function, so that adequate and appropriate modulation of dysfunctional neurotransmission requires a deep understanding of the neurobiology of the brain, especially how neurotransmission is altered in a given illness (Harvey, 2008). Furthermore, a psychiatric illness is not a single neurotransmitter disorder, but represents a continuum of environmental, genetic and neurochemical determinants that occupy a variable yet distinct role in the aetiology, progression and treatment response of the disorder. We have already highlighted in the previous section how intrasynaptic and intracellular cross-talk can blur the lines with respect to predicting a cellular response. To affect a proper response with minimal side effects and complications, we therefore have to know how the drug acts at the synaptic and the subcellular level (Brink *et al.*, 2003; Stahl, 2013).

The scope of this chapter prevents an extended discussion on the complex molecular aspects of drug-receptor pharmacology. At the most basic level it can be said that most drugs bind with specific receptors (functional binding sites) to either initiate a cascade of subcellular events that culminate in a particular response (**agonist**), or to prevent other drugs (or the endogenous agonist) from binding to the receptor, without themselves initiating the cascade (competitive **antagonist**). Drug-receptor binding is a precise physicochemical and steric interaction between chemical groupings of the drug and the three-dimensional structure of the receptor. Typically an agonist, such as an endogenous physicochemical like 5-HT, or a molecule (drug) that mimics the endogenous **ligand** will both bind to specific binding sites on the receptor molecule and also interact with an **activation site** to elicit a physiological response (see 'activation site' in Figure 4.8). While interaction with the activation site is necessary to evoke a response, binding to a variable number of associated binding sites allows the molecule to lock onto the receptor, thereby allowing it to occupy the receptor with sufficient **affinity** (tightness of binding). In the case of an agonist, this would be sufficient to allow adequate interaction with the activation site (see 'binding sites' in Figure 4.8). Typical examples in this scenario could for example be: 5-HT (endogenous agonist), sumatriptan (5-HT1D agonist), ritanserin (5-HT2A antagonist), buspirone (a partial 5-HT1A agonist or DA (endogenous agonist), bromocryptine (D2 agonist), haloperidol (D2 antagonist) and aripiprazole (partial D2 agonist).

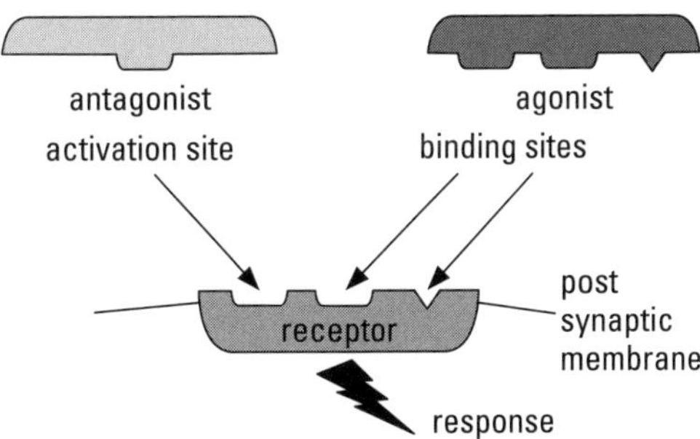


**Figure 4.8** Diagrammatic representation of agonist (e.g. endogenous transmitter or a drug) and antagonist binding to a postsynaptic receptor leading to a cellular response

Antagonists bind to the receptor in a manner that precludes interaction with the activation site, thus having the capacity to bind to the receptor without evoking a response (see Figure 4.8). Depending on competition with the endogenous ligand (e.g. NA, DA, 5-HT), antagonists will prevent binding of the endogenous ligand to produce receptor blockade. Receptor blockade, in turn, is dependent on the binding of the antagonist to the receptor (termed *affinity*). Receptor occupancy, or the number of receptors bound by the drug, is dependent on both affinity and pharmacokinetic factors, such as tissue distribution and **half-life (t½)**. The concept of receptor occupancy has great importance in pharmacotherapeutics, especially in psychiatry. For example, a strong correlation exists between $D_2$ receptor binding and response to an antipsychotic, a $D_2$ antagonist. Indeed, a minimum 70% receptor occupancy is necessary for antipsychotic action, while $D_2$ occupancy beyond this threshold is associated with an increasing risk of **extrapyramidal side effects**. Due to their specific interactions with the receptor, **partial agonists** are less effective at activating the receptor. Under conditions of excessive endogenous agonist activity, however, partial agonists act as antagonists ('**dualism**'). Importantly, one drug molecule occupies one receptor in a reversible manner, with the magnitude of response proportional to the fraction of total receptor sites occupied by drug molecules. Drug response is thus dose dependent.

If drugs bind to their receptor within minutes of being taken up by a biological system, why do **psychotropic** agents such as antidepressants often take so long to attain clinical effectiveness *in vivo*? Importantly, there is a differential response following acute versus chronic exposure to a drug. An acute response is described by an immediate effect on receptor activation via rapid synaptic changes in neurotransmitter levels acting on ionotropic and metabotropic receptors (Leonard, 2003). However, chronic states of deficient neurotransmission (e.g. in major depression) or excessive neurotransmission (e.g. following chronic cocaine abuse) will induce slowly developing subcellular-directed changes in protein synthesis which eventually culminate in receptor **up-regulation** (e.g. depression) or **down-regulation** (e.g. cocaine abuse) that underlie the behavioural symptoms of these conditions (Leonard, 2003; Stahl, 2013). Gradual reversal of these changes over time is proposed to underlie the delay in onset of action of various psychotropic drugs, which often complicates timeous and effective management of the illness (Stahl, 2013). Some of these insidious changes also underlie the behavioural manifestations of non-compliance, such as that following inappropriate antidepressant **discontinuation**, that have acute manifestations ('antidepressant discontinuation syndrome') but if repeated over time (i.e. habitual non-compliance) may have long-term neurobiological effects that compromise a successful outcome (Harvey *et al.*, 2003; Harvey and Slabbert, 2014).

## 4.5 Neurotransmitters in psychiatry and psychopharmacology I: Monoamines (norepinephrine, epinephrine, dopamine and serotonin)

The monoamines are neurotransmitters that are important in psychiatric illnesses. There are different classes of neurotransmitter chemicals and we will pay special attention to some of these, including DA, 5-HT and NE.

Monoamine neurotransmitters are divided into two groups: indoleamines and catecholamines. Indoleamines, such as serotonin and melatonin, have an amine group in common and play a role in sleep and mood. Catecholamines such as dopamine, norephinephrine and epinephrine share a benzene ring with two hydroxyl groups and play a major role in the'fight or flight' response.

It is important for clinicians to be familiar with the actions of neurotransmitters, since dysfunction involving them has been implicated in several disorders. Dopamine dysregulation, for example, is implicated in conditions such as

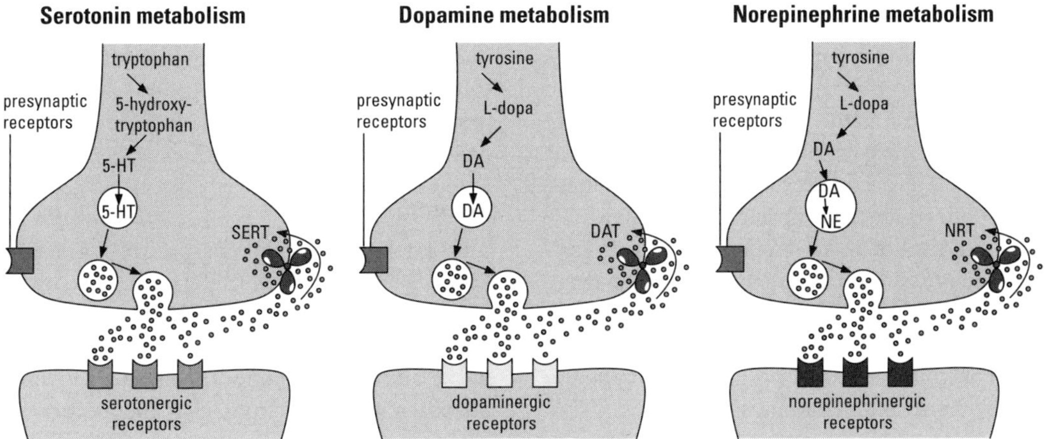


**Figure 4.9** Pre- and postsynaptic neurons showing the storage, release, reuptake and metabolism of dopamine, norepinephrine and serotonin neurotransmitters

schizophrenia, drug addiction and Parkinson's disease, while the 5-HT system plays a role in anxiety and mood disorders. To facilitate a better understanding of the roles of these neurotransmitters, we will briefly look at each of them in terms of synthesis, storage and termination of action, receptor types, pathways along which they act, and important clinical implications.

## 4.5.1 Synthesis, storage and terminating action

### 4.5.1.1 Synthesis

Since the presynaptic neuron is the one that sends the message, it also is the neuron that produces the neurotransmitters. Since neuronal signals originate in the presynaptic nerve terminals, neurotransmitters are manufactured in the presynaptic neurons.

**Dopamine (DA)**

The amino acid tyrosine is transported actively (by using energy) from the plasma into the brain tissue. A tyrosine pump (or transporter) then pumps it into the dopaminergic cell, after which the enzyme tyrosine hydroxylase catalyses the rate-limiting step (the speed of this step determines the speed of dopamine production) in its conversion to DOPA. Finally, DOPA is converted into DA by the enzyme dopa decarboxylase.

**Norepinephrine (NE) and epinephrine**

Dopamine can be further converted into NE by the enzyme dopamine beta hydroxylase. If the neuron is making NE it will be taken up into vesicles by action of the pump vesicular monoamine transporter 2 (VMAT2) for storage and later use. If epinephrine is being made, the NE is converted into epinephrine. This step occurs if the required enzyme is present in the neuron. As with DA, the rate-limiting step is controlled by the enzyme tyrosine hydroxylase.

**Serotonin**

Serotonin, or 5-hydroxytryptamine (5-HT) is synthesised in the intestinal chromaffin cells and in central and peripheral neurons from L-tryptophan, an essential amino acid. Two enzymes are involved in this biochemical process: tryptophan hydroxylase and an aromatic L-amino acid decarboxylase. Tryptophan hydroxylase catalyses the rate-limiting step in the transformation of L-tryptophan to 5-HT.

### 4.5.1.2 Storage and release

DA, NE and epinephrine must be available for release into the **synapse** when an action potential arrives, so that they can signal transmission of the impulse to the next nerve cell. To prevent them from being released into the synapse in the absence of an action potential, neurotransmitters, once formed, are taken up into vesicles by VMAT2.

On arrival of an action potential, these vesicles merge with the cell membrane of the nerve terminal, and the neurotransmitter molecules are released into the synapse where they can interact with receptors on the postsynaptic or presynaptic cell membranes.

### 4.5.1.3 Terminating action

Once the neurotransmitter has performed its function in the synaptic cleft, it must be removed to prevent it from constantly interacting with its receptors, causing changes at those receptors. This is achieved in three ways:

1 by being recycled back into the presynaptic cell
2 by DA and NE being metabolised by various enzymes
3 by monoamines being taken up by transporters.

1 It can be recycled back into the presynaptic cell.

**Dopamine**

The DA transporter (DAT) pumps it back into the presynaptic cell where it is again taken up into vesicles by VMAT2 or broken down by MAO-A or MAO-B (monoamine oxidase A or B). DAT is inhibited by some antidepressants (e.g. buproprion) and by illicit stimulant drugs (e.g. methylphenidate, metamphetamine and cocaine) thereby increasing dopamine concentrations in the synaptic cleft. Amphetamine also targets VMAT. You may be surprised to learn that psychotropic medications and drugs of abuse act at similar sites, but since drugs of abuse act much faster and on a greater number of receptors than medications do, their potential for abuse is much greater.

**Norepinephrine**

Reuptake into the presynaptic neuron occurs under the action of the NE reuptake transporter (NRT). Once inside the neuron it is pumped into vesicles and reused or broken down by the enzyme MAO-A or MAO-B.

**Serotonin**

5-HT is taken back up into the presynaptic neuron by the 5-HT transporter (SERT). Once inside the neuron it is reused or broken down by MAO-A.

2 DA and NE can be metabolised by various enzymes. In the synaptic cleft this occurs via catechol-O-methyl-transferase (COMT; see Figure 4.6). If it occurs in the presynaptic cell or in surrounding glial cells (supporting cells in the brain), the relevant enzyme is MAO-A or MAO-B (see Figure 4. 6). 5-HT is metabolised by MAO-A to 5-hydroxyindole acetic acid (5-HIAA). Further metabolic excretory pathways via aldehyde dehydrogenase and aldehyde reductase also exist. 5-HIAA is excreted via the kidneys.

3 The monoamines can also drift away from the synaptic cleft and be taken up by transporters such as SERT and NRT. The latter transporter can also take up DA (which acts as a false substrate in this case). Once inside the neuron, the monoamines can be pumped into vesicles and reused or broken down by the enzyme MAO-A or MAO-B (see Figure 4.6).

The main brain metabolites of NE, DA and 5HT are 3-methoxy-4-hydroxy-phenylglycol (MHPG), homovanillic acid (HVA) and 5-hydroxyindole acetic acid (5-HIAA), respectively.

## 4.5.2 Receptors

As described above, VMAT2 and DAT are forms of DA receptors. Other receptors include $D_1$, $D_2$, $D_3$ and $D_4$. DA can have different effects depending on the receptor on which it acts. $D_1$ receptors are excitatory while $D_2$ receptors are inhibitory, thus making the neuron less likely to fire an action potential. $D_2$, the best-known

DA receptor, is the receptor subtype targeted in the treatment of Parkinson's disease (where it is stimulated) and in schizophrenia (in which case all antipsychotics currently used block the receptor). $D_2$ can also function as an autoreceptor by binding to the presynaptic membrane, thus creating a negative feedback loop controlling further release of dopamine.

Similarly, VMAT2 and NET are types of NE receptor. In addition, we find $\alpha_1$ (excitatory and found in the brain), $\alpha_2$ (inhibitory), $\beta_1$ (excitatory and also in the brain) and $\beta_2$ receptors (excitatory in the brain and inhibitory in other settings).

More than 15 5-HT receptors have been identified. These receptors are grouped into seven families. Most of the receptor subtypes are found in the nervous system and the gastrointestinal tract. Of the receptor subtypes, the 5-$HT_3$ subtype is ionotropic (a ligand-gated ion channel), whereas the other subtypes are metabotropic (G-protein coupled receptors with intra-cellular second messenger pathways) (see Section 4.3). The following 5-HT receptors are currently of interest in the study of psychiatric conditions such as anxiety, aggression, disorders of appetite control and mood disturbances: 5-$HT1_A$, 5-$HT1_B$, 5-$HT1_D$, 5-$HT2_A$, 5-$HT2_B$, 5-$HT2_C$, 5-HT3 and 5-HT7. Of these 5-$HT1_A$, 5-$HT2_A$, 5-$HT2_B$, 5-$HT2_C$, 5-HT3 and 5-HT7 are of particular importance in the mechanism of action of antidepressants.

## 4.5.3 Pathways in the brain

### Dopamine

The nerve cells that produce DA as their principal neurotransmitter are called dopaminergic neurons. The cell bodies of these neurons lie predominantly in the midbrain, specifically the ventral tegmental area and the substantia nigra. There are five main dopaminergic pathways (groups of dopaminergic neurons which travel together) in the brain.

### Norepinephrine

In the brain, the majority of NE cell bodies are found in the locus coeruleus in the brainstem (more specifically the upper end of the pons under the floor of the fourth ventricle). They project to all parts of the brain and to the spinal cord. In the peripheral nervous system, NE is found in sympathetic neurons, mostly in the cardiovascular system. It is the key neurotransmitter in the fight-or-flight response.

### Epinephrine

Epinephrine-secreting neurons in the brain are far more limited in number, the cell bodies being found in the medulla oblongata of the brainstem. These neurons project to the hypothalamus and spinal cord. In the spinal cord they synapse with sympathetic neurons. In the peripheral nervous system epinephrine is produced by the adrenal medulla and released into the blood as a hormone.

### Serotonin

5-HT is widely distributed throughout the human body and plays an important role in many physiological processes. Among other functions, serotonin is intricately involved in the gastrointestinal system, vascular system and coagulation, cardiovascular system, respiratory system, urogenital system and in the perception of **nociceptive** stimuli.

Neurologically, serotonin neurons send projections from the brainstem to specific areas within the cortical, limbic, midbrain and hindbrain regions. These serotonergic neurons form the largest and most complex efferent system in the brain. Most of these neurons are located in the median raphae nuclei, with a number also found in the paramedian reticular formation. Efferent projections originate from the raphae nuclei and terminate in the lateral cortex, hypothalamus, basal forebrain, septum, basal ganglia, amygdala, cingulum and hippocampus. Additionally, efferent serotonergic projections also pass laterally to the reticular formation and caudally to the spinal column.

## 4.5.4 Clinical implications

The integrated DA hypothesis of schizophrenia assumes dysregulation of key DA pathways. In schizophrenia, the hypothesis states that there is too much DA released in the mesolimbic pathway and too little in the mesocortical pathway. The effects of this can be seen in Table 4.1. Thus the therapeutic challenge is to find a drug that targets both these pathways at the same time. Typical antipsychotics treat the positive symptoms of psychosis relatively well by blocking DA action in the mesolimbic system, but the negative and cognitive symptoms are relatively poorly addressed as these drugs also block DA in the mesocortical pathways (see Chapter 11: Schizophrenia spectrum and other psychotic disorders, for further discussion). It was hoped that the arrival of **atypical antipsychotics** would overcome this problem, but this has not been fully realised in practice. Table 4.1 also shows how antipsychotics may cause hyperprolactinaemia and extrapyramidal side effects.

An important consideration is that the release of each monoamine does not occur in isolation: rather, the release of one can influence the release of others. Each of the monoamines can have overlapping and complementary functions (see Figure 4.5 and Figure 4.7). They are all implicated to varying degrees in mood disorders – in both unipolar and bipolar depression. While antidepressants are known to act by increasing the concentrations of one or more of the monoamines, the exact pathophysiology of depression, or pharmacological action of antidepressants, remains to be established. The clinical implications of the better-known neurotransmitters are discussed briefly below.

NE is targeted in the treatment of various psychiatric conditions. In depressed patients the levels of NE (as well as other neurotransmitters)

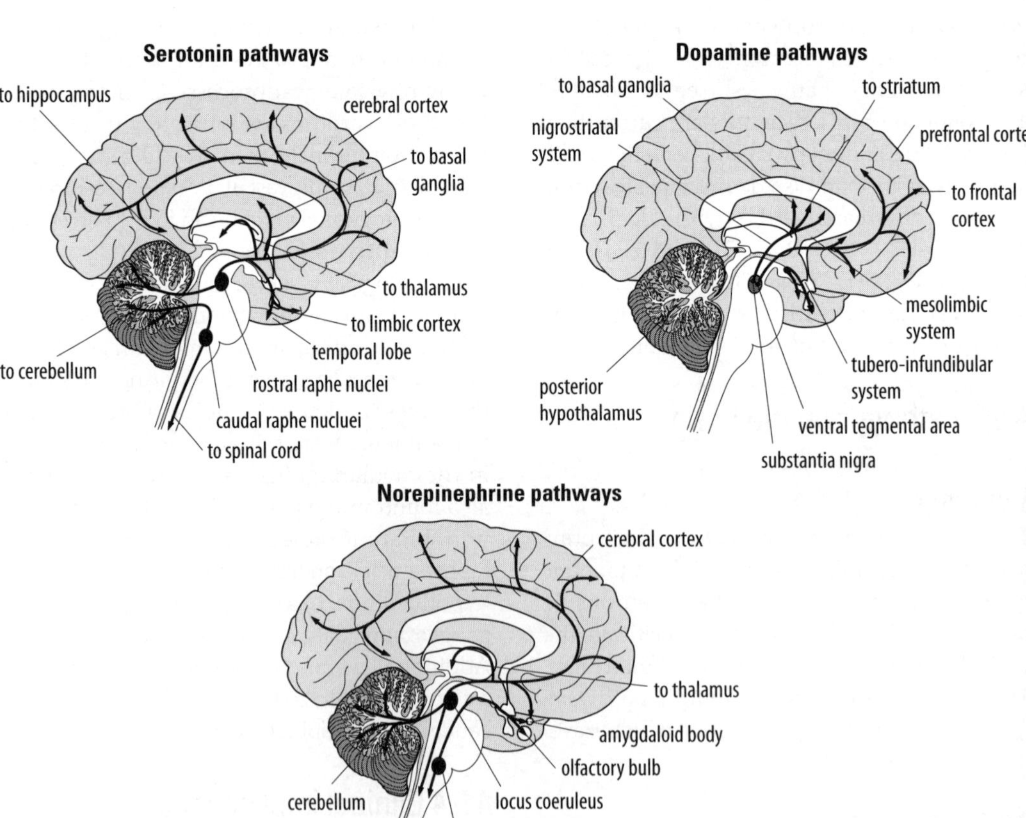


**Figure 4.10** The brain pathways of dopamine, norepinephrine and serotonin

**Table 4.1** Main dopaminergic pathways and their clinical correlates

| Name | Pathway | Function | Dysfunction | Medications and their effects |
|---|---|---|---|---|
| nigrostriatal | From the substantia nigra to the striatum (part of the basal ganglia). | Part of the extrapyramidal system controlling motor function. | Degeneration of neurons in substantia nigra causes Parkinson's disease.<br>Hyperactivity of DA function here thought to underlie some hyperkinetic movement disorders (e.g. **chorea**, **tics**) | Antipsychotics decrease DA here and cause extrapyramidal side effects. These include **parkinsonism**, acute **dystonia**, **akathisia** and, with chronic blockade, **tardive dyskinesia**. |
| mesolimbic | Extends from the ventral tegmental area in the midbrain to the limbic area, specifically the nucleus accumbens. | DA release results in pleasurable feelings. Forms key component of reward pathway, encouraging behaviours necessary for survival (eating, sex, socialising). | An excess of DA here, as found in primary mental illness (e.g. schizophrenia) and illicit drug use (e.g. phencyclidine, amphetamine), can produce psychosis (delusions and **hallucinations**).<br>When drugs are abused, the reward pathway is hijacked. Long-term changes here are associated with the pathophysiology of drug addiction. | **Euphoria** when drugs of abuse used.<br>Antipsychotics block dopamine action here and treat psychosis (or alleviate psychotic symptoms). |
| mesocortical | Extends from ventral tegmental area to prefrontal cortex. | Mediates cognitive functions, **executive functioning** and emotions. | A deficiency of DA here is implicated in negative symptoms (e.g. alogia, affective flattening) and cognitive dysfunction in schizophrenia and possibly also in depression. | A focus of current schizophrenia research is to find medications which optimise function here. |
| tubero-infundibular | From hypothalamus to the anterior pituitary gland | Dopamine inhibits prolactin secretion. | Hyperprolactinaemia and decreased **libido**, menstrual irregularities, decreased fertility, galactorrhoea, decreased bone mass | Certain antipsychotics (specifically the typicals, risperidone, and amisulpiride) cause dopamine blockade. Thus this inhibition is removed and hyperprolactinaemia may result. |
| fifth dopamine pathway | Arises from multiple sites and projects to the thalamus | Exact function not known | Unknown | Unknown |

can be increased by using agents such as the tricyclic antidepressants. Antidepressants such as phenelzine also increase NE levels by inhibiting MAO, but these are used far less frequently due to their side effects.

NE also plays a role in arousal. The pathophysiology of attention deficit hyperactivity disorder (ADHD) probably involves a deficiency of NE and DA in the arousal system. Thus, treatment for ADHD includes stimulants (e.g.

methylphenidate) that boost these neurotransmitters. Atomoxetine is a selective NE reuptake inhibitor used in ADHD. NE inhibition is useful in treating chronic pain such as fibromyalgia and neuropathic pain. NE may also play a role in the effects of antipsychotics, and may, by virtue of a cross-over effect on other monoamine systems, interact with them in the pathogenesis of many mental disorders.

5-HT is most commonly implicated in the pathology of depression. This is commonly referred to as the monoamine hypothesis of mood disorders, which states that a 5-HT deficiency is associated with depression, and an excess of 5-HT is associated with mania. The simplified view proposed by the monoamine hypothesis has been proven to be not entirely accurate. The more tenable permissive hypothesis proposes that low 5-HT levels enable either depressed or elevated mood. In addition to the association of 5-HT with depression, its role in the pathophysiology of schizophrenia is becoming an exciting field of study. The newer atypical antipsychotic drugs, which exhibit serotonergic antagonism, have become the drugs of choice in the treatment of many mood and psychotic disorders.

## 4.6 Neurotransmitters in psychiatry and psychopharmacology II: Acetylcholine

Acetylcholine (Ach) acts as a neuromodulator in both the peripheral and central nervous systems. What makes it unique is that it is the only neurotransmitter found in the motor division of the somatic nervous system and is the dominant neurotransmitter in the autonomic nervous system. While Ach causes excitatory responses in the peripheral nervous system, it seems to be more inhibitory in the CNS as part of the cholinergic system.

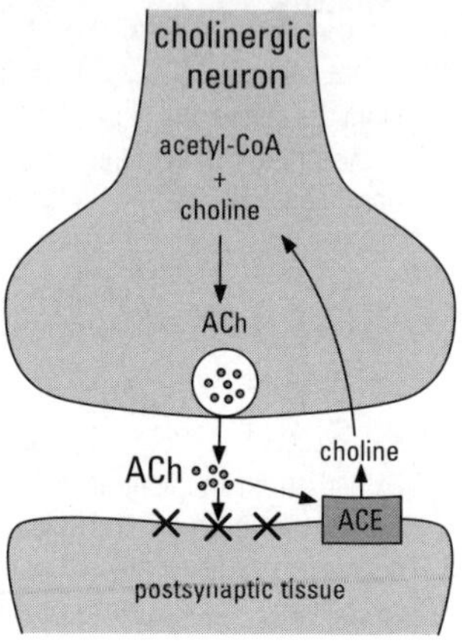


**Figure 4.11** Pre- and postsynaptic neurons showing the storage, release, reuptake and metabolism of acetylcholine

### 4.6.1 Synthesis, storage and terminating action of acetylcholine

#### 4.6.1.1 Synthesis and storage

Cholinergic neurons (in, for example, the nucleus basalis of Meynert) produce Ach from choline and acetyl-CoA by means of the enzyme choline acetyltransferase.

#### 4.6.1.2 Terminating action

Ach is inactivated in the synaptic cleft by conversion to choline and acetate by acetylcholinesterase (AChE).

### 4.6.2 Receptors

Ach acts on two groups of receptors, namely nicotinic and muscarinic. Nicotinic receptors, which can be stimulated by nicotine and Ach, are ionotropic receptors located on muscle or nerve cells which allow the influx of sodium, potassium and calcium ions into cells. Muscarinic receptors are metabotropic and are stimulated by muscarine and Ach and blocked by atropine.

When Ach binds to its receptors on, for example, skeletal muscle fibres, ligand-gated sodium channels open up, causing sodium ions to flow into the cells, leading to the contraction of muscles. However, in the case of the heart, Ach binding to muscarinic receptors inhibits these contractions.

In the brain, Ach has its effect via a neuromodulatory mechanism. Ach can have different effects on postsynaptic neurons depending on factors such as duration of activation. It is outside the scope of this textbook to provide a detailed account of the complexities of Ach function.

### 4.6.3 Pathways in the brain and their clinical application

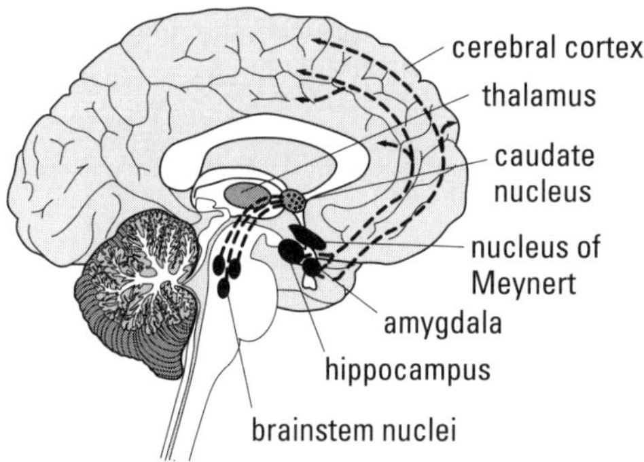


**Figure 4.12** The brain pathways of acetylcholine

The CNS effects of Ach include effects on arousal, sustained attention, plasticity and reward. Ach is released by all parasympathetic neurons, all preganglionic sympathetic neurons and selected postganglionic sympathetic fibres (those linked to sweat glands). In the CNS there are three Ach pathways of note where especially type 1 muscarinic receptors play an important role:

- from the pons to the thalamus and cortex
- from the magnocellular forebrain nucleus to the cortex
- the septohippocampal pathway.

Medical conditions in which Ach is implicated include myasthenia gravis and Alzheimer's disease. Myasthenia gravis, characterised by muscular weakness, is an autoimmune disorder caused by the destruction of muscular nicotinic receptors by the body's immune system. Alzheimer's disease is also closely linked to deficits in Ach function and treatment of this condition relies heavily on inhibition of the rate-limiting enzyme in Ach metabolism, AChE, thereby increasing the available Ach. Recent evidence also highlights the possible role of Ach in depression, with cholinergic hyperfunction a suggested mechanism in depression.

## 4.7 Neurotransmitters in psychiatry and psychopharmacology III: Amino acids (glutamate, GABA, glycine)

Aside from serving as building blocks for proteins, certain amino acids are also neurotransmitters in the brain, most notably as excitatory signals (glutamate and aspartate) and as inhibitory signals (glycine (GLY) and GABA). Although structurally GABA is an amino acid, it is not classified as such since it does not partake in protein synthesis. These amino acids are central to higher-order functioning, including emotion and cognition, and the regulation of muscle tone. Disorders characterised by excessive neuronal **excitation**, such as epilepsy, are due to an excess glutamate transmission in certain cortical regions. Huntington's disease, a disorder of GABA-neuron degeneration, presents with incontrollable movements. Similarly anxiety disorders are characterised by a paucity of GABA-ergic signalling, while excessive glutamatergic transmission underlies psychosis (or mania) and epilepsy (Stahl, 2013). Excessive glutamate-nitric oxide signalling is also suggested to mediate depression (Harvey *et al.*, 2003; Harvey, 2008). GABA-glutamate interactions have importance in **kindling**, a mechanism implicated in the association between prior depressive or psychotic episodes, and treatment discontinuation, as well as how stressful life events impact on the development and long-term outcome of a psychiatric illness (Emsley *et al.*, 2013). GABA pathways exert essentially a permissive role on the kindling action of glutamate (Harvey *et al.*, 2003; Harvey and Shahid, 2012). Excessive glutamatergic activity is associated with synaptic remodelling and neurodegenerative effects. Indeed, glutamate receptor modulators and inhibitors are attracting a great deal of interest in the treatment of a number of psychiatric disorders, such as resistant depression, obsessive compulsive disorder, schizophrenia, post-traumatic stress disorder and others (Harvey and Shahid, 2012).

## 4.7.1 Glutamate

Glutamate receptors can be subdivided into (Harvey and Shahid, 2012):

- ionotropic receptors, including N-methyl-D-aspartate (NMDA), alpha-amino-3-hydroxy-5-methyl-4- isoxazole-propionic acid (AMPA) and kainate receptors
- metabotropic glutamate (mGlu) receptors (see Figure 4.13), of which there are a number of sub-families).

Presynaptic release of glutamate can either bind to presynaptic or postsynaptic ionotropic NMDA and AMPA receptors, or to metabotropic mGlu receptors (mGluR), or can be taken up by the glutamate transporter (GluT) into neighbouring glia or into the presynaptic terminal (see Figure 4.13). Presynaptic mGluR's also play an important part in regulating glutamate release.

Excitatory ionotropic receptor-gated ion channels promote the movement of $Na^+$, $Ca^{2+}$ (inwards) and $K^+$ (outwards) ions across the membrane. While NMDA receptor activation promotes many beneficial changes in the brain (e.g. memory), overstimulation is neurotoxic and related to the damaging effects of brain trauma and stroke. Moreover, the degenerative aspects of many psychiatric illnesses, such as in

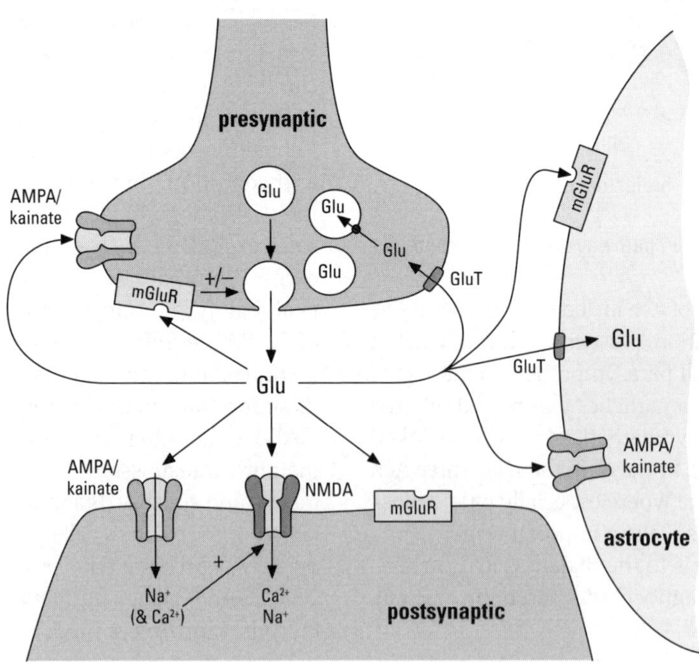


**Figure 4.13** Glutamatergic neuron and synapse

**Source:** Adapted figure, Martha I. Dávila-García, Department of Pharmacology, Howard University

depression (hippocampal shrinkage), may also involve glutamate excitotoxicity (Cooper *et al.*, 2003; Savitz and Drevetts, 2009), usually as a sequelae to hypercortisolemia present in the disorder. On the other hand, hypoglutamatergia is also detrimental being implicated in cell death as well as underlying the neuro-pathology of schizophrenia.

Consequently NMDA ion channels are under multiple regulatory mechanisms: $Mg^{2+}$ blocks the channel at rest to prevent inappropriate activation, GLY increases ion channel opening to facilitate excitatory glutamatergic actions and zinc inhibits channel opening. Presynaptic and glial glutamate transporters (GluT) also ensure stability of glutamatergic networks (see Figure 4.13) and prevent excitotoxicity. In addition, the NMDA ion channel also binds drugs such as phencyclidine, ketamine, memantine, and dizocilpine that are associated with potent central nervous system actions, in particular **psychomimetic**, psychotropic and neuroprotective properties, while positive and negative **allosteric** receptor modulators of the NMDA and AMPA receptor represent an attempt at regulating glutamate signalling in a more physiologically compatible manner (e.g. ampakines).

Metabotropic glutamate receptors engender a slower but more sustained effect on glutamatergic networks and are gaining in recognition as targets for novel drug development (Harvey and Shahid, 2012). Glutamate receptors are essential for learning and memory, neurodevelopment, neuronal plasticity and **apoptosis** (spontaneous cell death), all of which are variably affected in a number of neuropsychiatric illnesses. Ionotropic and metabotropic glutamate receptors, together with GABA, are responsible for regulating muscle tone and are useful in certain forms of epilepsy (e.g. topiramate, an AMPA receptor blocker). Moreover, the subcellular cascades set in motion by the activation of glutamatergic receptors, such as the NMDA-nitric oxide-cyclic guanosine monophosphate (cGMP) cascade, are also receiving attention as possible targets for novel psychotropic drug development (Dhir and Kulkarni, 2011; Bernstein *et al.*, 2011).

### 4.7.2 GABA

GABA receptors are classified into ligand-gated $GABA_A$ receptors and metabotropic $GABA_B$ receptors that use G protein-linked couplings to open or close ion channels. $GABA_A$ receptors are predominantly supra-spinal while $GABA_B$ receptors are located in the spinal cord. GABA binding to presynaptic and postsynaptic $GABA_A$ receptors allows $Cl^-$ influx or $K^+$ efflux (see Figure 4.14), in both cases decreasing membrane potential causing **hyperpolarisation** (inhibition). If we consider Figure 4.14 we can examine the process of GABA'ergic transmission. Especially pertinent here is the metabolic link between GABA and glutamate.

GABA (denoted as a square in Figure 4.14) is synthesized from glutamate using the enzyme L-glutamic acid decarboxylase via the GABA shunt, which converts the principal excitatory neurotransmitter, glutamate, into the principal inhibitory neurotransmitter, GABA. Depolarisation of the pre-synaptic terminal provokes the release of GABA into the synapse where it can either bind to post-synaptic ionotropic $GABA_A$ or metabotropic $GABA_B$ receptors, or be taken up into the pre-synaptic terminal by the GABA transporter. $GABA_A$ receptors are ligand-activated chloride ($Cl^-$) channels, with GABA activation leading to influx of $Cl^-$ into the cell leading to hyperpolarisation and neuronal inhibition.

Modulation of the GABA system may ensue via a number of ways, including positive or negative allosteric modulation of GABA receptors, inhibition of GABA metabolism by GABA transaminase and inhibition of GABA reuptake transporters.

The GABA ionophore is allosterically regulated by a number of endogenous chemicals, foremost among these being neurosteroids (e.g. progesterone, allopregnanolone and dehydroepiandrosterone) and benzodiazepine-like chemicals (endozepines) (see Figure 4.14). Such binding increases the frequency of the $Cl^-$ channel opening to enhance the inhibitory actions of GABA, although their action still requires endogenous GABA for full function. Benzodiazepine compounds (e.g. diazepam, denoted by a triangle in Figure 4.14) are positive allosteric modulators of the $GABA_A$ receptor and function as indirectly acting GABA-mimetics. Importantly, barbiturates (e.g. amobarbital) and neurosteroids (denoted by a double triangle in Figure 4.14) bind to *non-benzodiazepine* receptors (see Figure 4.14) so that their action is *independent* of GABA binding to the $GABA_A$ receptor, making them far more likely to induce general central nervous system depression, coma and death. $GABA_A$-mimetics, such as the benzodiazepines, valproate, tiagabine and vigabactin, are used extensively for their anxiolytic, sedative, muscle relaxant and antiepileptic properties, while non-benzodiazepine GABA-mimetics that target specific subunits of the $GABA_A$ receptor, such as zopiclone and zolpidem, are used more exclusively as sedative-hypnotics. $GABA_B$-mimetics, such as baclofen, are used for their muscle relaxant properties. Flumazenil is an example of *negative* allosteric $GABA_A$ modulator, and is used to reverse the action of benzodiazepines and itself is anxiogenic.

## 4.8 Neurotransmitters in psychiatry and psychopharmacology IV: Histamine

Histamine is an organic nitrogen-containing compound that acts not only as a neurotransmitter, but also performs a wide variety of functions, including a critical role in local immune responses.

Histamine is produced in and released by basophils and mast cells in response to specific triggers. Histamine release is associated with increased capillary permeability to white blood cells and other substances, thus allowing the body to mount an immune response to foreign invaders. Histamine is produced by decarboxylation of the amino acid histidine, a process that is under the control of the enzyme L-histidine decarboxylase. Histamine is then either stored or is inactivated by the enzyme

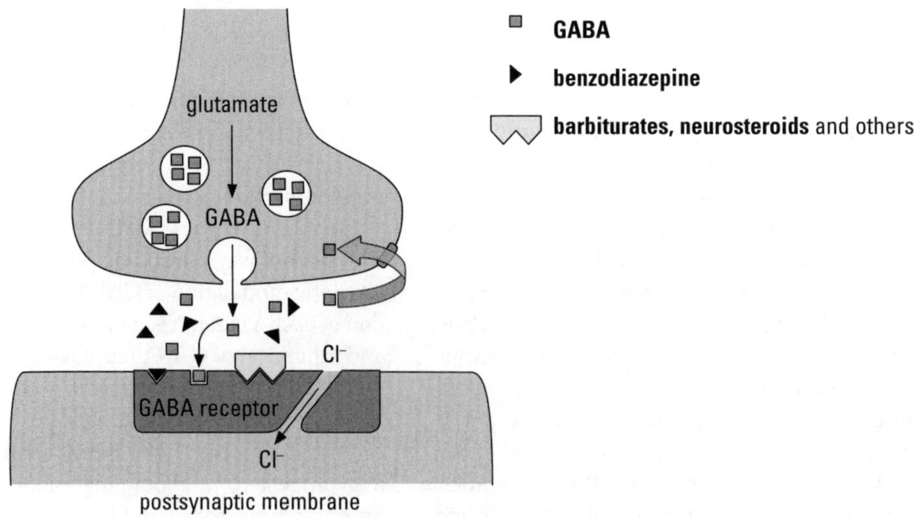


**Figure 4.14** GABA'ergic neuron and synapse showing GABA interaction with postsynaptic ionotropic $GABA_A$ receptors (metabotropic $GABA_B$ receptor not shown)

**Source:** Adapted figure, Martha I. Dávila-García, Department of Pharmacology, Howard University

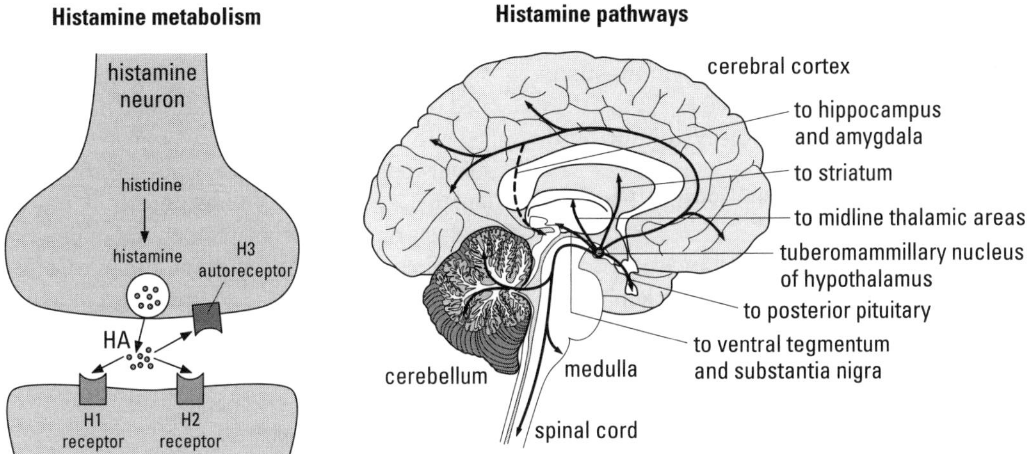


**Figure 4.15** Pre- and postsynaptic neurons showing the storage, release, reuptake and metabolism of histamine as well as the pathways in the brain

histamine-N-methyltransferase (the enzyme responsible for the breakdown of histamine in the central nervous system) or diamine oxidase. The products are then further metabolised by MAO-B and aldehyde dehydrogenase 2 (ALDH2). Histamine exerts its actions via four types of G protein-coupled histamine receptors (H1-H4). H3 is found in the CNS, where it inhibits the release of histamine, Ach, NE, epinephrine and 5-HT. The neurons releasing histamine in the CNS are found in the posterior hypothalamus. The cortical projections of these neurons are widespread, thus accounting for histamine's impact on sleep. Indeed, histamine receptor fire rates are closely related to wakefulness; H3 antagonists increase wakefulness. Clinically, antihistamines (H1 histamine receptor antagonists) are known to induce sleep and changes in appetite. The effect on appetite is important as later on we describe how atypical antipsychotics (such as olanzepine and clozapine) and antidepressants such as mirtazapine, beyond their primary impact on DA and 5-HT respectively, also affect histamine and thus have a significant effect on appetite and weight (Harvey, 1999; Harvey and Bouwer, 2000).

## 4.9 Neurotransmitters in psychiatry and psychopharmacology V: Neuroactive peptides

Neuroactive peptides (or neuropeptides), are small protein-like molecules that function as neurotransmitters and/or neuromodulators in the brain. While typical neurotransmitters affect the excitability of neurons, neuropeptides are released via a $Ca^{2+}$-dependent mechanism to exert diverse effects on gene expression, local blood flow, synaptogenesis and glial cell morphology. Because they act via metabotropic G protein-coupled receptors, they tend to have late-onset but prolonged actions. As neuronal signalling molecules, they are invariably co-localised with monoaminergic or aminergic transmitters, although are two to three orders of magnitude lower in concentration, and in so doing modulate the activity of monoaminergic/aminergic receptors.

Neuropeptides are thus active in modulating a number of neurotransmitter systems of importance to neuronal function and neuropharmacology:

- NE co-exists with galanin, enkephalin and neuropeptide Y (NPY)

- GABA co-exists with somatostatin, cholecystokinin and NPY
- Ach co-exists with vaso-active intestinal peptide (VIP) and substance P
- DA co-exists with cholecystokinin and neurotensin
- epinephrine co-exists with NPY and neurotensin
- 5-HT co-exists with substance P, thyroid releasing hormone (TRH) and enkephalin.

Other neuropeptides of importance in psychiatry include vasopressin, dynorphin, corticotrophin releasing factor (CRF) and oxytocin. Neuropeptides are involved in a number of specific brain functions, most notably analgesia, reward, anxiety, food intake, motor function, learning and memory. Five peptide families are recognised:

- vasopressin and oxytocin
- tachykinins (e.g. substance P)
- VIP-related peptides (e.g. orexin A and B)
- pancreatic polypeptides (e.g. NPY)
- opioid peptides (e.g. leu-enkephalin and met-enkephalin, β-endorphin, dynorphin).

A select number of the more widely recognised neuro-active peptides are discussed briefly below, although the reader is encouraged to read more broadly on the subject.

## 4.9.1 Opioid peptides

The endogenous opioid systems play a critical role in modulating sensory, motivational, emotional and cognitive functions (Brunton *et al.*, 2011). As inhibitory neuropeptide transmitters, opioid peptides fine-tune neurotransmission. Three principal G protein-coupled opioid receptors are defined: μ-, δ- and κ-opioid receptors.

Their density and diverse distribution in the brain and spinal cord mediates profound effects in the brain, although they are also widely distributed in cardiovascular, lung, gut and immune-inflammatory tissue (Brunton *et al.*, 2011). Their analgesic effects arise from direct inhibition of ascending nociceptive information from the spinal cord, and by activating descending pain control circuits from the midbrain.

μ-agonists are invariably antinociceptive, whereas κ-agonists can be either antinociceptive or pro-nociceptive, the latter hyperalgesia mediated by a functional antagonism of μ-receptors.

The δ-receptor plays a more prominent role in spinal analgesia. Analgesics, such as morphine, fentanyl, and methadone, act predominantly as agonists on μ-receptors while compounds such as nalbuphine display more pronounced κ-receptor activity. Agonists of δ-opioid receptors are less analgesic but have a lower risk of respiratory depression (Brunton *et al.*, 2011).

## 4.9.2 Tachykinins

The best-known members of the tachykinin family – substance P and neurokinins A and B – act on specific G protein-PLC coupled tachykinin NK1, NK2 and NK3 receptors (Brunton *et al.*, 2011). Tachykinin NK1 receptors are involved in nociceptive transmission, basal ganglia function or anxiety and depression, while NK1 receptor antagonists show promise as antidepressants and treating chemotherapy-induced emesis. Substance P is especially rich in sensory fibres projecting from the dorsal root ganglia to the spinal cord, and is an important dual transmitter with DA in the substantia nigra.

## 4.9.3 Neuropeptide Y

NeuropeptideY (NPY) mostly co-exists with NE or epinephrine, where it increases the sensitivity of response to these transmitters. It is also a highly potent vasoconstrictor. Central actions of NPY include appetite stimulation and anxiolysis (Brunton *et al.*, 2011). NPY has been linked to insulin resistance in brain regions associated with appetite regulation, especially stress-related changes (namely, amygdala). Considering the high comorbidity of obesity, diabetes and metabolic disorders in psychiatric disorders such as schizophrenia and depression, NPY is likely to play a notable role here as well as the metabolic effects of psychotropics (e.g. antipsychotics).

### 4.9.4 Vasoactive intestinal peptide (VIP)

VIP is structurally related to glucagon, secretin, gastric inhibitory peptide (GIP) and growth hormone-releasing hormone (GHRH). VIP is a co-transmitter with nitric oxide and carbon monoxide, of nonadrenergic-noncholinergic relaxation of vascular and nonvascular smooth muscle, and with Ach in exocrine glands. VIP may also promote neuronal survival and regulates glycogen metabolism in the cerebral cortex (Harmar *et al.*, 2012). VIP is involved in the control of circadian rhythms in the suprachiasmatic nuclei of the hypothalamus.

Orexin, or hypocretins, expressed exclusively in the lateral hypothalamic area, are essentially two neuropeptides (Hcrt1, Hcrt2) that act in a G protein dependent manner. Orexin neurons are inactive during sleep but become activated during wakefulness and arousal and are a prominent player in regulating negative and positive emotional valence, and facilitating adaptive and maladaptive responses to stressful or rewarding environmental stimuli (Giardino and De Lecea, 2014). Its actions are mediated by CRF, the prototypical stress neuropeptide that in turn activates the hypothalamic–pituitary–adrenal (HPA) stress axis, resulting in increased levels of adrenocorticotropin hormone (ACTH) and cortisol, as well as DA, the primary monoamine involved in reward processing.

As a consequence of the above actions, orexin enhances anxiety-like behaviour and decreases brain reward function, and is thus of relevance for disorders characterised by chronic stress and compulsive drug-seeking states. Moreover, since the tight regulation of sleep/wake states is critical for mental and physiological well-being, orexin dysregulation is implicated in various metabolic and mood-related disorders such as depression, particularly co-morbidity of these states.

### 4.9.5 Oxytocin

Apart from its well-known stimulating effects on uterine contraction and milk ejection, oxytocin has prominent effects in the brain, having been found to be an important regulator of trust and attachment and of autonomic systems linked to fear and anxiety. In fact, while cortisol and adrenaline are associated with the 'fight or flight' response, research on the role of oxytocin has revealed its central role in how females cope with adversity, namely, the 'tend and befriend' response. Importantly, brain regions intimately involved in the fear response, such as the amygdala, are inhibited by oxytocin. Indeed, both oxytocin and vasopressin are gaining increasing recognition as important players in mental disorders characterised by social dysfunction, such as autism, social anxiety disorder, borderline personality disorder and schizophrenia (Meyer-Lindenberg *et al.*, 2011).

## 4.10 Neurotransmitters in psychiatry and psychopharmacology VI: Other neuromodulators

A number of less well-recognised endogenous substances are gaining in importance with respect to their putative role as neuromodulators, and indeed in the neurobiology of disease. Some that are attracting a great deal of attention as possible novel therapeutic targets in neuropsychiatry are discussed briefly below.

### 4.10.1 Adenosine

Adenosine is an endogenous purine **nucleoside** that acts via four G protein coupled receptors: A1, A2A, A2B, and A3. Most notably it exerts an inhibitory effect on the CNS, probably by suppressing DA and glutamate transmission. Indeed, adenosine agonists are **anxiolytic**, while antagonists, such as caffeine, are **anxiogenic** (Brunton *et al.*, 2011). Adenosine A2 receptor modulation of Ach, DA and glutamate neurons play an important role in the functioning of the basal ganglia where A2 antagonists can augment DA activity with therapeutic potential in Parkinson's disease (Brunton *et al.*, 2011).

## 4.10.2 Nitric oxide

Nitric oxide is a gaseous, paramagnetic molecule with important brain, cardiovascular and immune functions (Bernstein *et al.*, 2011). It is synthesised de novo from the semi-essential amino acid, L-arginine, via the enzyme nitric oxide synthase (NOS). In nervous tissue this conversion invariably follows activation of the glutamate NMDA receptor (Harvey, 2006). Upon release, it rapidly moves within and between cells to stimulate soluble guanylate cyclase leading to an increase in cGMP. Cyclic cGMP is terminated by phosphodiesterase (PDE), (e.g. PDE 5; see Figure 4.1). Nitric oxide plays a role in memory and cell survival and is implicated in anxiety disorders, depression and schizophrenia, as well as neurodegenerative disorders such as Alzheimer's disease. Nitric oxide is also involved in inflammation via activation of the immunologically induced nitric oxide synthase (NOS) (Bernstein *et al.*, 2011). Although clinically safe and effective NO-cGMP modulators have not yet been synthesised. Preliminary studies with PDE5 inhibitors (e.g. sildenafil) and the NOS-guanylyl cyclase inhibitor methylene blue are promising (Harvey *et al.*, 2010; Liebenberg *et al.*, 2010).

## 4.10.3 Brain-derived neurotrophic factor

Brain-derived neurotrophic factor (BDNF) is a member of the neurotrophin family. It plays a vital supportive role in the survival of existing neurons, and encourages the growth and differentiation of new neurons and synapses, especially in the hippocampus, cortex and basal forebrain where it is involved in learning, memory, and mood regulation (Castren, 2005; 2007). Disturbances in BDNF release are implicated in a number of psychiatric illnesses, especially depression, schizophrenia and posttraumatic stress disorder (Dwivedi, 2009). Most often its release is inhibited under the aforementioned conditions leading to compromised neuroplastic and neuroprotective processes. Indeed, the above disorders present with atrophy of a number of brain regions involved in regulating mood, cognition and the stress response (Savitz and Drevets, 2009; Martinez *et al.*, 2012). Chronic antidepressant use and recovery from these illnesses is associated with an increase in BDNF release (Dwivedi, 2009).

## 4.10.4 Endogenous cannabinoids

The medicinal value of the hemp plant (*Cannabis sativa*) was first documented by the Chinese more than 2 000 years ago. The principal **psychoactive** ingredient of cannabis extract is the alkaloid tetra-hydrocannabinol (THC), although a number of cannabinoids have been identified ((Brunton *et al.*, 2011). Endogenous cannabinoids, or endocannabinoids, confirm the physiological importance of this signalling system. The brain contains mainly CB1 receptors that are widely distributed in areas involved with motor activity (basal ganglia, cerebellum), memory and cognition (cortex, hippocampus), emotion (amygdala, hippocampus), sensory perception (thalamus) and endocrine function (pons, hypothalamus). The immunological actions of cannabinoids are mediated by CB2 receptors. The best-known endocannabinoid is anandamide, derived from arachidonic acid metabolism ((Brunton *et al.*, 2011). It appears that the endocannabinoids are not released into the synaptic cleft and are not involved in interneuronal communication, being more involved in modulating neuronal excitability via cannabinoid heteroreceptors. The anandamide system is involved in thermoregulation and sleep induction, although THC-related cannabinoids also demonstrate effects on cognition, mood, coordination, perception and appetite.

## 4.10.5 Melatonin

Melatonin is an endocrine secretion of the pineal gland. Melatonin receptors are widely distributed in the brain, with the highest density of $MT_1$ and $MT_2$ receptors found in the suprachiasmatic nucleus (SCN) of the hypothalamus and pars tuberalis (Racagni *et al*, 2011). However, their presence in the frontal and prefrontal cortex, cerebellar cortex, basal ganglia, substantia nigra, hippocampus, ventral tegmental area, nucleus accumbens and thalamus suggest a broad impact on brain function.

In the SCN, interaction between $5HT_{2c}$ receptors and melatonergic input from the pineal gland is responsible for establishing the biorhythms of the master clock, the expression of both receptors showing a diurnal rhythmicity. The resulting balance between light-mediated effects on serotonin versus melatonin synthesis in the SCN-pineal complex are felt in a number of biochemical, metabolic and behavioural processes, in particular changes in the release of hormones of the HPA- and thyroid axis, sex hormones etc., but also monoamine changes via SCN connections to the brainstem monoaminergic nuclei (Harvey *et al.*, 2003). It is the latter actions that link melatonin and altered circadian rhythms to a number of psychiatric illnesses, foremost being depression. Indeed, depression is associated with significant disturbances in melatonin release.

Agomelatine is an antidepressant that acts via a delicate synergy between $MT_1/MT_2$ receptor agonism and $5\text{-}HT_{2C}$ antagonism, thereby allowing it to re-entrain altered biological rhythms (Racagni *et al.*, 2011). Given the important role for dysregulation of the HPA-axis in depression and the role of the circadian system in regulating HPA-axis hormones and peptides, these actions emphasise the importance of circadian rhythms in psychiatry and, indeed, in psychotropic drug action.

## Conclusion

Most psychotropic agents currently in use in psychiatry were discovered by chance. Although their introduction into clinical medicine can be regarded as one of the most significant advances in medical science, a general lack of understanding of their mechanisms of action and the neurobiology behind the illnesses themselves led to many iatrogenic complications in the years and decades to follow.

Illnesses such as depression (reduced 5-HT and NE levels) and schizophrenia (DA dysfunction) were considered to be exclusively disturbances of monoamine concentrations, leading to the development and marketing of monoamine reuptake inhibitors for depression and dopamine $D_2$ receptor blockers for treating schizophrenia. Given that signalling in the brain involves many different cross-talk interactions across all transmitter systems, such a non-specific action on, for example, 5-HT not only lays the foundation for a host of adverse serotonergic effects, but also for adverse effects mediated by its actions on other signalling systems. Similarly, non-specific antagonism of DA receptors has set the scene for the current plague of psychotropic adverse effects experienced with antipsychotic drugs, including neuroleptic deficit syndrome, and metabolic, endocrine and cardiovascular disturbances. Moreover, these illnesses (and most psychiatric illnesses) do not constitute a single neurotransmitter disorder, but involve a large number of environmental, genetic and neurochemical determinants that together determine the aetiology and progression of the disorder. It is therefore critical that clinicians realise that this complexity extends to treatment response as well, with the choice of treatment tailored to a specific clinical presentation and the underlying biology.

Clinicians must be aware of the importance of long-term **compliance**, especially since psychiatric patients all too often discontinue their medication prematurely (Harvey *et al.*, 2003). Clinicians must consider that, while treatment onset and response is an end result of a distinct pharmacodynamic process that produces the desired therapeutic response, abrupt, premature and repeated treatment discontinuation follows the same precepts. However, in the case of habitual treatment discontinuation, there are more salient adverse effects caused by non-compliance that must be considered and that will negatively influence long-term treatment outcome, including break-through symptoms, **relapse**, discontinuation syndrome and treatment resistance (Harvey *et al.*, 2003; Harvey and Slabbert, 2014).

As has been described in earlier sections, drug treatment is rarely selective for a given process, making it imperative that clinicians closely consider the pharmacological profile of a psychotropic drug. Being mindful of this will assist in avoiding potentially harmful adverse reactions and drug-drug interactions (especially those related to many psychotropic drugs being either inhibitors and/or substrates of **cytochrome P450** in the liver), while also allowing for appropriate counselling of patients with regards to expected adverse effects (Harvey, 1997). Thus, most antipsychotic and antidepressant drugs are multi-potent antagonists, therefore blocking histamine, muscarinic cholinergic, $\alpha_1$-adrenergic and other receptors to a clinically relevant degree. Clinicians should be aware of relevant contraindications, such as heart failure, postural hypotension, drowsiness during driving, cardiac arrhythmias etc., as well as the risk of combining psychotropic drugs with other drugs acting on the above-mentioned systems (e.g. antihypertensives, sedative-hypnotics). Interaction at certain peripheral and central neuro-receptors, for example, will confer a risk for the following adverse effects:

- Ach antagonism: blurred vision, dry mouth, constipation, sinus tachycardia, urinary retention, memory dysfunction
- H1 antagonism: sedation/drowsiness, weight gain
- DA reuptake inhibition: psychomotor activation, psychosis, abuse
- 5-$HT_2$ agonism: anxiety, sexual dysfunction, sleep disturbances
- 5-$HT_3$ agonism: nausea
- 5-HT reuptake inhibition: gastrointestinal side effects, headache, activating effects
- NE reuptake inhibition: dry mouth, urinary retention, activating effects, **tremor**, tachycardia, hypertension
- $\alpha_2$ antagonism: postural hypotension, dizziness, reflex tachycardia
- $\alpha_1$ antagonism: **priapism**.

This section has covered many important pharmacodynamic principles that must be considered. However, apart from acquiring a deeper knowledge of the pharmacological profile of psychotropic drugs, the clinician must also be mindful of a number of important pharmacokinetic characteristics. Indeed, plasma t½ is a significant parameter to consider, even within the same drug class. For example, while all SSRIs have a t½ of 15-30 hours, fluoxetine has an active metabolite that extends its therapeutic t½ to 9 days, with both advantages and disadvantages that must be considered (Harvey, 1997). Since treatment **adherence** remains a problem, issues of t½ and the risk of developing a discontinuation syndrome or even breakthrough psychiatric symptoms using short half-life agents must be considered (Harvey and Slabbert, 2014). Further discussion on this is beyond the scope of this chapter, and more specialised articles and textbooks on neuro- and psychopharmacology should be consulted.

# References


Bernstein H, Keilhoff G, Steiner J, Dobrowolny H, Bogerts B (2011) Nitric oxide and schizophrenia: Present knowledge and emerging concepts of therapy. *CNS and Neurological Disorders - Drug Targets* 10: 792–807

Brink CB, Harvey BH, Bodenstein J, Venter DP, Oliver DW (2004) Understanding drug action and therapeutics: Relevance of G-protein-coupled receptors and signal transduction. *British Journal of Clinical Pharmacology* 57: 373–87

Brunton LL, Chabner BA, Knollmann BC (Eds) (2011) *The Pharmacological Basis of Therapeutics*, 12th ed. New York: McGraw-Hill

Castrén E. Is mood chemistry? (2005) *Nature Reviews Neuroscience* 6: 241–6

Castrén E, Võikar V, Rantamäki T (2007) Role of neurotrophic factors in depression. *Current Opinion in Pharmacology* 7: 18–21

Cooper JR, Bloom FE, Roth RH (2003) *The Biochemical Basis of Neuropharmacology*, 8th ed. Oxford: Oxford University Press

Davila-Garcia M I, Department of Pharmacology, Howard University, available at http://www.slideshare.net/bhatti106/antiepiliptic-drugs

Dhir A, Kulkarni SK (2011) Nitric oxide and major depression. *Nitric Oxide* 24: 125–31

Dwivedi Y (2009) Brain-derived neurotrophic factor: Role in depression and suicide. *Neuropsychiatric Diseases Treatment* 5: 433–49

Emsley R, Chiliza B, Asmal L, Harvey BH (2013) The nature of relapse in schizophrenia. *BMC Psychiatry* 8(13): 50

Giardino WJ, de Lecea L (2014) Hypocretin (orexin) neuromodulation of stress and reward pathways. *Current Opinion in Neurobiology* 29: 103–8

Harmar AJ, Fahrenkrug J, Gozes I, Laburthe M, May V, Pisegna JR, Vaudry D, Vaudry H, Waschek JA, Said SI (2012) Pharmacology and functions of receptors for vaso-active intestinal peptide and pituitary adenylate cyclase-activating polypeptide: IUPHAR review 1. *British Journal of Pharmacology* 166(1): 4–17

Harvey BH (1997) The neurobiology and pharmacology of depression: A comparative overview of serotonin-selective anti-depressants. *South African Medical Journal* 87: 540–52

Harvey BH (2006) Adaptive plasticity during stress and depression and the role of glutamate-nitric oxide pathways. *South African Psychiatry Review* 9: 132–9

Harvey BH, Bouwer CD (2000) Neuropharmacology of paradoxical weight gain with selective serotonin reuptake inhibitors. *Clinical Neuropharmacology* 23: 90–7

Harvey BH, McEwen BS, Stein DJ (2003) Neurobiology of anti-depressant withdrawal: implications for the longitudinal outcome of depression. *Biological Psychiatry* 54: 1105–17

Harvey BH, Stein DJ, Emsley RA (1999) The new-generation anti-psychotics: integrating the neuro-pathology and pharmacology of schizophrenia. *South African Medical Journal* 89: 661–72

Harvey BH, Shahid M (2012) Metabotropic and ionotropic glutamate receptors as neurobiological targets in anxiety and stress-related disorders: Focus on pharmacology and preclinical translational models. *Pharmacology Biochemistry and Behavior* 100: 775–800

Harvey BH, Slabbert FN (2014) New insights on the anti-depressant discontinuation syndrome. *Human Psychopharmacology*. 29: 503–16

Krishnan V, Nestler EJ (2008) The molecular neurobiology of depression. *Nature* 455: 894–902

Leonard BE (2003) *Fundamentals of Psychopharmacology*, 3rd ed. Chichester: John Wiley & Sons.

Liebenberg N, Harvey BH, Brand L, Brink CB (2010). Antidepressant-like properties of phosphodiesterase type 5 inhibitors and cholinergic dependency in a genetic rat model of depression. *Behavioural Pharmacology*. 21: 540–7

Lundbeck Institute, https://www.cnsforum.com/

Martinez JM, Garakani A, Yehuda R, Gorman JM (2012) Proinflammatory and 'resiliency' proteins in the CSF of patients with major depression. *Depression and Anxiety* 29: 32–8

McClung CA (2013) How might circadian rhythms control mood? Let me count the ways. *Biological Psychiatry* 74: 242–9

Meyer-Lindenberg A, Domes G, Kirsch P, Heinrichs M (2011) Oxytocin and vasopressin in the human brain: social neuropeptides for translational medicine. *Nature Reviews Neuroscience* 12: 524–38

Oosthuizen F, Wegener G, Harvey BH (2005) Role of nitric oxide as inflammatory mediator in post-traumatic stress disorder (PTSD): Evidence from an animal model. *Neuropsychiatric Disease and Treatment* 1: 109–24

Racagni G, Riva MA, Molteni R, Musazzi L, Calabrese F, Popoli M, Tardito D (2011) Mode of action of agomelatine: Synergy between melatonergic and 5-HT (2C) receptors. *World Journal of Biological Psychiatry* 12: 574–87

Savitz J, Drevets WC (2009) Bipolar and major depressive disorder: Neuroimaging the developmental-degenerative divide. *Neuroscience & Biobehavioral Reviews* 33: 699–771

Stahl SM (2013) *Stahl's Essential Psychopharmacology: Neuroscientific basis and practical applications*. Cambridge: Cambridge University Press.

## Additional reading

Areiasa MFC, Prada PO (2015). Mechanisms of insulin resistance in the amygdala: Influences on food intake. *Behavioural Brain Research* (in Press), doi:10.1016/j.bbr.2015.01.003

FitzGerald MJT, Gruener G, Mtui E. (2012) *Clinical Neuroanatomy and Neuroscience*, 4th ed. Edinburgh: Saunders/Elsevier

Harvey BH (2008). Is major depressive disorder a metabolic encephalopathy? *Human Psychopharmacology* 23: 371–84

Harvey BH, Duvenhage I, Viljoen F, Scheepers N, Malan SF, Wegener G, Brink CB, Petzer JP (2010). Role of monoamine oxidase, nitric oxide synthase and regional brain monoamines in the antidepressant-like effects of methylene blue and selected structural analogues. *Biochemical Pharmacology* 80: 1580–91

Hodges JR. (2007) *Cognitive assessment for clinicians*, 2nd ed. Oxford: Oxford University Press

Lindsay KW, Bone I. (2011) *Neurology and Neurosurgery* (illustrated), 5th ed. Edinburgh: Churchill Livingstone Elsevier

Prats-Galino A, Soria G, De Notaris M, Puig J, Pedraza S (2012) Functional anatomy of subcortical circuits issuing from or integrating at the human brain stem. *Clinical Neurophysiology* 123: 4–12

Sapolski RM (2004) *Why zebras don't get ulcers*, 3rd ed. New York: Henry Holt and Co

Shams TA, Müller DJ (2014). Antipsychotic induced weight gain: genetics, epigenetics, and biomarkers reviewed. *Current Psychiatry Reports* 16: 473

Stein DJ, Daniels WM, Savitz J, Harvey BH (2008). Brain-derived neurotrophic factor: the neurotrophin hypothesis of psychopathology. *CNS Spectrums* 13: 945–9

Van den Pol AN (2012). Neuropeptide transmission in brain circuits. *Neuron* 76: 98–115

# CHAPTER 5 Psychosocial determinants of mental disorders

*Jonathan Burns*

## 5.1 Introduction

The link between psychological and social features of the environment and risk for mental disorders is complex and has a long history. With the emergence of clear evidence for genetic, neurodevelopmental and other biological factors underpinning all psychiatric disorders, the challenge is to understand the relative roles of nature and nurture and to integrate biological, psychological and social risk factors into a coherent theory of causation.

## 5.2 Early developments

For nearly a century scientists and sociologists have demonstrated a robust relationship between features of the psychosocial environment and mental health. Founding sociological theorists such as Marx, Weber and Durkheim focused on social problems, including class distinctions, unequal distribution of wealth and health inequalities, in their efforts to understand how social structures and processes impacted on the welfare of individuals (Morgan and Kleinman, 2010). In terms of mental health, Durkheim's classic work on suicide reveals how differences in the frequency of suicide were explained by differences in social structure (Durkheim, 1938; Durkheim, 1952). Specifically, rates of suicide are higher in neighbourhoods characterised by low social cohesion and low respect for social norms. The philosopher Michel Foucault, author of *Madness and Civilization*, maintains that psychiatry was a product of the Enlightenment, emerging as a political institution designed to safeguard reason, suppress dissent, and enforce the boundary between normality and abnormality (Foucault, 2001).

During the 1960s and 1970s, the Anti-psychiatry movement (represented by Foucault, Thomas Szasz and RD Laing) argued that mental illness was a social construct and that psychiatry was an agent of social control (Szasz, 1961; Laing and Estersen, 1964). Defenders of psychiatry struck back, arguing that such theories were unscientific and naïvely ignored and minimised the suffering associated with mental illness. The divide between psychiatry and social sciences was so great by the end of the 1970s that Leon Eisenberg commented that the gap was almost unbridgeable (Eisenberg, 1977; Morgan and Kleinman, 2010).

The origins of a constructive collaboration between psychiatry and the social sciences can be traced to the late 1930s, with the seminal work of Faris and Dunham in Chicago (Faris and Dunham, 1939). These sociologists showed that first-admission rates for schizophrenia were 102 per 100 000 in the slums of central Chicago and diminished steadily to less than 25 per 100 000 in the affluent neighbourhoods on the outskirts of the city (Gottesman, 1991). While the **social drift** hypothesis (according to which people with schizophrenia drift down in social class as a result of the illness) was strongly supported for a long time (Goldberg and Morrison, 1963) more recent research indicates that features of the city (impoverished slums, overcrowding, etc.) play a causal role in the disorder (March *et al.*, 2008a). Faris and Dunham had postulated that the high incidence inner-city neighbourhoods were characterised by social fragmentation, a concept that has re-emerged in relation to mental disorders with recent interest in the social capital construct (McKenzie and Harpham, 2006).

New statistical approaches such as multilevel modelling have strengthened research efforts to untangle the relative roles of individual level and macro or environmental level factors in the aetiology of mental disorders. Likewise, the emergence of research methods that incorporate a focus on gene-environment interactions and epigenetic mechanisms have moved psychiatric research forward. Where previously genetics and environment were investigated in isolation from each other, we now have the ability to study the biological and **psychosocial causation** of mental disorders in an integrated manner. With such approaches we are more likely to discover the causes and pathological processes that give rise to mental disorders.

## 5.3 Social determinants of health

The World Health Organization (WHO) has defined the social determinants of health as 'the conditions in which people are born, grow, live, work and age, including the health system' (World Health Organization, 2013). WHO goes on to state: 'These circumstances are shaped by the distribution of money, power and resources at global, national and local levels. The social determinants of health are mostly responsible for health inequities – the unfair and avoidable differences in health status seen within and between countries' (World Health Organization, 2013). The social determinants of health can be seen as the economic and social conditions – and their distribution among the population – that influence individual and group differences in health status. Marmot notes that there is a range of life expectancy of 48 years among countries (and more than 20 years within some countries) and that 'research identifies social factors at the root of much of these inequalities in health' (Marmot, 2005).

In 2005, WHO established the Commission on Social Determinants of Health (CSDH) and tasked it to provide guidance on how best to address social determinants and reduce health disparities. Some of the major social determinants that have been identified include:

- poverty and material deprivation
- inequality
- unemployment
- conditions of the work environment
- social and political policies
- poor social cohesion
- social exclusion of minorities
- gender and ethnic/racial disparities
- migration
- globalisation
- urbanisation
- housing
- the structuring of health systems.

Marmot points out that the social determinants of health apply to all health conditions and should be addressed in efforts to improve population health and bring about social justice (Marmot, 2005).

## 5.4 Psychosocial risk factors for mental disorders

There is good evidence supporting the role played by many of the above social and economic factors in establishing risk for mental disorders. In addition a number of important psychological factors operate throughout the lifespan to increase or decrease vulnerability to mental disorders. The next section of this chapter will review the evidence for psychosocial determinants of mental disorders. Adopting a developmental approach, we will first examine factors during childhood and adolescence, followed by exposures during adulthood. Finally we will review the role of macro-environmental factors (that is factors operating at the level of the general environment, relating to features of the neighbourhood, geographical region and country).

### 5.4.1 Childhood adversity

Childhood adversity is a major risk factor for the development of mental disorders throughout the lifespan. Amongst the various forms of early adversity, direct experiences of trauma and abuse and loss of parents appear to have the most negative impact. In Hungary, for example, parental health events, death of a close relative and intra-familial events between the ages of seven and nine were significantly associated with major depressive disorder (MDD) in 434 children between the ages of seven and 14 (Mayer *et al.*, 2009). Children of parents with psychiatric disorders are particularly at risk of mental disorders. This is partly related to inherited genetic vulnerability but has also been shown to relate to negative aspects of the family environment and parent-child interaction (Manning and Gregoire, 2008). For example, children of parents with schizophrenia may be exposed not only to the trauma of witnessing psychosis in the parent, but also to more subtle deficits, such as impaired maternal sensitivity and responsiveness to the infant's signals, a lack of emotional warmth or emotional intrusiveness. Children of mothers with depression often experience insecure attachment, anxiety problems and subtle cognitive deficits (Melchior *et al.*, 2012). Mood and anxiety disorders, behavioural problems and substance abuse are common consequences of parental psychiatric disorder. Parental antisocial behaviour, hostility and substance abuse place the child at significant risk of later developing behavioural and conduct disorders, substance abuse and mood disorders (Manning and Gregoire, 2008).

The impact of experiencing parental loss, maltreatment and parental maladjustment was investigated in a US national sample of 6 483 adolescents-parent pairs (adolescents aged 13–17 years) (McLaughlin *et al.*, 2012). Maladaptive family functioning was significantly associated with adolescent onset of psychiatric disorders (especially behavioural disorders) and there was a linear relationship between increasing numbers of childhood adverse events and increased risk for adolescent onset of psychiatric disorder.

The consequences of childhood adversity may only manifest later in life during adulthood. In a Canadian study of 34 653 adults, childhood experiences of abuse or neglect (physical, sexual and emotional abuse, physical and emotional neglect) were associated with increased risk for substance use disorders in adulthood (Afifi *et al.*, 2012). In Chile, women who had experienced psychological violence during childhood had more than a threefold increased risk of depression in adulthood (Illanes *et al.*, 2007). Psychological trauma also predisposes adolescents to subsequent psychosis. A Dutch study of 2 524 adolescents and young adults showed that psychological trauma almost doubled the risk of psychotic symptoms four years later (OR: 1,89) (Spauwen *et al.*, 2006).

Finally, direct experiences of physical violence and trauma may precipitate post-traumatic stress disorder (PTSD) in a proportion of individuals regardless of their age. A Palestinian study of 179 boys aged 12-18 years who had been injured with permanent physical disability during the Al-Aqsa *intifada*, reported that 77% had PTSD (Khamis, 2008). Those with PTSD had an increased risk of co-morbid depression and anxiety disorders, while negative coping and fatalism were associated with the chronicity of PTSD symptoms.

### 5.4.2 Family environment and social support

The quality of the family environment and immediate availability of social support is vitally important for mental health.

The negative effects of a strained family environment can be seen in very young children. The EDEN Study in France examined the family environment in 1 903 mother-child pairs, and showed that family socioeconomic disadvantage (low family income) was associated with high emotionality scores in children as young as 12 months (Melchior *et al.*, 2012). Older children and adolescents are particularly vulnerable to negative family environments and poor social support. In Western Australia (Shepherd *et al.*, 2012), it was found that parenting quality, overcrowding and family functioning was associated with the risk of emotional and behavioural disorders in 3 993 indigenous children between the ages of four and 17, while Mao and Zhao (2012) showed that poor social cohesion was associated with an increased risk of depression in adolescents in Shanghai, China.

In adulthood, the availability of strong social support is a key contributor to resilience against mental disorders. For example, in the Gulf Coast Child and Family Health Study, 1 077 households in Louisiana and Mississippi that were greatly affected or displaced by Hurricane Katrina were surveyed. Two years after the disaster, the greatest predictors of poor mental health included lack of informal social support networks as well as greater numbers of children in the household (Abramson *et al.*, 2008).

Finally, older adults who live alone and are socially isolated are at particular risk of suicide (Conwell *et al.*, 2002).

## 5.4.3 Socioeconomic status

Low socioeconomic status and domestic income have long been recognised as risk factors for mental disorders. For example, among 3 738 adults surveyed in rural China, family socioeconomic status was associated with depression (Liang *et al.*, 2012). In our own context, the nationally representative South African Stress and Health (SASH) study, which surveyed 4 351 adults between 2002 and 2004, reported that low socioeconomic status was associated in logistic **regression** models, with a more than twofold increased risk of recent psychological distress (Myer *et al.*, 2008).

Women in low- and middle-income countries (LAMICs) appear to be especially vulnerable to the effects of living in poverty. Household poverty was associated with **common mental disorders (CMDs)** in 2 814 Ghanaian women living in Accra (De Menil *et al.*, 2012) and in 2 494 women in India (Patel *et al.*, 2006). Pregnant women in Qatar who experienced financial difficulties were at a twofold increased risk of developing post-partum depression (OR: 2.04) (Bener *et al.*, 2012).

In the UK, Weich and Lewis (1998) demonstrated that household income and housing tenure were associated with CMDs in a linear fashion. Interestingly, and with great relevance to the recent global economic recession, it appears that the experience of a recent decrease in personal or household income may be a potent risk factor for CMDs. For example, in Santiago, Chile (Araya *et al.*, 2003), it was found that a recent decrease in income was associated with a twofold increased risk of CMDs (OR: 2,14). A meta-analysis ($n$=5 179) on CMDs and social mobility in migrants reported that migrants to higher income countries who experienced downward mobility or under-employment were more likely to screen positive for CMDs (Das-Munshi *et al.*, 2012). It has long been recognised that financial and legal difficulties are potent risk factors for suicide in young and middle adulthood (Conwell *et al.*, 2002).

As with other forms of early adversity, family socioeconomic status during childhood is a powerful determinant of adult mental health (Poulton *et al.*, 2002). In a Swedish adoption study of 13 163 children, those reared in families with a disadvantageous socioeconomic position had an increased risk of later developing psychosis (Wicks *et al.*, 2010). This has particularly worrying implications for South Africa and indeed for most of sub-Saharan Africa (SSA). Fifty-seven per cent of the South African population live below the poverty line (where household income is not sufficient to sustain that household) (Human Sciences Research Council, 2004). This means that more than half the population of children in South Africa is at increased risk of developing mental disorders during adolescence and early adulthood. Unfortunately we do not have data from SSA; clearly there is an urgent need for a prospective longitudinal study of the effects of childhood poverty on subsequent risk of adolescent and adult mental disorders in this region.

## 5.4.4. Education, employment and the work environment

Limited education, unemployment and a stressful work environment are well-recognised risk factors for mental disorders in both high-income country (HIC) and LAMIC contexts. In developing countries, low levels of education and unemployed status have been associated with CMDs in Brazil, Chile, Ghana and South Africa.

A study conducted in a sample of 2 814 Ghanaian women living in Accra showed strong associations with these risk factors (De Menil *et al.*, 2012). In Campinas, Brazil, the risk of CMDs in adults with less than five years of schooling was 5½ times greater than in those with more schooling (Marin-León *et al.*, 2007). A study of 3 870 adults in Santiago, Chile, found that those with less education were almost 2½ times more likely to have CMDs than those with more education (OR: 2,44) (Araya *et al.*, 2001; 2003). In the same study in Chile, unemployment increased adults' risk for CMDs, while in the Brazilian study, unemployment or under-employment was associated with a twofold increased risk of CMDs.

In the South African SASH study, Myer *et al.* (2008) found that tertiary education (OR: 0,59) and being employed (OR: 0,59) was protective against life events during the preceding year in adults. Notably, multiple life events were strongly associated with recent psychological distress in this study. Given that the 2011 national census in South Africa reported that only 38% of adults have completed secondary education and that unemployment rates average 29.8% across the country, the associations between lower education, unemployed status and poor mental health are a major concern.

Finally, a stressful work environment impacts negatively on mental health and has been associated with increased risk for depression. In the UK, 7 732 British civil servants were assessed three times over 10 years for levels of work stress and the presence of Major Depressive Disorder (MDD) (Stansfield *et al.*, 2012). Repeated job strain was associated with increased risk for MDD (OR: 2,19); while repeated low work social support was also associated with MDD (OR: 1,61). In Ibadan, Nigeria, Collins *et al.* (1996) reported an association between job distress in men and acute brief psychosis.

## 5.4.5 Adult adversity

While early experiences of adversity in childhood and adolescence set up individuals for later risk of mental disorders, negative life experiences during adulthood itself also increase the likelihood of individuals requiring mental health care. Some of the major negative events associated with mental disorders include:

- relationship status and relationship quality
- family conflict and violence
- lack of social support
- exposure to interpersonal violence.

In Santiago, Chile, single or separated marital status and single parenting were associated with CMDs in 3 870 adults (Araya *et al.*, 2001), while a survey of 3 738 adults in rural China found that recent negative life events were significant risk factors for depression (Liang *et al.*, 2012).

Women appear to be particularly at risk for CMDs in homes characterised by conflict and a lack of social support. In northern Sweden, gender inequity in adult relationships correlated with depressive mood (Hammarström and Phillips, 2012); while poor family support (OR: 1,52) and poor marital relationships (OR: 1,13) were associated with an increased risk of post-partum depression in women in Qatar (Bener *et al.*, 2012). In Temuco, a low-income neighbourhood in Chile, risk factors for depression or anxiety in women included physical violence against children in the home (OR: 14.3), being a victim of sexual violence (OR: 9.7) and lack of a family support network (OR: 2.7) (Illanes *et al.*, 2007).

Interpersonal violence and crime also increase the risk of mental disorders. In a household survey of 5 037 adults in São Paulo, Brazil, exposure to crime was associated with anxiety disorders, mood disorders, impulse-control disorders and substance use disorders (Andrade *et al.*, 2012).

Finally, recent stressful life events are one of the major precipitants of suicide in the elderly (Conwell *et al.*, 2002).

## 5.4.6 Macro-environmental level risk factors

Dating back from Durkheim's observations on suicide (Durkheim, 1938; Durkheim, 1952) and Faris and Dunham's findings on schizophrenia (Faris and Dunham, 1939), sociologists, geographers and more recently, social, economic and health scientists, have laboured to unravel the complex relationships that exist between features of the wider environment (ecological factors) and the risk of mental disorders. In recent times, disciplines such as social geography, social epidemiology and social psychiatry have built on earlier work in order to overcome some of the methodological challenges and potholes that have frustrated and undermined the field. A major criticism of earlier work was that it was subject to the 'ecological fallacy' – that is, generalising ecological level results to the individual level. Failure to control for individual-level factors in ecological level association studies leaves any conclusions reached open to severe critique. Thus, approaches that adopt multilevel analytic statistical methods are now the gold standard.

The evidence for risk effects for CMDs in large geographical areas (e.g.at the level of the UK electoral wards with average populations of 5 500) is mixed and difficult to interpret (Wainwright and Surtees, 2004; Weich *et al.*, 2003). Effect sizes are small in these studies. Electoral wards (or their equivalent) may be too large an area and have a too heterogenous population. On the other hand, the neighbourhood level may be better, but is notoriously hard to define and is arguably a highly subjective measure (Stansfield *et al.*, 2008). In a large national household survey in Britain, 10% of the variance in scores on the General Health Questionnaire occurred at household level (Weich *et al.*, 2003).

More recently, the evidence seems to be swaying in favour of the wider socioeconomic environment having an impact on individual risk for CMDs. For example, in Santiago, Chile, living in a better built environment (with adequate green spaces) was associated with a lower risk of CMDs, after adjusting for individual level factors (Araya *et al.*, 2007), while in Australia, individuals who perceived their neighbourhoods as highly green, had 1,6 times higher odds of better mental health (Sugiyama *et al.*, 2008). In London, UK, the significant factors negatively affecting mental well-being included neighbour noise, a sense of overcrowding in the home, and reduced access to green spaces and community facilities (Guite *et al.*, 2006). A multilevel study conducted in 59 neighbourhoods in New York City found that residence in neighbourhoods characterised by a poor quality built environment was associated with a greater individual likelihood of lifetime depression and depression during the previous six months (Galea *et al.*, 2005). The neighbourhood built environment in New York City has also been associated with the prevalence of fatal drug overdoses in various parts of that city (Hembree *et al.*, 2005).

#### 5.4.6.1 Urbanicity, urban birth, and urban upbringing

The majority of research on urbanicity and mental disorders has been in relation to schizophrenia and other psychoses. High rates of schizophrenia have long been observed in urban areas (Faris and Dunham, 1939). The rates were originally ascribed to social drift, whereby individuals with incipient psychosis tend to drift to cities, giving rise to a situation of social selection (Goldberg and Morrison, 1963). However, subsequent research (Dohrenwend *et al.*, 1992; Mortensen *et al.*, 1999; McGrath *et al.*, 2004) disproved the social drift theory, lending support for urbanicity playing a social causative role.

With respect to schizophrenia, early work focused on residence in urban versus rural areas. However, over the last 20 years, this focus has shifted to urban birth and upbringing, rather than mere residence. What has become increasingly apparent is the fact that the urban effect is largely to do with being born in a city and raised in a city (Lewis *et al.*, 1992; Marcelis *et al.*, 1999; March *et al.*, 2008a; Mortensen *et al.*, 1999). Furthermore, a review of the literature found that one-third of studies report a 'dose-response' relationship between level of urbanicity and risk of psychosis (March *et al.*, 2008a). Urban birth and upbringing are associated with exposure from *in utero* to childhood to a host of potential environmental threats, including:

- high rates of perinatal infection in crowded low income city neighbourhoods
- increased exposure to toxins such as leaded gasoline

- a lack of vitamin D due to a clear urban-rural gradient in dietary availability of this neurodevelopmental nutrient
- various sociocultural factors (Brown, 2011).

Much of the evidence on urban birth and upbringing comes from large population studies conducted in Scandinavia. Lewis *et al.* (1992) used data from a cohort of more than 49 000 Swedish conscripts and showed a linear trend with highest rates in those who mostly grew up in cities. A particularly large Danish study (with a cohort of 1,75 million persons) identified the overall increased risk of developing schizophrenia for those born in urban areas as being twofold (Mortensen *et al.*, 1999). Subsequently, in an extensive study on the effects of urbanicity in Denmark, this research group clarified the relative importance of urban birth versus urban upbringing in conferring risk (Pedersen and Mortensen, 2001). They demonstrated that the timing of the effect is important. Specifically, for those individuals born versus raised in an urban area:

- the greater the amount of time spent living in an urban area during upbringing, the greater the risk of later developing schizophrenia
- the effect of urban birth disappeared when adjusted for confounding factors, while the effect of urban residence during upbringing persisted.

Thus, their conclusion was that being raised in an urban area is the main risk factor. Nevertheless, urban birth alone is still associated with a risk for schizophrenia – the population attributable risk due to urban birth is estimated at 30% (Mortensen *et al.*, 1999).

The urban effect also appears to play a role in risk across the whole psychotic spectrum. In the Netherlands, the effect of cannabis on the risk for new onset of psychotic symptoms in those aged 14-24 was much stronger for those who grew up in an urban environment (Kuepper *et al.*, 2011). Van Os and colleagues (2001) reported that psychosis-like experiences occur in 23% of urban residents but in only 13% of rural residents in the Netherlands. A survey of 646 young adult Ugandans found that urban birth was associated with more lifetime psychotic experiences and more recent symptoms of psychosis, depression and anxiety (Lundberg *et al.*, 2009).

Urbanicity has also been associated with risk for CMDs. A higher prevalence of CMDs was reported among urban residents in the UK (Paykel *et al.*, 2000; Weich *et al.*, 2006), while higher rates of depression were reported in urban women in a large pan-European study (Lehtinen *et al.*, 2003). Sundquist *et al.*, (2004) found a linear association between increasing population density (as a proxy for urbanicity) and rates of first admission for depression amongst the Swedish adult population.

Finally, urban residence is associated with both personality and impulse-control disorders. A large nationally representative study in the UK reported an association between urban residence and rates of personality disorder (Coid *et al.*, 2006), while the risk for impulse-control disorders was associated with high urbanicity in a household survey of 5 037 adults in São Paulo, Brazil (Andrade *et al.*, 2012).

Suicide may be the exception. Many studies show increased rates of suicide in rural areas compared with urban areas, especially in males (Rost *et al.*, 1998; Singh and Siahpush, 2002; Yip and Liu, 2006; Caldwell *et al.*, 2004; Levin and Leyland, 2005). This may relate to social isolation, lack of social networks and poorer access to services.

### 5.4.6.2 Social capital and social cohesion

Social capital refers to the ability of individuals to draw on collective resources at group level. Social capital describes aspects of social networks, relations, trust and power and can be studied as a property of individuals or as a property of groups (ecological). The latter is most commonly measured by aggregating individual social capital at a particular spatial level, such as a city neighbourhood.

It is a concept that emerged from the social, economic and political sciences (Putnam, 1993) but in recent years has also entered the health domain as a possible explanatory factor for variations in health (Whitely and McKenzie, 2005).

There is a large amount of literature on the relationship between social capital and mental health (Henderson and Whiteford, 2003; Almedon, 2005; De Silva *et al.*, 2005). Hypothetically, social capital reduces negative life events and long-term difficulties and is protective against mental disorders (Harpham *et al.*, 2002). For example, in Maastricht in the Netherlands, strong neighbourhood trust and social cohesion were associated with a reduced use in mental health care services by children from socioeconomically deprived neighbourhoods (Van der Linden *et al.*, 2003).

There is evidence from both HICs and LAMICs that social capital is protective against CMDs. In a large study conducted in 234 communities in Peru, Ethiopia, Vietnam and Ahdhra Pradesh (India), 6 909 mothers of 1-year-old infants were assessed for CMDs (De Silva *et al.*, 2007). Ecological social capital was calculated by aggregating individual measures to community level. Multilevel modelling showed that social capital is associated with a reduced risk of CMDs in mothers across all four countries. A household survey in South Wales found that positive perceptions of neighbourhood social capital was associated with better mental health (Araya *et al.*, 2006), while a study of 9 000 residents in 239 neighbourhoods in England and Scotland reported a protective effect for social capital against CMDs for people living in deprived circumstances only (Stafford *et al.*, 2008). In South Africa, in the SASH household study (Myer *et al.*, 2008) showed that low-level social capital was associated with an almost twofold increased risk for psychological distress (OR: 1,73). Tomita and Burns (2013) analysed data from the National Income Dynamics Study and showed that lower neighbourhood social capital predicted higher individual depression scores.

Social capital and social cohesion (versus social fragmentation) may explain how urbanicity increases the risk of schizophrenia (Brown, 2011; March *et al.*, 2008a). Social capital is inversely related to incidence of psychosis, adjusting for individual-level factors and neighbourhood-level deprivation (Kirkbride *et al.*, 2007; Lofors and Sundquist, 2007). Social fragmentation, which is particularly associated with inner city urban life, has been associated with an increased risk of schizophrenia (Allardyce *et al.*, 2005). This hearkens back to Faris and Dunham (1939) who linked social fragmentation in inner-city Chicago to higher rates of schizophrenia in those areas. A review (March *et al.*, 2008a) of 44 studies of urbanicity, neighbourhood and psychosis, suggest that since social pathways emphasise place over space, they could explain the urbanicity effect: one's natural and built environment could give rise to 'a multitude of social, economic, and biological risk factors which interact with one another at different levels, thereby increasing schizophrenia risk' (Brown, 2011). March *et al.* (2008b) describe social pathways as 'cascades of social processes across multiple levels that produce a variety of conditions in a given place, which shape exposures more proximal to the individual'.

#### 5.4.6.3 Deprivation and inequality

It appears that socioeconomic deprivation is a risk factor for mental illness not just at the level of the individual and household but also at the level of the neighbourhood. In the 1930s, Faris and Dunham had observed the links between neighbourhood deprivation and squalor in Chicago and higher rates of schizophrenia. Contemporary research using modern multilevel statistical methods confirm these early findings. For example, in a study including 3 993 indigenous children (aged 4–17) in Western Australia, housing quality and neighbourhood-level disadvantage were associated with the risk of emotional and behavioural disorders (Shepherd *et al.*, 2012). In a household survey of 5 037 adults in São Paulo, Brazil, neighbourhood social deprivation was associated with an increased prevalence of substance use disorders (Andrade *et al.*, 2012), while neighbourhood-level deprivation and social **disorganisation** were associated with increased risk for substance related disorders in the adult population of Malmö, Sweden (Chaix *et al.*, 2006).

The question whether the effects of socioeconomic privation can operate at the level of large regions such as cities and states remains controversial and many authors argue that large-scale effects are confounded by too many intermediate factors (at neighbourhood, household and individual level) to be confident regarding their role. Nevertheless, in a multilevel study of 88 of the largest metropolitan areas in the US, an association was demonstrated between political economy at the metro-level and risk for injection drug use (Roberts *et al.*, 2010). In this study, a one-percentage point worsening of political economy was associated with greater risk of injection drug use (RR: 1,10). However, a systematic review of the incidence of schizophrenia found no relationship between schizophrenia incidence and economic status of countries (Saha *et al.*, 2006).

Income inequality is a relatively neglected concept in the study of macro-level socioeconomic risk factors for mental disorders. Income inequality is a measure of the gap between rich and poor in any given society and reflects the extent to which a society is unequal in terms of income distribution. This is a concept of great relevance to South Africa, which ranks among the most inequitable in the world (Leibbrandt *et al.*, 2010). There are multiple associations between income inequality and health status. In the 1980s and 1990s, Wilkinson (1992; 1996) demonstrated that the relative distribution of income in a society matters in its own right for population health. This has been supported by subsequent research (Kawachi *et al.*, 2002; Subramanian and Kawachi, 2004).

There is growing evidence that income inequality at the macro level is associated with an increased risk of a range of mental disorders. Pickett and Wilkinson (2010) showed that greater income inequality is associated with a threefold increase in prevalence of mental disorders and substance use disorders, and that this is likely due to the impact of inequality on the quality of social relationships and social cohesion. In a US state-level study of the Gini coefficient (a measure of income inequality) versus prevalence of depression, higher income inequality in a state was associated with a higher prevalence of depression (Messias *et al.*, 2011). In a second US study, Ahern and Galea (2006) investigated the effects of neighbourhood-level income inequality on risk for depression in New York City during the six months after 9/11. High income inequality was associated with an increased prevalence of depression among low-income individuals. Interestingly, an earlier British household study of 8 191 adults had reported that a high income inequality was associated with a higher prevalence of CMDs among the most affluent individuals (Weich *et al.*, 2001).

The association between ecological level income inequality and the incidence of schizophrenia and psychosis has been investigated in three studies to date. In the most deprived electoral wards in South London, the incidence of schizophrenia increased with increasing inequality (Boydell *et al.*, 2004). Since this finding emerged from a *post hoc* analysis of the primary results, this finding should be treated with some caution. A second study, conducted in seven mixed urban and rural municipalities in KwaZulu-Natal in South Africa, found a significant association between increasing income inequality and treated incidence of first-episode psychosis (FEP) after controlling for urbanicity (Burns and Esterhuizen, 2008). In a recent systematic review of schizophrenia incidence rates and national Gini coefficients, multilevel methods were used to demonstrate a significant relationship between incidence rates of schizophrenia and country-level measures of income inequality (Burns *et al.*, 2014).

The role of income inequality is controversial because there are many potential intermediary confounders between this macro-level societal characteristic and an individual risk for mental disorders. Yet, research to date, using appropriate statistical methods, appears to support an association. Clearly further research is indicated to confirm the role of income inequality. If income inequality does play a role, it is likely that economic disparities have their effects by damaging social capital and reducing social cohesion at neighbourhood and household levels.

### 5.4.6.4 Migration, ethnicity and discrimination

One of the most striking – and perhaps disturbing – observations in recent decades regarding the role of macro-level factors in enhancing risk for mental illness is that relating to migration, ethnicity and **discrimination**. While most of the interest has focused on risks of migration and ethnic status for psychosis and schizophrenia, associations have also been reported for CMDs. Migration is a stressful experience in its own right, but it appears that the process of settling in a host country is further complicated by major stresses related to the extent to which host neighbourhoods welcome immigrants and particularly ethnic-minority immigrants in their midst. (Note: the terms 'migrant' and 'immigrant' are used interchangeably in this chapter). Furthermore, as will be discussed in more detail below, the risk of mental disorder is often greater in second-generation immigrants: children born in the host country to immigrant parents appear to be at an even greater risk than their parents of developing mental disorders.

There is now a large literature confirming that migration is a risk factor for schizophrenia (McGrath *et al.*, 2004; Cantor-Graae and Selten, 2005). Studies show this in Afro-Caribbeans and Africans in the UK, migrants from Surinam, Morocco and the Dutch Antilles in Netherlands, as well as in migrants to Denmark. Age at migration also matters, with younger migrants experiencing greater risk. In a seven-year first-contact incidence study of psychosis in the Netherlands, age at migration was associated in a linear fashion with risk for psychosis: from birth to four years, the risk ratio was 2,96; at 5–9 years, it was 2,31; and at 10–14 years, it was 1,51 (Veling *et al.*, 2011).

As stated above, risk is greater in second-generation immigrants compared with first-generation migrants. In a Danish case-controlled study (including 892 individuals with schizophrenia), second-generation immigrants had an almost twofold increased risk of schizophrenia (RR: 1,94) (Pedersen *et al.*, 2012). Cantor-Graae and Selten (2005) showed in their meta-analysis that the relative risk in first-generation immigrants was 2,7, while the relative risk in second-generation immigrants was 4,5. Importantly, rates of schizophrenia in the countries of origin are similar to those in the native populations of host countries.

Rates also differ depending on country of origin, and migrants from developing countries show a greater risk than those from developed countries. In the Netherlands, for example, the risk of schizophrenia was highest in migrants from Morocco (RR: 5,8), intermediate in migrants from Surinam (RR: 2,9) and lowest in migrants from Turkey (RR: 2,3) (Veling *et al.*, 2006). Re-analysis of data demonstrated that the risk was five-fold higher if migrants came from countries with predominantly black populations (Cantor-Graae and Selten, 2005). Dealberto (2010) also reported an increased risk in black immigrants (compared with other races) while a two-fold increased risk of schizophrenia was reported in African-Americans in a birth cohort study in the USA (Bresnahan *et al.*, 2007). This suggests that discrimination may be a potent risk factor for schizophrenia as well as ethnic disadvantage, so that ethnic minority migrants are not able to realise their goals and adapt as easily in a new environment (Brown, 2011). Cantor-Graae and Selten (2005) have postulated a social-defeat hypothesis, based on animal studies, whereby repeated failure to realise goals due to social barriers and social marginalisation leads to alterations in monoamine levels and a subsequent risk of psychosis.

Attempts to understand the social mechanisms that may underlie the increased risk of schizophrenia experienced by migrants and ethnic minorities have led to a focus on the ethnic density of neighbourhoods. Researchers have explored whether risk varies according to the extent to which an ethnic-minority individual is in fact a minority (or is actually part of the majority ethnic group) within his or her immediate neighbourhood of residence. A recent review of meta-analytic findings on risk for schizophrenia and other psychoses in migrants, found that variations in neighbourhood-level ethnic density did, in fact, correspond to variations in the risk for schizophrenia. (Bourque *et al.*, 2012). Several studies confirm this variability.

Boydell *et al.* (2001) reported that the incidence of schizophrenia was higher in ethnic minorities living in low ethnic-density neighbourhoods in London (i.e. in neighbourhoods where the predominant population was of another ethnic group) (Boydell *et al.*, 2001). In the Netherlands the incidence of psychotic disorders amongst migrants varied according to the ethnic density of their neighbourhoods of residence (Veling *et al.*, 2008). Ethnic-minority status also seems to have an impact on risk across the psychotic spectrum, including psychotic-like experiences and **at-risk mental states** (Bourque *et al.*, 2012). Thus it appears that one's social context can modify the effect of individual-level risk factors (such as immigrant status and ethnicity) (Brown, 2011).

A possible explanation for the ethnic-density finding is that living in a high ethnic-density neighbourhood may be protective against the negative effects of discrimination on risk for schizophrenia (Brown, 2011). Supporting this hypothesis is evidence from the Netherlands where Veling *et al.* (2007) showed a clear association between the experience of discrimination and increased risk for schizophrenia and psychotic symptoms.

A recent review of ethnic density and mental disorders confirms the findings for psychosis, and also suggests that high ethnic density may be protective against depression and anxiety in African-American and Hispanic adults in the US (Shaw *et al.*, 2012). Certainly, the negative effects of migration have been demonstrated in relation to CMDs in a variety of contexts. Migrant adolescents in Shanghai, China, for example, reported significantly higher levels of depression and had fewer social connections (Mao and Zhao, 2012), while a study of Latino immigrants to the US showed that depression was associated with high poverty prior to migration, stressful experiences during migration and racial problems or ethnic discrimination post-migration (Ornelas and Perreira, 2011). In the US, Mexican migrants to the US had a significantly higher risk for first onset of any depressive or anxiety disorder (OR: 1,42) compared with non-migrant family members still residing in Mexico (Breslau *et al.*, 2011b). A recent meta-analysis (*n*=5 179) on CMDs and social mobility in migrants, found that migrants to higher-income countries who experienced downward mobility or underemployment on arrival were more likely to screen positive for CMDs (Das-Munshi *et al.*, 2012). Finally, surveys conducted in Mexico and the US show that migration is associated with increased risk for both conduct disorder (Breslau *et al.*, 2011a) and binge-eating disorder (Swanson *et al.*, 2012). Conduct disorder was more than four times more common in the children of Mexican immigrants raised in the USA (OR: 4,12), while an even higher risk was detected amongst second-generation children of Mexican migrants (OR: 7,64) (Breslau *et al.*, 2011a). Interestingly, the association with migration was particularly strong for the non-aggressive form of conduct disorder (the aggressive form is under substantial genetic influence). The risk of binge-eating disorder was 2-3 times higher in second-generation Mexican migrants compared to Mexicans in their families of origin (OR: 2,58) (Swanson *et al.*, 2012).

## 5.4.7 Concluding comments on risk factors

In concluding this section on psychosocial risk factors for mental disorders, it is apparent that features of the personal, family and wider neighbourhood and societal environment impact considerably on the risk for a wide range of mental disorders. Unravelling the respective contribution of different factors, and establishing the relative contribution of factors at different levels, requires two broad approaches, both calling for innovative research methods:

- the use of carefully designed social epidemiological methods that account for multiple levels of effect and allow for the fact that risk factors interact reciprocally within and between different levels
- the study of how features of the social environment impact on the individual at the neurobiological level to either enhance risk for, or enhance resilience against, the development of psychiatric disorder.

The former approach is discussed in some detail in Chapter 3: Psychiatric epidemiology and genetics, while the latter is the subject of the next section of this chapter.

## 5.5 Psychosocial processes and neurobiological mechanisms

In recent years there has emerged a fascinating literature on the question of how aspects of the social environment impact on individuals at the neurobiological level. In an excellent review of the topic, Toyokawa asks the question:'How does the social environment "get into the mind?"' (Toyokawa *et al.*, 2012). This is the subject of the following discussion and the focus of the burgeoning fields of social and affective neuroscience as well as epigenetics.

As discussed in Chapter 3: Psychiatric epidemiology and genetics, most psychiatric disorders result from an interaction between genetic vulnerability factors and psychosocial exposures. In addition to their common role as precipitants of illness in genetically vulnerable individuals, psychosocial factors may also operate early on, impacting on neurodevelopmental processes and causing vulnerability to later mental disorder. An example of the latter mechanism is the manner in which exposure to childhood abuse and neglect can have lasting neurobiological effects that render the individual highly vulnerable to later depression, PTSD and even psychosis (Varese *et al.*, 2012). Here two particular mechanisms are hypothesised, with growing evidence to support them.

### 5.5.1 Hypothalamo-pituitary-adrenal axis dysregulation

The first mechanism involves the hypothalamo-pituitary-adrenal (HPA) axis. Chronic, recurrent exposure to childhood abuse leads to both HPA over-reactivity through behavioural **sensitisation** (Read *et al.*, 2001) and to HPA dysregulation (De Bellis *et al.*, 1994), with evidence of elevated baseline cortisol and adrenocorticotropic hormone (ADH) levels and increased cortisol response to pharmacological stressors in individuals with a history of childhood abuse (Walker *et al.*, 2008; Van Winkel *et al.*, 2008). In patients with schizophrenia, those abused as children (especially emotionally abused) had greater HPA axis dysregulation, measured by cortisol levels, compared with their non-abused counterparts (Braehler *et al.*, 2005).

### 5.5.2 Dopaminergic dysregulation

The other mechanism (which is likely to operate in parallel) relates to the dopaminergic system.

Laruelle (2000) suggested that psychosis is associated with mesolimbic dopamine (DA) sensitisation characterised by hyperactivity of DA neurons to environmental stimuli, with even exposure to moderate levels of stress being associated with an excessive DA response. Girls who have been sexually abused show elevated DA levels (De Bellis *et al.*, 1994). Psychotic patients with a history of early abuse show marked reactivity to stressors in normal life resulting in stronger increases in negative emotions and psychosis intensity in reaction to daily life stressors (Myin-Germys *et al.*, 2001; Myin-Germys *et al.*, 2005). Thus, early exposure to stressful adverse experiences or traumas leads to a state of vulnerability whereby individuals show greater negative reactivity to later environmental stressors. In this way, childhood adversity may, in part, mediate the relationship between adult adversity and mental health disorders.

These chronic abnormalities in HPA and DA function, in response to stress and trauma, give rise to neuro-anatomical changes in structures involved in regulation of these systems such as the hippocampus. Hippocampal volume reduction, particularly on the left side, is consistently found in adult victims of childhood maltreatment and may include all hippocampal subfields (Teicher *et al.*, 2012). In schizophrenia, decreased (left) hippocampal volume is associated with childhood adversity (Hoy *et al.*, 2012), increased emotional stress reactivity (Collip *et al.*, 2013) and diurnal cortisol levels (Mondelli *et al.*, 2010).

### 5.5.3 Neurotransmitters and neurotrophins

Early exposure to environmental stress has also been associated with other neurobiological disruptions, for example in neurotransmitters and in neurotrophins. Rhesus macaques reared apart from their mothers (by peers only) consistently exhibit significantly lower concentrations of the primary central serotonin metabolite 5-hydroxyindoleacetic acid (5-HIAA) than mother-reared monkeys from early infancy to early adulthood (Shannon *et al.*, 2005). They also exhibit significantly different developmental trajectories of peripheral measures of the neurotrophic factors NGF and BDNF (Cirulli *et al.*, 2009). Notably, BDNF, which is involved in brain development and plasticity, is thought to play a role in mediating the effects of stress and HPA hyperactivity on the hippocampus and depression (Kunugi *et al.*, 2010); while low serum BDNF levels correlate with cumulative trauma exposure and psychotic symptoms in patients with first-episode psychosis (Fawzi *et al.*, 2013).

### 5.5.4 Neurobiological correlates of urbanicity, ethnic minority and social or socioeconomic status

Exposure to ecological level stressors is likely to operate through similar mechanisms. For example, using functional magnetic resonance imaging (fMRI) in three independent experiments, Lederbogen and colleagues (2011) showed that urban upbringing and city living have dissociable impacts on social evaluative stress processing in humans. Current city living was associated with increased amygdala activity, whereas urban upbringing affected the perigenual anterior cingulate cortex (pACC), a key region for regulation of amygdala activity, negative affect and stress (Lederbogen *et al.*, 2011). The same researchers recently showed similar results in a study comparing ethnic-minority individuals with local German individuals (Akdeniz *et al.*, 2014). During fMRI stress induction, the ethnic-minority individuals showed increased activation and functional connectivity in the pACC, which correlated with perceived group discrimination, which in turn was mediated by chronic social stress. The authors propose that this social stress results from experiences of social threat and chronic **social defeat**.

Similar experiences of social stress are likely to underlie the increased risk for mental disorders associated with low social and socioeconomic status, especially as experienced during childhood. A key concept here is subjective or perceived status, which is strongly related to negative emotionality and health outcomes (Gallo and Matthews, 2003; Sapolsky, 2004). Neuro-imaging studies provide insights into the biological effects of such experiences. Structural changes (decreased grey matter volume) in the pACC have been demonstrated in individuals with lower perceived social standing (Gianaros *et al.*, 2007). fMRI studies indicate that lower perceived personal and parental social standing is associated with increased reactivity in limbic structures including the amygdala, anterior cingulate gyrus (ACC) and striatum (Zink *et al.*, 2008; Gianaros *et al.*, 2008).

### 5.5.5 Epigenetics

This section would be incomplete without a brief mention of the rapidly growing field of epigenetics, which is likely to shed further light on how environmental factors impact on neurobiological processes, thereby giving rise to mental illnesses. A full discussion of this would require a chapter on its own; thus just a few examples of important findings will be presented to illustrate this mechanism.

As was mentioned in Chapter 3: Psychiatric epidemiology and genetics, the term epigenetics, first coined by Waddington (1940), refers to a mechanism by which gene expression is modified without any change to the primary DNA sequence. This regulation of gene function, which is heritable and also modifiable, occurs through several chemical processes including DNA methylation, histone modification and the more recently identified non-protein coding micro-RNAs (Toyokawa *et al.*, 2012).

DNA methylation occurs when a methyl group is added to a cytosine residue in the promotor region of DNA, typically reducing the level of expression of neighbouring coding regions (genes). Histone is the main protein component of chromatin, around which DNA is wound. Histone regulates the degree to which the chromatin relaxes to allow gene transcription to take place. Histone acetyltransferases add acetyl groups to the histone, causing relaxation of chromatin and increased gene transcription (expression), while histone deacetylases remove acetyl groups from histone, causing chromatin to condense, thus preventing gene transcription (Tsankova *et al.*, 2007).

Epigenetic mechanisms have been shown to be involved in schizophrenia, MDD, PTSD, **anorexia** nervosa and substance use disorders (Toyokawa *et al.*, 2012). It is likely that they occur in most psychiatric disorders. Hypermethylation of the *reelin* gene (*RELN*) promotor is associated with down-regulation of *RELN* expression in several brain regions in schizophrenia (Costa *et al.*, 2002). Importantly, *RELN* is expressed during neurodevelopment and is critical for proper positioning of neurons and healthy connectivity (Tissir and Goffinet, 2003). Reduced dietary intake of nutrients such as methionine and folate (for example in poverty or famine conditions) alters methylation rates of various genes such as *RELN* and the insulin-like growth factor (*IGF2*) gene (which plays a key role in the regulation of cellular proliferation and growth) and may thus negatively affect neurodevelopmental processes (Toyokawa *et al.*, 2012). Prenatal exposure to deficiencies of nutrients such as methionine and folate (such as during the Dutch 'hunger winter' of 1944–45 and the Chinese famine of 1959–1961) may well explain the increased rates of schizophrenia observed in birth cohorts from these two events (Susser *et al.*, 1996; Hoek *et al.*, 1998; St Clair *et al.*, 2005). In support of this hypothesis was the finding from the Dutch 'hunger winter' cohort that prenatal exposure to famine was associated with reduced methylation of *IGF2* six decades after the famine exposure (Heijmans *et al.*, 2008).

Epigenetic mechanisms have also been implicated in depression and PTSD. Prenatal exposure to third trimester maternal depression has been associated with increased methylation of the glucocorticoid receptor gene (*NR3C1*) promotor in infants, and with increased infant cortical stress reactivity at three months (Oberlander *et al.*, 2008). This suggests a potential epigenetic process linking antenatal maternal mood to altered HPA stress reactivity in neonates (Toyokawa *et al.*, 2012).

Other research indicates that child abuse is associated with hypermethylation of the 5-hydroxytryptamine transporter (5-HTT or *SLC6A4*) gene (Beach *et al.*, 2010), which in turn is associated with depression (Philibert *et al.*, 2008). Finally, epigenetic investigations on participants in the Detroit Neighborhood Health Study, where levels of exposure to violence and rates of PTSD where markedly high, reported a correlation between number of reported traumatic events and methylation levels at multiple gene sites in those with PTSD (Uddin *et al.*, 2010). Importantly, epigenetic changes in many of these genes have been confirmed in an independent cohort of traumatised adults from Atlanta (Smith *et al.*, 2011).

## Conclusion

There is indisputable evidence that psychological, social, economic and even spatial factors in the environment contribute to risk for most – if not all – psychiatric disorders. Psychosocial determinants act at multiple levels including the levels of the individual, the family and the neighbourhood and society. The genetic and neurobiological mechanisms underlying these interactions between environmental exposures and the brain are complex and fascinating. Some of the fastest-growing fields of scientific research are those concerned with understanding these links: social epidemiology, affective neuroscience, epigenetics and genetic epidemiology. It is likely that the next few decades will bring a host of remarkable new findings and increasingly astounding insights to our understanding of how our environment actively shapes our mental health.

# References

Abramson D, Stehling-Ariza T, Garfield R, Redlener I (2008) Prevalence and predictors of mental health distress post-Katrina: Findings from the Gulf Coast Child and Family Health Study. *Disaster Medicine and Public Health Preparedness* 2(2): 77–86

Afifi TO, Henriksen CA, Asmundson GJ, Sareen J (2012) Childhood maltreatment and substance use disorders among men and women in a nationally representative sample. *Canadian Journal of Psychiatry* 57(11): 677–86

Ahern J, Galea S (2006) Social context and depression after a disaster: The role of income inequality. *Journal of Epidemiology and Community Health*. 60(9): 766–70

Akdeniz C, Tost H, Streit F, Haddad L, Wüst S, Schäfer A, Schneider M, Rietschel M, Kirsch P, Meyer-Lindenberg A (2014.) Neuroimaging evidence for a role of neural social stress processing in ethnic minority-associated environmental risk. *Journal of the American Medical Association, Psychiatry* 71(6): 672–80. DOI: 10.1001/jamapsychiatry.2014.35.

Allardyce J, Gilmour H, Atkinson J, Rapson T, Bishop J, McCreadie RG (2005) Social fragmentation, deprivation and urbanicity: Relation to first-admission rates for psychoses. *British Journal of Psychiatry* 187: 401–6

Almedon AM (2005) Social capital and mental health: An interdisciplinary review of primary evidence. *Social Science and Medicine* 61: 943–64

Andrade LH, Wang YP, Andreoni S, Silveira CM, Alexandrino-Silva C, Siu ER, Nishimura R, Anthony JC, Gattaz WF, Kessler RC, Viana MC (2012) Mental disorders in megacities: Findings from the São Paulo megacity mental health survey, Brazil. *Proceedings of the Library of Science One* 7(2): e31879

Araya R, Dunstan F, Playle R, Thomas H, Palmer S, Lewis G (2006) Perceptions of social capital and the built environment and mental health. *Social Science and Medicine* 62(12): 3072–83

Araya R, Lewis G, Rojas G, Fritsch R. (2003) Education or income: Which is more important for mental health? *Journal of Epidemiology and Community Health* 57(7): 501–5

Araya R, Montgomery A, Rojas G, Fritsch R, Solis J, Signorelli A, Lewis G. (2007) Common mental disorders and the built environment in Santiago, Chile. *British Journal of Psychiatry* 190: 394–401

Araya R, Rojas G, Fritsch R, Acuña J, Lewis G (2001) Common mental disorders in Santiago, Chile: Prevalence and socio-demographic correlates. *British Journal of Psychiatry* 178: 228–33

Beach SR, Brody GH, Todorov AA, Gunter TD, Philibert RA (2010) Methylation at *SLC6A4* is linked to family history of child abuse: An examination of the Iowa adoptee sample. *American Journal of Medical Genetics. Part B: Neuropsychiatric Genetics* 153B(2): 710–3

Bener A, Burgut FT, Ghuloum S, Sheikh J (2012) A study of postpartum depression in a fast developing country: Prevalence and related factors. *International Journal of Psychiatry and Medicine* 43(4): 325–37

Bourque F, Van der Ven E, Fusar-Poli P, Malla A (2012) Immigration, social environment and onset of psychotic disorders. *Current Pharmaceutical Design* 18(4): 518–26

Boydell J, Van Os, J, McKenzie K, Allardyce J, Goel R, McCreadie RG, Murray RM (2001) Incidence of schizophrenia in ethnic minorities in London: Ecological study into interactions with environment. *British Medical Journal* 323: 1336–8

Boydell J, Van Os J, McKenzie K, Murray RM (2004) The association of inequality with the incidence of schizophrenia – an ecological study. *Social Psychiatry and Psychiatric Epidemiology* 39: 597–9

Braehler C, Holowka D, Brunet A, Beaulieu S, Baptista T, Debruille JB, Walker CD, King S (2005) Diurnal cortisol in schizophrenia patients with childhood trauma. *Schizophrenia Research* 79: 353–354

Breslau J, Borges G, Saito N, Tancredi DJ, Benjet C, Hinton L, Kendler KS, Kravitz R, Vega W, Aguilar-Gaxiola S, Medina-Mora ME (2011a) Migration from Mexico to the United States and conduct disorder: A cross-national study. *Archives of General Psychiatry* 68(12): 1284–93

Breslau J, Borges G, Tancredi D, Saito N, Kravitz R, Hinton L, Vega W, Medina-Mora ME, Aguilar-Gaxiola S (2011b) Migration from Mexico to the United States and subsequent risk for depressive and anxiety disorders: A cross-national study. *Archives of General Psychiatry* 68(4): 428–33

Bresnahan M, Begg MD, Brown A, Schaefer C, Sohler N, Insel B, Vella L, Susser E (2007) Race and risk of schizophrenia in a US birth cohort: Another example of health disparity? *International Journal of Epidemiology* 36: 751–8

Brown AS (2011) The environment and susceptibility to schizophrenia. *Progress in Neurobiology* 93: 23–58

Burns, JK, Esterhuizen, T (2008) Poverty, inequality and the treated incidence of first-episode psychosis – an ecological study from South Africa. *Social Psychiatry and Psychiatric Epidemiology* 43 (4): 331–5

Burns JK, Tomita MA, Kapadia AS (2014) Income inequality and schizophrenia: Increased schizophrenia incidence in countries with high levels of income inequality. *International Journal of Social Psychiatry* 60(2): 185–19

Caldwell TM, Jorm AF, Dear KB (2004) Suicide and mental health in rural, remote and metropolitan areas in Australia. *Medical Journal of Australia* 181: S10–S4

Cantor-Graae E, Selten JP (2005) Schizophrenia and migration: A meta-analysis and review. *American Journal of Psychiatry* 162: 12–24

Chaix B, Leyland AH, Sabel CE, Chauvin P, Råstam L, Kristersson H, Merlo J (2006) Spatial clustering of mental disorders and associated characteristics of the neighbourhood context in Malmö, Sweden, in 2001. *Journal of Epidemiology and Community Health* 60(5): 427–35

Cirulli F, Francia N, Brachi I, Antonucci M, Aloe L, Suomi SJ, Alleva E (2009) Changes in plasma levels of BDNF and NGF reveal a gender-selective vulnerability to early adversity in rhesus macaques. *Psychoneuroendocrinology* 34: 172–80

Coid J, Yang M, Tyrer P, Roberts A, Ullrich S (2006) Prevalence and correlates of personality disorder in Great Britain. *British Journal of Psychiatry* 188: 423–31

Collins PY, Wig NN, Day R, Varma VK, Malhotra S, Misra AK, Schanzer B, Susser E (1996) Psychosocial and biological aspects of acute brief psychoses in three developing country sites. *Psychiatric Quarterly* 67(3): 177–93

Collip D, Habets P, Marcelis M, Gronenschild E, Lataster T, Lardinois M, Nicolson NA, Myin-Germeys I (2013) Hippocampal volume as a marker of daily life stress sensitivity in psychosis. *Psychological Medicine* 43: 1377–87

Conwell Y, Duberstein PR, Caine ED (2002) Risk factors for suicide in later life. *Biological Psychiatry* 52: 193–204

Costa E, Chen Y, Davis J, Dong E, Noh JS, Tremolizzo L, Veldic M, Grayson DR, Guidotti A (2002) *REELIN* and schizophrenia: a disease at the interface of the genome and the epigenome. *Molecular Interventions* 2(1): 47–57

Das-Munshi J, Leavey G, Stansfield SA, Prince MJ (2012) Migration, social mobility and common mental disorders: Critical review of the literature and meta-analysis. *Ethnicity and Health* 17(1–2): 17–53

Dealberto MJ (2010) Ethnic origin and increased risk for schizophrenia in immigrants to countries of recent and longstanding immigration. *Acta Psychiatrica Scandinavia* 121: 325–39

De Bellis MD, Chrousos GP, Dorn LD, Burke L, Helmers K, Kling MA, Trickett PK, Putnam FW (1994) Hypothalamic-pituitary-adrenal axis dysregulation in sexually abused girls. *Journal of Clinical Endocrinology and Metabolism* 78(2): 249–55

De Menil V, Psei A, Douptcheva N, Hill AG, Yaro P, De-Graft Aikins A (2012) Symptoms of common mental disorders and their correlates among women in Accra, Ghana: A population-based survey. *Ghana Medical Journal* 46(2): 95–103

De Silva MJ, Huttly SR, Harpham T, Kenward MG (2007) Social capital and mental health: A comparative analysis of four low-income countries. *Social Science and Medicine* 64(1): 5–20

De Silva MJ, McKenzie K, Harpham T, Huttly SRA (2005) Social capital and mental illness: A systematic review. *Journal of Epidemiology and Community Health* 59: 619–27

Dohrenwend BP, Levav I, Shrout PE, Schwartz S, Naveh G, Link BG, *et al.* (1992) Socioeconomic status and psychiatric disorders: The causation-selection issue. *Science* 255: 946–52

Durkheim E (1938) *The Rules of Sociological Method*. New York: The Free Press

Durkheim E (1952) *Suicide*. Glencoe, Illinois: The Free Press

Eisenberg L (1977) Psychiatry and society: A sociobiological synthesis. *New England Journal of Medicine* 296: 903–10

Faris R, Dunham H (1939) *Mental Disorders in Urban Areas*. Chicago, Illinois: University of Chicago Press

Fawzi M, Kira I, Fawzi M Jr, Mohamed H, Fawzi M (2013) Trauma profile in Egyptian adolescents with first-episode schizophrenia: Relation to psychopathology and plasma brain-derived neurotrophic factor. *Journal of Nervous and Mental Diseases* 201: 23–9

Foucault M (2001) *Madness and Civilisation*. London: Routledge

Galea S, Ahern J, Rudenstine S, Wallace Z, Vlahov D (2005) Urban built environment and depression: A multilevel analysis. *Journal of Epidemiology and Community Health* 59(10): 822–27

Gallo LC, Matthews KA (2003): Understanding the association between socioeconomic status and physical health: Do negative emotions play a role? *Psychological Bulletin* 129(1): 10–51

Gianaros PJ, Horenstein JA, Cohen S, Matthews KA, Brown SM, Flory JD, Critchley HD, Manuck SB, Hariri AR (2007) Perigenual anterior cingulate morphology covaries with perceived social standing. *Social and Cognitive Affective Neuroscience* 2(3): 161–73. DOI: 10.1093/scan/nsm013

Gianaros PJ, Horenstein JA, Hariri AR, Sheu LK, Manuck SB, Matthews KA, Cohen S (2008) Potential neural embedding of parental social standing. *Social and Cognitive Affective Neuroscience* 3(2): 91–6. DOI: 10.1093/scan/nsn003

Goldberg EM, Morrison SL (1963) Social class and schizophrenia. *British Journal of Psychiatry* 190: 785–802

Gottesman II (1991) *Schizophrenia Genesis: The Origins of Madness*. New York: WH Freeman and Company

Guite HF, Clark C, Ackrill G (2006) The impact of the physical and urban environment on mental well-being. *Public Health* 120(12): 1117–26

Hammarström A, Phillips SP (2012) Gender inequity needs to be regarded as a social determinant of depressive symptoms: Results from the Northern Swedish cohort. *Scandinavian Journal of Public Health* 40(8): 746–52

Harpham T, Grant E, Thomas E (2002) Measuring social capital within health surveys: Key issues. *Health Policy and Planning* 17(1): 106–11

Heijmans BT, Tobi EW, Stein AD, Putter H, Blauw GJ, Susser ES, Slagboom PE, Lumey LH (2008) Persistent epigenetic differences associated with prenatal exposure to famine in humans. *Proceedings of the National Academy of Sciences USA* 105(44): 17046–49

Hembree C, Galea S, Ahern J, Tracy M, Markham Piper T, Miller J, Vlahov D, Tardiff KJ (2005) The urban built environment and overdose mortality in New York City neighborhoods. *Health and Place* 11(2): 147–56

Henderson S, Whiteford H (2003) Social capital and mental health. *The Lancet* 362: 505–6

Hoek HW, Brown AS, Susser E (1998) The Dutch famine and schizophrenia spectrum disorders. *Social Psychiatry and Psychiatric Epidemiology* 33(8): 373–9

Hoy K, Barrett S, Shannon C, Campbell C, Watson D, Rushe T, Shevlin M, Bai F, Cooper S, Mulholland C (2012) Childhood trauma and hippocampal and amygdalar volumes in first-episode psychosis. *Schizophrenia Bulletin* 38: 1162–9

Human Sciences Research Council (2004) *Fact Sheet: Poverty in South Africa*. http://www.sarpn.org/documents/d0000990/ (Accessed on 19 March 2013)

Illanes E, Bustos L, Vizcarra MB, Muñoz S (2007) Social and familial determinants of anxiety and depressive symptoms in middle to low income women. *Revista Médica de Chile* 135(3) 326–234

Kawachi I, Subramanian SV, Almeida-Filho N (2002) A glossary of health inequalities. *Journal of Epidemiology and Community Health* 56: 647–52

Khamis V. (2008) Post-traumatic stress and psychiatric disorders in Palestinian adolescents following intifada-related injuries. *Social Science and Medicine* 67(8): 1199–207

Kirkbride JB, Morgan C, Fearon P, Dazzan P, Murray RM, Jones PB (2007) Neighbourhood-level effects on psychoses: re-examining the role of context. *Psychological Medicine* 37: 1413–25

Kuepper R, Van Os J, Lieb R, Wittchen HU, Henquet C (2011) Do cannabis and urbanicity co-participate in causing psychosis? Evidence from a 10-year follow-up cohort study. *Psychological Medicine* 41(10): 2121–129

Kunugi H, Hori H, Adachi N, Numakawa T (2010) Interface between hypothalamic–pituitary–adrenal axis and brain-derived neurotrophic factor in depression. *Psychiatry and Clinical Neurosciences* 64: 447–59

Laing RD, Esterson D (1964) *Sanity, Madness and the Family*. New York: Basic Books

Laruelle M (2000) The role of endogenous sensitization in the pathophysiology of schizophrenia: Implications from recent brain imaging studies. *Brain Research and Brain Research Reviews* 31(2–3): 371–84

Lederbogen F, Kirsch P, Haddad L, Streit F, Tost H, Schuch P, Wüst S, Preussner JC, Rietschel M, Deuschle M, Meyer-Lindenberg A (2011) City living and urban upbringing affect neural social stress processing in humans. *Nature* 474(7352): 498–501

Lehtinen V, Michalak E, Wilkinson C, Dowrick C, Ayuso-Mateos JL, Dalgard OD, Casey P, Vázquez-Barquero JL, Wilkinson G, ODIN Group (2003) Urban-rural differences in the occurrence of female depressive disorder in Europe. *Social Psychiatry and Psychiatric Epidemiology* 38: 283–89

Leibbrandt M, Woolard I, Finn A, Argent J (2010) Trends in South African income distribution and poverty since the fall of apartheid. *OECD Social, Employment and Migration Working Papers* No. 101, OECD Publishing http://oberon.sourceoecd.org/vl=1072615/cl=23/nw=1/rpsv/cgi- bin/wppdf?file=5kmms0t7p1ms.pdf (Accessed on 22 March 2013)

Levin KA, Leyland AH (2005) Urban/rural inequalities in suicide in Scotland, 1981-1999. *Social Science and Medicine* 60: 2877–90

Lewis G, David A, Andreasson S, Allebeck P (1992) Schizophrenia and city life. *The Lancet* 340: 137–40

Liang Y, Gong YH, Wen XP, Guan CP, Li MC, Yin P, Wang ZQ (2012) Social determinants of health and depression: A preliminary investigation from rural China. *Proceedings of the Library of Science One* 7(1): e30553

Lofors J, Sundquist K (2007) Low-linking social capital as a predictor of mental disorders: A cohort study of 4.5 million Swedes. *Social Science and Medicine* 64: 21–34

Lundberg P, Cantor-Graae E, Rukundo G, Ashaba S, Ostergren PO (2009) Urbanicity of place of birth and symptoms of psychosis, depression and anxiety in Uganda. *British Journal of Psychiatry* 195(2): 156–62

Manning C, Gregoire A (2008) Effects of parental mental illness on children. *Psychiatry* 8(1): 7–9

Mao ZH, Zhao XD (2012) The effects of social connections and self-rated physical and mental health among internal migrant and local adolescents in Shanghai, China. *BMC Public Health* 12: 97

Marcelis M, Takei N, Van Os J (1999) Urbanization and risk for schizophrenia: does the effect operate before or around the time of illness onset? *Psychological Medicine* 29: 1197–203

March D, Hatch SL, Morgan C, Kirkbride JB, Bresnahan M, Fearon P, Susser E (2008a) Psychosis and place. *Epidemiological Reviews* 30: 84–100

March D, Morgan C, Bresnahan M. (2008b) Conceptualising the social world. In: Morgan C, McKenzie K, Fearon P (Eds) *Society and Psychosis*. Cambridge, UK: Cambridge University Press

Marín-León L, Oliveira HB, Barros MB, Dalgalarrondo P, Botega NJ (2007) Social inequality and common mental disorders. *Revista Brasileira de Psiquiatria* 29(3): 250–3

Marmot M (2005) Social determinants of health inequalities. *Lancet* 365: 1099–104

Mayer L, Lopez-Duran NL, Kovaks M, George CJ, Baji I, Kapornai K, Kiss E, Vetró A (2009) Stressful life events in a clinical sample of depressed children in Hungary. *Journal of Affective Disorders* 115(1–2): 207–14

McGrath J, Saha S, Welham J, El Saadi O, MacCauley C, Chant D (2004) A systematic review of the incidence of schizophrenia: The distribution of rates and the influence of sex, urbanicity, migrant status and methodology. *BMC Medicine* 2(13): 1–22

McKenzie K, Harpham T (Eds) (2006) *Social Capital and Mental Health*. London: Jessica Kingsley

McLaughlin KA, Greif Green J, Gruber MJ, Sampson NA, Zaslavsky AM, Kessler RC (2012) Childhood adversities and first onset of psychiatric disorders in a national sample of US adolescents. *Archives of General Psychiatry* 69(11): 1151–160

Melchior M, Chastang JF, de Lauzon B, Galéra C, Saurel-Cubizolles MJ, Larroque B; EDEN Mother-Child Cohort Study Group (2012) Maternal depression, socioeconomic position, and temperament in childhood: the EDEN Mother-Child Cohort. *Journal of Affective Disorders* 137(1–3): 165–9

Messias E, Eaton WW, Grooms AN (2011) Economic grand rounds: income inequality and depression prevalence across the United States: An ecological study. *Psychiatric Services* 62(7): 710–2

Mondelli V, Pariante C, Navari S, Aas M, D'Albenzio A, Di Forti M, Handley R, Hepgul N, Marques TR, Taylor H, Papadopoulos AS, Aitchison KJ, Murray RM, Dazzan P (2010) Higher cortisol levels are associated with smaller left hippocampal volume in first-episode psychosis. *Schizophrenia Research* 119: 75–8

Morgan C, Kleinman A (2010) Social science perspectives: A failure of the sociological imagination. In: Morgan C and Bhugra D (Eds) *Principles of Social Psychiatry*, 2nd Ed. Chichester, UK: Wiley-Blackwell

Mortensen PB, Pedersen CB, Westergaard T, Wohlfahrt J, Ewald H, Mors O, Andersen PK, Melbye M (1999) Effects of family history and place and season of birth on the risk of schizophrenia. *New England Journal of Medicine* 340: 603–8

Myer L, Stein DJ, Grimsrud A, Seedat S, Williams DR (2008) Social determinants of psychological distress in a nationally-representative sample of South African adults. *Social Science and Medicine* 66: 1828–40

Myin-Germeys I, Delespaul P, Van Os J (2005) Behavioural sensitization to daily life stress in psychosis. *Psychological Medicine* 35(5): 733–41

Myin-Germeys I, Van Os J, Schwartz JE, Stone AA, Delespaul PA (2001) Emotional reactivity to daily life stress in psychosis. *Archives of General Psychiatry* 58(12): 1137–44

Oberlander TF, Weinberg J, Papsdorf M, Grunau R, Misri S, Devlin AM (2008) Prenatal exposure to maternal depression, neonatal methylation of human glucocorticoid receptor gene (*NR3C1*) and infant cortisol stress responses. *Epigenetics* 3(2): 97–106

Ornelas IJ, Perreira KM (2011) The role of migration in the development of depressive symptoms among Latino immigrant parents in the USA. *Social Science and Medicine* 73(8): 1169–77

Patel V, Kirkwood BR, Pednekar S, Weiss H, Mabey D (2006) Risk factors for common mental disorders in women. Population-based longitudinal study. *British Journal of Psychiatry* 189: 547–55

Paykel ES, Abbott R, Jenkins R, Brugha TS, Meltzer H. (2000) Urban-rural mental health differences in great Britain: Findings from the national morbidity survey. *Psychological Medicine* 30(2): 269–80

Pedersen CB, Demontis D, Pedersen MS, Agerbo E, Mortensen PB, Børglum AD, Hougaard DM, Hollegaard MV, Mors O, Cantor-Graae E. (2012) Risk of schizophrenia in relation to parental origin and genome-wide divergence. *Psychological Medicine* 42(7): 1515–21

Pedersen CB, Mortensen PB (2001) Evidence of a dose-response relationship between urbanicity during upbringing and schizophrenia risk. *Archives of General Psychiatry* 58: 1039–46

Philibert RA, Sandhu H, Hollenbeck N, Gunter T, Adams W, Madan A (2008) The relationship of *5HTT* (*SLC6A4*) methylation and genotype on mRNA expression and liability to major depression and alcohol dependence in subjects from the Iowa Adoption Studies. American Journal of Medical Genetics. Part B: *Neuropsychiatric Genetics* 147B(5): 543–49

Pickett KE, Wilkinson RG (2010) Inequality: An underacknowledged source of mental illness and distress. *British Journal of Psychiatry* 197(6): 426–28

Poulton R, Caspi A, Milne BJ, Thomson WM, Taylor A, Sears MR, Moffitt TE (2002) Association between children's experience of socioeconomic disadvantage and adult health: A life-course study. *Lancet* 360: 1640–5

Putnam R (1993) *Making Democracy Work: Civic Traditions in Modern Italy*. Princeton, NJ: Princeton University Press

Read J, Perry B, Moskowitz A, Connolly J (2001) The contribution of early traumatic events to schizophrenia in some patients: A traumagenic neurodevelopmental model. *Psychiatry* 64: 319–45

Roberts ET, Friedman SR, Brady JE, Pouget ER, Tempalski B, Galea S (2010) Environmental conditions, political economy, and rates of injection drug use in large US metropolitan areas 1992–2002. *Drug and Alcohol Dependence* 106(2–3): 142–53

Rost K, Zhang ML, Fortney J, Smith J, Smith GR (1998) Rural-urban differences in depression treatment and suicidality. *Medical Care* 36: 1098–107

Saha S, Welham J, Chant D, McGrath J (2006) Incidence of schizophrenia does not vary with economic status of the country: Evidence from a systematic review. *Social Psychiatry and Psychiatric Epidemiology* 41: 338–40

Sapolsky RM (2004) Social status and health in humans and other animals. *Annual Review of Anthropology* 33: 393–418

Shannon C, Schwandt ML, Champoux M, Shoaf SE, Suomi SJ, Linnoila M, Higley JD (2005) Maternal absence and stability of individual differences in CSF 5-HIAA concentrations in rhesus monkey infants. *American Journal of Psychiatry* 162: 1658–64

Shaw RJ, Atkin K, Bécares L, Albor CB, Stafford M, Kiernan KE, Nazroo JY, Wilkinson RG, Pickett KE (2012) Impact of ethnic density on adult mental disorders: A narrative review. *British Journal of Psychiatry* 201(1): 11–9

Shepherd CC, Li J, Mitrou F, Zubrick SR (2012) Socioeconomic disparities in the mental health of indigenous children in Western Australia. *BMC Public Health* 12: 756

Singh GK, Siahpush M (2002) Increasing rural-urban gradients in US suicide mortality, 1970–97. *American Journal of Public Health* 92: 1161–7

Smith A, Conneely KN, Kilaru V, Mercer KB, Weiss TE, Bradley B, Tang Y, Gillespie CF, Cubells JF, Ressler KJ (2011) Differential immune system DNA methylation and cytokine regulation in post-traumatic stress disorder. *American Journal of Medical Genetics. Part B: Neuropsychiatric Genetics* 156B(6): 700–8

Spauwen J, Krabbendam L, Lieb R, Wittchen HU, Van Os J (2006) Impact of psychological trauma on the development of psychotic symptoms: Relationship with psychosis proneness. *British Journal of Psychiatry* 188: 527–33

Stafford M, De Silva M, Stansfield S, Marmot M (2008) Neighbourhood social capital and common mental disorder: Testing the link in a general population sample. *Health and Place* 14(3): 394–405

Stansfield S, Weich S, Clark C, Boydell J, Freeman H (2008) Urban-rural differences, socio-economic status and psychiatric disorder. In: Freeman H and Stansfield S (Eds) *The Impact of the Environment on Psychiatric Disorder*. East Sussex, UK: Routledge

Stansfeld SA, Shipley MJ, Head J, Fuhrer R (2012) Repeated job strain and the risk of depression: longitudinal analyses from the Whitehall II study. *American Journal of Public Health* 102(12): 2360–6

St Clair D, Xu M, Wang P, Yu Y, Fang Y, Zhang F, Zheng X, Gu N, Feng G, Sham P, He L (2005) Rates of adult schizophrenia following prenatal exposure to the Chinese famine of 1959–1961. *Journal of the American Medical Association* 294(5): 557–62

Subramanian SV, Kawachi I (2004) Income inequality and health: What have we learned so far? *Epidemiological Reviews* 26: 78–91

Sugiyama T, Leslie E, Giles-Corti B, Owen N (2008) Associations of neighbourhood greenness with physical and mental health: Do walking, social coherence and local social interaction explain the relationships? *Journal of Epidemiology and Community Health* 62(5): e9

Sundquist K, Frank G, Sundquist J (2004) Urbanisation and incidence of psychosis and depression: Follow-up study of 4.4 million women and men in Sweden. *British Journal of Psychiatry* 184: 293–8

Susser E, Neugebauer R, Hoek HW, Brown AS, Lin S, Labovitz D, Gorman JM (1996) Schizophrenia after prenatal famine. Further evidence. *Archives of General Psychiatry* 53(1): 25–31

Swanson SA, Saito N, Borges G, Benjet C, Aguilar-Gaxiola S, Medina-Mora ME, Breslau J (2012) Change in binge eating and binge eating disorder associated with migration from Mexico to the US. *Journal of Psychiatric Research* 46(1): 31–7

Szasz T (1961) *The Myth of Mental Illness: Foundations of a Theory of Personal Conduct*. New York: Harper and Row

Teicher M, Anderson C, Polcari A (2012) Childhood maltreatment is associated with reduced volume in the hippocampal subfields CA3, dentate gyrus, and subiculum. *Proceedings of the National Academy of Science* 109: e563–e572

Tissir F, Gossinet AM (2003) *Reelin* and brain development. *Nature Reviews Neuroscience* 4(6): 496–505

Tomita A, Burns JK (2013) A multilevel analysis of association between neighborhood social capital and depression: Evidence from the first South African National Income Dynamics Study. *Journal of Affective Disorders* 144(1–2): 101–5. DOI: 10.1016/j.jad.2012.05.066

Toyokawa S, Uddin M, Koenen KC, Galea S (2012) How does the social environment 'get into the mind'? Epigenetics at the intersection of social and psychiatric epidemiology. *Social Science and Medicine* 74: 67–74

Tsankova N, Renthal W, Kumar A, Nestler EJ (2007) Epigenetic regulation in psychiatric disorders. *Nature Reviews Neuroscience* 8(5): 355–67

Uddin M, Aiello AE, Wildman DE, Koenen KC, Pawelec G, de Los Santos R, Goldmann E, Galea S (2010) Epigenetic and immune function profiles associated with post-traumatic stress disorder. *Proceedings of the National Academy of Sciences USA* 107(20): 9470–5

Van der Linden J, Drukker M, Gunther N, Feron F, van Os J. (2003) Children's mental health service use, neighbourhood socioeconomic deprivation, and social capital. *Social Psychiatry and Psychiatric Epidemiology* 38(9):507-14

Van Os J, Hanssen M, Bijl RV, Vollebergh W (2001) Prevalence of psychotic disorder and community level of psychotic symptoms – an urban-rural comparison. *Archives of General Psychiatry* 58: 663–8

Van Winkel R, Stefanis NC, Myin-Germeys I (2008) Psychosocial stress and psychosis. A review of the neurobiological mechanisms and the evidence for gene-stress interaction. *Schizophrenia Bulletin* 34(6): 1095–105

Varese F, Smeets F, Drukker M, Lieverse R, Lataster T, Viechtbauer W, Read J, van Os J, Bentall RP (2012) Childhood adversities increase the risk of psychosis: A meta-analysis of patient-control, prospective- and cross-sectional cohort studies. *Schizophrenia Bulletin* 38(4): 661–71

Veling W, Hoek HW, Selten JP, Susser E (2011) Age at migration and future risk of psychotic disorders among immigrants in the Netherlands: A 7-year incidence study. *American Journal of Psychiatry* 168(12): 1278–85

Veling W, Selten JP, Susser E, Laan W, Mackenbach JP, Hoek HW (2007) Discrimination and the incidence of psychotic disorders among ethnic minorities in the Netherlands. *International Journal of Epidemiology* 36: 761–8

Veling W, Selten JP, Veen N, Laan W, Blom JD, Hoek HW (2006) Incidence of schizophrenia among ethnic minorities in the Netherlands: A four-year first-contact study. *Schizophrenia Research* 86(1–3): 189–93

Veling W, Susser E, Van Os J, Mackenbach JP, Selten JP, Hoek HW (2008) Ethnic density of neighborhoods and incidence of psychotic disorders among immigrants. *American Journal of Psychiatry* 165: 66–73

Waddington C (1940) *Organisers and Genes*. Cambridge: Cambridge University Press

Wainwright NW, Surtees PG (2004) Area and individual circumstances and mood disorder prevalence. *British Journal of Psychiatry* 185: 227–32

Walker E, Mittal V, Tessner K (2008) Stress and the hypothalamic pituitary adrenal axis in the developmental course of schizophrenia. *Annual Review of Clinical Psychology* 4: 189–216

Weich S, Holt G, Twigg L, Jones K, Lewis G (2003) Geographic variation in the prevalence of common mental disorders in Britain: A multilevel investigation. *American Journal of Epidemiology* 157: 730–7

Weich S, Lewis G (1998) Material standard of living, social class, and the prevalence of the common mental disorders in Great Britain. *Journal of Epidemiology and Community Health* 52: 8–14

Weich S, Lewis G, Jenkins SP (2001) Income inequality and the prevalence of common mental disorders in Britain. *British Journal of Psychiatry* 178: 222–7

Weich S, Twigg L, Lewis G (2006) Rural/non-rural differences in rates of common mental disorders in Britain: prospective multilevel cohort study. *British Journal of Psychiatry* 188: 51–7

Whitely R, McKenzie MD (2005) Social capital and psychiatry: Review of the literature. *Harvard Review of Psychiatry* 13(2): 71–84

Wicks S, Hjern A, Dalman C (2010) Social risk or genetic liability for psychosis? A study of children born in Sweden and reared by adoptive parents. *American Journal of Psychiatry* 167(10): 1240–6

Wilkinson RG (1992) Income distribution and life expectancy. *British Medical Journal* 304: 165–8

Wilkinson RG (1996) *Unhealthy Societies: The Afflictions of Inequality*. London: Routledge

World Health Organization (2013) *Social Determinants of Health*. http://www.who.int/social_determinants/en/ (Accessed on 7 March 2013.)

Yip PSF, Liu KY (2006) The ecological fallacy and the gender ratio of suicide in China. *British Journal of Psychiatry* 189: 465–6

Zink CF, Tong Y, Chen Q, Bassett DS, Stein JL, Meyer-Lindenberg A (2008) Know your place: Neural processing of social hierarchy in humans. *Neuron* 58(2): 273–83. DOI: 10.1016/j.neuron.2008.01.025

CHAPTER

# 6 Culture and psychiatry

*Elizabeth Weiss, Thebe Madigoe*

## 6.1 Introduction

The interaction of culture and psychiatry deals with the phenomenology and the management of symptoms and behaviour as conceptualised by a population group of which the client is a member by birth, affiliation or choice. It recognises the impact of a person's cultural background on the expression of symptoms, and the person's understanding of the cause of the symptoms.

In the past fifty years the attitude and language around culture in psychiatry have been dramatically revised, abandoning **stereotypes** such as primitive and native, and doing away 'with this notion many authors believed, that insanity tends to become more prevalent as civilization evolves' (Raimundo Oda *et al.*, 2005). However, progress in incorporating culture into mainstream psychiatric teaching has been slow.

In the wake of a rapidly changing world with accelerated movements of people of many different cultural backgrounds into unfamiliar environments, mental health aspects across cultures and continents have been treated more seriously and realistically. This change has been aided by psychiatrists from a multitude of cultural backgrounds sharing their expertise and producing research. This has stimulated the continuing discussions and controversies about a range of manifestations and symptoms that are defined by cultural variations.

The importance of culture in psychiatry was recognised in the DSM-IV which introduced a section on culture-bound syndromes and guidelines towards a cultural formulation. There was significant discussion, consultation and controversy about cultural aspects of diagnostic criteria in the DSM-5. The outcome was that the DSM-5 has aimed for a greater cultural sensitivity by updating criteria to reflect cross-cultural variations in presentations, giving more detailed and structured information about cultural concepts of distress and including a clinical interview tool to facilitate comprehensive, person-centred assessments.

The World Psychiatric Association (WPA) has recognised the importance of culture in psychiatry by creating a Transcultural Psychiatry Section, supporting and enabling exchange of information by specialists in this field.

## 6.2 What is cultural psychiatry?

The word culture is used in many different ways in the 21st century: it is applied to minorities, religious sects or cults, music genres, the business world and to lifestyle orientations, often also called 'subcultures'.

Cultural psychiatry includes cultural variations as they emerge over time in a population group. Subcultures deserve the same attention when clinicians engage with any patient to formulate diagnosis, treatment and management.

As the world has become a melting pot of cultures, as new ideas have been disseminated, and as electronic media have penetrated even remote areas, an acceleration has taken place forcing people to shift mind sets, beliefs and practices rapidly and continuously. Immigration and emigration, by choice or through **displacement**, for economic or political reasons, within a continent, a country or even a village, destabilise cultural mind sets and require adaptation to new environments, values and ways of life.

## 6.3 Definition of culture

It is necessary to understand the complexities of culture before engaging in an analysis of the impact of culture on mental health or mental illness.

In the absence of a single definition of culture, various authors have attempted to cover the concept as comprehensively as possible.

- 'The word culture refers to the sum total of the learned behaviour of a group of people that is generally considered to be the tradition of that people and is transmitted from generation to generation' (Hofstede, 1997)
- 'Culture is a set of behavioral norms, meanings, and values or reference points utilized by members of a particular society to construct their unique view of the world, and ascertain their identity' (Group for the Advancement of Psychiatry, Committee on Cultural Psychiatry, 2001)
- 'Culture is manifested in the core of behaviour and in the various ways in which life is regulated, such as rituals, customs, etiquette, taboos, and laws. It is reflected in such things as common sayings, legends, drama, art, philosophical thought, and religions' (Tseng, 2001)
- 'Culture shapes people's behaviour, but at the same time it is moulded by the ideas and behaviour of the members of the culture. Thus, culture and people influence each other reciprocally and interactionally' (Tseng, 2001)

These definitions provide a framework for understanding the concepts of culture and create a platform from where to embrace similarities and differences in humankind and enjoy the challenge of making sense of it all.

## 6.4 Application of culture in mental health

Culture is ubiquitous and not a concept defining the difference between the West and the rest of the world. There is no homogeneous European, American or other culture. There are few –if any – unadulterated cultures anywhere in the world.

The concept of culture is present in every encounter between a health professional and a client, and even more so when mental health is at stake. Such encounters are consciously and unconsciously defined by similarities and differences between the two parties concerned and must lead to a situation where both world views meet and where exchanges that are accessible to both parties can take place. This means it is necessary to take cognizance of the culture of the physician and the client, the medical culture that dictates the actions of the physician or psychiatrist, and the culture of the environment where the interaction takes place.

Cultural sensitivity is a necessary attribute in the physician and his or her team, since it is hardly possible to be familiar with every culture or belief system in the world. Cultural sensitivity could relate to:

- **confidentiality** when making use of an interpreter
- an awareness of gender issues in certain cultures
- religious considerations
- respect for certain ritual obligations.

Western attire, education and degrees do not necessarily indicate that traditional or cultural practices have been replaced.

Cultural sensitivity includes efforts to learn and gain an appreciation of the communication styles of the population being served. Getting to the point quickly might not be possible with an elderly grandmother from a rural area who is giving collateral information about her mentally ill grandson.

### 6.4.1 Culture is not a static concept

Culture change has been present since time immemorial, mostly slow and pedantic, but has accelerated as information and knowledge have become available through access to the media and better education. Since people move at a different pace, clusters or groups have emerged, choosing different directions. The old and the new (and versions between the two) are co-existing, creating greater insight or greater confusion.

It is the task of the interviewer to establish the client's beliefs and cultural and/or religious reality.

In most societies, including African ones, there has been a growth in cultural and religious syncretism, which refers to the integration of previously disparate belief systems in an individual, a family or a group. Families are often divided around belief systems, which results in conflict. Clinical assessment and management will therefore have to prioritise the needs of the individual patient, while taking into account his or her family or group affiliation.

## 6.4.2 Cultural change and cultural disintegration

A clash of cultures can ultimately lead to conflict. This may apply to migrant groups, religious groups with strict codes of conduct and isolated groups. Some cultures defend and maintain their boundaries longer than others, but in mixed societies, as is the case in most parts of the world, boundaries have become blurred. One such an example is arranged marriages, which have become a source of conflict for many young people in certain communities. Reports still emerge in the media of forced abduction of young girls for marriage, as happened in KwaZulu-Natal in 2012 (News 24, 2012). In 2011, legislation was passed in Germany to outlaw forced marriages, which mostly affected Muslim girls from immigrant families (www.spiegel.de/international/germany, 2011). These influences are powerful stressors, since older generations do not accept the rapidly changing cultural parameters and still hold on to traditional patterns.

Social and cultural disintegration have been a phenomenon through time and history. This is vividly experienced in South Africa, with the breakdown of the extended family system due to various factors. The migrant labour system still plays a large part in this, since there are limited employment opportunities in rural areas. As in many parts of the world, urbanisation has contributed to a redefinition of the family. Many children grow up with grandparents, an absent father figure, or do not know their fathers at all. Marriage must be contextually defined during interviews, due to the various configurations of families. HIV/Aids has accelerated the breakdown of family structures.

These factors all interfere with the execution of customary traditions, ancestral rituals or culturally prescribed milestones, such as initiation rites, lobola negotiations and more.

## 6.4.3 Culture and technology

Electronic media have penetrated even the remotest areas, making information rapidly accessible and shaping the perceptions and reactions of communities previously deprived of such communication. In South Africa, for example, it can be assumed that nowadays almost everybody has a cellphone. This has become a fixture in people's lives, from the very old to the very young; even illiteracy finds its way past the complexities of the cellphone. Being able to communicate has an impact on peoples' lives, creates better links with family over distance, improves security for people living in remote areas, and also brings with it new needs. Resources must be diverted to pay for this new acquisition (and new lifestyle) and this has its own challenges.

The technological advancements referred to above also influence the symptomatic content of psychopathology. It thus becomes increasingly common for a psychotic patient to experience **delusions** of microchips having been implanted in the brain, or that a cellphone is being used to monitor the person's movements. In South Africa, television has become available to many people. Programmes have influenced positive and negative behaviour, and have found their way into the content of hallucinations and delusions of psychotic patients.

Sexually explicit TV programmes and DVDs have become easily accessible, as has the access to sexually explicit images on cellphones and computers. This has in some instances affected young or intellectually disabled persons, who have presented with sexually inappropriate behaviour and may be referred for forensic psychiatric observation.

## 6.5 Healers and mental health

Every culture has its healers, and it is useful to keep in mind that many African patients, before seeking help from the mental health services, will have consulted and sometimes even exhausted traditional treatment, faith healing, and performed rituals considered necessary for recovery. In some instances traditional healers bring patients to medical health services or churches refuse further treatment for some patients when they can no longer cope with their behaviour. Whereas the cause of the illness might still be explained by the family and the patient in cultural terms, improving the patient's condition by medical means may serve to stabilise the condition and the situation for the family and community.

Some people have proposed that traditional healers be integrated into national health care systems. Others have raised concerns, citing reservations with regards to norms, standards and empirical evidence in traditional health systems. It has been noted that traditional healers are often able to address existential questions (e.g. Why me?) whereas Western medicine typically cannot. The culturally sensitive mental health professional should acknowledge and respect the choice of patients to receive traditional or faith healing when desired. However, releasing a dangerous psychiatric patient to fulfil ritual obligations in the name of culture sensitivity, for example, would be professionally and ethically irresponsible. In such an instance, it would be more appropriate to negotiate the timing of the traditional consultation, within the context of mental health legislation, in a way that minimises clinical risk.

## 6.6 The South African context

### 6.6.1 South Africa is a truly multicultural society

The political past, which emphasised segregation to the extreme, did not allow for a natural progression of cultures meeting and **acculturation** processes taking place. Most research has been done in the black population, which is in itself not cohesive, with vast differences in cultural perceptions and ritual expressions.

Stereotypes and **prejudice** abound and, unless the individual cultural background of that patient is defined, can easily find their way into assessments of patients.

Spirituality and religion play a major part in most peoples' lives in South Africa, with great variations in rules, regulations, taboos and expression. Considering the great variety of migrant workers from neighbouring countries, political and economic refugees, and other transient or permanent immigrants seeking a life in South Africa from all over the world, cultural sensitivity is a must.

## 6.7 Culture in the sector of general medicine

Whereas a violent psychotic patient eventually finds his or her way to the psychiatrist, most 'soft psychiatry' patients end up in outpatient departments of general hospitals and primary health care clinics, and are seldom referred for a specialist psychiatric assessment. Soft psychiatry patients include people with stress-related conditions, anxiety, depression, adjustment disorders and somatoform disorders.

Health professionals must be familiar with how the client expresses symptoms that do not immediately indicate severe physical or mental illness. Somatic complaints are universal, and in both Western and non-Western cultures anxiety and depression are not easily expressed by sufferers or recognised by practitioners.

The following general complaints should arouse suspicion:

- sleep difficulties
- palpitations
- pains moving all over the body
- headaches
- backache, waist pain and lower abdominal pains
- tingling sensation in the brain
- burning sensation on the scalp
- other complaints that have no palpable explanation.

Most are expressed in specific ways, and the exact meaning must be explored with an interpreter.

## 6.8 Examination of mental state across cultures

### 6.8.1 Interpersonal contact

The clinician must be sensitive to differences in acceptable expressions of non-verbal communication, including eye contact, hand shaking, and the relative importance of personal space, tone of voice, etc.

### 6.8.2 Appearance

Much is given away by appearance across cultures. Starting with tattoos, which can have a meaning (like gang tattoos and prison tattoos), or be decorative, indicating association with a specific ethnic group. Scarification, either as decoration or as an indication of traditional healing, is an important observation. Prophets and traditional healers are often recognisable due to their colourful clothing or ornaments around the wrists, ankles and necks. In some cultures beads or leather bracelets are often worn on the wrist after a ritual – usually relating to ancestors – has been performed. Among the amaXhosa, persons undergoing ***ukuthwasa*** (training to become a traditional healer) typically wear white beads in their ears, on the head, wrists and ankles.

Any unusual attire or adornment in any culture or religion is worth exploring. Rastafarians may be recognisable by their long braided hair and ornamental colours of red, yellow and green. Goths will be noticeable by their dark, often torn clothes, with leather and other accessories. Muslim and Jewish headgear and dress must be explored as to the specific significance in culture and religion for the individual.

### 6.8.3 Interpreter pitfalls

Cross-cultural communication frequently requires the navigation of a language barrier. Given the multi-lingual setting, the clinician is often unable to understand or speak the patient's language, thus needing the help of interpreters. This is fraught with many potential pitfalls.

Most health facilities in South Africa do not have trained interpreters. As a result, reliance is often placed on any health worker (such as a nurse, a health sciences student, a general assistant or a security officer), or even a relative or friend accompanying the patient. Such a person may not be adequately proficient in the examiner's language or the medical jargon being used.

The ethical aspects of such a consultation could be compromised if the patient cannot give informed **consent** to the presence of a non-professional person. This must be explored prior to the interview with the patient and the family. When delicate topics are broached, the patient must be comfortable with the topic, the context and the presence of other persons in the room. If necessary, discussing some issues could be postponed until a satisfactory environment has been created to deal with them.

Untrained interpreters often misunderstand their role. For example, the interviewer asks a question, the interpreter engages in a lengthy conversation with the client, then conveys the answers as a 'yes' or 'no', without elaborating on the details of the conversation. It some cases the person interpreting starts his or her own line of questioning – and sometimes even provides counselling – without giving details to the interviewer.

Language has its own pitfalls: the same word can have many meanings. For example, when asking a patient about visual hallucinations, the interviewer must be aware that the word for 'vision' and 'dream' could be the same when translated, requiring clarification through follow-up questions.

Another source of confusion is the use of gender-neutral personal pronouns as is the case with many African languages. As a result, there may not be a clear differentiation between 'he' and 'she', requiring alertness during any verbal or written communication.

The clinician should also consider how an untrained interpreter may be emotionally adversely affected and even traumatised by the clinical material he or she is exposed to during patient interviews.

## 6.8.4 The role of the clinician's cultural beliefs

The clinician should be aware of his or her own belief system and ensure that this does not adversely affect the assessment and management of patients. The cultural and religious beliefs of mental health workers may arouse strong emotions during clinical encounters, which may in turn undermine accuracy in diagnostic assessment.

The following case studies serve as illustrations:

Culture-related experiences such as those described above can be traumatic and therefore associated with overwhelming emotions by both clinicians and patients. Such emotions can be effectively managed by exploring the beliefs of the community, showing respect for both those who believe and those who don't, and adopting a collaborative approach by which the clinical team, the patient and the patient's family effectively address the patient's condition.

## 6.8.5 Delusion vs. belief

Pathological beliefs can be classified as delusions and as **overvalued ideas**. A delusion is commonly defined as a fixed, false belief not in

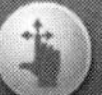

### Case study 6.1

A 15-year-old girl, who proclaimed herself a witch, was brought to a psychiatric unit by the police, who did not know what to do with her. Her mother was intellectually disabled and could not look after her. Her relatives had removed her from a semi-urban environment to a deeply rural one, using her for chores and child care. She had not yet reached puberty and had the physical appearance of a nine-year-old child. A school principal in her rural area had been forced to leave the community, and several houses had been burnt down following her admission that she was a witch and her naming fellow witches. She presented a detailed account of her activities, elicited and written down by a social worker. The content of this account was described in gruesome detail. Her presentation created a three-way split in the unit among those adhering to traditional belief systems, Christians, and a non-African team member who pointed out what could be regarded as impossibilities and discrepancies in the girl's account. The other patients did not appear at all perturbed by her presentation and she fitted in easily. She only became distressed when she was challenged about her story. However, it took the laborious process of allowing the members of the team to overcome their own anxieties and to analyse her account and compare it with what they knew and believed about witchcraft, and then to acknowledge that her account was not in keeping with cultural beliefs. Her presentation was interpreted as her way to seek an escape from her difficult and unfamiliar living conditions. An assessment of ***Pseudologia phantastica*** was made, and the girl was released into the care of her uncle and aunt in an urban environment. Having grown up in a semi-urban area, she felt out of place in the rural community: returning to a more urbanised setting was her primary goal when concocting her presentation. She also felt exploited by her rural relatives who used her as a domestic servant.

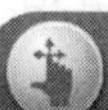

### Case study 6.2

A student who had grown up in a rural community became very excited and felt traumatised when she became involved in a situation where the community had identified a woman who was keeping zombies. There also were reports of things flying around in the woman's house. The student photographed the zombie – a very emaciated naked woman – as she was loaded into a police van. The student's friends quickly became as emotionally excited as she was. They had never believed that such things existed, but now had sleepless nights. After a detailed analysis of what zombies are within their belief system, calm returned. The student was asked to follow up the incident and learnt that the zombie was actually a mentally ill person.

keeping with a person's culture or religion. In the overvalued idea, a false belief is held but with less intensity and can be shifted. Given that no practitioner will be familiar with all the belief systems that his or her various patients subscribe to, it can at times be very difficult to distinguish religious and cultural beliefs from pathological ones. A belief could be delusional if it:

- is disputed by the patient's family, religious or (sub)cultural group
- results in functional impairment or inappropriate or **maladaptive behaviour**
- is associated with other psychiatric symptoms (e.g. other psychotic or mood features)

Nonetheless, the differentiation between belief and delusion can be difficult, and in the end it often becomes necessary to treat the symptoms and to leave the question as to the validity of the belief to the family, community or traditional and faith healers. Exercise caution when the delusion is shared by the family and/or the community (Grobler *et al.*, 2011).

## 6.8.6 Hallucinations

Language presents a major obstacle, since it does not always accurately clarify what the interviewer is looking for, and the same word may be used for very different experiences. As discussed in Section 6.8.3, this poses a particular challenge when one is using an interpreter. For example, the isiZulu word *imibono*, commonly used to elicit visual hallucinations, is also used to describe visions and dream images. It is therefore important to clarify with the interpreter what is being asked. Visions are very commonly described in a number of cultures in South Africa, and are not necessarily associated with psychopathology. Seeing a deceased person, for example, especially after a recent and traumatic death, can be a very vivid experience for somebody who has no other pathology. Reports that God or the ancestors are talking to the patient require careful interpretation to determine if they reflect the patient's religious or cultural experience or are hallucinations. As is the general rule in psychiatry, the clinician has to rely on the associated symptoms to formulate a diagnosis.

## 6.8.7 Cognitive assessment

Educational achievements are not a measurement of the actual levels of intellectual or cognitive performance of a patient. One must understand the way the educational system works, and find or invent a way in which a patient can be assessed. This has an impact on assessment tools, including the Mini Mental State Examination (Folstein *et al.*, 1975), which have not been standardised for many culturally differing population groups.

## 6.8.8 Diagnosis

Culture in psychiatry is not only about a Western-trained practitioner making a diagnosis or treating a patient from a different culture adequately. It is about any mental health professional shifting into a mode of cultural awareness and sensitivity, becoming investigative rather than making diagnostic assumptions, and about admitting that we do not have answers for all clinical scenarios.

## 6.8.9 Summary

In summary, working across cultures means:

- becoming observant (noticing outward appearance, tattoos, clothing and accessories) and asking the patient or relatives for the meaning of such observations
- asking for an explanation of unknown terms or explanations
- accepting that some patients very likely have already been treated by traditional or faith healers and will continue doing so once leaving your care, or will be doing so parallel with conventional treatment
- acknowledging that ultimately the family will influence what will happen with the patient.

When a decision must be made about potentially dangerous or forensic patients, the safety of the community supersedes the wishes and cultural preferences of the patient or family, as provided for by relevant legislation.

## 6.9 Culture and phenomenology in psychiatry

Phenomenology refers to descriptions of what people experience and how it is that they experience what they experience (Patton,1990). Culture substantially influences psychopathology (Tseng and Streltzer, 1997). It has less influence on organic mental disorders and major (functional) psychiatric disorders than on minor psychiatric disorders (neuroses) or substance abuse. Culture has a profound influence on culture-related specific syndromes or epidemic mental disorders (Tseng, 2001).

Phenomenology is bound to be coloured by the experiences of the patient. As these experiences and the exposure of the patient to new influences undergo changes, so do perceptual disturbances. It is ultimately the quality of the disturbance – and not the content - that guides the interviewer towards an integrated assessment.

## 6.10 Cultural syndromes - an international perspective

### 6.10.1 Cultural syndromes

Cultural syndromes (CS, previously referred to as culture-bound syndromes) are conditions recognised in specific cultures as a group of symptoms indicating a cause embedded in the belief system of that particular culture. According to the DSM-5 (APA, 2013) cultural syndromes are 'clusters of symptoms and attributions that tend to co-occur among individuals in specific cultural groups, communities, or contexts... that are recognized locally as coherent patterns of experience' (p. 758).

These syndromes have been recognised through time immemorial and have been acted upon in a way prescribed by cultural healing practices. As the frequency of occurrence diminishes over time there are changes in the description and manifestation of the conditions, the interpretation and the cure.

There are numerous such syndromes, with many localised syndromes being described as mental health professionals reach areas that previously did not have access to these services (Aina and Morakinyo, 2011). Many of these syndromes are extremely localised, while others are universally recognisable under different names, and some have only historical value. Some conditions that were thought to belong to this category have since been found to have organic causes.

We shall now briefly look at some of the more commonly known cultural syndromes.

#### 6.10.1.1 Amok

A dissociative episode characterised by an outburst of violent, aggressive, or homicidal behaviour directed at people and objects. Such episodes are also referred to as 'running amok'. The episode is often accompanied by **persecutory** ideas, **automatism**, **amnesia**, exhaustion and a return to the premorbid state after the episode. The episode is usually preceded by a period of brooding and may at times end in suicide. Originally described in the Far East (mainly Malaysia and Indonesia), the condition has also been seen in other countries.

#### 6.10.1.2 *Bouffée délirante*

***Bouffée délirante*** is a syndrome observed in West Africa and Haiti. This French term refers to a sudden outburst of agitated and aggressive behaviour, marked confusion and **psychomotor excitement**. It may sometimes be accompanied by visual and auditory hallucinations or paranoid ideation. The term has long been used in France for brief psychotic episodes. An equivalent term used in the ICD-10 is 'acute transient psychotic disorder' (World Health Organization, 1992). Duration can be from a few days to a few months.

#### 6.10.1.3 Brain fag

**Brain fag** is a term initially used in West Africa to refer to a condition experienced by high school or university students in response to the challenges of schooling (Prince, 1960). Symptoms include difficulty in concentrating, remembering and thinking. Students often state that their brains are fatigued. Brain tiredness or fatigue from 'too much thinking' is an idiom of distress in many cultures, and resulting syndromes can resemble certain anxiety, depression, and somatoform disorders. This syndrome has been described in South Africa as *isimnyama esikolweni* (bad luck or bewitchment in school) (Ensink and Robertson, 1996; Peltzer *et al.*, 1998).

## 6.11 Cultural syndromes in South Africa

### 6.11.1 Syndromes of bewitchment

The belief in witchcraft is an omnipresent persistent belief that has a variety of expressions. Witchcraft is defined as magic (in the form of material substances or familiars), used to inflict harm upon an individual or on those whom one considers an enemy, and spring from envy, greed, hate, malevolence or other evil intentions. (The term *umona*, meaning 'envy' is used in several indigenous languages.) A witch is a person who possesses the power to use witchcraft.

A witchdoctor (the more acceptable terms being traditional healer or *sangoma*) is not a witch but is a healer or diviner who is consulted to identify the cause of misfortune or illness. The traditional healer may identify witchcraft as a cause of misfortune or illness and also provides protection against witchcraft. (This pointing out of witchcraft may sometimes indirectly support accusations against individuals.)

Belief in witchcraft is a reality for many communities in South Africa and all over the world. It is pervasive and may be associated with depression, somatisation and anxiety. It is unabating, despite suppression by law and Christian teachings. Witchcraft often becomes a chronic stressor, leading to feelings of hopelessness and helplessness. Communities no longer have means to deal with alleged witches, and although persecution of witches occur regularly in South Africa and accusations are still frequently made (especially by mentally ill persons), there is no sanctioned way to deal with it. Charging an accuser with 'imputing witchcraft' is one way for an alleged witch to defend himself or herself. People accused of this are sometimes sent for forensic observation. In South Africa, police are familiar with this problem and are on the alert to defuse witchcraft-related situations quickly and efficiently. The Witchcraft Suppression Act (No. 3 of 1957), as amended by the Witchcraft Suppression Amendment Act (No. 50 of 1970), makes the following punishable offences:

- accusing a person of witchcraft
- naming of witches
- sniffing out of witches
- attempting to practice witchcraft
- claiming to have knowledge of witchcraft.

#### 6.11.1.1 Bewitchment

Witchcraft remains a common explanation for unexplained misfortunes, illnesses, disasters, unfortunate coincidences and sudden or premature deaths (including those associated with HIV/Aids). Witchcraft accusations occur commonly for many reasons and witchcraft beliefs are a potent inducer of unexplained somatic and neurotic symptoms (Weiss, 2004)

Below and on the next page are several case studies from a forensic setting that serve as illustrations.

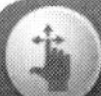

**Case study 6.3**

Mr A was a 45-year-old male with a long history of psychiatric treatment. He had accused seven women in his village of being witches during the years of his illness. He was cared for by his father up to the time of his father's death. During the wake he saw two of the women and killed both. He was declared a State Patient.

## Case study 6.4

Mr B was a 34-year-old male., At the onset of his mental illness, he was diagnosed with bipolar disorder, manic episode, with psychotic features. Three years later he was declared a State Patient after he smashed someone's car in a hypomanic state. After his release from hospital he experienced occasional mild relapses and his functioning at work deteriorated. Subsequently his newborn child was diagnosed HIV-positive. He was, naturally, very upset about this. The following year the child died and his wife returned to her maternal home where she later died. He had refused an HIV test after the child had died. His employer became concerned about his behaviour at work following these events. He was closely monitored, and then was arrested for killing his aunt. He was referred for psychiatric observation He stated that he was restless, depressed, hearing voices, ruminating about his condition and wondering why and who was responsible. He explained that he had decided to go and see his uncle, with whom he had had no contact for the previous 15 years. He found his uncle in the house ill with Aids. The uncle complained that his wife did not allow him hospital treatment. Mr B now 'knew' that his aunt was responsible for 'everything' and killed her with a piece of wood. Mr B had lost his whole family in car accidents 15 years earlier, something the doctors treating him did not know about. The aunt had been the main witch suspect following that tragedy and this was the reason Mr B had had no contact with his uncle and aunt for 15 years. He was declared a State Patient, but never stabilised and committed suicide a few years later.

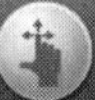

## Case study 6.5

Mr C was a 45-year-old man, with little education, single, and had an alcohol problem. He lived in a rural area. He had experienced a number of events, including falling from his bicycle many times, hitting a cow with his bicycle when he came home at night from the tavern, and generally not being very successful. He had consulted a traditional healer who told him that two women were bewitching him. Just before Christmas one year, he was selling beer from his home when two rural women approached and asked for beer for free. Although it was still morning, he was already drunk. He refused them. They left, but one returned later, again asking for beer. He refused, and she left him saying that he would not see the sun set. He now 'knew' that these two women were the witches who had caused him misfortune. He walked two kilometres to their homes and killed both. There was no evidence of psychosis; he was tried in court and sentenced.

As stated earlier, if a delusion is isolated, coherent, in keeping with cultural beliefs, and occurs in the absence of other psychotic features, it can be difficult to diagnose. Delusions about witchcraft in psychosis can be persistent or only emerge during a psychotic episode. It is important to understand that delusions and cultural beliefs can co-exist. All witchcraft accusations must be taken seriously. The anxiety and fear that surround witchcraft is usually underestimated as a source of somatic complaints. It is difficult for communities to effectively resolve accusations of witchcraft. For many people, this means living with the suspicion or knowledge or information that a person is the victim of witchcraft or that oneself is a victim.

### 6.11.1.2 *Amafufunyane*

***Amafufunyane*** is a broad construct used by black South Africans to describe a combination of symptoms including hallucinations, delusions, outbursts of aggression, hysterical behaviour, disorientation and violent madness (Mkhize, 1998). It is conceptualised as a manifestation of spirit possession (in the form of mealie stalk borers and ants collected from graves), mediated through witchcraft. The term *amafufunyane* has largely lost its original context. A variety of psychiatric symptoms are now attributed to *amafufunyane,* without the patient being familiar with the symptoms described here.

The attacks are frightening and often victims, who are typically adolescent or young adult women, have to be restrained in order not to inflict or sustain injury. The talking *amafufunyane* are particularly dangerous because they name the person who 'owns' them. Outbreaks of *amafufunyane* affecting groups of children in schools have been reported across South Africa and neighbouring countries, usually labelled as 'mass hysteria' in the media in some instances leading to injury and even the death of those accused.

Useful mental health interventions in such cases are to:

- engage with the affected children by isolating them from others
- reduce attention to the phenomena
- empathetically facilitate expression of their fears
- desensitise them to their fears.

This approach also allows the victims to concurrently engage in any cultural or religious interventions they deem necessary for their recovery.

## 6.11.2 Syndrome of ancestral calling

### 6.11.2.1 *Ukuthwasa*

The calling to become a traditional healer, or *ukuthwasa*, has been widely described (Buhrmann, 1986; Broster, 1982) and is a condition related to ancestral beliefs.

The condition is associated with dreams of an ancestor who was a traditional healer handing over beads or paraphernalia needed by a traditional healer to the chosen person. Another belief associated with *ukuthwasa* involves disappearing into the river to be in contact with the ancestors, and emerging again after some time. Mood symptoms are the prominent symptoms presented before a diagnosis is made. These can include manic states, depressive states, dissociative states and somatic symptoms. *Umoya* (spirit) or *amadlozi* (benevolent ancestral spirits) are terms used to indicate that the person is in communication with ancestral spirits. *Umoya* and *amadlozi* may be expressed in brief emotional outbursts associated with loud noises. The diagnosis is made by a traditional healer.

The length of the *ukuthwasa* process varies. It requires animal sacrifices from those undergoing the *ukuthwasa* process. It usually is expensive for the family since in most cases all rituals required traditionally must be performed before the training process can even begin. Since the process can take weeks, months or years, and can be continuous or interrupted, it demands a strong commitment from the person undergoing *ukuthwasa*.

*Ukuthwasa* requires the initiate (*umkwetha*) to move away from the family and submit himself or herself to training by an experienced traditional healer. *Ukuthwasa* practices are too numerous to cover in detail, but include:

- steam inhalations
- vigorous dancing
- slaughtering and besmearing with blood of ritual animals
- collecting herbal medicines.

In some instances, the ritual of *ukuvum'ukufa* (accepting the condition) can provide a reprieve from symptoms. Should an illness (physical or mental) occur, the cause of the condition may be attributed to the incomplete process. The Xhosa variation is extremely lengthy; initiates may return to the process again and again as they suffer relapses of mental illness, blaming the incomplete *ukuthwasa* process. White beads amongst the Xhosa are the outward manifestation of an initiate who has not completed the process. Any unusual adornment should raise the question of whether the person is undergoing the *ukuthwasa* process or is a traditional healer.

Many of the symptoms described above also occur within the context of being called to become a prophet, sometimes in clients who have abandoned traditional practices or are affiliated with African indigenous religions.

Familiarity with the way of life of patients is useful when trying to understand the link between ancestral beliefs and illness. With increasing urbanisation, lack of family cohesion and scarce resources, rituals are omitted. As physical or mental illnesses arise, these may be attributed to ancestral wrath and to the need to perform those rituals, which can become a complicated process if the family is dysfunctional or heads of households are absent.

In southern Africa, most discussions of local cultural factors in mental health involve a consideration of the influence of the traditional African world view and cosmology, as reflected in the two main language groupings, the Nguni (including the Zulu, Xhosa, Swazi, and Ndebele) and the Sotho (including the North and South Sotho and Tswana) groups. Harriet Ngubane (1977) and Vera Buhrmann (1986) led the way with their extensive writings and exposure to the Nguni culture. Robertson (2006) looked at the collaboration between healers and psychiatry, while Swartz (1998) also contributed. Many other eminent psychiatrists, psychologists, sociologists, political analysts and anthropologists have contributed to a better understanding of the different cultural groups in South Africa.

## 6.12 Culture and migration

Migration is a process of social change where an individual, alone or accompanied by others, leaves one geographical area for a prolonged stay or a permanent settlement in another geographical area. The reasons for migrating are varied: economic betterment, political upheaval, education or other purposes. Migration is not only a trans-national process but can also be rural–urban (Bhugra, 2004), as has been and remains common in South Africa.

Acculturation is a process when groups of individuals from different cultures come into continuous first-hand contact with each other, with subsequent changes in the original cultural patterns of either one or both groups (Redfield *et al.*, 1936).

When two cultures come in contact, either **assimilation**, where cultural differences disappear (Berry, 1992) or rejection, where the individual or the group withdraws from the larger society, takes place.

When the individual has to negotiate alien customs while experiencing economic hardship, communication difficulties and social isolation, the likelihood of experiencing adjustment problems is increased. People who experience adjustment problems as a result of displacement can respond to the process of acculturation in one or more of these four ways (Drennan, 2000)

- integration: aspects of the culture of origin are retained while adopting aspects of the new culture
- assimilation: the culture of origin is largely rejected, and the new culture is adopted as a replacement.
- separation: recreating a familiar environment through seeking out people from the same background and grouping together, with the minimum adoption of the host culture's features
- marginalisation: the person is unable to sustain identification with the culture of origin, but also does not adopt the new cultural environment (Berry *et al.*, 1992)

South Africa's migrant labour system has been a powerful contributor to a range of unhealthy developments, mainly due to the political situation during apartheid, and this pattern has persisted with some modifications. Segregation was not a choice but a political idea, and in many ways this has persisted in townships, squatter camps, peri-urban settlements and the so-called independent states (Transkei, Bophuthatswana, Venda and Ciskei) and homelands created during the apartheid era.

Though people take their cultural beliefs with them when migrating, a dilution occurs in the face of so many challenges, with a powerful emergence of their cultural beliefs during regression and in crisis situations.

With refugees from other countries entering South Africa, a host of new potential adjustment problems have arisen in a cultural context similar to, yet different from, the South African population. Xenophobia and its results on immigrants cannot be ignored as a major stressor. (See Chapter 5: Psychosocial determinants of mental disorders, for further discussion of the stressors associated with migration and implications for mental illness.)

## 6.13 Cultural formulation

Mental health workers can no longer be satisfied with the bio-psycho-social formulation when addressing the needs of their patients. This must be expanded to the bio-psycho-social-cultural formulation, to be able to conceptualise a holistic understanding of a person's world.

The cultural formulation, suggested by the DSM-5 through guidelines, and modified by other authors, is not only relevant but essential in the South African context. Especially in the teaching and training situation, where cultural competency should be encouraged and nurtured, this will provide a basis from where cultural similarities and differences can be explored.

### 6.13.1 Guidelines for a cultural formulation

The cultural formulation is a process that helps the clinician to recognise key aspects of a patient's identity that have a significant impact on their diagnosis and management. Its main components can be outlined as follows:

#### 6.13.1.1 Cultural reference group

A person's cultural reference group is multifaceted, and includes:

- language, ethnicity, upbringing, cultural and religious belief systems
- family system and composition
- impact of those systems on the individual
- current involvement with original cultural background
- impact of religion on the original cultural background
- preferred identification with a culture
- support system.

#### 6.13.1.2 Stressors

Stressors take on many forms, including:

- life events and reactions/adjustments
- social stressors
- economic stressors
- occupational stressors
- current levels of functioning.

#### 6.13.1.3 Patient's view of the illness

- Understanding of the illness and perceived cause
- Available or preferred treatment modalities
- Previous treatment experiences
- Who will influence the patient's choices?

#### 6.13.1.4 Cultural issues and the therapeutic relationship

The clinician should identify ways in which cultural differences with the patient can affect the therapeutic alliance.

#### 6.13.1.5 Culture sensitive diagnostic and management plan

Diagnosis and management should be broad and holistic and should allow for aspects that may not be adequately addressed by Western diagnostic labels and interventions.

## Conclusion

This chapter provides an overview of cultural issues relevant to psychiatry from a South African perspective. Selected examples provided as illustrations highlight aspects of some of the indigenous belief systems, while recognising the reality of similar and dissimilar Western and other non-African cultural constructs.

As a culturally diverse society, South Africa provides a great opportunity for mental health professionals to develop cultural sensitivity and apply it to their work. Attaining this proficiency is a life-long endeavour which begins by acknowledging one's own cultural affiliation, and respectfully learning to understand the cultural affiliation of one's patients, irrespective of their racial, language or geographical origins. Such an appreciation will ultimately assist the mental health professional to gain rapport and establish a therapeutic alliance with patients, and to identify cultural factors pertinent to diagnosis and management.

# References


Aina OF, Morakinyo O (2011) Culture-bound syndromes and the neglect of cultural factors in psychopathologies among Africans. *African Journal of Psychiatry14*(4) : 278–85

American Psychiatric Association (2013) *Diagnostic and Statistical Manual of Mental Disorders* (5th edition). Arlington, VA: American Psychiatric Association

Berry JW (1992) Acculturation and adaptation in a new society. *International Migration* 30(Supplement 1): 69–85.

Berry JW (1997) Immigration, acculturation and adaptation. *Applied Psychology: An International Review* 46(1): 5–68.

Bhugra D (2004) Migration, distress and cultural identity. *British Medical Bulletin* 69(1): 129–41

Broster JA, HC Bourn (1982) *Amagqirha: Religion, Magic, and Medicine in Transkei*. Cape Town: Via Afrika Limited

Buhrmann MV (1986) *Living in Two Worlds: Communication Between a White Healer and Her Black Counterparts.* Illinois: Chiron Publications

Drennan G (2000) Cultural Psychiatry. In: Robertson B, Allwood C, Gagiano C (Eds) *Oxford Textbook of Psychiatry for Southern Africa.* Cape Town: Oxford University Press

Ensink K, Robertson B (1996) Indigenous categories of distress and dysfunction in South African Xhosa children and adolescents as described by indigenous healers. *Transcultural Psychiatry* 33: 137–72

Folstein MF, Folstein SF, McHugh PR (1975) 'Mini-mental state': A practical method for grading the cognitive state of patients for the clinician. *Journal of Psychiatric Research* 12(3): 189–198

Grobler C, Weiss EA, Lebelo E, Malerotho E (2011) Culture, religion and psychosis – a case study from Limpopo Province, South Africa. *African Journal of Psychiatry* 14: 239–40

Group for the Advancement of Psychiatry: Committee on Cultural Psychiatry (2001) *Cultural assessment in clinical psychiatry.* Washington: American Psychiatric Publishing

Hofstede G (1997) Cultures and Organizations: *Software of the mind.* New York: McGraw-Hill

News 24 (2012) *KZN task team to probe child marriages* http://www.news24.com/SouthAfrica/News/KZN-task-team-to-probe-child-marriages-20121121 (Accessed 2 February 2015)

Mkhize DL (1998) *Amafufunyane* — is it a culture-bound syndrome? *South African Medical Journal* 88: 329–31

Ngubane H (1977) *Body and Mind in Zulu Medicine: An Ethnography of Health and Disease in Nyuswa-Zulu Thought and Practice.* London: Academic Press

Patton MQ (1990) *Qualitative Evaluation and Research Methods* (2nd ed) Newbury Park, CA: Sage

Peltzer K, Cherian VI, Cherian L (1998) Brain fag symptoms in rural South African secondary school pupils. *Psychological Reports* 83: 1187- 96

Prince R (1960) The 'brain fag' syndrome in Nigerian students. *British Journal of Psychiatry* 106: 559–70

Raimundo Oda AM, Banzato CE, Dalgalarrondo P (2005) Some origins of cross-cultural psychiatry. *History of Psychiatry* 16(62 Pt 2): 155–69

Redfield R, Linton R, Herskovit M (1936) Memorandum on the study of acculturation. *American Anthropologist* 38: 149–52

Republic of South Africa. The Witchcraft Suppression Act, No. 3 of 1957. Pretoria: Government Printers

Republic of South Africa. The Witchcraft Suppression Amendment Act, No. 50 of 1970. Pretoria: Government Printers

Robertson BA (2006) Does the evidence support collaboration between psychiatry and traditional healers? Findings from three South African studies. *South African Psychiatry Review* 9: 87–90

Spiegel Online (2011) *New abuse figures: Forced marriages in Germany more prevalent than thought* http://www.spiegel.de/international/germany/new-abuse-figures-forced-marriages-in-germany-more-prevalent-than-thought-a-796760.html (Accessed 11 February 2015)

Swartz L (1998) *Culture and Mental Health: A Southern African View.* Cape Town: Oxford University Press

Tseng WS (2001) *Handbook of Cultural Psychiatry.* San Diego, CA: Academic Press. Quotations on page 92 reprinted with permission from Elsevier

Tseng WS, Streltzer J (1997) *Culture and Psychopathology: A Guide to Clinical Assessment.* New York: Brunner/Mazel

Weiss EA (2004) *Witchcraft and criminal responsibility.* World Association of Social Psychiatry Conference. March 2004.

World Health Organization (1992) *International Statistical Classification of Diseases and Related Health Problems* (tenth revision). Geneva: World Health Organization

# PART 3

# Assessment of psychiatric disorders

CHAPTER

# 7 Clinical assessment in psychiatry

*Orlando Alonso Betancourt*

## 7.1 Introduction

Psychiatric diagnosis relies heavily on the quality of the clinician's observations and interview of the patient. This chapter offers a basic structure to the clinical assessment.

Throughout the chapter the reader will navigate from a setting where the interview could take place to the different components of the clinical assessment in psychiatry.

## 7.2 Clinical assessment

A psychiatric assessment is a process whereby a trained health professional determines the presence of psychiatric symptoms and signs in a patient. This assessment usually proceeds as a semi-structured conversation between the clinician and the patient. Medical students must learn the structure as part of their training. This process has several objectives (Lingard, 1999):

- to understand the patient as an individual and within various contexts
- to establish a working diagnosis that leads to specific investigations (biological, psychological and social) at the end of the examination and that directs the clinician to an initial pragmatic treatment plan
- a final and clinically sound diagnosis and a full comprehensive management plan.

A secondary – and important – aim is that this psychiatric assessment will be available to colleagues who will also be in contact with the patient.

Medical students often find a psychiatric assessment challenging, since psychiatric terminology is usually a new language for them. The assessment is fundamentally based on three elements:

- a clinical interview
- direct observation of the patient
- gathering collateral information (which may not always be available).

A good understanding of psychiatric symptoms and signs is crucial to obtain a good psychiatric history. Even though psychiatric assessments have been standardised many times within a framework of the structured interview, it remains primarily a subjective measurement that begins the moment the patient enters the consulting room. Observe his or her personal grooming and hygiene and, on a deeper level, factors such as whether the patient is dressed appropriately for the weather and his or her culture. For example, note whether the patient is wearing colourful and flamboyant clothes: this type of observation will tell you more about the patient's mood and insight into his/her illness. Other behaviour to note may include a patient talking to himself or herself in the waiting area or smiling inappropriately or pacing outside the office door. Record all observations.

### 7.2.1 The examiner's style

It is crucial for the good development and outcome of the assessment to establish adequate rapport with the patient. The first step is for the interviewer to make an introduction in a friendly, calm and appropriate manner. Speak directly to the patient during this introduction, and pay attention to the patient's body language and whether he or she maintains eye contact.

Making mental notes of such things may aid in guiding the interview later. If a patient appears uneasy when he or she enters the office, attempt to relax the situation by making small talk or offering something to drink.

Patients, including psychiatric patients, expect physicians to look and act like 'the doctor'. The biological aetiology of most psychiatric disorders is undeniable and the care of those affected requires a solid foundation in medicine. One view is that psychiatrists in hospitals and clinical settings should wear the traditional white hospital coat: this subtly communicates to the patient that he or she has a medical condition and that the clinician is there to help.

A psychiatric history is incomplete without a full physical examination: it is crucially important to rule out any medical condition in the presence of psychiatric symptoms. Furthermore, co-morbidity of medical conditions like HIV/Aids and TB and psychiatric disorders is common in the South African context.

Politeness and respect are essential in establishing a good doctor-patient relationship. Compassion, respect and sympathy will enhance the patient's positive feelings towards the clinician and improve the history taking process. Later, this rapport will assist to increase compliance with treatment.

Open-ended questions (e.g.,'Tell me about your childhood') are used to elicit the patient's own perceptions about his or her problems and to gather general information. Close-ended questions (e.g. 'What is your highest level of education?') elicit specific details and clarifies patient information.

### 7.2.2 Examination setting

Safety in emergency rooms and when interviewing a new or unknown psychiatric patient should be your primary concern for you (and by extension the rest of the staff indirectly involved in the examination) and the patient. Before engaging with the patient, you must have an idea of the potential for violence and your possible escape route. Never put yourself in a position where escape is difficult or impossible.

When the threat of violence is evident, the rules of safety supersede the need for privacy, and the patient is seen in an open area or with other staff members present. If needed, you should have trained security personnel present.

## 7.3 The structured clinical assessment

There are several valid formats of a psychiatric clinical history. For the purpose of this publication, we will follow the format used in the Eastern Cape for teaching medical students, which includes recent modifications suggested by the College of Psychiatrists of South Africa. This format corresponds closely to that used throughout South Africa. Although this format mainly refers to inpatients, it could easily be modified to be used in an outpatient setting.

### 7.3.1 Psychiatric history

In this section, we shall look at the specific components of the psychiatric history.

#### 7.3.1.1 Identifying data or demographics

The objective is to get a first impression of the person in context, which means gathering personal information. It is also used as a first attempt to establish contact and rapport and to prepare the field for collecting data that are important in later management of the patient. The items to record are:

- full names and surname
- date of birth (if not available, estimated age)
- marital status and children (if any)
- living where, with whom, and for how long
- highest level of education
- employment/source of income
- religious affiliation (note whether practising or not).

#### 7.3.1.2 Referral data

This section, which is sometimes underestimated, will give you crucial information about who referred the patient, what the problem was, when the patient arrived at the referral place and under which section of the Mental Health Care Act (MHCA) this patient was referred.

The following information is needed:
- name and contact details of referral source
- reason for referral
- which section of MHCA applies
- history provided
- date of first admission to referral clinic or hospital
- date of admission to current facility
- treatment given so far.

You can usually obtain this information from the patient's referral sheet.

### 7.3.1.3 Presenting problem

The presenting problem or complaint is a chronological narrative of the facts that brought that patient to the clinic or to be admitted. It typically consists of two parts: the chief complaint and the history of the presenting complaint.
- Chief complaint: This is a verbatim statement from the patient, which is very important as it will alert you to the patient's understanding of the reason for his/her admission. The question could be 'Why are you here?', or 'Why were you admitted in this hospital?', asked in a friendly, simple and clear manner.
- History of the presenting complaint:
  - what is the problem?
  - when did it start?
  - how did it develop?
  - what triggered it?
  - modifying factors (medication, etc.)?

Remember that this part is a narrative of symptoms and signs describing in a chronological order, in your own words and the patient's own words, what happened. Some clinicians prefer to describe the symptom and, in brackets, add the technical name, for example 'The patient referred to hearing the voice of a neighbour insulting him even though he couldn't see the person talking; he is the only one who can hear this voice…' (complex auditory hallucinations).

It is also useful to establish the patient's and his or her family's view of what has caused the current symptoms/illness.

Although a good examination resembles a conversation, it is systematic, methodical and exhaustive.

### 7.3.1.4 Past psychiatric history

Discover as much about previous treatment as possible, by asking:
- if the patient had been hospitalised before or whether he or she had been treated as an outpatient
- if any previous diagnosis is available
- if there is a history of previous suicide attempts
- if the patient has any untreated conditions
- what treatment the patient had received in the past (e.g. psychotropic medications and response to them, benefits and side effects, compliance and dosages).

This information may offer clues as to which class of medication the patient is likely to respond. If possible, try to obtain old psychiatric records.

### 7.3.1.5 Medical and surgical history

The patient's medical and surgical history should include information about:
- illnesses (e.g. infections, including tuberculosis (TB) and sexually transmitted diseases (STDs)
- cardiac conditions
- metabolic illnesses
- surgical interventions
- injuries, in particular head injuries
- neurological illnesses, in particular epilepsy (in which case, enquire in detail about type of seizures and treatment)
- neurocysticercosis.

Obstetric and gynaecological history should include information about:
- parity and gravida
- last normal menstrual period
- currently breastfeeding or not

- contraception
- post-partum mental health problems.

Obtain information about current medication, including psychiatric, medical and traditional medicines prescribed. Enquire about allergies and adverse drug reactions experienced. Finally, ask whether other forms of health provider have been consulted for this illness (e.g. traditional healers).

#### 7.3.1.6 Substance use

Get a thorough description of the use of drugs (both legal and illegal). Start with alcohol and over the counter medication use, time spent consuming drugs, associated symptoms, **tolerance**, **withdrawal** symptoms and patterns of drug use.

#### 7.3.1.7 Forensic history

Enquire whether the patient has a history of any of the following forensic matters:

- cautions, charges or convictions for criminal behaviour
- prison sentences, including information on charges, duration and probation
- current court cases pending
- screening for antisocial behaviour.

#### 7.3.1.8 Family history

A thorough family history is essential.

- Establish a **genogram** that includes parents, siblings, spouse or partner and children.
- Note deaths in the family, with specific causes, age and time as far as possible.
- Ask about medical illness.
- Ask about mental illness, specifically suicides, admissions to psychiatric institutions, treatments, use of substances and known diagnosis.
- Ask about the quality of the relationships with the family, especially with primary caregivers.

#### 7.3.1.9 Personal history

When asking the patient about his or her personal history, obtain information on:

- birth history and perinatal complications
- ages at which developmental milestones were reached
- childhood illness, trauma, behaviour
- schooling
- further training and work history
- sexual history
- children
- social activities
- current socioeconomic circumstances.

#### 7.3.1.10 Personality

It is important to determine the person's view of self. Try to identify obvious personality traits according to clusters (keep in mind that you will need collateral information to confirm any hypothesis).

### 7.3.2 Mental status examination (MSE)

The mental status examination (MSE) is the core of the psychiatric examination. The clinician looks for the presence of current symptoms; the assessment is done throughout the whole interview from the moment the patient comes into contact with the clinician (American Psychiatric Association, 2006). Observe the following:

- state of consciousness: alert, hyper-alert, lethargic
- appearance: physical appearance (is the patient neatly dressed with attention to detail and well groomed?) as well as emotional appearance
- general behaviour and psychomotor activity: **mannerisms**, gestures, combative, rigid, twitching, psychomotor activity (increased, reduced, agitated, abnormal movements), **compulsions** and other perseverative actions and movements
- attitude towards clinician: cooperative, hostile, defensive, seductive, evasive, ingratiating

- mood and affect: observed current emotional state (full, **labile**, elated, euthymic, restricted, flat, inappropriate, irritable)
- language and speech: rate (increased, pressured, slow), tone (soft, angry) volume, articulation, language (aphasia)
- **thought flow**: normal, accelerated, retarded
- **thought form**: circumstantial, tangential, **flight of ideas**, evasiveness, **loosening of associations**, perseverance, blocking
- **thought content**: main theme, **suicidal ideation**, **preoccupations**, **obsessions**, **phobias**, delusions (bizarre and non-bizarre)
- perceptions: **misperceptions**, **illusions**, hallucinations, **depersonalization** and **derealization**
- cognition:
  - **orientation**: time, place and person
  - attention and **concentration**: evaluate by doing the serial-sevens test or asking the patient to name the months of the year or days of week backwards
  - memory: short-term (repeat and later recall the names of three unrelated objects), recent (recount recent sporting or political events) and remote memory (provide dates of distant personal or newsworthy events)
  - judgement: this refers to how the mental illness impacts on the patient's ability to assess daily life situations or make decisions that have safety implications. To assess judgement, present the patient with an everyday situation where he or she has to exercise judgement (e.g. 'if you find a baby alone crying on the street, what would you do?') and assess the answer
  - intellectual functioning (**intelligence** is the ability to think and act rationally and logically)
  - insight: assess insight according to an awareness of the illness, e.g. the capacity to identify psychotic experiences as abnormal or to accept the necessity of treatment.

## 7.3.3 More important symptoms

There are many ways of grouping symptoms. For the purposes of this chapter we'll follow the same order used during the MSE. The most important symptoms will be briefly discussed below. (Symptom descriptions are extracted mainly from Taylor and Vaidya (2009).)

### 7.3.3.1 Symptoms related to the level of consciousness

Consciousness is probably the highest function of the brain. According to Fish (Casey and Kelly, 2007) consciousness 'is a state of awareness of the self and the environment'.

A short description of the most important symptoms in this sphere is given below:

- alertness: the normal state of consciousness defined by the capacity to think clearly, to notice things in one's surrounding and to have a timeous response
- hyper-alertness: the individual is excessively aware of small details happening in the surroundings
- lethargy: the individual looks indifferent, apathetic and sluggish, with no energy
- **dissociation**: both the DSM-5 and ICD-10 (WHO, 1993) recognise several types of **dissociative disorders**. 'Dissociative disorders are characterized by a disruption of and/or discontinuity in the normal integration of consciousness, memory, identity, emotion, perception, body representation, motor control, and behavior. Dissociative symptoms can potentially disrupt every area of psychological functioning' (American Psychiatric Association, 2013).
- confusion: inability to think clearly and quickly. The term 'acute mental confusion' is often used interchangeably with delirium in different classifications to describe a pathological condition in which it usually presents with a loss of orientation (ability to place oneself correctly in the world by time, location and/or personal identity) and

sometimes accompanied by disordered consciousness (loss of linear thinking) and loss of memory (the inability to correctly recall previous events or learn new material).

- coma: a state of unconsciousness in which a person cannot be awakened, fails to respond normally to painful stimuli, light or sound, lacks a normal sleep-wake cycle and does not initiate voluntary actions (Taylor and Vaidya, 2009). There are different degrees of it but these are not discussed in this chapter
- physical appearance: the way people dress, their degree of grooming and general hygiene are related to social class and culture, but it could also reflect some level of psychopathology. Typically the histrionic person dresses more flamboyantly, wears colourful clothes and appears sexually alluring. Being clean and neat is expected in most cultures; when these standards are lacking for no reason it may indicate mental disorder. Pockets or bags full of garbage could point to severe psychotic disorders.

### 7.3.3.2 General behaviour and psychomotor activity

The person's general appearance, behaviour both in the waiting room and in the interview room as well as the quality and type of movements (particularly motor symptoms) should all be observed and assessed.

- hyperactivity: excessive or abnormally increased motor function or activity; the activity is goal directed, however, and the patient is able to explain what he or she is trying to do
- hypoactivity: abnormally decreased motor and cognitive activity, with slowing of thought, speech, and movement. All stuporous patients are hypoactive but not all hypoactive patients are stuporous
- agitation: increased frequency of non-goal-directed movements (as opposed to hyperactivity). It usually is associated with an intense mood or psychotic disorder. It could coincide with hypoactivity like in melancholic depression
- akathisia: motor restlessness, ranging from a subjective feeling of jitteriness to inability to lie or sit quietly or to sleep; a common extrapyramidal side effect of neuroleptic drugs
- gait problems: gait reflects general medical health and/or the presence of a neurological or psychiatric disorder. Slowed gait is seen in depressive patients, hypothyroidism or in highly sedated patients
- fine motor coordination (difficulty with handwriting, cutting food, buttoning clothes, sewing, typing, playing an instrument or a sport). Cerebellar **ataxia** is seen in intoxicated patients and patients with degenerative diseases of the cerebellum. 'A spastic gait is seen in myelopathies and upper motor neuron disease. A wide-based gait suggests peripheral nerve disease or proprioception problems' (Taylor and Vaidya, 2009). Generally, both are a consequence of alcohol abuse
- **catatonia**: a syndrome with symptoms that include **mutism**, immobility, patient staring off into space and keeping the same posture for a prolonged period of time. The syndrome has different degrees or variations, including episodes of agitation (catatonic excitement) to cases that show extreme rigidity where the patient is frozen in the same position for some time. Catatonia is usually due to toxic metabolic and drug-induced disorders, disease or trauma to frontal lobe circuits and psychotic disorders like schizophrenia (Brannon, 2010). Severe forms of catatonia are associated with sudden withdrawal of dopaminergic drugs or inappropriate prescription of antipsychotic medication (neuroleptic malignant syndrome, or NMS), such as high dosages of haloperidol IMI or IV. In such cases the above-mentioned symptoms are accompanied by fever, muscle rigidity, unstable vital signs and elevated serum creatinine phosphokinase. 'Serotonin syndrome is identical but may also be associated with cramping and diarrhoea' (Taylor and Vaidya, 2009)
- **stupor**: extreme unresponsiveness and hypoactivity. The patient fails to respond to questions or commands and usually seems unaware of his or her surroundings. Psychiatric

causes of stupor include depression, catatonic schizophrenia and dissociative disorders. Metabolic conditions, infections and drug **intoxication** could also present with stupor

- mutism: verbal unresponsiveness, which could be a symptom on its own or accompanied by other motor symptoms like **bradykinesia** (slow movements)
- **negativism**: resistance to stimulation. A patient with this symptom will resist with the opposite movement when somebody tries to move any of his or her limbs
- **waxy flexibility**: also known as ***cerea flexibilitas***, it forms part of catatonic symptoms. The patient initially offers some resistance to movement but gradually allows himself or herself to be repositioned as if made of wax, sometimes in abnormal positions
- **catalepsy** and **posturing**: keeping the same position for prolonged periods of time
- posturing: ordinary or bizarre positions maintained by patients
- **stereotypy** movements: automatic repetition of ordinary movements like grooming, rubbing the face or the head, or gesturing
- automatic obedience: an exaggerated co-operation with instructions given by the clinician, as if the patient were an automaton
- mannerisms: odd and unnecessary movements done while completing a task.

#### 7.3.3.3 Symptoms related to mood and affect

The clinician should look for symptoms related to emotions. While normal emotions are impermanent and related to a specific context, abnormal emotional experiences are out of context or exaggerated in terms of duration and intensity.

- mood: prolonged or pervasive emotional state. Affect is inferred objectively and is used to describe the overall emotional state. Terms used to describe mood and affect include depression, elation, emotional lability, euphoria, ecstasy, apathy, affective flattening, anxiety and irritability. **Blunted affect** refers to a significantly diminished emotional response to a stimulus or experience
- **flat affect**: the extreme form of diminished affect, where the patient shows no emotional response at all
- **inappropriate affect**: an emotional response that does not correspond with the experience that triggers it, such as laughing for no reason at all during a serious conversation
- elated mood: exaggerated happiness, optimism and self-satisfaction that do not reflect the patient's actual circumstances; it usually is infectious and the clinician and people around the patient are able to feel it.

#### 7.3.3.4 Symptoms related to thought

The only way to know about thoughts is listening to the patient's speech and assessing it. We shall study the use of words, its syntax and ways of association.

- thought flow: this is the speed and smoothness of thought. Thoughts are accelerated when they occur rapidly and uninhibited. In retarded thinking thoughts are slowed down and the number of ideas entering consciousness is decreased
- thought form: this is the structure of thoughts, i.e. how thoughts proceed logically to form phrases, sentences, etc. Abnormalities include:
  - **circumstantiality**: speech is very indirect and delayed in reaching its goal due to the inclusion of tedious detail (sometimes also referred to as over-inclusiveness)
  - flight of ideas occurs when the thoughts follow each other rapidly. The connections between successive thoughts are still understandable. Flight of ideas often occurs in the context of pressured speech
  - loosening of associations: here the connections between words, phrases or sentences are broken so that the form or structure of thought is disturbed and often illogical
  - perseverance or **perseveration** refers to the adherence of an individual to the same concepts and words beyond the point of relevance, i.e. representing the same thing

  - blocking (**thought blocking**): complete interruption of speech before a thought or an idea has been completely expressed
- thought content: this refers to the actual subjects, topics, ideas and beliefs that make up the thoughts themselves. Abnormalities include:
  - suicidal ideation: recurrent ideas about committing suicide are typical of depressive disorders
  - obsessions: recurrent ideas, thoughts, impulses or images that are experienced as being intrusive and senseless but are recognised as the person's own thoughts
  - phobias: irrational fear of objects, animals or situations
  - delusions: fixed, false beliefs that are out of keeping with the patient's social or cultural background. They are classified as bizarre or non-bizarre. **Bizarre delusions** are defined as clearly implausible
  - overvalued ideas: these have a real core, but the interpretation of it is exaggerated or distorted and accompanied by intense emotional response.

#### 7.3.3.5 Symptoms related to perceptions

'Perceptual distortions are alterations in the perception of external stimuli' (Taylor & Vaidya, 2009).

- dysmegalopsia: distortion of the size and shape of objects and body parts. In the case of **micropsia** objects look smaller while with **macropsia** they appear bigger. These symptoms could be associated with epilepsy or visual problems; they are very rare in other types of psychiatric disorder
- illusions: false perception or misinterpretation of an external stimulus that really exist (e.g. mistaking the silhouette of a tree for a person at night). Illusions could be triggered by anxiety and are not necessarily an expression of a mental disorder
- hallucinations: false perceptions of an object that doesn't exist in the perceptual field at the time. Typically they are classified according to the specific sense involved, for example auditory (the most common), olfactory, tactile, visual and gustative. Simple hallucinations refer to sounds, colours and lights while complex auditory hallucinations are voices talking to the patient. Perceptual disturbances like hallucinations could be the source of delusions.

#### 7.3.3.6 Cognition

Assessment of cognitive status should always be included and should, as a minimum, include the following:

- attention and concentration: evaluate by doing the serial-sevens test or asking the patient to name the months of the year or days of week backwards
- memory: consists of short-term memory (repeat and later recall the names of three unrelated objects), recent memory (recount recent sporting or political events) and remote memory (provide dates of distant personal or newsworthy events)
- intellectual functioning: the ability to think and act rationally and logically.

#### 7.3.3.7 Insight and judgement

Mental illness very often impairs the individual's capacity to recognise his or her illness (insight) and also may interfere with his or her judgement (ability to make sound choices and decisions).

- insight: limited or lost insight typically occurs in psychosis and is evident in the patient's limited ability or complete inability to recognise that he or she is ill, that psychotic symptoms are not real and that treatment is necessary
- judgement: poor judgement occurs in severe mental illness and is evident in the patient's inability to assess daily life situations or make decisions about common situations. Typically the clinician presents one or two mundane situations where the patient has to exercise his or her judgement.

## 7.3.4 Physical examination

This refers to a full and comprehensive physical examination. Without one, the psychiatric evaluation is incomplete.

## 7.3.5 Summary

The summary consists of a specific and brief review of all the important findings of the history, the MSE and the physical examination, presented as clusters or syndromes. The summary should not consist of a detailed repetition of every symptom and sign; rather cluster symptoms and signs into syndromes, for example, 'Marked anxiety symptoms were present, together with features of a major depressive episode. No psychotic features were present.'

## 7.3.6 Differential diagnosis

Your hypothesis should be ranked from the most probable to the least probable diagnosis. It is based on all information, especially on the data contained in your summary and formulation. If psychiatric and medical co-morbidities are present, you should include them. Usually there are no more than five and no less than three hypotheses/diagnoses. You should explain which factors are in favour and against each of them. A common error is the omission of co-morbid differentials: a patient with a psychotic disorder may have five differential diagnoses (including substance-induced psychotic disorder) while a separate diagnosis of substance use disorder may be present as a co-morbid psychiatric disorder.

## 7.3.7 Disabilities

Comment briefly on any difficulties the patient could have on the following activities:

- understanding and communicating
- getting around
- self-care
- getting along with people
- household/school/work activities
- participation in society.

## 7.3.8 Risk assessment

A risk assessment should be included in every patient evaluation and should be repeated at every encounter. It is important to consider risk in terms of the following issues or circumstances:

- medical risk
- risk of self-harm or suicide
- risk of violence (verbal, physical, sexual)
- other risks (e.g. non-compliance, escape, being vulnerable to victimisation, manipulation or abuse).

## 7.3.9 Aetiological formulation

Present the aetiological formulation as brief narrative, discussing the biological, psychological, social and cultural predisposing factors. In similar style, also consider the precipitating, perpetuating and protective factors.

## 7.3.10 Management plan

The management plan should clearly set out your short-term and long-term management plan of the patient in the biological, psychological and social sphere.

### 7.3.10.1 Acute management

Acute management centres on how you will treat the patient at the moment of admission and during the first days. Consider the following:

- goals
- treatment setting: inpatient, outpatient, section of the MHCA
- investigations:
  - biological: blood tests, urine analysis, radiology, electroencephalogram (EEG), lumbar puncture (LP) and other
  - psychological: psychological testing (if possible at this high time)
  - social: collateral information, home visits, etc.
- treatment interventions
  - biological
  - psychological

- social
- nursing
- occupational therapy.

#### 7.3.10.2 Long-term management

1 Goals
2 Treatment settings
3 Critical review
4 Psycho-education.

### 7.3.11 Prognosis

When making a prognosis, you have to consider the nature of the disorder itself (diagnosis, severity of illness, co-morbidity) and the patient's age, gender, social and family support, access to services, etc. Try to indicate a short-term and a long-term prognosis based upon all the information you have available.

### 7.3.12 Managing challenging situations during the clinical assessment

Table 7.1 gives guidance on how to manage specific situations that may be present at the outset of a clinical psychiatric assessment or develop during its course.

## 7.4 Principles of diagnosis

One of the goals of a psychiatric assessment is to make a sound diagnosis, but this is a process that requires experience, the necessary clinical skills to identify specific signs, symptoms and syndromes, as well as knowledge regarding epidemiological data on the incidence and prevalence of disorders. Taylor and Vaidya (2009) mention three principles that could help the diagnostic process: the Duck Principle, Sutton's Law, and the Rule of Parsimony.

### 7.4.1 The Duck Principle

'If it looks and walks like a duck and quacks like a duck, it is a duck!' When applied to the diagnostic situation, this principle means that if the patient shows signs and symptoms that make you think of disorder A, the patient is likely to have disorder A.

Case study 7.1 illustrates this principle.

The 'duck' for schizophrenia is an insidious onset of a psychotic episode with bizarre delusions and inappropriate affect in a healthy young man who has no history of drug use and is in good physical health. Admission and treatment with risperidone 4 mg daily managed to control this episode within a few weeks. Further interviews and investigations confirmed the diagnosis of schizophrenia.

### 7.4.2 Sutton's Law: Go where the money is

Sutton's Law, when applied to the process of making a diagnosis, is a reminder that under most circumstances the patient will have a

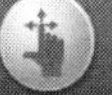

**Case study 7.1**

SP is 22 years old and a final-year law student. During his final block examination his friends realise that he has become peculiar during the past six weeks. He seems to have strange ideas about politics and religion, doesn't appreciate normal jokes any more, laughs inappropriately in social situations and seems to have difficulty concentrating. He also accuses his friends of stealing his notes. On the day of his oral examination he informs the professor that his friends have put a transmitter inside his computer that broadcasts his thoughts to other students and that God has spoken to him about this matter. He wants to take immediate legal action. There is no history of previous mental disorders, and family and friends confirm he has never used drugs of any kind; he has a history of good physical health. During the admission interview he admits to having odd ideas about political issues for more than six months, but refrained from sharing them with his friends.

**Table 7.1** Managing challenging situations

| Situation | What to do and what not to do |
|---|---|
| Agitated patient | Don't overwhelm the patient with your questions; conduct several short interviews rather than one long one that upsets the patient.<br>Don't engage the patient in controversial topics.<br>Stay in control all the time.<br>Speak calmly and in a low voice.<br>Proceed with initial sedation if necessary. |
| Manic patient with elated mood, **pressure of speech** and flight of ideas | Be kind and friendly and try to keep the focus of your interview.<br>Redirect the patient to the main topic of the conversation with short phrases like 'We'll talk about that specific topic later but now please let me know…'.<br>Speed up the rhythm of the interview. |
| Distrustful patient with paranoid delusions | Be aware of any signs of irritation and offer help.<br>Carefully listen to the patient's story and show trust.<br>Avoid being judgemental. |
| Demented patient | The scope of the interview is limited by the level of cognitive decline.<br>Ask brief, clear and concrete questions and repeat them if necessary.<br>There are specific bedside tests that are useful in such cases (also see Chapter 30: Psychogeriatrics). |
| Patient with antisocial personality traits or disorder | This type of patient may be aggressive and even dangerous. Antisocial personality disorder is sometimes associated with mood or psychotic disorders and it is important to identify underlying personality traits.<br>Avoid confrontation.<br>Defer responsibility to 'hospital policies' when unreasonable demands cannot be met.<br>See the patient with other members of the multidisciplinary team: remember that safety supersedes confidentiality. |
| Patient in a panic attack | Talk to the patient calmly and in a low voice. Do not hesitate to administer 2–4 mg of Lorazepam IMI.<br>Reassure the patient that he or she is not dying and try to calm his or her breathing.<br>Explain your understanding of the situation and your management plan. |

common, rather than a rare, disorder. Taylor and Vaidya (2009) mention a corollary of Sutton's Law, the Zebra Principle, which states that outside of sub-Saharan Africa, if you hear hoof beats it will likely be a horse, not a zebra.Both principles refer to the same phenomenon: think of the commonest conditions first.

The scenario in case study 7.2 illustrates this principle.

In this case, Sutton's Law tells us that the commonest diagnosis is that of postpartum depression and that the obsessive-compulsive symptoms are merely part of the clinical picture and not the main diagnosis. After a month on venlafaxine 150 mg/day and psychotherapy she showed significant improvement.

### 7.4.3 The rule of parsimony: The simplest explanation is usually the best explanation

Instead of thinking of five different conditions affecting the same patient at the same time, think of one condition that could give the five different types of manifestations.

The scenario in case study 7.3 illustrates this principle.

The patient's attacks were typical panic attacks, suggesting a diagnosis of a panic disorder. The symptoms and the physical examination, however, indicate the characteristic features of a vitamin B12 deficiency caused by pernicious anaemia. Instead of making two separate diagnoses, the diagnosis of anxiety disorder due to pernicious anaemia covers the full clinical presentation of this patient.

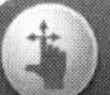

## Case study 7.2

A 24-year-old woman who was learning to take care of her two-month-old infant was deeply distressed by thoughts that she might accidentally kill the baby by dropping her. She felt tired and on edge, crying frequently, and complained of **insomnia** and being unable to cope with her maternal duties. She found herself constantly checking the floor to see if there was a soft area in case the baby fell. She also found herself washing her hands excessively because of her concern that she might transmit an infection of some sort to the baby, who would then die from the transmitted agent. When she was evaluated for treatment, she adamantly denied any hostile thoughts toward the child. However, when the clinician explained to her that wishes to harm the child and hostile feelings towards the child are part of the normal mothering experience, the patient's defensiveness decreased and she was able to acknowledge that she harboured such thoughts. She immediately condemned herself for having them and was deeply worried that the interviewer would be just as harsh on her as she was on herself.

## Case study 7.3

A 57-year-old retired teacher, mother of two, sought help for the onset of a series of attacks in which she experienced intense apprehension, edginess and the need to move to an open place to relieve her sense of discomfort. The most recent episode happened the day before, around 5:00 a.m., the time she usually wakes up every day. After walking for ten minutes in fresh air she felt much better, but a residual feeling of anxiety remained for the whole day. During the examination the patient denied palpitations, dyspnoea, paraesthesia or other somatic complaints. She also denied changes in appetite or weight, feeling depressed or lack of energy. She admitted to taking Lorazepam 2,5 mg b.d. (prescribed by a general practitioner) for the past four weeks. She also noted mild memory problems of late. Further inquiry established she had an intermittent pain in the right arm and sometimes felt unstable waking; she said she had stomach problems and frequent diarrhoea for the past year. During the physical examination, she presented with pale skin, a sore tongue and bleeding gums. Laboratory investigations revealed a macrocytic anaemia and vitamin B12 deficiency. Treatment with vitamin B12 replacement solved the problem and the attacks did not recur in six months after treatment.

## Conclusion

The guidelines, rules and principles discussed here are a good starting point when examining a patient, but the art of diagnosis remains closely linked to experience and a sound knowledge of clinical psychiatry and psychiatric epidemiology.

Patients do not read textbooks, so do not expect to see all the typical symptoms in any one patient. Use all your resources and don't hesitate to ask for a second opinion from another colleague or from your seniors.

# References


American Psychiatric Association (2013) *Diagnostic and Statistical Manual of Mental Disorders* (5th edition). Arlington, VA: American Psychiatric Association

American Psychiatric Association (2000) *Diagnostic and Statistical Manual of Mental Disorders* (4th edition, text revision). Washington DC: American Psychiatric Association

American Psychiatric Association (2006) *Practice guideline for the psychiatric evaluation of adults* (2nd edition). Washington (DC): American Psychiatric Association

Brannon G. *History and Mental Status Examination.* http://emedicine.medscape.com/ (Accessed 21 November 2010)

Casey P, Kelly B (2007) *Fish's Clinical Psychopathology* (3rd edition). London: RCPsych Publications

Lingard L, Haber R (1999) What do we mean by 'relevance'? A clinical and rhetorical definition with implications for teaching and learning the Case Presentation format. *Academic Medicine* 74(10): 124–7

Taylor M, Vaidya N (2009) *Descriptive Psychopathology. The Signs and Symptoms of Behavioral Disorders.* Cambridge: Cambridge University Press

World Health Organization (1993) *The ICD-10 Classification of Mental and Behavioural Disorders.* Geneva: World Health Organization

CHAPTER

# 8 Person-centred psychiatry

*Manfred Böhmer*

## 8.1 Introduction

The explosion of knowledge and rapid scientific developments have contributed immensely to progress in medicine and psychiatry and the possibility of better treatment and care. This has, however, also led to increased specialisation with a resultant fragmentation and **compartmentalisation** of service, an over-dependency on technology and often a materialistic orientation. A present danger is that the focus is on symptoms and illness and not on the person, with the physician becoming a technologist and the patient an object whose resources are not recognised. In response to these limitations of modern medicine, a person-centred approach has emerged.

## 8.2 Person-centred psychiatry

Person-centred psychiatry is an initiative to place the whole person, rather than the disease, at the centre of mental health care (Mezzich *et al.*, 2010). In 2005 the World Psychiatric Association established an Institutional Program of Psychiatry for the Person, aimed at promoting a psychiatric approach with the following characteristics (Mezzich *et al.*, 2010; Mezzich *et al.*, 2011; Miles and Mezzich, 2011):

- of the person: the totality of the person's health is addressed, including both the illness and the positive aspects
- by the person: psychiatrists and other health professionals extend themselves as total human beings and not merely as technicians
- for the person: the focus is not merely on the management of disease, but the fulfilment of the person's health aspirations and life project is promoted
- with the person: working respectfully and in an empowering manner.

Person-centred psychiatry is contingent on the quality of the therapeutic relationship and an integrative approach to the mind, the body and the spirit. It is an approach that combines science with a concern for the dignity, autonomy, values and responsibility of every person involved – including the patient, his or her family members and the physician. The whole person is treated, since it is impossible for a part to be well if the whole is not well (Mezzich *et al.*, 2010). This fits into the World Health Organization's definition of health as a complete state of physical, emotional and social well-being, and not merely the absence of disease (Mezzich, 2005). There is no health without mental health.

Evidence-based treatments and algorithms are valuable, but not enough for the complex needs of people with a mental illness. The bio-psycho-social-spiritual model is an attempt to address these complex needs and to take cognizance of all the possible contributors to the illness of the patient and of the different aspects of patient care. Even in this model there is the danger of fragmentation and of not engaging with the patient as person. Person-centred psychiatry is aware of this danger and tries to address it by emphasising that a bio-psycho-social-spiritual model must be embedded in a relationship approach and that a personalised approach is needed for each patient. The illness of the patient has to be understood in the context of his or her life story and current illness narrative. Health is more than the **remission** of disease: it requires the reduction of vulnerability to disease and the cultivation of **positive health**, of life satisfaction and virtues such as kindness and patience (Allen, 2007; Cloninger, 2011). The core hypothesis of positive health is that the experience of well-being contributes to the effective functioning of multiple biological systems, which may keep the person from succumbing to disease or may help promote recovery (Ryff *et al.*, 2004). The goal is to promote wellness and quality of life (Mezzich, 2005; Allen, 2007).

Table 8.1 shows the differing approaches of the traditional view of mental health versus the positive health model.

**Table 8.1** Views of mental health

| Traditional view | Positive health |
| --- | --- |
| The focus is on illness and its burdens, diagnosing disorders and grading disability | The focus is on well-being, with recovery, wellness and functioning being emphasised |
| Experience of illness | Experience of health, e.g. self-awareness, resilience, fulfilment |
| The contributors to illness are researched | Contributors to health are identified |
| The mind and belief system of the patient is not seen as something to understand and address | The mind and belief system of the patient is seen as critical to the desired outcome |
| The inner attitude of the patient is not addressed | The inner attitude of the patient towards his or her illness and life is very important |
| Health is defined as the absence of illness | Health is seen as something that must be created; the strengths of the patient must be identified to facilitate this |
| Fragmentary | Integrative |

**Source:** Adapted from Mezzich *et al.*, 2010. Reprinted with permission from the Canadian Psychiatric Association.

## 8.3 Diagnosis

The conventional purpose of diagnosis is to classify an illness, to link it to an existing understanding of the illness and in this process to elucidate potential causes, underlying mechanisms and the likely course, and to plan appropriate treatment.

In a person-centred approach, diagnosis can be seen as an attempt to understand what goes on in the body and mind of the patient (Mezzich *et al.*, 2010). Since health involves the ability to pursue one's goals in life, the person's life context must be assessed. An understanding of an illness involves understanding the interactive aspects of a bio-psycho-social-spiritual framework, the interaction between patient and others, patient and culture, as well as environment.

## 8.4 Models of practising medicine

A physician can operate from within three different models of practising medicine (Charles *et al.*, 1997; Moreau *et al.*, 2012):

- a paternalistic model, in which the physician decides what is best for the patient
- a consumerist-informative model, in which the autonomous patient makes a decision after having been informed of the options
- a shared decision-making model, in which decisions are reached through discussions between physician and patient and where the patient plays an active role in this decision-making process.

Although these models overlap to a certain degree, the shared decision-making model is often considered the ideal approach. The physician must be flexible in moving between them, since an elderly patient, for example, may prefer the paternalistic model. In person-centred psychiatry such preferences should be noted and respected.

Patients have a huge need for information, regardless of the model. Information exchange by question-response reinforces the therapeutic alliance and allows the patient to develop a better understanding of the treatment options available to him or her (Moreau *et al.*, 2012). Physicians who are emotionally involved and give more information achieve greater patient involvement (Van den Brink-Muinen *et al.*, 2006).

There is more and more evidence that suggests that non-pharmacological factors and non-specific factors in the pharmacological treatment of patients are at least as potent as the accepted active ingredients in the medication and that **empathy** plays a role in the outcome of treatment (Mintz and Flynn, 2012). One study showed that diabetic patients of physicians who scored high on empathy had a significantly lower rate of acute metabolic complications (Del Canale *et al.*, 2012).

The treatment process requires a high-quality relationship in which trust, the quality of non-verbal communication and allowing the patient time to think, are facilitating factors. Obstacles to this process include:

- serious and emergency situations
- a patient having trouble making requests
- a perception of the physician as not being competent
- the fear of knowing about one's potentially serious medical condition (Moreau *et al.*, 2012).

The physician must keep in mind that this is a process of information exchange with a layperson: simple language and a need for repeated explanations are often necessary. Table 8.2 compares the bio-medical and person-centred models of medicine.

## 8.5 Dynamic psychiatry

The classification systems used in psychiatry, whether the American Diagnostic and Statistical Manual of Mental Disorders (DSM) or the World Health Organization's International Statistical Classification of Diseases and Related Health Problems (ICD), are descriptive systems based on phenomenology. The diseases described are defined as syndromes not linked to a specific aetiology.

Descriptive psychiatry categorises patients according to clusters of symptoms and common behavioural and phenomenological features. The patient's subjective experience is less important. When diagnosing a patient according to the DSM-5 system with a major depressive disorder, for example, the physician will look for features that a patient has in common with others who suffer from a similar problem and provide a summary label. The diagnosis in descriptive psychiatry, however, cannot and does not indicate the complexity of the different factors and chain of events leading to the development of a mental illness in a specific individual: it is reductionist

**Table 8.2** Models of medicine

| Bio-medical model | Person-centred model |
|---|---|
| Focus on symptoms, the patient as carrier of illness | Focus on the person<br>The patient as person comes first<br>Value and dignity of patient emphasised |
| Diagnosis of an illness | Diagnosis of an illness in the context of the life history and current illness narrative<br>Illness experience explored |
| Relationship between physician and patient not important | Patient-physician relationship central to treatment |
| Person of physician not important; impersonal provider of care | Person of physician very important |
| Non-verbal communication not seen as important | Non-verbal communication very important |
| Treating illness | Treating illness while simultaneously promoting prevention and emphasising positive health |
| Patient not recognised as an expert and partner | Patient competence and expertise (acquired from having a specific illness, e.g. type 1 diabetes mellitus) recognised |
| Knowledge of people not important | Knowledge of people important |

and does not provide any information about the person suffering from the disease.

In descriptive psychiatry the question asked when categorising patients is,'How are patients similar to each other?' (Gabbard, 2005). Taken to the extreme, a psychiatrist using this approach could treat a patient based purely on the symptoms and behaviour displayed, without any knowledge of the patient's life history.

**Dynamic psychiatry** (or psychodynamic psychiatry) is a different and person-centred approach (Schmolke, 2011). It looks at what is unique about each patient and how a particular patient differs from others as a result of their specific life history (Gabbard, 2005). Symptoms and behaviour are seen as an expression of underlying psychological and biological forces with a hidden logic and meaning. Dynamic psychiatry encompasses descriptive psychiatry, but is furthermore interested in the subjective and personal experiences of the individual. A basic **psychological mindedness** is fostered, meaning that a patient is not just seen as someone with only a descriptive diagnosis, but as a person whose difficulties and problems must be understood in relation to events and how the person interpreted these events and reacted to them.

Dynamic psychiatry also addresses the question of how a person continually recreates his or her internal conflicts in external situations. Patients can, for example, unconsciously recreate their internal world and their inner conflicts in the interpersonal field, in the interaction between themselves and their psychiatrist. Internal conflicts are then played out in the therapeutic relationship (Gabbard, 2005; Böhmer, 2011).

The question in dynamic psychiatry is therefore how one patient differs from another with a similar descriptive diagnosis, who this person is, what makes him or her unique, what happened in his or her life, why he or she now presents with this problem, and what the meaning of this is for him or her (Böhmer, 2011).

## Conclusion

A constant danger in medical practice is to treat disorders and not persons. In such an approach the therapeutic relationship is not recognised as important; the mistaken belief is that the ability to diagnose and prescribe or operate is enough. There is, however, substantial evidence to the contrary and it is important to take cognisance of the person-centred and dynamic models in psychiatry. A sophisticated knowledge of important dynamic concepts such as resistance, **transference** and **counter-transference** can be helpful in clinical work and **pharmacotherapy** (see Chapter 37: Psychological interventions).

# References


Allen D, Carlson D, Ham C (2007) Well-being: New paradigms of wellness – inspiring positive health outcomes and renewing hope. *American Journal of Health Promotion* 21(3): 1–9

Böhmer MW (2011) Dynamic psychiatry and the psychodynamic formulation. *African Journal of Psychiatry* 14: 273–7

Charles C, Gafni A, Whelan T (1997) Shared decision-making in the medical encounter: What does it mean (or it takes at least two to tango), *Social Science and Medicine* 44(5): 681–92

Cloninger CR, Abou-Saleh MT, Mrazek DA, Möller HJ (2011) Biological perspectives on psychiatry for the person. *The International Journal of Person Centered Medicine* 1(1): 137–9

Del Canale S, Louis DZ, Maio V, Wang X, Rossi G, Hojat M, Gonella JS (2012) The relationship between physician empathy and disease complication: An empirical study of primary care physicians and their diabetic patients in Parma, Italy. *Academic Medicine* 87: 1243–9

Gabbard GO (2005) *Psychodynamic psychiatry* (4th edition). Arlington: American Psychiatric Publishing

Mezzich JE (2005) Positive health: Conceptual place, dimensions and implications. *Psychopathology* 38: 177–9

Mezzich JE, Christodoulou GN, Fulford KWM (2011) Introduction to the conceptual bases of psychiatry for the person. *The International Journal of Person Centered Medicine* 1(1): 121–4

Mezzich JE, Salloum IM, Cloninger CR, Salvador-Carulla L, Kirmayer LJ, Banzato CEM, Wallcraft J, Botbol M (2010) Person-centred integrative diagnosis: Conceptual bases and structural model. *Canadian Journal of Psychiatry*, 55(11): 701–8.

Miles M, Mezzich JE (2011) Advancing the global communication of scholarship and research for personalized healthcare (Editorial). *The International Journal of Person Centered Medicine* 1(1): 1–5

Mintz DL, Flynn DF (2012) How (not what) to prescribe: Nonpharmacologic aspects of psychopharmacology. *Psychiatric Clinics of North America* 35: 143–63

Moreau A, Carol L, Dedianne MC, Dupraz C, Perdrix C, Lainé X, Souweine G (2012) What perception do patients have about decision making? Toward an integrative patient-centred care model. A qualitative study using focus-groups interviews. *Patient Education and Counseling* 87: 206–11

Ryff CD, Singer BH, Love GD (2004) Positive health: Connecting well-being with biology. *Philosophical Transactions of the Royal Society* 359: 1383–94

Schmolke M (2011) Person-centred psychodynamic perspectives. *The International Journal of Person Centered Medicine1* (1): 105–8

Van den Brink-Muinen A, Van Dulmen S, de Haes H, Visser A, Schellevis F, Bensing J (2006) Has patients' involvement in the decision-making process changed over time? *Health Expectations* 9(4): 333–42

CHAPTER

# 9 Investigating psychiatric disorders

*John Joska, James Warwick*

## 9.1 Introduction

Psychiatry as a field relies primarily on clinical assessment for diagnosis. This is underscored by the structure of the commonly used diagnostic systems: the DSM-5 and the ICD-10. These publications base the main criteria of disorders on clinical observation and report, while exclusion criteria, such as for general medical conditions (GMC), are considered later. In this way, laboratory and imaging investigations have been used mainly to exclude or diagnose physical abnormalities or to monitor psychotropic levels or adverse effects. Psychiatry has not yet entered the era where investigations are used to include or confirm diagnosis, but this may happen with the incremental development of newer technologies.

In this chapter, we will present a rational approach to using investigations to augment the diagnostic and therapeutic process in psychiatry. Two factors must be considered when requesting and subjecting patients to undergo investigation: patient care and safety as well as cost effectiveness and cost utility. There is no generic approach that can be applied to all cases: each must be considered individually. The principles that apply are explored below. We then proceed to discuss the role and use of individual investigations. Several commonly encountered syndromes are presented for discussion of a rational approach to investigation. Finally we discuss the potential utility of risk categories as a consideration in investigating patients.

## 9.2 Considerations when performing investigations

A current dilemma facing psychiatrists and mental health professionals is the **splitting** of disorders based on primary and secondary causes. In this view, a psychiatric disorder is caused either by a primary (or functional) disorder or by an underlying (or secondary) physical one. The reality is likely to be more complex – some disorders occur without there being overt secondary causes, some occur when triggered or aggravated by an underlying factor, while others may be driven mainly by the secondary cause (and disappear when the offending cause is removed). A case in point is the co-existence of psychosis and substance abuse, for example; cannabis. Some individuals may develop psychosis in the absence of cannabis abuse, others will abuse cannabis and psychosis will be triggered and persist (in some cases for longer or shorter periods) and still others might abuse cannabis and display psychotic behaviour only whilst using the substance. (Note: the diagnostic interplay between intoxication and psychosis is not debated here.) Any psychiatric disorder or symptom, therefore, may be precipitated or aggravated by a physical factor, and these must be sought by thorough history taking, physical examination and directed investigation. The nature of the investigation will be guided by the findings across a number of domains, which we will discuss now.

### 9.2.1 Likelihood of secondary cause

Many highly prevalent psychiatric disorders, such as major depression, tend to follow a typical pattern of onset, course and outcome. Furthermore, while major depressive disorder (MDD) may indeed be associated with secondary causes, these occur much less commonly than primary MDD. In this way, major depression in a 30-year-old patient may be less intensively investigated than MDD presenting for the first time in a 60-year-old patient. Using another example, post-traumatic stress disorder (PTSD) occurs following a particular type of life event, and the diagnosis is made based on clinical phenomena. PTSD is an example of a disorder where medical causes are usually not considered. Despite the role of underlying biological vulnerability factors, such as genetic predisposition, clinicians pursue investigations only when unusual features or outcomes ensue.

### 9.2.2 Abnormal clinical findings on history or examination

Symptom patterns in psychiatric disorders may raise flags for the potential presence of underlying physical causes. These include late onset of some disorders, more rapid or fluctuating course, organic flags such as non-auditory hallucinosis and poor or non-response to medications.

### 9.2.3 Cost-effectiveness, availability and sensitivity or specificity of the investigation

Clinicians must be guided by the principles of targeting investigations and considering whether the diagnostic yield justifies its routine use. Examples include the requesting of a full blood counts when a haemoglobin (HB) would suffice, or requesting brain magnetic resonance imaging (MRI) when computed tomography (CT) is adequate (and sometimes preferable). There is also a difference between screening and targeted or directed investigations.

In screening, the investigation is used to detect subclinical disease across a wide patient group. The benefits of screening – detection and improved management – are true positives and must be weighed against the costs (that is, direct financial cost and cost of further unnecessary investigations, or false positives and false negatives).

Directed investigations are used when there is a clinical symptom or indicator. The distinction may become blurred when the mere presence of a psychiatric disorder is regarded as a symptom indicator to perform, for example, thyroid function tests or syphilis serology. Depression, for example, may be regarded as a disorder for which it is important to screen for thyroid disease. The thyroid stimulating hormone (TSH) is a relatively expensive test. In practice, hypothyroidism is uncommon in patients younger than 50, and is usually accompanied by other physical signs.

### 9.2.4 Presence of medical co-morbidity

Medical conditions contribute in varying degrees to psychiatric symptoms. Their effects may be direct or indirect (through the stress of having the physical condition). They may be quiescent or in remission or they may be more or less commonly associated with psychiatric disorder (e.g. hypertension is less commonly associated with a psychiatric disorder on its own than hypothyroidism). Investigations in these instances are directed towards the involvement of the relevant organ.

### 9.2.5 Need for monitoring

Almost all psychotropic treatments are associated with adverse physiological effects, and many of these can be measured by the use of laboratory and other tests, including haematological, renal, liver and metabolic effects. In many cases, some tests must be performed prior to initiating medication. In women of childbearing age, in addition to education and counselling, it may be necessary to perform urine or serum pregnancy tests, especially when **teratogenicity** of agents has been reported. The use of pretreatment physiological measurements is based on the expected side-effect profile of the prescribed agent. Baseline thyroid and renal function tests, for example, are important in patients starting lithium therapy, but liver function tests are not. Similarly, drug level monitoring is most useful when agents have narrow therapeutic ranges or when clinical toxicity develops.

## 9.3 Utility and cost-effectiveness of screening tests in psychiatry

The potential benefit of laboratory investigations to detect physical disease must be weighed against the cost of their widespread use. This refers to cost:benefit ratio.

In psychiatry, in patients previously diagnosed and investigated, there is little evidence of any benefit of tests other than serum glucose estimation (using a finger-prick or other means), urea and creatinine measurement. The rationale for excluding impaired glucose metabolism or low glucose is clear: hypoglycaemia and hyperglycaemia are associated with an impaired level of consciousness, due to the brain's dependence on glucose for its metabolism. The role of renal function as a measure of acute or chronic disease is less well established and may not be warranted in resource-limited settings. In patients older than 50, a urine analysis is both cost-effective and associated with a high yield. In women in this age group, the increased incidence of hypothyroidism may support performing a TSH investigation.

Further laboratory tests are only requested if specifically indicated and when the cost of performing the investigation is justified, such as when there are clinical grounds to suspect that a particular condition may be present.

There is no place for proxy testing (e.g. using the white cell count to establish compromised immunity in HIV infection).

## 9.4 Specific investigations

### 9.4.1 Renal and liver function tests

The use of renal function tests in routine screening in resource-limited settings is controversial. Some texts recommend the use of urea and creatinine, but their diagnostic value is uncertain (Korn *et al.*, 2000). In instances where hydration is clinically low or medical co-morbidity (such as hypertension) is present, they may be justified. Sodium and potassium levels are useful only when indicated, for example, when hyponatraemia is suspected due to medication.

Liver function tests may be divided into measures of inflammation (trans-aminases), obstruction (gamma glutamyltransferase (GGT)), bilirubin and alkaline phosphatase (ALP) and nutrition (albumin and protein). Different medical conditions may affect one or all of these enzyme systems. Liver function tests are usually only requested if an indication or medical cause is present and should not be used for undirected screening. For standard assessment of liver function, testing of ALP, albumin and alanine aminotransferase (ALT) is sufficient. If alcohol abuse is suspected, it may be useful to test for GGT, which usually remains elevated for 24 to 48 hours after alcohol intake has ceased.

### 9.4.2 Thyroid function tests

Hypothyroidism is present in only 0,1% of individuals younger than 50, and so should only be tested for when two or more symptoms of clinical hypothyroidism are present. In older individuals, the increased incidence of hypothyroidism warrants TSH screening in the absence of **physical symptoms**. These include weakness, stiffness, poor appetite, constipation, menstrual irregularities, slowed speech, apathy, impaired memory and even hallucinations and delusions.

A regular evaluation of thyroid function is indicated in patients who receive lithium therapy. Thyroid hormone tests (T3 and T4) are only indicated when TSH is abnormal or supplementation is being used. Special endocrine tests, such as the thyrotropin-releasing hormone stimulation test, are indicated in patients who have marginally abnormal thyroid test results with suspected subclinical hypothyroidism. These should be requested in consultation with an endocrinologist.

## 9.4.3 Syphilis tests

A wide variety of mental disorders are caused by neurosyphilis, including depressive illness, **hypomania**, delirium, dementia and personality change (e.g. frontal lobe syndrome). Neurological signs, such as pupillary changes, may only be present in 25–50% of cases (Hutto, 2001). The serum rapid plasma regain (RPR) is the most common screening test for syphilis, and we recommend screening all first-episode individuals with severe mental illness. The RPR confirms exposure to syphilis, and treatment to prevent progression and onward transmission is indicated. If the RPR is positive, it is followed up with the specific fluorescent treponema antibody-absorption (FTA-ABS) or TPHA test, which uses the spirochaete *treponema pallidum* as the antigen, and is generally a very reliable test.

If neurosyphilis is suspected (through the presence of atypical psychiatric features or neurologic signs) a treponemal test is recommended, even if the RPR is not done or is negative. In cases where the serum RPR and/or treponemal test is positive, a lumbar puncture must be performed. A cerebro-spinal fluid (CSF) RPR is then usually performed, as this establishes past or present treponemal activity and the need for intravenous penicillin therapy. It is usual in cases of neurosyphilis to find other typical CSF findings, such as elevated CSF protein and leucocytes. In this way a positive RPR with clear and acellular CSF suggests that neurosyphilis is either treated or inactive, while a positive TPHA/FTA and a high-protein and cellular CSF suggest more active disease. The presence of HIV (human immunodeficiency virus) infection, however, may change the findings, so consultation may be necessary when interpreting results.

## 9.4.4 HIV tests

Psychiatric syndromes commonly encountered in HIV-infected patients are dementia and delirium. Two assay techniques, the enzyme-linked immunosorbent assay (ELISA) and the Western blot assay are widely used to detect the presence of HIV antibodies in human serum. The ELISA is used as a screening test only, as false-positive results may occur. If the result is positive, the Western blot test is used to confirm positivity. A negative HIV test indicates that either the person has not been infected with the HIV virus, or has been infected but has not yet developed antibodies. Seroconversion (the point at which the HIV antibody test becomes positive) usually occurs six to 12 weeks after infection but can take six to 12 months in some cases. Appropriate counselling before the test is necessary, and must also be given in the case of positive test results. The ethics of testing patients with severe mental illness for HIV has been debated; tests may be performed according to certain guidelines and in consultation with a senior clinician (Joska *et al.*, 2008).

## 9.4.5 Haematological tests

The tests making up the full blood count (FBC) form an important aspect of investigation of a patient with suspected medical disorders. In young healthy adults, use of the FBC for screening is not necessary. The FBC becomes useful when older age, medical disorders or specific psychotropic treatments are considered. Older patients with neurocognitive disorders need a screening FBC, as do patients who are being initiated on therapy with clozapine, valproate and carbamazepine.

Other haematological tests include the erythrocyte sedimentation rate (ESR), which is used as a screening tool for inflammatory disease in the elderly, and the serum vitamin B12 and folate tests. Vitamin B12 deficiency gives rise to pernicious anaemia, which is associated with dementia, depression, delirium, fatigue, agitation and psychosis. In some cases, mental symptoms precede the megaloblastic anaemia and subacute combined degeneration of the spinal cord by many months. The neuropsychiatric manifestations usually disappear or improve following parenteral vitamin B12 therapy (hydroxycobalamin). The typical cause of vitamin B12 deficiency is the absence of intrinsic factor in the stomach, which prevents absorption of the vitamin. Other causes include carcinoma of the stomach and gastric surgery. As folic acid deficiency can cause similar mental syndromes, it should be measured together with vitamin B12 levels.

## 9.4.6 Inflammatory disease tests

Systemic lupus erythematosus (SLE) is a connective tissue disease and is relatively common in South Africa. Psychiatric complications include psychosis, depression, delirium, dementia and changes in personality. Most of the mental disturbances appear to be transient, usually remitting within a couple of weeks, but episodes are often recurrent. The ESR is raised in most of the cases. Other laboratory tests for SLE include the antinuclear antibody and anti-DNA tests. Some patients have a false-positive venereal diseases research laboratories (VDRL) test.

## 9.4.7 Substance abuse tests

Substance abuse is frequently co-morbid with psychotic and other psychiatric disorders. Where the history clearly reveals substance use, there is little value in performing toxicology for diagnostic purposes. However, urine and serum screening may be helpful where the history is unclear. It should be noted that substances are present in urine for varying periods: amphetamines (including methamphetamine) and cocaine for two days, benzodiazepines and opiates for three days, and cannabis for two to four weeks.

## 9.4.8 Cerebro-spinal fluid tests

CSF analysis is usually conducted as a second-tier investigation when a neurological disease is suspected. These include infections (virus, bacteria, fungus), inflammation (multiple sclerosis, lupus, non-infective encephalitis), vascular (sub-arachnoid haemorrhage), tumours (primary or secondary brain tumours), or pressure (pseudo-tumour cerebri). Patients who present with psychiatric disorders that are considered secondary to medical conditions (e.g. HIV or early-onset dementia) require CSF sampling. CSF investigations for diagnostic biomarkers (such as beta-amyloid for Alzheimer's disease) do not yet form part of routine practice.

## 9.4.9 Electroencephalograms

Electroencephalograms (EEGs) are not regarded as routine investigations, but they are often requested in psychiatric settings. They are of use in the clinical syndromes of first-episode psychosis (FEP), episodic behavioural disturbance, or altered levels of alertness. Abnormal EEG findings may be grouped into:

- paroxysmal activity seen in seizures (approximately 20% of EEGs are normal in epilepsy)
- non-paroxysmal slowing seen in delirium
- asymmetric activity seen in focal lesions of stroke or tumours
- sleep abnormalities, as seen in REM sleep disorder or sleep apnoea.

Specialised EEG and related investigations, including polysomnography and evoked potentials are generally requested after consultation with a neurologist. They are useful to confirm the diagnosis of a seizure disorder or when delirium is suspected but clinically uncertain. An EEG may also be useful in distinguishing between impaired levels of alertness due to delirium or catatonia: a normal EEG pattern is usually observed in catatonia.

## 9.4.10 Chest X-rays

From a cost-benefit point of view, chest X-rays have no place in routine screening. They should, however, be considered when respiratory symptoms are present and in the patient with a history of smoking and a late-onset cognitive disorder or an atypical psychiatric disorder.

## 9.4.11 Electrocardiograms

The use of electrocardiograms (ECGs) has become more controversial with the increased vigilance surrounding the complications of antipsychotics and the QT interval. It is recommended that patients with a history of cardiac disease or a family history of sudden death or arrhythmia undergo routine ECG screening prior to commencing treatment with tricyclic antidepressants or antipsychotics.

## 9.4.12 Neuro-imaging

Neuro-imaging is providing important new insights into our understanding of the pathology underlying most psychiatric conditions (Capote, 2009). Neuro-imaging can be broadly divided into structural and functional imaging. Modalities used to image the structure of the brain are more familiar to the majority of clinicians and include CT and MRI. In psychiatry, functional imaging is used more commonly in the research realm, although some clinical applications exist. These include techniques such as single photon emission computed tomography (SPECT), positron emission tomography (PET) and a number of functional techniques based on MRI.

Given its higher cost and limited availability, particularly in resource-limited environments, the use of neuro-imaging in clinical psychiatry must be evidence based and justified by careful evaluation of its costs and benefits.

### 9.4.12.1 Structural brain imaging

CT and MRI provide exquisitely detailed structural information about the brain. CT is based on the tomographic reconstruction of a three-dimensional volume from X-rays obtained rotating 360 degrees around the patient's head. The image depicts the differential attenuation of X-rays by different brain tissues. Interpretation of the images may be improved by the use of an intravenous contrast agent.

Structural MRI is based on the principle of nuclear magnetic resonance. Protons in the patient's body are aligned in a strong magnetic field and then exposed to an electromagnetic field at a specific frequency which results in the protons changing to a higher-energy state by flipping their orientation. When the electromagnetic field is turned off, the protons return to their rest state, thereby generating an electromagnetic signal that is detected by the scanner to produce an image of these emissions. These studies are sensitive for the detection of pathology that results in anatomical changes and/or alterations of the tissue properties being measured (e.g. in tumour, haemorrhage or infarction). Generally these studies are not routinely indicated for the majority of psychiatric patients, except when a specific underlying medical condition is suspected clinically.

### 9.4.12.2 Functional brain imaging

Functional brain imaging has undergone exciting developments in the research context in the last 30 years. While these studies have contributed much to our understanding of the pathophysiology of many psychiatric conditions, their role in routine clinical settings is currently limited to a few indications. SPECT is currently the most widely available functional brain imaging technique and is also relatively less expensive. However, PET is becoming more available and affordable due to rapid growth in its applications in oncology. PET has the advantages of more accurate quantification and better spatial resolution. SPECT and PET are both based on the tomographic imaging of gamma rays emitted by radiopharmaceuticals that are injected intravenously. The image provides an in-vivo measurement of the biodistribution of the radiopharmaceutical in the brain. The information provided by the image is therefore dependent on the radio-labelled molecule that is administered and how it is handled biochemically in the brain: $^{99m}$Tc-HMPAO provides information about brain perfusion, while $^{123}$I-FP-CIT is used for dopamine transporter density, $^{18}$F-FDG for glucose metabolism and $^{11}$C-PiB for beta-amyloid plaque density.

Molecular imaging using these techniques has the potential to provide vast amounts of information about brain function that are already showing their value in research, but are likely to have an expanding clinical role in future. A number of functional techniques based on MRI technology include functional MRI (fMRI), which can detect changes in blood oxygen **utilisation** in response to different mental paradigms, and magnetic resonance spectroscopy, which is able to provide information about the relative density of different molecules in brain tissue.

The measurement of functional changes in the brain using these techniques may result in further blurring of the distinction between primary and secondary causes of psychiatric conditions set out in the beginning of this chapter, as both have been shown to alter brain function. Conditions where brain SPECT and PET have an established role include dementias, SLE, trauma, and epilepsy (Warwick, 2004).

While these techniques are very sensitive, they are not specific in the majority of psychiatry scenarios. Generally brain perfusion or metabolism patterns do not correspond to clinical diagnoses as set out in the DSM or the ICD. This problem can be reduced if findings are interpreted in the light of all clinical and laboratory information. Some groups include functional imaging for clinical psychiatry in a multidisciplinary context. This can provide objective information of regional brain function that can facilitate decision-making by supporting or contradicting other information available to clinicians. The development of molecular brain scanning may play a greater role in clinical psychiatry in the future.

## 9.5 Pharmacogenetics and pharmacogenomics

It is now widely accepted that individuals metabolise drugs at different rates. This may lead to high (toxic) or low (non-therapeutic) drug levels. Human drug metabolism is handled by the cytochrome P450 system, with six enzymes being responsible for about 90% of metabolism (Streetman *et al.*, 2000).

Pharmacogenetics refers to the study of genetic variation in drug response and metabolism. This includes understanding the genes responsible for how drugs work (transporters and receptor proteins) and how drugs are metabolised (cytochromes). For cytochromes, polymorphisms (gene variants) may result in more or less effective metabolism, and accordingly more or less available drug.

The types of metabolism that occur are generally grouped into ultra-rapid, extensive, intermediate and poor. Extensive metabolisers have two normal copies of the gene, while ultra-rapid metabolisers have more than two and poor metabolisers have no effective copies.

## 9.6 Psychotropic monitoring

Monitoring of psychotropic medication is useful to determine whether drug levels are sub-normal (in individuals with poor adherence, or ultra-rapid metabolism), normal (for drugs with narrow **therapeutic index**), or above normal (for suspected overdose or poor metabolisers). To determine normal or therapeutic drug levels, it is usual to sample the trough (or prior to the next dose), while a random sample is drawn for toxicity or compliance testing.

### 9.6.1 Mood stabilisers

Laboratory investigations are used prior to initiation of therapy to screen for end-organ disease (and the risk of toxicity) with most mood stabilisers. Dosing intervals during treatment is also an important consideration. In addition, drug levels are needed for lithium therapy, but probably not for valproate and carbamazepine. There is no consensus on how to perform screening and monitoring, but the following guidelines apply:

- lithium: pretreatment renal function and TSH levels are measured, with an ECG if there is history of cardiac disease; then lithium levels are obtained every five to seven days after a dose change; once the dose is stable, levels are measured after a month, and then every six months
- valproate and carbamazepine: pre-treatment liver functions and full blood count are obtained, and then monitored every six to 12 months.

Symptom screening is probably equally important.

**Table 9.1** A comparison of physical and biochemical properties measured using structural and functional imaging techniques

| **Structural imaging techniques** | |
|---|---|
| CT | X-ray attenuation = tissue density |
| MRI – T1 | Spin-lattice relaxation time (varies for different tissues e.g. grey and white matter; water has a darker appearance and fat looks brighter/whiter) |
| MRI – T2 | Spin-spin relaxation time (varies for different tissues e.g. grey and white matter; fat is darker and water is brighter/whiter)<br>Fluid attenuation inversion recovery scans (FLAIR): the bright signal from water is suppressed, providing good differentiation for acute haemorrhage and solid masses |
| MRI – DTI | Principle direction of water diffusion provides information on white matter connectivity, allows exquisitely detailed 3D images of white matter tracts to be generated |
| **Functional imaging techniques** | |
| SPECT – $^{99m}$Tc-HMPAO or $^{99m}$Tc-ECD | cerebral blood flow (surrogate for neuronal function) |
| SPECT – $^{123}$I-FP-CIT (Datscan®) | dopamine transporter density (decreased in Parkinson's disease) |
| PET – $^{18}$F-FDG | neuronal glucose metabolism |
| PET – $^{11}$C-PiB | amyloid plaque density (increased in Alzheimer's disease) |

## 9.6.2 Antipsychotic medication

Drug levels are not routinely monitored for antipsychotics. A pretreatment ECG is needed in patients with a cardiac history or family history of sudden death. Baseline lipogram and glucose are advisable, and should be repeated with patient weight at least annually. The development of a metabolic syndrome in patients who use atypical antipsychotics has prompted the need for an approach to screen for the associated chronic diseases. In general, there are within-class differences, with clozapine and olanzapine being associated with the greatest risk of clinically significant weight gain and other agents producing lower levels of risk. Risperidone, quetiapine, amisulpride and zotepine generally show low to moderate levels of weight gain (Newcomer, 2005). Similarly, these agents may aggravate glycaemic and lipid dyscontrol in the same pattern. While weight gain is most often a clinical marker of underlying hyperglycaemia and dyslipidaemia, it is normal in about 25% of patients with metabolic syndrome. Since metabolic syndrome may be associated with considerable morbidity, screening and monitoring are advised. Given resource limitations, a rational approach is needed.

All patients who are started on an antipsychotic treatment should have their baseline weight recorded. In addition, all patients who are started on an atypical agent should have a fasting glucose and lipogram. Some guidelines suggest that this applies to all antipsychotics. Patients on clozapine and olanzapine should have these measures repeated after six months and then annually. Patients on other agents may have random finger-prick glucose done annually and fasting glucose and lipogram tests done after one year and then annually if weight gain is marked, there are other risk factors or if other symptoms emerge.

## 9.7 Psychological testing

Formal neuropsychological, intelligence and personality testing can assist with both the diagnosis and monitoring of the treatment progress. Bedside neuropsychological testing usually forms part of the neuropsychiatric assessment, while formal referral to a registered psychologist for formal batteries of tests may be helpful in some cases.

## 9.7.1 Neuropsychological testing

Neuropsychology is the study of the relationship between brain function and cognition, behaviour and personality.

Neuropsychological tests use standardised methods that are quantifiable and reliable. They assess cognitive and behavioural changes secondary to a range of brain pathologies, such as injury, disease or developmental abnormalities. These tests can aid in identifying cognitive defects, in diagnostic dilemmas (such as differentiating between depression and dementia), in evaluating and planning treatment programmes, in evaluating learning abnormalities and in the localisation of lesions.

Brain damage will affect cognition; the pattern of the deficit will vary with the nature and site of the injury. A hierarchical and anatomical approach is a useful method. In this way, the clinician tests diffuse brain functions (or domains) first: alertness, attention/concentration and memory. This is followed by the cortical functions in hierarchical order: speech and language functions (left hemisphere), recognition/gnosis (mainly right but also both hemispheres), **praxis** (mainly right hemisphere) and executive functions (both frontal lobes). Subcortical function is assessed by performance speed and behavioural apathy tests. Bedside approaches to neuropsychology must be brief and cover most of these domains (which they do to varying degrees). The Mini-Mental State Examination (MMSE) (Folstein *et al.*, 1975) is the most commonly used but does not test executive functions well. Other short tests, such as the Montreal Cognitive Assessment (MOCA) improve on this (www.mocatest.org). Additional bedside tests, such as clock-drawing, verbal fluency, trail-making and go-no-go tests, may be added to a battery as needed (Huntzinger *et al.*, 1992; Lezak, 1995). Formal neuropsychological batteries are compiled from an array of tests intended to measure the different neuropsychological domains that may be affected by the disorder in question. It is usual to include at least two tests of each domain in a battery.

In neuropsychiatric disorders, clinicians are interested mainly in frontal lobe functions, and these are typically measured by tests of executive function, such as the Wisconsin Card Sorting Test (Milner, 1963), the Stroop Color and Word Test, and the Color Trails 2 tests (Golden, 1978). Problem-solving, abstraction and **impulsivity** tests are also useful.

Neuropsychological tests are affected by differences in language, culture and education.

## 9.7.2 Intelligence testing

Intelligence can be defined as a person's ability to assimilate knowledge, to recall events, to reason logically, to synthesise forms and to deal with problems and priorities. A score (intelligence quotient or IQ) of 100 corresponds to the 50th percentile in intellectual ability for the general population. The normal IQ range is considered to be 85 to 115, which falls between the 25th and 75th percentiles. IQ testing does not differentiate learned from innate abilities and is not free of cultural bias.

There are also types of intelligence that are not specifically measured by standard tests, such as linguistic, musical, interpersonal, and logical or mathematical abilities.

The most widely used intelligence test is the Wechsler Adult Intelligence Scale (WAIS, 2008), which has validated versions for children and pre-schoolers. A South African version is also available. The WAIS is divided into verbal and non-verbal components. The verbal component has six subscales and the non-verbal five subscales. The reliability of the scale is high. The verbal scale measures retention of information and is more sensitive to education than the performance scale. The non-verbal performance scale measures visuospatial capacity and speed and is more sensitive to ageing than the verbal scale. Performance anxiety tends to lower scores on the arithmetic and memory for digits subscales.

### 9.7.3 Personality tests

There are a number of structured, standardised measurement instruments for the assessment of personality. These are mostly self-report questionnaires or inventories that use direct questions to probe a range of personality variables. These include the Minnesota Multiphasic Personality Inventory (MMPI) (Ben-Porath *et al.*, 2009), the Millon Clinical Multi-axial Inventory (MCMI), which has the advantage of being correlated with DSM diagnoses (Framingham, 2011), and the 16 Personality Factor Questionnaire (Cattell *et al.*,1993). They must be administered and interpreted by a trained technician; the results must be interpreted in the context of the clinical assessment.

## 9.8 Low and high risk for physical disorder

There are no published guidelines on which investigations to use in specific psychiatric disorders, so clinicians must be guided by each individual case. In the absence of a known or overt physical disorder – for which clinicians would then clearly be able to target investigations – decisions must be made regarding which tests are needed for screening. A convenient approach is to consider firstly whether the patient is at high or low risk of having an underlying physical condition and secondly to consider which investigations are needed as a routine (tier 1) and which are only required after indications emerge (tier 2).

### 9.8.1 Routine screening investigations

Essential first tier investigations include a thorough physical examination, with pulse, blood pressure and temperature measurement and a finger-prick glucose test. The addition of urea and creatinine and urine dipstick testing may demonstrate significantly increased yield when used to screen all patients. A TSH is required in women older than 50.

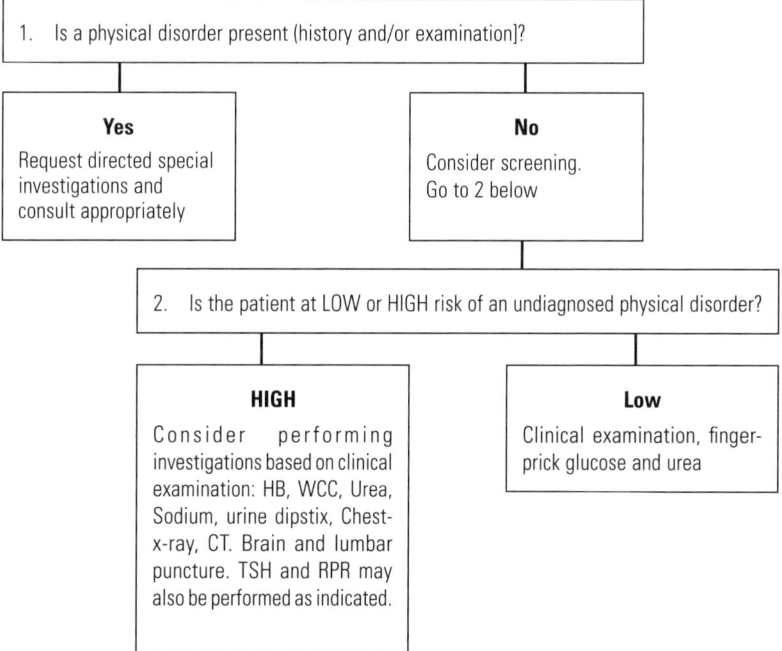


**Figure 9.1** Decision tree for investigating the psychiatric patient

**Table 9.2** Low risk and high risk of physical illness

| | Low risk | High risk |
|---|---|---|
| Course | Previous accurate diagnosis<br>Onset typical for age and duration | Unknown or uncertain history and onset<br>Age > 60 |
| Active medical condition | Medical condition excluded on history and examination | Medical (especially neurological) condition present and active |
| Symptom pattern | Typical | Atypical (e.g. visual hallucinations) |
| Cognition | Orientated to month and day | Not orientated |

# 9.9 Investigations in common psychiatric disorders

## 9.9.1 First-episode psychosis (FEP)

First-episode psychosis (FEP) occurs in widely differing contexts and the decision on how to investigate must be guided by the principles outlined above. Young men with a strong history of cannabis abuse will be investigated differently from older women who present with psychosis. Clinicians may consider performing tests of electrolytes, liver functions, TSH, full blood count, syphilis serology and HIV testing. Note that these tests are not necessarily urgent or required before a referral to a psychiatric facility. Structural imaging, such as CT brain scanning, is often regarded as part of the work-up of first-episode patients; a different view is that these should only be performed when indications are present. In women of childbearing age, a pregnancy test should be performed to manage risk to the foetus. Further investigation depends on the clinical picture and setting and may include CSF analysis, ESR and tests for auto-immune diseases (antinuclear antibodies and rheumatoid factor).

## 9.9.2 Mood disorders

New-onset major mood disorders (major depression and mania) require a similar approach to that used in FEP patients. The choice of medication may also influence which investigations are performed: ECG, renal function and thyroid tests become imperative prior to initiating lithium therapy, and a full blood count and liver function prior to initiating valproate therapy. These mood stabilisers, in addition to carbamazepine, require ongoing monitoring (see Chapter 13: Bipolar disorders). In general terms, while the monitoring of lithium levels is imperative due to its narrow therapeutic index, valproate levels are used mainly to establish whether the individual has been non-compliant, or whether toxicity is present.

## 9.9.3 Anxiety disorders

In addition to considering the investigations discussed above, the clinician must consider that many anxiety symptoms may arise from either cardiac or respiratory causes. Thyroid dysfunction may be a cause and thus careful history must be taken to exclude this or a TSH performed. Due consideration must be given to whether any such disorder exists and an ECG and/or chest X-ray may be helpful.

## 9.9.4 Neurocognitive disorders (dementias)

Laboratory investigations in neurocognitive disorders are aimed at excluding so-called reversible causes. As these patients are usually either older than 60 or medically unwell, a greater number of tests – including urea and electrolytes, liver function tests, ESR, full blood count, serum B12 and folate, calcium, magnesium, phosphate, TSH and syphilis serology – are regarded as routine. HIV testing should also be considered.

The decision whether to conduct CSF analysis depends on the clinical picture: in patients with typical features of Alzheimer's disease, CSF is unlikely to be useful, while CSF analysis is imperative in HIV-dementia. In addition to routine microbiology, the CSF should be examined for tuberculous bacilli and Cryptococcus yeasts.

Patients with HIV-dementia or encephalopathy and who have a headache and fever should also be investigated for Epstein-Barr, cytomegalovirus, herpes simplex and John Cunningham (JC) viruses using the polymerase chain reaction (PCR).

While not recommended routinely, neuro-imaging can play a role in some individuals with neurocognitive disorders.

In patients with a clinical dementia SPECT and PET can assist with the differentiation of different types of dementia, for example Alzheimer's disease, fronto-temporal, vascular and Lewy-Body. Similarly structural imaging, especially MRI, is useful to detect underlying vascular pathology. Particularly in clinically challenging cases this may provide useful prognostic information and assist in planning treatment. In addition it may be useful to distinguish dementias from conditions such as pseudo-dementia and mild cognitive impairment. These scans can also detect subclinical disease in genetically predisposed individuals. The development of radiopharmaceuticals to image amyloid plaques using PET may have important implications for the management of dementias in the future.

## Conclusion

Special investigations include a wide range of laboratory, imaging and clinical measures that are an adjunct to clinical diagnosis, treatment monitoring and adverse event reporting. There are differences between screening and diagnostic tests, as well as tests regarded as critical or supportive. In deciding on which investigations to use, the clinician must consider what is in the best interests of the individual patient, whether a local or published algorithm or guideline must be followed (or when deviation is justified), and the cost of the specific investigation. There is no substitute for good clinical judgement and sound reasoning. When an investigation is required, its use should always be supported by a good reason. In this way, we will be able to utilise the limited resources we have in a way that all who need them may benefit.

# References

Ben-Porath YS, Graham JR, Tellegen A (2009) FBS Test Monograph (The Minnesota Multiphasic Personality Inventory-2 (MMPI-2) Minesota: University of Minnesota Press

Capote HA (2009) Neuroimaging in psychiatry. *Neurologic Clinics* 27: 237–49

Cattell RB, Cattell AK, Cattell HEP (1993) *16 PF Fifth Edition Questionnaire*. Champaign, IL: Institute for Personality and Ability Testing

Folstein MF, Folstein SE, McHugh PR (1975) 'Mini-mental state'. A practical method for grading the cognitive state of patients for the clinician. *Psychiatric Research* 12(3): 189–98

Framingham J. (2011) Millon Clinical Multiaxial Inventory (MCMI-III). Psych Central. http://psychcentral.com/lib/millon-clinical-multiaxial-inventory-mcmi-iii/0006106 (Accessed 12 January 2015)

Golden, C. J. (1978). *The Stroop Color and Word Test: A manual for clinical and experimental uses*. Chicago, IL: Stoelting

Huntzinger JA, Rosse RB, Schwartz BL, Ross LA, Deutsch SI (1992) Clock drawing in the screening assessment of cognitive impairment in an ambulatory care setting: A preliminary report. *General Hospital Psychiatry* 14(2): 142–4

Hutto, B. (2001) Syphilis in clinical psychiatry: A review. *Psychosomatics* 42(6): 453–60

Joska JA, Kaliski SZ, Benatar SR (2008) Patients with severe mental illness: A new approach to testing for HIV. *South African Medical Journal* 98(3): 213-7

Korn CS, Currer, GW, Henderson, SO (2000) Medical clearance of psychiatric patients without medical complaints in the Emergency Department, *Journal of Emergency Medicine*, 18(2):173–6

Lezak, MD (1995) *Neuropsychological assessment*. Oxford: Oxford University Press

Milner, B (1963). Effects of different brain lesions on card sorting: The role of the frontal lobes. *Archives of Neurology*, 9: 100–10

Newcomer, JW (2005) Second-generation (atypical) antipsychotics and metabolic effects: a comprehensive literature review. *CNS Drugs*, 19 (Supplement 1):1–93

Streetman DS, Bertino JS (Jr), Nafziger AN (2000) Phenotyping of drug-metabolizing enzymes in adults: A review of in-vivo cytochrome P450 phenotyping probes. *Pharmacogenetics* 10(3): 187–216

Wechsler Adult Intelligence Scale, Fourth edition. Website: http://www.pearsonassessment.com/(Accessed 20 March 2012)

Warwick JM (2004) Imaging of brain function using SPECT. *Metabolic Brain Disease* 19: 113–23

www.mocatest.org (Accessed 15 June 2015)

# PART 4

# Psychiatric disorders

CHAPTER

# 10 Cognitive disorders

*Bonginkosi Chiliza, Laila Asmal*

## 10.1 Introduction

This chapter provides the reader with a framework for understanding neurocognitive disorders (NCDs), and must be read together with the chapters on Neuropsychiatry (Chapter 32), HIV and mental health (Chapter 33), Psychogeriatrics (Chapter 30) and Clinical assessment in psychiatry (Chapter 7).

In this chapter, the concept of cognition and what is meant by it in neuroscience is introduced. Approaches to help identify deficits in cognitive functioning are also discussed. The chapter closes with an overview of the three NCDs described in the DSM-5 (American Psychiatric Association, 2013), namely delirium, major neurocognitive disorder and mild neurocognitive disorder.

## 10.2 Cognition and neurocognitive disorders

There are many ways to define cognition. In psychiatry and psychology, the term is used to refer to a wide range of mental processes, such as:

- attention and concentration
- language comprehension and production
- memory and learning
- calculation
- problem solving
- reasoning
- decision-making.

Neurocognitive disorders have two defining characteristics: a cognitive deficit and a decline from previous levels of cognition. We shall now look at these two aspects.

### 10.2.1 Cognitive deficit

With neurocognitive disorders, cognitive problems are the core feature of the disorder and are directly due to structural or metabolic brain disease. Cognitive problems can occur in many mental disorders: people with depression, for example, can have memory problems that present as pseudo-dementia. However, cognitive problems are not the primary manifestations of these mental disorders.

### 10.2.2 Decline in cognitive functioning

Cognitive deficits can be present at birth or from early development, for example intellectual disability and autism. These neurodevelopmental disorders do not imply that a person's cognition has deteriorated. Instead, these conditions affect the development of a person's baseline level of cognitive function. However, it is possible for a person with a neurodevelopmental disorder to also develop a neurocognitive disorder: a patient with developmental delay due to Down's syndrome, for example, can later develop Alzheimer's disease.

## 10.3 Classification of neurocognitive disorders

The following NCDs are described in the DSM–5:

- delirium
- major neurocognitive disorder
- mild neurocognitive disorder.

### 10.3.1 Delirium

Delirium is a syndrome caused by underlying physiological disturbances that lead to disturbances in attention and awareness. Patients with delirium are unable to focus or shift their attention and are unaware of their surroundings. Delirium usually develops over a short period of time (hours to days) and fluctuates during the course of the day. It is very common in up to 80% of critically ill patients who require treatment in an intensive care unit (ICU). It is also common in elderly patients in medical and surgical wards, particularly in post-operative patients after major surgery.

It is important to recognise delirium as it often signifies a serious underlying medical illness, and it has been described as a medical emergency.

#### 10.3.1.1 Key features of delirium

Patients with delirium show a sudden change in their cognitive abilities of attention and awareness. These disturbances are accompanied by other cognitive deficits, including disorientation (particularly to time and place), recent memory difficulties, language impairment and perceptual disturbances. The perceptual disturbances range from misinterpretations to illusions and visual hallucinations. Some patients with delirium will have severely impaired arousal or a decreased level of consciousness. Delirium disturbs the sleep-wake cycle: patients appear drowsy during the day, yet become agitated at night. Most patients describe the experience of delirium as frightening and may scream or swear. Other emotional disturbances, such as irritability, anger and apathy, can also accompany delirium.

**Clinical subtypes**

Delirium is classified according to psychomotor activity into hyperactive, hypo-active and mixed subtypes.

Hyperactive delirium is characterised by increased psychomotor activity and agitation.

Hypo-active delirium is characterised by reduced psychomotor activity, apathy and lethargy. Hypoactive delirium often goes unrecognised, as patients are 'quietly delirious', yet they still have serious medical illnesses.

The mixed subtype alternates unpredictably between the above two.

#### 10.3.1.2 Assessment of delirium

**History**

In order to make a diagnosis of delirium, good collateral information is needed. Nurses who care for the patients are usually the best placed to give information about any fluctuations in the state of the patient and whether the patient becomes worse at night (so-called sun-downing). History taking should focus on medical and substance history, as well as getting as much information as possible on the presenting complaints. The disturbances are usually of acute onset and fluctuate during the course of the day.

**Mental state examination**

The mental state examination (MSE) is particularly important in delirium, as delirium is a clinical diagnosis. There are no specific laboratory tests that can definitively prove a diagnosis of delirium. The focus of the MSE must be on the cognitive examination of the patient.

The core feature of delirium is a problem of attention, thus one looks for inattentiveness, distractibility or difficulty in maintaining attention on a particular topic. Most patients with delirium lack awareness of their surroundings, which will manifest as disorientation. Short-term memory is also often impaired. Language disturbances often manifest as **dysphasia** or incoherence. Patients will also have disorganised thinking and impaired reasoning. Perceptual disturbances are commonly the reason for misdiagnosis of a psychotic disorder. The perceptual disturbances, however, are usually misinterpretations or illusions where, for example, a patient may misinterpret shadows cast by a curtain being blown in the breeze. Visual hallucinations are the most common type of hallucinations in delirium. Psychomotor changes are common, with lethargy or hyperactivity; sometimes patients switch

**Table 10.1** DSM-5 Diagnostic Criteria for Delirium

| Diagnostic Criteria |
|---|
| A. A disturbance in attention (i.e., reduced ability to direct, focus, sustain, and shift attention) and awareness (reduced orientation to the environment). |
| B. The disturbance develops over a short period of time (usually hours to a few days), represents a change from baseline attention and awareness, and tends to fluctuate in severity during the course of a day. |
| C. An additional disturbance in cognition (e.g., memory deficit, disorientation, language, visuospatial ability, or perception). |
| D. The disturbances in Criteria A and C are not better explained by another preexisting, established, or evolving neurocognitive disorder and do not occur in the context of a severely reduced level of arousal, such as coma. |
| E. There is evidence from the history, physical examination, or laboratory findings that the disturbance is a direct physiological consequence of another medical condition, substance intoxication or withdrawal (i.e., due to a drug of abuse or to a medication), or exposure to a toxin, or is due to multiple etiologies. |
| *Specify* whether: |
| **Substance intoxication delirium**: This diagnosis should be made instead of substance intoxication when the symptoms in Criteria A and C predominate in the clinical picture and when they are sufficiently severe to warrant clinical attention. |
| **Substance withdrawal delirium**: This diagnosis should be made instead of substance withdrawal when the symptoms in Criteria A and C predominate in the clinical picture and when they are sufficiently severe to warrant clinical attention. |
| **Medication-induced delirium**: This diagnosis applies when the symptoms in Criteria A and C arise as a side effect of a medication taken as prescribed. |
| **Delirium due to another medical condition**: There is evidence from the history, physical examination, or laboratory findings that the disturbance is attributable to the physiological consequences of another medical condition. |
| **Delirium due to multiple etiologies**: There is evidence from the history, physical examination, or laboratory findings that the delirium has more than one etiology (e.g., more than one etiological medical condition; another medical condition plus substance intoxication or medication side effect). |
| *Specify* if: |
| **Acute**: Lasting a few hours or days. |
| **Persistent**: Lasting weeks or months. |
| *Specify* if: |
| **Hyperactive**: The individual has a hyperactive level of psychomotor activity that may be accompanied by mood lability, agitation, and/or refusal to cooperate with medical care. |
| **Hypoactive**: The individual has a hypoactive level of psychomotor activity that may be accompanied by sluggishness and lethargy that approaches stupor. |
| **Mixed level of activity**: The individual has a normal level of psychomotor activity even though attention and awareness are disturbed. Also includes individuals whose activity level rapidly fluctuates. |

**Source:** Reprinted with permission from the *Diagnostic and Statistical Manual of Mental Disorders*, Fifth Edition, (Copyright 2013). American Psychiatric Association.

between the two quite suddenly. Finally, patients frequently appear fearful, angry, or agitated.

#### 10.3.1.3 Common causes of delirium

Delirium does not usually have a single cause but rather multiple, often interacting, causes. DIMTOP (Drugs Infection Metabolic Trauma Oxygen Postictal) is an easy mnemonic for the causes of delirium:

- Drugs – commonly used medications that have effects on the central nervous system can cause delirium in vulnerable patients. These include sedatives like benzodiazepines, anticholinergics, antihypertensives and oral hypoglycaemic agents. Severe alcohol intoxication and alcohol withdrawal can also cause delirium.
- Infections – any infection can cause delirium in a vulnerable patient. Infections in

the central nervous system, such as meningitis, are more likely to cause delirium in younger patients.

- **M**etabolic – any change in the metabolic profile, such as hyperglycaemia, hypoglycaemia, hyponatraemia, uraemia, dehydration due to diarrhoea or diuretic use can cause delirium.
- **T**rauma – traumatic brain injury, particularly from motor vehicle accidents, is common in South Africa and is a common cause of delirium in younger patients.
- **O**xygen deficit – any cardiovascular or respiratory cause that leads to oxygen deficits can cause delirium.
- **P**ostictal – epilepsy is also common in the South African context and can often lead to delirium after particularly prolonged seizures.

### 10.3.1.4 Pathophysiology of delirium

Acetylcholine is the principal neurotransmitter of the reticular formation, which is the key area involved in delirium. The reticular formation is the most important brain system that regulates consciousness and includes the dorsal tegmental pathways.

A deficit of acetylcholine in the brain is associated with delirium. It thus follows that drugs that reduce the action of acetylcholine may precipitate or worsen delirium. These drugs (usually in higher dosages) are antidepressants, antipsychotics (chlorpromazine) and anticholinergic agents (biperiden and orphenadrine).

### 10.3.1.5 Differential diagnosis of delirium

Delirium can present with many different symptoms and signs are often mistaken for other psychiatric disorders.

#### Major NCD

The key features that distinguish between delirium and a major NCD is the acute onset, fluctuating and reversible course of delirium coupled with disturbed consciousness, attention deficit, reversal of the sleep-wake cycle and altered motor activity.

#### Schizophrenia

Some schizophrenic patients demonstrate severe disordered behaviour that may be confused with the hyperactivity found in delirium. These patients, being floridly psychotic, will also have impaired attention and concentration spans.

#### Depression

Distinguish between patients who are severely depressed with **psychomotor retardation** and hypo-active patients who suffer from delirium.

#### Factitious disorder and malingering

These patients demonstrate contradictions in symptoms and signs.

### 10.3.1.6 Relationship between delirium and dementia

Since delirium and dementia are cognitive disorders that commonly occur in the elderly, clinicians are often called to make a distinction

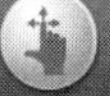

### Case study 10.1

Whilst on call, you are called to see a 45 year-old-male patient in the orthopaedic ward who is talking to himself, is agitated, and has just pulled out his drip. The nurses say that he is on Day 3 post-op (he had an open reduction and internal **fixation** of his right ankle). He was fine during the day and has been well for the last three days, but now is acting 'crazy'. During the MSE, the patient is frightened. He is unable to have a proper conversation as he keeps looking around the room and cannot concentrate on what you are saying. He does not know where he is, and thinks that you are his uncle. He occasionally derails (goes off the point) when you speak to him and you find it difficult to follow his thoughts. He suddenly laughs and then cries. He cannot explain why he removed his drip. On physical examination he appears dehydrated. His pulse is 120 beats per minute. He has a raised temperature and the wound on his right ankle smells suspiciously of infection. You suspect that the patient has delirium and proceed to do investigations to determine the cause.

**Table 10.2** Clinical differences and similarities between delirium and dementia

| | Delirium | Dementia |
|---|---|---|
| **Onset** | abrupt (hours to a few days) | insidious (months) |
| **Course** | fluctuating | progressive |
| **Duration** | days to weeks | months to years |
| **Level of consciousness** | clouded, fluctuating | alert |
| **Initial symptoms** | difficulty with attention | memory deficits |
| **Orientation** | impaired | initially intact, later impaired |
| **Attention/concentration** | prominently impaired | initially intact, later impaired |
| **Memory** | markedly impaired out of keeping | impaired in keeping with stage of dementia |
| **Language impairment** | incoherent | naming difficulties |
| **Executive function** | markedly impaired | relatively preserved |
| **Thinking** | disordered | decreased in amount |
| **Perceptual disturbances** | commonly illusions and visual hallucinations | less common |
| **Sleep** | disturbed sleep-wake cycle | occasional worsening of symptoms at night |
| **Restlessness** | worse at night | worse during the day |
| **Psychomotor** | agitated, retarded or mixed | initially unchanged later impaired |
| **Affect** | anxious, agitated irritable (labile) | various but stable bouts of irritability |
| **Reversibility** | reversible | irreversible |
| **Prognosis** | relatively good | poor |

between the two disorders. Management of the disorders differs markedly and it is important to be able to accurately differentiate the two.

### Dementia following delirium

There is growing evidence of long-term cognitive impairment following delirium. Up to 25% of patients admitted to an ICU for a critical illness have long-term cognitive impairment. The cognitive impairment includes disturbances in attention, memory and executive dysfunction. It is not yet clear whether these impairments improve with time or lead to the more severe illness of dementia. It is important to be aware of the possibility of long-term cognitive impairment, since ICU survivors often struggle to rebuild their lives and go back to meaningful employment.

## 10.3.1.7 Management of delirium

### Prevention of delirium

It is important for clinicians to be vigilant for the development of delirium in vulnerable patients. Patients with advanced age, dementia, a high medical co-morbidity burden, visual impairment, malnutrition, alcohol abuse and depression are particularly vulnerable to delirium.

A number of simple, cost-effective measures can be undertaken to prevent the onset of delirium. Small changes in the patient's environment can make a significant difference in prevention. Ensure that there are wall calendars and wall clocks, call the patient by his or her name, and avoid moving the patient from one ward to another. Address any sensory impairment, such as by providing patients with their glasses. Promote good sleep by avoiding unnecessary nursing procedures, reducing noise to a minimum and by providing some lighting at night. Encourage patients to become mobile soon after surgery with appropriate aid.

Medical management that can also prevent delirium includes ensuring adequate hydration and analgesia and avoiding introducing iatrogenic infection by inserting unnecessary urinary catheters.

The implementation of non-pharmacological multi-component interventions in patients prone to delirium can not only reduce the incidence rate of delirium by 33% but also reduce the number of episodes and the duration of delirium (Inouye *et al.*, 1999; Flaherty and Little, 2011).

**Medical management**

The most important principle in the management of delirium is to find the underlying cause and treat it. If the delirium is caused by an infection, then treating the infection will lead to an improvement in the symptoms of delirium. If the delirium is caused by medication, stopping the medication will also resolve the delirium. However, in the majority of cases, the aetiology is multi-factorial and often not easily identifiable. The symptoms of delirium must be managed whilst the more specific treatment of the underlying disorder is being sought.

Haloperidol has been shown to be effective in the treatment of delirium: it is the first-line treatment for delirium without a known cause. Haloperidol can be administered intraveneously (IV) or intramuscularly (IM) in delirium. IV administration is often the preferred route, as absorption is less erratic and has been shown to produce less extrapyramidal symptoms than IM or orally administered haloperidol. Haloperidol has a favourable cardiopulmonary side effect profile, which is important in the treatment of medically ill patients with delirium.

Benzodiazepines, such as lorazepam, can be used in the treatment of delirium due to alcohol and other drug withdrawal states. Benzodiazepines can also be used as second-line agents in calming agitated patients with delirium. Benzodiazepines can cause respiratory depression and monitoring is thus important. Lorazepam can also be combined with haloperidol if the agitation is difficult to control, but must be used cautiously in elderly patients where benzodiazepines may worsen the delirium. One of the positive effects of combining lorazepam with haloperidol is that lower doses of each drug can be used.

Newer antipsychotics can also be used as second-line treatment. Risperidone has been used in low doses where haloperidol is not available or contraindicated. Intramuscular ziprasidone and olanzapine have also been used as second-line agents.

## 10.3.2 Major and mild neurocognitive disorders

Major and mild NCDs are generic terms to describe the deterioration in cognition compared to baseline ability, in a setting of clear consciousness. Major and mild NCDs are not disease processes themselves, but rather umbrella terms that encompass a number of different conditions.

### 10.3.2.1 Key features of major and mild NCDs

Patients with major and mild NCDs show a decline in cognitive functioning compared to their baseline ability in at least one cognitive area (or cognitive domain) (American Psychiatric Association, 2013). Cognitive domains affected by NCDs include complex attention, executive function, learning and memory, language, perceptual-motor and **social cognition**.

The decline in cognitive functioning in NCDs is established by:

- history taking, done when the patient, the clinician or someone who knows the patient well raises a concern that there is a decline in cognitive functioning
- clinical assessment, undertaken when there is an impairment in cognitive functioning according to a measured clinical assessment. Ideally, this assessment should be performed using standardised neuropsychological tests, such as the Mini-Mental Status Examination (MMSE).

Importantly, this cognitive decline should not be accounted for by a delirium, which, as discussed, also has a disturbance in cognitive functioning. The cognitive decline should also not be accounted for by another mental disorder. Although patients with other mental disorders (such as depression or schizophrenia) can have cognitive deficits, cognitive problems are not the primary feature of those disorders.

### 10.3.2.2 Distinguishing between major and mild neurocognitive disorders

The key differentiating factors between major and mild NCDs are severity and impact on functioning. Major NCDs have more severe cognitive impairment and therefore a greater impact on daily functioning. Clinically, when we say that a patient has dementia, we mean that the patient has a major NCD.

In mild NCDs, the fall-off in neuropsychological testing results is relatively modest compared to major NCDs. The cognitive deficits of mild NCDs still allow the patient to remain fairly independent in his or her everyday activities, although it does take more effort to do so. For example, while the patient may have previously been an excellent driver who found his or her way around easily, he or she may now need to use maps more often, may need to ask for directions more frequently or may find parking more difficult.

### 10.3.2.3 Co-morbidity with mild and major NCDs

**Psychotic symptoms**

Psychotic features are common, especially in the early stages of major NCDs. **Paranoia** is common, as are hallucinations. It can be difficult to differentiate an NCD from a primary psychotic disorder, such as schizophrenia (see Section 10.3.2.8).

**Mood and anxiety symptoms**

Mood symptoms occur commonly in NCDs, especially in the earlier stages. These symptoms can include elevated mood, apathy and depression. Elevated mood and apathy occur more frequently with NCDs that affect the frontal lobe. Anxiety symptoms are common and are frequently due to the NCD itself or to changes in environment, for example, discharge from hospital.

> **Key points 10.1 Dementia versus major NCD**
>
> The term dementia instead of NCD is used by the ICD-10 in textbooks and by clinicians, patients, carers or the lay press. Dementia is almost exactly the same as a major NCD, but there are subtle differences:
>
> - amnestic disorders (e.g. Korsakoff's syndrome) are separate categories according to the ICD-10 but are incorporated under major NCD in the DSM-5.
> - younger patients (e.g. HIV positive) or patients with non-progressive cognitive impairment (e.g. traumatic brain injury) may prefer the term major NCD instead of dementia due to the stigma associated with the term dementia.

**Other behavioural symptoms**

Agitation is more likely to occur as the NCD progresses in severity. Other behavioural symptoms include disinhibition, sleep disturbances, hoarding, vocalisations, apathy and wandering.

**Delirium**

Major and mild NCDs increase the risk of delirium and it can be difficult to assess if delirium is superimposed on an underlying cognitive decline. Careful history taking and serial assessments are important.

### 10.3.2.4 Prevalence of mild and moderate NCDs

Prevalence of major NCDs (or dementias) varies widely according to age and cause. For those NCDs associated with the ageing process (e.g. Alzheimer's disease, vascular disease), it makes sense that prevalence increases with age. There are some NCDs that can occur almost throughout the lifespan (e.g. traumatic brain injury), while others peak in age of onset under the age of 60 years, for example HIV, frontotemporal degeneration and Huntington's disease.

**Table 10.3** DSM-5 Diagnostic Criteria for Major Neurocognitive Disorder

| **Diagnostic Criteria** |
|---|
| A. Evidence of significant cognitive decline from a previous level of performance in one or more cognitive domains (complex attention, executive function, learning and memory, language, perceptual-motor, or social cognition) based on:<br>1. Concern of the individual, a knowledgeable informant, or the clinician that there has been a significant decline in cognitive function; and<br>2. A substantial impairment in cognitive performance, preferably documented by standardized neuropsychological testing or, in its absence, another quantified clinical assessment. |
| B. The cognitive deficits interfere with independence in everyday activities (i.e., at a minimum, requiring assistance with complex instrumental activities of daily living such as paying bills or managing medications). |
| C. The cognitive deficits do not occur exclusively in the context of a delirium. |
| D. The cognitive deficits are not better explained by another mental disorder (e.g., major depressive disorder, schizophrenia). |
| *Specify* whether due to:<br>**Alzheimer's disease** (pp. 611–614)<br>**Frontotemporal lobar degeneration** (pp. 614–618)<br>**Lewy body disease** (pp. 618–621)<br>**Vascular disease** (pp. 621–624)<br>**Traumatic brain injury** (pp. 624–627)<br>**Substance/medication use** (pp. 627–632)<br>**HIV infection** (pp. 632–634)<br>**Prion disease** (pp. 634–636)<br>**Parkinson's disease** (pp. 636–638)<br>**Huntington's disease** (pp. 638–641)<br>**Another medical condition** (pp. 641–642)<br>**Multiple etiologies** (pp. 642–643)<br>**Unspecified** (p. 643)<br>*Specify*:<br>**Without behavioral disturbance**: If the cognitive disturbance is not accompanied by any clinically significant behavioral disturbance.<br>**With behavioral disturbance** *(specify disturbance)*: If the cognitive disturbance is accompanied by a clinically significant behavioral disturbance (e.g., psychotic symptoms, mood disturbance, agitation, apathy, or other behavioral symptoms).<br>*Specify* current severity:<br>**Mild**: Difficulties with instrumental activities of daily living (e.g., housework, managing money).<br>**Moderate**: Difficulties with basic activities of daily living (e.g., feeding, dressing).<br>**Severe**: Fully dependent. |

**Source:** Reprinted with permission from the *Diagnostic and Statistical Manual of Mental Disorders*, Fifth Edition, (Copyright 2013). American Psychiatric Association.

### 10.3.2.5 Cortical and subcortical dementias

The brain is not uniformly affected in dementia. A commonly used categorisation of dementia is into a cortical form (mostly involving the cerebral cortex) and a subcortical form (mostly affecting deeper brain structures like the deep white matter, basal ganglia and thalamus) (Cummings and Benson, 1984). Since specific brain areas are in charge of specific cognitive functions, this categorisation into cortical and subcortical forms of dementia is an important method to link clinical symptoms and signs with underlying brain pathology (Cooper and Greene, 2005). The differentiating clinical features of cortical and subcortical dementias are summarised in Table 10.5.

Cortical dementias typically involve progressive deterioration of memory and higher-order cortical dysfunction that affects language (aphasia), motor activity (apraxia) and interpreting sensory stimuli (agnosia).

**Table 10.4** DSM-5 Diagnostic Criteria for Mild Neurocognitive Disorder

| Diagnostic Criteria |
|---|
| A. Evidence of modest cognitive decline from a previous level of performance in one or more cognitive domains (complex attention, executive function, learning and memory, language, perceptual motor, or social cognition) based on:<br>1. Concern of the individual, a knowledgeable informant, or the clinician that there has been a mild decline in cognitive function; and<br>2. A modest impairment in cognitive performance, preferably documented by standardized neuropsychological testing or, in its absence, another quantified clinical assessment. |
| B. The cognitive deficits do not interfere with capacity for independence in everyday activities (i.e., complex instrumental activities of daily living such as paying bills or managing medications are preserved, but greater effort, compensatory strategies, or accommodation may be required). |
| C. The cognitive deficits do not occur exclusively in the context of a delirium. |
| D. The cognitive deficits are not better explained by another mental disorder (e.g., major depressive disorder, schizophrenia). |
| *Specify* whether due to:<br>**Alzheimer's disease** (pp. 611–614)<br>**Frontotemporal lobar degeneration** (pp. 614–618)<br>**Lewy body disease** (pp. 618–621)<br>**Vascular disease** (pp. 621–624)<br>**Traumatic brain injury** (pp. 624–627)<br>**Substance/medication use** (pp. 627–632)<br>**HIV infection** (pp. 632–634)<br>**Prion disease** (pp. 634–636)<br>**Parkinson's disease** (pp. 636–638)<br>**Huntington's disease** (pp. 638–641)<br>**Another medical condition** (pp. 641–642)<br>**Multiple etiologies** (pp. 642–643)<br>**Unspecified** (p. 643) |
| *Specify*:<br>**Without behavioral disturbance**: If the cognitive disturbance is not accompanied by any clinically significant behavioral disturbance.<br>**With behavioral disturbance** *(specify disturbance)*: If the cognitive disturbance is accompanied by a clinically significant behavioral disturbance (e.g., psychotic symptoms, mood disturbance, agitation, apathy, or other behavioral symptoms). |

**Source:** Reprinted with permission from the ***Diagnostic and Statistical Manual of Mental Disorders***, Fifth Edition, (Copyright 2013). American Psychiatric Association.

## Key points 10.2 Summary of major and mild neurocognitive disorders

- The key feature of major and mild NCDs is a decline from baseline in at least one cognitive domain, in clear consciousness.
- Major and mild NCDs are differentiated by severity and impact on functioning.
- Dementia is also known as major NCD.
- Diagnosis is based on history taking, clinical assessment (ideally using a standardised psychometric tool) and select special investigations.
- There are a number of different major and mild NCD subtypes, based on aetiology or underlying pathology.
- The main differential diagnoses are depression, delirium, normal ageing and differentiating major from mild NCDs.

Subcortical dementias typically involve slower speed and rigidity of thinking (**bradyphrenia**), difficulty in retrieving stored memory (memory impairment is generally not severe), poor problem-solving skills and personality changes (apathy, depression, anxiety).

Some disorders may even have signs of both cortical and subcortical dysfunction (e.g. multiple infarcts in cortical and subcortical regions, Lewy-Body dementia).

### 10.3.2.6 Causes of major and minor NCDs

There are many different causes of major and mild NCDs. It is especially important to recognise causes that occur commonly as well as those that are reversible. Interestingly, NCDs are the only conditions in psychiatry where the diagnostic criteria are based on aetiology or underlying pathology. In some cases, the cause is clear, for example HIV or traumatic brain injury. In others, characteristic typical symptoms cluster together and help to make a diagnosis. In Alzheimer's disease or frontotemporal lobar degeneration, for example, the occurrence of certain behavioural, functional and cognitive symptoms make the diagnosis.

The various causes of NCDs are addressed in other chapters of this book:

- Alzheimer's disease, vascular disease, frontotemporal degeneration, Lewy-Body disease and Prion disease: see Chapter 30: Psychogeriatrics
- Parkinson's disease, Huntington's disease, traumatic brain injury, normal pressure hydrocephalus and multiple aetiologies: see Chapter 32: Neuropsychiatry
- HIV infection: see Chapter 33: HIV and mental health
- substance or medication-induced NCDs: see Chapter 20: Alcohol-related disorders.

**Other medical conditions**

A considerable number of medical conditions can lead to cognitive impairment. Although many of these conditions are uncommon and in some cases quite rare, some may be treatable. It is therefore important to keep potentially treatable causes in mind when considering a patient with cognitive decline. Table 10.6 summarises medical and substance related causes of dementia that are potentially reversible.

Also see Chapter 32: Neuropsychiatry for other medical conditions.

**Table 10.5** Clinical features of cortical and subcortical dementias

| Affected domain | Cortical dementia | Subcortical dementia |
|---|---|---|
| Complex attention | present, but not a key early feature | key feature |
| Learning and memory | amnestic (abnormal memory storage) | forgetful (abnormal memory retrieval) |
| Language | aphasic (word finding and comprehension difficulty) | intact |
| Speech | intact | slow, dysarthric |
| Visuospatial | often present | often present |
| Agnosia | often present | not usually seen |
| Personality | intact till late, unless frontal type | apathetic, depressed, anxious |
| Motor speed | intact till late, unless frontal type | tremor, rigid, slow |
| Thinking speed | intact till late, unless frontal type | slow, rigid thinking |
| Causes | Alzheimer's disease, fronto-temporal dementia | vascular dementia, (deep white matter infarcts) HIV dementia, Parkinson's disease, Wilson's disease |

### 10.3.2.7 Reversible causes of dementia

Causes of dementia that are potentially reversible are listed in Table 10.6.

There are some clues as to whether the cognitive impairment is due to another identified medical condition. Treatment of the medical condition (e.g. hypothyroidism) could lead to a improvement in the cognitive decline (although the decline is generally not completely reversible). Alternatively, progression and fluctuation in the cognitive impairment can mirror progression and fluctuation in the medical symptoms (e.g. in SLE). The assessment of whether there is a major or mild NCD may be complicated by the occurrence of a delirium, which is common in people with serious medical conditions. Patients with other major and mild NCDs (such as Alzheimer's disease, HIV, vascular disease) are also at risk of other medical conditions that can also cause NCDs (e.g. nutritional disorders, infections, metabolic derangements). In many cases the patient presents with a multitude of medical problems and it is difficult to identify a single cause of the cognitive decline.

This brings us to the last, but by no means least, important cause of NCDs: multiple aetiologies.

**Table 10.6** Potentially reversible causes of dementia

| Category | Condition |
|---|---|
| Infectious causes | HIV (primary infection and related opportunistic infections)<br>neurosyphilis<br>neurocysticercosis<br>tuberculous meningitis |
| Endocrine and metabolic conditions | recurrent hypoglycaemia<br>chronic hypocalcaemia and hypercalcaemia<br>hypothyroidism<br>Cushing's disease<br>Addison's disease<br>Wilson's disease |
| Nutritional disorders | vitamins $B_{12}$, $B_1$ (thiamine), $B_6$ deficiencies<br>niacin (pellagra) |
| Space-occupying lesions | brain tumours<br>subdural haematoma |
| Normal-pressure hydrocephalus | |
| Auto-immune disorders and vasculitis | discoid or systemic lupus erythematosis (SLE) neurosarcoidosis<br>giant cell arteritis |
| Hypoxia | suicide attempts<br>heart failure<br>repeated status epilepticus |
| Multiple sclerosis | |
| Chronic substance intoxication | alcohol<br>stimulants (e.g. cocaine, methamphetamines)<br>carbon monoxide poisoning<br>heavy metals |

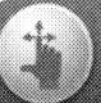

## Case study 10.2

Mr. Adams (69) comes to your office complaining of no energy, and memory problems for the past six months. His daughter reports that Mr. Adams moved in with his younger brother after the death of his wife in 2006 and he has aged fast after his brother died eight months earlier. For the past six months, Mr. Adams has been exhibiting significant withdrawal from his usually active social life and expects family members to do all his daily chores, including cooking and cleaning. Mr. Adams is on medication for hypertension and hypercholesterolaemia as well as paracetamol for back pain. He has never smoked or drank alcohol. He has lost three kilograms since his last doctor's visit but there are no other significant findings in the physical examination. On psychiatric examination, he had a flat affect. Answers were limited to 'yes' and 'no' with poor eye contact. He had a mini-mental status examination score of 20/30, but seemed to put in little effort and had many 'I don't know' answers. A CT scan of the brain shows cortical atrophy, in keeping with his age. You make the diagnosis of major depressive disorder.

#### Multiple aetiologies

It is not uncommon for evidence from the history, physical examination and special investigations to point to more than one aetiological process. In the elderly, vascular disease and Alzheimer's disease frequently co-exist. In the younger patient, risk factors for NCD overlap, for example the same individual who experiences a traumatic brain injury is potentially also at risk of HIV infection and illicit substance use.

### 10.3.2.8 Differential diagnosis of a major or mild NCD

Neurocognitive disorders can be mimicked by a number of different conditions.

#### Delirium

See Section 10.3.1.5 for a discussion of delirium.

#### Other neurocognitive disorders

The cause of major and mild NCDs is generally established by clinical assessment, supported by special investigations. There are cases where the underlying aetiology of cognitive decline is fairly clear, for example Huntington's disease verified by genetic testing, HIV infection with a low CD4 count. However, even with very careful assessment, in most other cases it is difficult to be completely certain of the diagnosis. In practice, NCDs mimic each other or co-exist, for example vascular NCD or frontotemporal NCD can look like Alzheimer's disease and vice versa.

#### Normal ageing

As a person ages, a progressive decline in functioning and performance occurs, and this may be accompanied by minor memory problems. This is not necessarily pathological and may simply be part of the ageing process. The ageing process can be associated with anxiety, **denial** and frustration that can be worsened by environmental stressors (e.g. financial stressors, loss of a partner) and physical illnesses. The role of the health professional in this case is, after careful evaluation, to reassure and help the person adapt to the changes.

#### Major depressive disorder

Some patients with depression show features of cognitive impairment (such as poor memory and difficulty concentrating) that are sometimes called pseudo-dementia. Although it can be difficult to distinguish between depression and dementia in the elderly, patients with depression frequently have a relatively abrupt decline in cognition that is associated with depressive symptoms while insight is generally preserved. Patients with depression may do poorly on cognitive testing such as the MMSE due to poor effort. However, up to half of elderly patients who are diagnosed and successfully treated for depression develop dementia within three years.

#### Intellectual disability

Intellectual disability is characterised by subaverage intelligence with an onset before the age of 18. Intellectual disability and dementia can co-exist (e.g. Alzheimer's disease is more common in Down's syndrome). In these cases there is a significant deterioration of memory and functioning from the patient's baseline.

**Schizophrenia**

Although cognitive impairment may be a clinical feature of schizophrenia, psychosis and negative symptoms tend to dominate acute presentations. NCDs usually have a later onset, and speech and behaviour are not disorganised until late in the disease. Visual hallucinations are also more likely to occur in NCDs than in a primary psychotic disorder.

**Factitious disorder and malingering**

In these patients, the signs and symptoms are not characteristic of those typically seen with dementia and are inconsistent over time.

## 10.3.2.9 Management of major and mild NCDs

The first task in managing major and mild NCDs is to fully assess the patient. This includes a history, mental state examination (including bedside neuropsychological testing), physical examination and special investigations. It is important to obtain collateral information from other sources, such as the carer, social worker and employer (with the patient's permission).

It is especially important to exclude other conditions that can mimic a major or mild NCD (see Section 10.3.1.5) and to try to identify the underlying cause of the NCD. It is essential to exclude treatable causes.

Also see Chapter 32: Neuropsychiatry, for further detail on managing major and mild NCDs.

**Where are patients managed?**

Most patients with major or mild NCDs are managed on an outpatient basis, although some do need hospitalisation. Most hospital admissions are for the evaluation and treatment of behavioural and psychological complications associated with major NCD (e.g. aggression, violence, wandering, psychosis, depression). Other reasons for hospitalisation include suicidal threats or behaviour, rapid weight loss, acute deterioration without apparent cause or a social situation that precludes adequate observation.

**Special investigations**

There is no routine set of special investigations used in the evaluation of a patient with cognitive decline. Choose tests carefully depending on the clinical profile of the patient. Frequently used special investigations are:

- full blood count
- serum electrolytes
- fasting glucose
- serum vitamin B12 levels
- lipid screening
- syphilis screening
- thyroid function
- HIV
- structural neuro-imaging (e.g. CT or brain MRI)
- lumbar puncture (if suspecting a CNS infection)
- Huntington genetics screening (if indicated)
- liver function
- urine dipsticks +- MC&S to exclude an urinary tract infection.

**Neuropsychological testing**

As a primary care physician, you can perform some bedside neuropsychological tests, such as the MMSE, international HIV dementia scale (IHDS) or the Montreal Cognitive Assessment (MOCA).

Referral to a clinical psychologist for comprehensive neuropsychological testing is indicated in certain instances, such as diagnostic uncertainty. Neuropsychological testing is useful for a number of reasons:

- it can help in the diagnosis of an NCD
- it can differentiate between major and mild NCD
- it can supply baseline data by which to measure change before and after treatment
- it can help to evaluate individuals suspected of having a mild NCD or an early major NCD

- when other test results (such as imaging studies) are ambiguous
- helps distinguish between delirium, dementia and depression.

### Who is involved in management?

In an acute setting, primary care physicians frequently manage co-morbid medical conditions as well as behavioural problems. Where necessary, patients are referred to psychiatrists or other medical specialists. Diagnosis frequently depends on information that occupational therapists obtain from the workplace, and psychologists acquire through neuropsychological testing. Once diagnosis and acute management are established, other members of the clinical team (e.g. psychologists, occupational therapists, social workers) play an even greater role.

### Medical management

While most causes of major or mild NCDs are progressive and cannot be cured, the treatable causes should, of course, be treated. Appropriate treatment may include antiretrovirals for HIV infection, supplements for vitamin and thyroid deficiencies as well as surgical treatment for hydrocephalus and subdural haematomas. Risk factors such as high blood pressure, diabetes and dyslipidaemia should also be treated. Cognitive enhancers, such as acetylcholinesterase inhibitors and memantine can be used for certain major or mild NCDs that cannot be treated (e.g. Alzheimer's disease).

Antipsychotics are often used to treat challenging behaviour such as hostility, agitation and aggression. These medications are ideally used for short periods only, and with caution, because they can increase the risk of a cardiovascular disease, particularly stroke and myocardial infarction.

Depression is a common co-morbidity with mild NCDs in any stage and with major NCDs in the early stages, and antidepressants are frequently prescribed.

### Psychological treatment

Some psychological treatments are available with variable degrees of success to help patients and carers cope with symptoms. These include cognitive stimulation (taking part in activities and exercises to improve memory, problem-solving ability and language skills), and reality orientation therapy (which reduces sense of disorientation and confusion) and behavioural therapy. Behavioural therapy is designed to try to change challenging behaviour (e.g. exercise to decrease wandering). Even severely affected patients are often responsive to familiar social activities and to music. Self-help groups for family members, where available, can provide educational and psychological support.

### Social management

The social consequences of major and mild NCDs are complex and frequently quite problematical by the time patients present for treatment. Patients may face job loss, financial ruin and break-ups with their romantic partners, particularly for major or mild NCDs in young patients or where the symptoms are largely behavioural. Psycho-education is therefore key.

Occupational therapists perform work assessments and liaise with employers to negotiate,

> **Key points 10.3 Checklist for major and mild NCDs**
>
> As a primary care physician, focus on:
>
> - ensuring that the cognitive problem is not better explained by delirium, intellectual disability, another mental disorder or simple ageing
> - if a neurocognitive disorder is present, deciding whether it is major or mild based on severity and impairment in functioning
> - using special investigations sensibly: a careful history and clinical examination often yields a diagnosis
> - keeping in mind common as well as rare, but treatable, causes
> - establishing if there are co-morbidities (e.g. another medical condition, depression, delirium)
> - identifying and treating symptoms of clinical, social and functional concern.

if possible, alternate tasks at work that are more in keeping with the patient's ability. This is especially important for mild NCDs or early major NCDs where it is still possible to work. Occupational therapists can also help with advice on activities of daily living (e.g. home safety).

Social workers can assist the family in identifying care options (e.g. home based carers, respite care, old-age home placements). Social workers also help with disability grant applications for younger patients with major NCD who are not yet eligible for an old-age pension.

## Conclusion

Neurocognitive disorders left unrecognised or poorly managed have a considerable impact on mortality and quality of life. Although NCDs frequently have complex presentations, by following the basic steps outlined in this chapter, the primary care doctor can optimise the assessment and management of these conditions.

# References

American Psychiatric Association (2013) *Diagnostic and Statistical Manual of Mental Disorders* (5th edition). Arlington, VA: American Psychiatric Association

Cooper S, Greene JD (2005) The clinical assessment of the patient with early dementia. *Journal of Neurology, Neurosurgery, and Psychiatry 76* (Supplement 5): 15–24

Cummings JL, Benson DF (1984) Subcortical dementia: Review of an emerging concept. *Archives of Neurology* 41(8): 874–9

Flaherty JH, Little MO (2011) Matching the environment for older hospitalized adults with delirium. *Journal of the American Geriatrics Society,* 59 (Suppl 2): S295–300

Inouye SK, Bogardus ST (Jr), Charpentier PA, Leo-Summers L, Acampora D, Holford TR, Cooney LM (Jr) (1999) A multicomponent intervention to prevent delirium in hospitalized older patients. *The New England Journal of Medicine,* 340: 669–76.

### Additional reading

Devlin JW, Al-Qadhee NS, Skrobik Y (2012) Pharmacologic prevention and treatment of delirium in critically ill and non-critically ill hospitalised patients: A review of data from prospective, randomised studies. *Best Practice & Research Clinical Anaesthesiology* 26(3): 289–309

Inouye SK. (2006) Delirium in older persons. *The New England Journal of Medicine,* 16;354(11): 1157–65.

CHAPTER 11

# Schizophrenia spectrum and other psychotic disorders

Louw Roos, Jonathan Burns

## 11.1 Introduction

Patients who suffer from schizophrenia spectrum and other psychotic disorders are usually very ill, and often lack insight into their illness and treatment. These patients are mostly admitted as involuntary mental health care users to tertiary hospitals. Primary care doctors must be able to diagnose these patients, perform risk assessments and manage these patients.

## 11.2 Schizophrenia

### 11.2.1 Introduction

Schizophrenia is a syndrome: a collection of signs and symptoms of largely unknown aetiology, predominantly defined by observed signs of psychosis. In its most common form schizophrenia presents with paranoid delusions and auditory hallucinations late in adolescence or early adulthood. Our present knowledge base is mostly based on clinical observation and has changed little over the past century. Its prevalence of 1% of the population and the disability that goes with the illness has remained unchanged over the past century. If we compare it with other major illnesses, such as tuberculosis and leprosy, where major progress has been made in the management of these illnesses, we lag behind in the management of schizophrenia because we still do not have a basic understanding of the pathophysiology of the disorder. Furthermore, we lack the tools for curative treatment or prevention needed for most people with schizophrenia.

### 11.2.2 One hundred years of schizophrenia

In 1908, Eugen Bleuler, a professor of psychiatry in Zurich, proposed the term 'schizophrenia' for what Emil Kraepelin had been calling 'dementia praecox'. Bleuler described the syndrome's four As – disturbances of association, affect, **ambivalence** and autistic isolation. The disease is characterised by often recurrent, sometimes chronic delusions, hallucinations and disordered thought. The term was an unfortunate choice, because it suggested some kind of splitting or divided consciousness. In schizophrenia, nothing is split: what Bleuler was attempting to describe was the dissociation between affect and thought content that is often evident in the disorder.

Freud's psychoanalysis appears as a pause in the evolution of biological approaches to the brain and mind, especially in the first half of the 20th century. Towards the end of the first half of the 20th century, Fromm-Reichman's description (1948) of the schizophrenogenic mother became the basis of the family systems theory in the treatment of schizophrenia. It became standard practice to believe that mothers were the cause of their children's psychosis (Neill, 1990).

Prior to the advent of neuroleptic drugs treatment for schizophrenia included sleep therapy, shock therapy and insulin coma therapy. In addition, lobotomies were carried out on thousands of chronic patients, especially in the USA. With the emergence of neuroleptic drugs in 1953, the focus turned to brain chemistry. Schizophrenia was considered a dopamine disorder, with the antipsychotic efficacy of drugs linked to blockade of the dopamine $D_2$ receptor. Early neuroleptic medications (e.g. chlorpromazine and haloperidol) transformed the treatment of psychosis. Increasingly, patients were treated outside of hospital, and in some cases, a remission of positive symptoms of the illness was possible.

Over the last two decades, the early neuroleptic medications have been replaced by second-generation antipsychotics. These drugs have fewer extrapyramidal side effects, but usually do not appear to be significantly more efficacious than the earlier neuroleptic medications. They do, however, have a new side-effect profile, including risk of metabolic syndrome. Neither conventional nor second-generation antipsychotics have enhanced functional recovery.

The disability of schizophrenia is largely due to cognitive deficits, which these drugs fail to improve. A focus on cognitive symptoms has led to a more recent hypothesis of schizophrenia as a glutamate disorder. The theory is that schizophrenia – and particularly the cognitive symptoms of the disorder – may result from low activity of the NMDA receptor on GABA inhibitory interneurons in the prefrontal cortex.

Little progress has been made in research into the pathophysiology of schizophrenia. One approach that could separate cause from effect is genetics. Just as neuropharmacology dominated schizophrenia research in the late twentieth century, genetics has been a leading focus in the first decade of the 21st century. The underlying architecture of the genetic risk of schizophrenia remains a contentious issue. Early linkage and candidate association studies led to largely inconclusive results. The role of rare genetic events, such as copy-number variants (CNVs) or point mutations, has become increasingly important in gene discovery of schizophrenia. Recent research has highlighted a de novo mutational paradigm as a major component of the genetic architecture of schizophrenia. Recent progress is bringing us closer to earlier intervention and new therapeutic targets (Rodriquez-Murillo *et al.*, 2012).

## 11.2.3 Epidemiology of schizophrenia

The lifetime prevalence of schizophrenia is approximately 0,55%; meta-analyses, however, show a wide range (0,12% to 1,6%) (Goldner *et al.*, 2002). One-year prevalence is estimated at 0,34% (range 0,2% to 0,9%). When one considers psychotic disorders in general, the lifetime prevalence is approximately 1,45% (range 0,4% to 2,2%), while the one-year prevalence is approximately 0,8% (range 0,2% to 2,6%) (Wittchen and Jacobi, 2005).

Incidence rates also vary considerably: the most influential study of incidence was the WHO 10 Nation Study: it reported a range of incidence rates from 16 to 42 per 100 000 of the population (Jablensky, 2003). A very comprehensive systematic review of incidence (McGrath *et al.*, 2004) found extensive variation in incidence with the distribution positive skewed; the mean incidence rate was 15,2 per 100 000 persons per year.

Although the prevalence of schizophrenia appears to be similar in men and women, there are gender differences in incidence rates. In their systematic review, McGrath *et al.* (2004) reported a predominance in men with a rate ratio median of 1,4. Some authors have suggested that rates are higher in men up to the mid-30s, and thereafter the male-female ratio reverses with increasing age (Jablensky, 2003). Other authors attribute the similar gender prevalence of schizophrenia to increased mortality rates in men (Harris and Barraclough, 1998). Males tend to have an earlier age of onset than females (23 years versus 26 years) and develop more severe illness.

Schizophrenia is associated with a higher mortality rate than that of the general population, ranging from a 1,5-fold increase to a 2,5-fold increase (Brown, 1997; Saha *et al.*, 2007). Increased mortality is mainly attributed to cardiovascular disease and suicide. Suicide accounts for 10–38% of deaths in schizophrenia and risk is greatest during the first year after diagnosis.

## 11.2.4 Diagnostic criteria, dimensional assessment and stages of schizophrenia

### 11.2.4.1 Diagnostic criteria

An important issue in the definition and diagnosis of schizophrenia is that of the approach to classification. Most sciences start with a categorical classification and then move towards a dimensional approach as more accurate measurement becomes possible (Jablensky, 2011). The classification of schizophrenia to date has been a categorical classification. Growing evidence for a spectrum of schizophrenia-like disorders as well substantial evidence for multiple diagnostic overlaps between schizophrenia, mood disorders, personality disorders and other psychiatric conditions, has generated a call for the development of a **dimensional classification** system of psychoses. The recently published DSM-5 (American Psychiatric Association, 2013) retained the categorical system and added a dimensional scale with which one can chart a patient's specific symptom profile. The future is likely to see further efforts to incorporate a dimensional approach to psychotic disorders that better reflects the clinical reality encountered in everyday practice.

Table 11.1 shows the DSM-5's (American Psychiatric Association, 2013) diagnostic criteria for schizophrenia.

### 11.2.4.2 Dimensional assessment

Dimensions are assessed on a 0–4 scale cross-sectionally, with severity assessment based on the past month) (see Table 11.2). There are distinct psychopathological domains in psychotic illnesses (most clearly noted in schizophrenia) with distinctive patterns of treatment response, prognostic implications and course. The relative severity of symptoms across these domains varies across the course of illness and among patients.

### 11.2.4.3 Stages of schizophrenia

If we conceptualise schizophrenia as a neurodevelopmental disorder then we may consider the notion of a trajectory of illness. As Insel (2010) states: 'If the disorder begins in prenatal or perinatal life, then the psychosis of late adolescence must be seen not as the onset but as a late stage of the disorder.' Insel (2010) describes four stages of schizophrenia: risk, **prodromal**, psychosis onset and chronic disability stage.

**Stage 1: Risk**

Features include genetic vulnerability and environmental exposure. A family history of schizophrenia must be taken into account. At present we do not know to what extent risk factors for schizophrenia might be modifiable. This earliest stage quite often does not involve distress or seeking help. Longitudinal studies provide evidence for subtle behavioural and cognitive problems in early childhood. There is no known intervention at this stage of the illness.

**Stage 2: Prodrome of schizophrenia**

The prodrome is characterised by changes in thoughts (e.g. bizarre ideas that are subthreshold for delusions), social isolation and impaired functioning. Features that suggest a high risk of psychosis can be elicited using the Structured Interview for Psychosis Risk Syndromes (SIPS) (McGlashan *et al.*, 2010). Not all individuals who seek help for prodromal symptoms will develop schizophrenia: some will develop other forms of psychopathology. Many authors argue that the best predictors of schizophrenia may turn out to be cognitive changes such as deficits in working memory (Insel, 2010). Disability during the prodrome may include change in school and social functioning. Possible interventions during this phase include cognitive training, polyunsaturated fatty acids as a supplement and family support.

**Table 11.1** DSM-5 Diagnostic Criteria for Schizophrenia

| **Diagnostic Criteria** |
|---|
| A. Two (or more) of the following, each present for a significant portion of time during a 1 -month period (or less if successfully treated). At least one of these must be (1), (2), or (3):<br>1. Delusions.<br>2. Hallucinations.<br>3. Disorganized speech (e.g., frequent derailment or incoherence).<br>4. Grossly disorganized or catatonic behavior.<br>5. Negative symptoms (i.e., diminished emotional expression or avolition).<br>B. For a significant portion of the time since the onset of the disturbance, level of functioning in one or more major areas, such as work, interpersonal relations, or self-care, is markedly below the level achieved prior to the onset (or when the onset is in childhood or adolescence, there is failure to achieve expected level of interpersonal, academic, or occupational functioning).<br>C. Continuous signs of the disturbance persist for at least 6 months. This 6-month period must include at least 1 month of symptoms (or less if successfully treated) that meet Criterion A (i.e., active-phase symptoms) and may include periods of prodromal or residual symptoms. During these prodromal or residual periods, the signs of the disturbance may be manifested by only negative symptoms or by two or more symptoms listed in Criterion A present in an attenuated form (e.g., odd beliefs, unusual perceptual experiences).<br>D. Schizoaffective disorder and depressive or bipolar disorder with psychotic features have been ruled out because either 1) no major depressive or manic episodes have occurred concurrently with the active-phase symptoms, or 2) if mood episodes have occurred during active-phase symptoms, they have been present for a minority of the total duration of the active and residual periods of the illness.<br>E. The disturbance is not attributable to the physiological effects of a substance (e.g., a drug of abuse, a medication) or another medical condition.<br>F. If there is a history of autism spectrum disorder or a communication disorder of childhood onset, the additional diagnosis of schizophrenia is made only if prominent delusions or hallucinations, in addition to the other required symptoms of schizophrenia, are also present for at least 1 month (or less if successfully treated).<br>*Specify* if:<br>The following course specifiers are only to be used after a 1-year duration of the disorder and if they are not in contradiction to the diagnostic course criteria.<br>**First episode, currently in acute episode**: First manifestation of the disorder meeting the defining diagnostic symptom and time criteria. An *acute episode* is a time period in which the symptom criteria are fulfilled.<br>**First episode, currently in partial remission**: *Partial remission* is a period of time during which an improvement after a previous episode is maintained and in which the defining criteria of the disorder are only partially fulfilled.<br>**First episode, currently in full remission**: *Full remission* is a period of time after a previous episode during which no disorder-specific symptoms are present.<br>**Multiple episodes, currently in acute episode**: Multiple episodes may be determined after a minimum of two episodes (i.e., after a first episode, a remission and a minimum of one relapse).<br>**Multiple episodes, currently in partial remission**<br>**Multiple episodes, currently in full remission**<br>**Continuous**: Symptoms fulfilling the diagnostic symptom criteria of the disorder are remaining for the majority of the illness course, with subthreshold symptom periods being very brief relative to the overall course.<br>**Unspecified**<br>*Specify* if:<br>**With catatonia** (refer to the criteria for catatonia associated with another mental disorder, pp. 119–120, for definition).<br>*Specify* current severity:<br>Severity is rated by a quantitative assessment of the primary symptoms of psychosis, including delusions, hallucinations, disorganized speech, abnormal psychomotor behavior, and negative symptoms. Each of these symptoms may be rated for its current severity (most severe in the last 7 days) on a 5-point scale ranging from 0 (not present) to 4 (present and severe). (See Clinician-Rated Dimensions of Psychosis Symptom Severity in the chapter 'Assessment Measures.')<br>**Note**: Diagnosis of schizophrenia can be made without using this severity specifier. |

**Source:** Reprinted with permission from the *Diagnostic and Statistical Manual of Mental Disorders*, Fifth Edition, (Copyright 2013). American Psychiatric Association.

**Table 11.2** Dimensional assessment of psychosis

| DOMAIN | 0 | 1 | 2 | 3 | 4 | SCORE |
|---|---|---|---|---|---|---|
| Hallucinations | Not present | Equivocal (severity or duration not sufficient to be considered psychosis) | Present, but mild (little pressure to act upon voices, not very bothered by voices) | Present and moderate (some pressure to respond to voices, or is somewhat bothered by voices) | Present and severe (severe pressure to respond to voices, or is very bothered by voices) | |
| Delusions | Not present | Equivocal (severity or duration not sufficient to be considered psychosis) | Present, but mild (delusions are not bizarre, or little pressure to act upon delusional beliefs, not very bothered by beliefs) | Present and moderate (some pressure to act upon beliefs, or is somewhat bothered by beliefs) | Present and severe (severe pressure to act upon beliefs, or is very bothered by beliefs) | |
| Disorganised speech | Not present | Equivocal (severity or duration not sufficient to be considered disorganisation) | Present, but mild (some difficulty following speech) | Present and moderate (speech often difficult to follow) | Present and severe (speech almost impossible to follow) | |
| Abnormal psychomotor behaviour | Not present | Equivocal (severity or duration not sufficient to be considered abnormal psychomotor behavior) | Present, but mild (occasional abnormal or bizarre motor behavior or catatonia) | Present and moderate (frequent abnormal or bizarre motor behavior or catatonia) | Present and severe (abnormal or bizarre motor behavior or catatonia almost constant) | |
| Negative symptoms (restricted emotional expression or **avolition**) | Not present | Equivocal decrease in facial expressivity, prosody, gestures or self-initiated behavior | Present, but mild decrease in facial expressivity, prosody, gestures or self-initiated behavior | Present and moderate decrease in facial expressivity, prosody, gestures or self-initiated behavior | Present and severe decrease in facial expressivity, prosody, gestures or self-initiated behavior | |
| Impaired cognition | Not present | Equivocal (cognitive function not clearly outside the range expected for age or SES, i.e., within 0.5 SD of mean) | Present, but mild (some reduction in cognitive function below expected for age and SES, b/w 0,5 and 1 SD from mean) | Present and moderate (clear reduction in cognitive function below expected for age and SES, b/w 1 and 2 SD from mean) | Present and severe (severe reduction in cognitive function below expected for age and SES, > 2 SD from mean) | |
| Depression | Not present | Equivocal (Occasionally feels sad, down depressed or hopeless; concerned about having failed someone or at something but not preoccupied) | Present, but mild (Frequent periods of feeling very sad, down, moderately depressed or hopeless; Concerned about having failed someone or at something with some preoccupation) | Present and moderate (Frequent periods of deep depression or hopelessness; preoccupation with guilt, having done wrong) | Present and severe (Deeply depressed or hopeless daily; Delusional guilt or unreasonable self reproach grossly out of proportion to circumstances) | |
| Mania | Not present | Equivocal (Occasional elevated, expansive or irritable mood or some restlessness) | Present, but mild (Frequent periods of somewhat elevated, expansive or irritable mood or restlessness) | Present and moderate (Frequent periods of extensively elevated, expansive or irritable mood or restlessness) | Present and severe (Daily and extensively elevated, expansive or irritable mood or restlessness) | |

**Stage 3: Onset of psychosis**

This phase is manifested by hallucinations, delusions, disorganised thinking and behaviour and psychomotor abnormalities. Negative symptoms and cognitive deficits are core features of the disorder and responsible for much of the long-term morbidity and poor functional outcomes. These features also represent major therapeutic needs and challenge. Despite pharmacological and psychotherapeutic interventions there is a relapse rate of approximate 80% (Insel, 2010).

**Stage 4: Chronic disability stage**

This stage is characterised by chronic social and occupational functional disability. Importantly, not all individuals progress to this chronic stage of the disease. Social disability manifests in the form of high rates of unemployment and homelessness. People with schizophrenia are over-represented within prisons in many countries. Life expectancy in schizophrenia is significantly reduced (by approximately 25 years) (Colton and Manderscheid, 2006). Smoking and obesity are very common among people with schizophrenia.

## 11.2.5 Clinical symptom domains of schizophrenia

The clinical symptom domains of schizophrenia are grouped into clusters.

The positive symptoms are delusions, hallucinations, disorganised speech and neuromotor abnormalities (catatonia). The negative symptoms are affective blunting, **alogia**, avolition, **anhedonia** and social withdrawal.

Cognitive deficits include attention deficits, memory impairment, executive function deficits (e.g. with abstraction) and social cognitive deficits. Mood symptoms are depression, hopelessness, **suicidality**, anxiety and agitation. Co-morbid substance abuse is also often present.

We shall now look at these symptoms in greater detail.

### 11.2.5.1 Positive symptoms

Auditory hallucinations are commonest in schizophrenia and may vary from indistinct simple noises to complex conversations in the third person, commentary or commands. Hallucinations may, however, occur in any sensory modality in schizophrenia. Common delusions include persecutory, **grandiose**, religiose and bizarre delusions, although all forms of delusions may occur. Delusions vary from simple isolated delusional beliefs to complex, highly **systematised delusions**. Disorganised speech and disturbances of the form of thought vary from slight **tangentiality** and circumstantiality to highly disorganised formal thought disorder with thought blocking, **neologisms** and incoherence. Catatonic excitement and stupor may occur although is uncommon in the modern era.

### 11.2.5.2 Negative symptoms

Negative symptoms include disturbances in affect ranging from slight restriction of expression to complete blunting. Patients with the disorder may show inappropriate affect, including **fatuousness**. Alogia may not be present, but if present it varies from a slight reduction in the flow and amount of speech to complete mutism. The patient manifests avolition in his or her lack of spontaneity: in its severest form the patient lacks complete motivation to interact with the environment and may require assistance with self-care. Anhedonia is apparent when the patient cannot experience normal feelings of pleasure in relation to his or her experiences. Social withdrawal commonly begins during the prodromal stage and may progress from slight hesitancy and apparent loss in social confidence to complete disengagement from the social environment. The social withdrawal associated with schizophrenia was termed 'autistic' by Bleuler and bears many similarities to that of autism itself. Social withdrawal is often accompanied by deficits in social cognition (see Section 11.2.5.3).

Negative symptoms are divided into primary negative symptoms (enduring negative symptoms) and secondary negative symptoms. The primary negative symptoms are present prior to the start of treatment and subtle symptoms are usually present during the prodromal phase. The powerful first-generation dopamine blockers contributed to the so-called secondary negative symptoms.

The negative symptoms can also be produced by depression. Depression and primary negative symptoms can look alike, especially the apathy and the withdrawal, anhedonia and **restricted affect**. Patients with schizophrenia often develop depression or get dysphonia from the dopamine blockade (antipsychotic treatment) that causes excessive loss of dopamine (the catecholamine needed for mood regulation). We can assist patients significantly by avoiding extrapyramidal symptoms (EPS). Managing EPS effectively may lead to a marked reduction in secondary negative symptoms. Enduring primary negative symptoms, however, are very difficult to treat.

### 11.2.5.3 Cognitive symptoms

More than 90% of patients with schizophrenia have significant deficits in executive functioning, attention, working memory and social cognition. These deficits may be evident at psychiatric assessment or even in normal conversation. Often, though, they are subtle and are only detectable during neuropsychological testing. Cognitive deficits are increasingly recognised as a core feature of the disorder. Notably, neurocognitive deficits appear to be relatively independent of clinical symptoms and are stable across varying clinical states. Thus they are not dependent on acute psychotic episodes and remain, despite remission of acute symptoms. Importantly, they are present prior to and at the time of the first psychotic episode and are thus not simply a feature of chronicity as was previously believed. Finally, milder neurocognitive deficits can be detected in first-degree relatives of patients with schizophrenia who have no evidence of psychosis, suggesting that certain neurocognitive deficits are likely to be components of genetic vulnerability to the disorder (Horan *et al.*, 2011; Mesholam-Gately *et al.*, 2009; Snitz *et al.*, 2006).

Social cognition refers to the evolved and normally developed ability to interact with other individuals as well as to reading and interpreting social signals and responding appropriately to them. Social cognition also includes the ability to perceive and interpret facial expressions, detect the intentionality of social signals, process the emotional content of interpersonal engagements, and formulate appropriate social and emotional responses (Grady and Keightley, 2002). Social cognition also includes a capacity termed 'theory of mind' (ToM) (see Box 11.1 for an overview). Patients with schizophrenia demonstrate a range of impairments of social cognition, for example, impaired judgement of the direction of eye gaze, altered face processing (both the processing of neutral faces and the perception of emotional expressions on faces), deficits in response and conflict monitoring, decision making and **affiliative behaviour** (Rosse *et al.*, 1994; Williams *et al.*, 1999; Gaebel and Wölwer, 1992; Mathalon *et al.*, 2002; Kirkpatrick, 1997). Social cognition is an important mediator in shaping a representation of oneself in relation to the social environment; impaired social cognition may result in aberrant representations and psychotic symptoms.

#### Box 11.1 Theory of Mind (ToM) deficits in schizophrenia

Social cognition includes the concept of theory of mind (ToM). This refers to the assumption one makes during communication that the other individual possesses a mind just like one's own. ToM is the ability to attribute mental states to others and thus forms the very basis of social interaction and communication. This is because it is critical to understand the beliefs and intentions of others in social discourse. ToM enables individuals to engage cognitively in the social arena, and thus is a core aspect of social cognition. The term ToM was used first in relation to chimpanzees' capacity for deception (Premack and Woodruff, 1978) and several authors have argued strongly for the existence of ToM or elements of ToM in the great apes (Premack and Woodruff, 1978; Russon, 1999; Van Schaik and Van Hoof, 1996). As for the development of full ToM in normal healthy children, it is generally accepted that this is achieved by the age of four (Perner, 1991; Wimmer and Perner, 1983).

ToM abnormalities have been demonstrated in people with schizophrenia using a range of experiments, which reveal their difficulty attributing mental states and detecting deception and false beliefs.

**Table 11.3** Neurocognitive domains assessed by the MATRICS Consensus Cognitive Battery (MCCB)

| Neurocognitive domain | MCCB test |
|---|---|
| Attention/vigilance | Continuous Performance Test – Identical Pairs version |
| Speed of processing | Trail Making Test – Part A<br>Brief Assessment of Cognition in Schizophrenia – Symbol Coding subtest<br>Category fluency – animal naming |
| Working memory | Letter-Number Span<br>Wechsler Memory Scale – III Spatial Span subtest |
| Verbal learning | Hopkins Verbal Learning Test – Revised |
| Visual learning | Brief Visuospatial Memory Test – Revised |
| Reasoning and problem solving | Neuropsychological Assessment Battery – Mazes subtest |
| Social cognition | Mayer-Salovey-Caruso Emotional Intelligence Test – Managing Emotions |

**Source:** Horan *et al.*, 2011. This material is reproduced with permission from John Wiley and Sons Inc.

**Table 11.4** Primary versus secondary cognitive deficits and mood symptoms in schizophrenia

| Primary and secondary cognitive deficits in schizophrenia |
|---|
| ▶ Primary cognitive deficits are present at the onset of schizophrenia and manifest several years before the first psychotic episode<br>▶ Secondary cognitive deficits are due to iatrogenic or metabolic factors, including:<br>1. Excessive dopamine blockade in the prefrontal cortex, usually concurrent with EPS (bradyphrenia accompanies bradykinesia)<br>2. Anticholinergic medications like benztropine given for EPS impair already poor memory in schizophrenia<br>3. Being overweight (body mass index (BMI)> 25kg/m2) or obese (BMI > 30kg/m2) is associated with memory dysfunction<br>4. Hypertension is associated with memory loss<br>5. Sedentary lifestyle, lack of exercise and lack of stimulation<br>▶ It is easier to reverse secondary than primary cognitive deficits |
| **Primary, secondary and comorbid mood symptoms in schizophrenia** |
| ▶ Primary depressive symptoms occur as an integral part of the schizophrenia disorder<br>▶ Secondary depressive symptoms are due to numerous iatrogenic, medical and stress factors, including:<br>1. Excessive dopamine antagonism; EPS is often accompanied by dysphoria<br>2. Post-traumatic stress disorder (PTSD) due to the overwhelming/frightening subjective experiences of psychosis. (Note: depressive symptoms are very common in PTSD.)<br>3. Medical disorders (infections, endocrinologic, neurologic, metabolic)<br>4. Severe nutritional deficiencies due to poor diet (e.g. a vitamin B12 deficiency)<br>5. Iatrogenic depression due to psychotropic or non-psychiatric medications (e.g. anti-hypertensive medications, central nervous system (CNS) depressants). (Note: iatrogenic agitation may occur due to EPS (akathisia) from antipsychotics.)<br>6. The treatment of second-degree depression is to recognise and treat causative condition.<br>Co-morbid mood disorders (e.g. post-psychotic depression) or anxiety disorders may occur in individuals with schizophrenia. |

An important development in recent years was the launch of the NIH-MATRICS initiative, a consensus process to identify key domains of cognition in schizophrenia as a foundation to establish a standardised assessment battery for clinical and research use (especially in trials to develop new treatments enhancing cognition in the disorder.) Seven domains were identified and ten tests were selected as a reliable and practical battery that would show a relationship with functional outcome. Table 11.3 summarises the seven domains and the final MATRICS Consensus Cognitive Battery (MCCB).

Several iatrogenic or metabolic factors can influence cognition. Anticholinergic medications to reduce EPS, for example, can further worsen memory – it has been demonstrated that they can reduce 50% of one's verbal memory after only a few doses. (See Table 11.4 for an overview of primary versus secondary cognitive symptoms in schizophrenia.)

#### 11.2.5.4 Mood symptoms

It is important to differentiate mood or affective symptoms that are primary in that they comprise part of the schizophrenia illness, from those that may occur as a co-morbid psychiatric diagnosis or as a secondary consequence of iatrogenic or medical causes. (See Table 11.4 for an overview of primary versus secondary versus co-morbid mood symptoms in schizophrenia.)

Mood symptoms in schizophrenia include depression, hopelessness and suicidality as well as anxiety, agitation and hostility. Symptoms may be present during the acute phase of the illness or occur after remission of psychotic symptoms (so-called post-psychotic depression). Post-psychotic depression is likely to relate to the individual, having regained partial or complete insight, struggling to come to terms with the fact that he or she has a severe disorder that typically disrupts quality of life and expectations for the future.

#### 11.2.5.5 Other clinical features of schizophrenia

During the psychotic phases of the illness (and sometimes during inter-psychotic periods of remission) individuals with schizophrenia very often lose insight and exhibit impaired judgement. If present, these features typically create a barrier to the development of a therapeutic relationship necessary to affect good adherence to treatment. Lack of insight and poor judgement are usually the basis for resistance to acute treatment, very often leading to the need for involuntary hospitalisation. Other clinical features that may or may not be present or apparent include minor physical anomalies, poor self-care and inappropriate behaviour at interview.

### 11.2.6 Aetiology and pathophysiology

There are few certainties regarding the aetiology of schizophrenia. Some facts about the aetiology are more robust, but their interpretation remains unclear.

Environmental factors interact with a genetic predisposition that leads to a neurodevelopmental disorder. There is likely a collection of neurodevelopmental disorders that involve alterations in brain circuits (Insel, 2010).

#### 11.2.6.1 Genetics and the neurodevelopmental basis of schizophrenia

The genetic architecture of schizophrenia is still unknown and currently there is no proven genetic risk factor that confers a significant risk of schizophrenia. One cannot assume that risk is synonymous with prediction where one would be able to determine who will become ill. Risk factors only elevate one's chances of becoming ill (DeLisi, 2014). Heritability in schizophrenia is relatively high (60 – 80%) and risk varies according to which relative is affected (see Table 11.5).

**Table 11.5** Schizophrenia liability based on affected relatives

| Family member(s) affected | Approximate risk |
|---|---|
| Identical (monozygotic) twin | 46%* |
| Fraternal (dizygotic) twin | 14%* |
| Sibling | 10%$ |
| Both parents | 46%$ |
| One parent | 13%$ |
| No relatives affected | 1%$ |

**Source:** Riley *et al.*, 2003* (Copyright 2008 John Wiley and Sons. This material is reprinted with permission of John Wiley and Sons Ltd); Gottesman and Shields$, 1967

There are two generally investigated major sets of risk factors in the genetics of schizophrenia. These are the common alleles that appear to confer a very small risk above the general population and the rare CNVs that have a high risk of conferring disease. CNVs that exist in the genome are either de novo or transmitted to offspring. CNVs are rare but, when pathogenic (i.e. occurring in a functional portion of a gene), are likely to have a high risk of conferring disease. Several have been found, such as the very large CNV on chromosome 22q11 and one on chromosome 7q36.3. Most of the CNVs associated with schizophrenia have been identified in large studies of unrelated patients and not yet proven to be causative of the disorder within families (DeLisi, 2014). They tend also to be more likely de-novo spontaneous mutations rather than run in families (Xu *et al.*, 2011).

Many of the structural variants associated with schizophrenia implicate neurodevelopmental genes involved in neural proliferation, migration or synapse formation. Even genes that are not exclusively developmental seem to influence schizophrenia by their early disruption. The genetics of schizophrenia also overlaps with the genetics of autism and other neurodevelopmental disorders (Insel, 2010). Genetic epidemiological studies have proposed that gene-environment interaction in schizophrenia and related diagnostic categories is common (Van Os *et al.*, 2010).

Although schizophrenia usually emerges in late adolescence or early adulthood, several longitudinal population-based studies indicate that the problems are evident much earlier. Early deviant behaviour patterns in children who go on to develop schizophrenia have been consistently reported in high-risk, prospective and retrospective behavioural studies of schizophrenia. Early behavioural deviance and the various neurodevelopmental anomalies may, in fact, be both a subtype and a disease-onset marker. Approximately two-thirds of patients who later develop schizophrenia report one or more forms of early non-psychotic deviance, including poor socialisation, extreme fears, chronic sadness and/or attention learning impairment (Sobin *et al.*, 2003). These findings support the hypothesis that psychosis does not emerge from a completely healthy brain.

The number of studies into the pathophysiological changes of schizophrenia has dramatically increased in the past ten years. Structural brain imaging studies have shown a subtle, almost universal, decrease in grey matter, enlargement of ventricles and focal alteration of white matter tracts (Ellison-Wright and Bullmore, 2009).

A mixture of dopamine dysregulation and aberrant assignment of **salience** to stimuli, together with a cognitive scheme that attempts to grapple with these experiences to give them meaning, may lead to the development of psychotic symptoms (Kapur, 2004). Alterations in affective state (depression or mania) and some ways of thinking, such as a tendency to jump to conclusions, might combine with the dopamine dysfunction to increase the risk of delusion formation (Fine *et al.*, 2007).

For contemporary reviews of the aetiology and conceptualisation of schizophrenia, see Van Os and Kapur (2009) and Insel (2010).

### 11.2.6.2 The environment and schizophrenia

Heritability, as an index of genetic influence, may have limited explanatory power unless viewed within the context of interaction with social effects. The onset of schizophrenia is often associated with environmental factors such as early-life adversity, growing up in an urban environment, minority group position and cannabis use. Longitudinal research is needed to uncover gene-environment interplay. It must be determined how expression on vulnerability in the general population may give rise to more severe psychopathology (Van Os *et al.*, 2010).

### Prenatal environmental factors

Rates of schizophrenia are increased in individuals who experienced obstetric complications, compared with their unaffected siblings or normal controls (Cannon *et al.*, 2002). Obstetric complications might be directly causal, a reflection of a pre-existing foetal abnormality, or even a reflection of maternal characteristics (e.g. the mother's antenatal health behaviour) (Nicodemus *et al.*, 2008).

Serological evidence of influenza infection during early pregnancy is associated with a sevenfold increase in risk of schizophrenia in the offspring (Brown *et al.*, 2004), although some studies have yielded negative results (Selten *et al.*, 2010). Other maternal (and childhood) infections have also been associated with schizophrenia, including toxoplasmosis, herpes simplex virus 2, and rubella (Brown *et al.*, 2010).

Children born to mothers who experienced famine early in their pregnancy have an increased risk of schizophrenia. This illness is also slightly more frequent among people born in winter than among those born in summer (Davies *et al.*, 2003). A replicated finding is that schizophrenia is associated with paternal age in sporadic cases. One large study found that the risk increased by almost 50% for each ten-year increase in paternal age (Sipos *et al.*, 2004).

### Growing up in an urban environment

The risk of schizophrenia and other psychoses increases linearly with the extent to which the environment in which children grow up is urbanised (Krabbendam and Van Os, 2005). Longitudinal studies of natural experiments show that changing the environmental exposure (e.g. moving from an urban to a rural environment in childhood) brings about a corresponding decrease in risk of a psychotic outcome. This argues against urbanicity representing merely a non-causal genetic epiphenomenon (Van Os *et al.*, 2010).

### Effects of migration and minority group position

Evidence exists that some immigrant ethnic groups have a higher risk of developing psychotic disorders than have native-born individuals (Cantor-Graae and Selten, 2005). This is particularly so when they live in a low ethnic-density area, or an area where there are fewer people of the same migrant group (Veling *et al.*, 2008). Findings suggest it is not ethnic group per se that increases risk, but rather the degree to which one occupies a minority position. This effect may be mediated by chronic social adversity and discrimination that result in social marginalisation or a state of social defeat (chronic experience of an inferior position or social exclusion) (Van Os *et al.*, 2010).

### Cannabis use

Individuals at genetic risk of psychotic syndrome display an exaggerated psychotic response when exposed to delta-9-tetrahydrocannabinol (THC). Meta-analytic work shows that the association between psychotic syndrome and cannabis is consistent, even after adjustment for a range of confounding factors. Cannabis use may reflect self-medication for early expression of psychotic vulnerability or symptoms; there is evidence that both self-medication (proneness to psychosis may induce cannabis use) and causation (cannabis induces proneness to psychosis) apply.

Studies addressing genetic confounding do not suggest that genetic confounding can explain much of the observed association between cannabis and psychotic syndrome. Early initiation of cannabis use correlates with an increased risk, as well as an earlier age of onset, of psychosis. In the Dunedin Study (a longitudinal birth cohort investigation from New Zealand) use of cannabis by the age of 15 was associated with a more than fourfold increase in risk of schizophreniform disorder by the age of 26 (Arseneault *et al.*, 2002). Thus, where cannabis use starts very early and continues into early adulthood, it is likely that there may be varying degrees of neurodevelopmental insult (possibly involving dopamine sensitisation and dysregulation) that places the individual at increased risk of later long-term psychotic disorders. Importantly, since younger age and male gender predominate amongst those who use cannabis, gender may be a powerful confounding factor in studies of the relationship between cannabis and early age of onset of psychosis. Gene-environment interactions clearly play a key role in determining the extent to which early cannabis use leads to psychosis. Several authors have shown how individuals homozygous or heterozygous for the COMTVal allele are at enhanced risk of developing psychosis later on if they have used cannabis during adolescence (Caspi *et al.*, 2005).

## 11.2.7 Management of schizophrenia

A bio-psycho-social approach towards the management of schizophrenia is emphasised. Each aspect of this approach is equally important. By giving attention to all these aspects the best outcome for an individual patient will be assured.

### 11.2.7.1 Antipsychotic medication

There is an ongoing debate whether – and which – first-generation antipsychotics (FGAs) or second-generation antipsychotics (SGAs) should be used. When considering individual adverse effect profiles of the antipsychotic, the differentiation into FGAs and SGAs as unified classes cannot be upheld and a more differentiated view and treatment selection are required. An individualised treatment approach is needed. The considerations to be taken into account include current symptoms, co-morbid conditions, past therapeutic response, adverse effects, patient choice and patient expectations.The acute and long-term goals and effects of medication treatment must be balanced.

A number of divergent interpretations have been offered regarding the comparative efficacy and effectiveness of FGAs and SGAs. This indicates that blanket statements do not do justice to the complex clinical situation and database. Although the CATIE (Lieberman *et al.*, 2005) and CUTLASS (Jones *et al.*, 2006) studies seemed to suggest that there are generally no differences between SGAs and FGAs, these conclusions have been challenged based on insufficient sample sizes to make non-inferiority claims as well as high drop-out rates.

Schizophrenia is a chronic remitting and relapsing disorder associated with shortened lifespan and significant impairments in social and vocational functioning. Comprehensive treatment entails a multi-modal approach, including medication, psychosocial interventions and assistance with housing and financial sustenance. The broad objectives of treatment are to reduce the mortality and morbidity of the disorder by decreasing the frequency and severity of episodes of psychotic exacerbation and improving the functional capacity and quality of lives of individuals affected with the illness.

Antipsychotic medication is the cornerstone in the pharmacological treatment of schizophrenia and three of these agents (chlorpromazine, fluphenazine and haloperidol) are included in the World Health Organization's list of Essential Medicines. To date, more than 60 antipsychotic medications have been developed; they are classified into groups of first- and second-generation agents. The one pharmacological property shared by all antipsychotic agents currently available is their ability to block the dopamine $D_2$ receptor; with the clinical antipsychotic potency found to correlate with their affinity for the receptor.

#### Comparative effectiveness of antipsychotics in the treatment of schizophrenia

FGAs are fairly effective in reducing positive symptoms (hallucinations and delusions) of the disorder in a large proportion of patients; they undoubtedly facilitated the de-institutionalisation of persons with schizophrenia in the 1960s.These medications are, however, minimally effective against primary negative and cognitive symptom domains that contribute to much of the illness-related disability. FGAs also cause a range of treatment burdens including acute EPS and tardive dyskinesia.

Clozapine, the first so-called atypical antipsychotic (subsequently labelled SGA) was introduced into clinical practice in the late 1960s. It does not cause EPS or tardive dyskinesia. Its other adverse effects, however, have substantially limited its use and the problem of **agranulocytosis** led to it being excluded in many parts of the world until the 1990s. The fact that it was found to be more effective than FGAs in **treatment-refractory** patients and in reducing suicidality and was devoid of significant short-term and long-term motor side-effects led to optimism that better antipsychotic treatments for schizophrenia were possible. Substantial efforts to develop a safer clozapine have led to the introduction of 12 additional SGAs into clinical practice over the past fifteen years. SGAs have progressively displaced the older agents in the treatment of schizophrenia. Results of recent large-scale studies comparing the effectiveness of FGAs versus SGAs in schizophrenia appear to indicate that SGAs are no more effective than FGAs and are not associated with better cognitive or social outcomes (Lieberman *et al.*, 2005).

Recent data obtained from first-episode and early-onset schizophrenia patients also suggest the absence of significant benefits of SGAs over FGAs (Zhang *et al.*, 2013).

### Summary of the effectiveness, safety and tolerability of antipsychotics

Antipsychotic medication is effective in reducing overall symptoms and risk of relapse in patients with schizophrenia, with their primary efficacy mainly against positive and disorganisation symptom domains. Except for the greater efficacy of clozapine in treatment-refractory schizophrenia patients, differences in efficacy among other antipsychotic agents are relatively minor. In contrast to small differences in efficacy, antipsychotic agents differ substantially in their side-effect profiles.

FGAs and SGAs both constitute very heterogeneous classes of antipsychotic medication without any definite categorical boundaries between them in terms of efficacy, safety tolerability or overall outcome. The broad distinction between SGAs and FGAs is the better ability of SGAs to provide an equivalent antipsychotic effect with a lower liability to cause EPS, although there is substantial variation within each class in this regard. Since there are no categorical differences between FGAs and SGAs, however, with reference to this or any other attribute, classification of antipsychotic agents into FGA and SGA classes has little value and should be abandoned. On the other hand, atypicality (the ability to provide a good antipsychotic effect without EPS) is an important attribute, with substantial variation across patients and different agents.

It should also be emphasised that broadly equivalent efficacy across patient groups does not translate into equal efficacy in individual patients. There is no best agent or a best dose of any agent for all patients. Despite limited data regarding antipsychotic dose-response relationships, these agents appear to have specific dose ranges for optimal effectiveness. It is not currently possible to predict which antipsychotic medication will be optimal for a given patient. Decisions about antipsychotic therapy consequently entail a trial-and-error process with a careful monitoring of clinical response and adverse effects and an on-going risk-benefit assessment and judicious switching if appropriate.

SGAs introduced into clinical practice during the past 20 years were initially considered to be much more effective than FGAs, with a broad spectrum of efficacy against the wide array of symptoms in schizophrenia and with a significantly better safety and tolerability profile. With continuing use and research, we now know that they do not differ substantially in efficacy from FGAs (with the exception of clozapine in treatment-refractory patients), are less likely to cause EPS than FGAs (but are not completely devoid of that adverse effect) and are associated with the same array of side-effects as FGAs (e.g. metabolic syndrome, anticholinergic effects).

Despite their shortcomings, the initial introduction of FGAs in the 1950s and the subsequent introduction of SGAs in the 1990s represented meaningful steps in our efforts to provide effective treatment for individuals with schizophrenia. Just as it is important not to exaggerate what existing treatments for schizophrenia can offer, however, it is equally important not to discount what they can do.

### 11.2.7.2 Specific treatment of cognitive deficits

Several pharmacological approaches to ameliorate cognitive impairments in schizophrenia are currently under study. (Harvey and Bowie, 2012). These include alpha-7 nicotinic receptor agonists, dopamine-1 receptor agonists, NMDA glutamate receptor agonists, modulators of the glutamergic AMPA receptor, metabotropic glutamate receptor agonists, muscarime receptor agonists, 5-HT1A agonist strategies, and phosphodiesterase 10 inhibitors.

### 11.2.7.3 Other pharmacological agents

In view of the limitations of antipsychotic agents in the pharmacotherapy of various symptom domains of schizophrenia, several other psychotherapeutic medications have been used in its treatment. These include various anticonvulsants, antidepressants, benzodiazepines and lithium. Whereas none of these treatments has been found to be consistently useful as **monotherapy**, some have provided modest benefits as adjuncts to antipsychotic medication in targeting specific symptom domains in some patients.

It is not precisely known how polyunsaturated fatty acids (PUFA) might be involved in schizophrenia, but several mechanisms have been suggested (Steullet *et al.*, 2006). The evidence is strong enough to have led to a membrane phospholipid hypothesis of schizophrenia (Horrobin, 1998). Fatty acids play critical roles in the cell membranes of neurons, and certain fatty acids appear to be abnormally low in the brains of patients with schizophrenia. The attempts to enhance endogenous levels thus seem a rational and worthwhile goal. The value of such intervention awaits the results of ongoing trials.

Given the low risk of harm, and despite the limited evidence that supplements ameliorate the symptoms of schizophrenia, some clinicians might decide to add eicosapentaenoic acid (EPA) to current drug regimens in hope of better symptomatic control in schizophrenia (Akter *et al.*, 2012).

### 11.2.7.4 Electroconvulsive therapy and repetitive transcranial magnetic stimulation

The role of electroconvulsive therapy (ECT) in the treatment of schizophrenia has diminished over the past two decades. Although recent data are limited, ECT may augment antipsychotic efficacy in some patients and may provide a more rapid onset of antipsychotic action. ECT is useful in treating catatonic symptoms in schizophrenia and as an adjunct to clozapine in some antipsychotic-refractory schizophrenia patients.

Repetitive **transcranial magnetic stimulation** (rTMS) is showing some promise in treating different symptom domains in schizophrenia (principally negative symptoms and auditory hallucinations) using different frequencies and targeting different cortical regions. Data are preliminary at this time.

### 11.2.7.5 Psychotherapy and social treatment

There is a need for multi-modal care (including psychosocial therapies) as adjuncts to antipsychotic medication to help alleviate symptoms and to improve adherence, social functioning and quality of life.

Research on psychosocial approaches to the treatment of schizophrenia has yielded incremental evidence of the efficacy of cognitive behaviour therapy (CBT), social skills training (SST), family psycho-education, assertive community treatment (ACT) and supported employment.

Psycho-educational interventions provide information about the disorder and its treatment to patients and their family members and also inform the patients and family members about strategies to cope with schizophrenic illness. Systematic reviews suggest that these interventions reduce high expressed emotion among relatives and decrease relapse and rehospitalisation rates (Xia *et al.*, 2011).

In general, interventions that include family members are more effective. Multi-family psycho-education group approaches (which provide psycho-education and offer an expanded social network) and peer-to-peer education programs for families and patients reduce rates of relapse.

About a third of patients with schizophrenia continue to suffer from persistent psychotic symptoms despite adequate pharmacotherapy. CBT, based on the hypothesis that psychotic symptoms stem from misinterpretations and irrational attributes caused by self-monitoring deficits, has emerged to address this need. CBT seeks to help patients rationally appraise their experience of disease symptoms and how they respond to them, thereby reducing symptoms and preventing relapse.

The goal of SST is to improve day-to-day living skills by focusing on components of social competence such as self-care, basic conversation, vocational skills and recreation.

ACT offers an approach to integrated delivery of clinical services to patients with schizophrenia using a multidisciplinary approach, high frequency of patient contact, low patient-to-staff ratios and outreach to the patient in the community.

These interventions are recommended for clinical application in the recently published Schizophrenia Patient Outcomes Research Team (PORT) guidelines which provide a comprehensive review of current evidence-based psychosocial interventions for schizophrenia. (Kreyenbuhl *et al.*, 2010)

There is little evidence of the efficacy of psychodynamic therapy in schizophrenia.

### 11.2.7.6 Management of first-episode psychosis

A growing body of evidence suggests that early and effective management in the critical early years of illness can improve long-term outcomes in schizophrenia (McGorry *et al.*, 2007). Furthermore, there is converging evidence to support the development of early and effective treatment from the earliest phases of psychotic disorders. Sustained symptomatic and functional remission and relapse prevention are key treatment targets, and the majority of psychotic patients require long-term continuous antipsychotic treatment (Kane and Correll, 2009). Poor medication adherence is common in schizophrenia, perhaps particularly after the first episode of psychosis (Coldham *et al.*, 2002).

The available evidence suggests that long-acting injectable antipsychotics can be used safely and effectively in the early stages of the illness and that they may be associated with better outcomes than with oral medications. However, this is largely supported by evidence from naturalistic cohort studies and a small number of controlled trials of risperidone long-acting injection. Evidence for olanzapine and paliperidone long-acting injectables in particular is limited (Emsley *et al.*, 2013).

### 11.2.7.7 Big picture view of the treatment of schizophrenia in the 21st century

Research in recent years has identified a number of key developments and targets in the treatment of schizophrenia. According to Insel (2010), these include:

- early intervention – prodrome
- focus of treatment on cognitive deficits and negative symptoms
- drug discovery beyond traditional dopamine-$D_2$ and serotonin $_2$A antagonism
- utility of several evidence-based psychotherapy modalities in combination with pharmacological approaches and even monotherapy
- a shift in focus of treatment towards disease-modifying approaches, quality of life and restoration of function
- outcome targets shift to states of remission and recovery
- deconstruct schizophrenia into gene-endophenotype elements linked to therapeutically meaningful clinical dimensions and offer novel targets for drug development
- advances in pharmacogenomics with better explanation of the extreme variability in treatment outcomes across patients and providing individualized predictive markers of response or adverse effects.

## 11.2.8 Recovery from schizophrenia

It emerges that one of the most robust findings (Emsley *et al.*, 2013) in relation to schizophrenia is that a substantial proportion of those who present with the illness will recover completely or with good functional capacity, with or without modern medical treatment. This is not the view of schizophrenia that was advanced by Emil Kraepelin a century ago or is currently held by many practising psychiatrists.

Practising mental health professionals do not have opportunities to follow patients who recover, as they drop out of treatment which results in a negative clinician bias regarding outcome. Based on the research data (Emsley *et al.*, 2013), however, it is reasonable to advise people who have recently developed schizophrenia and their relatives that the illness may have a good outcome.

Several authors have mounted a challenge to the famous finding of the World Health Organization's multi-country studies (Jablensky *et al.*, 1992) that people with schizophrenia in the developing world have a better course and outcome than their counterparts in developed countries. Significant political, social and economic ills characterise many countries in Africa, Latin America and Asia; this reality militates against a better outcome for individuals who live with this disorder in these contexts. The belief that community and family life in the developing world are widely intact and that these factors provide a nurturing environment that facilitates recovery and promotes social and economic empowerment of seriously mentally ill individuals, is dispelled as a myth. It is reasoned that **idealisation** of the under-developed South as a haven for schizophrenia sufferers will only add to the already heavy burden experienced by these individuals, their families and these societies in coping with this disabling disease (Burns, 2009).

The recovery model refers both to subjective experiences of optimism, empowerment and interpersonal support, and to the creation of positive, recovery-orientated services (Warner, 2009). Although remission has been precisely defined, recovery is a more diffuse concept that includes such factors as being productive, functioning independently and maintaining satisfying relationships. Optimism regarding outcome is supported by research data showing that many recover completely and many more regain good social functioning (Emsley *et al.*, 2013). The evidence suggests that working helps people recover from schizophrenia, and advances in vocational rehabilitation have made this more feasible (Emsley *et al.*, 2013). Empowerment is certainly an important component of the recovery process. User or consumer-driven services together with a focus on reducing internalised stigma are valuable strategies to empower those with schizophrenia and improve the outcome of the illness.

## 11.3 Schizophreniform disorder

Schizophreniform disorder appears as a diagnosis in both the DSM-5 and the ICD-10. It is a serious condition that requires early and effective identification and management.

In terms of diagnosis, the disorder manifests with symptoms identical to schizophrenia. In terms of the DSM-5, criterion A must be met in order to diagnose schizophreniform disorder. However, unlike schizophrenia, all phases of schizophreniform disorder (prodromal, active and residual phases) must last longer than one month but less than six months. Unlike schizophrenia, schizophreniform disorder requires a rather rapid period from the onset of prodromal symptoms to the point at which all the criterion A features of schizophrenia are met. In addition, criterion B of schizophrenia, namely deterioration in social and occupational functioning, is not required in schizophreniform disorder. Importantly, the illness must not be due to the direct physiological effects of a substance (e.g. an abused drug, a medication) or a general medical condition.

The prevalence of schizophreniform disorder is equal in men and women with a peak onset between the age of 18–24 in men and 24–35 in women.

In terms of course and outcome, approximately two-thirds of patients with schizophreniform disorder progress to a diagnosis of schizophrenia. Within two years, 50% of individuals will have a repeat psychotic episode (Fraguas *et al.*, 2008). The presence of negative symptoms is a predictor of poorer outcome of schizophreniform disorder. A significant risk of suicide exists in this condition, especially with the development of post-psychotic depression. Drake *et al.* (2004) report that patients who develop a better insight into their illness are less likely to experience relapse.

Good prognostic factors in schizophreniform disorder include:

- onset of prominent psychotic symptoms within four weeks of the first noticeable change in usual behaviour and functioning
- **perplexity** and thought disorganisation at the height of the psychotic episode
- good premorbid social and occupational functioning
- absence of blunted or flat affect (Perkins *et al.*, 2004).

Differential diagnosis includes:

- brief psychotic disorder
- schizophrenia
- schizo-affective disorder
- mood disorders with psychotic features
- psychotic disorder associated with another medical condition
- substance induced psychotic disorder.

Pathophysiological findings in schizophreniform disorder overlap considerably with those in schizophrenia. Neuropsychological deficits as well as structural and functional impairment have been reported (Crespo-Facorro *et al.*, 2009).

The management of schizophreniform disorder entails the use of antipsychotic medication in combination with early comprehensive psychological and social interventions. CBT, psycho-education and aggressive treatment of depression are recommended.

## 11.4 Brief psychotic disorder and acute transient psychotic disorder

The DSM-5 and the ICD-10 differ in their respective approaches to brief psychosis. The DSM-5's diagnosis of a brief psychotic disorder (BPD) refers to an illness that lasts less than one month and is manifested by hallucinations and/or delusions. While other symptoms, such as disorganised thinking, speech and behaviour, often occur, the emphasis in BPD is on a brief, non-affective type psychotic illness. The ICD-10, on the other hand, includes a diagnostic category termed acute transient psychotic disorder (ATPD). In the ICD-10 there are a number of subtypes of ATPD, although it is likely that the distinction between subtypes of ATPD will disappear in ICD-11. With ATPD, the emphasis is on a rapid onset of symptoms that fluctuate in intensity and nature over a period of up to a month, with rapid remission. These symptoms include hallucinations, delusions, disorganised thinking and behaviour, affective symptoms and cognitive symptoms (e.g. inattention, brief confusion). Systematic reviews of ATPD suggest a female predominance and a later age of onset than schizophrenia – typically in middle adulthood in both men and women (Castagnini and Berrios, 2009). Reviews also indicate a much higher prevalence of ATPD in low- and middle-income countries.

ATPD and BPD have historical antecedents in the French diagnosis of *bouffée délirante*, the German concept of cycloid psychoses and the Scandinavian psychogenic and schizophreniform psychoses (Castagnini and Berrios, 2009). Jaspers (1913) had described reactive psychosis, which later found a place within the DSM classification system as brief reactive psychosis in the DSM-III (American Psychiatric Association, 1987) and brief psychotic disorder in the DSM-IV (American Psychiatric Association, 1994) and the DSM-5 (American Psychiatric Association, 2013).

Interestingly, research shows that BPD and ATPD show modest degrees of diagnostic overlap. Concordance rates vary with between 30% and 62% of ATPD cases meeting criteria for BPD (Pillmann *et al.*, 2002).

A stressful event may or may not precede the onset of BPD and ATPD. In the DSM-5 the specifiers are with and without marked stressor(s), as well as with post-partum onset.

The differential diagnosis of BPD includes delirium, psychotic disorder due to a general medical condition, a substance-induced psychotic disorder or a mood disorder with psychotic features.

The management of BPD and ATPD entails excluding a medical or substance-related cause and brief treatment with antipsychotics and/or benzodiazepines. Hospitalisation is often indicated.

## 11.5 Schizo-affective disorder

Schizo-affective disorder was described in 1933 by Jacob Kasanin and referred to an illness characterised by concurrent features of schizophrenia and a mood disorder. In the last 80 years it has evoked considerable controversy as an independent diagnosis, with some authors regarding it as a form of schizophrenia, others as a form of bipolar disorder and – probably the majority – viewing it as an intermediate form of psychosis on a continuum between schizophrenia and affective disorder. The fact that the three disorders show considerable clinical, genetic and neurobiological overlap supports the last view.

The DSM-5 defines schizo-affective disorder as an uninterrupted period of illness during which there is, at some point, a major depressive, manic or mixed episode concurrent with the characteristic symptoms of schizophrenia (i.e. criterion A for schizophrenia). In addition there must be a period of at least two weeks during which delusions or hallucinations are present, with the absence of symptoms that meet the criteria for a major mood episode. A major mood episode, however, must be present for the majority (> 50%) of the total duration of the illness. Notably there are two subtypes: a bipolar subtype and a depressive subtype. The bipolar subtype is diagnosed if a manic or mixed episode is present while the depressive subtype is diagnosed if a major depressive episode is present.

Lifetime prevalence of schizo-affective disorder is approximately 0.5–0.8%.

Perhaps the most difficult differential diagnosis is a mood disorder with psychotic features. The inclusion of a period of at least two weeks of psychotic symptoms in the absence of mood symptoms for schizo-affective disorder is intended to differentiate this condition from a mood disorder with psychotic features where psychotic symptoms occur only in the context of mood symptoms.

The course and prognosis are intermediate between schizophrenia and mood disorder, although significant variability exists and many consider the outcome to be similar to that of schizophrenia.

Management is similar to that of schizophrenia, although mood stabilisers are often used in addition to antipsychotics to stabilise mood symptoms and are often continued into the maintenance phase of treatment.

In concluding this section on schizo-affective disorder, it is worth noting that many authors (e.g. Jäger *et al.*, 2011) advocate the omission of this diagnosis from our classification systems on the basis of the following arguments:

- the diagnostic category of schizo-affective disorder has a low reliability
- there are no clear boundaries between schizophrenia, schizo-affective disorder and affective disorders with respect to psychopathological syndromes
- common neurobiological factors are found across the traditional diagnostic categories
- outcome appears to approximate that of most cases of schizophrenia and many cases of bipolar disorder.

## 11.6 Schizotypal personality disorder

Schizotypal personality disorder (SPD) is classified in both the DSM and the ICD systems within the schizophrenia spectrum disorders.

In the case of the DSM-5 this marks a shift in thinking, since SPD was grouped with personality disorders in the DSM-IV. The authors of the DSM-5 concluded that research evidence strongly supports the inclusion of SPD within the spectrum of psychotic illness. According to Semple *et al.* (2005) there are considerable overlaps in terms of genetics, neurobiological findings and phenomenology between SPD and schizophrenia:

- **monozygotic twin** studies show an increased risk of schizotypy in the unaffected twin, where the other twin has schizophrenia
- **schizotypy** is more common in the first-degree relatives of people with schizophrenia than in the general population
- relatives of schizotypal individuals have an increased risk of schizophrenia
- schizotypy shares many clinical features of schizophrenia, but without delusions and hallucinations.

Typical clinical features include **ideas of reference**, excessive social anxiety, odd beliefs or **magical thinking**, unusual perceptions (e.g. illusions), odd eccentric behaviour or appearance, few or no close friends or confidants, odd speech, inappropriate or even constricted affect, suspiciousness and paranoid ideas.

Frank psychosis is not present in SPD. In some cases, clinically significant psychotic symptoms may develop that meet the criteria for brief psychotic disorder, schizophreniform disorder, delusional disorder or schizophrenia. It is important to differentiate SPD from schizophrenia, autism, language disorders and other personality disorders.

Estimates are that SPD affects approximately 3% of the population.

## 11.7 Delusional disorder

Delusional disorder is an uncommon disorder characterised by the presence of one or more non-bizarre **circumscribed delusions**, usually in the absence of other psychotic features. The DSM-5 requires symptoms to have been present for a minimum of one month, while the ICD-10 requires a period of three months for the diagnosis to be made. Formerly recognised under the term paranoia and first described by Kalhbaum in 1863, delusional disorder received its current name in 1977 (Winokur, 1977).

Prevalence is estimated at approximately 0.03%, with a mean age of onset between 40–49 years. Prevalence is equal in men and women, although men are more likely to develop **delusional jealousy** while **erotomania** is more common in women. Function is usually preserved, with most individuals being employed and married. In general the illness does not impact on psychosocial functioning unless the delusions intrude on social and occupational life.

The onset is usually insidious, although acute onset may occur. Individuals with delusional disorder usually do not present for treatment as they typically lack insight into their illness.

The DSM-5 diagnostic criteria for delusional disorder include a further classification of subtypes (see Table 11.6).

Clinical judgement is necessary to distinguish between delusions and overvalued ideas, culturally sanctioned beliefs and beliefs substantiated by fact. Delusions may be wholly plausible; the clinician must take various factors into account when making a diagnosis of delusional disorder. According to Manschreck (1996) some of these factors include:

- the degree of plausibility
- evidence of systematisation, complexity and persistence
- the impact of the beliefs on behaviour
- considering whether these may be culturally sanctioned beliefs
- presence of other symptoms e.g. hallucinations
- a history of morbid change.

It is important to differentiate delusional disorder from the following conditions:

- other functional psychotic disorders
- substance-induced delusional disorder
- delusional disorder due to another medical condition
- dementia and delirium
- body dysmorphic disorder
- obsessive-compulsive disorder (OCD)

**Table 11.6** DSM-5 Diagnostic Criteria for Delusional Disorder

| **Diagnostic Criteria** |
|---|
| A. The presence of one (or more) delusions with a duration of 1 month or longer.<br>B. Criterion A for schizophrenia has never been met.<br>**Note:** Hallucinations, if present, are not prominent and are related to the delusional theme (e.g., the sensation of being infested with insects associated with delusions of infestation).<br>C. Apart from the impact of the delusion(s) or its ramifications, functioning is not markedly impaired, and behavior is not obviously bizarre or odd.<br>D. If manic or major depressive episodes have occurred, these have been brief relative to the duration of the delusional periods.<br>E. The disturbance is not attributable to the physiological effects of a substance or another medical condition and is not better explained by another mental disorder, such as body dysmorphic disorder or obsessive-compulsive disorder.<br>*Specify* whether:<br>**Erotomanic type:** This subtype applies when the central theme of the delusion is that another person is in love with the individual.<br>**Grandiose type:** This subtype applies when the central theme of the delusion is the conviction of having some great (but unrecognized) talent or insight or having made some important discovery.<br>**Jealous type:** This subtype applies when the central theme of the individual's delusion is that his or her spouse or lover is unfaithful.<br>**Persecutory type:** This subtype applies when the central theme of the delusion involves the individual's belief that he or she is being conspired against, cheated, spied on, followed, poisoned or drugged, maliciously maligned, harassed, or obstructed in the pursuit of long-term goals.<br>**Somatic type:** This subtype applies when the central theme of the delusion involves bodily functions or sensations.<br>**Mixed type:** This subtype applies when no one delusional theme predominates.<br>**Unspecified type:** This subtype applies when the dominant delusional belief cannot be clearly determined or is not described in the specific types (e.g., referential delusions without a prominent persecutory or grandiose component).<br>*Specify* if:<br>**With bizarre content:** Delusions are deemed bizarre if they are clearly implausible, not understandable, and not derived from ordinary life experiences (e.g., an individual's belief that a stranger has removed his or her internal organs and replaced them with someone else's organs without leaving any wounds or scars).<br>*Specify* if:<br>The following course specifiers are only to be used after a 1 -year duration of the disorder:<br>**First episode, currently in acute episode:** First manifestation of the disorder meeting the defining diagnostic symptom and time criteria. An acute episode is a time period in which the symptom criteria are fulfilled.<br>**First episode, currently in partial remission:** Partial remission is a time period during which an improvement after a previous episode is maintained and in which the defining criteria of the disorder are only partially fulfilled.<br>**First episode, currently in full remission:** Full remission is a period of time after a previous episode during which no disorder-specific symptoms are present.<br>**Multiple episodes, currently in acute episode**<br>**Multiple episodes, currently in partial remission**<br>**Multiple episodes, currently in full remission**<br>**Continuous:** Symptoms fulfilling the diagnostic symptom criteria of the disorder are remaining for the majority of the illness course, with subthreshold symptom periods being very brief relative to the overall course.<br>**Unspecified**<br>*Specify* current severity:<br>Severity is rated by a quantitative assessment of the primary symptoms of psychosis, including delusions, hallucinations, disorganized speech, abnormal psychomotor behavior, and negative symptoms. Each of these symptoms may be rated for its current severity (most severe in the last 7 days) on a 5-point scale ranging from 0 (not present) to 4 (present and severe). (See Clinician-Rated Dimensions of Psychosis Symptom Severity in the chapter "Assessment Measures.")<br>**Note:** Diagnosis of delusional disorder can be made without using this severity specifier. |

**Source:** Reprinted with permission from the *Diagnostic and Statistical Manual of Mental Disorders*, Fifth Edition, (Copyright 2013). American Psychiatric Association.

- **hypochondriasis**
- paranoid personality disorder
- delusional **misidentification syndromes** (e.g. **Capgras syndrome** and **Frégoli syndrome**)
- induced or shared psychotic disorder (e.g. **folie à deux**).

Delusional disorder is notoriously difficult to treat and management includes a thorough psychiatric and cognitive assessment and investigation, exclusion of medical or substance-related causes, gathering collateral information from third parties to confirm evidence and a thorough documented assessment of risk. Outpatient treatment is preferable unless the risk is assessed as significant. There is evidence of some benefit from antipsychotics (especially pimozide) and, given the overlaps with OCD spectrum symptomatology, from selective serotonin re-uptake inhibitors (SSRIs). The judicious use of benzodiazepines is justified to reduce anxiety in the acute phase. Psychotherapeutic treatment depends on developing a therapeutic alliance (which is often difficult) and mainly entails supportive, educational and cognitive behavioural approaches.

Outcome is variable, but generally the condition is unremitting with 40–60% of patients showing little improvement. There is a better prognosis if the onset was acute. Research indicates that 3–22% of patients are later reclassified as schizophrenia (Manschreck, 1996).

## 11.8 Psychotic disorder associated with another medical condition

Many medical conditions may manifest with psychotic symptoms and it is important for the clinician to have a high index of suspicion for underlying medical causes. This is true always and for every patient, regardless of the stage of his or her illness. However, particular attention should be paid to exclude a medical cause in the following cases:

- the first episode of psychiatric disorder
- onset of psychiatric disorder for the first time (or a different psychiatric diagnosis) in older persons
- associated symptoms (or history of symptoms) of other medical conditions or physical ill health
- the presence of physical signs or laboratory evidence for other medical conditions
- a history of injury or trauma (note this need not be very recent as in the case of a subdural haematoma in an elderly individual with a fall within the last few months)
- a strong family history of another medical condition that has a familial basis
- any other factors that lead to suspicion of another medical condition.

### 11.8.1 Medical causes of psychotic illness

Neurological causes of psychotic illness are epilepsy, head injury, brain tumour, dementia, encephalitis (e.g. herpes simplex encephalitis), HIV, neurosyphilis, brain abscess, cerebro-vascular accident, demyelinating disorders, Huntington's disease and Parkinson's disease.

Endocrine causes are hyperthyroidism, hypothyroidism, Cushing's syndrome, hyperparathyroidism and Addison's disease.

Uraemia, electrolyte imbalances, porphyria, pellagra and a vitamin B12 deficiency are metabolic causes of psychotic illness.

Systemic lupus erythematosis (SLE or lupus psychosis) also play a role in psychotic illness.

## 11.9 Catatonic disorder associated with another medical condition

Formerly, catatonia was classified as a subtype of schizophrenia. However, in the DSM-5 it is now de-linked from an exclusive relationship with schizophrenia, as clinical and research evidence overwhelmingly show that this is a syndrome that may be associated with a variety of both psychiatric and other medical conditions (see Table 11.7). More than 50% of patients with

**Table 11.7** DSM-5 Diagnostic Criteria for Catatonic Disorder Due to Another Medical Condition

| Diagnostic Criteria |
|---|
| A. The clinical picture is dominated by three (or more) of the following symptoms:<br>1. Stupor (i.e., no psychomotor activity; not actively relating to environment).<br>2. Catalepsy (i.e., passive induction of a posture held against gravity).<br>3. Waxy flexibility (i.e., slight, even resistance to positioning by examiner).<br>4. Mutism (i.e., no, or very little, verbal response [**Note:** not applicable if there is an established aphasia]).<br>5. Negativism (i.e., opposition or no response to instructions or external stimuli).<br>6. Posturing (i.e., spontaneous and active maintenance of a posture against gravity).<br>7. Mannerism (i.e., odd, circumstantial caricature of normal actions).<br>8. Stereotypy (i.e., repetitive, abnormally frequent, non-goal-directed movements).<br>9. Agitation, not influenced by external stimuli.<br>10. Grimacing.<br>11. Echolalia (i.e., mimicking another's speech).<br>12. Echopraxia (i.e., mimicking another's movements). |
| B. There is evidence from the history, physical examination, or laboratory findings that the disturbance is the direct pathophysiological consequence of another medical condition. |
| C. The disturbance is not better explained by another mental disorder (e.g., a manic episode). |
| D. The disturbance does not occur exclusively during the course of a delirium. |
| E. The disturbance causes clinically significant distress or impairment in social, occupational, or other important areas of functioning. |

**Source:** Reprinted with permission from the *Diagnostic and Statistical Manual of Mental Disorders*, Fifth Edition, (Copyright 2013). American Psychiatric Association.

prominent catatonic features do not have schizophrenia. At the same time, 15–30% of patients diagnosed with schizophrenia do present with prominent catatonic features. The simple truth about catatonia is that not all is schizophrenia, but some is (Fink *et al.*, 2009).

Importantly, catatonia is always caused by an underlying medical, neurological or psychiatric illness. Identification of the symptoms of catatonia must be made while at the same time determining the cause.

Syndromes and symptoms to be differentiated from catatonia include coma, **akinetic** mutism, **abulia**, hypoactive delirium and locked-in syndrome. An accurate diagnosis can change the treatment and prognosis dramatically.

In order to identify thoroughly and monitor signs and symptoms of catatonia, it can be helpful to use a standardised examination and rating scale for catatonia. History from family and friends will be particularly important as catatonic patients are often mute.

The number of medical causes that can underlie catatonia demands an extensive work-up, including a thorough history taking, physical and neurological exam.

Medical causes of catatonia include:

- infections: HIV, syphilis, encephalitis, meningitis
- metabolic/endocrine: diabetes mellitus, thyroid illness, low serum iron, vitamin B deficiency, folate deficiency
- substance abuse: phencyclidine exposure, disulfuram toxicity
- non-psychiatric medication: sibutramine, clarithromycin, azithromycin, amoxcillion
- liver pathology following liver transplantation
- SLE
- diffuse cerebral dysfunction causes: encephalitis, seizures, corticosteroids, SLE

- focal disturbances: CNS structural damage, infections, focal seizures
- cancer: CNS masses, leptomeningeal disease, paraneoplastic encephalitis
- neuroleptic malignant syndrome (NMS) or malignant catatonia.

It is very important to quickly rule out the following causes in a patient who presents with catatonia: NMS, epilepsy, encephalitis, mass lesions or cerebral infarctions (seizures suspected with episodic bradycardia).

## 11.10 Substance induced psychotic disorder (SIPD)

A host of substances, both recreational and prescribed, may produce symptoms of psychosis. It is important that the clinician be aware of these potential causes in every patient presenting with psychotic symptoms. Psychotic symptoms may occur during intoxication or withdrawal from a substance or against a background of harmful or dependent use. It is often difficult to differentiate SIPD from a primary psychotic disorder with a co-morbid substance use disorder. Clinical and research evidence confirm a high prevalence of co-morbid substance use in individuals with primary psychosis (Wisdom *et al.*, 2011). The clinician should be wary of assuming that substances are directly aetiological in patients presenting with psychosis and a history of substance use: in many contexts there is over-use of the provisional diagnosis of SIPD, meaning that patients too often fail to receive appropriate treatment for underlying psychiatric disorders.

Table 11.8 lists the common substances associated with psychosis in the South African context.

**Table 11.8** Substances that cause psychotic features

| Recreational drugs | Medications |
|---|---|
| cannabis | steroids |
| alcohol | antiviral agents (e.g. Efavirenz) |
| tik (methamphetamine) | INH |
| other amphetamines | anxiolytics |
| whoonga/**nyaope** | sedatives |
| cocaine | L-Dopa |
| PCP | |
| hallucinogens | |
| inhalants | |
| opioids | |

See Chapter 21: Other substance-related and addictive disorders, for further information on SIPD.

## Conclusion

Despite pharmacologic advances, the treatment of schizophrenia spectrum and other psychotic disorders remains a challenge. Suboptimal outcomes are still too frequent. However, an individualised treatment approach must consider current symptoms, co-morbid conditions, past therapeutic response and adverse effects, as well as patient choice and expectations. Acute and long-term goals and effects of medication must be balanced (Kane and Correll, 2010). Although new treatment options are needed that act on non-dopaminergic targets, with the aim of symptom reduction, relapse prevention, enhanced efficacy for non-responders, and reduction of adverse effects, physicians should remain optimistic when treating these patients who suffer from a serious psychiatric illness.

# References

Akter K, Gallo DA, Martin SA, Myronyuk N, Roberts RT, Steraila K, Raffa RB (2012) A review of the possible role of essential fatty acids and fish oils in the aetiology, prevention or pharmacotherapy of schizophrenia. *Journal of Clinical Pharmacy and Therapeutics* 37: 132–9

American Psychiatric Association (2013) *Diagnostic and Statistical Manual of Mental Disorders* (5th edition). Arlington, VA: American Psychiatric Association

American Psychiatric Association (1994) *Diagnostic and Statistical Manual of Mental Disorders* (4th edition). Arlington, VA: American Psychiatric Association

Arseneault L, Cannon M, Poulton R, Murray R, Caspi A, Moffitt TE (2002) Cannabis use in adolescence and risk for adult psychosis: Longitudinal prospective study. *British Medical Journal* 325: 1212–3

Brown AS, Begg MD, Gravenstein S, Schaefer CA, Wyatt RJ, Bresnahan M, Babulas VP, Susser ES (2004) Serologic evidence of prenatal influenza in the etiology of schizophrenia. *Archives of General Psychiatry* 61: 774–780

Brown S (1997) Excess mortality of schizophrenia: A meta-analysis. *British Journal of Psychiatry* 171: 502–8

Burns J (2009) Dispelling a myth: Developing world poverty, inequality, violence and social fragmentation are not good for outcome in schizophrenia. *African Journal of Psychiatry* 12: 200–5

Cannon M, Jones PB, Murray RM (2002) Obstetric complications and schizophrenia: Historical and meta-analytic review. *American Journal of Psychiatry* 159(7): 1080–92

Cantor-Graae E, Selten JP (2005) Schizophrenia and migration: A meta-analysis and review. *American Journal of Psychiatry* 162: 12–24

Caspi A, Moffitt TE, Cannon M, McLay J, Murray R, Harrington H, Taylor A, Arseneault L, Williams B, Braithwaite A, Poulton R, Craig IW (2005) Moderation of the effect of adolescent-onset cannabis use on adult psychosis by a functional polymorphism in the catechol-O-methyltransferase gene: Longitudinal evidence of a gene x environment interaction. *Biological Psychiatry* 57: 1117–27

Castagnini A, Berrios GE (2009) Acute and transient psychotic disorders (ICD-10 F 23): A review from a European perspective. *European Archives of Psychiatry and Clinical Neurosciences* 259(8): 433–43

Coldham EL, Addington J, Addington D (2002) Medication adherence of individuals with a first episode of psychosis. *Acta Psychiatrica Scandinavica* 106: 286–90

Colton CW, Manderscheid RW (2006) Congruencies in increased mortality rates, years of potential life lost, and causes of death among public mental health clients in eight states. *Preventing Chronic Disease* 3: A42

Crespo-Facorro B, Roiz-Santiáñez R, Pérez-Iglesias R, Tordesillas-Gutiérrez D, Mata I, Rodríguez-Sánchez JM, de Lucas EM, Vázquez-Barquero JL (2009) Specific brain structural abnormalities in first-episode schizophrenia. A comparative study with patients with schizophreniform disorder, non-schizophrenic non-affective psychoses and healthy volunteers. *Schizophrenia Research* 115(2–3): 191–201

Davies G, Welham J, Chant D, Torrey EF, McGrath J (2003) A systematic review and meta-analysis of Northern Hemisphere season of birth studies in schizophrenia. *Schizophrenia Bulletin* 29(3): 587–93

DeLisi LE (2014) Ethical issues in the use of genetic testing of patients with schizophrenia and their families. *Current Opinion in Psychiatry* 27(3): 191–6

Drake RJ, Pickles A, Bentall RP Kinderman P, Haddock G, Tarrier N, Lewis SW (2004) The evolution of insight paranoia and depression during early schizophrenia. *Psychological Medicine* 34(2): 285–92

Ellison-Wright J, Bullmore E (2009) Meta-analysis of diffusion tensor imaging studies in schizophrenia. *Schizophrenia Research* 108: 3–10

Emsley R, Chiliza B, Asmal L, Mashile M, Fusar-Poli P (2013) Long-acting injectable antipsychotics in early psychosis: A literature review. *Early Intervention in Psychiatry* 7(3): 247–54

Fine C, Gardner M, Craigie J, Gold I (2007) Hopping, skipping or jumping to conclusions? Clarifying the role of JTC bias in delusions. *Cognitive Neuropsychiatry* 12: 46–77

Fink M, Shorter E, Taylor M (2010) Catatonia is not schizophrenia: Kraepelin's error and the need to recognize catatonia as an independent syndrome in medical nomenclature. *Schizophrenia Bulletin* 36(2): 314–20

Fraguas D, De Castro MJ, Medina O, Parellada M, Moreno D, Grael M, Merchan-Naranjo J, Arango C (2008) Does diagnostic classification of early-onset psychosis change over follow-up? *Child Psychiatry and Human Development* 39: 137–45

Fromm-Reichman F (1948) Notes on the development of treatment of schizophrenics by psychoanalytic psychotherapy. *Psychiatry* 11: 263–73

Gaebel W, Wölwer W (1992) Facial expression and emotional face recognition in schizophrenia and depression. *European Archives of Psychiatry and Clinical Neurosciences* 242: 46–52

Goldner E, Hsu L, Waraich P, Somers JM. (2002) Prevalence and incidence studies of schizophrenic disorders: A systematic review of the literature. *Canadian Journal of Psychiatry* 47: 833–43

Gottesman IL & Shields J (1967) A polygenic theory of schizophrenia. Proceedings of the National Academy of Sciences of the USA 58: 199–205

Grady CL, Keightley ML (2002) Studies of altered social cognition in neuropsychiatric disorders using functional neuroimaging. *Canadian Journal of Psychiatry* 47: 327–36

Harris E, Barraclough B (1998) Excess mortality of mental disorder. *British Journal of Psychiatry* 173: 11–53

Harvey PD, Bowie CR (2012) Cognitive enhancement in schizophrenia. Pharmacological and cognitive remediation approaches. *Psychiatric Clinics of North America* 35: 683–98

Horan WP, Harvey PO, Kern RS, Green MF (2011) Neurocognition, social cognition and functional outcome in schizophrenia. In: Hirsch SR, Weinberger DR (Eds) *Schizophrenia*. Oxford: Blackwell

Horrobin DF (1998) The membrane phospholipid hypothesis as a biochemical basis for the neurodevelopmental concept of schizophrenia. *Schizophrenia Research* 30: 193–208

Insel TR (2010) Rethinking schizophrenia. *Nature* 468: 187–93

Jablensky A (2011) Diagnosis and revision of the classification systems. In: Gaebel W (Ed) *Schizophrenia: Current Science and Clinical Practice*. Chichester, UK: Wiley-Blackwell

Jablensky A (2003) The epidemiological horizon. In: Hirsch SR, Weinberger DR (Eds) *Schizophrenia*. Oxford: Blackwell

Jablensky A, Sartorius N, Ernberg G, Anker M, Korten A, Cooper JE, Day R, Bertelsen A. (1992) Schizophrenia: Manifestations, incidence and course in different cultures. A World Health Organization ten-country study. *Psychological Medicine* (Monograph Supplement) 20: 1–97

Jäger M, Haack S, Becker T, Frasch K (2011) Schizoaffective disorder – an ongoing challenge for psychiatric nosology. *European Psychiatry* 26: 159–65

Jaspers K (1913) *Allgemeine Psychopathologie*. Berlin, Germany: Springer

Jones PB, Barnes TR, Davies L, Dunn G, Lloyd H, Hayhurst KP Murray RM, Markwick A, Lewis SW (2006) Randomized controlled trial of the effect on quality of life of second vs first generation antipsychotic drugs in schizophrenia: Cost Utility of the Latest Antipsychotic drugs in Schizophrenia Study (Cutlass I). *Archives of General Psychiatry* 63: 1079–87

Kane J, Correll CU (2010) Past and present progress in the pharmacological treatment of schizophrenia. *Journal of Clinical Psychiatry* (9): 1115–24

Kane JM, Garcia-Ribera C (2009) Clinical guideline recommendations for antipsychotic long-acting injections. *British Journal of Psychiatry* (Supplement) 52: S63–7

Kapur S (2004) How antipsychotics become 'anti-psychotic' – from dopamine to salience to psychosis. *Trends in Pharmacological Sciences* 25: 402–6

Kirkpatrick B (1997) Affiliation and neuropsychiatric disorders: The deficit syndrome of schizophrenia. *Annals of the New York Academy of Sciences* 807: 455–68

Krabbendam L, Van Os J (2005) Schizophrenia and urbanicity: A major environmental influence – conditional on genetic risk. *Schizophrenia Bulletin* 31: 795–9

Kreyenbuhl J, Buchanan RW, Dickenson FW, Dixon LB (2010) The Schizophrenia Patient Outcomes Research Team (PORT): Updated treatment recommendations 2009. *Schizophrenia Bulletin* 36(1): 94–103

Lieberman JA, Stroup TS, McEvoy JP, Swartz MS, Rosenheck RA, Perkins DD (2005) Clinical Antipsychotic Trials of Intervention Effectiveness (CATIE) investigators. Effectiveness of antipsychotic drugs in patients with chronic schizophrenia. *New England Journal of Medicine* 353: 1209–23

Manschreck T (1996) Delusional disorder: The recognition and management of paranoia. *Journal of Clinical Psychiatry* 57(Supplement 3): 32–8

Mathalon DH, Fedor M, Faustman WO, Gray M, Askari N, Ford JM (2002) Response monitoring dysfunction in schizophrenia: An event-related brain potential study. *Journal of Abnormal Psychology* 111: 22–41

McGlashan T, Walsh BC, Woods SW (2010) *The Psychosis Risk Syndrome: Handbook for Diagnosis and Follow-up*. New York: Oxford University Press

McGorry PD, Killackey E, Yung AR (2007) Early intervention in psychotic disorders: Detection and treatment of the first episode and the critical early stages. *Medical Journal of Australia* 187(7 Supplement): S8–10

McGrath JJ, Saha S, Welham J, El Saadi O, MacCauley C, Chant D. (2004) A systematic review of the incidence of schizophrenia: The distribution of rates and the influence of sex, urbanicity, migrant status and methodology. *BMC Medicine* 2: 1–22

Mesholam-Gately RI, Giuliano AJ, Goff KP, Faraone SV, Seidman LJ (2009) Neurocognition in first-episode schizophrenia: A meta-analytic review. *Neuropsychology* 23(3): 315–336

Neill J (1990) Whatever became of the schizophrenogenic mother? *American Journal of Psychotherapy* 44: 499–505

Nicodemus KK, Marenco S, Batten AJ, Vakkalanka R, Egan MF, Straub RE, Weinberger DR (2008) Serious obstetric complications interact with hypoxia-regulated/vascular-expression genes to influence schizophrenia risk. *Molecular Psychiatry* 13(9): 873–7

Perkins DA, Lieberman JA, Gu H, Tohen M, McEvoy J, Green AI, Zipursky RB, Strakowski SM, Sharma T, Kahn R, Gur R, Tollefson G (2004) Predictors of antipsychotic treatment response in patients with first-episode schizophrenia, schizoaffective and schizophreniform disorder. *British Journal of Psychiatry* 185: 18–24.

Perner J (1991) *Understanding the Representational Mind*. Boston, MA: MIT Press

Pillmann F, Haring A, Balzuweit S, Bloink R, Marneros A (2002) The concordance of ICD-10 acute and transient psychosis and DSM-IV brief psychotic disorder. *Psychological Medicine* 32: 525–33

Premack D, Woodruff G (1978) Does the chimpanzee have a 'theory of mind'? *Behavioral and Brain Sciences* 4: 515–26

Riley B, Asherson PJ, McGuffin P (2003) Genetics and schizophrenia. In: Hirsch SR and Weinberger DR, (Eds) *Schizophrenia* (2nd edition) Oxford, UK: Blackwell Publishing

Rodriquez-Murillo L, Gogos JA, Karayiorgou M (2012) The genetic architecture of schizophrenia: New mutations and emerging paradigms. *Annual Review of Medicine* 63: 63–80

Rosse RB, Kendrick K, Wyatt RJ, Isaac A, Deutsch SI (1994) Gaze discrimination in patients with schizophrenia: Preliminary report. *American Journal of Psychiatry* 151: 919–21

Russon AE (1999) Orangutans' imitation of tool use: A cognitive interpretation. In: Taylor Parker S, Mitchell RW, Miles HL, (Eds) *The Mentalities of Gorillas and Orangutans: Comparative Perspectives*. Cambridge: Cambridge University Press

Saha S, Chant D, McGrath J (2007) A systematic review of mortality in schizophrenia. *Archives of General Psychiatry* 64: 1123–31

Selten JP, Frissen A, Lensvelt-Mulders G, Morgan VA (2010) Schizophrenia and 1957 pandemic of influenza: Meta-analysis. *Schizophrenia Bulletin* 36(2): 219–28

Semple D, Smyth R, Burns J, Darjee R, McIntosh A (2005) *Oxford Handbook of Psychiatry*. Oxford: Oxford University Press

Sipos A, Rasmussen F, Harrison G, Tynelius P, Lewis G, Leon DA, Gunnell D (2004) Paternal age and schizophrenia: A population based cohort study. *British Medical Journal* 329(7474): 1070

Snitz BE, MacDonald AW, Carter CS (2006) Cognitive deficits in unaffected first-degree relatives of schizophrenia patients: A meta-analytic review of putative endophenotypes. *Schizophrenia Bulletin* 32: 179–94

Sobin C, Roos JL, Pretorius HW, Lundy LS, Karayiorgou M (2003) A comparison study of early non-psychotic deviant behaviour in Afrikaner and US patients with schizophrenia and schizoaffective disorder. *Psychiatry Research* 117: 113–25

Steullet P, Neijt HC, Cuenod M, Do KQ (2006) Synaptic plasticity impairment and hypofunction of NMDA receptors induced by glutathione deficit: Relevance to schizophrenia. *Neuroscience* 137: 807–19

Van Os J, Kapur S (2009) Schizophrenia. *Lancet* 374: 635–45

Van Os J, Kenis G, Rutten BPF (2010) The environment and schizophrenia. *Nature* 468: 203–212

Van Os J, Rutten BPF, Poulton R (2008) Gene-environment interactions in schizophrenia: Review of epidemiological findings and future directions. *Schizophrenia Bulletin* 34: 1066–82

Van Schaik CP, Van Hoof JA (1996) Towards an understanding of the orangutan's social system. In: McGrew WC, Marchant LF, Nishida T (Eds) *Great Ape Societies*. Oxford: Oxford University Press

Veling W, Susser E, Van Os J, Mackenbach JP, Selten JP, Hoek HW (2008) Ethnic density of neighborhoods and incidence of psychotic disorders among immigrants. *American Journal of Psychiatry* 165: 66–73

Warner R (2009) Recovery from schizophrenia and the recovery model. *Current Opinion in Psychiatry* 22: 374–80

Williams LM, Loughland CM, Gordon E, Davidson D (1999) Visual scanpaths in schizophrenia: Is there a deficit in face recognition? *Schizophrenia Research* 40:189–99

Wimmer H, Perner J (1983) Beliefs about beliefs: Representation and constraining function of wrong beliefs in young children's understanding of deception. *Cognition* 13: 103–28

Winokur G (1977) Delusional disorder (paranoia). *Comprehensive Psychiatry* 18: 511–21

Wisdom JP, Manuel JI, Drake RE (2011) Substance use disorder among people with first-episode psychosis: A systematic review of course and treatment. *Psychiatric Services* 62(9): 1007–12

Wittchen HU, Jacobi F (2005) Size and burden of mental disorders in Europe – a critical review and appraisal of 27 studies. *European Neuropsychopharmacology* 15: 357–76

Xia J, Merinder LB, Belgamwar MR (2011) Psychoeducation for schizophrenia. *Cochrane Database Systematic Reviews* 15(6): CD002831.

Xu B, Roos JL, Dexheimer P, Boone B, Plummer B, Levy S, Gogos JA, Karayiorgou M (2011) Exome sequencing supports a de novo mutational paradigm for schizophrenia. *Nature Genetics* 43(9): 864–8

Zhang JP, Gallego JA, Robinson DG, Malhotra AK, Kane JM, Correll CU (2013) Efficacy and safety of individual second-generation vs. first-generation antipsychotics in first-episode psychosis: a systematic review and meta-analysis. *International Journal of Neuropsychopharmacology* 16(6): 1205–18

CHAPTER

# 12 Depressive disorders

*Gian Lippi, Janus Pretorius*

## 12.1 Introduction

The fifth edition of the *Diagnostic and Statistical Manual of Mental Disorders*, or DSM-5, classifies depressive disorders into eight disorders (see Table 12.1). All of these disorders include symptoms of sadness, irritability and feelings of emptiness, and accompanying somatic and cognitive changes can cause functional impairment. (American Psychiatric Association, 2013).

**Table 12.1:** DSM-5 Depressive Disorders

| |
|---|
| 1. Major depressive disorder |
| 2. Persistent depressive disorder (dysthymia) |
| 3. Disruptive mood dysregulation disorder |
| 4. Premenstrual dysphoric disorder |
| 5. Substance / medication-induced depressive disorder |
| 6. Depressive disorder due to another medical condition |
| 7. Other specified depressive disorder |
| 8. Unspecified depressive disorder |

## 12.2 Major depressive disorder (American Psychiatric Association, 2013)

Major depressive disorder (MDD) is characterised by discrete episodes of at least two weeks' duration involving clear-cut changes in affect, cognition, and **neurovegetative** functions and inter-episode remissions. The disorder is recurrent in the majority of cases.

### 12.2.1 Epidemiology

Traditionally, a MDD was considered a rare disorder in Africa. During the 1950s, studies identified depression as an important problem but not as prevalent as in developed countries. By the 1970s, it was accepted that depression was as common in developing countries as in developed countries, but manifested with a different symptom profile. Modern studies dispute all of the above views and indicate prevalence rates and clinical presentations similar to those in developed countries.

Depression affects about 121 million people worldwide, and an estimated 5,8% of men and 9,5% of women will experience a depressive episode every year. The South African Stress and Health (SASH) study (Tomlinson *et al.*, 2009) reports that approximately 10% of South Africans experience a major depressive episode during their lifetime. Some international studies indicate lifetime prevalence rates of up to 25% (Tomlinson *et al.*, 2009).

This condition is a major cause of disability and distress and is expected to become the second commonest cause of loss of disability-adjusted life years globally by 2020 (World Bank, 1993).

Although viewed traditionally as a disease affecting the brain, it is now clear that MDD is a whole-body disease that affects multiple organ systems including the brain, endocrine system and the immune system. Through its effects on the hypothalamic-pituitary adrenal (HPA) axis and immune system, major depressive disorder has widespread effects on the central nervous, cardiovascular and gastrointestinal systems. If left untreated, MDD can contribute to deleterious long-term physical consequences. It is therefore not surprising that patients who suffer from MDD have higher rates of co-morbid chronic physical illnesses such as coronary heart disease, asthma, diabetes and rheumatoid arthritis. It is unclear whether these conditions are linked through a common genetic susceptibility or whether the physical abnormalities outside the central nervous system (CNS) result from changes secondary to the major depressive disorder. When depression and physical illness co-exist, the conditions interact and result in worse outcomes (Belmaker and Agam, 2008; Krishnadas and Cavanagh, 2012; Nemeroff, 2008).

Improvement of depression has been shown to improve outcomes in co-morbid chronic physical illnesses like ischaemic heart disease. Notably, untreated depression after coronary artery bypass surgery increases the risk of reinfarction 3 to 4 times.

Given its prevalence and morbidity, major depressive disorder deserves due attention and treatment. The majority of depressed patients who seek treatment do so from their general practitioner, followed by complementary service providers and human services providers. Only a minority seek help from mental health care specialists and it is therefore important that primary care practitioners screen for and manage depression correctly (Seedet *et al.*, 2009).

## 12.2.2 Factors contributing to under-diagnosis

### 12.2.2.1 Lack of awareness and recognition

Patients are often unaware that they have depression and may regard their symptoms as a result of normal suffering.

Many patients are unaware that they are suffering from a medically treatable condition and often present with symptoms related to depression, such as insomnia or other somatic complaints (e.g. fatigue, headache, abdominal distress, change in weight). Often patients don't complain of low mood or sadness but more of irritability or difficulty concentrating. Potentially, this could lead to misdiagnosis if the physician does not screen for underlying depression appropriately.

### 12.2.2.2 Shame and stigma

Patients often believe that their symptoms result from a character flaw or weakness that must be overcome. They may attempt to hide their symptoms from others or present with somatic complaints, which in their view is more acceptable.

### 12.2.2.3 Clinician factors

Clinicians often hold a normalising understanding of depression, where it is difficult to distinguish between normal human distress in response to the environment and a state of illness. Clinicians may also worry about medicalising social problems. This may lead to an under-diagnosis of depression.

### 12.2.2.4 Lack of professional responsibility and patient load

Doctors often regard primary nurses or other professionals as responsible for the identification and management of depression and thus do not take responsibility for screening or managing these patients. Most depressive patients can be identified using a few screening questions or even a self-administered rating scale that can be completed in the waiting room.

## 12.2.3 Pathogenesis of major depressive disorder

MDD is a heritable psychiatric syndrome in which the underlying pathophysiology has not been clearly defined. It is feasible that the pathophysiological mechanisms vary amongst individual patients with MDD. MDD appears to be a heterogeneous group of disorders resulting from complex interactions between biological vulnerability and psychosocial stressors. The contribution of these different factors may vary considerably among individual patients. The overall genetic contribution in depression is approximately 40%.

First-degree relatives of patients with depression are three times more likely than the general population to develop depression.

Psychosocial influences seem to play a more significant role than genetics in pre-pubertal depression, while heritability is a more important factor in adolescent-onset and adult-onset depression where the interaction between genes and psychosocial stressors become increasingly important (Saveanu and Nemeroff, 2012).

#### 12.2.3.1 Biological vulnerability

Biological vulnerability is determined by **genetic loading** as well as by abnormalities in neural networks in brain regions that are normally involved in regulation of emotions. Multiple genes are likely to influence the susceptibility to depression.

Neural circuits involving the medial prefrontal cortex and network (medial and caudolateral orbital cortex), the amygdala, hippocampus and ventromedial parts of the basal ganglia are implicated (Price and Drevets, 2012).

These areas:

- have widespread connections with other areas of the brain responsible for regulation of dopamine (DA), noradrenalin (NA) and serotonin (5-HT). Disturbances in CNS 5-HT, NA and DA activity are important factors in the pathogenesis of depression
- display adaptations to endocrine and immunologic stimuli arising from within and outside the CNS (Price and Drevets, 2012).

Over-activity of the HPA-axis and increased cortisol secretion have been well documented in patients with MDD and have been linked to hippocampal and left prefrontal neuronal loss (Nemeroff, 2008).

Approximately one-third of patients with MDD have elevated inflammatory biomarkers (pro-inflammatory cytokines) indicative of a hyper-inflammatory state (Gardner and Boles, 2011; Krishnadas and Cavanagh, 2012).

More modern theories support the role of increased oxidative stress as well as decreased neuronal plasticity and neurogenesis in the pathogenesis of MDD. Stress may play an important role in the slowing down of neurogenesis in the CNS; antidepressants have been shown to stimulate neurogenesis (Gardner and Boles, 2011).

#### 12.2.3.2 Psychosocial stressors

Although depression can arise without precipitating stressors, the risk of it is increased by stress and interpersonal losses. Poor social support, a lack of social skills and a disruption of normal social, marital, parental or familial relationships are correlated with high rates of depression and are risk factors for recurrence. Early losses, like parental death before the age of 10, sexual abuse, other adverse childhood experiences or chronic stressors may influence the sensitivity of individuals to later stressful events. (See Chapter 5: Psychosocial determinants of mental disorders, for more on psychosocial factors and risk of depression.)

Negative cognitions (negative view of self, others and the world) and all-or nothing **schemata** contribute to and perpetuate depressed mood.

Chronic pain, medical illness and disruption of natural biorhythms (i.e. sleep disruption) or exposure to certain pharmacologic medications or substances (see Table 12.4) can also precipitate a major depressive episode.

### 12.2.4 Clinical presentation

In many instances, patients with MDD present with somatic complaints like fatigue, headache, general body pains or insomnia. Irritability, difficulty in concentrating or excessive stress may also be presenting complaints. Some patients deny feeling depressed, even if a clearly dysphoric mood is observed, but on questioning, usually acknowledge the presence of the other symptoms associated with depression. Minor or **subsyndromal** depression may precede an episode of MDD as prodromal symptoms, occur after an episode of MDD as residual symptoms or persist without ever meeting the full criteria for MDD. The Quick Inventory of Depressive Symptomatology-Self-Report version (QIDS-SR

**Table 12.2** Biological abnormalities associated with a major depressive disorder

| Hypothesis | Supporting evidence | Explanation |
|---|---|---|
| Genes | ▶ Multiple genes are likely to influence susceptibility<br>▶ Genes that control production or utilisation of 5-HT are linked to depression<br>▶ HPA-axis<br>▶ Mu-opioid receptor | Genes have been identified that play an important role in the response and adverse effects of class of pharmacological treatment |
| Abnormal brain circuitry | ▶ Hypometabolic state of cortical structures<br>▶ Hypermetabolic state of limbic structures | Abnormal brain circuitry is implicated in the pathogenesis of MDD |
| Mono-amine hypothesis | ▶ 5-HT<br>▶ NA<br>▶ DA<br>Acute induced depletion of 5-HT and NA in a laboratory setting induces a depressed mood in genetically predisposed individuals | Antidepressants normalise synaptic monamines<br>Short allele of 5-HT transporter gene is associated with risk of depression |
| Inflammatory hypothesis | Depression is associated with a broad-spectrum inflammatory state affecting multiple systems (HPA-axis, 5-HT) | Antidepressants exert at least some antidepressant effects through anti-inflammatory properties |
| Neuroprogressive hypothesis | ▶ Structural brain changes<br>▶ **Neurodegeneration**<br>▶ Decreased neurogenesis<br>▶ Apoptosis | Antidepressants support **synaptic plasticity** and axonal growth (BDNF–Brain Derived Neurotropic Factor) |
| Oxidative and nitrosative stress | ▶ Damage to lipids<br>▶ Lowered levels of anti-oxidants<br>▶ Decreased levels of poly-unsaturated fatty acids<br>▶ Abnormal endothelial function | MDD is associated with ischaemic heart disease and endothelial dysfunction |
| Mitochondrial dysfunction | ▶ Experimental modalities strongly suggest components of mitochondrial dysfunction in the pathogenesis of MDD<br>▶ 'Major categories of drugs used to treat depression have been demonstrated to exert effects on mitochondria' (Gardner and Boles, 2011)<br>▶ Commonly used mitochondrial-targeted treatments are increasingly being shown to demonstrate efficacy in the treatment of MDD | The development of MDD may involve mitochondrial dysfunction |

**Source:** Gardner and Boles, 2011; Belmaker and Agam, 2008; Nemeroff, 2008; Krishnadas and Cavanagh, 2012; Price and Drevets, 2012; Saveanu and Nemeroff, 2012; Ghaemi *et al.*, 2015

(http://www.ids-quids.org/index2.html)) or the Beck Depression Inventory II (BDI-II) (Beck *et al.*, 1996)) can easily be incorporated into clinical practice and can be used to periodically measure symptom severity and improvement (Beck *et al.*, 1996; American Psychiatric Association, 2013; Labbate *et al.*, 2010; Sadock BJ and Sadock VA, 2014).

#### 12.2.4.1 Mood or affect

In order to diagnose a MDD, either a depressed or irritable mood or diminished interest or loss of ability to experience pleasure must be present. A depressed mood may be reflected in speech, facial expression and posture. A patient may look dispirited but still respond to environmental stimuli, appear unhappy or sad most of the time or look miserable all the time when severely depressed.

In milder forms, depressed patients report feeling sad or low but still have the ability to brighten up in response to stimuli. In severe depression, the ability to experience pleasure in response to positive environmental stimuli is usually diminished or absent (anhedonia), resulting in pervasive feelings of sadness, gloominess and despondency. Patients report a reduced interest in their surroundings or activities that previously gave them pleasure. The reduction in ability to enjoy activities usually correlates with the severity of the depression. The ability to react emotionally to circumstances or people is reduced or even absent and patients may feel emotionally paralysed with an inability to feel anger, grief or pleasure.

Feelings of guilt may include self-reproach or a conviction that they have let people down with **rumination** about past errors or sinful deeds. Patients sometimes view their illness as punishment and delusions of guilt may be present.

#### 12.2.4.2 Psychomotor behaviour

Behaviour may appear normal or may range from slight to obvious psychomotor retardation to complete stupor. Alternatively, patients may display psychomotor agitation in the form of fidgeting, playing with hands and hair or inability to sit still.

#### 12.2.4.3 Work and activities

A lack of energy may manifest in patients experiencing difficulty in starting even simple routine everyday activities. Typically patients spend less time on these activities or hobbies because of loss of interest, fatigue, listlessness or indecision. Much effort is required to conduct these activities; at worst, patients may be unable to do anything without assistance.

#### 12.2.4.4 Vegetative features (hypothalamic dysfunction)

Sleep abnormalities may include reduced duration or depth of sleep and should always be measured against the patient's own normal sleeping pattern. Insomnia can range from a slight difficulty in dropping off to sleep or slightly reduced or fitful sleep to less than two hours of sleep per night. Middle or terminal insomnia (i.e. early waking) are characteristic of MDD.

Appetite can be either decreased or increased with symptoms ranging from slightly reduced appetite to complete loss of appetite and sense of taste.

Libido may be decreased or absent.

#### 12.2.4.5 Cognitive functions

Concentration difficulties range from occasional difficulty in collecting one's thoughts to an incapacitating lack of concentration where a patient is unable to read or converse.

Negative thinking about the self, such as inferiority, failure, self-reproach or self-deprecation, is often present. Patients also have pessimistic thoughts about the future and the world in general.

#### 12.2.4.6 Suicide and thinking about death

Suicidal thoughts may be absent or range from fleeting suicidal thoughts to a conviction that suicide or death is the solution to, or means of escape from, their situation. They may have no intention to harm themselves or have specific plans with the intention or a desire to die with active preparations.

#### 12.2.4.7 Other symptoms frequently associated with major depressive disorder

The following symptoms are also commonly present in MDD sufferers:

- anxiety or nervousness: patients may describe feelings of ill-defined discomfort, edginess, inner turmoil or even panic
- bodily self-absorption and preoccupation or excessive concern with health, frequent doctor's visits or even hypochondriacal delusions (American Psychiatric Association, 2013; Hales *et al.*, 2014; Gagiano, 2001)
- insight may range from acknowledgment of the fact that one is depressed to attribution of symptoms to poor diet, climate, overwork or a need for rest; in some cases patients may deny being ill at all.

**Table 12.3** DSM-5 Diagnostic Criteria for Major Depressive Disorder

| **Diagnostic Criteria** |
|---|
| A. Five (or more) of the following symptoms have been present during the same 2-week period and represent a change from previous functioning: at least one of the symptoms is either (1) depressed mood or (2) loss of interest or pleasure.<br>**Note:** Do not include symptoms that are clearly attributable to another medical condition.<br>1. Depressed mood most of the day, nearly every day, as indicated by either subjective report (e.g., feels sad, empty, hopeless) or observation made by others (e.g., appears tearful). (**Note:** In children and adolescents, can be irritable mood.)<br>2. Markedly diminished interest or pleasure in all, or almost all, activities most of the day, nearly every day (as indicated by either subjective account or observation).<br>3. Significant weight loss when not dieting or weight gain (e.g., a change of more than 5% of body weight in a month), or decrease or increase in appetite nearly every day.<br>(**Note:** In children, consider failure to make expected weight gain.)<br>4. Insomnia or hypersomnia nearly every day.<br>5. Psychomotor agitation or retardation nearly every day (observable by others, not merely subjective feelings of restlessness or being slowed down).<br>6. Fatigue or loss of energy nearly every day.<br>7. Feelings of worthlessness or excessive or inappropriate guilt (which may be delusional) nearly every day (not merely self-reproach or guilt about being sick).<br>8. Diminished ability to think or concentrate, or indecisiveness, nearly every day (either by subjective account or as observed by others).<br>9. Recurrent thoughts of death (not just fear of dying), recurrent suicidal ideation without a specific plan, or a suicide attempt or a specific plan for committing suicide. |
| B. The symptoms cause clinically significant distress or impairment in social, occupational, or other important areas of functioning. |
| C. The episode is not attributable to the physiological effects of a substance or to another medical condition.<br>**Note:** Criteria A-C represent a major depressive episode.<br>**Note:** Responses to a significant loss (e.g., bereavement, financial ruin, losses from a natural disaster, a serious medical illness or disability) may include the feelings of intense sadness, rumination about the loss, insomnia, poor appetite, and weight loss noted in Criterion A, which may resemble a depressive episode. Although such symptoms may be understandable or considered appropriate to the loss, the presence of a major depressive episode in addition to the normal response to a significant loss should also be carefully considered. This decision inevitably requires the exercise of clinical judgment based on the individual's history and the cultural norms for the expression of distress in the context of loss.[1] |
| D. The occurrence of the major depressive episode is not better explained by schizoaffective disorder, schizophrenia, schizophreniform disorder, delusional disorder, or other specified and unspecified schizophrenia spectrum and other psychotic disorders. |
| E. There has never been a manic episode or a hypomanic episode.<br>**Note:** This exclusion does not apply if all of the manic-like or hypomanic-like episodes are substance-induced or are attributable to the physiological effects of another medical condition. |

*Specify*:

**With anxious distress** (p. 184)

**With mixed features** (pp. 184–185)

**With melancholic features** (p. 185)

**With atypical features** (pp. 185–186)

**With mood-congruent psychotic features** (p. 186)

**With mood-incongruent psychotic features** (p. 186)

**With catatonia** (p. 186).

**With peripartum onset** (pp. 186–187)

**With seasonal pattern (recurrent episode only)** (pp. 187–188)

[1] In distinguishing grief from a major depressive episode (MDE), it is useful to consider that in grief the predominant affect is feelings of emptiness and loss, while in MDE it is persistent depressed mood and the inability to anticipate happiness or pleasure. The dysphoria in grief is likely to decrease in intensity over days to weeks and occurs in waves, the so-called pangs of grief. These waves tend to be associated with thoughts or reminders of the deceased. The depressed mood of MDE is more persistent and not tied to specific thoughts or preoccupations. The pain of grief may be accompanied by positive emotions and humor that are uncharacteristic of the pervasive unhappiness and misery characteristic of MDE. The thought content associated with grief generally features a preoccupation with thoughts and memories of the deceased, rather than the self-critical or pessimistic ruminations seen in MDE. In grief, self-esteem is generally preserved, whereas in MDE feelings of worthlessness and self-loathing are common. If selfderogatory ideation is present in grief, it typically involves perceived failings vis-a-vis the deceased (e.g., not visiting frequently enough, not telling the deceased how much he or she was loved). If a bereaved individual thinks about death and dying, such thoughts are generally focused on the deceased and possibly about 'joining' the deceased, whereas in MDE such thoughts are focused on ending one's own life because of feeling worthless, undeserving of life, or unable to cope with the pain of depression.



## 12.2.5 Specifiers

Specifiers (see Table 12.3) give a clearer indication of the severity and longitudinal aspects of the disease process. They should be applied when formulating a diagnosis as they have implications for the choice of treatment as well as planning of treatment. For more detailed information about the specifiers please refer to the DSM-5.

**Table 12.4** Differential diagnosis of a major depressive episode

| **A) Psychiatric conditions** |
|---|
| ▶ Other depressive disorders.<br>▶ **Bereavement** or sadness (also see Chapter 15: Acute reactions to adverse life events).<br>▶ Adjustment disorder with depressed mood (also see Chapter 15: Acute reactions to adverse life events).<br>▶ Bipolar disorder, depressive or mixed episode or manic episode with irritable mood (also see Chapter 13: Bipolar disorders).<br>▶ Schizoaffective disorder (if psychotic features are present) (also see Chapter 11: Schizophrenia spectrum and other psychotic disorders). |
| **B) Major depressive episode due to the direct pathophysiological effects of:** |
| **i. Another medical condition**<br>▶ sleep abnormalities (e.g. sleep apnoea)<br>▶ endocrinopathies that affect the HPA-axis:<br>– hyperthyroidism or hypothyroidism<br>– Cushing's syndrome or Addison's disease |

- diseases affecting the CNS:
  - cerebrovascular accident, subdural hematoma, trauma, neoplastic lesions
  - Alzheimer and other degenerative and vascular dementias
  - Parkinson's disease
  - epilepsy
  - multiple sclerosis, systemic lupus erythamatosis (auto-immune)
- infectious diseases (e.g. HIV encephalopathy, Lyme disease, mononucleosis and syphilis)
- malignancies (e.g. carcinoid syndrome, lymphoma and pancreatic cancer)
- diabetes mellitus
- metabolic disturbances
  - hypercalcaemia or hypocalcaemia
  - hyponatraemia
- nutritional deficiencies (vitamin B12, pellagra, folate deficiency) and anaemia.

**ii. Substances or medication**

**Substances of abuse**

*Frequent association with:*

- alcohol
- sedatives, **hypnotics**, or anxiolytics (long term use)
- opioids (over the counter analgesics)
- amphetamines or other stimulants
- cocaine
- phencyclidine and other hallucinogens
- inhalants

**Medication**

*Frequent association with:*

- corticosteroids (long-term use)
- anticonvulsants (e.g. topiramate, phenobarbital, and vigabatrin)
- antimalarials (e.g. mefloquine)
- antiretrovirals (e.g. efavirenz)
- central acting antihypertensives (e.g reserpine, methyldopa)
- medication for migraine (e.g flunarizine)
- interferon

*Infrequentl association with:*

- cardiovascular medications i.e. β-blockers
- antibiotics and anti-tuberculosis medications
- levodopa
- chemotherapy agents
- isotretinoin.

**Source:** Celano *et al.*, 2011; Sadock BJ and Sadock VA, 2014; Hales *et al.*, 2014

## 12.2.6 Co-morbidity

Nearly three-quarters of persons with MDD have at least one other co-morbid psychiatric disorder. Most common are anxiety disorders (59%), impulse-control disorders and substance use disorders. People with co-morbid disorders seek help more often and experience greater functional impairment than depressed patients without co-morbid conditions. Psychiatric disorders that are commonly co-morbid with MDD are listed in Table 12.5. (Sadock BJ and Sadock VA, 2007; American Psychiatric Association, 2013)

**Table 12.5** Common co-morbid psychiatric disorders

**Anxiety disorders**
- separation anxiety disorder
- specific phobia
- social anxiety disorder (social phobia)
- panic disorder
- **agoraphobia**
- generalised anxiety disorder.

**Disruptive, impulse control and conduct disorders**
- conduct disorder
- intermittent explosive disorder
- pyromania
- kleptomania.

**Substance-related and addictive disorders**
- alcohol-use disorder
- caffeine intoxication
- caffeine withdrawal
- cannabis use disorder
- hallucinogen persisting perception disorder
- opioid use disorder
- sedative, hypnotic or anxiolytic use disorder
- tobacco use disorder
- **gambling** disorder

**Obsessive-compulsive and related disorders**
- obsessive-compulsive disorder
- body dysmorphic disorder
- hoarding disorder
- **trichotillomania** (hair-pulling disorder)
- excoriation (skin-picking) disorder

**Somatic symptom and related disorders**
- somatic symptom disorder
- illness anxiety disorder
- conversion disorder (functional neurological symptom disorder)

**Feeding and eating disorders**
- anorexia nervosa
- bulimia nervosa
- binge-eating disorder

**Personality disorders**
- antisocial personality disorder
- borderline personality disorder
- avoidant personality disorder
- dependent personality disorder
- obsessive-compulsive personality disorder

**Trauma and stressor-related disorders**
- post-traumatic stress disorder
- adjustment disorders

**Depressive disorders**
- persistent depressive disorder (dysthymia)
- premenstrual dysphoric disorder

**Neurocognitive disorders**
- mild neurocognitive disorders
- major neurocognitive disorders

**Neurodevelopmental disorders**
- intellectual disability (intellectual developmental disorder)
- autism spectrum disorder
- attention-deficit/hyperactivity disorder
- specific learning disorder
- tic disorders

**Dissociative disorders**
- dissociative amnesia
- depersonalisation/derealisation disorder

**Sleep-wake disorders**
- insomnia disorder
- hypersomnolence disorder
- narcolepsy
- circadian rhythm sleep-wake disorders
- non-rapid eye movement sleep arousal disorders
- nightmare disorder
- restless legs syndrome

**Sexual dysfunctions**
- delayed ejaculation
- female orgasmic disorder
- female sexual interest/arousal disorder
- male hypoactive sexual desire disorder

**Gender dysphoria**

**Paraphilic disorders**
- voyeuristic disorder
- exhibitionistic disorder
- frotteuristic disorder
- paedophilic disorder

## 12.2.7 Management

Complete remission of depressive symptoms should be seen as the primary goal of treatment. Long-term outcomes among patients who achieve full symptom remission are significantly higher compared to patients who report only symptomatic improvement over an equivalent period of treatment. Approximately 40% of patients with MDD achieve full remission (one year remission rate) with first-line or second-line treatment. It is therefore imperative that the optimal treatment options and management plans are implemented as early as possible, preferably from the time of first contact with medical or mental health services. The recent advances in modern treatment options for MDD, including newer antidepressants and innovative new treatment modalities, such as transcranial magnetic stimulation (TMS), are worth noting (Sadock BJ and Sadock VA, 2007; Weihs and Wert, 2011; Gagiano, 2001).

Psychosocial factors associated with the disorder such as social isolation, stressful life circumstances and long-term deterioration in general levels of functioning must be addressed to maintain treatment gains and achieve remission. Resources permitting, referral to social work, psychology or occupational therapy services should be considered in the long-term treatment plan.

Psycho-education involving both patient and family is an important component of the treatment programme. Psycho-education should include:

- the nature of the disorder
- identification of symptoms and signs
- treatment options
- response to treatment
- dosages and side-effects of medication
- avoidance of alcohol and illicit substances
- course of the disorder
- prognosis
- relapse prevention
- the role of the family in managing the disorder
- emotional impact of the disorder on the patient and family, including children
- information about local resources, such as self-help groups and caregiver support groups (Gagiano, 2001).

Even though a multi-disciplinary approach in the management of MDD is preferable, many cases are uncomplicated and can be treated by the primary care doctor and primary care team. Complicated or **treatment-resistant** cases must be identified so that appropriate referrals can be made to psychiatrists or, in emergency situations or when admission is required as part of the short-term treatment plan, to mental health care facilities. Hospitalisation may be necessary for suicidal or other severely depressed patients (including those who develop psychotic symptoms secondary to the depression) who require close monitoring or invasive procedures (Sadock BJ and Sadock VA, 2007; Gagiano, 2001). Hospitalisation may also be required in the case of **crisis intervention**, for complex diagnostic evaluation and for initiation of electroconvulsive therapy (ECT) or other treatment modalities.

Primary care doctors need basic knowledge and skills, not only to be able assess the risk for suicide and refer appropriately, but also to implement the first-line treatment options for MDD, namely pharmacotherapy and psychotherapy (Gagiano, 2001).

Research has shown that a combination of pharmacotherapy and psychotherapy results in better outcomes than any one of these modalities alone. Combination treatment is therefore preferable where appropriate, although feasibility and patient-preference issues must be taken into account. Monotherapy with any one of these treatment modalities is better than no treatment at all (Sadock BJ and Sadock VA, 2007; IsHak *et al.*, 2011).

### 12.2.7.1 Pharmacotherapy

The mainstay pharmacotherapeutic treatment of MDD is with antidepressants. First-line antidepressants for use in MDD are selective serotonin reuptake inhibitors (SSRIs). Serotonin noradrenalin reuptake inhibitors (SNRIs) can also be considered as first-line treatment options but their unavailability in certain primary care settings limits their use as first-line agents. Tricyclic antidepressants (TADs) are effective agents, even though their side effects are less tolerable than those of SSRIs. They are readily available in primary health care settings and can be used as a first-line treatment option, especially if SSRIs are unavailable. Even though SSRIs are recommended as first-line agents, the choice of medication should be made in conjunction with the patient. Age, gender, weight, pregnancy and breastfeeding, patient preference, specific symptoms experienced, cost, medication side-effect profile and co-morbid medical conditions such as epilepsy are factors that influence the prescription decision-making (Dupuy *et al.*, 2011; Sadock BJ and Sadock VA, 2007; Taylor *et al.*, 2012; Weihs and Wert, 2011; Gartlehner *et al.*, 2011, Soleimani *et al.*, 2011).

The potential benefits for the patient must be weighed up against the potential side effects when a particular medication is considered. Certain adverse effects of a particular medication may be potentially dangerous if prescribed for a patient with a particular medical condition. An example would be prescribing a tricyclic antidepressant, which has a known association with cardiac arrhythmia, to a patient on anti-arrhythmic medication (Taylor *et al.*, 2012; Sadock BJ and Sadock VA, 2007; Stahl, 2008).

Side-effect profiles of medications can also be used as therapeutic tools. If a patient presents with prominent melancholic depressive features such as insomnia and anorexia or weight loss, for example, consideration might be given to prescribing an antidepressant such as mirtazapine which is known, as part of its side-effect profile, to cause sedation and weight gain. Specific indications of a medication can be used in a similar way when deciding on which antidepressant to prescribe for a patient. If a patient is known to suffer from a painful peripheral neuropathy, an appropriate antidepressant might be the SNRI duloxetine, which is also routinely used in the treatment of neurological pain. In so doing one can attempt to treat two conditions with one medication and thus minimise the risk of **polypharmacy** (Sadock BJ and Sadock VA, 2007; Gagiano, 2001).

Even though SSRIs are correctly prescribed as first-line antidepressants on a routine basis, having a solid knowledge of all the antidepressants will enable one to prescribe the most appropriate medication, thereby having a potentially positive effect on response and adherence to treatment.

Also see Chapter 36: Pharmacological and other treatments in psychiatry, where all the available antidepressants are listed and classified, and matters such as indications, contra-indications, side effects and dosing are discussed in detail.

Basic principles of pharmacotherapy apply when first prescribing an antidepressant for the treatment of a case of MDD. One should start with the minimum effective dose and aim for monotherapy as opposed to polypharmacy. Even though some patients may experience a positive effect within a week of starting on an antidepressant, some will only respond after a month on treatment. Patients should therefore be advised not to discontinue medication if they do not experience improved mood soon after starting treatment. A proper course of 4–6 weeks at the appropriate dose of an antidepressant is necessary before it can be regarded as being ineffective (Sadock BJ and Sadock VA, 2007; Weihs and Wert, 2011; Soleimani *et al.*, 2011; Gagiano, 2001).

If, as is the goal, remission is achieved on a prescribed antidepressant, it is advised that the patient not stop taking the medication but continue treatment for at least another six months after a first major depressive episode (MDE) to decrease the risk of relapse. Only thereafter should an antidepressant be discontinued. Good practice dictates slowly tapering the dose over at least a four-week period before it is stopped, depending on the type of antidepressant and its half-life (the shorter the half-life, the more slowly it should be tapered). If a patient has achieved remission after a second MDE it is advised that antidepressant treatment be continued for at least another 18 months on the therapeutic dose before it is tapered and stopped (once again in an effort to prevent relapse). If a patient experiences a third

MDE life-long treatment with the antidepressant is advised. Some research suggests that life-long treatment should be advised after a second MDE to try to prevent relapse.

In conjunction with first-line antidepressant treatment, symptomatic treatment may be required to target certain prominent symptoms. Insomnia is a common complaint in depression and can be treated using a short course of low-dose sedative antidepressants like amitriptyline, trazodone, mirtazapine or agomelatine or with hypnotics like zopiclone or zolpidem.

Short-acting benzodiazepines like oxazepam can also be prescribed for insomnia, whilst the long-acting variety can be used in the treatment of agitation, restlessness and anxiety which is either part of the symptom complex of the disorder or secondary to the effects of a prescribed SSRI in the first few weeks of treatment. It is essential that the patient understands that the use of benzodiazepines in MDD is for short-term use only and that long-term use could lead to dependence. It is the prescriber's responsibility to ensure that the benzodiazepine is tapered and discontinued before dependence develops (Gagiano, 2001).

Antipsychotics are used in MDD when patients develop a psychosis secondary to the depression. The use of a second-generation antipsychotic (SGA) is preferred since some commonly used first-generation antipsychotics (FGAs) like haloperidol, can worsen dysphoric symptoms (Taylor *et al.*, 2012).

At specialist level, SGAs like aripiprazole and quetiapine can also be prescribed along with an antidepressant as an **augmentation** strategy in cases of treatment refractory major depressive disorder. Research is ongoing into the use of SGAs as monotherapy with quetiapine possibly having a beneficial effect (Rothchild, 2010; Stahl, 2008; Taylor *et al.*, 2012; Chen *et al.*, 2011; Dupuy *et al.*, 2011).

Also see Section 12.2.7.3 where poor response is discussed as well as Chapter 36: Pharmacological and other treatments in psychiatry, where all the available antipsychotics, sedatives, hypnotics and anxiolytics are listed and classified, and such matters as indications, contraindications, side-effects and dosing are discussed in detail.

### 12.2.7.2 Psychotherapy

Cognitive behavioural therapy (CBT) and interpersonal therapy have the most evidence for efficacy in the treatment of MDD and are seen as first-line psychotherapeutic treatment options. Supportive psychotherapy, short-term psychodynamic and emotion-focused psychotherapies may also be efficacious, but there is less compelling evidence supporting the use of these strategies for the treatment of depressed patients.

Family therapy examines the role of the depression in the overall well-being of the family and the role of the family in the maintenance of the patient's symptoms. Although it is not a first-line treatment option for MDD, there is evidence that it can help some patients cope with stress, which can lessen the chance of relapse. This form of psychotherapy is best indicated when the disorder jeopardises a patient's marriage or the family functioning (Sadock BJ and Sadock VA, 2007; Soleimani *et al.*, 2011; Jakobsen *et al.*, 2011; Jakobsen *et al.*, 2012; Hollon, 2011; Gagiano, 2001).

#### Cognitive behavioural therapy

CBT consists of a cognitive and a behavioural component. The patient is an active participant in the therapeutic process, which is very practical in nature and contains elements such as relaxation training. The intervention seeks to link thoughts, feelings and behaviour, and relates these to the depressive symptoms.

Patients with depressive symptoms present with **cognitive distortions** (errors in logical thought). Depression leads to negative thoughts. When these thoughts become instant and reflexive they are known as negative **automatic thoughts**. CBT aims to identify, record and correct these cognitive distortions and negative automatic thoughts and how they relate to the depressive symptoms by replacing them with positive ones. This process is known as cognitive restructuring. The patient is taught alternative, positive methods of thinking related to the depressive symptoms (Sadock BJ and Sadock VA, 2007).

Daily behaviour is influenced by mood. Maladaptive behavioural patterns as seen in

MDD result in negative feedback from society. The behavioural component of CBT similarly seeks to record and correct behavioural patterns related to depression by teaching patients alternative methods of behaviour that will lead to positive reinforcement from society (Sadock BJ and Sadock VA, 2007).

CBT is undertaken face-to-face, either individually or in a group.

**Mindfulness**-based cognitive therapy is a group-based clinical intervention programme designed to reduce relapse or recurrence of MDD by means of systematic training in mindfulness meditation combined with cognitive-behavioural methods. Recent research points to some efficacy in reducing relapse rates in MDD (Piet and Hougaard, 2011).

**Interpersonal therapy**

Interpersonal therapy focuses on one or two of the patient's current interpersonal problems (which are likely to be associated with childhood dysfunctional relationships) that precipitate or perpetuate the depressive symptoms. The therapy programme is characterised by an active therapeutic approach that is undertaken face-to-face, either individually or in a group (Sadock BJ and Sadock VA, 2007).

Also see Chapter 37: Psychological interventions, where different forms of psychotherapy are discussed in more detail.

### 12.2.7.3 Approaches to poor response

If the response of a patient's symptoms to the prescribed antidepressant is poor, certain scenarios must be excluded or considered before drawing a conclusion that the medication is ineffective.

- Make sure that adherence to medication is good. Is the patient actually taking the treatment and taking it correctly as prescribed?
- Make sure that the diagnosis is correct. Is it truly a case of MDD or may the patient be suffering from another psychiatric disorder like a bipolar disorder?
- Make sure that there are no co-morbid medical conditions that have an influence on the patient's mood. If there are, treat them effectively before re-evaluating the effects of the antidepressant.
- Make sure there are no co-morbid psychiatric disorders that have an influence on the patient's mood. If there are, incorporate the treatment of these disorders into the overall treatment plan. Once the treatment of other psychiatric disorders is optimised, re-evaluate the effects of the antidepressant or refer to a psychiatrist for specialist management of the complex or multiple psychiatric disorders.
- Make sure that the patient is not abusing alcohol or illicit substances with psychoactive properties known to have a causal effect on depressive symptoms. If so, the use of these substances must be discontinued before the effects of the antidepressant can be properly evaluated.
- Make sure that the patient has received a proper course of the antidepressant of at least 4–6 weeks before evaluating its effects.
- Make sure that the patient has been prescribed the optimum dose of the antidepressant. If not, adjust the dose first and evaluate the effects of the antidepressant after a proper course on the optimum dose (Sadock BJ and Sadock VA, 2007; Dupuy *et al.*, 2011; Gagiano, 2001).

Once all of these scenarios have been excluded, considered or addressed and it has been concluded that response to an antidepressant has been poor, evaluate whether there has been only a partial response of the symptoms to the antidepressant or no response at all, because this will influence the decision as to further management of the patient (see Advanced reading block 12.2). Always consider adding psychotherapy to the management plan in an attempt to improve the patient's symptoms. It is advised that patients with treatment-resistant cases of MDD be referred to a psychiatrist for further management if such a resource is available. It is therefore important that the concept of the management of these cases is understood (Sadock BJ and Sadock VA, 2007).

Despite the availability of the varied pharmacotherapeutic treatment options for the management of treatment-resistant MDD, ECT remains a proven effective treatment for this purpose and is considered a first-line treatment option. Clinicians should familiarise themselves with ECT and be able to present it to patients as a viable treatment option for severe depression through proper psycho-education (Brunoni *et al.*, 2010; Sadock BJ and Sadock VA, 2007).

Along with ECT, other forms of **neuromodulation** treatments (see Advanced reading block 12.1) are either available or being studied for the treatment of severe depression.

## 12.1 Advanced reading block

**Treatment strategies for managing poor response to initial antidepressant treatment**

A general guide is that if there has been a partial but incomplete response of the symptoms to the antidepressant, then one should:

- optimise the dose of the antidepressant if not already done

or

- augment by adding a medication not classified as an antidepressant to enhance the effect of the prescribed antidepressant

or

- use combination antidepressant treatment by adding an antidepressant from another class to the prescribed antidepressant

or

- consider ECT (Sadock BJ and Sadock VA, 2007).

If there has been no response of the symptoms to the antidepressant then one should:

- optimise the dose of the antidepressant if not already done

or

- switch to another antidepressant using the correct switching strategy (Sadock BJ and Sadock VA, 2007).

**Antidepressant augmentation**

Lithium has long been used as an augmenting agent. Research about its efficacy is mostly in the context of augmentation of TCAs, which are no longer being used as first-line antidepressants. Nevertheless, lithium remains the augmentation option with the most robust research backing and may be particularly useful in suicidal patients where there is evidence of it being helpful in the prevention of suicidal behaviour (Anderson *et al.*, 2008; Stahl, 2008; Taylor *et al.*, 2012; Sadock BJ and Sadock VA, 2007; Chen *et al.*, 2011; Dupuy *et al.*, 2011; Weihs and Wert, 2011; Soleimani *et al.*, 2011; Gagiano, 2001).

Triiodothyronine (T3) is another augmentation option. The strength of evidence of efficacy is similar to that of lithium. It has long been used as an augmenting agent (Anderson *et al.*, 2008; Stahl, 2008; Taylor *et al.*, 2012; Sadock BJ and Sadock VA, 2007 Chen *et al.*, 2011; Dupuy *et al.*, 2011; Weihs and Wert, 2011; Soleimani *et al.*, 2011; Gagiano, 2001).

Second-generation antipsychotics are the most well-researched augmentation strategy for treatment resistant major depressive disorder. There is evidence of the efficacy of aripiprazole and quetiapine. There is less compelling evidence of the efficacy of olanzapine and risperidone (Komossa *et al.*, 2012; Stahl, 2008; Taylor *et al.*, 2012; Weihs and Wert, 2011).

Most of the recent research has focused on the addition of second-generation antipsychotics (SGAs) as an augmenting strategy in the management of treatment-resistant MDD. These medications have proven to be effective in combination with antidepressants for short-term treatment in MDD, with the most compelling evidence for the use of aripiprazole. Augmentation with SGAs is now an accepted treatment strategy, even though their long long-term effects in this population is unclear (Rothchild, 2010; Stahl, 2008; Taylor *et al.*, 2012; Chen *et al.*, 2011; Dupuy *et al.*, 2011, Soleimani *et al.*, 2011).

Researched medications that have shown positive results in the augmentation of antidepressants in MDD are lamotrigine and modafinil. More research is still required before their use for this purpose. The same is true of buspirone which has long been used as an augmenting agent but for which there is currently no compelling evidence of efficacy (Dupuy *et al.*, 2011; Taylor *et al.*, 2012).

**Combination antidepressants**

Even though there is as yet insufficient evidence to conclude that combination antidepressant therapy be recommended for treatment-resistant MDD, most studies suggest that combining antidepressants with dissimilar structures or mechanisms of action may be of benefit. There is some evidence for adding mirtazipine or mianserin to an SSRI (adding an antidepressant with a different mechanism of action). Combination antidepressant strategies that target both noradrenalin and serotonin are more effective that those that target only one type of monoamine neurotransmitter, hence the commonly used combinations of a SSRI plus a TCA, or a SSRI plus a SNRI. A commonly used combination is that of a SSRI and bupropion, a noradrenalin dopamine reuptake inhibitor (NDRI). There is some evidence for the efficacy of this treatment strategy that targets all three monoamine neurotransmitters (Dupuy *et al.*, 2011; Connolly and Thase, 2011; Thase, 2011; Rocha *et al.*, 2012; Sadock BJ and Sadock VA, 2007; Taylor *et al.*, 2012; Stahl, 2008; Soleimani *et al.*, 2011).

**Switching antidepressants**

Even though it makes pharmacodynamic sense to switch from an SSRI to an SNRI, NDRI or a TCA in an attempt to target the noradrenergic neurotransmitter system (or to a lesser extent the dopaminergic neurotransmitter system), there is no consistent evidence in the literature to suggest that switching from a medication in one class to a medication in another class results in superior efficacy than when a medication is switched to another within the same class (Dupuy *et al.*, 2011; Connolly and Thase, 2011; Stahl, 2008).

The message is that one can switch to any other antidepressant of one's choice.

**Note**: In the event of one of these treatment strategies being unsuccessful, it is recommended that a switch be made to one of the other treatment strategies for treatment resistant MDD or to consider ECT, or another form of neuromodulatory treatment.

## 12.3 Other depressive disorders

The DSM-5 describes a range of depressive disorders that should be considered in patients presenting with symptoms of low mood or irritability.

### 12.3.1 Persistent depressive disorder (dysthymia)

Persistent depressive disorder is characterised by a chronic and persistent depressed mood that has been present for at least two years. Symptoms include poor appetite or overeating, insomnia or hypersomnia, decreased energy or fatigue, low **self-esteem**, poor concentration or difficulty making decisions, and feelings of hopelessness. Symptoms should be present for most of the day, on more days than not.

Major depression may precede persistent depressive disorder and major depressive episodes may occur during persistent depressive disorder. Patients whose symptoms meet criteria for MDD for two years should be given a diagnosis of persistent depressive disorder as well as a MDD.

Individuals can only be diagnosed with the condition in the absence of current or previous manic or hypomanic episodes, or if the symptoms are not better explained by the presence of schizophrenia, schizo-affective disorder, delusional disorder, or another psychotic disorder.

#### 12.3.1.1 Treatment

Patients may respond best to a combination of antidepressants and psychotherapy and should be referred for specialist care if possible.

### 12.3.2 Disruptive mood dysregulation disorder

Disruptive mood dysregulation disorder is characterised by severe recurrent temper outbursts with persistently irritable or angry mood between outbursts. Onset of this disorder is during childhood (American Psychiatric Association, 2013).

Also see Chapter 27: Child and adolescent psychiatry 1: Assessment and the young child, where this disorder is discussed in more detail.

### 12.3.3 Premenstrual dysphoric disorder

Patients with premenstrual dysphoric disorder present with mood symptoms that occur at a specific time in their menstrual cycles (American Psychiatric Association, 2013).

Also see Chapter 26: Women's mental health, where this disorder is discussed in more detail.

### 12.3.4 Substance-induced or medication-induced depressive disorder

Symptoms of substance induced or medication induced depressive disorder can occur due to the direct pathophysiological effects of prescription, recreational or illicit substances (American Psychiatric Association, 2013). (See Table 12.4 for a list of substances associated with depression.)

**Information box**

**Neuromodulation treatments for severe MDD**

**ECT**

ECT has longstanding proven efficacy in the treatment of depression. Several guidelines support the role of ECT as a first-line treatment of MDD, especially in psychotic and/or suicidal patients, or those with catatonia or treatment-resistant depression (Brunoni *et al.*, 2010; Sadock BJ and Sadock VA, 2007; Stahl, 2008; Weihs and Wert, 2011; Soleimani *et al.*, 2011; Gagiano, 2001).

**TMS**

TMS has been approved in many countries for the management of treatment-resistant MDD. Its efficacy is comparable to that of antidepressant medications (Brunoni *et al.*, 2010; Weihs and Wert, 2011; Soleimani *et al.*, 2011).

**Transcranial direct current stimulation (tDCS)**

Further research is needed to establish the role of tDCS in MDD treatment (Brunoni *et al.*, 2010).

**Deep brain stimulation (DBS)**

DBS is an invasive treatment option with a possible role in the management of treatment-resistant MDD. Although further research is needed, initial results are promising. It should still be seen as an experimental treatment option (Brunoni *et al.*, 2010; Blomstedt *et al.*, 2011).

**Vagus nerve stimulation (VNS)**

VNS is an invasive treatment option with a possible role in the management of treatment-resistant MDD (Brunoni *et al.*, 2010; Sadock BJ and Sadock VA, 2007; Stahl, 2008; Weihs and Wert, 2011; Soleimani *et al.*, 2011).

Also see Chapter 36: Pharmacological and other treatments in psychiatry, where neuromodulation treatments are discussed in more detail.

Successful management of a substance-induced depression depends on successful management of the substance use problem. In certain substance rehabilitation centres where professional management for both problems are available the substance use problem and the depression can be treated concurrently if needed.

The depressive symptoms may remit once the substance use is discontinued. If not, the depression should, as with MDD, be appropriately treated with psychotherapy and/or pharmacotherapy.

### 12.3.5 Depressive disorder due to another medical condition

Depressive symptoms can appear secondary to any number of different underlying medical conditions (see Table 12.4 for a list of medical conditions associated with depression). In order to pick up underlying medical conditions it is essential that clinicians do a thorough physical examination and appropriate special investigations as part of the psychiatric evaluation (American Psychiatric Association, 2013).

Management of depression secondary to another medical condition is appropriate management of the underlying medical condition. If depressive symptoms persist (even after the medical condition has been appropriately treated or is being well managed) the depression, as with MDD, should be suitably managed with psychotherapy and/or pharmacotherapy. In certain circumstances – such as when a patient is suicidal – it may be necessary to introduce antidepressant treatment before the underlying medical condition has been optimally managed.

### 12.3.6 Other specified depressive disorder

Occasionally patients present with a clinically significant depressed mood that warrants attention and professional intervention but does not necessarily fulfil the criteria of one of the depressive disorders discussed above. A diagnosis of 'other specified depressive disorder' can then be made followed by specification of the reason for not fulfilling the particular criteria.

Examples of such presentations include recurrent brief depression, short-duration depressive episode and depressive episode with insufficient symptoms (American Psychiatric Association, 2013).

### 12.3.7 Unspecified depressive disorder

When a patient presents with a clinically significant depressed mood that warrants attention and professional intervention but does not necessarily fulfil the criteria of one of the depressive disorders discussed above, and the reason for not fulfilling the criteria cannot be specified, a diagnosis of 'unspecified depressive disorder' is made. An example would be that of a patient who is clinically depressed but where there is not yet sufficient information available to determine whether the depressed mood is due to another medical condition, substance or medication induced or neither (American Psychiatric Association, 2013).

## Conclusion

Depressive disorders are very common in the general population. It is important to be able to recognise depressive symptoms in patients and to make a proper differential diagnosis. Once substances and other medical or psychiatric conditions have been excluded, the proper, most appropriate, patient-specific management must be commenced. While holistic management of depressive disorders is advocated, psychotherapy and pharmacotherapy form the basis of effective treatment of these disorders. If the correct psychotherapeutic intervention is commenced and/or the appropriate antidepressant prescribed, a positive outcome in terms of morbidity, mortality and quality of life is reasonably common.

# References


American Psychiatric Association (2013) *Diagnostic and Statistical Manual of Mental Disorders* (5th edition). Arlington, VA: American Psychiatric Association

Anderson IM, Ferrier IN, Baldwin RC, Cowen PJ, Howard L, Lewis G, Matthews K, McAllister-Williams RH, Peveler RC, Scott J, Tylee A (2008) Evidence-based guidelines for treating depressive disorders with antidepressants: A revision of 2000 British Association for Psychopharmacology guidelines. *Journal of Psychopharmacology* 22(4): 343–96

Beck AT, Steer RA, Ball R, Ranieri W (1996) Comparison of Beck Depression Inventories IA and II in psychiatric outpatients. *Journal of personality assessment* 67(30): 588–97

Belmaker RH, Agam G (2008) Mechanism of disease major depressive disorder. *New England Journal of Medicine* 358(1): 55–68

Blomstedt P, Sjöberg RL, Hansson M, Bodlund O, Hariz MI (2011) Deep brain stimulation in the treatment of depression *Acta Psychiatrica Scandinavica* 123: 4–11

Brunoni AR, Teng CT, Correa C, Imamura M, Brasil-Neto JP, Boechat R, Rosa M, Caramelli P, Cohen R, Del Porto JA, Boggio PS, Fregni F(2010) Neuromodulation approaches for the treatment of major depression: Challenges and recommendations from a working group meeting. *Arquivos de neuro-psiquiatria* 68(3): 433–51

Celano CM, Freudenreich O, Fernandez-Robles C, Stern TA, Caro MA, Huffman JC (2011) Depressogenic effects of medications: A review. *Dialogues in Clinical Neuroscience* 13(1): 109–26

Chen J, Gao K, Kemp DE (2011) Second-generation antipsychotics in major depressive disorder: Update and clinical perspective. *Current Opinion in Psychiatry* 24: 10–7

Connolly KR, Thase ME (2011) If at first you don't succeed: A review of the evidence for antidepressant augmentation, combination and switching strategies. *Drugs* 71(1): 43–64

Dupuy JM, Ostacher MJ, Huffman J, Perlis RH, Nierenberg AA (2011) A critical review of pharmacotherapy for major depressive disorder. *International Journal of Neuropsychopharmacology* 14: 1417–31

Gagiano C (2001) Mood disorders. In: Robertson B, Allwood C, Gagiano C (Eds). *Textbook of Psychiatry for Southern Africa*. Cape Town: Oxford University Press

Gardner A, Boles RG (2011) Beyond the serotonin hypothesis: Mitochondria inflammation and neurodegeneration in major depression and affective spectrum disorders. *Progress in neuro-psychopharmacology and biological psychiatry* 35(3): 730–43

Gartlehner G, Hansen RA, Morgan LC, Thaler K, Lux L (2011) Comparative benefits and harms of second-generation antidepressants for treating major depressive disorder. *Annals of internal medicine* 155: 772–85

Ghaemi SN, Raison C, McIntyre RS How the mind affects the body and the body affects the mind: inflammation, depression, drugs and disease. Program and abstracts of the American Psychiatric Association 168th Annual Meeting viewed on 1 July 2015, from http://medscape.com/viewarticle/846594

Hales RE, Yudofsky SC, Roberts LW (2014) *The American Psychiatric Publishing Textbook of Psychiatry*. Washington DC: American Psychiatric Association

Hollon SD (2011) Cognitive and behaviour therapy in the treatment and prevention of depression. *Depression and anxiety* 28: 263–66

IsHak WW, Ha K, Kapitanski N, Bagot K, Fathy H, Swanson B, Vilhauer J, Balayan K, Bolotaulo NI, Rapaport MH (2011) The impact of psychotherapy pharmacotherapy and their combination on quality of life in depression. *Harvard Review of Psychiatry* 19: 277–89

Jakobsen JC, Hansen JL, Simonsen S, Simonsen E, Gluud C (2012) Effects of cognitive therapy versus interpersonal psychotherapy in patients with major depressive disorder: A systemic review of randomized clinical trials with meta-analyses and trial sequential analyses. *Psychological Medicine* 42: 1343–57

Jakobsen JC, Hansen JL, Storebø OJ, Simonsen E, Gluud C (2011) The effects of cognitive therapy versus 'treatment as usual in patients with major depressive disorder. *PLoS ONE* 6(8):e22890 DOI:10.1371/journal.pone.0022890 from: http://www.plosone.org/article/info%3Adoi%2F10.1371%2Fjournal.pone.0022890 (Accessed 18 October 2012)

Komossa K, Depping AM, Gaudchau A, Kissling W, Leucht S (2012) Second-generation antipsychotics for major depressive disorder and dysthymia (Review). *The Cochrane Collaboration* 2: 1–230

Krishnadas R, Cavanagh J (2012) Depression: an inflammatory illness? *Journal of Neurology, Neurosurgery and Psychiatry* 83(5): 495–502

Labbate LA, Fava M, Rosenbaum JF (2010) *Handbook of psychiatric drug therapy* (6th edition). Philadelphia: Wolters Kluwer/Lippincott Williams and Wilkins

Nemeroff CB (2008) Recent findings in the pathophysiology of depression. *Journal of Lifelong Learning in Psychiatry* 4(1): 3–14

Piet J, Hougaard E (2011) The effect of mindfulness-based cognitive therapy for prevention of relapse in recurrent major depressive disorder: A systematic review and meta-analysis. *Clinical Psychology Review* 31: 1032–40

Price JL, Drevets WC (2012) Neural circuits underlying the pathophysiology of mood disorders. *Trends in Cognitive Science* 161(1): 61–7

Rocha FL, Fuzikawa C, Riera R, Hara C (2012) Combination of antidepressants in the treatment of major depressive disorder: A systematic review and meta-analysis. *Journal of Clinical Psychopharmacology* 32: 278–81

Rothchild AJ (2010) *The Evidence-Based Guide to Antipsychotic Medications*. Arlington, VA: American Psychiatric Publishing

Sadock BJ, Sadock VA (2007) *Kaplan & Sadock's synopsis of psychiatry: Behavioural sciences/clinical psychiatry* (10th edition). Philadelphia: Lippincott Williams and Wilkins

Sadock BJ & Sadock VA (2014) *Kaplan & Sadock's synopsis of psychiatry: Behavioural sciences/clinical psychiatry* (11th edition). Philadelphia: Wolters Kluwer

Saveanu RV, Nemeroff CB (2012) Etiology of depression: genetic and environmental factors. *Psychiatric Clinics of North America* 35(1): 51–71

Seedat S, Williams DR, Herman AA, Moomal H, Williams SL, Jackson PB, Myer L, Stein DJ (2009) Mental health service use among South Africans for mood, anxiety and substance use disorders. *South African Medical Journal* 99(5): 346–52

Soleimani L, Lapidus KAB, Iosifescu DV (2011) Diagnosis and treatment of major depressive disorder. *Neurologic clinics* 29: 177–93

Stahl SM (2008) *Stahl's Essential Psychopharmacology: Neuroscientific Basis and Practical Applications* (3rd edition). New York: Cambridge University Press

Taylor D, Paton C, Kapur S (2012) *Prescribing Guidelines in Psychiatry* (11th edition). Chichester: Wiley-Blackwell

Thase ME (2011) Antidepressant combinations: Widely used but far from empirically validated. *Canadian Journal of Psychiatry* 56(6): 317–23

Tomlinson MT, Grimsrud AT, Stein DJ (2009) The epidemiology of major depression in South Africa: Results from the South African stress and health study. *South African Medical Journal* 99(5): 368–73

Weihs K, Wert JM (2011) A primary care focus on the treatment of patients with major depressive disorder. *The American Journal of the Medical Sciences* 342(4): 324–30

World Bank (1993) World development report 1993: Investing in health. New York: Oxford University Press

# CHAPTER 13 Bipolar disorders

Franco Colin

## 13.1 Introduction

Every person experiences variations of mood, mostly in response to environmental stimuli. These variations are seen as normal and part of being human. However, when these variations become more severe, impair the various aspects of daily functioning and cause distress to the person experiencing the variations, then they constitute psychopathology and become the field of study of psychiatry.

Mood variations constitute two possibilities: firstly depression in which the persons mood is experienced as sad, anxious, empty, hopeless, worried, helpless, worthless, guilty, irritable, hurt or restless and secondly hypomanic or manic with euphoric, elevated, expansive or irritable mood. These variations are often referred to in lay terms as being'down or low'and'up or high'. When seen together, these pathological variations, when occurring consecutively, constitute what is referred to as bipolar disorder (often also referred to as the bipolar spectrum disorders when the term includes the wider definitions of the pathological spectrum of mood variations) (bi = Latin for'two', polar = indicating polar opposites of mood variations, i.e. happy and sad). Bipolar disorder (BD) was previously referred to as manic-depressive illness. This term has been replaced with the term bipolar disorder, as not all patients exhibiting mood variations become'manic'.

Bipolar disorder constitutes the one major part of the mood disorders, the other being the depressive disorders (i.e. major depressive disorder). These disorders constitute the spectrum of possible mood pathologies: bipolar disorder versus unipolar depression (i.e. major depressive disorder).

## 13.2 Epidemiology

The most comprehensive and contemporary epidemiological study of bipolar disorder was conducted in a representative sample of 9 282 English-speaking adults in the United States, aged 18 years or older (Merinkangas *et al.*, 2007). The researchers found the lifetime (and twelve-month) prevalence estimates are 1,0% (0,6%) for bipolar I (BP I) disorder, 1,1% (0,8%) for bipolar II (BP II) disorder, and 2,4% (1,4%) for subthreshold bipolar disorder. The study also detected a high lifetime co-morbidity with other Axis I disorders, particularly anxiety disorders. Clinical severity and role impairment was greater for threshold than for subthreshold bipolar disorder, and for bipolar II disorder than for bipolar I disorder episodes of major depression. Subthreshold cases still have moderate to severe clinical severity and role impairment. A high level of co-morbidity with substance use disorders was also found.

## 13.3 The aetiology of bipolar disorder

### 13.3.1 Genetics

Genome-wide linkage scans conducted to identify loci harbouring rare mutations or variants that increased susceptibility to familial schizophrenia identified loci on almost every chromosome, but only a few regions had been replicated across studies. One such region was near the telomere of chromosome 13q. Across studies the region of peak linkage was broad, from 13q12 to 13q34. This region has also been linked to bipolar disorder (Xu *et al.*, 2009).

Piletz (2011) gives a recent summary of genetic findings in bipolar disorder. Bipolar disorder is known to be highly heritable. The relative risk for bipolar I in first-degree relatives has been estimated at about seven times that in the general population. Several studies have found that the risk for bipolar II is increased in the relatives of **probands** with bipolar I disorder. The risk for bipolar II disorder is also increased in the relatives of probands with bipolar II disorder. It is important to note a significant genetic overlap of bipolar disorder, schizophrenia, schizo-affective disorder and possibly major depressive disorder.

Up to 93% of the risk for bipolar I disorder is attributable to heritable factors (Piletz, 2011). These factors have fuelled an intense search for the genes that predispose for bipolar disorder. However, given the highly complex and diverse phenotype (clinical presentation) of bipolar disorder, it is extremely unlikely that single-gene causes will be found. At best, one can probably infer a polygenic, multifactorial genetic basis in bipolar disorder, with environmental influences playing an important role in the onset of the disorder. The opposing view might be that a polygenic model, involving thousands of variants of weak effects, is not likely to contribute to the heightened relative risks observed for bipolar disorder in families (Piletz, 2011). It has been documented that aberrant gene expression patterns, some involving neurotransmission pathways, have been found in tissues from patients with bipolar disorder. However, exactly which gene variants underlie the heritability of this disorder remains elusive. There might be hundreds, or even thousands, of different alleles that compose the **polygenic inheritance** of these illnesses. Proposed candidate genes possibly implicated in the pathogenesis of bipolar disorder include genes associated with following functions:

- neural growth factors
- neurotransmitters and associated signal transduction
- clock genes and transcription factors
- neuronal metabolism, proliferation and apoptosis
- cell connectivity and adhesion (Le-Nicolescu *et al.*, 2008).

## 13.3.2 Neurobiology

Bipolar I disorder arises from abnormalities in the structure and function of key emotional control networks in the human brain. The hypothesis is that disruption in early development (e.g. white-matter connectivity and prefrontal pruning) within brain networks that modulate emotional behaviour leads to decreased connectivity between ventral prefrontal networks and limbic brain structures, including (perhaps especially) the amygdala. This loss of connectivity is associated with abnormal functional responses of emotional networks to various cognitive and emotional tasks in imaging studies, as well as abnormal development of the component brain regions (e.g. failure of the amygdala to mature normally with the resulting disruption of prefrontal modulation of limbic structures). Dysregulation of the limbic brain then leads to loss of emotional homeostasis, which results in mood instability. In the absence of healthy prefrontal-striatal-pallidal-thalamic-limbic brain networks that can restore this homeostasis, individuals with bipolar disorder are at risk of developing extreme mood states and switching among mood states as well as developing mixed states as different unregulated systems oscillate in the absence of homeostatic control. During **euthymia**, recovery of prefrontal function, along with compensation from other brain regions, temporarily restores homeostasis. Nonetheless, the underlying functional neuro-anatomic abnormalities leave the person with bipolar disorder at risk of disruption of this fragile homeostasis under even minor stress. In short, it is hypothesised that a developmental failure to establish healthy ventral prefrontal–amygdala networks underlies the onset of mania and ultimately, with progressive changes throughout these networks over time, a bipolar course of illness (Strakowski *et al.*, 2012).

The data on bipolar II disorder and related conditions are relatively sparse. Recent results of an MRI-study (Hauser *et al.*, 2000)) provide evidence for the involvement of the dentate gyrus (DG) and fimbria in BD II. DG-dependent inhibition of the stress response might play an important role in mood disorders. During stress, hippocampal projections that traverse the fimbria (a white-matter bundle on the hippocampal surface) inhibit the hypothalamic–pituitary–adrenal (HPA) axis.

Literature suggests that structural neuro-anatomical abnormalities are quite common in bipolar disorder. Subtle structural abnormalities in basal ganglia structures may be a primary focus of anatomical change in mood disorders (Bearden *et al.*, 2001):

- White-matter hyperintensities appear to be the most consistently reported abnormality thus far, though they have also been the most researched. They occur particularly in periventricular white matter, subcortical grey matter and deep white-matter brain regions, and are associated with cognitive impairment, particularly in functions that require complex processing. These may represent astrogliosis, demyelination and loss of axons, or arteriosclerotic disease of arteries that supply subcortical brain regions. These changes would be expected to cause slowed mental processing, which could affect encoding and retrieval processes in memory. Post-mortem studies have reported a variety of histological abnormalities in these areas, including minute brain cysts, infarctions, small vascular malformations and necrosis. It is unknown which of these aetiologies is implicated in bipolar disorder.
- Abnormalities of cortical and subcortical structures, in particular, the temporal lobes, amygdala, basal ganglia and caudate. Whether bipolar patients show enlargement or reduction of many of these structures is controversial.
- Findings of a reduced volume of the temporal lobe have been inconsistent in bipolar disorder (Bearden *et al.*, 2001). It is highly variable and may only be present in a small subgroup of patients.

The aetiology of the structural abnormalities of bipolar illness and their corresponding functional manifestations, remains unknown. It is possible that neurodevelopmental anomalies may play a role, but that there is also some pathophysiological progression that occurs with repeated illness episodes.

### 13.3.3 Cognitive impairment and structural abnormalities in bipolar disorder

There does not appear to be a pattern of deficit that is unique to bipolar disorder. While some researchers (Bearden *et al.*, 2001) have reported similarities between the profile of bipolar patients and that of patients with disorders of the subcortical structures, bipolar patients generally do not exhibit the same degree of deficit, although they often show a similar pattern of attenuated performance on tasks of speeded information processing, immediate and delayed memory and executive functions. Given that studies (Bearden *et al.*, 2001) of the cognitive sequelae of white-matter abnormalities in normal, non-affectively ill adults show a similar pattern of impairment, it is proposed that these abnormalities may mediate the cognitive impairments seen in bipolar patients or in the bipolar subtype of schizo-affective disorder.

## 13.4 Diagnosis and clinical presentation

The diagnosis of bipolar disorder is rooted in criteria of the DSM-5 (American Psychiatric Association, 2013).

It is important that the diagnosis is made rigorously and that bipolar disorder is not over-diagnosed. It must be stressed that the diagnosis is often made over time as the full spectrum of the disorder obviously does not present itself at one point in time only. It is therefore critical to compile a detailed mood chart that represents the variations in mood that the patient has experienced since onset of symptoms.

Clinical evaluation of the signs and symptoms of the illness remains the definitive means for achieving diagnosis. Once the diagnosis of bipolar disorder has been established,

## 13.1 Advanced reading block

**Bipolar disorder: Changes in the DSM-5**

The following changes have been made from DSM-IV to DSM-5 in the diagnosis of bipolar disorder (Angst, 2013):

- The base definition of a major depressive episode (inherent to both bipolar and major depressive disorder) is still basically the same: presence of five of nine diagnostic symptoms with a minimum duration of two weeks and a change from previous functioning.
- It is, however, now diagnostically possible to diagnose bipolar disorders with mixed features: a new specifier, 'With mixed features' has been added that can be applied to episodes of mania or hypomania when depressive features are present, and to episodes of depression in the context of major depressive disorder or bipolar disorder when features of mania/hypomania are present.
- The criteria for the diagnosis of manic and hypomanic episodes have been revised. Criterion A states that in addition to elation/euphoric or irritable mood, 'the mood change must be accompanied by persistently increased activity or energy levels'. This can be seen as restrictive. Angst (2013) is severely critical of this change and states: 'Thus, for no apparent reason, DSM-5 classifies some patients as having subthreshold bipolar disorders who would formerly have been diagnosed with manic episodes or bipolar I or II disorders. This strict new rule is not based on data, indeed it contradicts available evidence.'
- Hypomanic or manic switches from depression is now included in the diagnosis of bipolar disorder, provided that the syndrome persists beyond the discontinuation of the antidepressant treatment.
- Two exclusion criteria have been left in DSM-5, namely 'Substance/medication-induced bipolar and related disorder' and 'Bipolar and related disorder due to another medical condition'. These so-called causal relationships can be questioned by the hypothesis of a genetic diathesis underlying bipolar disorder.
- The poorly circumscribed group of DSM-IV's bipolar disorder 'Not Otherwise Specified' has been partially clarified by defining 'Major Depressive Episode' with several subthreshold conditions of bipolarity, for instance, allowing a duration of two to three days for hypomanic episodes, or fewer than four symptoms of hypomania during four days, or, for cyclothymia, specifying shorter manifestations (<24 months).
- DSM-5 recognises that dysthymia can co-occur with hypomania (thus a co-morbid condition). It is unclear why this co-morbidity has not been allocated to cyclothymic disorder.

A specifier for anxious distress is delineated. This specifier is intended to identify patients with anxiety symptoms that are not part of the bipolar diagnostic criteria.

the diagnostic formulation should specify the episode type and the longitudinal course of illness. Rating scales serve as a valuable clinical tool that informs assessment, assists monitoring and quantifies treatment response. Consider using:

- mood disorders questionnaire
- Bipolar Inventory of Symptoms Scale (BISS)
- Structured Clinical Interview for Mood Spectrum (SCI-MOOD)
- Young Mania Rating Scale (YMRS) for mania
- Bipolar Depression Rating Scale (BDRS) for bipolar depression.

Where possible, obtain collateral information from the family and other sources of information about the diagnosis and longitudinal course of illness. Assess medical and psychiatric co-morbidities. Finally, evaluate the social, occupational and cognitive functioning in detail.

A medical examination at the time of psychiatric assessment is important to identify co-morbidities and differential diagnoses. The following are recommended baseline blood investigations:

- screen/test:
  - full blood count

blood chemistry
  - electrolytes
  - serum creatinine
  - thyroid stimulating hormone
  - liver function tests
  - prolactin levels (if indicated)
  - substance use
  - urine toxicology (if indicated)
  - polycystic ovarian syndrome
  - reproductive endocrine abnormalities (if prescribing valproate to a woman of childbearing age)
  - pregnancy test (if indicated, especially if prescribing valproate or carbamazepine)
  - test for infectious diseases (if indicated)
- perform
  - ECG (electrocardiogram) (if prescribing lithium and age >40 years)
  - EEG (electroencephalograph) (if indicated)
  - MRI (preferred)/CT – indicated in suspected organic etiology (HDL, high-density lipoproteins; LDL, low-density lipoproteins; ECG, electrocardiogram; EEG, electroencephalograph; MRI, magnetic resonance imaging; CT, computerized tomography).

Some medication used for bipolar disorder can have significant adverse effects and require ongoing medical monitoring.

It is often very difficult for the inexperienced clinician to understand the difference between the types or disorders in contrast to the phases of bipolar disorder. The phases of bipolar disorder are:

- manic or hypomanic phase
- depressive phase
- rapid cycling phase
- mixed phases or states.

It must be stated that anxiety and severe agitation are frequent co-occurring phenomena with these phases, and some clinicians speculate that anxiety actually constitutes another recognisable phase.

Within the bipolar spectrum of disorders, bipolar I disorder, bipolar II disorder and cyclothymic disorder have been identified.

The diagnosis of bipolar I disorder (type) rests on a clinical course characterised by the occurrence of one or more manic episodes or mixed episodes (phase). It is also frequently found that individuals with bipolar disorder have often had one or more major depressive episode before the diagnosis is made.

The diagnosis of bipolar II disorder rests on the clinical course and is characterised by the occurrence of one or more major depressive episodes accompanied by at least one hypomanic episode. The key to diagnosis is the recognition of past hypomania. Depression is the typical presenting feature of the illness. This predominantly depressive presentation is responsible for a significant proportion of missed diagnoses, and consequent management according to unipolar guidelines.

The diagnosis of cyclothymic disorder rests on the occurrence of frequent hypomanic episodes and frequent depressive symptoms, both insufficient in duration, number, severity or pervasiveness to meet the full criteria of the above disorders.

## 13.4.1 Clinical features of the respective phases or episodes of bipolar disorder

### 13.4.1.1 Manic episode

The manic episode is defined as a distinct period during which there is a persistently and abnormally elevated, expansive or irritable mood. This should last at least one week (or less if the patient is hospitalised). This distinctive mood must be accompanied by at least three additional symptoms from the following list:

- Inflated self-esteem, ranging from an overinflated sense of self-value or ability, to marked **grandiosity** or even delusions of grandeur. Individuals may often embark on activities that do not reflect personal experience or ability.
- Decreased need for sleep: the person often feels refreshed after only a few hours of sleep, goes to sleep much later than usual,

experiences interrupted sleep or wake much earlier than usual.

- Speech is often characterised by being more talkative and/or the subjective experience of a pressure to keep on talking. Speech has increased volume, can be loud and rapid and difficult to interrupt. Speech can be characterised by punning, joking, or irrelevant facetious comments. Speech may be characterised by complaints and angry outbursts during an irritable mood.
- Flight of ideas or subjective experience that thoughts are racing: patients often report that the rate of thinking outstrips the ability to verbalise. Flight of ideas is characterised by an almost continuous flow of accelerated speech with abrupt changes of topics.
- Distractability: attention is often deviated by irrelevant stimuli. There is an inability to screen out irrelevant external stimuli. There can be an inability to focus on the question at hand and a tendency to deviate to irrelevant topics, losing the line of thought.
- Increase in goal-directed activity, including activities that involve sexual, occupational, political and religious pursuits.
- Excessive involvement in pleasurable activities that have a high potential for painful consequences, including buying sprees, sexual disinhibition or unwise business ventures. This aspect can lead to financial problems, unemployment and divorce.

#### 13.4.1.2 Hypomanic episode

The features of a hypomanic episode are in many respects similar to that of a manic episode. The important difference, however, lies in the degree and severity of symptoms and the degree and severity to which social, occupational and interpersonal functioning are impaired. (Impairment is to a lesser degree compared with a manic episode.) A further confusing distinction is often made that hypomanic episodes do not require hospitalisation, while manic episodes frequently do.

#### 13.4.1.3 Depressive episode

A characteristic feature of a depressive episode is a mood state that can be characteristically and variously described as:

- painful arousal
- hypersensitivity to unpleasant events
- insensitivity to present events
- insensitivity to unpleasant events
- reduced anticipatory pleasure
- anhedonia
- affective blunting
- apathy.

Subjectively, the mood in a major depressive episode can be described as depressed, sad, hopeless or discouraged (down in the dumps). For a major depressive episode, at least a two-week period during which there is either depressed mood or the loss of interest or pleasure in nearly all activities (or both) must be recorded.

Note: an irritable mood rather than a depressed mood may be seen in children and adolescents.

In addition to the above two features, four of the following features must be present:

- sleep: insomnia or hypersomnia can be found in bipolar disorder
- interest: is usually reduced in depression
- guilt: individuals can experience an excessive feeling of guilt, often related to minor problems or transgressions in the past. Unrealistically negative evaluations of the self may be present. The most common form is guilt about being ill and failure to perform role functions due to depression. In its most severe form, guilt can assume a psychotic character (i.e. delusions of guilt). A sense of extreme worthlessness often accompanies the experience of guilt or can in itself be present
- energy: patients can suffer from extreme fatigue or reduced psychic energy
- cognitive dysfunction: patients with depression can experience various forms of cognitive dysfunction, including disturbances of memory and concentration. Patients can report an inability to think or make decisions, which can lead to poorer academic

functioning. This symptom can assume the quality of dementia in the elderly, often referred to as a **pseudodementia**

- appetite: patients can experience loss of appetite, at times accompanied by weight loss of various degrees, or increased appetite (hyperphagia)
- psychomotor agitation or retardation: patients can experience various degrees of listlessness, or various degrees of restlessness. Psychomotor retardation can be present in that patients have a reduced level of movement, or slow response times, or speech that is reduced in content, inflection and amount or even muteness. In its extreme form this can assume the clinical picture of catatonia. Psychomotor agitation includes the inability to sit still or pacing, wringing the hands or pulling or rubbing the skin, clothing, or other objects
- suicidal ideation: during a major depressive episode patients can experience various degrees of suicidal ideation. This can include a feeling that life doesn't make sense any more, thoughts of death, active planning of methods of suicide, writing of suicide notes, suicide attempts or **completed suicide**
- atypical features in a depressive episode: it is often found that the symptoms of the major depressive episode, as part of a bipolar disorder, show atypical features. This includes hypersomnia, hyperphagia, and an extreme form of tiredness (referred to as leaden paralysis), increased stress or conflict sensitivity (often referred to as rejection sensitivity). The detection of these features in any patient who present with a major depressive episode should induce the clinician to search diligently for the possible presence of the mood variations characteristic of bipolar disorder.

Other accompanying features of a depressive episode include:

- decreased sexual functioning, such as erectile dysfunction, loss of libido or anorgasmia
- tearfulness, irritability, brooding, obsessive rumination, anxiety, phobias, excessive worry over physical health, complaints of pain, such as joint, abdominal, and other pains or headache
- marital problems and divorce
- occupational difficulties, such as unemployment
- substance abuse
- increased use of medical services
- increased rates of premature death from general medical conditions.

#### 13.4.1.4 Rapid cycling phase

Normal cycling in the context of bipolar disorder has not been defined, but the definition of rapid cycling most frequently cited in the literature is that of Dunner and Fieve (1974): at least four major depressive, manic, hypomanic or mixed episodes are required to have occurred during a twelve-month period. This definition is in keeping with the criteria adopted by the DSM-5, but not all investigators have been consistent in defining episode duration and periods of inter-episode remission. The time lines of rapid cycling range from illness-free spells of many years' duration, with apparent peaks at multiples of one year to mood variations of an extreme form occurring over the course of hours or minutes. Various terms have been used to describe these time lines:

- rapid cycling: four or more episodes of significant mood disturbance in a year
- ultra-rapid cycling: cycle frequencies in the range of weeks to days
- ultradian cycling: significant mood variation within a day
- continuous cycling: the absence of illness-free spells between episodes
- mixed states: may be seen either as co-existing depressive and (hypo)manic symptoms or as an extreme of rapid cycling.

#### 13.4.1.5 Mixed-episode phase

A mixed episode phase is characterised by a period of time, lasting at least one week, in which the features of a manic episode and a major depressive episode are experienced nearly every day. These conditions can be difficult to detect if one is not alert to the various ways of clinical presentation. The following aspects should alert one to the presence of a mixed state:

- unrelenting dysphoria or irascibility
- severe agitation: patients describe a sense of restless agitation during a severe depressive episode
- refractory anxiety: in very severe forms, anxiety often constitutes a mixed state, especially if accompanied by agitation and restlessness
- unendurable sexual excitement: patients describe increased libido or impulsive sexual behaviour during a depressed mood
- intractable insomnia: patients often describe very severe insomnia that often is unresponsive to hypnotics
- suicidal obsessions: suicidal ideation is experienced as near constant and intrusive for hours on end
- histrionic demeanour yet with genuine expressions of intense suffering: the excessive expression of emotion accompanying a depressed mood.

## 13.4.2 Other associated and clinically relevant features

Various studies have identified what is now commonly referred to as soft signs of bipolar disorder. These do not constitute diagnostic features but are clinical clues highly suggestive of the diagnosis of bipolar disorder:

- repeated episodes of major depressive disorder (>4)
- first episode of major depressive disorder before the age of 25 (some even suggest 18 to 20 years)
- first-degree relative with bipolar disorder
- when not depressed, mood and energy is found to be higher than normal (i.e. hyperthymic)
- atypical features in depressive episode
- episodes of major depressive disorder are brief (i.e. shorter than three months)
- rapid onset and offset of major depressive disorder
- major depressive disorder with psychosis
- postpartum onset of major depressive disorder
- frequent or repetitive loss of antidepressant effect in the treatment of major depressive disorder or three or more antidepressants tried with no effect or worsening of agitation
- seasonal mood shifts.

## 13.4.3 Cognitive deficits

Cognitive deficits involve attention, executive function and verbal memory, and are evident across all phases of bipolar disorder. Circumscribed cognitive deficits may be both iatrogenic and intrinsic to bipolar disorder. Differentiating between medication-induced and illness-induced cognitive dysfunction requires comprehensive assessment with an appreciation for the cognitive domains most affected by specific medications.

## 13.4.4 Course of illness

### 13.4.4.1 Bipolar I disorder

Bipolar I disorder is, by its very nature, a recurrent disorder: after a single manic episode, more than 90% of individuals will go on to have future episodes. Sixty to 70% of manic episodes will take place immediately before or after a major depressive episode. Furthermore, if taken together, manic and major depressive episodes will have a higher frequency in bipolar disorder than in major depressive disorder. Of patients with bipolar I disorder, 5–15% will have multiple (more than four) mood episodes within one year, constituting a rapid cycling pattern. This pattern is associated with a worse prognosis. The majority of individuals return to normal functioning between mood episodes, but 20–30% of patients continue to show severe mood lability, interpersonal and occupational problems. During a manic episode patients may develop psychotic symptoms (even after a non-psychotic onset). If psychosis forms part of a particular episode of mania, future episodes of mania are likely to be psychotic as well.

#### 13.4.4.2 Bipolar II disorder (Berk and Dodd, 2005)

Bipolar II disorder has a complex course and outcome and presents several difficulties for the treating doctor.

Depression is most often the presenting symptom. If not specifically explored by the examining psychiatrist, hypomania is only rarely reported during an initial interview. This is often due to the fact that most patients do not see elevated mood as abnormal. This makes collateral information mandatory as it is often the collateral history of the family that reveals the mood cycling. Behaviour and personality can also cloud mood symptomatology. Hypomania is frequently denied. The clinical presentation is further complicated by the frequent co-morbidity of anxiety disorders and substance use disorders (in up to 80% of patients).

Mixed states are often even more difficult to recognise as they constitute anxious dysphoric states accompanied by agitated restless behaviour, suicidal obsessions and intractable insomnia.

The disorder tends to start in adolescence or occasionally pre-adolescence, with a mean age of onset of 18 years. It is often initially misdiagnosed as unipolar depression, an adjustment disorder or a personality disorder, especially borderline personality disorder. The onset of the illness often presents with mild mood swings, which then slowly increase in amplitude until a diagnostic threshold is reached. The disorder is furthermore characterised by severe functional impairment and co-morbidity. In a naturalistic study (Judd *et al.*, 2003) patients were found to be symptomatic (versus euthymic) for 53,9% of the time studied. Of this 53,9% symptomatic time, depressive symptoms comprised 50,3%, and hypomania 1,3%.

Bipolar II disorder is therefore a predominantly depressive illness, further obscuring the diagnosis and frequently misdiagnosed as major depressive disorder. Substantial suicide risk is present.

#### 13.4.4.3 Cyclothymic disorder

The precise course of this disorder is not clear. The disorder begins in early adolescence or early adulthood. It has an insidious onset and follows a chronic course. Between 15–50% of patients develop bipolar I or II disorder in the course of the illness, suggesting that cyclothymic disorder may be an initial presentation of these.

### 13.4.5 Bipolar disorder and borderline personality disorder

The relationship between bipolar disorder and borderline personality disorder (BPD) is complex. The two disorders resemble each other, especially in terms of mood instability, impulsivity and identity disturbance.

#### 13.4.5.1 Mood instability

- In borderline personality disorder, the instability is frequently in response to negative interpersonal events (which cause frequent, short-lived depressive episodes) and positive events (which lead to feelings of happiness).
- Irritability frequently accompanies the mood swings in borderline personality disorder.
- In bipolar disorder the mood swings may also be reactive but are far more frequently spontaneous and not so short lasting or rapidly shifting.
- Bipolar disorder patients are depressed for longer periods.

#### 13.4.5.2 Impulsivity

- Patients with borderline personality disorder often show impulsive behaviour driven by the need to be closer to loved ones or fears of abandonment, with increased, impulsive sexual encounters.
- In bipolar disorder the hypersexual behaviour is often driven by increased libido and takes place often with little interpersonal needs expressed.

#### 13.4.5.3 Identity disturbance

- In borderline personality disorder, self-esteem can fluctuate rapidly between self-depreciation and self-idealisation. These fluctuations can be directly related to the experience of closeness or distance in interpersonal relationships.
- Grandiosity in bipolar disorder is often unrelated to interpersonal functioning. Patients with bipolar disorder seldom demonstrate the other areas of identity disturbance such as 'personal sense of who I am', sexual identity or orientation.

Further adding the confusion is the fact that anticonvulsant or antipsychotic treatments are effective in both conditions. Up to 30% of patients demonstrate co-morbid bipolar disorder and borderline personality disorder. This co-morbidity is often associated with earlier age of onset of bipolar disorder, a worse prognosis linked to worse compliance with treatment and increased rates of suicide.

## 13.5 Treatment of bipolar disorder

The treatment of bipolar disorder can be divided into the following components (Berk and Dodd, 2005):

- acute treatment of mania and hypomania
- acute treatment of depression
- maintenance treatment
- treatment of complex bipolar presentations (i.e. rapid cycling and mixed states)
- management of partial or no treatment responses
- treatment of co-morbidities (i.e. anxiety disorders and substance use disorders).

### 13.5.1 Treatment of acute symptoms of mania

Table 13.1 shows the appropriate treatment for acute symptoms of mania.

When targeting the acute symptoms of mania, taper and cease any antidepressants or agents with mood-elevating properties (e.g. stimulants). Where possible, institute general measures:

- reduce stimulation
- lower activity level
- delay individual from making important decisions
- maintain a structured routine.

Commence treatment with an antimanic agent (level I). In selecting an agent, consider its antimanic efficacy and tolerability; also factor in the likelihood of continuing acute treatment into the maintenance phase.

When combining therapy, lithium or valproate combined with short-term administration of an atypical antipsychotic are superior compared with monotherapy with either lithium or valproate alone. If symptoms and/or behavioural disturbance are severe or protracted, consider electroconvulsive therapy (ECT) (level II).

Discontinue lithium during ECT. It is advisable to stop anticonvulsants during ECT, although recent studies have indicated that anticonvulsants may be continued during ECT without losing the therapeutic efficacy of ECT.

Gabapentin, lamotrigine, topiramate, phenytoin and oxcarbamazepine are not recommended for the treatment of acute mania.

#### 13.5.1.1 Treatment of behavioural disturbances

Treatment of behavioural disturbance in acute mania include the following:

- Short-term use of a benzodiazepine (e.g. lorazepam) or an antipsychotic may be required to manage acute behavioural disturbance. (Note that the concurrent use of two antipsychotics is not recommended.)
- Oral administration is preferable; however, if intramuscular (IM) administration is necessary, an injectable atypical antipsychotic or a combination of an injectable typical antipsychotic and benzodiazepine is recommended.
- Treatment of acute agitation: randomised controlled trial data (Yatham, 2013) support the use of IM aripiprazole or IM olanzapine (Level II).

**Table 13.1** Treatment of mania symptoms

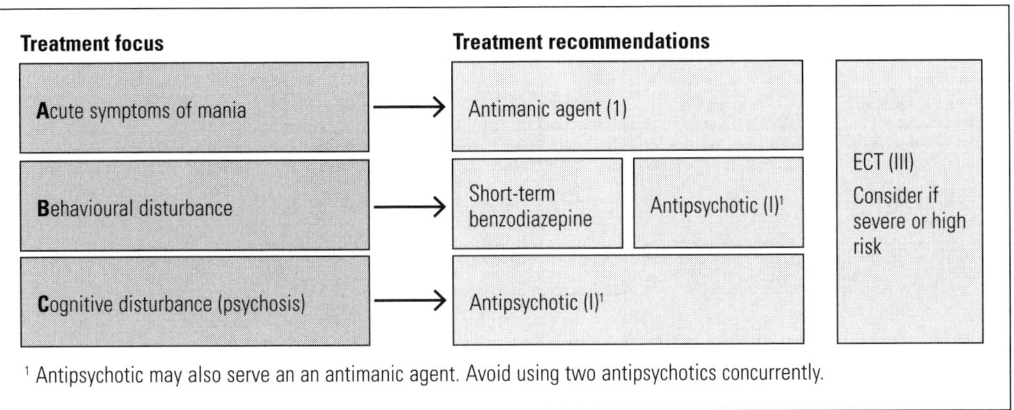


**Source:** Reproduced from Malhi *et al.*, 2009. This material is reproduced with permission from John Wiley and Sons Inc.

**Table 13.2** Recommendations for pharmacological treatment of acute mania

| | |
|---|---|
| **First line** | Monotherapy: lithium, divalproex, ***divalproex ER***[a], olanzapine[b], risperidone, quetiapine, quetiapine XR, aripiprazole, Ziprasidone, ***asenapine***[a], ***paliperidone ER***[a]<br>Adjunctive therapy with lithium or divalproex: risperidone, quetiapine, olanzapine, aripiprazole, ***asenapine***[a] |
| **Second line** | Monotherapy: Carbamazepine, carbamazepine ER, ECT, ***haloperidol***[a]<br>Combination therapy: lithium + divalproex |
| **Third line** | Monotherapy: Chlorpromazine, clozapine, oxcarbazepine, tamoxifen, ***cariprazine***[a] (not yet commercially available)<br>Combination therapy: lithium or divalproex + haloperidol, lithium + carbamazeoine, adjunctive tamoxifen |
| **Not recommended** | Monotherapy: gabapentin, topiramate, lamotrigine, verapamil, tiagabine<br>Combination therapy: risperidone + carbamazeoine, olanzapine + carbamazepine |

ECT = electroconvulsive therapy; XR or ER = extended release.

[a] ***New or change to recommendation.***

[b] Given the metabolic side effects, use should be carefully monitored.

**Source:** Yatham *et al.*, 2013. This material is reproduced with permission from John Wiley and Sons Inc.

- IM aripiprazole (9,75 mg and 15 mg) is superior to placebo and comparable with IM lorazepam (2 mg).
- In a double-blind randomised controlled trial, IM olanzapine 10 mg was superior to placebo and showed a trend toward greater improvement than IM lorazepam 2 mg.

▸ Do not combine olanzepine and benzodiazepines as there is a risk of respiratory failure.

Psychosis occurs in approximately 60% of episodes of acute mania. Antipsychotics may be used as an adjunctive treatment for acute psychotic symptoms (if not already being administered as an antimanic agent). Atypical antipsychotics are preferred to typical antipsychotics because of better tolerability.

**Table 13.3** Treatment options for acute bipolar depression

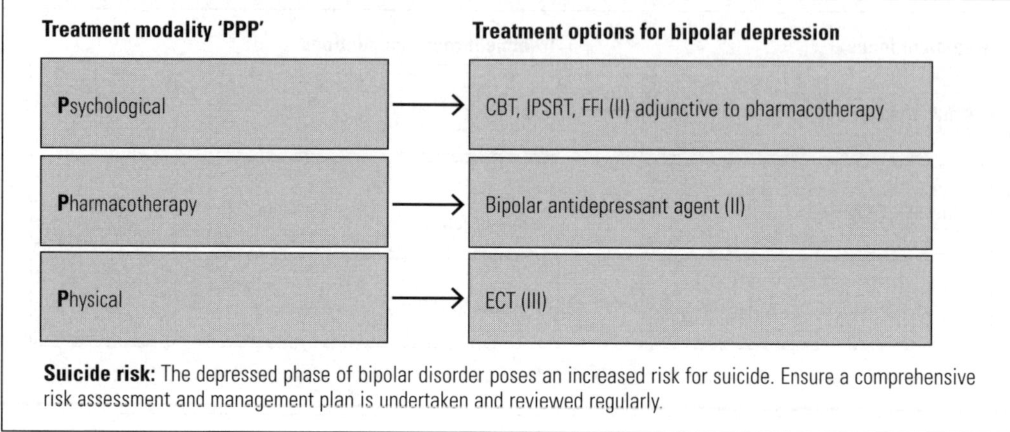

| Treatment modality 'PPP' | Treatment options for bipolar depression |
|---|---|
| **P**sychological | CBT, IPSRT, FFI (II) adjunctive to pharmacotherapy |
| **P**harmacotherapy | Bipolar antidepressant agent (II) |
| **P**hysical | ECT (III) |

**Suicide risk:** The depressed phase of bipolar disorder poses an increased risk for suicide. Ensure a comprehensive risk assessment and management plan is undertaken and reviewed regularly.

**Source:** Malhi, 2009. This material is reproduced with permission from John Wiley and Sons Inc.

## 13.5.2 Acute treatment of bipolar depression

Treatment options for acute bipolar depression include psychological interventions, pharmacotherapy and physical treatments.

### 13.5.2.1 Psychological interventions

See Section 13.5.6 for more information on psychological interventions.

### 13.5.2.2 Pharmacotherapy

Where practical, screen for and discontinue any agents that may exacerbate depression (e.g. typical antipsychotics such as chlorpromazine, antihypertensive agents, corticosteroids). Initiate and/or optimise a bipolar depression agent.

- First-line monotherapy treatment options include:
  - quetiapine 300–600 mg/day
  - lamotrigine 200–500 mg/day;
  - olanzapine 5–15 mg/day
  - lithium at therapeutic blood levels
  - valproate at therapeutic blood levels
- Second-line options for bipolar depression include adjunctive or combination therapies:
  - adjunctive risperidone 2–4 mg/day
  - lithium and antidepressant combinations
  - olanzapine and fluoxetine combination
  - valproate and lithium
  - lamotrigine as add-on to lithium.

If concurrent psychotic symptoms are present, augment with an atypical antipsychotic agent. However, avoid combining two antipsychotic medications.

- Conventional antidepressants: Efficacy of tricyclic antidepressants (TCAs), selective serotonin reuptake inhibitors (SSRIs) and serotonin and noradrenaline reuptake inhibitors (SNRIs) in the treatment of bipolar depression remain unclear. If a conventional antidepressant is to be used to treat bipolar depression, it should be administered in combination with an antimanic maintenance agent so as to diminish the likelihood of switching and then be gradually tapered after two to three months of sustained recovery. Antidepressants should not be prescribed in rapid-cycling bipolar disorder. TCAs (7–11%) and venlafaxine (13–15%) are associated with a relatively higher risk of inducing a switch to mania than SSRIs (0–4%); other agents can also precipitate switching (e.g. psychostimulants) (Malhi *et al.*, 2009).
- Physical treatments: ECT is an effective treatment (level III) and should be considered if

risk to self or others is high, if psychotic features are present or there has been a previous response to ECT (Yatham *et al.*, 2013).

## 13.5.3 Maintenance treatment of bipolar I disorder

Once a diagnosis of bipolar disorder has been established, ongoing treatment is necessary. Indications include:

- prior mood episode in the previous five years
- two previous mood episodes over any time period
- severe acute episode with suicide risk or psychotic features
- ongoing functional disability.

It is important to re-evaluate the treatment plan and consider co-morbid conditions, psychosocial stressors and other factors that may increase risk of relapse. Maintenance treatment should provide a collaborative approach to continued care. Pharmacological and psychological treatment strategies should be used to:

- eliminate subsyndromal depressive symptoms (disability is closely related to the depressive component of the illness)
- address psychosocial stressors
- develop the patient's problem-solving skills
- develop the patient's social support networks (especially with chronic depressive symptoms)
- encourage a healthy lifestyle (good **sleep hygiene**, exercise, regular routine)
- treat co-morbidities, particularly substance misuse
- monitor clinical response to medications, adherence and side effects
- monitor social and occupational functioning
- provide psycho-education for the family
- provide caregiver support.

### 13.5.3.1 Psychological interventions

Psychological interventions – adjunctive to medication – during the maintenance phase appear to have the greatest benefit in reducing risk of relapse and can improve functioning. The therapeutic effect can be optimised by targeting euthymic patients in the maintenance phase of illness. This, however, is likely to be less effective in those with a high number of prior mood episodes (>12 episodes). Strong evidence exists for interventions focused on the recognition of early warning signs. Evidence for specific therapies includes (see details below):

- cognitive behaviour therapy (CBT)
- family-focused therapy (FFT)
- interpersonal and social rhythm therapy (IPSRT)
- group psycho-education.

### 13.5.3.2 Pharmacotherapy

Initially, it is important to withdraw any adjunctive agents that have been used to manage behavioural disturbance associated with an acute mood episode. In practice, maintenance agents are often used in combination, even though there is a paucity of evidence for this strategy. Monotherapy is preferable. Medications that have been shown to be effective maintenance agents include:

- lithium (level I) particularly at preventing manic episodes
- lamotrigine (level II) particularly for preventing depressive episodes
- valproate (level II)
- atypical antipsychotics: olanzapine (level II)
- aripiprazole (level II)
- quetiapine adjunctive to lithium or valproate (level II).

Other atypical antipsychotics have a limited evidence base, restricted to small trials or retrospective data:

- ziprasidone (level III)
- risperidone (level III)
- adjunctive depot risperidone (level III)
- adjunctive clozapine (level III).

When selecting maintenance agents, consider their efficacy and tolerability profiles along with individual patient factors including preference, past response and safety factors. In this regard, lithium must be monitored regularly to maintain therapeutic blood levels (0,6–1,2 mmol/l).

Carbamazepine has a mixed evidence base as a maintenance treatment. The efficacy of conventional antidepressants (e.g. TCAs, SSRIs and SNRIs) in the maintenance of bipolar disorder is not established for maintenance treatment. However, if depressive episodes are recurrent, antidepressant treatment in combination with a bipolar maintenance agent may be considered only after weighing up the benefits of prevention against the risk of precipitating mania or rapid cycling.

## 13.5.4 Treatment of complex bipolar presentations

### 13.5.4.1 Rapid cycling

Rapid cycling is associated with poorer long-term response to treatment, higher rates of morbidity and increased suicide risk. Screen for and, where possible, exclude factors that may precipitate or exacerbate rapid cycling, such as antidepressants, substance misuse, medication and medical illness such as hypothyroidism.

The evidence base for rapid-cycling is limited and treatment appears to be less effective in countering depressive symptoms than manic symptoms.

**Pharmacological monotherapy**

Consider the following:

- valproate (level II)
- lithium (level II)
- olanzapine (level II)
- lamotrigine (level II) (primarily for bipolar II patients)
- quetiapine (level III).

**Combination therapies**

Consider adjunctive psychological interventions (level V) as outlined in the maintenance section (see Section 15.5.3).

There is limited evidence to support combination treatment, but clinical needs may warrant a trial of combinations, such as:

- lithium and valproate (level III)
- lithium and carbamazepine (level III)
- adjunctive lamotrigine (level V).

Physical treatments, in the form of an ECT should be considered for level III.

### 13.5.4.2 Mixed states

Mixed states are notoriously difficult to diagnose and distinguish from both mania and agitated depression. Few treatment studies have specifically examined mixed states, with most including patients with mixed states in studies of acute mania and acute bipolar depression. Therefore, treatment recommendations for mixed states also overlap with those for acute episodes. Initially, taper and then discontinue substances with a mood-elevating effect or those that may induce inter-episode switching (e.g. antidepressants, stimulants). Treatment options include:

- olanzapine (level II)
- quetiapine or valproate (in monotherapy)
- olanzapine and fluoxetine in combination
- valproate in combination with olanzapine (level II).

There is an overall paucity of evidence for adjunctive treatments in mixed states. Lamotrigine adjunctive to an antimanic agent may be a useful option for mixed states to treat depressive symptoms. However, treatment effect is likely to be delayed as this requires slow titration, especially in conjunction with valproate.

If symptoms and/or behavioural disturbance are severe or protracted, consider ECT (level III). Lithium may have a reduced efficacy for treating mixed states. Antidepressants are not recommended as they can worsen or induce rapid cycling.

## 13.5.5 Management of partial or no treatment response

Berk and Dodd (2005) graphically depict the approach to a partial or a no-treatment response in bipolar disorder. They divide the approach into a clinical management (read evaluation) phase, and a therapeutic strategy (read treatment)

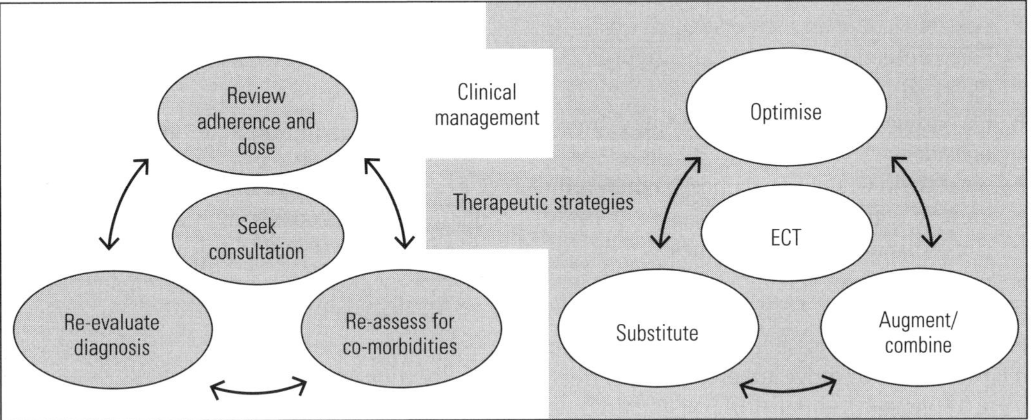


**Figure 13.1** Clinical management and therapeutic strategies in partial or no-treatment response

**Source:** Malhi, 2009. This material is reproduced with permission from John Wiley and Sons Inc.

phase (see Figure 13.1). Clinical management of partial or no-treatment responses includes:

- always use structured rating scales, along with clinical assessment, as they assist in gauging treatment response and quantifying change in clinical profile
- review adherence and dosage: reassess adherence and satisfaction with treatment plan. If the patient is using an antidepressant, ensure a therapeutic dose is prescribed and that adequate blood levels of medications are attained
- re-evaluate diagnosis: reassess for psychosocial stressors that maintain symptoms and consider alternative causes (e.g. organic causes)
- re-assess for co-morbidities, especially anxiety disorders, drug-use and alcohol-use disorders, personality disorders, or medical co-morbidities
- seek consultation with a psychiatrist when prescribing novel treatments, in complex cases, or where there has been a partial or no response to multiple treatment trials. Also consider specialist consultation or referral to a specialist clinic.

## 13.5.6 Psychotherapy for bipolar disorder

There are five general categories of psychotherapy for the treatment of bipolar disorder (Berk and Dodd, 2005).

### 13.5.6.1 Psycho-education

Psycho-education can be applied in individual or group formats or in combination with what is referred to as systematic care. The approach of Colom and Vieta (2006) is the most comprehensive; the following aspects are dealt with in a systematic way during psycho-education:

- what is bipolar illness?
- causes and triggers
- symptoms of mania and hypomania
- symptoms of depression and mixed episodes
- course and outcome
- treatment with mood stabilisers
- treatment with antimanic agents
- treatment with antidepressants
- monitoring of drug-serum levels
- pregnancy and genetic counselling
- psychopharmacology versus alternative treatments
- risks associated with treatment withdrawal

- risks of alcohol and street drugs
- early detection of manic and hypomanic episodes
- early detection of depression and mixed episodes
- what to do when a new phase is detected
- lifestyle regularity
- stress management techniques
- problem-solving techniques.

Psycho-education has been shown to prevent relapses and to improve adherence in the treatment of bipolar disorder (Rucci *et al.*, 2002).

### 13.5.6.2 Family-focused therapy

In family-focused therapy, including family psycho-education, the standard themes of psycho-education (Colom and Vieta, 2006) (see Section 13.5.6.1) are applied in addition to:

- training in communication and problem-solving skills
- developing a relapse-prevention plan
- examining the attitudes toward medication
- communication exercises (e.g. active listening and constructive feedback) aimed at reducing high expressed-emotion interchanges.

### 13.5.6.3 Cognitive behavioural therapy

CBT is applied in a standard way. It has been shown to be effective in improving several parameters of bipolar disorder, including relapse prevention, medication adherence, early detection of illness and improvement of depressive symptomatology. It has not been shown to be effective during the hypomanic or manic phases of the illness (Miklowitz, 2008).

### 13.5.6.4 Interpersonal Social Rhythm Therapy

The aims of IPSRT are to stabilise daily and nightly routines or social rhythms, and to resolve interpersonal problems that co-existed with the most recent illness episode. This involves stabilising social rhythms by tracking daily routines and sleep-wake cycles and keeping to routines even during events that would ordinarily change routines (e.g. preparing for an exam or taking a transatlantic flight) (Miklowitz, 2008).

### 13.5.6.5 Constructive psychotherapy

Constructive psychotherapy of bipolar disorder (Mahoney, 2003) is an integrated technique that consists of the following basic components:

- construction of representations related to the disease
- symptom monitoring
- identification of prodromal symptoms and activation of an early-intervention plan
- cognitive restructuring
- acquisition of problem-solving, communication and social skills.

### 13.5.6.6 General principles of psychotherapy of bipolar disorder

- Models of psychotherapy with 12 or more sessions consistently perform better than comparison treatments of three or fewer sessions.
- No particular modality emerges as superior to others; this suggests that the modalities operate through different change mechanisms and in turn affect different outcome variables.
- Active treatments are associated with a 30–40% reduction in relapse rates over a period of 12 to 30 months.
- Intensive psychosocial treatments have better functional outcomes than routine pharmacological care over a period of one to two years.
- The beneficial effects of psycho-education, systematic care, full-family therapy, CBT and IPSRT can be observed for at least one year after their termination.

### 13.5.6.7 Cognitive rehabilitation

Various research institutions are now attempting to compile cognitive rehabilitation programs for bipolar disorder. Cognitive impairment forms large parts of the dysfunctional state of even euthymic bipolar disorder patients. Although these trials are at very early stages, results are promising; further development and refinement still have to take place.

## 13.6 Specific issues in the management of bipolar disorder

### 13.6.1 Bipolar disorder and pregnancy

There are excellent resources for reference on the management of bipolar disorders related to reproductive issues in women (see Additional reading, at the end of the chapter).

The Canadian Network for Mood and Anxiety Treatments (CANMAT) and International Society for Bipolar Disorders (ISBD) (CANMAT/-ISBD) guidelines suggest the following with regards to bipolar disorder and pregnancy:

- The management of pregnant women with BD should incorporate careful planning.
- During the first trimester the risk of teratogenicity associated with use of psychotropic medication should be carefully weighed against the risks of an untreated mood episode to the mother and the foetus (risk-benefit ratio).
- Psychotropic medication can be used in the second and third trimester if necessary.
- If lithium is used during the second and third trimester, the serum-lithium levels should be monitored closely because of changes in blood volume during pregnancy. The dose should be adjusted accordingly to maintain levels in the therapeutic range.
- Teratogenic risk associated with sodium valproate, divalproex and carbamazepine during pregnancy must be considered.
- Topiramate has been associated with reduced birth weight but not with a decrease in gestational age or an increase in structural defects.
- Antidepressants during pregnancy do not confer an increased risk of major congenital anomalies compared to unexposed. (Note: in one analysis (Reis and Kallen, 2010), antidepressant use was associated with increased rates of pregnancy complications, including induced delivery, caesarean section, preterm birth and an increased risk of persistent pulmonary hypertension of the newborn.)
- Prenatal exposure to typical or atypical antipsychotics drugs: The Food and Drug Administration (2011) issued a safety alert regarding the risks to newborns associated with antipsychotic drugs, including potential risk for abnormal muscle movements and withdrawal symptoms including agitation, abnormal muscle tone, tremor, sleepiness, breathing, and feeding difficulties in newborns.

**Table 13.4** Psychiatric medications in pregnancy and lactation

| Agent | Pregnancy risk category[a] | American Academy of Pediatrics rating | Lactation risk category[b] |
|---|---|---|---|
| **Anxiolytic medications** | | | |
| *Benzodiazepines* | | | |
| Alprazolam | D | Unknown, of concern | L3 |
| Chlordiazepoxide | D | N/A | L3 |
| Clonazepam | D | N/A | L3 |
| Clorazepate | D | N/A | L3 |
| Diazepam | D | Unknown, of concern | L3, L4 if used chronically |
| Lorazepam | D | Unknown, of concern | L3 |
| Oxazepam | D | N/A | L3 |

| Agent | Pregnancy risk category[a] | American Academy of Pediatrics rating | Lactation risk category[b] |
|---|---|---|---|
| *Benzodiazepines for insomnia* | | | |
| Estazolam | X | N/A | L3 |
| Flurazepam | X | N/A | L3 |
| Quazepam | X | Unknown, of concern | L2 |
| Temazepam | X | Unknown, of concern | L3 |
| Triazolam | X | N/A | L3 |
| *Non-benzodiazepine anxiolytics and hypnotics* | | | |
| Buspirone | B | N/A | L3 |
| Chloral hydrate | C | Compatible | L3 |
| Eszoplicone | C | N/A | N/A |
| Zaleplon | C | Unknown, of concern | L2 |
| Zolpidem | B | N/A | L3 |
| **Antiepileptic and mood-stabilizing medications** | | | |
| Lithium carbonate | D | Contraindicated | L4 |
| Valproic acid | D | Compatible | L2 |
| Carbamazepine | D | Compatible | L2 |
| Lamotrigine | C | Unknown | L3 |
| **Antidepressants** | | | |
| *Tricyclic and heterocyclic antidepressants* | | | |
| Amitriptyline | C | Unknown, of concern | L2 |
| Amoxapine | C | Unknown, of concern | L2 |
| Clomipramine | C | Unknown, of concern | L2 |
| Desipramine | C | Unknown, of concern | L2 |
| Doxepin | C | Unknown, of concern | L5 |
| Imipramine | C | Unknown, of concern | L2 |
| Maprotiline | B | N/A | L3 |
| Nortriptyline | C | Unknown, of concern | L2 |
| Protriptyline | C | N/A | N/A |
| *Selective serotonin reuptake inhibitors* | | | |
| Citalopram | C | N/A | L3 |
| Escitalopram | C | N/A | L3 in older infants |
| Fluoxetine | C | Unknown, of concern | L2 in older infants, L3 if used in neonatal period |
| Fluvoxamine | C | Unknown, of concern | L2 |
| Paroxetine | D | Unknown, of concern | L2 |
| Sertraline | C | Unknown, of concern | L2 |
| *Other antidepressants* | | | |
| Bupropion | B | Unknown, of concern | L3 |
| Duloxetine | C | N/A | N/A |
| Mirtazapine | C | N/A | L3 |
| Nefazodone | C | N/A | L4 |
| Trazodone | C | Unknown, of concern | L2 |
| Venlafaxine | C | N/A | L3 |

| Agent | Pregnancy risk category[a] | American Academy of Pediatrics rating | Lactation risk category[b] |
|---|---|---|---|
| **Antipsychotic medications** | | | |
| *Typical antipsychotic agents* | | | |
| Chlorpromazine | C | Unknown, of concern | L3 |
| Fluphenazine | C | N/A | L3 |
| Haloperidol | C | Unknown, of concern | L2 |
| Loxapine | C | N/A | L4 |
| Perphenazine | C | Unknown, of concern | N/A |
| Pimozide | C | N/A | L4 |
| Thioridazine | C | N/A | L4 |
| Thiothixene | C | N/A | L4 |
| Trifluoperazine | C | Unknown, of concern | N/A |
| *Atypical antipsychotic agents* | | | |
| Aripiprazole | C | N/A | L3 |
| Clozapine | B | Unknown, of concern | L3 |
| Olanzapine | C | N/A | L2 |
| Quetiapine | C | Unknown, of concern | L4 |
| Risperidone | C | N/A | L3 |
| Ziprasidone | C | Unknown, of concern | L4 |

N/A = not available.

[a] The US Food and Drug Administration classifies drug safety using the following categories: A = controlled studies show no risk; B = no evidence of risk in humans; C = risk cannot be ruled out; D = positive evidence of risk; X = contraindicated in pregnancy.

[b] Lactation risk categories are listed as follows: L1 = safest; L2 = safer; L3 = moderately safe; L4 = possibly hazardous; L5 = contraindicated.

**Source:** Yatham *et al.*, 2013; American Congress of Obstetricians and Gynecologists, 2008. Reprinted with permission from Wolters Kluwer Health.

## 13.6.2 Postpartum period

Distinguishing bipolar depression from major depressive disorder can be challenging in the postpartum period because of a lack of screening instruments designed specifically for use during this period. The Mood Disorder Questionnaire (MDQ) (Hirschfeld *et al.*, 2000) is a useful screening instrument for bipolar disorder in the postpartum period.

Although hypomanic symptoms are common in early puerperium, they are often overlooked, leading to a misdiagnosis of major depressive disorder. One study showed a more than eight-fold increase in hypomanic symptoms in the early postpartum period (11,7%) compared to the first trimester (1,4%) and to eight weeks postpartum (4,9%) (Heron, 2009). A previous diagnosis of bipolar disorder was the strongest predictor of readmissions 10–19 days postpartum, with 27% of women with bipolar disorder being readmitted within the first year. Psychotic illness has been shown to peak immediately following a first childbirth.

## 13.6.3 Childhood-onset bipolar disorder

Up to two-thirds of adults with bipolar disorder report onset occurring during childhood or adolescence. In these cases of early onset, the course and outcome of bipolar disorder is worse than for later onset. There is still controversy surrounding the presence and presentation of bipolar disorder in children. Early recognition and treatment is critical to prevent the tremendously negative impact on development and brain function. Concerns exist about over-diagnosis and under-diagnosis. Misdiagnosis is common, with 47% of patients being diagnosed with depressive disorder and 37% with disruptive behaviour disorder in the previous year (McClellan *et al.*, 2007).

It is generally advised to use the standard presentations of bipolar I disorder, bipolar II disorder or bipolar disorder 'Not otherwise specified' among children and adolescents. It is obviously important to obtain collateral information on family history of bipolar disorder, or from multiple sources of information (e.g. child, parent and teacher), and information gleaned from questionnaires, checklists and diagnostic interviews.

First episodes in patients aged +12 years are generally depressive, while those in patients <12 years are more likely to be subsyndromal manic or hypomanic. Non-suicidal self-injury has also been reported in more than 20% of children and adolescents with bipolar disorder.

Symptoms that are relatively specific to bipolar disorder include pathological elation, decreased need for sleep and hypersexuality. Increased energy and distractibility have the greatest sensitivity to BD.

The American Academy of Child and Adolescent Psychiatry (AACAP) practice parameter (McClellan *et al.*, 2007) provides four recommendations as part of the minimal standard of assessment:

- include screening questions for bipolar disorder during psychiatric assessments of children and adolescents
- use unmodified DSM-5 criteria, including duration, when diagnosing mania or hypomania in youth
- if bipolar disorder is suspected, evaluate for suicidality, co-morbidities (including substance abuse and medical problems) and evaluate for psychosocial stressors
- be cautious when diagnosing preschool children with bipolar disorder, owing to uncertain validity.

Co-morbidities and mimics of BD:

- Studies (Swartz *et al.*, 2009) indicate that 44% of youth with bipolar disorder have at least one lifetime anxiety disorder and nearly 20% have two or more, with the most prevalent being separation anxiety (24%) and generalised anxiety disorder (GAD) (16%).
- There are extremely high rates of co-morbid attention-deficit hyperactivity disorder (ADHD) (85%), oppositional defiant disorder (90%), two or more anxiety disorders (64%), conduct disorder (51%), and substance use disorders (SUD) (12%).
- Early bipolar disorder onset (age <12 years) has been associated with ADHD. Later onset later (age ± 12 years) is associated with panic, conduct, and SUD.
- Psychotic symptoms have been reported in about one-third of youths with bipolar disorder (Muzina *et al.*, 2011), and confer a significantly greater likelihood of lifetime GAD, agoraphobia, social phobia, and obsessive-compulsive disorder (OCD).

#### 13.6.3.1 Acute and maintenance treatment of paediatric bipolar disorder

Most randomised controlled trials in youths with BD have investigated the acute treatment of manic or mixed symptoms (Yatham *et al.*, 2013), with few assessing maintenance therapy. Guidelines developed for adults with bipolar disorder should thus be cautiously applied to youths. Relatively little is known regarding the pharmacological treatment of the depressive phase of bipolar disorder, the maintenance and/or continuation of treatment or other bipolar disorder subtypes.

The second-generation antipsychotic agents (SGAs) appear to be more efficacious than the non-SGA mood stabilisers (divalproex sodium, lithium carbonate, and oxcarbazepine) among youths. The SGAs are associated with greater weight gain, greater **somnolence** and less akathisia among youths than among adults. Monitoring for metabolic syndrome is crucial.

For children with co-morbid ADHD and bipolar disorder, AACAP treatment guidelines recommend treating first with mood-stabilising medication and only subsequently treating ADHD pharmacologically if there are residual clinically impairing symptoms of ADHD.

Similarly, it is advisable to first stabilise mood prior to initiating treatment with a SSRI for the depressive phase of bipolar disorder or for co-morbid anxiety.

Several psychosocial treatments, adjunctive to pharmacotherapy, have been studied for paediatric bipolar disorder (Yatham *et al.*, 2013).

These include:

- psycho-education and multifamily group psycho-education to increase acceptance of the diagnosis and adherence to medications, improving the ability to manage stress, bolstering the protective effects of the family and enhancing functioning
- family-focused therapy has been most rigorously examined for the treatment of adolescents with BD
- after dialectical behaviour therapy (which primarily targets emotion regulation and communication skills) participants demonstrated significant improvements in depressive symptoms, emotion dysregulation, suicidality and non-suicidal self-injury
- interpersonal and social rhythm therapy (focusing on social and circadian rhythms)
- cognitive behavioural therapy.

See Chapter 28: Child and adolescent psychiatry 2: The older child and adolescent, for a further discussion of bipolar disorder in children and adolescents.

## 13.6.4 Managing bipolar disorder in older patients

Depp and Jeste (2004) discuss the issues in the management of older patients with bipolar disorder:

Presentation and course: The two-year EMBLEM study (Reed *et al.*, 2010) included 475 patients aged 60 years or older with acute bipolar disorder (mania or mixed), and found that older patients:

- had a history of more rapid cycling
- had fewer suicide attempts
- showed less severe manic and psychotic symptoms
- showed no difference in depressive symptomatology.

Older patients with late-onset bipolar disorder (age +50 years) experienced a better 12-week outcome with a faster recovery and earlier discharge compared to older patients with early-onset bipolar disorder (age <50 years). The prevalence of mixed episodes was reported in 10% of patients aged ± 60 years. A greater burden from vascular risk factors has been associated with poorer outcomes on some cognitive measures. No significant association between dementia or cognitive performance in older patients and the use of lithium has been found.

There seems to be a higher prevalence of the following co-morbidities in older patients with bipolar disorder:

- diabetes mellitus (27%)
- atopical diseases (20%)
- smoking (24%)
- unfavourable social functioning (22%)
- greater levels of cognitive dysfunction than age-matched mentally healthy control subjects when compared to age-matched controls
- a 20% increased risk of fracture compared to those without bipolar disorder, independent of the use of anticonvulsants.

### 13.6.4.1 Treatment of bipolar disorder in older patients

Data assessing pharmacotherapy specifically in older patients with BD remain scarce. Studies of quetiapine monotherapy in older patients with acute bipolar disorder mania suggest a significant improvement in manic symptoms as early as day four, with improvement sustained at 12-week follow-up (Sajatovic *et al.*, 2008).

Results from an open-label study of adjunctive lamotrigine in older patients with bipolar I disorder or bipolar II disorder, indicated an overall decline at 12-week follow-up in depressive symptoms, with a 65% response rate and a low rate (10%) of discontinuations because of adverse events (Sajatovic *et al.*, 2011).

## Conclusion

Patients with bipolar disorder can be amongst the most complex to manage in medicine. The practising doctor should have a sound working knowledge of the major issues in bipolar management, since appropriate treatment can have a huge impact on reducing the morbidity and mortality associated with this serious illness.

# References


American Congress of Obstetricians and Gynecologists Practice Bulletin: Clinical management guidelines for obstetrician-gynecologists number 92, April 2008 (replaces Practice Bulletin number 87, November 2007). Use of psychiatric medications during pregnancy and lactation. *Obstetrics and Gynecology* 111: 1001–1020

American Psychiatric Association (2013) *Diagnostic and Statistical Manual of Mental Disorders* (5th edition). Arlington, VA: American Psychiatric Association

Angst J (2013) Bipolar disorders in DSM-5: Strengths problems and perspectives. *International Journal of Bipolar Disorders* 1: 12

Bearden CE, Hoffman KM, Cannon TD, (2001) Bipolar disorders. The neuropsychology and neuroanatomy of bipolar affective disorder: A critical review. *Bipolar Disorders* 3: 106–50

Berk M, Dodd S (2005) Bipolar II disorder: A review. *Bipolar Disorders* 7: 11–21

Colom F, Vieta E (2006) *Psychoeducation Manual for Bipolar Disorder*. London: Cambridge University Press

Depp CA, Jeste DV (2004) Bipolar disorder in older adults: A critical review. *Bipolar Disorders* 6: 343–67

Dunner DL, Fieve RR (1974) Clinical factors in lithium carbonate prophylaxis failure. *Archives of General Psychiatry* 30(2): 229–33

Food and Drug Administration (2011) *Antipsychotic Drugs: Class Labeling Change – Treatment During Pregnancy and Potential Risk to Newborns*. Silver Spring MD: Food and Drug Administration

Hauser P, Matochik J, Altshuler LL, Denicoff KD, Conrad A, Li X, Post RM (2000) MRI-based measurements of temporal lobe and ventricular structures in patients with bipolar I and bipolar II disorder. *Journal of Affective Disorders* 60 1 25–32

Heron J, Haque S, Oyebode F, Craddock N, Jones I (2009) A longitudinal study of hypomania and depression symptoms in pregnancy and the postpartum period. *Bipolar Disorders* 11: 410–17

Hirschfeld RMA, Williams JBW, Spitzer RL, Calabrese JR, Flynn L, Keck PE, Lewis L, McElroy SL, Post RM, Rapport DJ, Russell JM, Sachs GS, Zajecka J (2000) Development and validation of a screening instrument for bipolar spectrum disorder: The Mood Disorder Questionnaire. *Psychiatry Online* 157(11): 1873–75

Judd LL, Akiskal HS, Schettler PJ, Coryell W, Endicott J, Maser JD, Solomon DA, Leon AC, Keller MB (2003) A prospective investigation of the natural history of the long-term weekly symptomatic status of bipolar II disorder. *Archives of General Psychiatry* 60: 261–9

Le-Niculescu H, McFarland MJ, Ogden CA, Balaraman Y, Patel S, Tan J, Rodd ZA, Paulus M, Geyer MA, Edenberg HJ, Glatt SJ, Faraone SV, Nurnberger JI, Kuczenski R, Tsuang MT, Niculescu AB (2008) Phenomic convergent functional genomic and biomarker studies in a stress-reactive genetic animal model of bipolar disorder and co-morbid alcoholism. *American Journal of Medical Genetics Part B* 134–66

Mahoney MJ (2003) *Constructive Psychotherapy: Theory and Practice*. New York: Guilford Press

Malhi GS, Adams D, Lampe L, Paton M, O'Connor N, Newton LA, Walter G, Taylor A, Porter R, Mulder RT, Berk M (2009) Clinical practice recommendations for bipolar disorder, *Acta Psychiatrica Scandinavia* 119 (Suppl 439): 27–46

McClellan J, Kowatch R, Findling RL, (2007) Practice parameters for the assessment and treatment of children and adolescents with bipolar disorder. *Journal of the American Academy of Child and Adolescent Psychiatry* 46: 107–25

Merinkangas KR, Akiskal HS, Angst J, Greenberg PE, Hirschfeld RMA, Petukhova M, Kessler RC (2007) Lifetime and 12-month prevalence of bipolar spectrum disorder in the national comorbidity survey replication. *Archives of General Psychiatry* 64: 543–52

Miklowitz DJ (2008) Adjunctive psychotherapy for bipolar disorder: State of the evidence. *American Journal of Psychiatry* 165: 1408–19

Muzina DJ, Gao K, Kemp DE, Khalife S, Ganocy SJ, Chan PK, Serrano MB, Conroy CM, Calabrese JR (2011) Acute efficacy of divalproex sodium versus placebo in mood stabilizer naive bipolar I or II depression: A double-blind randomized placebo-controlled trial. *Journal of Clinical Psychiatry* 72: 813–9

Piletz JE, Zhang X, Ranade R, Liu C (2011) Database of genetic studies of bipolar disorder. *Psychiatric Genetics* 21(2): 57–68.

Reed C, Goetz I, Vieta E, Bassi M, Haro JM (2010) Work impairment in bipolar disorder patients – results from a two-year observational study (EMBLEM). *European Psychiatry* 25: 338–44

Reis M, Kallen B (2010) Delivery outcome after maternal use of antidepressant drugs in pregnancy: An update using Swedish data. *Psychological Medicine* 2010; 40: 1723–1733

Rucci P, Frank E, Kostelnik B, Fagiolini A, Mallinger AG, Swartz HA, Thase ME, Siegel L, Wilson D, Kupfer DJ (2002) Suicide attempts in patients with bipolar I disorder during acute and maintenance phases of intensive treatment with pharmacotherapy and adjunctive psychotherapy. *American Journal of Psychiatry* 159: 1160–4

Sajatovic M, Calabrese JR, Mullen J (2008) Quetiapine for the treatment of bipolar mania in older adults. *Bipolar Disorders* 10: 662–71

Sajatovic M, Gildengers A, Al Jurdi RK, Gyulai L, Cassidy KA, Greenberg RL, Bruce ML, Mulsant BH, Ten Have T, Young RC (2011) Multisite open-label prospective trial of lamotrigine for geriatric bipolar depression: A preliminary report. *Bipolar Disorders* 13: 294–302

Strakowski SM, Adler CM, Almeida J, Altshuler L, Blumberg HP, Chang KC, DelBello MP, Frangou S, McIntosh A, Phillips ML, Sussman JE, Townsend JD (2012) The functional neuroanatomy of bipolar disorder: A consensus model. *Bipolar Disorders* 14: 313–25

Swartz HA, Frank E, Frankel DR, Novick D, Houck P (2009) Psychotherapy as monotherapy for the treatment of bipolar II depression: A proof of concept study. *Bipolar Disorders* 11: 89–94

Xu B, Woodroffe A, Rodriquez-Murillo L, Roos JL, Van Rensburg E, Abecasis G, Gogos J, Karayiorgou M (2009) Elucidating the genetic architecture of familial schizophrenia using rare copy number variant and linkage scans. Proceedings of the National Academy of Sciences of the United States of America 106(39): 16746–751

Yatham LN, Kennedy SH, Parikh SV, Schaffer A, Beaulieu S, Alda M, O'Donovan C, MacQueen G, McIntyre RS, Sharma V, Ravindran A, Young TR, Milev R, Bond DJ, Frey BN, Goldstein BI, Lafer B, Birmaher B, Ha K, Nolen WA, Berk M (2013) Canadian Network for Mood and Anxiety Treatments (CANMAT) and International Society for Bipolar Disorders (ISBD) collaborative update of CANMAT guidelines for the management of patients with bipolar disorder: update. *Bipolar Disorders* 15(1): 1–44

## Additional reading

ACOG Practice Bulletin: Clinical management guidelines for obstetrician-gynecologists number 92, April 2008 Use of psychiatric medications during pregnancy and lactation. *Obstetrics and Gynecology* 111: 1001–1020

Canadian Hospital for Sick Children (http://www.motherisk.org/ )

CHAPTER

# 14 Anxiety, fear and panic

Nastassja Koen, Dan Stein

## 14.1 Introduction

Anxiety disorders are a major contributor to the overall burden of psychiatric disease in both South Africa and abroad. In a number of large community surveys (Kessler *et al.*, 1994; Kessler *et al.*, 2005; Herman *et al.*, 2009) assessing the lifetime and 12-month population prevalence of common mental disorders, anxiety disorders have been consistently among the highest ranked. In a primary care setting, although these conditions are a common reason for seeking care and are a major contributor to the burden of disease, they are under-diagnosed. Underdiagnosis reflects a range of barriers, including low **mental-health literacy** and lack of screening for psychiatric disorders. If undiagnosed or mismanaged, individuals with anxiety disorders may incur a range of direct and indirect health costs and may suffer significant social, occupational and interpersonal impairment (Dupont *et al.*, 1996; Murray and Lopez, 1996).

Fortunately, there have been a number of noteworthy advances in understanding the pathogenesis and treatment of anxiety disorders. Structural, functional and molecular imaging methods have provided insight into the neurocircuitry that underpins these conditions and into the relevant neurochemistry. Advances in animal models and in cognitive-affective neuroscience have gradually allowed researchers to take laboratory knowledge and apply this in clinical settings. A range of pharmacotherapies and psychotherapies has proven efficacious for the treatment of these conditions.

In this chapter, six major categories of anxiety will be discussed, namely normal anxiety, generalised anxiety disorder, panic disorder, social anxiety disorder, specific phobias and anxiety disorders secondary to general medical conditions or substance abuse. The phenomenology, pathogenesis and treatment of these disorders will be outlined. For a more comprehensive understanding, this chapter should be studied in conjunction with Chapter 16: Trauma, and Chapter 17: Obsessive-compulsive and related disorders. While the Diagnostic and Statistical Manual of Mental Disorders IV Text Revision (DSM IV-TR) (American Psychiatric Association, 2000) classified both PTSD (post-traumatic stress disorder) and OCD (obsessive-compulsive disorder) as anxiety disorders, DSM-5 (American Psychiatric Association, 2013) has separate chapters on trauma and stress-related disorders (including acute stress disorder, adjustment disorders and dissociative disorders) (Friedman *et al.*, 2011), obsessive-compulsive and related disorders (including body dysmorphic disorder, hoarding disorder, trichotillomania (hair pulling disorder) and excoriation (skin picking) disorder) (Stein *et al.*, 2010). Separation anxiety disorder and selective mutism are covered in the chapters on child and adolescent disorders.

## 14.2 Fear and normal anxiety

### 14.2.1 Phenomenology

At one point or another, everyone will experience symptoms of fear or anxiety – tension prior to an examination, fear of an overdue visit to the dentist, stress over relationship conflicts and so forth. However, these experiences of fear and normal anxiety are significantly different from

**Case study 14.1**

Paul, a fourth-year medical student, was preparing for his final clinical examination, due to take place the following week. He had underestimated the amount of dedicated study time he would need, and was thus far behind schedule. Realising that he was ill-prepared, he began to feel exceedingly worried, irritable and on edge, struggling to concentrate on his work. Over the next few days, he had difficulty falling asleep at night, sometimes waking with a racing heart. These symptoms peaked in intensity the night before his examination. However, the following day, having completed his assessment, he felt immediate relief and treated himself to a long nap.

what is now conceptualised as an anxiety disorder. The DSM-5 defines fear as 'An emotional response to perceived imminent threat or danger associated with urges to flee or fight', while anxiety is described as 'The apprehensive anticipation of future danger or misfortune accompanied by a feeling of worry, distress, and/or somatic symptoms of tension. The focus of anticipated danger may be internal or external.' From an evolutionary perspective, fear and anxiety serve as protective mechanisms, enabling us to cope with potentially harmful stimuli (Hofer, 1995; Stein and Bouwer, 1997; Etkin, 2010). For example, when faced with his clinical examiner, Paul may have chosen to flee, freeze or fight (although in more realistic terms, his options would have been far more limited!). This is the crux of the classic fight-or-flight response (Cannon, 1915). Individuals experience a number of well-described anxiety and fear responses, including increased vigilance, startle reaction and autonomic heart rate and blood pressure changes (Rosen and Schulkin, 1998; Cannon, 1915). While the fear response is often characterised by autonomic fight-or-flight symptoms, individuals who experience normal anxiety will more likely complain of muscle tension and **hypervigilance** in anticipation of an impending danger (American Psychiatric Association, 2013).

Fear and normal anxiety are generally viewed as transient physiological and psychological adaptive responses to external stressors. An anxiety disorder is diagnosable when symptoms are present in excess or for a longer period than is deemed developmentally appropriate, resulting in multidimensional functional impairment (American Psychiatric Association, 2013; Hoehn-Saric and McLeod, 1988). Pathological anxiety may thus be described in either quantitative terms (i.e. excessive normal anxiety) or as a qualitative variation (Belzung and Griebel, 2001).

### 14.2.2 Pathogenesis

Fear and normal anxiety may be mediated by specific cognitive-affective systems involved in memory, perception and planning of motor activities. Neurobiological circuits, comprising a number of cortical and sub-cortical components, may also play a role. Neuro-anatomical structures integral to these circuits include the amygdala and insula (which are responsible for registering negative stimuli and processing fear and anxiety-relevant negative emotions) and the peri-aqueductal (PA) grey matter and hypothalamus (which contribute to autonomic regulation) (Etkin, 2010). Genetic and environmental factors play a role in establishing susceptibility to both pathological and normal anxiety. Specific candidate genetic polymorphisms (variants) may lead to neuro-anatomical and physiological changes that increase individual vulnerability to environmental risk factors and ultimately to normal anxiety traits and disorders (Gross and Hen, 2004).

### 14.2.3 Treatment

In the clinical setting, it is important to differentiate between the signs and symptoms of normal anxiety and those of adjustment disorder (AD) with anxiety features. The major distinction between these two conditions is the degree of distress or impairment: adjustment disorder is, by definition, associated with clinically significant distress or functional impairment (Strain and Friedman, 2011).

In general, non-pharmacological strategies should be the first-line option for individuals with symptoms of normal anxiety. In particular, preventative coping strategies, including improved nutrition, exercise, relaxation techniques and appropriate time management, have been found to be helpful (Godbey and Courage, 1994; Shapiro *et al.*, 2000). Typically, psychotherapeutic agents should be avoided in these cases, given risk-benefit ratio considerations.

# 14.3 Generalised anxiety disorder

## 14.3.1 Phenomenology

### 14.3.1.1 Epidemiology

Of all the anxiety disorders, generalised anxiety disorder (GAD) is the condition most likely to be seen at the primary health care level. In international and local population surveys, this disorder has been shown to have a lifetime prevalence of approximately 2, 5-5% (Herman *et al.*, 2009; Kessler *et al.*, 2005; Tyrer and Baldwin, 2006) with females more commonly affected (Wittchen and Jacobi, 2005). Onset of symptoms of generalised anxiety disorder is earlier than with other common psychiatric conditions (e.g. depression and substance-use disorders), but is later than certain other anxiety disorders (e.g. social anxiety disorder).

### 14.3.1.2 Clinical signs and symptoms

Diagnostic criteria for individuals with generalised anxiety disorder are outlined in both the International Classification of Diseases (ICD-10) (World Health Organization, 1993; World Health Organization, 2007) and the DSM-5 guidelines (American Psychiatric Association, 2013). Table 14.1 provides a comparison of these widely-used diagnostic criteria.

### 14.3.1.3 Assessment

Individuals with generalised anxiety disorder may experience a wide range of symptoms, including psychic and somatic manifestations. In a primary care setting, it would be easy to miss or misdiagnose the somatic symptoms of generalised anxiety disorder (e.g. tension headaches, dry mouth and epigastric discomfort as in Jessica's case in Case study 14.2). Differential diagnoses that should be considered include panic disorder, PTSD and social anxiety disorder. To distinguish between these disorders, one should aim to identify the most pervasive presenting symptomatology. For example, if Jessica were to report a history of repeated, unexpected panic attacks with persistent fear of recurrence, a diagnosis of panic disorder would be most likely. By comparison, as her chief complaint seems to be anxiety that is free-floating (ubiquitous) in any or all environments, generalised anxiety disorder should be high on the list of diagnostic considerations (World Health Organization, 1993; World Health Organization, 2007).

In addition, one should always bear in mind the high rate of co-occurrence of generalised anxiety disorder with other anxiety, mood and substance use disorders. In particular, by the time individuals present to a psychiatrist for care, they are very likely also to have co-morbid major depression (Kessler *et al.*, 2008; Kessler *et al.*, 2005; Grant *et al.*, 2005). There are a number

**Case study 14.2**

Jessica, a 40-year-old divorced mother of two presents to her GP with a nine-month history of feeling 'nervous and ill at ease'. She feels that she is not in control of her life, and constantly worries about her financial problems, her job, her children and her inability to 'find a good man'. She is often restless during the day, struggles to concentrate at work and occasionally has tension headaches. In addition, she has noticed exacerbation of a number of physical symptoms – her mouth is often dry and she sometimes has a vague feeling of discomfort in her upper abdomen. Her relationship with her children is being strained by her constant worry, which prompted her to seek medical care.

**Table 14.1** Generalised Anxiety Disorder

<table>
<tr><th>DSM-5 Diagnostic Criteria for Generalized Anxiety Disorder</th><th>ICD-10</th></tr>
<tr><td>A. Excessive anxiety and worry (apprehensive expectation), occurring more days than not for at least 6 months, about a number of events or activities (such as work or school performance).</td><td rowspan="2">The essential feature is anxiety, which is generalised and persistent but not restricted to, or even strongly predominating in, any particular environmental circumstances (i.e. it is free-floating).<br>The individual must have primary symptoms of anxiety most days for at least several weeks at a time, and usually for several months.</td></tr>
<tr><td>B. The individual finds it difficult to control the worry.</td></tr>
<tr><td>C. The anxiety and worry are associated with three (or more) of the following six symptoms (with at least some symptoms having been present for more days than not for the past 6 months):<br>Note: Only one item is required in children.<br>1. Restlessness or feeling keyed up or on edge.<br>2. Being easily fatigued.<br>3. Difficulty concentrating or mind going blank.<br>4. Irritability.<br>5. Muscle tension.<br>6. Sleep disturbance (difficulty falling or staying asleep, or restless, unsatisfying sleep).</td><td>Symptoms should usually involve elements of:<br>a) apprehension (worries about future misfortunes, feeling on edge, difficulty in concentrating, etc. )<br>b) motor tension (restless fidgeting, tension headaches, trembling, inability to relax)<br>c) autonomic over-activity (lightheadedness, sweating, tachycardia or tachypnoea, epigastric discomfort, dizziness, dry mouth, etc. ).<br>In children, frequent need for reassurance and recurrent somatic complaints may be prominent.</td></tr>
<tr><td>D. The anxiety, worry, or physical symptoms cause clinically significant distress or impairment in social, occupational, or other important areas of functioning.</td><td rowspan="3">The transient appearance (for a few days at a time) of other symptoms, particularly depression, does not rule out generalised anxiety disorder as a main diagnosis, but the individual does not meet the full criteria for depressive episode, phobic anxiety disorder, panic disorder or obsessive-compulsive disorder.</td></tr>
<tr><td>E. The disturbance is not attributable to the physiological effects of a substance (e.g., a drug of abuse, a medication) or another medical condition (e.g., hyperthyroidism).</td></tr>
<tr><td>F. The disturbance is not better explained by another mental disorder (e.g., anxiety or worry about having panic attacks in panic disorder, negative evaluation in social anxiety disorder [social phobia], contamination or other obsessions in obsessive-compulsive disorder, separation from attachment figures in separation anxiety disorder, reminders of traumatic events in posttraumatic stress disorder, gaining weight in anorexia nervosa, physical complaints in somatic symptom disorder, perceived appearance flaws in body dysmorphic disorder, having a serious illness in illness anxiety disorder, or the content of delusional beliefs in schizophrenia or delusional disorder).</td></tr>
</table>

**Source:** Reprinted with permission from the *Diagnostic and Statistical Manual of Mental Disorders*, Fifth Edition, (Copyright 2013). American Psychiatric Association; World Health Organization, 1993; World Health Organization 2007

of standardised, reliable and validated tools to assess the severity of generalised anxiety disorder. For example, the Hamilton Anxiety Rating Scale (Hamilton, 1959) – a 14-item screen for both psychic and somatic symptoms of anxiety – may be useful in stratifying individuals into mild, moderate and severe cases, and so informing treatment decisions.

### 14.3.2 Pathogenesis

#### 14.3.2.1 Cognitive-affective factors

Early cognitive-affective paradigms of anxiety hypothesised that dysfunctional cognitive biases are at the root of generalised anxiety disorder and other anxiety disorders (Beck *et al.*, 1985).

More recently, evidence has emerged in support of these early models, showing that individuals with cognitive-affective biases are more likely to misinterpret ambiguous situations as threatening rather than as innocuous, and are thus predisposed to developing generalised anxiety disorder (Tyrer and Baldwin, 2006).

#### 14.3.2.2 Neurobiological factors

Despite the high prevalence of this disorder, there is a paucity of functional brain imaging studies of generalised anxiety disorder. Nonetheless, it has been suggested that dysfunctions in the limbic-medial prefrontal circuits may be implicit in dysfunctional emotional regulation – a hallmark of generalised anxiety disorder (Etkin, 2010; Stein, 2005). Work with children and adolescents also suggests involvement of the ventrolateral prefrontal cortex (VLPFC), amygdala and anterior cingulate cortex (Monk *et al.*, 2006; Monk *et al.*, 2008; McClure *et al.*, 2007).

Abnormalities in the serotonin (5-HT), noradrenaline (NA) and GABA/glutamate molecular systems may be seen in individuals with generalised anxiety disorder. The role of these neurotransmitters is given some credence by the efficacy of common pharmacotherapeutic agents (e.g. selective serotonin reuptake inhibitors (SSRIs), serotonin and noradrenaline reuptake inhibitors (SNRIs) and benzodiazepines) in the treatment of generalised anxiety disorder (Baldwin *et al.*, 2005; Baldwin and Polkinghorn, 2005; Paris, 2006; Bandelow *et al.*, 2008).

#### 14.3.2.3 Genetic predisposition and environmental factors

While there is evidence to suggest a genetic basis to the pathogenesis of generalised anxiety disorder (Hettema *et al.*, 2001), environmental stressors (e.g. childhood abuse) may increase the risk of developing this disorder (see Chapter 15: Acute reactions to adverse life events, and Chapter 16: Trauma). There is also a neuro-evolutionary understanding that generalised anxiety disorder and all other anxiety disorders result from a dysregulation of normal defensive arousal mechanisms (Marks and Nesse, 1994).

### 14.3.3 Treatment

#### 14.3.3.1 Pharmacotherapy

Having taken a comprehensive history from Jessica (see Case study 14.2), performed a physical examination, excluded other biomedical and psychiatric causes of her symptoms and arrived at your definitive diagnosis of generalised anxiety disorder, you must now decide how best to treat her. To aid in this decision, there is a vast array of treatment guidelines, consensus statements and expert recommendations available. Despite the daunting magnitude of this literature, most guidelines agree that SSRIs or SNRIs should be the first choice in the acute setting (Baldwin *et al.*, 2005; Baldwin and Polkinghorn, 2005; Paris, 2006; Bandelow *et al.*, 2008; Nutt, 2005). SSRIs (e.g. escitalopram, paroxetine) and SNRIs (e.g. venlafaxine, duloxetine) have been registered for use in individuals with generalised anxiety disorder. While there have been few head-to-head comparisons of these agents, factors such as tolerability, co-morbidity, stage of life, patient preference and personal or family history of drug response should be taken into consideration (Zetin *et al.*, 2006). These would be helpful to bear in mind in the management of most anxiety disorders. In most cases, one should aim to initiate a low-dose SSRI or SNRI therapy, which can then be increased gradually to the maximum dose tolerated ('start low, go slow').

There are relatively few maintenance studies of SSRIs and SNRIs in the longer-term treatment of generalised anxiety disorder (Baldwin and Polkinghorn, 2005). However, clinical trials have indicated consistently that early discontinuation of these agents is associated with a high risk of relapse. Thus, once an initial improvement in symptoms has been observed, Jessica's treatment should be continued for at least 12 months. Thereafter, treatment can be discontinued gradually (Baldwin *et al.*, 2005; Baldwin and Polkinghorn, 2005; Paris, 2006; Bandelow *et al.*, 2008).

However, it may be that Jessica does not respond adequately to her initial SSRI/SNRI prescription. In this case, the first step should be a re-assessment to ensure that her diagnosis is correct. A next step would be to ensure that a drug trial of sufficient duration (at least 12 weeks) and dosage have been undertaken. Should her resistance to SSRI or SNRI therapy persist, switching to a different agent or augmentation therapy may be considered (Baldwin *et al.*, 2005; Bandelow *et al.*, 2008). While the literature on augmentation strategies in refractory generalised anxiety disorder is limited, these may include the addition of an atypical antipsychotic (Pollack *et al.*, 2009) or buspirone (Tyrer and Baldwin, 2006). However, due to the unfavourable side effect profile and potential drug-drug interactions of these agents, referral for more specialised psychiatric care may be warranted.

#### 14.3.3.2 Psychotherapy

Cognitive behavioural therapy (CBT) is generally considered as first-line psychotherapy for individuals with generalised anxiety disorder (Baldwin *et al.*, 2005; Paris, 2006; Bandelow *et al.*, 2008; Ballenger *et al.*, 2001). While research has not as yet demonstrated an added benefit of combined pharmacotherapeutic and psychotherapeutic interventions, it may be useful to use techniques such as cognitive restructuring, exposure therapy and controlled relaxation (Tyrer and Baldwin, 2001) to ensure a longer-term effect after initial drug treatment.

## 14.4 Panic disorder

Recently, however, Fatima has experienced a recurrence and increase in the severity of her 'asthma attacks', with the additional symptoms of stabbing chest pain and dizziness. During the most recent episode that occurred at home, she also noted a brief 'out-of-body' experience, just prior to feeling as if she would suffocate and die. Despite the severity of these symptoms, they began to diminish spontaneously after about 10 minutes, and had resolved completely within 20 minutes. Fatima and her mother are deeply concerned about these attacks. Fatima feels that she is losing control of her life and claims to live in constant fear of recurrent episodes. She has significantly restricted her social activities and exercise regimen, as she is uncertain when her next attack will occur.

### 14.4.1 Phenomenology

#### 14.4.1.1 Epidemiology

Panic disorder (PD) is a common psychiatric condition, with a population prevalence of about 1-5% (Kessler *et al.*, 2005; Herman *et al.*, 2009; Roy-Byrne *et al.*, 2005). Females are more likely to be afflicted than males (Kessler *et al.*, 1994). The peak period of onset is early adulthood. Panic disorder usually follows a chronic relapsing and remitting course. Notably, panic disorder is highly co-morbid with disorders such as major depression (Kessler *et al.*, 1997; Roy-Byrne *et al.*, 2000) and substance-use disorders (Cox *et al.*, 1990; Crowley, 1992). As these co-morbidities significantly affect the course of illness and choice of treatment in panic disorder, it is essential to perform a comprehensive assessment on these individuals.

#### 14.4.1.2 Clinical signs and symptoms

As in Fatima's case (see Case study 14.3) the essential clinical feature of panic disorder is the occurrence of repeated panic attacks – sudden, recurrent and unexpected episodes that reach maximal intensity after one to two minutes and usually last for 10 to 20 minutes (World Health

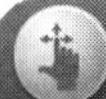

**Case study 14.3**

Fatima, a 20-year-old university student, presents to her general practitioner with her mother after having experienced her fourth 'asthma attack' in the past month. Since being diagnosed with mild asthma and allergic rhinitis in childhood, Fatima has been hospitalised only once, for nebulisation, when she was 7 years old. Her symptoms improved substantially during adolescence, and she has not needed to use her inhaler since the age of 15.

Organization, 1993; World Health Organization, 2007). Although variable, the physical symptoms of a panic attack include dyspnoea, dizziness, palpitations, chest pain, choking sensations, nausea, sweating and paraesthesia of the fingers and lips. **Psychological symptoms** include depersonalisation, derealisation and fear of dying, losing control or going mad (World Health Organization, 1993; World Health Organization, 2007). It has been suggested that the heterogeneous clinical presentation of panic disorder may warrant its distinction into subtypes (e.g. respiratory, nocturnal, non-fearful, cognitive, vestibular) (Kircanski *et al.*, 2009).

These attacks are not restricted to specific situations or circumstances (World Health Organization, 2007). Panic attacks may be situationally bound (occurring exclusively in particular situations) or situationally predisposed (more likely to occur in particular situations) (Nutt and Ballenger, 2005; American Psychiatric Association, 1994). Importantly, while these cued panic attacks may be a feature of other anxiety disorders (e.g. PTSD, social phobia), mood disorders (e.g. depression) or schizophrenia (Nutt and Ballenger, 2005), it is the un-cued (spontaneous) panic attack that is the hallmark of panic disorder. Conventionally, a panic attack that occurs in a particular phobic situation is categorised as an expression of that phobia.

Table 14.2 provides a comparison of the definitive diagnostic criteria for this disorder, as outlined in the DSM-5 (American Psychiatric Association, 2013) and the ICD-10 (World Health Organization, 1993; World Health Organization, 2007).

### 14.4.1.3 Assessment

Cases such as Fatima's are not uncommon. At a primary health care level, it is not uncommon to encounter individuals with panic disorder presenting with somatic manifestations of their disorder (and who, like Fatima and her mother, may incorrectly attribute their symptoms to a biomedical condition). The association between obstructive respiratory illnesses (e.g. asthma, chronic obstructive pulmonary disease) and panic disorder is particularly interesting, and is often discussed with reference to Klein's theory of 'false suffocation alarm' (Klein, 1993). Persons with panic disorder are hypothesised to be hypersensitive to arterial carbon dioxide ($CO_2$) due to hyperactivity of the locus coeruleus. Subtle increases in $CO_2$ levels are thus misperceived as asphyxia, and compensatory hyperventilation occurs. Therefore, individuals with pre-existing asthma or chronic obstructive pulmonary disease are at increased risk of developing panic disorder due to intermittent hypercapnia (Zandbergen *et al.*, 1991; Nutt and Ballenger, 2005; Yellowlees *et al.*, 1987; Shavitt *et al.*, 1992).

Once the diagnosis of panic disorder has been made, the frequency, timing and severity of the panic attacks should be elicited, as well as their concordance with certain settings. Also, the presence of sequelae (e.g. anticipatory anxiety and functional impairment) should be assessed (Wilson, 2007). Individuals who suffer from recurrent panic attacks will soon grow concerned about the occurrence and consequences of future attacks (Nutt and Ballenger, 2005). As this concern intensifies, anticipatory anxiety may develop. Unfortunately, this pervasive worry may then lead to extreme **avoidance** behaviour or agoraphobia, with individuals avoiding specific situations from which, they believe, escape would be difficult or embarrassing (World Health Organization, 2007; Nutt and Ballenger, 2005). Ultimately, such agoraphobia may lead to individuals becoming housebound in an effort to avoid all potential triggers of future panic attacks. Fatima has already begun to exhibit avoidance behaviour, so it would be essential to diagnose and manage her anxiety disorder timeously.

Panic disorder also tends to co-occur with other psychiatric disorders, in particular major depressive disorder (MDD). Overall, individuals with co-morbid panic disorder and major depressive disorder tend to have more severe symptomatology, poorer prognosis, poorer response to treatment, increased health service utilisation and greater long-term functional impairment and disability (Nutt and Ballenger, 2005; Brown *et al.*, 1996; Kessler *et al.*, 1994; Roy-Byrne *et al.*, 2000). One should also screen for

**Table 14.2** Panic Disorder

| DSM-5 Diagnostic Criteria for Panic Disorder | ICD-10 |
|---|---|
| A. Recurrent unexpected panic attacks. A panic attack is an abrupt surge of intense fear or intense discomfort that reaches a peak within minutes, and during which time four (or more) of the following symptoms occur;<br>**Note:** The abrupt surge can occur from a calm state or an anxious state.<br>1. Palpitations, pounding heart, or accelerated heart rate.<br>2. Sweating.<br>3. Trembling or shaking.<br>4. Sensations of shortness of breath or smothering.<br>5. Feelings of choking.<br>6. Chest pain or discomfort.<br>7. Nausea or abdominal distress.<br>8. Feeling dizzy, unsteady, light-headed, or faint.<br>9. Chills or heat sensations.<br>10. Paresthesias (numbness or tingling sensations).<br>11. Derealization (feelings of unreality) or depersonalization (being detached from oneself).<br>12. Fear of losing control or 'going crazy.'<br>13. Fear of dying.<br>**Note:** Culture-specific symptoms (e.g., tinnitus, neck soreness, headache, uncontrollable screaming or crying) may be seen. Such symptoms should not count as one of the four required symptoms. | For a definite diagnosis, several severe attacks of autonomic anxiety should have occurred within a period of about one month:<br>▶ in circumstances where there is no objective danger<br>▶ without being confined to known or predictable situations<br>▶ with comparative freedom from anxiety symptoms between attacks (although anticipatory anxiety is common). |
| B. At least one of the attacks has been followed by 1 month (or more) of one or both of the following:<br>1. Persistent concern or worry about additional panic attacks or their consequences (e.g., losing control, having a heart attack, 'going crazy').<br>2. A significant maladaptive change in behavior related to the attacks (e.g., behaviours designed to avoid having panic attacks, such as avoidance of exercise or unfamiliar situations). | |
| C. The disturbance is not attributable to the physiological effects of a substance (e.g., a drug of abuse, a medication) or another medical condition (e.g., hyperthyroidism, cardiopulmonary disorders). | |
| D. The disturbance is not better explained by another mental disorder (e.g., the panic attacks do not occur only in response to feared social situations, as in social anxiety disorder; in response to circumscribed phobic objects or situations, as in specific phobia; in response to obsessions, as in obsessive-compulsive disorder; in response to reminders of traumatic events, as in posttraumatic stress disorder; or in response to separation from attachment figures, as in separation anxiety disorder). | A panic attack that occurs in an established phobic situation is regarded as an expression of the severity of the phobia, which should be given diagnostic precedence. Panic disorder should be the main diagnosis only in the absence of any specific phobia. |

**Source:** Reprinted with permission from the *Diagnostic and Statistical Manual of Mental Disorders*, Fifth Edition, (Copyright 2013). American Psychiatric Association; World Health Organization, 1993; World Health Organization 2007

the misuse of cannabis and/or **sympathomimetic** drugs (e.g. cocaine, methamphetamines, caffeine), alcohol dependence and withdrawal from benzodiazepines (Wilson, 2007; Cox *et al.*, 1990; Crowley, 1992; Brown *et al.*, 1996).

## 14.4.2 Pathogenesis

### 14.4.2.1 Cognitive-affective factors

Work with animal models suggests that phobic avoidance associated with panic disorder may be due, in part, to dysfunctional contextual **conditioning** (Gorman *et al.*, 2000; Phillips and LeDoux, 1992). In these experiments, animal subjects demonstrated the same behavioural and autonomic responses to artificial fear-conditioning as they had to the actual fear-stimuli themselves. Gorman and colleagues (2000) suggest that this analogy may be applied to persons with panic disorder. Individuals, such as Fatima, experience anticipatory anxiety and exhibit avoidance behaviour in the same setting in which panic attacks had previously occurred. These authors hypothesise that dysfunctional contextual fear-conditioning may account for the hypersensitivity to minor physical discomfort that individuals with panic disorder exhibit. Thus, somatic sensation functions as a fear context, which may induce panic over time.

### 14.4.2.2 Neurobiological factors

The major components of panic disorder (i.e. the acute panic attack, anticipatory anxiety, maladaptive avoidance behaviour) are thought to be reflected in specific neuro-anatomical alterations in the brainstem, amygdala and PFC. In the normal circuit of fear conditioning, the amygdala receives cortical sensory input via the anterior thalamus and disseminates this information by way of innervations to a number of efferent brain structures. These targets include:

- brainstem nuclei, for example, the parabrachial nucleus (which increases respiratory rate) and the locus coeruleus (LC) (which increases noradrenaline release)
- the hypothalamus, which causes an increase in corticosteroid secretion and autonomic sympathetic activity
- the peri-aqueductal grey matter, which is involved in motor-defensive behaviour and postural freezing (Gorman *et al.*, 2000).

However, in persons with panic disorder there seems to be dysfunctional activation of the amygdala, possibly due to in-coordinate upstream (cortical) and downstream (brainstem) sensory information (Gorman *et al.*, 2000). There is thus inadequate control of the efferent targets of the fear circuit, leading to paroxysmal activation of central and peripheral organs. This cascade of events ultimately manifests as a panic attack.

There is also evidence suggesting that, while the amygdala is responsible for the so-called positive symptoms of anxiety (e.g. autonomic hyperarousal), it is the hippocampus that accounts for the negative symptoms of avoidance (Stein, 2006). The hippocampus paralimbic circuit is affected by amygdala hyperactivation, thus contributing to the agoraphobic tendencies that may follow panic attacks. Animal models show that stimulation of the LC provokes symptoms of anxiety, which mimic those of a panic attack (Redmond and Haung, 1979).

From an evolutionary perspective, it is hypothesized that panic disorder represents a false alarm (Klein, 1993). Individuals with panic disorder may have a lowered threshold for detecting cerebral hypoxia (false suffocation alarm). Thus, with increasing levels of $PCO_2$ and brain lactate, there is a physical adaptation that leads to the symptom of dyspnoea. This dyspnoea develops to compensate for worsening hypercapnia.

Within these neuro-anatomical and neuro-physiological circuits, key molecular systems include serotonin and noradrenaline, as well as various neuropeptides. For example, recent neuro-imaging studies have found reduced 5-HT receptor binding in persons with panic disorder versus normal controls (Neumeister *et al.*, 2004; Nash *et al.*, 2008), thus supporting the theory that abnormal 5-HT functioning plays a significant role in the neurobiological pathogenesis of panic disorder. In addition, abnormalities in the β- and α2-adrenergic systems (Charney and Heninger, 1986; Charney *et al.*, 1987; Nutt and Ballenger, 2005) and neuropeptidergic (e.g. cholecystokinin) systems (Kennedy *et al.*, 1999; Lydiard *et al.*, 1992; Rehfeld, 2000) may play a role in PD.

#### 14.4.2.3 Genetic predisposition and environmental factors

Panic disorder appears to be partly heritable, with risk ratios for first-degree relatives of individuals with this disorder ranging from 3,4% to 14% (Nutt and Ballenger, 2005). However, while PD is no doubt highly familial, the data that support a genetic predisposition are less definitive. Although twin studies have found a higher concordance of panic disorder between monozygotic and **dizygotic twins**, this concordance is far lower than 50% (Togersen, 1983; Gorman *et al.*, 2000). Thus, although monozygotic twins are more likely to have panic disorder than their dizygotic counterparts, there are many cases (i.e. >50%) in which only one identical twin has panic disorder (Gorman *et al.*, 2000). It is thus likely that individuals inherit a certain vulnerability to fearfulness and anxiety, rather than to panic disorder itself. While this susceptibility may be mediated by a hypersensitive fear circuit (involving the central nucleus of the amygdala), environmental factors also play a role. For example, individuals exposed to childhood adversity such as abuse or disrupted emotional attachments from primary caregivers may go on to develop panic disorder later in life (Gorman *et al.*, 2000; Pine *et al.*, 1998).

### 14.4.3 Treatment

#### 14.4.3.1 Pharmacotherapy

Initially, antidepressant treatment of panic disorder comprised the tricyclic antidepressant (TCA), imipramine and the monoamine oxidase inhibitor (MAOI), phenelzine (Nutt and Ballenger, 2005). While both agents were shown to be effective in providing symptomatic relief (Sheehan *et al.*, 1980), most guidelines currently recommend SSRIs seeing that they have shown equal efficacy in treating panic disorder and a better side-effect profile than earlier classes of antidepressants (Baldwin *et al.*, 2005; Paris, 2006). These agents may inhibit amygdala hyperactivity (thus modulating the conditioned fear network) and have a secondary effect of decreasing noradrenergic action (Gorman *et al.*, 2000). This relieves the cardiovascular symptoms of a panic attack, including tachycardia and palpitations. SSRIs currently registered for use in panic disorder include fluoxetine, paroxetine and sertraline. In Fatima's case, she should be started on a SSRI treatment at a low dose (e.g. fluoxetine 5 mg or 10 mg), which may then be titrated slowly upwards to avoid adverse effects such as agitation. A trial period of six to eight weeks should also be undertaken to achieve optimal effect. Thereafter, her medication should be tapered slowly, as abrupt discontinuation may be associated with rebound anxiety, relapse or a discontinuation syndrome.

A benzodiazepine (e.g. alprazolam, clonazepam) may also be co-prescribed for the first two weeks of treatment (Kasper and Resinger, 2001; Paris, 2006). Once Fatima's symptoms are adequately controlled, this benzodiazepine should be discontinued slowly (while the antidepressant therapy is continued).

Once Fatima has showed an initial response to SSRI treatment, maintenance therapy should be continued for a prolonged period of time (Paris, 2006; Rickels and Schweizer, 1998). In a number of long-term follow-up studies, fluoxetine (Tiller *et al.*, 1999), paroxetine (Lecrubier and Judge, 1997) and sertraline (Lepola *et al.*, 2003) have shown ongoing benefits over 6–12 months of treatment.

Should Fatima not respond adequately to first-line SSRI treatment, there is only limited evidence in support of increasing dosage (Baldwin *et al.*, 2005). Switching between agents may be helpful (National Institute for Clinical Excellence (NICE), 2004). That being said, a switch strategy should only be considered once initial drug dosage has been optimised, adherence to treatment has been established and a thorough assessment for co-morbid biomedical or psychiatric disorders has been performed (Paris, 2006). Second-line choices in this case may then include a different SSRI or SNRI, a TCA (clomipramine, imipramine) or a benzodiazepine (alprazolam, clonazepam, lorazepam, diazepam) (Paris, 2006). However, due to their unfavourable side-effect profile and potential for drug interactions, initiation of these second-line agents warrants referral to more specialised psychiatric care.

#### 14.4.3.2 Psychotherapy

Fatima may also benefit from CBT. This form of psychotherapy may be useful in combating the false alarm underlying her panic disorder (Gorman *et al.*, 2000; Roy-Byrne *et al.*, 2005; Landon and Barlow, 2004). Interventions include relaxation therapy (muscle and breathing exercises) and **desensitisation** (i.e. gradual, graded exposure to feared situations until tolerance develops (Wilson, 2007). There is controversy surrounding the routine use of combined pharmacotherapy and psychotherapy for individuals with panic disorder (Paris, 2006; Baldwin *et al.*, 2005), with most reviews of efficacy yielding mixed results (Van Balkom *et al.*, 1997; Clum and Surls, 1993; Mitte, 2005; Barlow *et al.*, 2000; Marks *et al.*, 1993). However, incorporating CBT into the treatment plan at the time of discontinuation of pharmacotherapy may lower Fatima's rate of relapse in the long-term (Otto and Deveney, 2005; Schmidt *et al.*, 2002).

## 14.5 Social anxiety disorder

### 14.5.1 Phenomenology

#### 14.5.1.1 Epidemiology

Social anxiety disorder (SAD, social phobia) is the second-most common anxiety disorder after the specific phobias. The lifetime prevalence of this disorder is estimated to be 12,1% (range 2,5 to 16%), with a 12-month prevalence of approximately 7,1% (Ruscio *et al.*, 2008; Kessler *et al.*, 2005; Herman *et al.*, 2009). Although men have been found to present more commonly for treatment than women, lifetime prevalence rates show a female preponderance (Weinstock, 1999). Symptoms usually appear early in life, during adolescence or childhood (Chavira *et al.*, 2004; Chavira and Stein, 2005) and may then persist throughout adulthood.

#### 14.5.1.2 Clinical signs and symptoms

Individuals with social anxiety disorder exhibit excessive fear and anxiety of social situations, often leading to avoidance of interpersonal contact. The range of settings that may evoke symptoms is vast. In fact, most affected individuals fear a number of social situations, with public speaking often identified as the most feared (Nutt and Ballenger, 2005; Faravelli *et al.*, 2000; Holt *et al.*, 1992; Turner *et al.*, 1992).

Should Vuyo be forced to interact with others (e.g. during a class presentation or group work

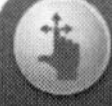

**Case study 14.4**

Vuyo is an 18-year-old first-year university student whose mother brings him to see her general practitioner. She mentions that Vuyo has always been shy, choosing to spend most of his free time alone. However, since starting university earlier the year, she has noticed that Vuyo has become increasingly withdrawn and makes every effort to avoid interacting with his peers outside of lectures. She is particularly worried, as she fears that Vuyo's disinterest is a symptom of depression. Upon further questioning, Vuyo denies feeling depressed, but admits that he feels that his classmates are constantly judging him in terms of his appearance, speech and mannerisms. He avoids conversation with his peers and lecturers whenever possible, as he fears that he will embarrass himself. Sometimes he feels that his concerns may be unwarranted, but is unsure how to cope with them.

assignment), he may well experience an array of intense physical or psychological symptoms. Somatic fear responses may include blushing, tachycardia, sweating or difficulty concentrating, while behavioural symptoms are usually dominated by patterns of social avoidance (Stein and Stein, 2008; Nutt and Ballenger, 2005; Amies *et al.*, 1983; Solyom *et al.*, 1986). Table 14.3 provides the full diagnostic criteria for this disorder, as outlined in the DSM-5 and the ICD-10.

### 14.5.1.3 Assessment

When assessing an individual like Vuyo, it is important to consider a wide range of differential diagnoses. A thorough history-taking, clinical examination and full psychiatric assessment should be completed in order to exclude other psychiatric conditions such as panic disorder, major depression, bipolar mood disorder, schizophrenia, personality disorders (schizoid and avoidant subtypes) as well as other medical

**Table 14.3** Social Anxiety Disorder (Social Phobia)

| DSM-5 Diagnostic Criteria for Social Anxiety Disorder (Social Phobia) | ICD-10 |
|---|---|
| A. Marked fear or anxiety about one or more social situations in which the individual is exposed to possible scrutiny by others. Examples include social interactions (e.g., having a conversation, meeting unfamiliar people), being observed (e.g., eating or drinking), and performing in front of others (e.g., giving a speech).<br>**Note:** In children, the anxiety must occur in peer settings and not just during interactions with adults. | All of the following criteria should be fulfilled for a definite diagnosis:<br>▶ the psychological, behavioural or autonomic symptoms must be primarily manifestations of anxiety and not secondary to other symptoms such as delusions or obsessional thoughts<br>▶ the anxiety must be restricted to or predominate in particular social situations<br>▶ the phobic situation is avoided whenever possible. |
| B. The individual fears that he or she will act in a way or show anxiety symptoms that will be negatively evaluated (i.e., will be humiliating or embarrassing: will lead to rejection or offend others). | |
| C. The social situations almost always provoke fear or anxiety.<br>**Note:** In children, the fear or anxiety may be expressed by crying, tantrums, freezing, clinging, shrinking, or failing to speak in social situations. | |
| D. The social situations are avoided or endured with intense fear or anxiety. | |
| E. The fear or anxiety is out of proportion to the actual threat posed by the social situation and to the sociocultural context. | |
| F. The fear, anxiety, or avoidance is persistent, typically lasting for 6 months or more. | |
| G. The fear, anxiety, or avoidance causes clinically significant distress or impairment in social, occupational, or other important areas of functioning. | |
| H. The fear, anxiety, or avoidance is not attributable to the physiological effects of a substance (e.g., a drug of abuse, a medication) or another medical condition. | |
| I. The fear, anxiety, or avoidance is not better explained by the symptoms of another mental disorder, such as panic disorder, body dysmorphic disorder, or autism spectrum disorder. | |
| J. If another medical condition (e.g., Parkinson's disease, obesity, disfigurement from burns or injury) is present, the fear, anxiety, or avoidance is clearly unrelated or is excessive.<br>*Specify* if:<br>**Performance only:** If the fear is restricted to speaking or performing in public. | |

**Source:** Reprinted with permission from the *Diagnostic and Statistical Manual of Mental Disorders*, Fifth Edition, (Copyright 2013). American Psychiatric Association; World Health Organization, 1993; World Health Organization 2007

disorders such as Parkinson's disease or stuttering (Nutt and Ballenger, 2005; Pallanti *et al.*, 2004; Simon *et al.*, 2004; Grant *et al.*, 2005; Schneier *et al.*, 2001; Stein *et al.*, 1996).

In particular, the overlap of social anxiety disorder and panic disorder should be borne in mind. In both disorders, avoidance is a common feature. In addition, a panic attack may occur in an individual with social anxiety disorder who is forced to confront his or her feared situation (Nutt and Ballenger, 2005; Seedat and Stein, 2007). However, these disorders may be distinguished by assessing the nature of the feared stimulus and outcomes, and the clinical symptomatology experienced during the panic attack (Page, 1994; Nutt and Ballenger, 2005). Persons with social anxiety disorder are more likely to fear humiliation and embarrassment as a result of social interaction (as compared to the fear of unexpected, recurrent panic attacks in panic disorder). The panic attacks of social anxiety disorder are more commonly associated with physical manifestations such as blushing, muscle twitching and stammering, as opposed to the dizziness, choking sensations and foreboding of a sense of dying often experienced during a panic attack of panic disorder (Nutt and Ballenger, 2005; Page, 1994; Amies *et al.*, 1983; Solyom *et al.*, 1986; Reich *et al.*, 1988). However, it may be that an individual suffers from both disorders concomitantly. In these cases, the onset of social anxiety disorder is likely to precede that of panic disorder by several years (Nutt and Ballenger, 2005; Moutier and Stein, 1999; Mannuzza *et al.*, 1990).

Most individuals with social anxiety disorder are likely to suffer from at least one co-morbid psychiatric disorder (Nutt and Ballenger, 2005; Magee *et al.*, 1996). Therefore, a high index of suspicion should be maintained while screening for other anxiety disorders (e.g. agoraphobia and specific phobias), mood disorders (e.g. major depression, bipolar mood disorder) and substance use disorders (Magee *et al.*, 1996; Kessler *et al.*, 1999; Regier *et al.*, 1998).

A number of assessment tools may be useful as diagnostic instruments and as measures of symptom severity. These include the Social Phobia Inventory (SPIN) – which may also be used for screening purposes – and its abridged version, the Mini-SPIN (Connor *et al.*, 2000; Connor *et al.*, 2001). Both questionnaires may be self-administered and have shown good sensitivity and specificity. The SPIN consists of 17 items focusing on symptoms such as embarrassment, avoidance and physical manifestations (e.g. sweating, palpitations). Each question may be answered on a rating scale from 0 (no symptoms) to 4 (severe symptoms). A score of 19 or more is highly suggestive of diagnostic status. The Mini-SPIN comprises just three questions focusing on avoidance and fear of embarrassment in the past week. Each item is scored in the same way as in the full SPIN.

## 14.5.2 Pathogenesis

### 14.5.2.1 Cognitive-affective factors

Dysfunctional cognitive-affective processes seem to play a role in the pathogenesis of social anxiety disorder. Affected individuals appear to misperceive social settings: they exaggerate their low status and overestimate external social threats (Stein and Bouwer, 1997; Stein 2006). This can be conceptualised as a display of false appeasement, indicating submission to the more dominant in society (Stein and Bouwer, 1997).

### 14.5.2.2 Neurobiological factors

Neuro-anatomical alterations may also play a role in the aetiology of this disorder. A number of structural and functional brain imaging studies have shown involvement of the amygdala-hippocampal (limbic) pathway (which contributes to memory processing and to acquiring and expressing conditioned fear responses) and of the cortico-striatal circuitry (which mediates cognition and affect) (Etkin and Wager, 2007; Phan *et al.*, 2006; Rapee and Spence, 2004; Nutt and Ballenger, 2005). Overall, these studies have shown a selective increase in amygdala action in persons with social anxiety disorder when exposed to feared stimuli. In addition, dysfunctions within the frontal and inferior cortices (including grey matter abnormalities) have been demonstrated (Syal *et al.*, 2012; Tupler *et al.*, 1997; Nutt *et al.*, 1998; MacDonald *et al.*, 2000).

Functional defects within the major neurotransmitter systems may also play a role (Nutt and Ballenger, 2005; Stein *et al.*, 2002). First, increased levels of serotonin have been demonstrated in dominant animal models, with a reduction in serotonergic function in socially inhibited primates (Raleigh *et al.*, 1991). Second, individuals with social anxiety disorder have shown evidence of dopaminergic dysfunction, (i.e. lower rates of striatal D2 receptor binding, decreased densities of striatal dopamine reuptake sites and mild atrophy of basal ganglia (Tiihonen *et al.*, 1997; Schneier *et al.*, 2001).

#### 14.5.2.3 Genetic predisposition and environmental factors

There seems to be an element of partial heritability in the pathogenesis of social anxiety disorder – the prevalence rate is higher in first-degree relatives of affected individuals than in the general population (Stein *et al.*, 1998; Stein *et al.*, 2002). Although evidence is inconclusive, there may be a genetic basis to this heritability, with particular involvement of chromosome 16 (Gelernter *et al.*, 2004). Susceptible genes may transmit an underlying heritable trait (e.g. behavioural inhibition) (Hirshfeld-Becker *et al.*, 2007). Learning and environmental conditioning may also contribute to the development of social anxiety disorder. For example, behavioural inhibition in childhood or prior traumatic events may predispose to social anxiety disorder later in life (Chavira and Stein, 2005).

### 14.5.3 Treatment

#### 14.5.3.1 Pharmacotherapy

As is the case in many of the anxiety disorders, SSRIs should be the first-line pharmacotherapy for persons with social anxiety disorder (Paris, 2006; Baldwin *et al.*, 2005; Ganasen and Stein, 2010; Stein *et al.*, 2010). Citalopram, escitalopram, fluoxetine and sertraline are all suitable choices (Lader *et al.*, 2004; Kobak *et al.*, 2002). The SNRI venlafaxine has also been shown to be effective (Rickels *et al.*, 2004). Once an initial improvement in symptomatology has been observed, treatment should be continued for at least twelve months at the dose at which a response was observed, in order to minimise the chance of relapse (Van Ameringen *et al.*, 2003; Paris, 2006). Thereafter, treatment should be tapered gradually (Stein *et al.*, 2010).

While MAOIs may also be effective (Liebowitz *et al.*, 1992), these pose a number of clinical problems. The older, irreversible agents have severe dietary restrictions and a range of potential adverse events while the newer reversible agents such as moclobemide (which do not have the disadvantages of the classical agents) have not proved consistently efficacious (Stein *et al.*, 2004; Stein *et al.*, 2010).

If, after initial SSRI or SNRI therapy, symptoms do not show an adequate improvement, there is a range of other pharmacotherapeutic options. While there is no clear evidence for dose escalation (Baldwin *et al.*, 2005), switching to a different SSRI or SNRI may prove helpful. While augmentation strategies analogous to those used in major depression have been investigated, there is very little supporting literature. Nonetheless, augmentation with a benzodiazepine, mirtazapine (another class of antidepressant), certain anticonvulsants (e.g. gabapentin), a MAOI (e.g. phenelzine) or a second-generation (atypical) antipsychotic agent in the case of partial or non-response to initial therapy may be considered (Stein *et al.*, 2010; Seedat and Stein, 2004; Muehlbacher *et al.*, 2005; Pande *et al.*, 1999). However, due to a problematic side-effect profile and potential for drug-drug interactions of many of these second-line agents, referral to more specialised psychiatric care may be warranted.

#### 14.5.3.2 Psychotherapy

Vuyo may benefit from CBT (Stein *et al.*, 2010; Blanco *et al.*, 2010). Performed in individual or group settings, this form of psychotherapy would expose him to situations that induce anxiety (either imaginal or in-vivo), such as public speaking, thereby desensitising him and reducing avoidance behaviour (Stein, 2006). Techniques include progressive muscle relaxation, social skills training, systematic desensitisation and cognitive restructuring to address and alter misperceptions about social embarrassment (Fedoroff and Taylor 2001; Huppert *et al.*, 2003; Schneier, 1991). Ultimately, CBT should facilitate improvement in symptoms and discontinuation of medication (Stein *et al.*, 2010; Singh and Hope, 2009).

## 14.6 Specific phobias

### 14.6.1 Phenomenology

#### 14.6.1.1 Epidemiology

Specific phobias (also known as simple or isolated phobias) are the most prevalent of the anxiety disorders, with a population prevalence of about 7-9% (Kessler *et al.*, 2005; Baldwin *et al.*, 2005). Age of onset is early, with symptoms often arising in childhood or adolescence and persisting into adulthood. If left undiagnosed and untreated, phobic fear and avoidance patterns can continue for decades and result in significant functional impairment (World Health Organization, 2007).

#### 14.6.1.2 Clinical signs and symptoms

When confronted with a phobic trigger, individuals with a specific phobia will experience an immediate anxiety response that may manifest as a situationally-bound panic attack (American Psychiatric Association, 2013). Table 14.4 provides an outline of the diagnostic criteria for this group of anxiety disorders. As mentioned earlier, the panic attack of panic disorder can be distinguished from that of social anxiety disorder or simple phobias by the type of trigger and the symptoms experienced (Page, 1994; Nutt and Ballenger, 2005). If the clinical presentation of two of our case studies (Thatho and Fatima) is compared, this distinction is clear. In general, the fear and avoidance response of individuals with specific phobia(s) does not fluctuate over time (World Health Organization, 2007). Thus, unless managed correctly, it is unlikely that Thatho will be able to receive her Gardasil® vaccine without experiencing significant anxiety and/or distress.

#### 14.6.1.3 Assessment

Specific fears are very common in the general population. However, the majority of these fears will not meet the diagnostic criteria for a simple phobia (Kessler *et al.*, 2005). Thus, when encountering a fearful individual, it is important to differentiate between subthreshold symptoms and a diagnosable (and treatable) anxiety disorder. In general, a person with a specific phobia will experience increasing and multi-dimensional functional impairment. However, he or she may be reluctant to seek treatment (often owing to phobias concerning blood, injection, injury or other medical procedures). Thus, it may be that individuals with specific phobias only present for health care when new occupational or household responsibilities override their routine coping mechanisms (Baldwin *et al.*, 2005).

A number of self-report tools may be of use to assess the presence and/or severity of a specific phobia. The Fear Questionnaire (Marks and Matthews, 1979) is a one-page, reliable

**Case study 14.5**

Thatho is a 21-year-old personal assistant who has always hated visiting the doctor. In particular, she dreads receiving injections. However, having recently been told of the merits of the recombinant human papillomavirus (HPV) vaccine (types 6, 11, 18) (Gardasil® vaccine) by her general practitioner, she has now agreed to receive it. Upon arriving at his office on the day of her appointment, she begins to feel flushed and sweaty. She then starts trembling uncontrollably, feeling that her heart is racing. She is overcome with dizziness, and feels that she might faint. She is helped to a seat by a nurse. After about 15 minutes, her symptoms have resolved and she prepares to leave the doctor's office. She declines his offer to reschedule her appointment, stating that she will need more time to think about it.

and validated inventory designed to monitor symptom change in phobic individuals. A total phobia score is obtained by summing sub-scores for social phobia, blood-injury phobia and agoraphobia. A number of more specific questionnaires have also been developed to assess individuals with particular phobic fears, such as the Acrophobia Questionnaire (AQ) (Cohen, 1977).

When assessing these individuals the high risk of co-morbidity – in particular major depression, substance use disorders and other anxiety disorders – should be borne in mind (Vythilingum and Stein, 2004). Thus, the clinical evaluation should be comprehensive and include both biomedical and psychiatric components.

**Table 14.4** Specific Phobia

<table>
<tr><th>DSM-5 Diagnostic Criteria for Specific Phobia</th><th>ICD-10</th></tr>
<tr><td>A. Marked fear or anxiety about a specific object or situation (e.g., flying, heights, animals, receiving an injection, seeing blood).<br>Note: In children, the fear or anxiety may be expressed by crying, tantrums, freezing, or clinging.</td><td rowspan="7">All of the following should be fulfilled for a definite diagnosis:<br>▶ the psychological or autonomic symptoms must be primary manifestations of anxiety, and not secondary to other symptoms such as delusion or obsessional thought<br>▶ the anxiety must be restricted to the presence of the particular phobic object or situation<br>▶ the phobic situation is avoided whenever possible.<br>Includes:<br>▶ acrophobia (fear of heights)<br>▶ animal phobias<br>▶ claustrophobia<br>▶ examination phobia<br>▶ simple phobia.</td></tr>
<tr><td>B. The phobic object or situation almost always provokes immediate fear or anxiety.</td></tr>
<tr><td>C. The phobic object or situation is actively avoided or endured with intense fear or anxiety.</td></tr>
<tr><td>D. The fear or anxiety is out of proportion to the actual danger posed by the specific object or situation and to the sociocultural context.</td></tr>
<tr><td>E. The fear, anxiety, or avoidance is persistent, typically lasting for 6 months or more.</td></tr>
<tr><td>F. The fear, anxiety, or avoidance causes clinically significant distress or impairment in social, occupational, or other important areas of functioning.</td></tr>
<tr><td>G. The disturbance is not better explained by the symptoms of another mental disorder, including fear, anxiety, and avoidance of situations associated with panic-like symptoms or other incapacitating symptoms (as in agoraphobia): objects or situations related to obsessions (as in obsessive-compulsive disorder); reminders of traumatic events (as in posttraumatic stress disorder); separation from home or attachment figures (as in separation anxiety disorder); or social situations (as in social anxiety disorder).<br>Specify if:<br>Code based on the phobic stimulus:<br>▶ 300.29 (F40.218) Animal (e.g., spiders, insects, dogs).<br>▶ 300.29 (F40.228) Natural environment (e.g., heights, storms, water).<br>▶ 300.29 (F40.23X) Blood-injection-injury (e.g., needles, invasive medical procedures).<br>▶ 300.29 (F40.248) Situational (e.g., airplanes, elevators, enclosed places).<br>▶ 300.29 (F40.298) Other (e.g., situations that may lead to choking or vomiting; in children, e.g., loud sounds or costumed characters).</td></tr>
</table>

**Source:** Reprinted with permission from the *Diagnostic and Statistical Manual of Mental Disorders*, Fifth Edition, (Copyright 2013). American Psychiatric Association; World Health Organization, 1993

## 14.6.2 Pathogenesis

### 14.6.2.1 Cognitive-affective factors

From an evolutionary perspective, many of the anxiety disorders, including the specific phobias, can be conceptualised as a dysfunctional alarm system (Klein, 1993). In other words, responses that initially developed to detect and avoid potentially harmful stimuli may now be triggered either inadequately or excessively (Stein and Matsunaga, 2006; Stein and Bouwer, 1997). It is thought that dysfunctional associative models and conditioned fear responses may also contribute to the cognitive-affective pathophysiology of specific phobias (Fyer, 1998; Stein and Matsunaga, 2006).

### 14.6.2.2 Neurobiological factors

In line with the cognitive-affective understanding of specific phobia, much work has been done on the neurobiological basis of fear conditioning. Neuro-imaging studies show that the amygdala, thalamus, insula, cingulate and dorsomedial prefrontal cortex (PFC) are significant components of the neurocircuitry of conditioned fear responses (i.e. the automatic processing of noxious stimuli) (Del Casale *et al.*, 2012; Linares *et al.*, 2011; Straube *et al.*, 2006; Wright *et al.*, 2003; Veltman *et al.*, 2004, Stein and Matsunaga, 2006). Activation of limbic/paralimbic structures (e.g. the insula and thalamus) has been found to be particularly associated with specific phobias with prominent autonomic symptoms (Del Casale *et al.*, 2012).

The main neurotransmitters involved in this neurocircuitry seem to include both monoamine (5-HT, noradrenaline) and amino acid receptors (glutamate, GABA), thus possibly accounting for the broad range of clinically efficacious pharmacotherapeutic agents, e.g. SSRIs and benzodiazepines for specific phobias (Stein and Matsunaga, 2006).

### 14.6.2.3 Genetic predisposition and environmental factors

It is estimated that the liability to suffer from a host of specific phobias is at least partially moderated by genetic factors (Kendler *et al.*, 1992; Kendler *et al.*, 1999), which may be related to variants in neuro-endocrine, monoamine and/or amino acid receptors (Smoller *et al.*, 2005; Stein and Matsunaga, 2006). According to the stress-diathesis model (Monroe and Simons, 1991), disorders arise when genetically vulnerable individuals are exposed to environmental adversity. In the context of specific phobias, these environmental stressors may include a traumatic event occurring to self or others, observation of fear in others, observation of avoidance in others and being taught to be afraid (fear learning) (Kendler *et al.*, 2002; Rachman, 1977).

## 14.6.3 Treatment

### 14.6.3.1 Psychotherapy

Psychotherapy is the generally recommended first-line option (Baldwin *et al.*, 2005; Paris, 2006). Exposure-based therapy (either in-vivo or virtual reality-type) has proved effective in many individuals with specific phobias (Paris, 2006; Antony and Barlow, 2002). In particular, therapeutic sessions in close succession over a prolonged period of time and involving real (rather than imagined) exposures in graded levels of intensity may be beneficial (Antony and McCabe, 2003; Ost *et al.*, 1997). Response to treatment may vary across different phobias. For example, individuals with acrophobia generally respond well to virtual reality-type therapy, while cognitive therapy is most helpful for those with claustrophobia (Choy *et al.*, 2007).

### 14.6.3.2 Pharmacotherapy

There has been very little work on the pharmacotherapeutic management of specific phobias, as most individuals respond well to first-line psychotherapy (Paris, 2006; Baldwin *et al.*, 2005). Nonetheless, in a clinical setting, short-course benzodiazepines are sometimes used in addition to exposure therapy when it is necessary for an individual to face a specific phobia (Paris, 2006). It is unclear whether this combined approach has a positive or deleterious effect.

There are even fewer data on the use of antidepressants in individuals with specific phobias.

While fluoxetine (Abene and Hamilton, 1998), fluvoxamine (Balon, 1999) and paroxetine (Benjamin *et al.*, 2000) have been investigated, results have been unconvincing. One study demonstrated that D-cycloserine, a partial NMDA (N-methyl-D-aspartate) receptor agonist, used in combination with exposure therapy, was beneficial in individuals with acrophobia (Ressler *et al.*, 2004; Choy *et al.*, 2007). Further research is needed before introduction into routine care.

## 14.7 Anxiety secondary to general medical conditions, substances or medication

### 14.7.1 Phenomenology

As discussed elsewhere in this chapter, symptoms of anxiety may be secondary to substance use or to a general medical condition. Thus, it is important to have a high index of suspicion for screening for these primary disorders, and for performing a thorough systemic enquiry and examination. However, it should also be noted that a primary substance use disorder or a general medical condition may be associated with an anxiety disorder in two ways: as an independent co-morbidity or as a causative precursor (Brown *et al.*, 1995; Goodwin and Guze, 1996). While some recent work suggests that this distinction may be insignificant (Bakken *et al.*, 2003), current clinical convention dictates that primary and secondary anxiety disorders should still be differentiated.

In the case study, thyrotoxicosis was the primary cause of Connie's panic attacks. Other medical conditions that may mimic panic disorder include cardiorespiratory disease, other endocrinopathies and neurological disorders (Wilson, 2007). Individuals using or abusing psycho-active substances may also present in this way. Thus, a recent history of sympathomimetic use (e.g. methamphetamine, cocaine, caffeine) or sedative use (e.g. benzodiazepine, alcohol) should also be elicited and the individual should be examined for signs of intoxication or withdrawal (Wilson, 2007). Common causes of anxiety secondary to general medical conditions or substances/medication can found in Table 14.5.

The diagnostic criteria as outlined in the DSM-5 and the ICD-10 can be seen in Table 14.6. In the clinical assessment of these individuals, you should pay close attention to temporality (i.e. onset of the general medical condition GMC or substance use related to the onset of anxiety symptoms) as well as to the history of symptom exacerbation or improvement. For example, substance induced anxiety generally develops in close temporal connection with substance use and/or withdrawal and should improve with abstinence (Akiskal, 1995; Kadden *et al.*, 1995).

### 14.7.2 Treatment

In general, the management of secondary anxiety disorders should be guided by the underlying primary condition. In Connie's case (see Case study 14.6) treatment with levothyroxine should lead to an improvement in her somatic and psychiatric symptoms (including her panic attacks). However, should the symptoms of anxiety not improve once the underlying general medical condition or substance abuse has been treated, an alternative diagnosis should be sought and managed accordingly.

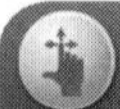

## Case study 14.6

Connie is a 42-year-old married mother of three who presents to her general practitioner with recurrent, unexpected panic attacks overs the past two months. She has never before experienced these episodes, and cannot identify any specific trigger. She does not consider herself to be a generally nervous or anxious person. She is particularly concerned now, as she has also been experiencing some weight loss (despite having an increased appetite), a fine hand tremor and intolerance to heat. She feels that she has become quite frenetic and irritable in her day-to-day activities, and fears that she may be experiencing early menopause. On clinical examination, she is found to be tachycardic with warm peripheries and a fine tremor. Ophthalmic examination reveals subtle lid lag with some lid retraction. Thyroid function tests (TFTs) show decreased thyroid stimulating hormone (TSH) with increased triiodothyronine (T3) and thyroxine (T4) levels. Full blood count and renal/liver function tests are normal. Having confirmed his suspicion of thyrotoxicosis, Connie's GP prescribes 40 mg oral carbimazole for 4 weeks, with a plan to reduce dosage according to her next TFT results.

**Table 14.5** Common causes of anxiety secondary to general medical conditions or substances/medication

| General medical conditions | Substances or medications |
|---|---|
| ▶ Endocrine disease (e.g. hyperthyroidism and hypothyroidism, pheochromocytoma, hypoglycaemia, hyperadrenocortisolism)<br>▶ Cardiovascular disease (e.g. congestive heart failure, pulmonary embolism, arrhythmia such as atrial fibrillation)<br>▶ Respiratory disease (e.g. chronic obstructive pulmonary disease, asthma, pneumonia)<br>▶ Metabolic disturbances (e.g. vitamin $B_{12}$ deficiency, porphyria)<br>▶ Neurological disease (e.g. neoplasms, vestibular dysfunction, encephalitis, seizure disorders). | ▶ Substance intoxication: alcohol, caffeine, cannabis, hallucinogens, amphetamine and related substances (including cocaine) and other (or unknown) substances<br>▶ Substance withdrawal: alcohol, cocaine, sedatives, hypnotics, anxiolytics and other (or unknown) substances<br>▶ Medication: anaesthetics and analgesics, sympathomimetics or other bronchodilators, anticholinergics, insulin, thyroid preparations, oral contraceptives, antihistamines, antiparkinsonian medication, corticosteroids, antihypertensive and cardiovascular medication, anticonvulsants, lithium carbonate, antipsychotic medication and antidepressant medication<br>▶ Heavy metals and toxins: organophosphate insecticide, nerve gases, carbon monoxide, carbon dioxide, volatile substances such fuel and paint. |

**Table 14.6** Diagnostic criteria for anxiety disorders secondary to a general medical condition, or to substances/medications

| **Anxiety Disorder Due to Another Medical Condition** | |
|---|---|
| **DSM-5 Diagnostic Criteria for Anxiety Disorder due to Another Medical Condition** | **ICD-10** |
| A. Panic attacks or anxiety is predominant in the clinical picture. | A disorder characterised by the essential descriptive features of a generalised anxiety disorder, a panic disorder, or a combination of both, but arising as a consequence of an organic disorder capable of causing cerebral dysfunction (e.g. temporal lobe epilepsy, thyrotoxicosis, phaechromocytoma). |

<table>
<tr><th colspan="2">Anxiety Disorder Due to Another Medical Condition</th></tr>
<tr><td>B. There is evidence from the history, physical examination, or laboratory findings that the disturbance is the direct pathophysiological consequence of another medical condition.</td><td rowspan="4">The decision to classify a clinical syndrome here is supported by the following:<br>▸ evidence of cerebral disease, damage or dysfunction of systemic physical disease known to be associated with one of the listed syndromes<br>▸ a temporal relationship (weeks or a few months) between the development of the underlying disease and the onset of the mental syndrome<br>▸ recovery from the mental disorder following removal or improvement of the underlying presumed cause<br>▸ absence of evidence to suggest an alternative cause of the mental syndrome (such as a strong family history or precipitating stress).<br>Conditions (a) and (b) justify a provisional diagnosis; if all four are present, the certainty of diagnostic classification is significantly increased.</td></tr>
<tr><td>C. The disturbance is not better explained by another mental disorder.</td></tr>
<tr><td>D. The disturbance does not occur exclusively during the course of a delirium.</td></tr>
<tr><td>E. The disturbance causes clinically significant distress or impairment in social, occupational, or other important areas of functioning.</td></tr>
</table>

<table>
<tr><th colspan="2">Substance/Medication-Induced Anxiety Disorder</th></tr>
<tr><th>DSM-5 Diagnostic Criteria for Substance/Medication-Induced Anxiety Disorder</th><th>ICD-10</th></tr>
<tr><td>A. Panic attacks or anxiety is predominant in the clinical picture.</td><td rowspan="5">While full diagnostic criteria for a substance induced anxiety disorder are not included in the ICD guidelines (World Health Organization, 1993; World Health Organization, 2007), it is required that the disorder be clearly related to the substance use in terms of temporality, symptomology and duration (Hasin et al., 2006).</td></tr>
<tr><td>B. There is evidence from the history, physical examination, or laboratory findings of both (1) and (2):<br>1. The symptoms in Criterion A developed during or soon after substance intoxication or withdrawal or after exposure to a medication.<br>2. The involved substance/medication is capable of producing the symptoms in Criterion A.</td></tr>
<tr><td>C. The disturbance is not better explained by an anxiety disorder that is not substance/ medication-induced. Such evidence of an independent anxiety disorder could include the following:<br>The symptoms precede the onset of the substance/medication use; the symptoms persist for a substantial period of time (e.g., about 1 month) after the cessation of acute withdrawal or severe intoxication: or there is other evidence suggesting the existence of an independent non-substance/medication-induced anxiety disorder (e.g., a history of recurrent non-substance/ medication-related episodes).</td></tr>
<tr><td>D. The disturbance does not occur exclusively during the course of a delirium.</td></tr>
<tr><td>E. The disturbance causes clinically significant distress or impairment in social, occupational, or other important areas of functioning.<br>Note: This diagnosis should be made instead of a diagnosis of substance intoxication or substance withdrawal only when the symptoms in Criterion A predominate in the clinical picture and they are sufficiently severe to warrant clinical attention.<br>Specify if (see Table 1 in the chapter 'Substance-Related and Addictive Disorders' for diagnoses associated with substance class):<br>▸ With onset during intoxication: This specifier applies if criteria are met for intoxication with the substance and the symptoms develop during intoxication.<br>▸ With onset during withdrawal: This specifier applies if criteria are met for withdrawal from the substance and the symptoms develop during, or shortly after, withdrawal.<br>▸ With onset after medication use: Symptoms may appear either at initiation of medication or after a modification or change in use.</td></tr>
</table>

**Source:** Reprinted with permission from the *Diagnostic and Statistical Manual of Mental Disorders*, Fifth Edition, (Copyright 2013). American Psychiatric Association; World Health Organization, 1993; World Health Organization 2007

## Conclusion

In this chapter, we have aimed to provide a user-friendly, practical guideline to six anxiety disorders that are likely to be seen in the clinical setting. We have included the most up-to-date diagnostic criteria, a range of neuroscientific and empirical research findings, and real-life case studies.

# References

Abene MV, Hamilton JD (1998) Resolution of fear of flying with fluoxetine treatment. *Journal of Anxiety Disorders* 12(6): 599–603

American Psychiatric Association (2000) *Diagnostic and Statistical Manual of Mental Disorders* (4th edition). Text Revision. Washington USA: American Psychiatric Press

American Psychiatric Association (2013) *Diagnostic and Statistical Manual of Mental Disorders* (5th edition). Arlington, VA: American Psychiatric Publishing

Amies PL, Gelder MG, Shaw PM (1983) Social phobia: A comparative clinical study. *British Journal of Psychiatry* 142: 1174–179

Antony MM, Barlow DH (2002) Specific phobias. In: Barlow D (Ed) *Anxiety and its disorders: the nature and treatment of anxiety and panic*. New York: Guilford Press

Antony MM, McCabe RE (2003) Anxiety disorders: Social and specific phobias. In: Tasman A, Kay J, Lieberman (Eds). *Psychiatry*. Chichester (UK): John Wiley & Sons

Akiskal HS (1995) Mood disorders: clinical features. In: Kaplan HI, Sadock BJ (Eds) *Comprehensive Textbook of Psychiatry* (6th edition, Vol 1 ) Baltimore: Williams and Wilkins

Bakken K, Landheim AS, Vaglum P (2003) Primary and secondary substance misusers: Do they differ in substance-induced and substance-independent mental disorders? *Alcohol Alcohol* 38(1): 54–9

Baldwin DS, Polkinghorn C (2005) Evidence-based pharmacotherapy of generalized anxiety disorder. *International Journal of Neuropsychopharmacology* 8(2): 293–302

Baldwin SA, Anderson IM, Nutt DJ, Bandelow B, Bond A, Davidson JR, den Boer JA, Fineberg NA, Knapp M, Scott J, Wittchen HU (2005) Evidence-based guidelines for the pharmacological treatment of anxiety disorders: Recommendations from the British Association for Psychopharmacology. *Journal of Psychopharmacology* 19(6): 567–96

Ballenger JC, Davidson JR, Lecrubier Y, Nutt DJ, Borkovec TD, Rickels K, Stein DJ, Wittchen HU (2001) Consensus statement on generalised anxiety disorder from the International Consensus Group on Depression and Anxiety. *Journal of Clinical Psychiatry* 62 (suppl 11):53–58

Balon R (1999) Fluvoxamine for phobia of storms. *Acta Psychiatrica Scandinavica* 100(3): 244–245; discussion: 245–246

Bandelow B, Zohar J, Hollander E, Kasper S, Möller HJ World Federation of Societies of Biological Psychiatry (FSBP) Task Force on Treatment Guidelines for Anxiety Obsessive-Compulsive and Post-Traumatic Stress Disorders Zohar J, Hollander E, Kasper S, Möller HJ, Bandelow B, Allgulander C, Ayuso-Gutierrez J, Baldwin DS, Buenvicius R, Cassano G, Fineberg N, Gabriels L, Hindmarch I, Kaiya H, Klein DF, Lader M, Lecrubier Y, Lépine JP, Liebowitz MR, Lopez-Ibor JJ, Marazziti D, Miguel EC, Oh KS, Preter M, Rupprecht R, Sato M, Starcevic V, Stein DJ, van Ameringen M, Vega J (2008) World Federation of Societies of Biological Psychiatry (WFSBP) guidelines for the pharmacological treatment of anxiety obsessive-compulsive and posttraumatic stress disorders – first revision. *World Journal of Biological Psychiatry* 9(4): 248–312

Barlow D, Gorman J, Shear M, Woods S (2000) Cognitive-behavioral therapy, imipramine, or their combination for panic disorder: A randomized controlled trial. *Journal of the American Medical Association* 283(19): 2529–36

Beck AT, Emery G, Greenberg RC (1985) Anxiety disorders and phobias: *A cognitive perspective*. New York USA: Basic Books

Belzung C, Griebel G (2001) Measuring normal and pathological anxiety-like behaviour in mice: A review. *Behavioural Brain Research* 125(1–2): 141–9

Benjamin J, Ben-Zion I, Karbofsky E, Dannon P (2000) Double-blind placebo-controlled pilot study of paroxetine for specific phobia. *Psychopharmacology* 149(2): 194–196

Blanco C, Heimberg RG, Schneier FR, Fresco DM, Chen H, Turk CL, Vermes D, Erwin BA, Schmidt AB, Juster HR, Campeas R, Liebowitz MR (2010) A placebo-controlled trial of phenelzine, cognitive behavioral group therapy, and their combination for social anxiety disorder. *Archives of General Psychiatry* 67(3): 286–95

Brown C, Schulberg H, Madonia M, Shear MK, Houck PR (1996) Treatment outcomes for primary care patients with major depression and lifetime anxiety disorders. *American Journal of Psychiatry* 153(10): 1293–300

Brown SA, Inaba RK, Gillin JC, Schuckit MA, Stewart MA, Irwin MR (1995) Alcoholism and affective disorder: Clinical course of depressive symptoms. *American Journal of Psychiatry* 152(1): 45–52

Cannon WB (1915) *Bodily changes in pain, hunger, fear and rage*. New York: Harper & Row

Charney DS, Heninger GR (1986) Abnormal regulation of noradrenergic function in panic disorders. Effects of clonidine in healthy subjects and patients with agoraphobia and panic disorder. *Archives of General Psychiatry* 43(11): 1042–1054

Charney DS, Woods SW, Goodman WK, Heninger GR (1987) Neurobiological mechanisms of panic anxiety: biochemical and behavioral correlates of yohimbine-induced panic attacks. *American Journal of Psychiatry* 144(8): 1030–1036

Chavira DA, Stein MB (2005) Childhood social anxiety disorder: From understanding to treatment. *Child*

*and Adolescent Psychiatric Clinics of North America* 14(4): 797–818
Chavira DA, Stein MB, Bailey K, Stein MT (2004) Child anxiety in primary care: Prevalent but untreated. *Depression and Anxiety* 20(4): 155–64
Choy Y, Fyer AJ, Lipsitz JD (2007) Treatment of specific phobia in adults. *Clinical Psychology Review* 27(3): 266–86
Clum GA, Surls R (1993) A meta-analysis of treatments for panic disorder. *Journal of Consulting and Clinical Psychology* 61(2): 317–326
Cohen DC (1977) Comparison of self-report and overt behavioral procedures for assessing acrophobia. *Behavior Therapy* 8: 17–23
Connor K, Kobak KA, Churchil E, Katzelnick D, Davidson JR (2001) Mini-SPIN: A brief screening assessment for generalized social anxiety disorder. *Depression and Anxiety* 14(2): 137–40
Connor KM, Davidson JR, Churchill LE, Sherwood A, Foa E, Weisler RH (2000) Psychometric properties of the Social Phobia Inventory (SPIN): a new self-rating scale. *British Journal of Psychiatry* 176: 379–86
Cox BJ, Norton GR, Swinson RP, Endler NS (1990) Substance abuse and panic-related anxiety: A critical review. *Behaviour Research and Therapy* 28(5) 385–93
Crowley D (1992) Alcohol abuse, substance abuse and panic disorder. *The American Journal of Medicine* 92(1A): 41S-48S
Del Casale A, Ferracuti S, Rapinesi C, Serata D, Piccirilli M, Savoja V, Kotzalidis GD, Manfredi G, Angeletti G, Tatarelli R, Girardi P (2012) Functional neuroimaging in specific phobia. *Psychiatry Research* July DOI: 10.1016/j.pscychresns.2011.10.009 (Epub ahead of print) (Accessed November 2014)
Dupont RL, Rice DP, Miller LS, Shiraki SS, Rowland CR, Harwood HJ (1996) Economic costs of anxiety disorders. *Anxiety* 2(4): 167–72
Etkin A (2010) Functional neuroanatomy of anxiety: A neural circuit perspective. *Current Topics in Behavioral Neurosciences* 2: 251–77
Etkin A, Wager TD (2007) Functional neuroimaging of anxiety: A meta-analysis of emotional processing in PTSD, social anxiety disorder and specific phobia. *American Journal of Psychiatry* 164(10): 1476–88
Faravelli C, Zucchi T, Viviani B (2000) Epidemiology of social phobia: A clinical approach. *European Psychiatry* 15(1): 17–24
Fedoroff IC, Taylor S (2001) Psychological and pharmacological treatments of social phobia: A meta-analysis. *Journal of Clinical Psychopharmacology* 21(3): 311–24
Friedman MJ, Resick PA, Bryant RA, Strain J, Horowitz M, Spiegel D (2011) Classification of trauma and stressor-related disorders in DSM-5. *Depression and Anxiety* 28(9): 737–49
Fyer AJ (1998) Current approaches to etiology and pathophysiology of specific phobia. *Biological Psychiatry* 44(12): 1295–304
Ganasen KA, Stein DJ (2010) Pharmacotherapy of social anxiety disorder. *Current Topics in Behavioral Neurosciences* 2: 487–503
Gelernter J, Page GP, Stein MB, Woods SW (2004) Genome-wide linkage scan for loci predisposing to social phobia: Evidence for a chromosome 16 risk locus. *American Journal of Psychiatry* 161(1): 59–66
Godbey KL, Courage MM (1994) Stress-management program: Intervention in nursing student performance anxiety. *Archives of Psychiatric Nursing* 8(3): 190–9
Goodwin DW, Guze SB (1996) *Psychiatric Diagnosis* (5th edition). New York: Oxford University Press
Gorman JM, Kent JM, Sullivan GM, Coplan JD (2000) Neuroanatomical hypothesis of panic disorder (revised). *American Journal of Psychiatry* 157(4): 493–505
Grant BF, Hasin DS, Stinson FS, Dawson DA, Patricia Chou S, June Ruan W, Huang B (2005) Co-occurrence of 12-month mood and anxiety disorders and personality disorders in the US: Results from the national epidemiologic survey on alcohol and related conditions. *Journal of Psychiatric Research* 39(1): 1–9
Gross C, Hen R (2004) Genetic and environmental factors interact to influence anxiety. *Neurotoxicity Research* 6(6): 493–501
Hamilton M (1959) The assessment of anxiety states by rating. *British Journal of Medical Psychology* 32(1): 50–5
Herman AA, Stein DJ, Seedat S, Heeringa SG, Moomal H, Williams DR (2009) The South African Stress and Health (SASH) study: 12-month and lifetime prevalence of common mental disorders. *South African Medical Journal* 99(5 Pt 2): 339–44
Hettema JM, Neale MC, Kendler KS (2001) A review and meta-analysis of the genetic epidemiology of anxiety disorders. *American Journal of Psychiatry* 158(10): 1568–78
Hirshfeld-Becker DR, Biederman J, Henin A, Faraone SV, Davis S, Harrington K, Rosenbaum JF (2007) Behavioural inhibition in preschool children at risk is a specific predictor of middle childhood social anxiety: A five-year follow-up. *Journal of Developmental and Behavioral Pediatrics* 28(3): 225–33
Hoehn-Saric R, McLeod DR (1988) The peripheral sympathetic nervous system: It's role in normal and pathologic anxiety. *Psychiatric Clinics of North America* 11(2): 375–86
Hofer MA (1995) An evolutionary perspective on anxiety In: Roose SP, Glick RK (Eds). *Anxiety as symptom and signal*. Hillsdale NJ: Analytic Press
Holt CS, Heimberg RG, Hope DA (1992) Avoidant personality disorder and the generalized subtype of social phobia. *Journal of Abnormal Psychology* 101(2): 318–325
Huppert JD, Roth DA, Foa EB (2003) Cognitive-behavioural treatment of social phobia: New advances. *Current Psychiatry Reports* 5(4): 289–96
Kadden RM, Kranzler HR, Rounsaville BJ (1995) Validity of the distinction between 'substance-induced' and 'independent' Depression and Anxiety disorders. *American Journal on Addictions* 4: 107–17
Kasper S, Resinger E (2001) Panic disorder: The place of benzodiazepines and selective serotonin reuptake inhibitors. *European Neuropsychopharmacology* 11(4): 307–21
Kendler KS, Karkowski LM, Prescott CA (1999) Fears and phobias: Reliability and heritability. *Psychological Medicine* 29(3): 539–53
Kendler KS, Myers J, Prescott CA (2002) The etiology of phobias: An evaluation of the stress-diathesis model. *Archives of General Psychiatry* 59(3): 242–8

Kendler KS, Neale MC, Kessler RC, Heath AC, Eaves LJ (1992) The genetic epidemiology of phobias in women: The inter-relationship of agoraphobia, social phobia, situational phobia and simple phobia. *Archives of General Psychiatry* 49(4): 273–281

Kennedy JL, Bradwejn J, Koszycki D, King N, Crowe R, Vincent J, Fourie O (1999) Investigation of cholecystokinin system genes in panic disorder. *Molecular Psychiatry* 4(3): 284–5

Kessler RC, Chiu WT, Demler O, Merikangas KR, Walters EE (2005) Prevalence, severity and comorbidity of 12-month DSM-IV disorders in the National Comorbidity Survey Replication. *Archives of General Psychiatry* 62(6): 617–627

Kessler RC, Crum RM, Warner LA, Nelson CB, Schulenberg J, Anthony JC, McGonagle KC, Zhao S (1997) Lifetime co-occurrence of DSM-III-R alcohol abuse and dependence with other psychiatric disorders in the National Comorbidity Survey Lifetime and 12-month prevalence of DSM-III-R psychiatric disorders in the National Comorbidity Survey. *Archives of General Psychiatry* 54(4): 313–21

Kessler RC, Gruber M, Hettema JH, Hwang I, Sampson N, Yonkers KA (2008) Comorbid major depression and generalized anxiety disorders in the national comorbidity survey follow-up. *Psychological Medicine* 38(3): 365–74

Kessler RC, McGonagle KC, Zhao S, Nelson CB, Hughes M, Eshleman S, Wittchen HU, Kendler KS (1994) Lifetime and 12-month prevalence of DSM-III-R psychiatric disorders in the United States: Results from the National Comorbidity Survey. *Archives of General Psychiatry* 51(1): 8–19

Kessler RC, Stang P, Wittchen HU, Stein M, Walters EE (1999) Lifetime co-morbidities between social phobia and mood disorders in the US National Comorbidity Survey. *Psychological Medicine* 29(3): 555–67

Kircanski K, Craske MG, Epstein AM, Wittchen HU (2009) Subtypes of panic attacks: A critical review of the empirical literature. *Depression and Anxiety* 26(10): 878–87

Klein DF (1993) False suffocation alarms, spontaneous panics, and related conditions: An integrative hypothesis. *Archives of General Psychiatry* April 50(4): 306–17

Kobak KA, Greist JH, Jefferson JW, Katzelnick DJ (2002) Fluoxetine in social phobia: A double-blind, placebo-controlled pilot study. *Journal of Clinical Psychopharmacology* 22(3): 257–62

Lader M, Stender K, Burger V, Nil R (2004) Efficacy and tolerability of escitalopram in 12- and 24-week treatment of social anxiety disorder: Randomised, double-blind, placebo-controlled, fixed-dose study. *Depression and Anxiety* 19(4): 241–8

Landon TM, Barlow DH (2004) Cognitive-behavioral treatment for panic disorder: Current status. *Journal of Psychiatric Practice* 10(4): 211–26

Lecrubier Y, Judge R (1997) Long-term evaluation of paroxetine, clomipramine and placebo in panic disorder. Collaborative Paroxetine Panic Study Investigators. *Acta Psychiatrica Scandinavica* 95(2): 153–60

Lepola U, Arato M, Zhu Y, Austin C (2003) Sertraline versus imipramine treatment of comorbid panic disorder and major depressive disorder. *Journal of Clinical Psychiatry* 64(6): 654–62

Liebowitz MR, Schneier FR, Campeas R, Hollander E, Hatterer J, Fyer A, Gorman J, Papp L, Davies S, Gully R (1992) Phenelzine vs atenolol in social phobia. *Archives of General Psychiatry* 49(4): 290–300

Linares IM, Trzesniak C, Chagas MH, Hallak JE, Nardi AE, Crippa JA (2012) Neuroimaging in specific phobia disorder: A systematic review of the literature. *Revista Brasileira de Psiquiatria* 34(1): 101–11

Lydiard RB, Ballenger JC, Laraia MT, Fossey MD, Beinfeld MC (1992) CSF cholecystokinin concentrations in patients with panic disorder and in normal comparison subjects. *American Journal of Psychiatry* 149(5): 691–3

Magee WJ, Eaton WW, Wittchen HU, McGonagle KA, Kessler RC (1996) Agoraphobia, simple phobia, and social phobia in the National Comorbidity Survey. *Archives of General Psychiatry* 53(2): 159–68

Mannuzza S, Fyer AJ, Liebowitz MR, Klein DF (1990) Delineating the boundaries of social phobia: Its relationship to panic disorder and agoraphobia. *Journal of Anxiety Disorders* 4(1): 41–59

Marks IM, Mathews AM (1979) Brief standard self-rating for phobic patients. *Behaviour Research and Therapy* 17: 263–7

Marks IM, Nesse RM (1994) Fears and fitness: An evolutionary analysis of anxiety disorders. *Ethnology and Sociobiology* 15: 247–61

Marks IM, Swinson RP, Basoglu M, Kuch K, Noshirvani H, O'Sullivan G, Lelliott PT, Kirby M, McNamee G, Sengun S (1993) Alprazolam and exposure alone and combined in panic disorder with agoraphobia. A controlled study in London and Toronto. *British Journal of Psychiatry* 162: 776–87

MacDonald AW, Cohen JD, Stenger VA, Carter CS (2000) Dissociating the role of the dorsolateral prefrontal and anterior cingulate cortex in cognitive control. *Science* 288(5472): 1835–8

McClure EB, Monk CS, Nelson EE, Parrish JM, Adler A, Blair RJ, Fromm S, Charney DS, Leibenluft E, Ernst M, Pine DS (2007) Abnormal attention modulation of fear circuit function in pediatric generalized anxiety disorder. *Archives of General Psychiatry* 64(1): 97–106

Mitte K (2005) A meta-analysis of the efficacy of psycho- and pharmacotherapy in panic disorder with and without agoraphobia. *Journal of Affective Disorders* 88(1): 27–45

Monk CS, Nelson EE, McClure EB, Mogg K, Bradley BP, Leibenluft E, Blair RJ, Chen G, Charney DS, Ernst M, Pine DS (2006) Ventrolateral prefrontal cortex activation and attentional bias in response to angry faces in adolescents with generalized anxiety disorder. *American Journal of Psychiatry* 163(6): 1091–7

Monk CS, Telzer EH, Mogg K, Bradley BP, Mai X, Louro HM, Chen G, McClure-Tone EB, Ernst M, Pine DS (2008) Amygdala and ventrolateral prefrontal cortex activation to masked angry faces in children and adolescents with generalized anxiety disorder. *Archives of General Psychiatry* 65(5): 568–76

Monroe SM, Simons AD (1991) Diathesis-stress theories in the context of life stress research: Implications for the depressive disorders. *Psychological Bulletin* 110(3): 406–25

Moutier CY, Stein MB (1999) The history, epidemiology, and differential diagnosis of social anxiety disorder. *Journal of Clinical Psychiatry* 60(Suppl 9): 4–8

Muehlbacher M, Nickel MK, Nickel C, Kettler C, Lahmann C, Gil, FP, Leiberich PK, Rother N, Bachler E, Fartacek R, Kaplan P, Tritt K, Mitterlehner F, Anvar J, Rother WK, Loew TH, Egger C (2005) Mirtazapine treatment of social phobia in women: A randomised, double-blind, placebo-controlled study. *Journal of Clinical Psychopharmacology* 25(6): 580–3

Murray CJL, Lopez AD (Eds) (1996) *The global burden of disease: A comprehensive assessment of mortality and morbidity from diseases injuries and risk factors in 1990 and projected to 2020* (Volume I) Harvard: World Health Organization

Nash JR, Sargent PA, Rabiner EA, Hood SD, Argyropoulos SV, Potokar JP, Grasby PM, Nutt DJ (2008) Serotonin 5-HT1A receptor binding in people with panic disorder: Positron emission tomography study. *British Journal of Psychiatry* 193(3): 229–34

National Institute for Clinical Excellence (NICE) (2004) *The management of panic disorder and generalised anxiety disorder in primary and secondary care*. London: National Collaborating Centre for Mental Health

Neumeister A, Bain E, Nugent AC, Carson RE, Bonne O, Luckenbaugh DA, Eckelman W, Herscovitch P, Charney DS, Drevets WC (2004) Reduced serotonin type 1A receptor binding in panic disorder. *Journal of Neuroscience* 24(3): 589–91

Nutt D (2005) Overview of diagnosis and drug treatment of anxiety disorders. *CNS Spectrums* 10(1): 49–56

Nutt D, Ballenger J (Eds) (2005) *Anxiety disorders: Panic disorder and social anxiety disorder*. Massachusetts: Blackwell Publishing

Nutt DJ, Bell CJ, Malizia AL (1998) Brain mechanisms of social anxiety disorder. *Journal of Clinical Psychiatry* 59(suppl 17): 4–11

Ost LG, Ferebee I, Furmark T (1997) One-session group therapy of spider phobia: Direct versus indirect treatments. *Behaviour Research and Therapy* 35(8): 721–32

Otto MW, Deveney C (2005) Cognitive-behavioral therapy and the treatment of panic disorder: Efficacy and strategies. *Journal of Clinical Psychiatry* 66(suppl 4): 28–32

Page AC (1994) Distinguishing panic disorder and agoraphobia from social phobia. *Journal of Nervous and Mental Disease* 182(11): 611–7

Pallanti S, Quercoli L, Hollander E (2004) Social anxiety in outpatients with schizophrenia: A relevant cause of disability. *American Journal of Psychiatry* 161(1): 53–8

Pande AC, Davidson JR, Jefferson JW, Janney CA, Katzelnick DJ, Weisler RH, Greist JH, Sutherland SM (1999) Treatment of social phobia with gabapentin: A placebo-controlled study. *Journal of Clinical Psychopharmacology* 19(4): 341–8

Paris J (2006) Clinical practice guideline: management of anxiety disorders. *Canadian Journal of Psychiatry* 51 (suppl 2):1–92

Phan KL, Fitzgerald DA, Nathan PJ, Tancer ME (2006) Association between amygdala hyperactivity to harsh faces and severity of social anxiety in generalized social phobia. *Biological Psychiatry* 59(5): 424–9

Phillips RG, LeDoux JE (1992) Differential contribution of amygdala and hippocampus to cued and contextual fear conditioning. *Behavioral Neuroscience* 106(2): 274–85

Pine DS, Cohen P, Gurley D, Brook J, Ma Y (1998) The risk for early-adulthood anxiety and depressive disorders in adolescents with anxiety and depressive disorders. *Archives of General Psychiatry* 55(1): 56–64

Pollack MH (2009) Refractory generalized anxiety disorder. *Journal of Clinical Psychiatry* 70 (suppl2):32–38

Rachman S (1977) The conditioning theory of fear-acquisition: A critical examination. *Behaviour Research and Therapy* 15(5): 375–87

Raleigh MJ, McGuire MT, Brammer GL, Pollack DB, Yuwiler A (1991) Serotonergic mechanisms promote dominance acquisition in adult male vervet monkeys. *Brain Research* 559(2): 181–90

Rapee RM, Spence SH (2004) The etiology of social phobia: Empirical evidence and an initial model. *Clinical Psychology Review* 24(7): 737–67

Redmond D, Huang Y (1979) Current concepts. II. New evidence for a locus coeruleus-norepinephrine connection with anxiety. *Life Sciences* 25(26): 2149–62

Regier DA, Rae DS, Narrow WE, Kaelber CT, Schatzberg AF (1998) Prevalence of anxiety disorders and their comorbidity with mood and addictive disorders. *British Journal of Psychiatry Supplement* 34: 24–8

Rehfeld JF (2000) Cholecystokinin and panic disorder – three unsettled questions. *Regulatory Peptides* 93(1–3): 79–83

Reich J, Noyes R, Yates W (1988) Anxiety symptoms distinguishing social phobia from panic and generalized anxiety disorders. *Journal of Nervous and Mental Disease* 176(8): 510–3

Ressler KJ, Rothbaum BO, Tannenbaum L, Anderson P, Graap K, Zimand E, Hodges L, Davis M (2004) Cognitive enhancers as adjuncts to psychotherapy: Use of D-cycloserine in phobic individuals to facilitate extinction of fear. *Archives of General Psychiatry* 61(11): 1136–344

Rickels K, Mangano R, Khan A (2004) A double-blind, placebo-controlled study of a flexible dose of venlafaxine ER in adult outpatients with generalized social anxiety disorder. *Journal of Clinical Psychopharmacology* 24(5): 488–96

Rickels K, Schweizer E (1998) Panic disorder: Long-term pharmacotherapy and discontinuation. *Journal of Clinical Psychopharmacology* 18(6 Suppl 2): 12S–18S

Rosen JB, Schulkin J (1998) From normal fear to pathological anxiety. *Psychological Review* April 105(2): 325–350

Roy-Byrne P, Stang P, Wittchen U, Ustun B, Walters EE, Kessler RC (2000) Lifetime panic-depression co-morbidity in the National Comorbidity Survey: Association with symptoms, impairment, course and help-seeking. *British Journal of Psychiatry* 176: 229–35

Roy-Byrne R, Wagner A, Schraufnagel T (2005) Understanding and treating panic disorder in the primary care setting. *Journal of Clinical Psychiatry* 66(Suppl 4): 16–22

Ruscio AM, Brown TA, Chiu WT, Sareen J, Stein MB, Kessler RC (2008) Social fears and social phobia in the USA: Results from the National Comorbidity Survey Replication. *Psychological Medicine* 38(1): 15–28

Schmidt NB, Wollaway-Bickel K, Trakowski JH, Santiago HT, Vasey M (2002) Antidepressant discontinuation in the context of cognitive behavioral treatment for panic disorder. *Behaviour Research and Therapy* 40(1): 67–73

Schneier FR (1991) Social phobia. *Psychiatric Annals* 21(6): 349–353

Schneier FR, Barnes LF, Albert SM, Louis ED (2001) Characteristics of social phobia among persons with essential tremor. *Journal of Clinical Psychiatry* 62(5): 367–72

Schneier FR, Liebowitz MR, Abi-dargham A, Zea-Ponce Y, Lin SH, Laruelle M (2001) Low dopamine D2 receptor binding potential in social phobia. *American Journal of Psychiatry* 157(3): 457–9

Seedat S, Stein D (2007) The anxious patient. In: Baumann SE (Ed). *Primary Health Care Psychiatry: A Practical Guide for Southern Africa*. Kenwyn: Juta & Co

Seedat S, Stein MB (2004) Double-blind, placebo-controlled assessment of combined clonazepam with paroxetine compared with paroxetine monotherapy for generalized social anxiety disorder. *Journal of Clinical Psychiatry* 65(2): 244–248

Shapiro SL, Shapiro DE, Schwartz GE (2000) Stress management in medical education: A review of the literature. *Academic Medicine* 75(7): 748–59

Shavitt RG, Gentil V, Mandetta R (1992) The association of panic/agoraphobia and asthma: Contributing factors and clinical implications. *General Hospital Psychiatry* 14(6): 420–3

Sheehan D, Ballenger JC, Jacobson G (1980) Treatment of endogenous anxiety with phobic hysterical and hypochondriacal symptoms. *Archives of General Psychiatry* 37(1): 51–9

Simon NM, Otto MW, Wisniewski SR, Fossey M, Sagduyu K, Frank E, Sachs GS, Nierenberg AA, Thase ME, Pollack MH (2004) Anxiety disorder comorbidity in bipolar disorder patients: Data from the first 500 participants in the Systematic Treatment Enhancement Program for Bipolar Disorder (STEP-BD). *American Journal of Psychiatry* 161(12): 2222–9

Singh JS, Hope DA (2009) Cognitive-behavioral approaches to the treatment of social anxiety disorder. *Israel Journal of Psychiatry and Related Sciences* 46(1): 62–9

Smoller JW, Yamaki LH, Fagerness JA, Biederman J, Racette S, Laird NM, Kagan J, Snidman N, Faraone SV, Hirshfeld-Becker D, Tsuang MT, Slaugenhaupt SA, Rosenbaum JF, Sklar PB (2005) The corticotropin-releasing hormone gene and behavioral inhibition in children at risk for panic disorder. *Biological Psychiatry* 57(12): 1485–92

Solyom L, Ledwidge B, Solyom C (1986) Delineating social phobia. *British Journal of Psychiatry* 149: 464–70

Stein DJ (2005) Generalized anxiety disorder: Rethinking diagnosis and rating. *CNS Spectrums* 10(12): 930–4

Stein DJ (2006) Advances in understanding the anxiety disorders: The cognitive-affective neuroscience of 'false alarms'. *Annals of Clinical Psychiatry* 18(3): 173–82

Stein DJ, Baldwin DS, Bandelow B, Blanco C, Fontenelle LF, Lee S, Matsunaga H, Osser D, Stein MB, van Ameringen M (2010) A 2010 evidence-based algorithm for the pharmacotherapy of social anxiety disorder. *Current Psychiatry Reports* 12(5): 471–7

Stein DJ, Bouwer C (1997) A neuro-evolutionary approach to the anxiety disorders. *Journal of Anxiety Disorders* 11(4): 409–29

Stein DJ, Fineberg NA, Bienvenu J, Denys D, Lochner C, Nestadt G, Leckman JF, Rauch SL, Phillips KA (2010) Should OCD be classified as an anxiety disorder in DSM-V? *Depression and Anxiety* 27(6): 495–506

Stein DJ, Ipser JC, Balkom AJ (2004) Pharmacotherapy for social phobia. *Cochrane Database of Systematic Reviews* 4 CD001206

Stein DJ, Matsunaga H (2006) Specific phobia: A disorder of fear conditioning and extinction. *CNS Spectrums* 11(4): 248–51

Stein DJ, Westenberg H, Liebowitz MR (2002) Social anxiety disorder and generalized anxiety disorder: Serotonergic and dopaminergic neurocircuitry. *Journal of Clinical Psychiatry* 63(Suppl 6): 12–9

Stein MB, Baird A, Walker JR (1996) Social phobia in adults with stuttering. *American Journal of Psychiatry* 153(2): 278–80

Stein MB, Chartier MJ, Hazen AL, Kozak MV, Tancer ME, Lander S, Furer P, Chubaty D, Walker JR (1998) A direct-interview family study of generalized social phobia. *American Journal of Psychiatry* 155(1): 90–7

Stein MB, Jang KL, Livesley WJ (2002) Heritability of social-anxiety related concerns and personality characteristics: A twin study. *Journal of Nervous and Mental Disease* 190(4): 219–24

Stein MB, Stein D (2008) Social anxiety disorder. *The Lancet* 371(9618): 1115–25

Strain JJ, Friedman MJ (2011) Considering adjustment disorders as stress response syndromes for DSM-5. *Depression and Anxiety* 28: 818–23

Straube T, Mentzel HJ, Miltner WH (2006) Neural mechanisms of automatic and direct processing of phobogenic stimuli in specific phobia. *Biological Psychiatry* 59(2): 162–70

Syal S, Hattingh CJ, Fouché JP (2012) Grey matter abnormalities in social anxiety disorder: A pilot study. *Metabolic Brain Disease* 27(3): 299–309

Tiihonen J, Kuikka J, Bergstrom K, Lepola U, Koponen H, Leinonen E (1997) Dopamine reuptake site densities in patients with social phobia. *American Journal of Psychiatry* 154(2): 239–42

Tiller JW, Bouwer C, Behnke K (1999) Moclobemide and fluoxetine for panic disorder. International Panic Disorder Study Group. *European Archives of Psychiatry and Clinical Neurosciences* 249(Suppl 1): 7S–10S

Togersen S (1983) Genetic factors in anxiety disorder. *Archives of General Psychiatry* 40(10): 1085–9

Tupler LA, Davidson JR, Smith RD, Lazeyras F, Charles HC, Krishnan KR (1997) A repeat proton magnetic resonance spectroscopy study in social phobia. *Biological Psychiatry* 42(6): 419–24

Turner SM, Beidel DC, Townsley RM (1992) Social phobia: A comparison of specific and generalized subtypes and avoidant personality disorder. *Journal of Abnormal Psychology* 101(2): 326–31

Tyrer P, Baldwin D (2006) Generalized anxiety disorder. *The Lancet* 368(9553): 2156–66

Van Ameringen M, Allgulander C, Bandelow B, Greist JH, Hollander E, Montgomery SA, Nutt DJ, Okasha A, Pollack MH, Stein DJ, Swinson RP. World Council of Anxiety (2003) WCA recommendations for the long-term treatment of social phobia. *CNS Spectrums* 8(8 Suppl 1): 40–52

Van Balkom AJ, Bakker A, Spinhoven P, Blaauw BM, Smeenk S, Ruesink B (1997) A meta-analysis of the treatment of panic disorder with or without agoraphobia: A comparison of psychopharmacological, cognitive-behavioral, and combination treatments. *Journal of Nervous and Mental Disease* 185(8): 510–6

Veltman DJ, Tuinebreijer WE, Winkelman D, Lammertsma AA, Witter MP, Dolan RJ, Emmelkamp PM (2004) Neurophysiological correlates of habituation during exposure in spider phobia. *Psychiatry Research* 132(2): 149–58

Vythilingum B, Stein DJ (2004) Specific phobia In: Stein DJ (Ed). *Clinical Manual of Anxiety Disorders.* Washington DC: American Psychiatric Publishing

Weinstock LS (1999) Gender differences in the presentation and management of social anxiety disorder. *Journal of Clinical Psychiatry* 60(Suppl 9): 9–13

Wilson D (2007) The problem of fear and panic. In: Baumann SE (Ed). *Primary Health Care Psychiatry: A Practical Guide for Southern Africa.* Kenwyn: Juta & Co

Wittchen H-U, Jacobi F (2005) Size and burden of mental disorders in Europe – a critical review and appraisal of 27 studies. *European Neuropsychopharmacology 15*(4): 357–76

World Health Organization (1993) *The ICD-10 Classification of Mental and Behavioural Disorders: Diagnostic Criteria for Research.* Available at: http://www.who.int/classifications/icd/en/GRNBOOK.pdf (Accessed 15 August 2011)

World Health Organization (2007) *International statistical classification of diseases and related health problems* 10th Revision Version for 2007. Available at: http://www.who.int/classifications/apps/icd/icd10online/ (Accessed 20 March 2011)

Wright CI, Martis B, McMullin K, Shin LM, Rauch SL, (2003) Amygdala and insular responses to emotionally valenced human faces in small animal specific phobia. *Biological Psychiatry* 54(10): 1067–76

Yellowlees P, Alpers J, Bowden J, Bryant GD, Ruffin RE (1987) Psychiatric morbidity in patients with chronic airflow obstruction. *Medical Journal of Australia* 146(6): 305–7

Zandbergen J, Bright M, Pols H, Fernandez I, de Loof C, Griez EJ (1991) Higher lifetime prevalence of respiratory diseases in panic disorder. *American Journal of Psychiatry* 148(11): 1583–5

Zetin M, Hoepner CT, Bjornson L (2006) Rational antidepressant selection: Applying evidence-based medicine to complex real-world patients. *Psychopharmacology Bulletin* 39(1): 38–104

CHAPTER

# 15 Acute reactions to adverse life events

*Werdie van Staden, Thebe Madigoe*

## 15.1 Introduction

There are various reactions that may follow in the weeks after an adverse life event. Many of the psychiatric disorders considered in the other chapters of this book may be triggered by an adverse life event, but this chapter considers reactions that are necessarily and primarily caused by an adverse life event. Not all reactions to an adverse life event are psychiatric disorders – consider, for example, bereavement. But all reactions are nonetheless clinically important for mainly the following reasons: people present to clinicians with them, clinicians have to understand and distinguish among these reactions in making a differential diagnosis and clinicians potentially have the clinical abilities to help people deal with these reactions irrespective of whether the reactions are psychiatric disorders or not.

The reactions to adverse life events on which the chapter will focus are:

- adjustment disorder
- bereavement
- acute stress disorder
- brief psychotic disorder (with a marked stressor), and
- culture-specific reactions in the southern African context.

There is an endless list of potential adverse life events, but Table 15.1 is helpful to appreciate the scope and nature of adverse life events.

## 15.2 Differential diagnoses of acute reactions to adverse life events

The reactions to adverse life events that we consider in this chapter are the following:

- An adjustment disorder is a reaction to a non-life-threatening adverse event or psychosocial stressor, usually with depressive and/or anxiety features, that causes

**Table 15.1** Examples of adverse life events

| Life-threatening adverse events | Non-life-threatening adverse events |
|---|---|
| natural disaster | the death of a significant other |
| bodily assault | severe illness of a significant other |
| threat of being killed or seriously injured | falling seriously ill |
| rape or sexual assault | separation or divorce from a spouse |
| motor vehicle accident | separation from a close family member |
| torture | termination of a significant relationship |
| war | major breach of trust in a relationship (e.g. infidelity) |
| trapped in a fire | losing one's livelihood, property or employment |
| animal attack (dog, wild cat, crocodile, snake, etc.) | a significant threat to one's livelihood, property or employment |

significant distress and/or functional impairment.

- Bereavement is the ordinary reaction to the death of a significant other and entails various distressing emotions, patterns of thinking, behaving and relating to others.
- Acute stress disorder is a reaction to a life-threatening event, which entails mainly anxiety and dissociative features.
- A brief psychotic disorder may be caused by an adverse event irrespective of whether it is life-threatening or not, and presents mainly with delusions and/or psychotic hallucinations (American Psychiatric Association, 2013).
- A culture-specific reaction may present as any one of these conditions or may fit into none of them.

The following aspects are critical to distinguish one reaction to an adverse life event from another: if the reaction to the adverse life event presents with psychotic features, then by definition it cannot be an adjustment disorder, a mere bereavement, an acute stress disorder or merely a culture-specific reaction. Whether the adverse life event is life-threatening typically differentiates an adjustment disorder from an acute stress disorder. If the adverse life event is the death of a significant other, it is by definition not an adjustment disorder. See Table 15.2 for a summary of these comparisons.

## 15.2.1 Adjustment disorder

The main features of an adjustment disorder are depressive features and/or anxiety features and/or disturbance of conduct.

Depressive features include tearfulness, sadness, feelings of hopelessness, insomnia, loss of appetite and energy, anhedonia, death ideation, suicidal ideation and behaviour.

Anxiety features include palpitations, jitteriness, agitation, insomnia, excessive concerns and worries.

Conduct disturbances include irritability, aggression and irresponsible behaviour.

The disorder begins within three months of an identifiable non-life-threatening adverse event or stressor(s) and persists for no longer than six months once the stressor(s) has terminated. It is specified as acute when it lasts less than six months and as chronic when it lasts longer.

In addition to distinguishing between an adjustment disorder and other reactions to adverse life events (see Table 15.2), it should also be distinguished from a major depressive episode (Despland *et al.*, 1995). A major depressive disorder takes precedence over an adjustment disorder. Both disorders may appear in the wake of an adverse life event. When a patient presents with symptoms caused by a non-threatening adverse event or stressor, a key clinical distinction between an adjustment disorder and a major depressive episode relates to

**Table 15.2** Differentiating features of reactions to adverse life events

| | **Psychotic features** | **Life-threatening event** | **Non-life-threatening event or psychosocial stressor** | **Following the death of a significant other** |
|---|---|---|---|---|
| **Adjustment disorder** | no | not typical | yes | no |
| **Bereavement** | no | no | yes | yes |
| **Acute stress disorder** | no | yes | no | not principally |
| **Brief psychotic disorder** | yes | possible | possible | possible |
| **Culture-specific reaction** | then not *merely* a culture-specific reaction, but necessarily a disorder too | possible | possible | possible |

the daily duration of the symptoms. Most symptoms of a major depressive episode are present most of the time each day and for most days; whereas most symptoms of an adjustment disorder do not adhere to this pattern (Van Staden and Kruger, 2002). Table 15.3 provides a comparison between the clinical features of the two disorders. Making this distinction is important as it determines the appropriate management and prognosis.

## 15.2.2 Bereavement

Bereavement is a culturally influenced, emotional and behavioural reaction to the death of a significant other, commonly referred to as grief. It is not a psychiatric disorder but may complicate into a major depressive episode or some other psychiatric disorder. It is typically self-limiting and may include feelings of intense sadness, rumination about the loss, insomnia, poor appetite and weight loss. It may include wishes to be dead and even suicidal ideation. The fifth edition of the Diagnostic and Statistical Manual of Mental Disorders (DSM-5) has recognised that bereavement usually lasts for one to two years (in most cultures), and has accepted that a major depressive episode can be diagnosed even during the first few weeks of bereavement, provided the diagnostic criteria are met (American Psychiatric Association, 2013).

When the following features are present after the death of a significant other, a major depressive episode should be considered in addition to the bereavement:

- catatonia
- psychomotor retardation that persists for days
- psychotic features (note the cautionary note in the next paragraph)
- morbid preoccupation with worthlessness of oneself
- the depressive thoughts are not about or not related to the deceased person.

Softer indications of a major depressive episode co-morbid with bereavement are prolonged and marked global functional impairment and/or a previous major depressive episode in circumstances other than bereavement.

If psychotic features present after the death of a significant other, a major depressive disorder with psychotic features or a psychotic disorder (including a possible brief psychotic disorder) should be considered. Note, however, that transient perceptions in which the deceased is heard, seen, smelled or felt are typical of bereavement and should not be regarded as psychotic experiences. Feelings of guilt about the death of the significant other should usually also not be construed as psychotic. In other words, disturbance of perceptions and thoughts should be about other things or people before they usually qualify as indicating psychosis in a bereaved patient.

## 15.2.3 Acute stress disorder

Most people do not develop an acute stress disorder following a life-threatening event. An acute stress disorder appears within four weeks and usually within a few days of the life-threatening event. Some patients suffer from persistent symptoms beyond one month in duration, in which case the diagnosis then changes to a post-traumatic stress disorder. Acute stress disorder may occur in response to an event that was directly experienced or witnessed or was experienced by another person in a significant relationship with the afflicted person.

The event involves actual or threatened death or serious injury or a threat to a person's physical integrity. During the event or thereafter, the person may experience dissociative symptoms such as a subjective sense of numbing, **detachment**, absence of emotional responsiveness, feeling 'in a daze', derealisation, depersonalisation or an inability to recall important aspects of the event. The traumatic event is persistently **re-experienced** through recurrent images, thoughts, dreams, **flashback** episodes, a sense of reliving the experience or distress on exposure to reminders of the event. The afflicted person shows marked avoidance of stimuli that arouse recollections of the event through thoughts, feelings, conversations, activities, places and/or people. He or she usually suffers from marked

**Table 15.3** Comparing clinical features of an adjustment disorder (with depressed mood) and a major depressive episode

| Symptom | | Major depressive episode | Adjustment disorder with depressed mood |
|---|---|---|---|
| **Depressed emotion** | **Duration** | ▶ necessarily more than 50% of the time | ▶ not necessarily more than 50% of the time<br>▶ likely less than 50% of the time |
| | **Diurnal variation** | ▶ more likely<br>▶ usually worse in the morning | ▶ unlikely<br>▶ usually worse later in the day |
| | **Content** | ▶ not necessarily about the adverse event<br>▶ also about other things<br>▶ poverty of thought may be present | ▶ necessarily and predominantly about the adverse event<br>▶ no poverty of thought |
| | **Intensity of emotion** | ▶ may be very intense or blunted | ▶ may be very intense, but unlikely to be blunted |
| **Anhedonia** | | ▶ necessarily more than 50% of time | ▶ not necessarily more than 50% of time<br>▶ likely less than 50% of time<br>▶ some interests or pleasurable activities remain |
| **Energy** | | ▶ usually lacking more than 50% of time | ▶ level of energy may be preserved<br>▶ if level of energy is reduced, likely less than 50% of the time |
| **Insomnia** | | ▶ any stage, most nights | ▶ more often during initial stage<br>▶ rarely early morning awakening<br>▶ not usually every night |
| **Feelings of guilt** | **Content** | ▶ also about things unrelated to adverse event | ▶ about things related to adverse event |
| | **Extent** | ▶ may be delusional | ▶ never delusional |
| | **Duration** | ▶ usually most of the time | ▶ likely less than 50% of time |
| **Psychomotor functions** | | ▶ may be impaired, even catatonic | ▶ at worst, only briefly affected (hours), never catatonic |
| **Weight** | | ▶ may be changed | ▶ may be changed |
| **Appetite** | | ▶ may be changed, usually most of the time | ▶ may be changed, but usually not every day |
| **Death or suicide ideation** | **Content** | ▶ not necessarily about the adverse event<br>▶ also about other things | ▶ usually about the adverse event |
| | **Intent or lethality** | ▶ may be very serious or high risk | ▶ may be very serious or high risk |
| **Concentration** | | ▶ may be objectively impaired<br>▶ most of the time | ▶ usually only subjectively impaired<br>▶ not most of the time |
| **Psychotic features** | | ▶ may be present | ▶ never |
| **Severity** | | ▶ more | ▶ less (e.g. less than five of nine criteria of a major depressive episode) |
| **Global functioning** | | ▶ necessarily and more significantly impaired | ▶ less impaired and likely to be less than half of the time |

anxiety or increased arousal such as insomnia, irritability, poor concentration, hypervigilance, exaggerated startle response or motor restlessness (American Psychiatric Association, 2013).

Acute stress disorder is distinguished from post-traumatic stress disorder in that the duration of an acute stress disorder is less than one month after a life-threatening event. Besides the other reactions to adverse life events (see Table 15.2), consider co-morbid disorders such as borderline personality disorder, dissociative disorders, factitious disorder, other anxiety disorders as well as alcohol and other substance use disorders. **Malingering** and a head injury should also be considered in a differential diagnosis.

## 15.2.4 Brief psychotic disorder (with a marked stressor)

Brief psychotic disorder is an illness characterised by the acute onset of at least one of the following positive psychotic symptoms: delusions, hallucinations, disorganised speech or grossly disorganised behaviour. The episode lasts at least one day, but less than one month, with eventual full remission of all symptoms (American Psychiatric Association, 2013).

The specifier 'With marked stressor' is used when the brief psychotic disorder occurs in response to an adverse life event or major stressor such as the loss of a loved one, domestic strife, employment problems, accidents, the psychological trauma of combat or other serious life stressors. These events, either singly or together, would be markedly stressful to almost anyone in similar circumstances in that person's culture. If a brief psychotic disorder occurs within one month postpartum it may also be specified as 'With postpartum onset'.

Associated features include the experience of emotional turmoil or overwhelming confusion. The level of impairment may be severe and patients with the disorder may be a danger to themselves or others. There appears to be an increased risk of suicide in younger patients. Brief psychotic disorder appears to be an uncommon condition. It is seen more often among persons with personality disorders (especially schizotypal, histrionic and borderline personality disorder). (See Chapter 11: Schizophrenia spectrum and other psychotic disorders, for further information on brief psychotic disorder.)

## 15.2.5 Cultural-specific reactions to adverse life events in the southern African context

Being necessarily embedded in culture, all of the reactions to adverse life events described above may be expected to have cultural content. Also, what counts as an adverse life event is, among other things, culturally influenced. For example, news that a traditional Xhosa man might be infertile may be devastating for him and result in an adjustment disorder. It might also present as an acute stress disorder or even as a brief psychotic disorder when the news is experienced as life-threatening. The appropriateness of conduct in bereavement depends on the culture within which the patient lives. The appropriate period of mourning, for example, varies among cultures, and in some cases last for more than a year.

A patient's culture can both protect against the effect of an adverse life event and also increase its likelihood. One may even consider 'culturogenic' reactions to adverse life events whereby certain cultural beliefs, values and practices are likely to increase the number of adverse life events to which the individual is exposed (Helman, 2000). For example, pursuit of the cultural value and expectation of 'keeping up with the Joneses' may lead to excessive debt and the eventual shattering loss of both esteem and property when the latter is re-possessed.

Certain folk beliefs in cultures, held in varying degrees, may be associated with reactions to adverse life events. Examples include beliefs of bad luck associated with Friday the 13th and reported experiences related to ghosts, aliens or elves. Also, the tokoloshe (described as a short man with magical powers sent to afflict others) in southern African folklore may be associated with presentations of emotional distress in some patients (Hadley *et al.*, 1993). Other cultural constructs commonly described in southern Africa include experiences of adverse life events attributed to witchcraft, the violation of societal taboos and ancestral displeasure.

The brain fag syndrome, first reported among African-Americans (Prince, 1960), was also observed among Nigerian students. In the southern African context, it was reported in Swaziland (Guinness, 1992), among the Xhosa people of the Eastern Cape (Ensink and Robertson, 1996) where it is called *isimnyama esikolweni* (which can be translated as bad luck or bewitchment at school), and in Limpopo Province (Peltzer *et al.*, 1998). It presents in the context of pressure to perform academically in school. The predominant symptoms are complaints of being unable to see the book or paper, the afflicted person's eyes being red or sore. Headaches are common. A few diviners have reported that their clients may present with difficulty in hearing, dizziness, weak fingers, and heart palpitations.

Case series of patients who present with acute anxiety and emotional distress following a culturally based realisation that they have been bewitched or that they have violated a sexual taboo have been described (Weiss, 2004; Madigoe and Weiss, 2004). Depending on the clinical picture, such presentations may or may not be classifiable as conditions such as acute stress disorder or adjustment disorder. The cultural context and meaning of such syndromes would nonetheless require attention in the clinical interface.

There are other commonly described southern African culture-bound 'syndromes' such as *amafufunyana* and *ukuthwasa*. These two kinds of experience do not arise necessarily as acute reactions to adverse life events, but they may. *Amafufunyana* is possession by evil spirits, which is believed to be caused by witchcraft. Those afflicted present acutely with hallucinations, disorganised and dissociative experiences as well as mood and anxiety features. *Ukuthwasa* is regarded as a calling by the ancestors to become a traditional healer. One aspect of ukuthwasa is its presentation with a variety of physical and psychological experiences, which may include anxiety, mood and dissociative experiences. Both *amafufunyana* and *ukuthwasa* may be difficult to distinguish from a psychotic episode. In some, but not all instances, *amafufunyana* and *ukuthwasa* may also be part of a psychotic episode. Congruently, in case it turns out to be a psychotic episode, an original cultural 'diagnosis' of *ukuthwasa* may be revised to become that of *ukuphambana* ('madness'). Neither *amafufunyana* nor *ukuthwasa* is necessarily a psychotic experience, however. Usually, their experiential aspects are dissociative and not psychotic in nature.

As illustrated by the above examples, patients who are affected by an adverse life event may present with disorders (such as those listed in the previous sections as defined by the DSM-5), or they may present with a culture-specific reaction: a recognised set of experiences and behaviour specific to their cultural context. Although some of these culture-specific reactions could resemble certain disorder defined in the DSM-5 or the International Classification of Diseases (ICD) to varying extents, the clinician should avoid the temptation to limit all clinical presentations to the labels proffered by these diagnostic classification systems (which could be termed diagnostic **reductionism**). Diagnostic reductionism could lead to an inaccurate representation of the condition as well as a clinical miscommunication with the patient, which could in turn undermine the therapeutic process.

The converse applies too. When a reaction to an adverse life event appears culture-specific in nature, that does not necessarily preclude the use of DSM or ICD diagnoses, including those listed above. A clinician who thinks dichotomously that a patient's condition is either a cultural condition or a psychiatric disorder will commit the clinical error of failing to make a critically important psychiatric diagnosis (and thereby failing to treat it appropriately) when it coincides with culture-specific reactions. The opposite mistake would be if the clinician does not account diagnostically for culture-specific aspects of a patient's presentation when a psychiatric disorder is diagnosed. (See Chapter 6: Culture and psychiatry, for further general discussion on cultural-specific reactions in the South African context.)

## 15.3 Management of reactions to adverse life events

The clinician should sensitively observe and enquire for the presence of the above reactions after a recent adverse life event, for it may be difficult for patients to reveal the adverse events and their reactions to them. The difficulty in, and hesitance about, talking about the adverse event and its related symptoms may already be an important clue, for this reticence may, in fact, be the manifestation of the avoidance symptoms that present in an acute stress disorder. A diagnosis should be reconsidered at subsequent consultations when emerging symptoms suggest so or when complications arise.

### 15.3.1 Practical crisis management

The safety of the patient and others is paramount in the practical crisis management of the above reactions to an adverse life event. Any of the reactions to an adverse life event attract a risk of suicide. Acute stress disorder pose a significant risk for suicide and the clinician should not infer that the risk for suicide is less simply because of a diagnosis of a disorder less severe than a major depressive disorder. The risk of suicide may be less apparent in a brief psychotic disorder owing to increased impulsivity, and the clinician should be sensitive for subtle cues. In a vulnerable individual, even bereavement may increase the risk for suicide.

Practical crisis management aims to assess the extent of the risk of suicide and harm to others and to then contain the risk by interventions appropriate to its extent. The clinician should seek the patient's participation in constructing a plan that would contain the risk. This may involve brief hospitalisation or the active involvement of the patient's social support network rather than leaving him or her alone (Greenberg *et al.*, 1995). If the patient is not hospitalised, regular consultations may form part of the plan to contain the risk. The particular risks and the availability of social support will determine how regular the consultations should be (which may even be daily). If there is a high risk of suicide and the patient is rendered incapable of making decisions pertaining to the management of the risk of suicide risk by the mental disorder, involuntary or assisted hospitalisation in terms of the Mental Health Care Act (No. 17 of 2002) should be considered. This is especially appropriate when a patient is suffering from a brief psychotic disorder.

Sedation may be appropriate if the risk to others or self is high, especially for a brief psychotic disorder. The clinician should, however, avoid sedation or hypnotics for other purposes, since their use delays the process of recovery in an adjustment disorder, bereavement and acute stress disorder (Forbes *et al.*, 2007a). Resorting to sedatives or hypnotics may be particularly tempting for the clinician and the patient in his or her desperation to numb the distress of these reactions, but they should be avoided as far as possible.

When there is a risk to the patient owing to a threat to his or her life, involving social services and/or the police should be considered. If there is such a threat, as may be the case in an imminent divorce or when the patient was victim of a criminal or civil offence, referring the patient for legal advice may also be appropriate.

### 15.3.2 Medication

A brief psychotic disorder should be treated with antipsychotic medication, beginning with a low dosage and continuing for at most a few months after recovery. Second-generation antipsychotic medication should pose less risk of extra-pyramidal side effects. A benzodiazepine may be an alternative, but clinicians should avoid using these for more than a few weeks.

Medication for the other reactions to an adverse life event plays at most an auxiliary role (Kavan *et al.*, 2012). Antidepressants have not been shown to be effective for an adjustment disorder with depressed mood, in contrast with a major depressive disorder for which an antidepressant is the mainstay of treatment.

While post-traumatic stress disorder is usually managed with antidepressant medication, these are not proven to be efficacious in acute stress disorder. If medication is used at all, it takes only an adjunctive place in the management of this disorder (Ursano *et al.*, 2004; Forbes *et al.*, 2007b). In general, medication should not be given in the first four weeks after a life-threatening event. Benzodiazepines are best avoided, because they may suppress the cognitive and emotional processing of the event, enhance avoidance behaviour, delay the recovery and even worsen the eventual outcome. The same applies for a bereavement reaction.

Although not adequately researched specifically for adjustment disorder, bereavement or an acute stress disorder, disruptive insomnia (for example, persisting for three consecutive days) may be treated adjunctively with a hypnotic like zolpidem or zopiclone.

## 15.3.3 Main therapeutic tasks

With medication playing at best an adjunctive role in adjustment disorder, bereavement and acute stress disorder, the clinician may feel without resources, especially when undervaluing the substantial worth of attending to the emotional needs of the patient and the provision of appropriate advice. The value of emotional support and psycho-education should not be underestimated or minimised (Ursano *et al.*, 2004; Forbes *et al.*, 2007a).

Emotional support should not be confused with psychotherapy. Psychiatrists and clinical psychologists may utilise an appropriate kind of psychotherapy that will extend beyond emotional support. Cognitive behavioural therapy (CBT) has been shown as being efficacious for acute stress disorder and adjustment disorder, and as being superior to supportive counselling (Bryant *et al.*, 1998; Bryant *et al.*, 1999; Bryant *et al.*, 2003; Forbes *et al.*, 2007a). However, a referral for psychotherapy may not be feasible considering the limited numbers and cost of psychiatrists and psychologists, as well as the large number of people who experience reactions to adverse life events. Emotional support should nonetheless be within the abilities of a generalist and primary care clinician.

### 15.3.3.1 Emotional support

The guiding objective in attending to the emotional needs of a patient who suffers from a reaction to an adverse life event is to create an opportunity for the adaptive integration of emotions with both the adverse life event and the subsequent challenges to his or her life and continued existence. A route to such integration is through the sharing of the story of the adverse life event and its consequences with another person.

The clinician may play an important role in facilitating this integration through adopting an attitude of sincere, profound and empathetic interest in the patient and how he or she experiences his or her situation. Practically, the patient should be given ample opportunity to tell about his or her situation while the clinician listens interestedly for as long and often as is required.

In the case of an acute stress disorder and a brief psychotic disorder, recounting a life-threatening event and ventilating feelings about it (as is often proposed in a so-called **debriefing**) should be approached with caution, since secondary trauma may result from the clinician's insistence or probing. Rather, the clinician should be sensitive and distinguish between patients who are ready and want to recount the life-threatening experience, those who are too distressed and impaired to do so and those who are not so inclined. Routine debriefings to prevent an acute stress disorder or a post-traumatic disorder should be discouraged: there are indications that these are ineffective and may worsen outcomes (Forbes *et al.*, 2007b).

The therapeutic telling of the story about the adverse life event and its consequences concerns not only matters of fact, but – critically important – the whole experience, including the inevitable upsetting emotions (typically anger, fear, sadness, turmoil, despair, attempts to avoid reminding stimuli or attempts to detach emotionally). If this is too overwhelming, it may be sensible to let the patient first talk about less distressing aspects of the adverse life event and then later introduce more distressing aspects.

Attending to the emotional needs of the patient who suffers from an adverse life event should preferably start when the patient presents during the first consultation – even before a diagnosis has been made. For this therapeutic purpose the clinician may initially postpone the systematic enquiry and deliberately avoid asking questions too soon. Instead, create the opportunity (or space) for the patient to talk openly about his or her experience of the adverse life event. If the patient wants to talk about the event, a genuinely interested remark like, 'I would like to hear what happened,' and, 'I wonder what it was like for you?' followed by an uninterrupted opportunity to talk may create just such an empathetic space.

Ideally, emotional support should not be a once-off event, but subsequent consultations should be offered. During further consultations, the empathetic space should be re-created (even if the clinician feels he or she already knows what happened). The difficulty is, after all, not merely with the factual content. Even when the patient does not take up the opportunity to talk about the event, the therapeutic space may be affirmed by, 'I wonder what it has been like for you since the event?' which would still invite emotional content, but at a less threatening stage emotionally.

The emotions that are brought about by the death of a significant other are well-known owing to the work of Elizabeth Kübler-Ross (Sadock and Sadock, 2007). The clinician's understanding and emotional support may be aided by expecting at least some of the usual reactions, these being shock and denial, anger, bargaining, depressive features, despair, guilt and, eventually, acceptance.

Emotional support entails also that the cultural beliefs of every patient affected by an adverse life event should be understood and explored emotionally in terms of their fit within their cultural framework. This should strengthen the therapeutic alliance with the patient and the therapeutic gains as well as help to ensure that salient clinical information relevant to a proper diagnostic assessment and formulation of a holistic management plan is not overlooked.

Sufficient consulting time to talk with the clinician should be scheduled as often as is needed by the patient. A patient without much social and emotional support may initially have to consult the clinician as often as daily, while weekly appointments may suffice for others.

The clinician may often find it challenging to provide emotional support, since many of the usual activities of the clinician, as well as the patient's expectations, may give priority to tangible interventions instead. Emotional support puts emotional demands on the clinician and may mean longer consultations.

Another factor that poses a challenge is the expectation of a prescription or medication. The clinician may be tempted to write a prescription as a way to terminate the consultation prematurely, especially when the emotional demands become too much. The clinician may also wrongly think that his or her clinical support is an inferior intervention when not accompanied by a prescription. The patient may expect a prescription simply because he or she has seen a physician. The patient may want antidepressants in the mistaken expectation that they will alleviate his or her depressive feelings, even when these feelings are not caused by a major depressive disorder.

These challenges require skilful management by the clinician.

### 15.3.3.2 Psycho-education and guidance: what the patient should and should not be told

**Provide hope**

Tell the patient that the upsetting emotions are usually transient and usually resolve within a month. Secondary to providing hope (Kavan *et al.*, 2012), reassure the patient of some safety in that the clinician and patient will jointly guard and act against further potential psychiatric complications.

**Say what would help**

Patients who are not too severely impaired and who do not suffer from a brief psychotic disorder may be encouraged to share their account of events and the subsequent emotions with trusted people in their circle of family and friends. Thus, say to these patients that it would help to share their experience. The patient could even ask a close relative or friend to kindly tolerate the re-telling of the story of the events again and again (within limits!).

#### Actively seek the support of relatives and/or friends

Discuss with the patient how to actively seek support from others more so than he or she usually does, considering his or her living circumstances, relationships with relatives and/or friends and whether they are in a position to support the patient. The purpose is for the patient to stay actively involved in his or her own life and to prevent social withdrawal and isolation or avoidance of dealing with the challenges that the adverse life event has brought about.

#### Say what would compromise recovery

Inform the patient about actions and behaviour that could compromise recovery. Advise the patient against social withdrawal and isolation. Advise also against the use of alcohol or other substances, emphasising that, although alcohol or other substances may apparently numb the distressing feelings and may appear to help with falling asleep, they are likely to delay recovery, disturb sleep architecture and counteract the restorative effects of sleep.

Explain to the patient that he or she is in a period during which his or her mental health is vulnerable more than usually to not only the adverse effects of alcohol but also to stressors. Additional stressors should be minimised by postponing making major decisions and by reducing responsibilities if at all feasible.

#### Do not dismiss or minimise symptoms

Clinicians may be tempted to reassure patients inappropriately that their reactions are 'normal' or understandable. This may suggest to patients that their distress is not serious, which may be very different from how they experience it, and for that reason be interpreted as not being empathic. By dismissing or minimising symptoms, furthermore, the clinician may disturbingly make an issue of whether a patient's reactions are normal, whereas the patient may have not doubted that until it was raised by the clinician. Doing so is ill-advised and may undermine recovery.

#### Do not give advice that reinforces avoidance

Exposure is key to recovery from reactions to life-threatening events, whereas avoidance maintains the symptoms. Advice that reinforces avoidance is therefore ill-advised. Examples of bad advice are, 'Try to forget about it and just go on with your life,' or, 'Go away for a while to get away from it all,' or, 'If you become anxious when you think about it, this sedative will calm you down.' Rather explain the limited role of medication (see Section 15.3.2) and the risks of prescribed and over-the-counter medication.

### 15.3.4 Preventing complications

Other than for emotional support, follow-up consultations should be scheduled with the patient to prevent complications. An adjustment disorder, a bereavement reaction and acute stress disorder may complicate into a major depressive disorder, substance misuse or abuse and even a brief psychotic disorder. An acute stress disorder may also complicate into a post-traumatic stress disorder when its symptoms persist for longer than a month.

A patient who suffers from a brief psychotic disorder or a post-traumatic stress disorder should ideally be referred to a psychiatrist for further management. Similarly, in situations where disruptive behaviour or the risk to the patient becomes too difficult to contain, a referral to, or consultation with, a psychiatrist is advisable.

## Conclusion

In approaching a person who experienced an adverse life event, a clinical examination should consider whether the reaction constitutes a potential mental disorder. Not all reactions to adverse life events are mental disorders, and some may present in a culture-specific way. A culture-specific presentation, however, does not preclude the diagnosis of a mental disorder.

A careful clinical examination should differentiate diagnostically between the reactions to an adverse life event. When an adverse event results in depressive features, the clinician should differentiate between an adjustment disorder with depressive features and a major depressive episode. This diagnostic precision is important for choosing appropriate interventions. For example, prescribing medication is appropriate for some reactions to adverse life events, but not all.

Clinicians should not underestimate the importance of emotional support, psycho-education and guidance as the mainstay of clinical care for most of the reactions to adverse life events. This means investing sufficient time with a patient and developing the requisite knowledge, skills and attitude for professionally competent health care in the aftermath of an adverse life event.

# References

American Psychiatric Association (2013) *Diagnostic and Statistical Manual of Mental Disorders* (5th edition). Arlington, VA: American Psychiatric Association

Bryant RA, Harvey AG, Dang ST, Sackville T, Basten C (1998) Treatment of acute stress disorder: A comparison of cognitive-behavioral therapy and supportive counselling. *Journal of Consulting and Clinical Psychology* 66 (5): 862–6

Bryant RA, Moulds ML, Nixon RV (2003) Cognitive behaviour therapy of acute stress disorder: A four-year follow-up. *Behaviour Research and Therapy* 41(4): 489–94

Bryant RA, Sackville T, Dang ST, Moulds M, Guthrie R (1999) Treating acute stress disorder: An evaluation of cognitive behavior therapy and supportive counseling techniques. *American Journal of Psychiatry* 156 (11): 1780–6

Despland JN, Monod L, Ferrero F (1995) Clinical relevance of adjustment disorders in DSM-III-R and DSM-IV. *Comprehensive Psychiatry* 36: 454–60

Ensink K, Robertson B (1996) Indigenous categories of distress and dysfunction in South African Xhosa children and adolescents as described by indigenous healers. *Transcultural Psychiatry* 33: 137–72

Forbes D, Creamer M, Phelps A, Bryant R, McFarlane AC, Devilly GJ, Matthews L, Raphael B, Doran C, Merlin T, Newton C (2007a) Australian guidelines for the treatment of adults with acute stress disorder and post-traumatic stress disorder. *Australian and New Zealand Journal of Psychiatry* 41: 637–48

Forbes D, Creamer MC, Phelps AJ, Couineau A-L, Cooper JA, Bryant RA, McFarlane AC, Devilly GJ, Matthews LR, Raphael B (2007b) Treating adults with acute stress disorder and post-traumatic stress disorder in general practice: A clinical update. *Medical Journal of Australia* 187: 120–3

Greenberg WM, Rosenfeld DN, Ortega EA (1995) Adjustment disorder as an admission diagnosis. *American Journal of Psychiatry* 152: 459–62

Guinness EA (1992) Social origins of the brain fag syndrome. *British Journal of Psychiatry* 16(Suppl): 53–64

Hadley GP, Bösenberg AT, Wiersma R, Grant H (1993) Needle implantation ascribed to 'tikoloshe'. *The Lancet* 342(8882): 1304

Helman C (2000) *Cultural Aspects of Stress. Culture, Health and Illness* (4th edition). London: Arnold

Kavan MG, Alsasser GN, Barone EJ (2012) The physician's role in managing acute stress disorder. *American Family Physician* 86: 643–9

Madigoe T, Weiss E (2004) The psychiatric sequelae of taboo sex. Paper presented at the Congress of the World Association of Social Psychiatry, Johannesburg, 22–26 March 2004

Peltzer K, Cherian VI, Cherian L, (1998) Brain fag symptoms in rural South African secondary school pupils. *Psychological Reports* 83: 1187–96

Prince R (1960) The 'brain fag' syndrome in Nigerian students. *British Journal of Psychiatry* 106: 559–70

Sadock BJ, Sadock VA (2007) Human development throughout the life cycle. In: Sadock BJ, Sadock VA (Eds). *Kaplan and Sadock's Synopsis of Psychiatry* (10th edition). Philadelphia: Lippincot Williams and Wilken

Ursano RJ, Bell C, Eth S, Friedman M, Norwood A, Pfefferbaum B, Pynoos RS, Zatnick DF, Benedek DM (2004) Practice guidelines for the treatment of patients with acute stress disorder and posttraumatic stress disorder. *American Journal of Psychiatry* 11(Suppl): 1–95

Van Staden CW, Krüger C (2002) 'I am depressed doctor': adjustment disorders in general practice. *The Medicine Journal/Geneeskunde* 44 (5): 10–3

Weiss E (2004) Witchcraft in forensic psychiatry. Paper presented at the Congress of the World Association of Social Psychiatry, Johannesburg, 22–26 March 2004

# CHAPTER 16 Trauma

Soraya Seedat, Belinda Bruwer

## 16.1 Introduction

World Trauma Day is commemorated on 17 October. South Africans of all socioeconomic classes are faced with traumatic experiences on a daily basis. The South African Burden of Disease study (Norman *et al.*, 2007), conducted in 2000, noted the exceptionally high burden of injuries in South Africa, especially injuries related to violence and road traffic accidents. These injuries contribute substantially to health care usage and cost. In addition to the high rates of injury-related deaths, trauma survivors exposed to a diverse range of traumas (e.g. interpersonal violence, accidents, natural disasters), are likely to present first to primary health care services for medical, surgical and psychological treatment of their injury-related sequelae. It is therefore crucial that medical students and doctors in South Africa have the requisite knowledge and skill to holistically manage patients with trauma-related presentations.

In the late 19th century, Pierre Janet and Sigmund Freud provided some of the first descriptions of the clinical manifestations of exposure to traumatic events in their writings on the aetiology of **hysteria**. They attributed hysteria largely to experiences of psychological trauma, particularly sexual trauma. Over the years, traumatic stress became a focus of attention, with descriptions of male soldiers negatively affected by the horrors of the World War I and II and the Vietnam War. Later, data from several studies of the mental health sequelae of combat trauma and other forms of interpersonal violence led to the inclusion of trauma and post-traumatic stress disorder (PTSD) in the DSM-III (Diagnostic and Statistical Manual of Mental Disorders, 3rd edition) in 1980 (American Psychiatric Association, 1980). The DSM-III classified trauma as an event that was 'outside the range of usual human experience' (American Psychiatric Association, 1980). PTSD was described as a normative response to an abnormal event that the individual had experienced or witnessed. This reflected the notion that traumatic events were rare. In the DSM-IV (American Psychiatric Association, 1994) and DSM-IV Text Revision (American Psychiatric Association, 2000), definitions of trauma and PTSD were revised. Trauma was considered to be more ubiquitous and a wide range of events (e.g. car accidents, learning about the death of a loved one, natural disasters) were recognised as traumatogenic. Furthermore, PTSD was considered as a pathological anxiety response (i.e. an anxiety disorder) characterised by 'intense fear, horror, or helplessness' (American Psychiatric Association, 1994; American Psychiatric Association, 2000) in the immediate aftermath of an event. This immediate response was accompanied by a symptom set comprising re-experiencing, avoidance and hyperarousal disturbances associated with distress and, often devastating, functional impairment.

## 16.2 What is trauma?

Globally, millions of people are exposed to traumatic events during their lifetime and suffer a range of trauma-related reactions of variable intensity and duration that are not necessarily abnormal. However, in a percentage of people exposed to a profoundly threatening event, a range of persisting psychopathological reactions may occur. Acute stress disorder (ASD) and PTSD are common sequelae in the aftermath of trauma and are psychiatric conditions associated with severe distress and/or functional impairment. These disorders are no longer categorised as anxiety disorders in the DSM-5 but are grouped in a new category known as trauma- and stressor-related disorders, in which the onset of every disorder is preceded by exposure to a traumatic or otherwise adverse environmental event. This category of trauma- and stressor-related disorders includes adjustment disorders, reactive attachment disorder, disinhibited social engagement disorder, other specified trauma- and stressor-related disorders and unspecified trauma- and stressor-related disorders.

Traumatic events can broadly be divided into two categories: interpersonal traumas and non-interpersonal traumas. Interpersonal traumas are traumas that involve interactions between individuals, such as sexual and physical abuse and intimate partner violence, while natural disasters are an example of non-interpersonal traumas. Individuals with interpersonal trauma histories are at a higher risk of experiencing interpersonal traumas again in the future. This is known as revictimisation and is especially applicable to individuals with a history of childhood maltreatment (Classen *et al.*, 2005).

## 16.2.1 Traumatic experiences

The following is a non-exhaustive list of traumatic experiences adapted from the National Child Traumatic Stress Network (2008):

- sexual abuse or assault: actual or attempted sexual contact, exposure to age-inappropriate sexual material or environment, sexual exploitation, unwanted or coercive sexual contact
- physical abuse or assault: actual or attempted infliction of physical pain with or without the use of an object or weapon, including severe corporal punishment
- emotional abuse/psychological maltreatment: including verbal abuse, emotional abuse, emotional neglect, intentional social deprivation and even excessive demands on a child's performance that may lead to negative self-image and disturbed behaviour
- neglect: failure by the caregiver(s) to provide needed age-appropriate care, including physical, medical or educational neglect, although financially able to do so or offered financial or other means to do so
- serious accident or illness/medical procedure: unintentional injury or accident, having a physical illness or experiencing medical procedures that are extremely painful and/or life threatening
- victim of, or witness to, domestic violence: exposure to emotional abuse, actual or attempted physical or sexual assault or aggressive control perpetrated between a parent or caregiver or adolescent and another adult in the home environment
- victim of, or witness to, community violence: extreme violence in the community, including exposure to gang-related violence
- school violence: violence that occurs within a school setting
- natural or man-made disasters: major accident or disaster that is an unintentional result of a natural or man-made event
- forced displacement: forced relocation to a new home due to political reasons, generally including political asylum seekers or immigrants fleeing political persecution
- war or terrorism or political violence: exposure to acts of war, terrorism or political violence, including incidents such bombing, shooting, looting or accidents that are a result of terrorist activity as well as actions of individuals acting in isolation if they are considered political in nature
- victim of, or witness to, extreme personal or interpersonal violence: including extreme violence by or between individuals, exposure to homicide, suicide and other similar extreme events
- traumatic grief or separation: death of a parent, primary caregiver or sibling, abrupt and/or unexpected, accidental or premature death or homicide of a close friend, family member or other close relative, abrupt,

unexplained and/or indefinite separation from a parent, primary caretaker or sibling due to circumstances beyond the victim's control
- system-induced trauma: traumatic removal from the home, traumatic foster placement, sibling separation or multiple placements in a short amount of time.

The fifth edition of the DSM (DSM-5) (American Psychiatric Association, 2013) has further revised the definition of trauma and the criteria set for PTSD. The DSM-5 defines trauma as death, threatened death, actual or threatened serious injury or actual or threatened sexual violence, which includes direct exposure, witnessing in person, indirect exposure (by learning from a close friend or relative) and repeated or extreme indirect occupational exposure (e.g. first responders who are repeatedly exposed to body parts and professionals who are repeatedly exposed to details of child abuse) (referred to as Criterion A in the DSM-5). A diagnosis of PTSD requires exposure to a traumatic event that meets these specific stipulations. Among all psychiatric disorders, PTSD represents a unique psychiatric condition because of the essential requirement of the aetiological agent – the traumatic event. The traumatic event is experienced (either objectively or subjectively) as a threat to life or bodily integrity or as a threat to the life or bodily integrity of a caregiver or family member (American Psychiatric Association, 2000), and the individual's capacity to process and integrate the fearful emotional response to the event is diminished. Several factors have been identified to play a role in increasing vulnerability to PTSD, as we discuss later in the chapter.

## 16.3 Acute stress disorder

Acute stress disorder refers to an acute stress reaction within the first four weeks after exposure to a traumatic event and is characterised by dissociative, re-experiencing, avoidance, negative mood and hyperarousal symptomatology. Symptoms typically begin immediately post-trauma and persist for at least three days and up to one month. The first-line treatment of ASD is trauma-focused CBT (cognitive behaviour therapy).

If the aforementioned symptoms last longer than four weeks, then a diagnosis of PTSD must be made (American Psychiatric Association, 2013).

Note: See Chapter 15: Acute reactions to adverse life events, for a further discussion of acute stress disorder.

## 16.4 Post-traumatic stress disorder

### 16.4.1 Introduction

Descriptions such as 'shell shock' and 'battle fatigue' were used to describe stress-related syndromes in World War I and II. It was only after the Vietnam War that psychiatrists systematically documented a stress-related disorder with a delayed onset and chronic course. Even though this condition was initially referred to as post-Vietnam syndrome, other professionals working in the trauma field described similar phenomena in victims of rape, natural disasters and the Holocaust. The inclusion of PTSD in the DSM-III provided validation of the diagnosis and filled an important gap as war veterans were able to receive treatment from the Veterans Administration as well as service-related disability payments.

The DSM-IV-TR diagnostic criteria for PTSD included a history of exposure to a traumatic event and symptoms from each of three symptom clusters: intrusive recollections, avoidant or numbing symptoms and **hyper-arousal** symptoms. A fifth criterion concerned the duration of symptoms (at least one month) and a sixth criterion required that PTSD symptoms must cause significant distress or functional impairment. In the DSM-5, a fourth symptom cluster (negative alterations in cognition and mood) has been added to the three symptom clusters mentioned above. All of these symptoms must have begun or worsened since the trauma.

## 16.4.2 Epidemiology

Rates of traumatic exposure and PTSD vary depending on the population studied (Edwards, 2005). The prevalence of PTSD is much higher in populations such as refugees, soldiers and rape survivors than in the general population.

In South Africa, PTSD remains a significant public health concern. This is against the backdrop of high rates of domestic and criminal violence. In the general adult population in the USA, the lifetime prevalence rate of PTSD is in the range of 6,8%–12,3% and one-year prevalence is in the range of 3,5%–6%. The lifetime prevalence of PTSD in the South African adult general population is 2,3% (Herman *et al.*, 2009). In a study of 1 050 black and white women who visited a general practitioner, 21,5% reported experiencing domestic violence, while PTSD was diagnosed in 35% of those exposed to domestic violence (Marais *et al.*, 1999). In a Xhosa-speaking population attending a primary health care clinic, 94% reported at least one traumatic life event and 20% of participants met the criteria of PTSD during the time of the study (Carey *et al.*, 2003). Trauma exposure and PTSD rates are remarkably high in adolescent populations, with more than 80% of adolescents reporting exposure to traumatic events and rates of PTSD in the range of 19–22% (Seedat *et al.*, 2004; Suliman *et al.*, 2005). In an earlier study in township children (10–16 years) in the Western Cape, all children experienced indirect exposure to significant violent events, with 56% experiencing direct violence and 17–27% meeting criteria for PTSD (Ensink *et al.*, 1997).

Although men experience more potentially traumatic events than women, women are more likely to develop PTSD than men. After traumatic exposure, about 20% of women and 8% of men develop PTSD. These gender differences are not explained by the likelihood of exposure or the type of event. Reasons that might explain the difference include gender differences in the appraisal of the traumatic event, gender differences in the perceptions of threat and the severity of exposure as well as gender differences in neurobiological and psychosocial characteristics.

## 16.4.3 Aetiology

In contrast to most other psychiatric disorders, PTSD has a clearly identifiable aetiological trigger. As not everyone exposed to a severe traumatic stressor develops PTSD, biological (e.g. genetic) factors, psychosocial factors, cultural, risk and resilience factors as well as the characteristics and proximity of the traumatic stressor can influence whether an individual develops PTSD. Over the past decade, there has been a greater emphasis on resilience, which is more than an absence of risk and represents an ability to bounce back after adversity.

The following risk factors may place someone at increased risk of being exposed to traumatic events: male gender, lower educational level, childhood history of conduct problems, family history of psychiatric illness, extroversion and **neuroticism**.

### 16.4.3.1 Nature and timing of the traumatic stressor

Interpersonal stressors (rape and violent assault), sudden and unexpected life-threatening events and exposure to death are more likely to result in the development of PTSD than accidental traumas or natural disasters. For women, rape and childhood physical abuse have the highest probability of giving rise to PTSD. Risk factors have been examined at different time points relative to the trauma. These include pre-trauma risk factors (factors before the trauma that make an individual more vulnerable to developing PTSD once they are exposed to trauma), peri-trauma risk factors (factors around the time of the trauma) and post-trauma risk factors (factors after the event that serve to increase risk) (Brewin *et al.*, 2000).

Pre-trauma risk factors for developing PTSD when exposed to traumatic events include female gender, younger age, neuroticism, lower intellectual capacity (intelligence quotient), lower socioeconomic class, pre-existing mood and anxiety disorders, previous PTSD, a history of mood, anxiety disorders or substance abuse disorders in family as well as non-specific central nervous system function abnormalities (neurological soft signs). Individuals with PTSD have increased neurological soft signs that are indicative of subtle nervous system dysfunction. In addition, they have more developmental problems, suggesting that these pre-existing impairments in neurodevelopment may serve as risk factors for the development of PTSD (Gurvits *et al.*, 2000).

Peri-traumatic factors include trauma severity, dissociative responses such as feeling disconnected from one's body or experiencing the traumatic event in slow motion, greater perceived life threat and the uncontrollability or unpredictability of the trauma.

Post-trauma risk factors include low social support and subsequent life stress. It is important to note that peri-traumatic and post-traumatic risk factors have a much stronger role in the development of PTSD than pre-trauma risk factors (Brewin *et al.*, 2000).

### 16.4.3.2 Psychobiological alterations in PTSD

A number of psychobiological alterations have been documented in PTSD. Firstly, the risk for PTSD is heavily influenced by genetic factors, as evidenced by data from family and twin studies. Genetic risk factors account for 30–40% of the heritability for PTSD. Several of the biological endophenotypes of PTSD, such as decreased hippocampal volume and exaggerated amygdala activity, may also be genetically heritable. Another example is cognitive ability, which has a strong genetic determinant. Increased cognitive ability seems to be associated with less trauma exposure and may be a protective factor against the development of PTSD. In addition, genetic and epigenetic variations in genes that code for stress responses in key neurobiological systems have been found in trauma-exposed individuals who develop PTSD. Family studies have also provided evidence for the intergenerational effects of stress, trauma and PTSD. Early developmental factors are also critical: individuals with a history of early childhood adversity exhibit sensitisation of both neuro-endocrine and autonomic stress responses that place them at much higher risk of developing PTSD (Yehuda and LeDoux, 2007).

Psychobiological alterations in PTSD involve both the central and autonomic nervous systems. These include, among others, the hypothalamic-pituitary-adrenal, noradrenergic, serotonergic, glutamatergic, thyroid and endogenous opioid systems. The hypothalamic-pituitary-adrenal axis and sympathetic nervous system appear to be hyper-responsive in PTSD. It is of interest that the biology of the acute stress response contrasts with that in chronic PTSD. While the acute stress response is characterised by glucocorticoid release and elevated peripheral cortisol levels, adult trauma survivors with PTSD have been found to have low ambient cortisol levels.

In PTSD there is an impairment of the normal checks and balances on amygdala activation (Charney, 2004; Vermetten and Bremner, 2002), such that the dampening-down influence of the amygdala on the medial prefrontal cortex (especially the anterior cingulate gyrus and orbitofrontal cortex) is impaired. Structural brain imaging studies of adults with PTSD have found reduced volumes of the hippocampus and the anterior cingulate, while functional brain imaging studies have documented excessive amygdala activity and reduced activation of the prefrontal cortex and hippocampus. Flashbacks of the traumatic events and associated increased physiological arousal may be explained by an underactive medial prefrontal cortex and/or an overactive amygdala. The over-reactivity of the amygdala results in recurrent fear conditioning, whereby ambiguous stimuli are more likely to be appraised as threatening. The mechanisms for extinguishing fear responses are disrupted and key limbic nuclei are sensitised which, in turn, lowers the threshold for fearful reactivity (Charney *et al.*, 1993).

Another region of the limbic system that is abnormal in PTSD is the hippocampus. The hippocampus is vital for autobiographical memory function. Elevated cortisol levels in response to stress may be neurotoxic and underlie the hippocampal atrophy seen in PTSD. Notably, reversal of neurotoxicity can be achieved with treatment that promotes neurogenesis. For example paroxetine, a selective serotonin reuptake inhibitor (SSRI), has been shown to increase hippocampal volume in PTSD patients (Vermetten *et al.*, 2003). The question is whether the reduced hippocampal volume is a consequence of PTSD or represents as a vulnerability marker for PTSD in individuals who are exposed to trauma. Twin studies have found hippocampal volume reduction to be a vulnerability factor for the development of PTSD in individuals exposed to trauma.

In summary, neurobiological changes identified in individuals with PTSD probably represent a combination of markers of neural risk for the development of PTSD following exposure to extreme stress and abnormalities that are acquired through exposure to trauma (Sherin and Nemeroff, 2011).

## 16.4.4 Clinical features

Most individuals exposed to trauma will manifest distress upon exposure to reminders of the event, especially in the days and weeks after the trauma. Patients with PTSD, however, repeatedly experience significant affective, cognitive and behavioural reactions to reminders of the traumatic event in the form of nightmares, flashbacks, intense anxiety and fight-or-flight behaviour; these symptoms persist over a prolonged period. Patients with PTSD attempt to compensate by avoiding stimuli that may trigger this hyperarousal, leading to reduced interest in daily activities, numbing of emotions and feeling detached from others. The symptom burden goes hand-in-hand with significant distress and impairment in social, occupational and interpersonal functioning. A diagnosis of PTSD is warranted if the duration of the aforementioned disturbance lasts more than four weeks (American Psychiatric Association, 2013).

## 16.4.5 Diagnosis

During the development of the DSM-5, the idea of a distinct category of disorders that was preceded or precipitated by an identifiable environmental stressor was conceptualised. PTSD, acute stress disorder, and adjustment disorders have been included in this category of trauma- and stressor-related disorders (Friedman *et al.*, 2011). In order to make a diagnosis of PTSD the patient must, in addition to a history of exposure to a traumatic event, present with symptoms from each of four symptom clusters: **intrusion**, avoidance, negative alterations in cognition and mood and alterations in arousal and reactivity. These symptoms must have been present for at least one month, be associated with distress or functional impairment and not be attributable to a substance or co-occurring medical condition. Two specifications to the diagnosis are stipulated: 'With dissociative symptoms' and 'With delayed onset'. These criteria apply to adults, adolescents and children older than six. A preschool subtype has been added to the DSM-5 for children younger than six.

The DSM-5 criteria for PTSD are listed in Table 16.1.

A subtype that has long been described but has not found its way into the DSM-5 is complex PTSD (complex trauma). Complex PTSD often refers to PTSD that results from exposure to long-term trauma (e.g. exposure to multiple or prolonged traumatic events in childhood or adulthood), often within a primary caregiving system or social environment, that impacts on development and leads to a complex mix of behavioural and emotional symptoms (Van der Kolk, 2005; Van der Kolk *et al.*, 2009; Blumenfeld, *et al.*, 2010). Other types of trauma associated with complex PTSD include exposure to long-term domestic violence, organised child exploitation rings and prisoner-of-war experience. Patients with complex PTSD have pervasive difficulties that are additional to the conventional PTSD symptom criteria.

Complex PTSD is characterised by deficits in attachment and forming trusting relationships, prominent dissociative symptoms, difficulties with emotional regulation (e.g. persistent sadness, suicidal thoughts and explosive anger outbursts) and self-perception (e.g. helplessness, shame, guilt, stigma, a sense of being completely different from others), and distorted perceptions of the perpetrator (e.g. preoccupation with relationship with the perpetrator, attributing total power to the perpetrator and preoccupation with revenge).

**Table 16.1** DSM-5 Diagnostic Criteria for Posttraumatic Stress Disorder

| Diagnostic Criteria |
|---|
| **Posttraumatic Stress Disorder**<br>**Note:** The following criteria apply to adults, adolescents, and children older than 6 years. For children 6 years and younger, see corresponding criteria below.<br>A. Exposure to actual or threatened death, serious injury, or sexual violence in one (or more) of the following ways:<br>1. Directly experiencing the traumatic event(s).<br>2. Witnessing, in person, the event(s) as it occurred to others.<br>3. Learning that the traumatic event(s) occurred to a close family member or close friend. In cases of actual or threatened death of a family member or friend, the event(s) must have been violent or accidental.<br>4. Experiencing repeated or extreme exposure to aversive details of the traumatic event(s) (e.g., first responders collecting human remains: police officers repeatedly exposed to details of child abuse).<br>**Note:** Criterion A4 does not apply to exposure through electronic media, television, movies, or pictures, unless this exposure is work related.<br>B. Presence of one (or more) of the following intrusion symptoms associated with the traumatic event(s), beginning after the traumatic event(s) occurred:<br>1. Recurrent, involuntary, and intrusive distressing memories of the traumatic event(s).<br>**Note:** In children older than 6 years, repetitive play may occur in which themes or aspects of the traumatic event(s) are expressed.<br>2. Recurrent distressing dreams in which the content and/or affect of the dream are related to the traumatic event(s).<br>**Note:** In children, there may be frightening dreams without recognizable content.<br>3. Dissociative reactions (e.g., flashbacks) in which the individual feels or acts as if the traumatic event(s) were recurring. (Such reactions may occur on a continuum, with the most extreme expression being a complete loss of awareness of present surroundings.)<br>**Note:** In children, trauma-specific reenactment may occur in play.<br>4. Intense or prolonged psychological distress at exposure to internal or external cues that symbolize or resemble an aspect of the traumatic event(s).<br>5. Marked physiological reactions to internal or external cues that symbolize or resemble an aspect of the traumatic event(s).<br>C. Persistent avoidance of stimuli associated with the traumatic event(s), beginning after the traumatic event(s) occurred, as evidenced by one or both of the following:<br>1. Avoidance of or efforts to avoid distressing memories, thoughts, or feelings about or closely associated with the traumatic event(s).<br>2. Avoidance of or efforts to avoid external reminders (people, places, conversations, activities, objects, situations) that arouse distressing memories, thoughts, or feelings about or closely associated with the traumatic event(s).<br>D. Negative alterations in cognitions and mood associated with the traumatic event(s), beginning or worsening after the traumatic event(s) occurred, as evidenced by two (or more) of the following:<br>1. Inability to remember an important aspect of the traumatic event(s) (typically due to dissociative amnesia and not to other factors such as head injury, alcohol, or drugs).<br>2. Persistent and exaggerated negative beliefs or expectations about oneself, others, or the world (e.g., "I am bad," "No one can be trusted," 'The world is completely dangerous," "My whole nervous system is permanently ruined").<br>3. Persistent, distorted cognitions about the cause or consequences of the traumatic event(s) that lead the individual to blame himself/herself or others.<br>4. Persistent negative emotional state (e.g., fear, horror, anger, guilt, or shame).<br>5. Markedly diminished interest or participation in significant activities.<br>6. Feelings of detachment or estrangement from others.<br>7. Persistent inability to experience positive emotions (e.g., inability to experience happiness, satisfaction, or loving feelings). |

E. Marked alterations in arousal and reactivity associated with the traumatic event(s), beginning or worsening after the traumatic event(s) occurred, as evidenced by two (or more) of the following:
   1. Irritable behavior and angry outbursts (with little or no provocation) typically expressed as verbal or physical aggression toward people or objects.
   2. Reckless or self-destructive behavior.
   3. Hypervigilance.
   4. Exaggerated startle response.
   5. Problems with concentration.
   6. Sleep disturbance (e.g., difficulty falling or staying asleep or restless sleep).

F. Duration of the disturbance (Criteria B, C, D, and E) is more than 1 month.

G. The disturbance causes clinically significant distress or impairment in social, occupational, or other important areas of functioning.

H. The disturbance is not attributable to the physiological effects of a substance (e.g., medication, alcohol) or another medical condition.

*Specify* whether:

**With dissociative symptoms:** The individual's symptoms meet the criteria for posttraumatic stress disorder, and in addition, in response to the stressor, the individual experiences persistent or recurrent symptoms of either of the following:

1. **Depersonalization:** Persistent or recurrent experiences of feeling detached from, and as if one were an outside observer of, one's mental processes or body (e.g., feeling as though one were in a dream; feeling a sense of unreality of self or body or of time moving slowly).
2. **Derealization:** Persistent or recurrent experiences of unreality of surroundings (e.g., the world around the individual is experienced as unreal, dreamlike, distant, or distorted).

**Note:** To use this subtype, the dissociative symptoms must not be attributable to the physiological effects of a substance (e.g., blackouts, behavior during alcohol intoxication) or another medical condition (e.g., complex partial seizures).

*Specify* if:

**With delayed expression:** If the full diagnostic criteria are not met until at least 6 months after the event (although the onset and expression of some symptoms may be immediate).

**Posttraumatic Stress Disorder for Children 6 Years and Younger**

A. In children 6 years and younger, exposure to actual or threatened death, serious injury, or sexual violence in one (or more) of the following ways:
   1. Directly experiencing the traumatic event(s).
   2. Witnessing, in person, the event(s) as it occurred to others, especially primary caregivers.

   **Note:** Witnessing does not include events that are witnessed only in electronic media, television, movies, or pictures.

   3. Learning that the traumatic event(s) occurred to a parent or caregiving figure.

B. Presence of one (or more) of the following intrusion symptoms associated with the traumatic event(s), beginning after the traumatic event(s) occurred:
   1. Recurrent, involuntary, and intrusive distressing memories of the traumatic event(s).

   **Note:** Spontaneous and intrusive memories may not necessarily appear distressing and may be expressed as play reenactment.

   2. Recurrent distressing dreams in which the content and/or affect of the dream are related to the traumatic event(s).

   **Note:** It may not be possible to ascertain that the frightening content is related to the traumatic event.

   3. Dissociative reactions (e.g., flashbacks) in which the child feels or acts as if the traumatic event(s) were recurring. (Such reactions may occur on a continuum, with the most extreme expression being a complete loss of awareness of present surroundings.) Such trauma-specific reenactment may occur in play.
   4. Intense or prolonged psychological distress at exposure to internal or external cues that symbolize or resemble an aspect of the traumatic event(s).
   5. Marked physiological reactions to reminders of the traumatic event(s).

C. One (or more) of the following symptoms, representing either persistent avoidance of stimuli associated with the traumatic event(s) or negative alterations in cognitions and mood associated with the traumatic event(s), must be present, beginning after the event(s) or worsening after the event(s):

**Persistent Avoidance of Stimuli**

1. Avoidance of or efforts to avoid activities, places, or physical reminders that arouse recollections of the traumatic event(s).
2. Avoidance of or efforts to avoid people, conversations, or interpersonal situations that arouse recollections of the traumatic event(s).

**Negative Alterations in Cognitions**

3. Substantially increased frequency of negative emotional states (e.g., fear, guilt, sadness, shame, confusion).
4. Markedly diminished interest or participation in significant activities, including constriction of play.
5. Socially withdrawn behavior.
6. Persistent reduction in expression of positive emotions.

D. Alterations in arousal and reactivity associated with the traumatic event(s), beginning or worsening after the traumatic event(s) occurred, as evidenced by two (or more) of the following:

1. Irritable behavior and angry outbursts (with little or no provocation) typically expressed as verbal or physical aggression toward people or objects (including extreme temper tantrums).
2. Hypervigilance.
3. Exaggerated startle response.
4. Problems with concentration.
5. Sleep disturbance (e.g., difficulty falling or staying asleep or restless sleep).

E. The duration of the disturbance is more than 1 month.

F. The disturbance causes clinically significant distress or impairment in relationships with parents, siblings, peers, or other caregivers or with school behavior.

G. The disturbance is not attributable to the physiological effects of a substance (e.g., medication or alcohol) or another medical condition.

*Specify* whether:

**With dissociative symptoms:** The individual's symptoms meet the criteria for posttraumatic stress disorder, and the individual experiences persistent or recurrent symptoms of either of the following:

1. **Depersonalization:** Persistent or recurrent experiences of feeling detached from, and as if one were an outside observer of, one's mental processes or body (e.g., feeling as though one were in a dream; feeling a sense of unreality of self or body or of time moving slowly).
2. **Derealization:** Persistent or recurrent experiences of unreality of surroundings (e.g., the world around the individual is experienced as unreal, dreamlike, distant, or distorted).

**Note:** To use this subtype, the dissociative symptoms must not be attributable to the physiological effects of a substance (e.g., blackouts) or another medical condition (e.g., complex partial seizures).

*Specify* if:

**With delayed expression:** If the full diagnostic criteria are not met until at least 6 months after the event (although the onset and expression of some symptoms may be immediate).

**Source:** Reprinted with permission from the *Diagnostic and Statistical Manual of Mental Disorders*, Fifth Edition, (Copyright 2013). American Psychiatric Association.

Standard evidence-based treatments for PTSD are also effective for treating complex PTSD. It is imperative to address interpersonal difficulties and the specific disturbances mentioned above when treating complex PTSD (Roth *et al.*, 1997).

## 16.4.6 Assessment

As is the case with other anxiety disorders, patients with PTSD are more likely to reach out to their GP or primary health care provider

**Table 16.2** Primary Care PTSD Screen (PC-PTSD)

| In your life, have you ever had any experience that was so frightening, horrible, or upsetting that, **in the past month**, you: |
|---|
| 1. Have had nightmares about it or thought about it when you did not want to? |
| YES NO |
| 2. Tried hard not to think about it or went out of your way to avoid situations that reminded you of it? |
| YES NO |
| 3. Were constantly on guard, watchful, or easily startled? |
| YES NO |
| 4. Felt numb or detached from others, activities, or your surroundings? |
| YES NO |
| If a patient answers 'yes' to any three items on the PC-PTSD, he/she has screened positive. This means that a patient may have PTSD or trauma-related problems, and further assessment and referral (if indicated) may be warranted. |

**Source:** Prins *et al.*, 2003

than to a psychiatrist. Patients who present to primary health care with PTSD have higher medical utilisation rates and longer hospital stays than patients without PTSD in primary care (Friedman and Schnurr, 1995). In addition, they are more likely to be currently unemployed and to have marital problems.

Screening tools such as the Primary Care PTSD Screen (PC-PTSD) (Prins *et al.*, 2003) may be useful as an initial screening of symptoms (see Table 16.2). Patients who screen positive on the PC-PTSD should be explicitly screened for the presence of suicidality. Screening should be followed up with a comprehensive psychiatric assessment in any patient who presents with PTSD symptoms and/or a history of traumatic exposure. In administering the PC-PTSD it is useful to clarify whether the reported symptoms are indeed trauma-related and whether the reported symptoms are disruptive to the patient's life. It is also important to ascertain whether the traumatic event is ongoing in the patient's life and if there are ongoing threats to the patient's safety. If there are ongoing threats, also determine if reporting is legally required and provide the patient with information about local resources that he or she can access. It is also important to screen for co-morbid psychiatric disorders, substance use disorders and physical illnesses. If the patient does have active PTSD symptoms, referral to a mental health professional is indicated. In screening patients, it is important to acknowledge any reported distress and to show empathic support.

Note: Patients may be reluctant to talk about the trauma or about their symptoms.

There are a number of other measures that can be used to assess trauma exposure, such as the Life Event Checklist for DSM-5 (LEC-5) (Weathers *et al.*, 2013a) and the Traumatic Events Questionnaire (TEQ) (Vrana and Lauterbach, 1994). Measures that can be used in the case of PTSD symptoms include the Davidson Trauma Scale (DTS) (Davidson *et al.*, 1997) and the PTSD Checklist for DSM-5 (PCL-5) (Weathers *et al.*, 2013b). There is no single best measure for the assessment of trauma or PTSD. Trauma and PTSD symptom measures vary in their length, level of detail and complexity, range of traumas and symptoms assessed and the form of administration (whether they are self-reporting or administered by a clinician). All measures have psychometric strengths and weaknesses; some have been better validated than others. Structured interviews, such as the Clinician Administered PTSD Scale for DSM-5 (CAPS-5) (Weathers *et al.*, 2013c) and the Structured Interview for PTSD (SI-PTSD) (Davidson *et al.*, 1990) generally yield a more valid diagnostic assessment of PTSD than other types of measures. The CAPS-5 measure is considered as the gold standard in PTSD assessment but it is a structured interview that takes 45–60 minutes to administer.

## 16.4.7 Co-morbidity

Approximately 75% of patients with PTSD have a co-morbid psychiatric disorder. The risk of suicide attempts is also increased two- to three-fold by the presence of PTSD (Nepon *et al.*, 2010). Rates of co-morbidity are particularly high for major depressive disorder (MDD), other anxiety disorders, borderline personality disorder, attention-deficit hyperactivity disorder (ADHD), oppositional defiant disorder, alcohol dependence and other substance use disorders. While it is important to screen for substance use disorders in a patient with a history of trauma or a diagnosis of PTSD, it is just as important to ask about traumatic experiences in patients who present with substance use disorders. Patients often use substances as self-medication for their PTSD symptoms, while patients who abuse substances often expose themselves to situations that place them at a high risk of traumatic exposure. Traumatic brain injury, other physical illnesses such as asthma and ischaemic heart disease as well as somatisation disorders are more common in patients with PTSD than in those without PTSD. Patients who present with somatic symptoms should, therefore, be asked about trauma exposure.

## 16.4.8 Differential diagnosis

The following conditions are important to consider in arriving at a diagnosis:

- Acute stress disorder: symptoms are similar to PTSD following a significant trauma, but the duration is less than four weeks.
- Adjustment disorders: symptoms such as mood and anxiety and/or disturbed behaviour following a less traumatic stressor in terms of the direct danger that it poses to oneself or others. These symptoms rarely resemble acute stress disorder and PTSD.
- Obsessive-compulsive disorder (OCD): OCD is characterised by recurrent intrusive thoughts about current and future threats.
- Major depressive disorder: insomnia, irritability, decreased interest in activities, unable to envision one's future, sleep disturbance and anhedonia are some of the non-specific symptoms that may be present in patients with PTSD or/and major depressive disorder. These symptoms should not be attributed to PTSD if other, more specific, symptoms of PTSD are absent.
- Other anxiety disorders, e.g. panic disorder, phobic disorders. Panic attacks sometimes may occur for the first time in the context of a traumatic event or shortly thereafter. In other instances it may be present before the onset of PTSD, with panic disorder continuing on a course of its own. Panic attacks may also become incorporated into PTSD as a reaction to exposure to traumatic reminders with symptoms of both conditions present at the same time. This can create diagnostic confusion. It is important to note that panic attacks in panic disorder typically occur in a variety of settings and are not restricted to situations, activities or places that remind the patient of the traumatic event. The distinction between phobic disorders and PTSD is largely based on the reasons for avoidance behaviour (which are not limited to the reminders of the trauma in phobic disorders) and the presence of other characteristic symptoms of PTSD. It is important to note that the onset of both agoraphobia and PTSD may be keyed to the specific traumatic event. Generalised anxiety disorder, on the other hand, is characterised by excessive, daily worries about future threats and some overlap in the symptoms of autonomic hyperactivity evident in PTSD.
- Dissociative disorders: a number of dissociative disorders (e.g. dissociative amnesia, depersonalisation disorder and dissociative identity disorder) may be difficult to distinguish from PTSD, particularly when their onset is preceded by the trauma, as is often the case. The absence of other characteristics of PTSD suggests a dissociative disorder.
- Malingering: malingering should be considered in the differential diagnosis, particularly if there is a legal process under way or if the patient is facing criminal charges. The goals of malingering may be to avoid

punishment, shift the blame to someone else or to elicit sympathy. Suspect malingering if the patient appears to exaggerate his or her symptoms and distress, when the clinical presentation is inconsistent or unusual or when there is a significant underlying personality disturbance.

## 16.4.9 Course and prognosis

The course of PTSD is quite variable and relapse is common. A third of patients will have a chronic course. In the US National Comorbidity Survey (Kessler *et al.*, 1995), there was a pattern of early disappearance of symptoms (within one year) in the majority of individuals with PTSD. The rates decreased sharply after this time, with an overall recovery rate of 60%. Thus, recovery rates tend to decline sharply one to two years after onset. One of the most important predictors of the course of PTSD is symptom duration – the longer the duration of symptoms, the less the likelihood of recovery. Similar rates of recovery (up to 66% of patients) have been reported in other studies (Blanchard *et al.*, 1997; Shalev *et al.*, 1997).

New traumas and negative life events can reactivate symptoms or exacerbate current symptoms. Patients with PTSD may also have a low tolerance for stressful situations and may have difficulty adjusting to any novelty or life change. They may react to these situations with anger or impulsive behaviour, by further withdrawal or by using alcohol, illicit drugs and medication such as benzodiazepines.

Chronic PTSD is associated with occupational problems, poor social support, increased rates of disability and suicidality as well as with a higher rate of intimate relationship difficulties. A substantial proportion of patients with chronic PTSD have a deteriorating course, with additional complications (most commonly depression, substance abuse or substance dependence), lasting impairments in several areas of functioning, greater likelihood of cardiovascular, respiratory, gastrointestinal and neurological disease and risky health behaviours (e.g. cigarette smoking).

An early appearance and long duration of symptoms is an indicator of poorer outcome.

War-related traumas and traumas related to physical and sexual assault are generally associated with a poorer prognosis than traumas associated with traffic accidents and natural disasters. Other factors associated with a poorer prognosis include female gender, early developmental (childhood) trauma, a history of other anxiety disorders, mood disorders, substance use disorders, co-occurring medical conditions and poor social support or social instability.

## 16.4.10 Treatment of PTSD

In treating patents, it is important to bear in mind that PTSD is a disorder with biological, psychological, social and cultural causes and implications. Trauma-focused CBT is an effective first-line therapy for the treatment of PTSD. The most effective form of CBT is prolonged exposure therapy (PE). Other effective approaches include cognitive processing therapy (CPT) and eye movement desensitisation and reprocessing (EMDR). The benefits of psychotherapy persist in the long-term, and studies show that benefits are maintained up to one to 10 years after treatment. For patients with PTSD who also have co-morbid depression, psychotherapy may be less effective than pharmacotherapy and, in this instance, pharmacotherapy could be used as a first-line treatment. If pharmacotherapy is used, begin with one of the first-line options which include a SSRI, such as fluoxetine, paroxetine or sertraline, or the serotonin-noradrenaline reuptake inhibitor (SNRI) venlafaxine extended release (XR) (SASOP Guidelines, Seedat, 2013).

### 16.4.10.1 Psychotherapy

**Prolonged exposure therapy**

Trauma-focused CBT in the form of exposure therapy has the best evidence for efficacy in PTSD. CBT is generally short-term, averaging 8–12 sessions in total, held once or twice a week. Patients are asked to relive the trauma in their imagination and describe the event and their thoughts and feelings during the traumatic event. Repeated imaginal exposure in a safe therapeutic environment typically leads to a decrease in distress when thinking or talking about the trauma. The therapist assists the patient to gradually confront fearful situations until distress is reduced, thereby addressing the avoidance behaviour associated with PTSD.

An interesting recent development is virtual reality exposure therapy, which is a technology-assisted CBT intervention where traumatic memories are stimulated via a head-mounted computer display. Internet-based therapist-assisted CBT (ICBT) is also increasingly being investigated for its efficacy in PTSD.

**Cognitive processing therapy (CPT)**

CPT combines cognitive therapy and written accounts of the trauma. During CPT, the patient writes a detailed account of the incident, which is read during consultation and at home. Thoughts and feelings triggered by reading the account are examined and problematic beliefs about themes (such as safety, control and intimacy) are challenged and corrected.

**Eye movement desensitisation and reprocessing**

Eye movement desensitisation and reprocessing (EMDR) is a manualised therapy that uses eye movements or other dual-attention stimuli to facilitate the kind of emotional processing that is needed to resolve traumatic memories and stress management/coping skills training (i.e. stress inoculation training or SIT).

### 16.4.10.2 Pharmacotherapy

PTSD treatment is aimed at reducing symptoms such as intrusive thoughts or images, avoidance, hyperarousal, hypervigilance, depression, anger and irritability (SASOP Guidelines, Seedat, 2013). Response to pharmacotherapy may be variable and polypharmacy is not uncommonly used in general psychiatric practice to treat persistent PTSD symptoms.

**Selective serotonin reuptake inhibitors**

SSRIs are considered first-line medication for PTSD treatment. It is advisable to start with a low dose and to increase slowly until a response or maximum tolerable dose is reached. Patients may need high doses of SSRIs: start with 20 mg paroxetine/fluoxetine/citalopram and increase with 10–20 mg after three to four weeks of no or minimal clinical response, up to 60 mg/day if needed. Give six to eight weeks on the maximum tolerable dose for an adequate trial before considering changing or augmenting medication. If there is no response to the first antidepressant, then consider switching to a second-line antidepressant, such as mirtazapine.

**Serotonin-noradrenaline reuptake inhibitors**

Although the evidence is less than for SSRIs, venlafaxine XR has been found to be more effective than placebo in reducing PTSD symptoms in a few studies.

> **Important:** All patients with PTSD who are a suicidal risk and all adolescents and young adults started on an antidepressant should be warned of, and closely monitored for, the emergence of suicidal ideation, suicidal behaviour and akathisia. Antidepressants may be particularly helpful in patients with PTSD with moderate to severe co-morbid depression National Institute for Clinical Excellence (NICE) Guidelines, 2005).

**Alpha-adrenergic receptor blockers**

Alpha-adrenergic receptor blockers, such as prazosin, may be useful in reducing nightmares and insomnia in PTSD patients. Orthostatic hypotension is a problematic side effect and medication should therefore be initiated at 1mg at night and slowly increased to 3–10 mg. Advise patients never to discontinue prazosin abruptly because of the risk of rebound hypertension.

**Atypical antipsychotics**

Evidence for the use of atypical antipsychotics as augmentation agents for SSRI/SNRI treatment is limited. However, some patients do seem to benefit from adjunctive use of atypical antipsychotics such as risperidone and olanzapine if the PTSD symptoms are persistent despite SSRI/SNRI treatment. There are a few, small trials to support this. The suggested starting dose of risperidone is 0,5 mg with weekly increases until adequate response or a maximum of 4 mg/day. Discontinue the medication slowly if there is no clinical improvement in PTSD symptoms after two to three weeks.

**Benzodiazepines and hypnotics**

Benzodiazepines and hypnotics should be used with caution and close monitoring in patients with acute or chronic PTSD owing to their risk of abuse and dependence.

### 16.4.10.3 Combining psychotherapy and pharmacotherapy

The benefit of combining psychotherapy and medication for PTSD is not known and requires further study.

### 16.4.10.4 Early intervention: can PTSD be prevented?

Several studies have assessed early intervention strategies (both psychological and pharmacological) for the prevention of PTSD. Meta-analyses do not support the use of either single session or multiple session psychological debriefing for the prevention of PTSD (or for symptom reduction) in the early aftermath of trauma. In fact, forcing people to talk about their experiences so soon after a traumatic event may negatively impact on recovery. Similarly, early use of benzodiazepines is not beneficial, and can increase the risk of developing PTSD. However, providing emotional, social and practical support to trauma survivors, ensuring that they are medically stable and providing a safe, secure environment where there is someone (such as a family member) available to talk to, if the patient expresses the wish to do so, can be helpful (NICE Guidelines, 2005). In addition, initial screening of patients is preferable so that preventive interventions can be administered to those individuals who may have difficulty recovering on their own.

Meta-analyses have also shown that multiple session trauma-focused CBT (TF-CBT) therapy in patients with ASD or acute PTSD is beneficial. In contrast, data on the benefits of pharmacotherapy (e.g. propranolol, SSRIs, pregabalin, gabapentin) for the prevention of PTSD have been disappointing and, to date, most pharmacotherapy studies have indicated no preventive benefit.

### 16.4.10.5 Summary

- Psychological debriefing in the immediate aftermath of a traumatic event should be avoided.
- High-risk patients (e.g. patients who are suicidal, need medical attention or lack social support) should be managed appropriately.
- If a person has mild symptoms that last less than four weeks, watchful waiting and follow-up within one month should be arranged.
- Routine use of a screening instrument for PTSD can help in the timeous identification of patients who require treatment (NICE Guidelines, 2005).
- If the patient shows severe post-traumatic symptoms (acute stress disorder symptoms) in the first four weeks, individual outpatient trauma-focused CBT by a competent professional should be offered.
- Individual, outpatient trauma-focused CBT (at least 8–12 sessions) by a competent professional is the treatment of choice for patients with PTSD.
- Trauma-focused CBT is a first-line treatment for PTSD. If extreme fear and avoidance are the prominent symptoms, exposure therapy is indicated. If extreme guilt and distrust is prominent, cognitive therapies may be more helpful. If there is no improvement after eight sessions, consider switching to another evidence-based CBT modality.
- Pharmacotherapy (SSRIs or SNRIs) can be considered if the patient has co-morbid depression, refuses psychotherapy, does not respond to trauma-focused CBT, or if CBT is not available.
- Start with a low dose, increase medication gradually and be prepared to end with a higher dose (SSRIs) if needed.

- Duration of effective medication treatment is at least 12 months to reduce the risk of relapse, after which treatment can be gradually discontinued if the decision is made to stop treatment (SASOP guidelines, Seedat, 2013; NICE Guidelines, 2005).
- If an adequate trial of monotherapy (psychotherapy or pharmacotherapy) fails, consider switching to the other modality or a combination of psychotherapy (exposure therapy) and pharmacotherapy if only a partial response to SSRIs or SNRIs (SASOP guidelines, Seedat, 2013).

## Conclusion

Exposure to trauma is common and the development of PTSD in those who have been exposed to trauma can have devastating consequences, particularly if the disorder goes unrecognised and untreated. Primary health care providers should have the basic skills and knowledge to manage trauma survivors effectively in the aftermath of trauma, and should be able to attend to the patient's immediate physical and mental health needs. This includes screening high-risk patients for the development of ASD and PTSD and referring, as needed. Debilitating symptoms of PTSD can potentially be prevented or limited if clinicians are able to diagnose and intervene in a timely manner.

# References


American Psychiatric Association (1980) *Diagnostic and Statistical Manual of Mental Disorders* (3rd edition). Arlington, VA: American Psychiatric Publishing. Washington, DC

American Psychiatric Association (1994) *Diagnostic and Statistical Manual of Mental Disorders* (4th edition). Arlington, VA: American Psychiatric Association

American Psychiatric Association (2000) *Diagnostic and Statistical Manual of Mental Disorders* (4th edition). Text Revision. Arlington, VA: American Psychiatric Association

American Psychiatric Association (2013) *Diagnostic and Statistical Manual of Mental Disorders* (5th edition). Arlington, VA: American Psychiatric Association

Blanchard EB, Hickling EJ, Forneris CA, Taylor AE, Buckley TC, Loos WR, Jaccard J, (1997) Prediction of remission of acute posttraumatic stress disorder in motor vehicle accident victims. *Journal of Traumatic Stress* 10(2): 215–34

Blumenfeld S, Groves BM, Rice KF, Weinreb M, (2010) *Children and trauma: A curriculum for mental health clinicians.* Chicago: The Domestic Violence and Mental Health Policy Initiative

Brewin CR, Andrews B, Valentine JD (2000) Meta-analysis of risk factors for posttraumatic stress disorder in trauma-exposed adults. *Journal of Consulting and Clinical Psychology* 68(5): 748–66

Carey D, Stein DJ, Zungu-Dirwayi N, Seedat S (2003) Trauma and post-traumatic stress disorder in an urban Xhosa primary care population. *Journal of Nervous and Mental Disease* 19: 230–6

Charney DS (2004) Psychobiological mechanisms of resilience and vulnerability: Implications for the successful adaptation to extreme stress. *American Journal of Psychiatry* 161: 195–216

Charney DS, Deutch AY, Krystal JH, Southwick SM, Davis M (1993) Psychobiologic mechanisms of posttraumatic stress disorder. *Archives of General Psychiatry* 50: 295–305

Classen CC, Palesh OG, Aggarwal R (2005) Sexual revictimization: A review of the empirical literature. *Trauma Violence & Abuse* 6(2): 103–29

Davidson JRT, Book SW, Colket JT, Tupler LA, Roth S, David D, Hertzberg M, Mellman T, Beckham JC, Smith R, Davison RM, Katz R, Feldman M (1997) Assessment of a new self-rating scale for post-traumatic stress disorder. *Psychological Medicine* 27: 153–60

Davidson JRT, Kudler HS, Smith RD (1990) Assessment and pharmacotherapy of posttraumatic stress disorder In: Giller JEL (Ed). *Biological assessment and treatment of posttraumatic stress disorder.* Washington DC: American Psychiatric Press

Edwards D (2005) Post-traumatic stress disorder as a public health concern in South Africa. *Journal of Psychology in Africa* 15(2):125–34

Ensink K, Robertson BA, Zissis C, Leger P (1997) Post-traumatic stress disorder in children exposed to violence. *South African Medical Journal* (97): 1526–30

Friedman MJ, Resick PA, Bryant RA, Strain J, Horowitz M, Spiegel MD (2011) Review: Classification of trauma and stressor-related disorders in DSM-5. *Depression and Anxiety* 28: 737–49

Friedman MJ, Schnurr PP (1995) The relationship between trauma, post-traumatic stress disorder, and physical health In: Friedman MJ, Charney DS, Deutch AY (Eds) *Neurobiological and clinical consequences of stress: From normal adaptation to post-traumatic stress disorder.* Philadelphia: Lippincott Raven

Gurvits TV, Gilbertson MW, Lasko NB, Tarhan AS, Simeon D, Macklin ML, Orr SP, Pitman RK (2000) Neurologic soft signs in chronic posttraumatic stress disorder. *Archives of General Psychiatry* 57(2):181–6

Herman AA, Stein DJ, Seedat S, Heeringa SG, Moomal H, Williams DR (2009) The South African Stress and Health (SASH) study: 12-month and lifetime prevalence of common mental disorders. *South African Medical Journal* 99(5 Part 2): 339–44

Kessler RC, Sonnega A, Bromet E, Hughes M, Nelson CB (1995) Posttraumatic stress disorder in the National Comorbidity Survey. *Archives of General Psychiatry* 52(12): 1048–60

Marais A, De Villiers PJT, Mšller AT, Stein DJ (1999) Domestic violence in patients visiting general practitioners: Prevalence phenomenology and association with psychopathology. *South African Medical Journal* 89: 635–40

National Child Traumatic Stress Network (2008) *Child Welfare Trauma Training Toolkit*. DOI: http://wwwnctsnetorg/nccts/navdo?pid=ctr_cwtool (Accessed: 20 August 2010)

National Institute for Clinical Excellence (NICE). Clinical Guideline 26: *The management of PTSD in adults and children in primary and secondary care* (2005) DOI: wwwniceorguk/CG026NICEguideline (Accessed 7 October 2014)

Nepon J, Belik SL, Bolton J, Sareen J (2010) The relationship between anxiety disorders and suicide attempts: Findings from the National Epidemiologic Survey on Alcohol and Related Conditions. *Depression and Anxiety* 27: 791–8

Norman R, Matzopoulos R, Groenewald P, Bradshaw D (2007) The high burden of injuries in South Africa. *Bulletin of the World Health Organization* 85(9): 649–732

Prins A, Ouimette P, Kimerling R, Cameron RP, Hugelshofer DS, Shaw-Hegwer J, Thrailkill A, Gusman FD, Sheikh JI (2003) The primary care PTSD screen (PC-PTSD): development and operating characteristics. *Primary Care Psychiatry* 9: 9–14

Roth S, Newman E, Pelcovitz D, Van der Kolk B, Mandel FS (1997) Complex PTSD in victims exposed to sexual and physical abuse: Results from the DSM-IV field trial for Posttraumatic Stress Disorder. *Journal of Traumatic Stress* 10: 539–55

Seedat S (2013) Post-traumatic stress disorder In: Emsley RA, Seedat S (Eds) The South African Society of Psychiatrists (SASOP) Treatment Guidelines for Psychiatric Disorders. *South African Journal of Psychiatry* 19(3): 187–91

Seedat S, Nyamai C, Njenga F, Vythilingum B, Stein DJ (2004) Trauma exposure and post-traumatic stress symptoms in urban African schools: Survey in Cape Town and Nairobi. *British Journal of Psychiatry* 184: 169–175

Shalev AY, Freedman S, Peri T, Brandes D, Sahar T (1997) Predicting PTSD in trauma survivors: Prospective evaluation of self-report and clinician-administered instruments. *British Journal of Psychiatry* 170: 558–64

Sherin JE, Nemeroff CB (2011) Post-traumatic stress disorder: The neurobiological impact of psychological trauma. *Dialogues in Clinical Neuroscience* 13(3): 263–78

Suliman S, Kaminer D, Seedat S, Stein DJ (2005) Assessing post-traumatic stress disorder in South African adolescents: Using the child and adolescent trauma survey (CATS) as a screening tool. *Annals of General Psychiatry* 31 4(1): 2

Van der Kolk B (2005) Developmental trauma disorder: Towards a rational diagnosis for children with complex trauma histories. *Psychiatric Annals* 35: 401–8

Van der Kolk B, Pynoos R, Cicchetti D, Cloitre M, D'Andrea W, Ford J, Liebermann A, Putnam F, Saxe G, Spinazolla J, Stolbach B, Teicher M (2009) *Proposal to include a developmental trauma disorder diagnosis for children and adolescents in DSM-V*. DOI: http://wwwtraumacenterorg/ (Accessed 24 September 2010)

Vermetten E, Bremner JD (2002) Circuits and systems in stress. II. Applications to neurobiology and treatment in posttraumatic stress disorder. *Depression and Anxiety* 16: 14–38

Vermetten E, Vythilingam M, Southwick SM, Charney DS, Bremner JD (2003) Long-term treatment with paroxetine increases verbal declarative memory and hippocampal volume in posttraumatic stress disorder. *Biological Psychiatry* 54: 693–702

Vrana SR, Lauterbach D (1994) Prevalence of traumatic events and post-traumatic psychological symptoms in a nonclinical sample of college students. *Journal of Traumatic Stress* 7: 289–302

Weathers FW, Blake DD, Schnurr PP, Kaloupek DG, Marx BP, Keane TM (2013a) *The Clinician-Administered PTSD Scale for DSM-5 (CAPS-5)*. DOI: www.ptsd.va.gov (Accessed 7 October 2014)

Weathers FW, Litz BT, Keane TM, Palmieri PA, Marx BP, Schnurr PP (2013b) *The PTSD Checklist for DSM-5 (PCL-5)*. Scale available from the National Center for PTSD at www.ptsd.va.gov

Weathers FW, Blake DD, Schnurr PP, Kaloupek DG, Marx BP, Keane TM (2013c) *The Life Events Checklist for DSM-5 (LEC-5)*. Instrument available from the National Center for PTSD at www.ptsd.va.gov

Yehuda R, LeDoux J (2007) Response variation following trauma: A translational neuroscience approach to understanding PTSD. *Neuron* 56:19–32

CHAPTER

# 17 Obsessive-compulsive and related disorders

Dan Stein, Christine Lochner

## 17.1 Introduction

There is growing interest in the concept of a nosologically distinct spectrum of obsessive-compulsive spectrum disorders (OCSDs), as evidenced in the DSM-5 (and likely in the ICD-11), where for the first time there is a separate section on obsessive-compulsive and related disorders (OCRDs). The current chapter in the DSM-5 reflects increasing evidence of how these disorders are related to, and overlap with, one another in terms of a range of diagnostic validators. There also is evidence of the clinical utility of grouping these disorders together. There are some crucial differences in the phenomenology, psychobiological underpinnings and treatment approaches across the OCRDs, which will also be discussed in this chapter.

The disorders covered here are obsessive-compulsive disorder, body dysmorphic disorder, hoarding disorder, trichotillomania (hair-pulling disorder), excoriation (skin-picking) disorder and body-focused repetitive behaviour disorder. The other condition that will be covered is Tourette's disorder: although not included in the OCRD section of the DSM-5, it has strong links and/or overlap with obsessive-compulsive disorder. The phenomenology, psychobiology, and treatment of each will be discussed.

The ICD-11 chapter on OCRDs will likely also make reference to hypochondriasis and olfactory reference syndrome.

## 17.2 Obsessive-compulsive disorder

### 17.2.1 Introduction

In the DSM-IV, obsessive-compulsive disorder (obsessive-compulsive disorder) was categorised as one of the anxiety disorders, along with generalised anxiety disorder (GAD), panic disorder, specific phobia, social anxiety disorder (SAD) and post-traumatic stress disorder (PTSD). In the DSM-5, OCD now falls under a grouping of obsessive-compulsive and related disorders.

Although there is some controversy about the prevalence of obsessive-compulsive disorder, it is generally assumed that the prevalence of obsessive-compulsive disorder in adult samples is between 2–3% of the population (Fontenelle *et al.*, 2006; Ruscio *et al.*, 2010). In an early analysis of data from a global burden of disease study obsessive-compulsive disorder was found to be the 10th most disabling of all medical disorders (Murray and Lopez, 1996).

Generally, studies of obsessive-compulsive disorder in adults have found either an equal distribution of men and women, or a slight predominance of women with this disorder. Epidemiological studies indicate that three times as many pre-adolescent boys as girls are diagnosed with OCD, but that the incidence of obsessive-compulsive disorder in females increases markedly after puberty (Karno *et al.*,

1988; Weissman *et al.*, 1994). The typical age-of-onset of obsessive-compulsive disorder is late adolescence or early adulthood (American Psychiatric Association, 2000). More recently, it has been argued that the prevalence of childhood-onset OCD has been underestimated, and that childhood-onset obsessive-compulsive disorder may be at least as common as onset in late adolescence or adulthood (Geller, 2006). Patients with obsessive-compulsive disorder seek therapeutic help 7-17 years after the first occurrence of symptoms (Grabe *et al.*, 2000; Rasmussen and Eisen, 1992; Stein *et al.*, 1996). Some years may pass after the first professional contact and before the diagnosis of obsessive-compulsive disorder is made (Stengler *et al.*, 2013).

## 17.2.2 Phenomenology

Obsessive-compulsive disorder is characterised by obsessions and/or compulsions. Obsessions are defined as recurrent and persistent thoughts, urges or images that are experienced, at some time during the disturbance, as intrusive and unwanted and that usually cause marked anxiety or distress. The person attempts to ignore or suppress such thoughts, urges or images, or to neutralise them with some other thought or action (i.e. by performing a compulsion or ritual). Compulsions are defined as repetitive behaviour (e.g. hand washing, ordering, checking) or mental acts (e.g. praying, counting, repeating words silently) that the person feels driven to perform in response to an obsession, or according to rules that must be applied rigidly. The behaviour or mental acts are aimed at preventing or reducing anxiety or distress or preventing some dreaded event or situation; however, these behaviours or mental acts are not connected in a realistic way with what they are designed to neutralise or prevent, or are clearly excessive (American Psychiatric Association, 2013).

The obsessions or compulsions are time consuming (for example, take more than one hour a day) or cause clinically significant distress or impairment in social, occupational or other important areas of functioning. The obsessive-compulsive symptoms are not due to the direct physiological effects of a substance (e.g. a drug of abuse or medication) or a general medical condition.

The content of the obsessions or compulsions is not restricted to:

- the symptoms of another mental disorder (e.g. excessive worries about real life problems in generalised anxiety disorder, or a preoccupation with food or ritualised eating behaviour in an eating disorder, or hair pulling in trichotillomania)
- stereotypies in stereotypic movement disorder
- preoccupation with appearance in body dysmorphic disorder
- preoccupation with drugs in a substance use disorder
- preoccupation with having a serious illness in hypochondriasis
- preoccupation with sexual urges or fantasies in a **paraphilia** or compulsive sexual behaviour
- preoccupation with gambling or other behaviours in behavioural addictions or impulse-control disorders
- guilty ruminations in major depressive disorder
- paranoia or **thought insertion** in a psychotic disorder
- restricted and repetitive patterns of behaviour in pervasive developmental disorders.

The symptoms used to define obsessive-compulsive disorder are diverse and include a range of obsessions and compulsions. The predominant symptoms in obsessive-compulsive disorder have been well documented and include:

- concerns about contamination or illness, along with compulsive cleaning or washing
- sexual or religious concerns or preoccupations and related behaviours such as praying and checking
- obsessions with symmetry, ordering and neatness along with ordering and arranging
- harm-related or aggression-related worries with behaviour like checking.

OCD patients also sometimes present with so-called obsessional slowness. Importantly, at any one time, OCD patients may have symptoms from more than one of these symptom constellations (symptom clusters) and symptoms may evolve over time from one symptom cluster to another (Rasmussen and Tsuang, 1986; Rettew *et al.*, 1992).

The course of obsessive-compulsive disorder may be episodic or chronic (Ravizza *et al.*, 1997; Tukel *et al.*, 2007) with obsessive-compulsive disorder symptoms being chronic in approximately 50% of cases (Thomsen and Mikkelsen, 1995). There seems to be much continuity between the clinical presentation of obsessive-compulsive disorder in childhood and in adulthood (Lochner and Stein, 2003). For example, one study (Rapoport *et al.*, 1992) suggests that obsessive-compulsive symptoms typically changed over time but that almost all patients with obsessive-compulsive disorder experienced excessive washing and cleaning as their main symptomatology at some time. On the other hand, there may also be differences, for example, children are less likely to have abstract obsessions that precede their washing. Despite advances in the short-term treatment of obsessive-compulsive disorder, a substantial number of individuals remain significantly impaired by their symptoms over the longer term. It has been suggested that obsessive-compulsive disorder is chronic in approximately half of all cases (Thomsen and Mikkelsen, 1995). If untreated, obsessive-compulsive disorder is mostly chronic with varying intensity of symptoms (Perugi *et al.*, 1998; G Skoog and I Skoog, 1999). If treated, however, outcome may be improved: in a 40-year repeated-measures study of a cohort of 251 individuals treated for obsessive-compulsive disorder, the researchers found that improvement was observed in 83% of the sample (G Skoog and I Skoog, 1999). Notably, fewer than half had "recovered" from obsessive-compulsive disorder (20% no longer had symptoms and 28% had subclinical symptoms). Factors that influence course (i.e. as episodic or chronic) include age, gender and severity of childhood obsessive-compulsive disorder symptomatology (Ravizza *et al.*, 1997).

Obsessive-compulsive disorder commonly presents with psychiatric co-morbidity, with depression the most frequent co-morbid illness (Pigott *et al.*, 1994). Other common lifetime co-morbid diagnoses include social anxiety disorder, specific phobia and generalized anxiety disorder. Co-morbidity with post-traumatic stress disorder (PTSD) has also been shown (Huppert *et al.*, 2005). OCD patients also often present with other OCRDs (Lochner and Stein, 2010). There is also a range of personality disorders that may present in OCD patients, with those of cluster C-like dependent and avoidant personality disorders highly prevalent (Torres *et al.*, 2006).

There is much evidence that points to the relative heterogeneity of this disorder. Indeed, although the core symptoms of obsessive-compulsive disorder are remarkably consistent across cultures, its specific features and course varies (Leckman *et al.*, 2001; G Skoog and I Skoog, 1999). It is likely that this heterogeneity has confounded clinical and biological investigation. The current trend in research is to rather use subtypes (e.g. specific-symptoms subtypes, or early-onset obsessive-compulsive disorder) as more homogenous foci for study.

The specifier 'With poor insight' was introduced in the DSM-IV. However, insight varies to a large extent in obsessive-compulsive disorder patients and therefore the DSM-5 requires that the clinician assess and indicate whether the patient's OCD beliefs are characterised by:

- good or fair insight (the patient recognises that his or her OCD beliefs are definitely or probably not true, or that they may or may not be true)
- poor insight (the patient thinks his or her OCD beliefs are probably true)
- delusional beliefs (the patient is completely convinced that his or her OCD beliefs are true.

It has been argued that this change may improve differentiation between OCD beliefs (even delusional OCD) and psychotic disorders (Thomsen, 2013).

In the DSM-5, tic-related obsessive-compulsive disorder is identified as a subtype, and the clinician has to specify whether the patient has a lifetime history of a chronic tic disorder. Tic-related obsessive-compulsive disorder seems to be less responsive to SSRIs alone and may need augmentation with antipsychotic medication. There is an overlap between cases of early-onset obsessive-compulsive disorder and tic-related obsessive-compulsive disorder in the form of a significant male predominance and high co-morbidity rates of other developmental disorders (such as attention-deficit hyperactivity disorder or ADHD) (Thomsen, 2013).

### 17.2.3 Psychobiology

Current models of obsessive-compulsive disorder emphasise the role of cortical-striatal-thalamic-cortical (CSTC) circuits in obsessive-compulsive disorder. Disruption of these circuits is supported by a range of data, including descriptions of patients with neurological disorders and obsessive-compulsive disorder, structural and functional brain imaging and neuropsychological testing. CSTC function is mediated by neurotransmitters including serotonin, dopamine and glutamate, and there is also a range of evidence that such transmitters play an important role in OCD.

One important strand within the neurological literature refers to obsessive-compulsive disorder and tic disorders as resulting from post-streptococcal auto-immunity (Allen *et al.*, 1995). The term **paediatric auto-immune neuropsychiatric disorders associated with streptococcal infections (PANDAS)** refers to patients with tics and obsessive-compulsive symptoms induced by streptococcal infections (Leonard and Swedo, 2001). However, this area remains controversial: several researchers have argued that a range of neurological insults can lead to acute onset of obsessive-compulsive disorder and/or tics, and the term paediatric acute-onset neuropsychiatric syndrome (PAN) has been proposed.

### 17.2.4 Pharmacotherapy and psychotherapy

Cognitive behavioural therapy (CBT) and serotonin reuptake inhibitors (SRIs) are considered safe and effective first-line treatments for obsessive-compulsive disorder. Whether to recommend monotherapy (i.e. either CBT or a SRI) or combined treatment, will depend on a number of factors, including the nature and severity of the patient's symptoms, the nature of any psychiatric and medical co-morbidities, the availability of CBT, the patient's past treatment history, and costs (American Psychiatric Association, 2007).

CBT for obsessive-compulsive disorder should be implemented by an appropriately trained clinician. CBT is mostly delivered in individual sessions, but group and family therapy sessions may be helpful, if available. Expert consensus recommends 13–20 weekly sessions for most patients (American Psychiatric Association, 2007). Preferably, a complete trial of CBT should be followed by monthly booster sessions for three to six months. CBT on its own, if available, is recommended as initial treatment for an OCD patient who is not too severely ill to co-operate with this treatment modality, is willing to do the extensive work that CBT requires during and after sessions, can afford it financially or who prefers not to use medication (American Psychiatric Association, 2007). Importantly, as noted above, if treatment response to CBT is unsatisfactory, it may be augmented with a SRI.

CBT entails behavioural techniques such as **exposure and response prevention (ERP)** and cognitive techniques. ERP involves prolonged exposure to, or confrontation with, stimuli that evoke obsessional fear, along with instructions to not engage in the typically conducted compulsive ritual (i.e. response prevention). ERP is based on the principle of systematic desensitisation (i.e. the patient's distress and anxiety naturally subsides over time) making compulsive behaviours unnecessary. The efficacy of ERP in OCD patients is supported by a large body of treatment outcome research (Rosa-Alcázar *et al.*, 2008).

SRIs (clomipramine, citalopram, escitalopram, fluoxetine, fluvoxamine, paroxetine, and sertraline) have all been shown efficacious in obsessive-compulsive disorder. Because the selective SRIs have a less troublesome side-effect profile than the non-selective SRI clomipramine, these are preferred for a first medication trial. A SRI alone is recommended for a patient who is not able to co-operate with CBT, has previously responded well to a given drug or who prefers treatment with an SRI alone. In terms of SRI use, most patients will not experience substantial improvement until four to six weeks after starting medication. Medication doses may be titrated up in small increments during the first month of treatment or when little or no symptom improvement is seen within four weeks of starting medication. Increments may be to a maximum dose that is comfortably tolerated. Treatment should then be continued at this dose for at least six weeks before the treatment trial is considered a failure.

Approximately 40-60% of patients with obsessive-compulsive disorder do not show adequate response to SRIs (Bloch *et al.*, 2006; Erzegovesi *et al.*, 2001). Patients who do not respond to their first SRI (even at maximum doses), may have their medication switched to a different SRI. Evidence suggests that patients who do not respond to the first trial of an SRI may respond to a second (Math and Janardhan Reddy, 2007). Clomipramine (a serotonergic tricyclic antidepressant) is generally recommended when treatment with at least two SRIs have failed (Math and Janardhan Reddy, 2007). Alternatively, SRIs can be augmented with trials of different antipsychotic medications. Relatively low doses of antipsychotic agents are used (Dold *et al.*, 2013; Skapinakis *et al.*, 2007). If pharmacotherapy is successful, it should be continued for at least one to two years before gradual tapering is considered.

Combined treatment should be considered for patients with an unsatisfactory response to either CBT or an SRI alone. It has been suggested that when treatment is combined, CBT may delay or prevent relapse when SRI treatment is discontinued. Initial treatment with an SRI alone may reduce symptom severity to such an extent that patients are able to start with CBT at a later stage.

Other treatments for OCD include transcranial magnetic stimulation (TMS), deep brain stimulation (DBS) and intensive residential treatment.

## 17.3 Tourette's disorder

### 17.3.1 Introduction

Tourette's disorder (TD) was categorised under Childhood Disorders in the DSM-IV-TR (American Psychiatric Association, 1994). In the DSM-5 however, it is considered as one of the neurodevelopmental disorders.

Note: see Chapter 25: Impulse-control disorders, for Tourette's disorder in children and adolescents.

### 17.3.2 Phenomenology

Tourette's disorder is characterised by both multiple motor tics and one or more vocal tics that have been present at some time during the illness, although not necessarily concurrently. A tic is a sudden, rapid, recurrent, non-rhythmic motor movement or vocalisation. Motor tics are divided into simple motor tics (e.g. blinking, nose twitching, grimacing) and complex motor tics, involving several muscle groups producing apparently purposeful movements. Similarly, vocal tics can also be divided into simple vocal tics (e.g. grunting, coughing) and complex vocal tics, where entire words or phrases are produced. These can be socially inappropriate words (e.g. swearing) or repetitions of the same phrase or words (echolalia). Tics may change in character, frequency and intensity over relatively short periods (Bruun and Budman, 1996). Generally, tics are distressing and can lead to a significant disruption of social functioning and quality of life. The tics may wax and wane in frequency. Simple tics may be disguised or suppressed (Banaschewski *et al.*, 2003) or occur less frequently in public. Tics are often more pronounced in an environment where the sufferer feels comfortable, such as when at home.

For a diagnosis of Tourette's disorder, the condition should have persisted for more than one year since first tic onset. The onset of the condition is before the age of 18 and is not due to the direct physiological effects of a substance (e.g. cocaine or methamphetamine) or a general medical condition (e.g. stroke, Huntington's disease or post-viral encephalitis). The onset of tics typically occurs between the ages of three to eight, with a mean onset between six and seven years); 93% of patients are symptomatic by the age of ten (Freeman *et al.*, 2000), which is also reported to be the average age of greatest tic severity (Leckman *et al.*, 1998).

Tourette's disorder is three to four times more common in males than in females (Freeman *et al.*, 2000) and the overall prevalence of Tourette's disorder is as high as 1%, as shown by studies conducted in mainstream schools (Robertson *et al.*, 2009). In one paediatric study, the prevalence of TD was 0,77%, with 1,06% of boys and 0,25% of girls affected (Knight *et al.*, 2012). The frequency and severity of tics reduce over time (Hassan and Cavanna, 2012). 'It is thus not surprising that in adults, the prevalence rate of Tourette's disorder is lower (0,05% (95% confidence interval, 0,03–0,08%)) than in younger individuals' (Knight *et al.*, 2012). The condition often remits by adulthood (Leckman *et al.*, 1998).

In the majority of patients, Tourette's disorder often co-occurs with other disorders, most notably obsessive-compulsive disorder and ADHD, and self-injurious behaviours (Cavanna *et al.*, 2009). Other conditions such as depression, sleeping disturbances and so-called rage attacks have also been documented in individuals with TD (Mol Debes, 2013).

## 17.3.3 Psychobiology

CSTC circuits play an important role in Tourette's disorder, with dopamine a particularly key mediating neurotransmitter. Nevertheless, the precise pathogenesis of Tourette's disorder is unknown. Genetic factors have received increased attention and a number of candidate genes have emerged as potentially important.

## 17.3.4 Pharmacotherapy and psychotherapy

Some consider pharmacotherapy to be the treatment of choice in patients with moderate to severe tics (Thomas and Cavanna, 2013). Antipsychotics, in particular, are used most often in the treatment of tics in Tourette's disorder and include haloperidol, pimozide and sulpiride. Before the development of atypical neuroleptics, haloperidol was the most commonly used medication for Tourette's disorder. Although this medication has shown good efficacy in the reduction of tics (AK Shapiro and E Shapiro, 1981; AK Shapiro and E Shapiro, 1982), other drugs are nowadays preferred, given haloperidol's high risk for extrapyramidal side effects (EPSEs) (Thomas and Cavanna, 2013). Like haloperidol, pimozide is another typical neuroleptic that has shown efficacy in the treatment of tics. Pimozide is also associated with EPSEs. A third typical neuroleptic, sulpiride, is also commonly used in the treatment of Tourette's disorder. Different studies have noted a significant decrease in tics as well as other symptoms such as obsessive-compulsive personality traits, aggression, subjective tension and low mood when treated with sulpiride (Robertson *et al.*, 1990). Low-dose sulpiride has also showed significant reduction of tics in children with Tourette's disorder or chronic tic disorder (Huys *et al.*, 2012).

Note: in children, treatment often begins with a different drug (i.e. clonidine) from that used to initiate treatment in adults.

Nowadays, atypical neuroleptics are used more often than the typical neuroleptics given their side-effect profile. Examples of atypical neuroleptics that have shown efficacy in Tourette's disorder are risperidone, aripiprazole, olanzapine, ziprasidone and quetiapine. Risperidone was found to be superior to placebo (Dion *et al.*, 2002; Scahill *et al.*, 2003) and similar in efficacy to haloperidol and pimozide (Huys *et al.*, 2012; Scahill *et al.*, 2006). Aripiprazole is another atypical neuroleptic that has shown efficacy in both adults and children with TD (Huys *et al.*, 2012). Olanzapine, another atypical neuroleptic, effectively reduces tics in adults (Budman *et al.*, 2001) and children (McCracken *et al.*, 2008). Ziprasidone and quetiapine have been found effective in the treatment of tics in children (Huys *et al.*, 2012; Roessner *et al.*, 2011).

Note: clozapine was found not to be useful in the treatment of tics and has, in fact, been implicated in the development of facial tics, stuttering and in increased tics (Roessner *et al.*, 2011).

Other drugs that have shown efficacy in the treatment of tics and Tourette's disorder symptoms are clonidine (Cavanna *et al.*, 2012; Leckman *et al.*, 1991), anticonvulsants like topiramate (Jankovic *et al.*, 2010), dopamine agonists (Goetz, 1992), nicotine (Thomas and Cavanna., 2013), and cannabinoids like tetrahydrocannabinol (THC) (Muller-Vahl, 2003; Muller-Vahl *et al.*, 2003; Muller-Vahl, 2013). The most convincing evidence seems to be for the use of clonidine.

It has recently been suggested that deep brain stimulation may help for severe tics that do not respond to other treatment, although more research is needed to determine the efficacy of deep brain stimulation for Tourette's disorder.

Overall, habit reversal training (HRT) is the best-studied and most widely-used behavioural intervention; there is evidence supporting its efficacy in patients with Tourette's disorder (Frank and Cavanna, 2013). There also is evidence – although somewhat less – for the use of ERP as a behavioural intervention for Tourette's disorder (Verdellen *et al.*, 2008). Both HRT and ERP are considered first-line behavioural treatments for tics for both children and adults with Tourette's disorder. Other treatments that are considered second-line or add-on behavioural treatments include contingency management and neurofeedback training (Frank and Cavanna, 2013; Verdellen *et al.*, 2011).

## 17.4 Body dysmorphic disorder

### 17.4.1 Introduction

Previously categorised as one of the somatoform disorders in the DSM-IV-TR, body dysmorphic disorder (BDD) is now classified under the rubric of OCRDs in the DSM-5.

### 17.4.2 Phenomenology

Body dysmorphic disorder is characterised by a preoccupation with a perceived defect(s) or flaw(s) in physical appearance that is not observable or appears slight to others. Concerns range in severity from mild (e.g. thoughts of looking unattractive or not right) to severe (e.g. looking hideous or like a monster).

The preoccupation focuses on one or more body areas, and any body area can be the focus point. Skin is the most common area of concern (e.g. perceived acne, scars, lines, wrinkles, paleness), with concerns with the appearance of hair (e.g. thinning hair or excessive body or facial hair), or nose (e.g. size or shape) also common (Phillips *et al.*, 2010b). The preoccupations are intrusive, unwanted, time-consuming (occurring, on average, three to eight hours per day), and are usually difficult to resist or control (Phillips *et al.*, 2010b). At some point during the course of the disorder, the person has performed repetitive behaviours (e.g. mirror checking, excessive grooming, excoriation or reassurance seeking) or mental acts (e.g. comparing with others) that he or she feels driven to perform in response to the preoccupation with the perceived appearance defects or flaws. The preoccupation causes clinically significant distress (e.g. depressed mood, anxiety or shame) or impairment in social, occupational or other important areas of functioning (e.g. at school, in relationships, in the household). The preoccupation with appearance is not restricted to symptoms of an eating disorder (i.e. concern with body fat or weight).

The clinician must specify if the patient presents with the muscle dysmorphia form of body dysmorphic disorder (i.e. the belief that one's body build is too small or is insufficiently muscular) which almost exclusively occurs in males. Insight should also be assessed in patients presenting with BDD: the clinician should specify whether the body dysmorphic beliefs are currently characterised by:

- good or fair insight (the patient recognises that his or her body dysmorphic disorder beliefs are definitely or probably not true, or that they may or may not be true)

- poor insight (he or she thinks the body dysmorphic disorder beliefs are probably true)
- delusional beliefs about appearance (he or she is completely convinced that the body dysmorphic disorder beliefs are true).

Body dysmorphic disorder with absent insight or delusional beliefs must be differentiated from delusional disorder and other psychotic disorders. Body dysmorphic disorder delusions, if present, relate only to appearance.

Body dysmorphic disorder usually starts during adolescence, with the most common age at onset 12–13 years (Phillips *et al.*, 2010a).

In general, the prevalence of body dysmorphic disorder among adults in the US is 2,4% (2,5% in females and 2,2% in males) (Koran *et al.*, 2008). In specific settings, however, rates are much higher: for example, current prevalence is 9–15% among dermatology patients, 7–8% among US cosmetic surgery patients, 3–16% among international cosmetic surgery patients, 8% among adult orthodontia patients and 10% among patients presenting for oral or maxillofacial surgery (Crerand and Sarwer, 2010). Although there is much overlap in the way that body dysmorphic disorder presents in males and females, there are some differences. Studies suggest that males are more likely to have genital preoccupations whereas females more likely to have a co-morbid eating disorder (Phillips *et al.*, 2010a). As noted above, muscle dysmorphia occurs almost exclusively in males (Phillips *et al.*, 2010a).

Individuals with body dysmorphic disorder often present with excoriation to correct perceived flaws or irregularities. Major depressive disorder is the most common co-morbid disorder in body dysmorphic disorder and usually presents after the onset of body dysmorphic disorder (Phillips *et al.*, 2010b). Psychiatric disorders that also often present in patients with body dysmorphic disorder include social anxiety disorder, obsessive-compulsive disorder, and substance-related disorders (Phillips *et al.*, 2010b; Phillips *et al.*, 2008). Personality traits often present in patients with body dysmorphic disorder are neuroticism, perfectionism, low extroversion and low self-esteem (Buhlmann *et al.*, 2008; Phillips and McElroy, 2000).

## 17.4.3 Psychobiology

There has been surprisingly little work on the neuro-imaging and neuropsychology of body dysmorphic disorder. The work that does exist suggests some overlap with obsessive-compulsive disorder, but also the involvement of different regions.

## 17.4.4 Pharmacotherapy and psychotherapy

There is evidence to support the efficacy of both pharmacotherapy and psychotherapy (Williams *et al.*, 2006).

Pharmacotherapy primarily involves SRIs. Overall, SRIs (e.g. clomipramine, fluvoxamine, fluoxetine, citalopram) have all shown efficacy or partial efficacy in the treatment of body dysmorphic disorder (Hollander *et al.*, 1994; Hollander *et al.*, 1999; Phillips *et al.*, 2002; Phillips and Najjar, 2003), particularly in terms of improving insight and reducing distress and the time spent on defect-focused behaviour (Phillips, 1996). High relapse rates after discontinuation of SRI treatment have also been reported (Phillips and Najjar, 2003), which suggest that longer-term treatment is appropriate. Neuroleptic drugs (e.g. aripiprazole, pimozide) have been used to augment SRIs in the treatment of treatment-refractory body dysmorphic disorder but efficacy rates vary, with some suggesting good response (Uzun and Ozdemir, 2010) and others not (Phillips, 2005).

Psychological interventions primarily involve behaviour therapy (BT) and CBT and can be implemented both in individual and group therapy format. BT for body dysmorphic disorder primarily consists of ERP. During ERP, the patient is instructed to confront their preoccupations by exposing themselves gradually to specific anxiety-provoking stimuli (e.g. the sight of a pimple), and to not engage in behaviours aimed at reducing the anxiety (e.g. covering it with his or her hand, using excessive make-up to cover up or avoidance of interaction with others who may notice the 'flaw'). Prolonged exposure will lead to anxiety reduction and therefore the exposure exercise should continue until the anxiety becomes manageable. CBT involves ERP, but also involves the implementation of cognitive techniques such as the identification of appearance-related automatic thoughts (e.g. the thought that one's nose is skew and ugly), identification of cognitive distortions (e.g. everyone gossips about it), and the disputing and modification of such cognitions.

## 17.5 Hoarding disorder

### 17.5.1 Introduction

Hoarding was not a separate disorder in the DSM-IV. In the DSM-IV, 'the inability to discard worn-out or worthless objects even when they have no sentimental value' was one of the eight criteria for obsessive-compulsive personality disorder (American Psychiatric Association, 1994). Hoarding obsessions and collecting compulsions were also previously considered as one of the OCD symptom dimensions. In the DSM-5, hoarding disorder is included as a separate disorder within the section on obsessive-compulsive and related disorders. Indeed, there now is much evidence to support the hypothesis of compulsive hoarding as a distinct clinical syndrome, highly co-morbid with obsessive-compulsive disorder as well as with other psychiatric disorders (Frost *et al.*, 2000; Samuels *et al.*, 2007).

### 17.5.2 Phenomenology

According to the DSM-5, hoarding disorder is characterised by the persistent difficulty discarding or parting with possessions, regardless of whether they are perceived by others to be valuable. This difficulty is due to strong urges to save items, distress and/or indecision associated with discarding them. The symptoms of this condition result in the accumulation of a large number of possessions that fill up and clutter the active living areas of the home or the workplace to the extent that the intended use of at least some of these areas is no longer possible (e.g. unable to cook in kitchen or sit in living room). Hoarding can pose dangers, for example fire in the home, falling (especially older people), poor sanitation and consequent health risks (Pertusa *et al.*, 2010). If some of the living areas are uncluttered, it is only because of the interventions of third parties (e.g. family members, cleaners, local authorities). The symptoms cause clinically significant distress or impairment in social, occupational or other important areas of functioning (including maintaining a safe environment for self and others). The hoarding symptoms are not due to a general medical condition (e.g. a brain injury, cerebrovascular disease). The symptoms are not restricted to the symptoms of another mental disorder (e.g. hoarding due to obsessions in OCD, decreased energy in major depressive disorder, delusions in schizophrenia or another psychotic disorder, cognitive deficits in dementia, restricted interests in autistic disorder or food storing in **Prader-Willi syndrome**).

If hoarding is accompanied by excessive acquisition (i.e. if symptoms are accompanied by the excessive collecting, buying or stealing of items that are not needed or for which there is no available space), this must be specified. Specification of the level of insight is also needed. Indicate whether hoarding beliefs and behaviours (pertaining to difficulty in discarding items, clutter or excessive acquisition) are currently characterised by:

- good or fair insight: recognising that hoarding-related beliefs and behaviour are problematic
- poor insight: mostly convinced that hoarding-related beliefs and behaviour are not problematic despite evidence to the contrary
- delusional: completely convinced that hoarding-related beliefs and behaviour are not problematic despite evidence to the contrary.

The prevalence of compulsive hoarding in the community ranges between 2-5% (Iervolino *et al.*, 2009; Samuels *et al.*, 2008). The condition seems to follow a chronic course, with age of onset usually in childhood or early adolescence (Frost and Gross, 1993; Samuels *et al.*, 2002).

In terms of gender distribution, it appears that females of all ages, including young girls and older women, are more prone to present with problematic hoarding.

Hoarding is also associated with significant psychiatric co-morbidity. Although there is some overlap between obsessive-compulsive disorder and hoarding disorder (with some OCD patients presenting with hoarding or collecting obsessions and compulsions) a substantial number of individuals with severe hoarding disorder do not present with other obsessive-compulsive disorder symptoms. In one community study, for example, 18% were diagnosed with co-morbid obsessive-compulsive disorder, whereas the concurrent co-morbidity rates with major depression (36%), social anxiety disorder (20%) and generalised anxiety disorder (24%) were much higher (Frost *et al.*, 2010). Hoarding is also associated with significant personality disorder co-morbidity (Frost *et al.*, 2000; Mataix-Cols *et al.*, 2002; Pertusa *et al.*, 2008; Samuels *et al.*, 2007).

## 17.5.3 Psychobiology

One of the reasons for distinguishing between obsessive-compulsive disorder and hoarding disorder in the DSM-5 is a small but growing literature indicating that the psychobiology of the two disorders is somewhat distinct. Neuroimaging studies have suggested that somewhat different neurocircuitry is responsible for hoarding disorder.

## 17.5.4 Pharmacotherapy and psychotherapy

Until recently, the literature on treatment response in compulsive hoarders suggested that treatment failures are frequent (Pertusa *et al.*, 2010). One study found that only 18% of hoarding patients responded to medication and CBT (Black *et al.*, 1998). More recently however, there is evidence that SRIs may be as effective for compulsive hoarders as for non-hoarding OCD patients. In an open-label study with paroxetine it was found that compulsive hoarders responded equally well to paroxetine as non-hoarding OCD patients (Saxena *et al.*, 2007). Response rate in the hoarding group was 50% and 49% in the obsessive-compulsive disorder group. Other medications may also be beneficial in hoarding: preliminary results from an open label-trial with extended-release venlafaxine suggest that venlafaxine may prove to be effective for treatment and appears better tolerated than paroxetine by individuals with hoarding disorder (Saxena, 2011).

In terms of psychotherapy, many studies have indicated poor response (Shafran and Tallis, 1996; Tolin *et al.*, 2007). Reasons for such poor response may arguably include patterns of poor insight, treatment refusal, lack of cooperation and lack of resistance to the hoarding behaviour (Christensen and Greist, 2001; Damecour and Charron, 1998; Fitzgerald *et al.*, 1997). However, there are now increasing data that suggest that some psychotherapeutic interventions (in individual and group format) do show promise (Gilliam *et al.*, 2011; Steketee *et al.*, 2010; Tolin *et al.*, 2007). Effective techniques include office and home visits that emphasise motivational interviewing, decision-making training, exposure, cognitive restructuring and efforts to reduce acquisition (Cermele *et al.*, 2001; Hartl *et al.*, 1999; Saxena *et al.*, 2002; Steketee *et al.*, 2000). The aim of these techniques is to increase insight and motivation, assist with problem-solving, build organisational skills, teach cognitive restructuring, assist with decision making and to expose the patient to acquiring and discarding (Tolin *et al.*, 2007). A commonly used manual emphasises cognitive restructuring relative to behavioural components, such as exposure (Steketee and Frost, 2007). One recent study that investigated the efficacy of CBT found that there were significant improvements on self-reported hoarding severity measures (Tolin *et al.*, 2007). Some clinicians feel that the combination of pharmacotherapy and CBT (adjusted for compulsive hoarding) may also be useful (Saxena, 2011).

## 17.6 Hair-pulling disorder

### 17.6.1 Introduction

Hair-pulling disorder (HPD or trichotillomania) was previously included under'Impulse control disorders not elsewhere classified'in the DSM-IV-TR. It is now categorised with the OCRDs.

### 17.6.2 Phenomenology

Hair-pulling disorder is characterised by recurrent pulling out of one's hair resulting in hair loss. There are repeated attempts to decrease or stop hair pulling. The hair pulling causes clinically significant distress or impairment in social, occupational or other important areas of functioning. The hair pulling or hair loss is not attributable to another medical condition (e.g. a dermatological condition) and the hair pulling is not better explained by the symptoms of another DSM-5 disorder (e.g. hair pulling due to preoccupation with appearance in body dysmorphic disorder).

Although large-scale epidemiological studies have yet to be conducted, hair-pulling disorder is estimated by smaller studies to affect 1–3,5% of late adolescents and young adults (Christenson *et al.*, 1991a). Rates among younger children are unclear.

In adult recruitment studies, female participants have typically outnumbered males by at least three to one or more.

Onset of pathological hair pulling generally appears to be in childhood or adolescence. Although not everyone agrees, it has been suggested that hair-pulling disorder can be subtyped according to the age of onset of pulling, with patients with early onset presenting with phenomenological and course differences compared with those with late onset of hair pulling (Sah *et al.*, 2008)). It seems that hair pulling in children younger than five years often remits spontaneously (Sah *et al.*, 2008; Tay *et al.*, 2004), whereas a later age of onset (pre-adolescence to young adulthood) is more common and may have a more chronic and relapsing course (Christenson *et al.*, 1991a; Cohen *et al.*, 1995).

Psychiatric co-morbidity is common, with anxiety disorders (mainly generalised anxiety disorder and specific phobias), mood disorders (major depressive disorder), substance-use disorders, eating disorders and personality disorders being the most prevalent in adults with hair-pulling disorder. Younger patients most often present with anxiety, disruptive behaviour disorders and OCRDs (particularly body-focused repetitive behaviours such as nail-biting, cheek-chewing and lip-biting) (Franklin *et al.*, 2011).

### 17.6.3 Psychobiology

Neuro-imaging and neuropsychological research suggest both overlaps and distinctions between hair-pulling disorder and obsessive-compulsive disorder. Thus, there is some involvement of CTSC circuitry in hair-pulling disorder. At the same time, other regions may also play an important role.

### 17.6.4 Pharmacotherapy and psychotherapy

A variety of treatments are currently available to alleviate the symptoms of hair-pulling disorder in patients of all ages. These include **habit reversal therapy** (HRT), online CBT, medications and a combination of these approaches (Franklin *et al.*, 2011). Further **randomised placebo-controlled trials** are required to assess the effects of these types of treatment and treatment combinations in larger samples of hair-pulling disorder patients of all ages.

HRT, a behavioural therapy technique, has been used over the years in the treatment of 'nervous' habits such as nail-biting and thumb-sucking (Azrin *et al.*, 1980a; Azrin *et al.*, 1980b). It involves three primary components: awareness training, competing response training and social support (Azrin and Nunn, 1973). HRT has also been found to be effective in the treatment of hair-pulling disorder (Franklin *et al.*, 2011). HRT and acceptance-enhanced behaviour therapy were found to be superior to waiting-list-control conditions (Woods *et al.*, 2006).

Seemingly effective in the treatment of habit disorders like thumb-sucking and nail-biting (Kohen, 1991; Kohen, 1996), hypnotherapy has also been tried in patients with hair-pulling disorder (Galski, 1981). However, there is an absence of randomised placebo-controlled trials.

In terms of pharmacotherapy, a number of different agents have been tried over the years. Clomipramine was found to be superior to the tricyclic desipramine in reducing hair-pulling symptoms (Swedo *et al.*, 1989). In another randomised placebo-controlled trial clomipramine was compared with placebo and CBT (including HRT) (Ninan *et al.*, 2000). It was found that CBT was superior to clomipramine and placebo in reducing HPD symptoms. Regarding SSRIs, two studies assessed the efficacy of fluoxetine in the treatment of patients with HPD (Christenson *et al.*, 1991b; Streichenwein and Thornby, 1995). Neither study found evidence for superiority of fluoxetine over placebo. Fluoxetine and CBT were also compared (Van Minnen *et al.*, 2003) and CBT, including stimulus-control and stimulus-response management techniques, was found to render better results than fluoxetine. In a group of patients who had not responded to sertraline monotherapy, sertraline in combination with HRT, showed superior outcomes (Dougherty *et al.*, 2006).

One randomised placebo-controlled trial suggested that olanzapine may be effective in HPD (Van Ameringen *et al.*, 2010). Significant symptom improvement has also been reached with other pharmacological agents, for example venlafaxine (Ninan *et al.*, 1998), topiramate (Lochner *et al.*, 2006), and olanzapine (Stewart and Nejtek, 2003). However, none of these were randomised placebo-controlled trials.

N-acetyl cysteine (NAC) has also been tried in the treatment of hair-pulling disorder. NAC, a precursor to the amino acid cysteine, has a role as a modulator of the glutamatergic system. NAC was found efficacious in a randomised placebo-controlled trial (Grant *et al.*, 2009).

## 17.7 Excoriation (skin picking disorder)

### 17.7.1 Introduction

Excoriation (skin-picking disorder) or SPD is characterised by skin lesions, distress and functional impairment (Grant and Odlaug 2009; Odlaug and Grant, 2010). Other labels for this condition are neurotic excoriation, compulsive picking and dermatillomania.

Skin-picking disorder was not previously included in the DSM. However, in recent years evidence suggested that it is a prevalent and disabling condition which has received increasing study. It is now included in the DSM-5, as one of the OCRDs (Lochner *et al.*, 2012a).

The condition is characterised by recurrent skin-picking, which results in skin lesions. Problematic skin-picking persists despite repeated attempts to decrease or stop. Clinically significant distress or impairment in social, occupational or other important areas of functioning characterises the condition. Skin-picking disorder is diagnosed only when skin-picking is not attributable to the direct physiological effects of a substance (e.g. cocaine) or another medical condition (e.g. scabies). Skin-picking is also not better explained by symptoms of another DSM-5 disorder (e.g. skin-picking due to delusions or tactile hallucinations in a psychotic disorder, preoccupation with appearance in body dysmorphic disorder, stereotypies in stereotypic-movement disorder, or intention to harm oneself in non-suicidal self-injury) (Grant *et al.*, 2012; Lochner *et al.*, 2012a).

### 17.7.2 Phenomenology

The literature on the prevalence of skin-picking disorder has increased in recent years, with community studies finding rates ranging from 1,2–5,4% in a variety of cohorts (Grant *et al.*, 2012). Most studies of skin-picking disorder thus far focused on college or university students. These suggest that skin-picking is relatively common. One study with 354 participants reported that 62,7% engaged in some form of skin-picking whereas 5,4% of those reported clinical levels of picking (Hayes *et al.*, 2009). In another community study of 2 513 participants, 16,5% reported skin-picking with noticeable skin damage whereas 1,4% of those satisfied criteria for skin-picking disorder (Keuthen *et al.*, 2010). In a recent university telephone survey in which 1 916 students participated, the overall prevalence of skin-picking disorder was 4,2% (Odlaug *et al.*, 2013).

Skin picking severity varies among the population from mild to severe, with most people engaging in some form of picking. Only a few engage in the pathological picking associated with clinically significant distress and functional impairment.

Patients with skin-picking disorder spend a significant amount of time picking per day, often leading to impaired functioning due to an absence from work or school. Patients report multiple reinforcement triggers and maintaining factors to picking. For example, picking can be triggered by the feel (e.g. unevenness) or appearance (e.g. a blemish) of the skin (Grant *et al.*, 2012). Other theories also exist: skin-picking disorder may be maintained by positive social reinforcement (e.g. reinforced or maintained by attention from others), positive non-social reinforcement (e.g. pleasure derived from picking), negative social reinforcement (e.g. escaping or avoiding unpleasant things, including studies or work) and negative non-social reinforcement (e.g. escaping or avoiding high levels of arousal or discomfort) (Iwata, 1994).

Although skin-picking disorder is more prevalent in females (Odlaug *et al.*, 2013; Odlaug and Grant, 2011), some studies suggest that the condition is equally common in both genders (Tucker *et al.*, 2011).

Skin-picking disorder can start at any age but frequently has its onset in childhood or adolescence (Arnold *et al.*, 2001; Keuthen *et al.*, 2000; Odlaug and Grant, 2007a) and often follows after a dermatological condition such as acne, eczema or psoriasis (Wilhelm *et al.*, 1999).

Evidence suggests that skin-picking disorder is associated with significant psychological and physical problems (Odlaug *et al.*, 2013). Skin-picking disorder occurs with a variety of other disorders, such as major depressive disorder (12,5–48%), anxiety disorders (8–23%) and substance-use disorders (14–36%) (Grant *et al.*, 2012). Co-morbidity with hair-pulling disorder and obsessive-compulsive disorder has been found to be fairly common in patients with skin-picking disorder (Christenson *et al.*, 1999; Odlaug and Grant, 2008; Snorrason *et al.*, 2012). In terms of medical sequelae, most individuals with skin-picking disorder will present with noticeable excoriations and some with severe ulcerations, scarring from previous picking and infections that requires oral, topical or intravenous antibiotics and in severe cases, skin grafting (Odlaug and Grant, 2008)).

## 17.7.3 Psychobiology

Little is known about the pathogenesis of skin-picking disorder. However, there is an emerging evidence base (as well as in associated neuropsychological tests) suggesting altered neurocircuitry.

## 17.7.4 Pharmacotherapy and psychotherapy

Relatively few studies have been published on treatment of skin-picking disorder. Nevertheless, given its overlap and co-morbidity with obsessive-compulsive disorder and other body-focused repetitive behaviours like hair-pulling disorder, treatment for skin-picking disorder would arguably involve medication (SRIs, NAC or naltrexone) and CBT (including HRT or acceptance-enhanced behaviour therapy).

Data on the efficacy of SRIs have been mixed. In two different double-blind placebo-controlled clinical trials in patients with skin-picking disorder it was found that fluoxetine was superior to placebo on some measures of picking (Bloch *et al.*, 2001; Simeon *et al.*, 1997). In an open-label trial with escitalopram, approximately half of the sample showed a good response and one-quarter were partial-medication responders (Keuthen *et al.*, 2007b). Citalopram has also been found to be effective in reducing picking behaviour (Arabi *et al.*, 2008). Efficacy of the anticonvulsant lamotrigine has also been investigated in skin-picking disorder, with one open-label study indicating that it may be efficacious (Grant *et al.*, 2007). Another study found lamotrigine not to be of greater benefit than placebo (Grant *et al.*, 2010). As in hair-pulling disorder, NAC has also demonstrated benefit for the treatment of skin-picking disorder, but randomised placebo-controlled trials remain to be undertaken (Odlaug and Grant, 2007b). Since naltrexone, an opioid receptor antagonist, is used to reduce the urge to engage in pleasurable (but pathological) behaviours, it has been reported useful in case series (Grant *et al.*, 2012). Larger scale treatment trials are needed to further explore the efficacy of opioid antagonists in SPD.

There is preliminary evidence for skin picking reduction with CBT including HRT (Kent and Drummond, 1989; Teng *et al.*, 2006; Twohig and Woods, 2001) and acceptance-enhanced behaviour therapy (Flessner *et al.*, 2008a; Twohig *et al.*, 2006).

## 17.8 Other obsessive-compulsive disorder spectrum disorders

The DSM-5 includes categories of substance-induced or medication-induced OCRDs, OCRDs secondary to other medical conditions, and OCRDs not elsewhere classified (NEC). OCRDs not elsewhere classified include individuals who present with distress and functional impairment but who do not meet diagnostic criteria for an OCRD. Examples include individuals with body dysmorphic disorder who have observable flaws, individuals with body-focused repetitive behavioural disorder (with symptoms such as nail-biting, cheek-chewing and lip-biting), and individuals with obsessional jealousy.

## Conclusion

OCRDs is a new diagnostic category in the DSM-5 and is likely to be included in ICD-11, and includes obsessive-compulsive disorder, body dysmorphic disorder, hoarding disorder, hair-pulling disorder, and skin-picking disorder. Given that many of these disorders have been under-recognised in the past and patients have endured much distress and inappropriate treatment as a result, clinicians must be more aware of these conditions. Clinicians are encouraged to screen for all of these conditions in individuals who present with one of them, keeping the overlaps (and differences) between the conditions in mind.

Treatment guidelines across these conditions overlap to some extent: for example, pharmacotherapy of the OCRDs often entails an SRI as first-line therapy, with antipsychotic medications used to augment the SRIs when their efficacy is less than optimal. Psychotherapy generally involves CBT, consisting of behavioural techniques such as ERP, HRT and cognitive therapy. At the same time, there are differences in pharmacotherapy approach across these disorders, and CBT treatments must be tailored to the specific OCRD.

In addition to the treatment options for OCRDs discussed above, patients and their significant others can also consider joining a support group, especially in areas where CBT specialists are not available. Information on these groups can be obtained from consumer groups such as the OCD Association of South Africa (http://www.ocfoundation.com/) or the OCD Foundation in the USA (http://www.ocfoundation.org/) or the Trichotillomania Learning Centre (www.trich.org). Locally, the Mental Health Information Centre (MHIC; www.mentalhealthsa.org.za) can be contacted for the contact information of suitable clinicians and/or therapy or support groups. There are online support groups for patients with OCRDs as well, such as www.ownocd.ning.com.

# References


Allen AJ, Leonard HL, Swedo SE (1995) Case study: A new infection-triggered autoimmunee subtype of pediatric OCD and Tourette's syndrome. *Journal of the American Academy of Child & Adolescent Psychiatry* (34): 307–311

American Psychiatric Association (1994) *Diagnostic and Statistical Manual of Mental Disorders* (4th edition). Arlington, VA: American Psychiatric Association

American Psychiatric Association (2000) *Diagnostic and Statistical Manual of Mental Disorders* (4th edition). Text Revision. Arlington, VA: American Psychiatric Association

American Psychiatric Association (2013) *Diagnostic and Statistical Manual of Mental Disorders* (5th edition). Arlington, VA: American Psychiatric Association

American Psychiatric Association (2007) *Practice guideline for the treatment of patients with obsessive-compulsive disorder*. Arlington VA: American Psychiatric Association

Arabi M, Farnia V, Balighi K, Mohammadi MR, Nejati-Safa AA, Yazdchi H, Golestan B, Darvish F (2008) Efficacy of citalopram in treatment of pathological skin picking: A randomized double blind placebo controlled trial. *Acta Medica Iranica* (46): 367–72

Arnold LM, Auchenbach MB, McElroy SL (2001) Psychogenic excoriation. Clinical features, proposed diagnostic criteria, epidemiology, and approaches to treatment. *CNS Drugs* (15): 351–59

Avalos L, Tylka TL, Wood-Barcalow N (2005) The Body Appreciation Scale: Development and psychometric evaluation. *Body Image* (2): 285–97

Azrin NH, Nunn RG (1973) Habit-reversal: A method of eliminating nervous habits and tics. *Behaviour Research and Therapy* (11): 619–28

Azrin NH, Nunn RG, Frantz SE (1980a) Habit reversal vs negative practice treatment of nailbiting. *Behaviour Research and Therapy* (18): 281–5

Azrin NH, Nunn RG, Frantz-Renshaw S (1980b) Habit reversal treatment of thumbsucking. *Behaviour Research and Therapy* (18): 395–9

Banaschewski T, Woerner W, Rothenberger A (2003) Premonitory sensory phenomena and suppressibility of tics in Tourette syndrome: Developmental aspects in children and adolescents. *Developmental Medicine & Child Neurology* (45): 700–703

Black DW, Monahan P, Gable J, Blum N, Clancy G, Baker P (1998) Hoarding and treatment response in 38 nondepressed subjects with obsessive-compulsive disorder. *Journal of Clinical Psychiatry* (59): 420–5

Bloch MH, Landeros-Weisenberger A, Kelmendi B, Coric V, Bracken MB, Leckman JF, (2006) A systematic review: Antipsychotic augmentation with treatment refractory obsessive-compulsive disorder. *Molecular Psychiatry* (11): 622–32

Bloch MR, Elliott M, Thompson H, Koran LM (2001) Fluoxetine in pathologic skin-picking: Open-label and double-blind results. *Psychosomatics* (42): 314–9

Brunhoeber S, Maes J (2007) Diagnostik der Körperdysmorphen Störung. *Diagnostica* (53): 17–32

Bruun RD, Budman CL (1996) Risperidone as a treatment for Tourette's syndrome. *Journal of Clinical Psychiatry* (57): 29–31

Budman CL, Gayer A, Lesser M, Shi Q, Bruun RD (2001) An open-label study of the treatment efficacy of olanzapine for Tourette's disorder. *Journal of Clinical Psychiatry* (62): 290–4

Buhlmann U, Etcoff NL, Wilhelm S (2008) Facial attractiveness ratings and perfectionism in body dysmorphic disorder and obsessive-compulsive disorder. *Journal of Anxiety Disorders* (22): 540–7

Cavanna AE, Selvini C, Termine C, Balottin U, Eddy CM (2012) Tolerability profile of clonidine in the treatment of adults with Tourette syndrome. *Clinical Neuropharmacology* (35): 269–2

Cavanna AE, Servo S, Monaco F, Robertson MM (2009) The behavioral spectrum of Gilles de la Tourette syndrome. *Journal of neuropsychiatry and clinical neurosciences* (21): 13–23

Cermele JA, Melendez-Pallitto L, Pandina GJ (2001) Pandina Intervention in compulsive hoarding: A case study. *Behavior Modification* (25): 214–32

Christensen DD, Greist JH (2001) The challenge of obsessive-compulsive disorder hoarding. *Primary Psychiatry* (8): 79–86

Christenson GA, Mackenzie TB, Mitchell JE (1991a) Characteristics of 60 adult chronic hair pullers. *American Journal of Psychiatry* (148): 365–70

Christenson GA, Mackenzie TB, Mitchell JE, Callies AL (1991b) A placebo-controlled, double-blind crossover study of fluoxetine in trichotillomania. *American Journal of Psychiatry* (148): 1566–71

Christenson G, Mansueto C (1999) Trichotillomania: Descriptive characteristics and phenomenology. In: Stein D, Christenson G, Hollander E (Eds). *Trichotillomania*. Washington DC: American Psychiatric Press

Cohen DJ, Detlor J, Young JG, Shaywitz BA (1980) Clonidine ameliorates Gilles de la Tourette syndrome. *Archives of General Psychiatry* (37): 1350–7

Cohen LJ, Stein DJ, Simeon D, Spadaccini E, Rosen J, Aronowitz B, Hollander E (1995) Clinical profile comorbidity and treatment history in 123 hair pullers: A survey study. *Journal of Clinical Psychiatry* (56): 319–26

Cooper PJ, Taylor MJ, Cooper Z, Fairburn CG (1987) The development and validation of the Body Shape Questionnaire. *International Journal of Eating Disorders* (6): 485–94

Crerand CE, Sarwer DB (2010) Cosmetic treatments and body dysmorphic disorder. *Psychiatric Annals* (40): 344–8

Damecour CL, Charron M (1998) Hoarding: A symptom not a syndrome. *Journal of Clinical Psychiatry* (59): 267–72

Diefenbach GJ, Tolin DF, Crocetto J, Maltby N, Hannan S (2005) Assessment of Trichotillomania: A psychometric evaluation of hair-pulling scales. *Journal of Psychopathology and Behavioral Assessment* (27): 169–78

Dion Y, Annable L, Sandor P, Chouinard G (2002) Risperidone in the treatment of Tourette syndrome: A double-blind placebo-controlled trial. *Journal of Clinical Psychopharmacology* (22): 31–9

Dold M, Aigner M, Lanzenberger R, Kasper S (2013) Antipsychotic augmentation of serotonin reuptake inhibitors in treatment-resistant obsessive-compulsive disorder: A meta-analysis of double-blind, randomized, placebo-controlled trials. *International Journal of Neuropsychopharmacology* (16): 557–574

Dougherty DD, Loh R, Jenike MA, Keuthen NJ (2006) Single modality versus dual modality treatment for trichotillomania: Sertraline, behavioral therapy or both? *Journal of Clinical Psychiatry* (67): 1086–92

Erzegovesi S, Cavallini MC, Cavedini P, Diaferia G, Locatelli M, Bellodi L (2001) Clinical predictors of drug response in obsessive-compulsive disorder. *Journal of Clinical Psychopharmacology* (21): 488–92

Evans C, Dolan B, (1993) Body Shape Questionnaire: Derivation of shortened 'alternate' forms. *International Journal of Eating Disorders* (13): 315–21

Fitzgerald PB (1997) The 'bowerbird symptom': A case of severe hoarding of possessions. *Australian and New Zealand Journal of Psychiatry* (31): 597–600

Flessner CA, Busch AM, Heideman PW, Woods DW (2008a) Acceptance-enhanced behavior therapy (AEBT) for trichotillomania and chronic skin picking: Exploring the effects of component sequencing. *Behavior Modification* (32): 579–94

Flessner CA, Woods DW, Franklin ME, Cashin SE, Keuthen NJ (2008b) The Milwaukee Inventory for Subtypes of Trichotillomania – Adult Version (MIST-A): Development of an instrument for the assessment of 'focused' and 'automatic' hair pulling. *Journal of Psychopathology and Behavioral Assessment* (30): 20–30

Flessner CA, Woods DW, Franklin ME, Keuthen NJ, Piacentini J, Cashin SE, Moore PS (2007) The Milwaukee Inventory for Styles of Trichotillomania – Child Version (MIST-C): Initial development and psychometric properties. *Behavior Modification* (31): 896–918

Foa EB, Kozak MJ, Salkovskis PM, Coles ME, Amir N (1998) The validation of a new obsessive compulsive disorder scale: The Obsessive Compulsive Inventory (OCI). *Psychological Assessment* (10): 206–14

Fontenelle LF, Mendlowicz MV, Versiani M (2006) The descriptive epidemiology of obsessive-compulsive disorder. *Progress in Neuro-Psychopharmacology & Biological Psychiatry* (30): 327–37

Frank M, Cavanna AE (2013) Behavioural treatments for Tourette syndrome: An evidence-based review. *Behavioural Neurology* (27): 105–117

Franklin ME, Zagrabbe K, Benavides KL (2011) Trichotillomania and its treatment: A review and recommendations. *Expert Review of Neurotherapeutics* (11): 1165–74

Freeman RD, Fast DK, Burd L, Kerbeshian J, Robertson MM, Sandor P (2000) An international perspective on Tourette syndrome: Selected findings from 3 500 individuals in 22 countries. *Developmental Medicine & Child Neurology* (42): 436–47

Frost RO, Gross RC, (1993) The hoarding of possessions. *Behaviour Research and Therapy* (31): 367–81

Frost RO, Steketee G, Grisham J (2004) Measurement of compulsive hoarding: Saving inventory revised. *Behavior Research and Therapy* (42): 1163–82

Frost RO, Steketee G, Tolin D, Glossner K (2010) Diagnostic comorbidity in hoarding and obsessive-compulsive disorder. World Congress of Behavioral and Cognitive Therapies. Boston, June 2–5

Frost RO, Steketee G, Tolin D, Renaud S (2008) Development and validation of the clutter image rating. Journal of *Psychopathology and Behavioral Assessment* (30): 193–203

Frost RO, Steketee G, Williams LF, Warren R (2000) Mood, personality disorder symptoms and disability in obsessive compulsive hoarders: A comparison with clinical and nonclinical controls. *Behaviour Research and Therapy* (38): 1071–81

Galski TJ (1981) The adjunctive use of hypnosis in the treatment of trichotillomania: A case report. *American Journal of Clinical Hypnosis* (23): 198–201

Geller D (2006) Obsessive-compulsive and spectrum disorders in children and adolescents. *Psychiatric Clinics of North America* (29): 353–70

Gilliam CM, Norberg MM, Villavicencio A, Morrison S, Hannan SE, Tolin DF (2011) Group cognitive-behavioral therapy for hoarding disorder: An open trial. *Behaviour Research and Therapy* (49): 802–7

Goetz CG (1992) Clonidine and clonazepam in Tourette syndrome. *Advances in neurology* (58): 245–51

Goodman WK, Price L, Rasmussen SA, Mazure C, Fleischmann R, Hill C, Heninger GR, Charney DS (1989a) The Yale-Brown Obsessive Compulsive Scale. I. Development, use, and reliability. *Archives of General Psychiatry* (46): 1006–11

Goodman W, Price L, Rasmussen S, Mazure C, Delgado P, Heninger G, Charney DS (1989b) The Yale-Brown Obsessive Compulsive Scale. II. Validity. *Archives of General Psychiatry* (46): 1012–6

Grabe HJ, Meyer C, Hapke U, Rumpf HJ, Freyberger HJ, Dilling H, John U (2000) Prevalence, quality of life and psychosocial function in obsessive-compulsive disorder and subclinical obsessive-compulsive disorder in northern Germany. *European Archives of Psychiatry and Clinical Neuroscience* (250): 262–8

Grant JE, Odlaug BL (2009) Update on pathological skin picking. *Current Psychiatry Reports* (11): 283–8

Grant JE, Odlaug BL, Chamberlain SR, Keuthen NJ, Lochner C, Stein DJ (2012) Skin picking disorder. *American Journal of Psychiatry* (169): 1143–9

Grant JE, Odlaug BL, Chamberlain SR, Kim SW (2010) A double-blind, placebo-controlled trial of lamotrigine for pathological skin picking: Treatment efficacy and neurocognitive predictors of response. *Journal of Clinical Psychopharmacology* (30): 396–403

Grant JE, Odlaug BL, Kim SW (2007) Lamotrigine treatment of pathologic skin picking: An open-label study. *Journal of Clinical Psychiatry* (68): 1384–91

Grant JE, Odlaug BL, Kim SW (2009) N-acetylcysteine, a glutamate modulator, in the treatment of trichotillomania: A double-blind, placebo-controlled study. *Archives of General Psychiatry* (66): 756–63

Hartl TL, Frost RO (1999) Cognitive-behavioral treatment of compulsive hoarding: A multiple baseline experimental case study. *Behaviour Research and Therapy* (37): 451–61

Hassan N, Cavanna AE (2012) The prognosis of Tourette syndrome: Implications for clinical practice. *Functional Neurology* (27): 23–7

Hayes SL, Storch EA, Berlanga L (2009) Skin picking behaviors: An examination of the prevalence and severity in a community sample. *Journal of Anxiety Disorders* (23): 314–9

Hollander E, Allen A, Kwon J, Aronowitz B, Schmeidler J, Wong C, Simeon D (1999) Clomipramine vs desipramine crossover trial in body dysmorphic disorder: Selective efficacy of a serotonin reuptake inhibitor in imagined ugliness. *Archives of General Psychiatry* (56): 1033–9

Hollander E, Cohen L, Simeon D, Rosen J, DeCaria C, Stein DJ (1994) Fluvoxamine treatment of body dysmorphic disorder. *Journal of Clinical Psychopharmacology* (14): 75–7

Huppert JD, Moser JS, Gershuny BS, Riggs DS, Spokas M, Filip J, Hajcak G, Parker HA, Baer L, Foa EB (2005) The relationship between obsessive-compulsive and posttraumatic stress symptoms in clinical and non-clinical samples. *Journal of Anxiety Disorders* (19): 127–36

Huys D, Hardenacke K, Poppe P, Bartsch C, Baskin B, Kuhn J (2012) Update on the role of antipsychotics in the treatment of Tourette syndrome. *Journal of Neuropsychiatric Disease and treatment* (8): 95–104

Iervolino AC, Perroud N, Fullana MA, Guipponi M, Cherkas L, Collier DA, Mataix-Cols D (2009) Prevalence and heritability of compulsive hoarding: A twin study. *American Journal of Psychiatry* (166): 1156–61

Iwata BA, Dorsey MF, Slifer KJ, Bauman KE, Richman GS (1994) Toward a functional analysis of self-injury. *Journal of Applied Behavior Analysis* (27): 197–209

Jankovic J, Jimenez-Shahed J, Brown LW (2010) A randomised, double-blind placebo-controlled study of topiramate in the treatment of Tourette syndrome. *Journal of Neurology Neurosurgery and Psychiatry* (81): 70–3

Karno M, Golding JM, Sorenson SB, Burnam MA (1988) The epidemiology of obsessive-compulsive disorder in five US communities. *Archives of General Psychiatry* (45): 1094–9

Kent A, Drummond LM (1989) Acne excoriée – a case report of treatment using habit reversal. *Clinical and Experimental Dermatology* (14): 163–4

Keuthen NJ, Deckersbach T, Wilhelm S, Hale E, Fraim C, Baer L, O'Sullivan RL, Jenike MA (2000) Repetitive skin-picking in a student population and comparison with a sample of self-injurious skin-pickers. *Psychosomatics* (41): 210–5

Keuthen NJ, Deckersbach T, Wilhelm S, Engelhard I, Forker A, O'Sullivan RL, Jenike MA, Baer L (2001a) The Skin Picking Impact Scale (SPIS): Scale development and psychometric analyses. *Psychosomatics* (42): 397–403

Keuthen NJ, Flessner CA, Woods DW, Franklin ME, Stein DJ, Cashin SE (2007a) Factor analysis of the Massachusetts General Hospital Hairpulling Scale. *Journal of Psychosomatic Research* (62): 707–9

Keuthen NJ, Jameson M, Loh R, Deckersbach T, Wilhelm S, Dougherty DD (2007b) Open-label escitalopram treatment for pathological skin picking. *International Clinical Psychopharmacology* (22): 268–74

Keuthen NJ, Koran LM, Aboujaoude E, Large MD, Serpe RT (2010) The prevalence of pathologic skin picking in US adults. *Comprehensive Psychiatry* (51): 183–6

Keuthen NJ, Wilhelm S, Deckersbach T, Engelhard IM, Forker AE, Baer L, Jenike MA (2001b) The Skin Picking Scale: Scale construction and psychometric analyses. *Journal of Psychosomatic Research* (50): 337–41

Kircanski K, Woods DW, Chang SW, Ricketts EJ, Piacentini JC (2010) Cluster analysis of the Yale Global Tic Severity Scale (YGTSS): Symptom dimensions and clinical correlates in an outpatient youth sample. *Journal of Abnormal Child Psychology* (38): 777–88

Knight T, Steeves T, Day L, Lowerison M, Jette N, Pringsheim T (2012) Prevalence of tic disorders: A systematic review and meta-analysis. *Pediatric Neurology* (47): 77–90

Kohen DP (1991) Applications of relaxation and mental imagery (self-hypnosis) for habit problems. *Pediatric Annals* (20): 136–4

Kohen DP (1996) Hypnotherapeutic management of pediatric and adolescent trichotillomania. *Journal of Developmental and Behavioral Pediatrics* (17): 328–34

Kollei I, Brunhoeber S, Rauh E, de Zwaan M, Martin A (2012) Body image, emotions and thought control strategies in body dysmorphic disorder compared to eating disorders and healthy controls. *Journal of Psychosomatic Research* (72): 321–7

Koran LM, Abujaoude E, Large MD, Serpe RT (2008) The prevalence of body dysmorphic disorder in the United States adult population. *CNS Spectrums* (13): 316–22

Leckman JF, Hardin MT, Riddle MA, Stevenson J, Ort SI, Cohen DJ (1991) Clonidine treatment of Gilles de la Tourette's syndrome. *Archives of General Psychiatry* (48): 324–8

Leckman JF, Riddle M, Hardin M, Ort S, Swartz K, Stevenson J, Cohen DJ (1989) The Yale Global Tic Severity Scale: Initial testing of a clinician-rated scale of tic severity. *Journal of the American Academy of Child & Adolescent Psychiatry* (28): 566–73

Leckman JF, Zhang H, Alsobrook JP, Pauls DL (2001) Symptom dimensions in obsessive-compulsive disorder: Toward quantitative phenotypes. *American Journal of Medical Genetics* (105): 28–30

Leckman JF, Zhang H, Vitale A, Lahnin F, Lynch K, Bondi C, Kim YS, Peterson BS (1998) Course of tic severity in Tourette syndrome: The first two decades. *Pediatrics* (102): 14–9

Leonard HL, Swedo SE (2001) Paediatric autoimmune neuropsychiatric disorders associated with streptococcal infection (PANDAS). *International Journal of Neuropsychopharmacology* (4): 191–8

Lochner C, Grant JE, Odlaug BL, Stein DJ (2012a) DSM-5 field survey: Skin picking disorder. *Annals of Clinical Psychiatry* (24): 300–4

Lochner C, Grant JE, Odlaug BL, Woods DW, Keuthen NJ, Stein DJ (2012b) DSM-5 field survey: Hair-pulling disorder (trichotillomania). *Depression and Anxiety* (29): 1025–31

Lochner C, Seedat S, Niehaus DJ, Stein DJ (2006) Topiramate in the treatment of trichotillomania: An open-label pilot study. *International Clinical Psychopharmacology* (21): 255–9

Lochner C, Stein DJ (2003) Heterogeneity of obsessive-compulsive disorder: A literature review. *Harvard Review of Psychiatry* (11): 113–32

Lochner C, Stein DJ (2010) Obsessive-compulsive spectrum disorders in obsessive-compulsive disorder and other anxiety disorders. *Psychopathology* (43): 389–96

Mataix-Cols D, Marks IM, Greist JH, Kobak KA, Baer L (2002) Obsessive-compulsive symptom dimensions as predictors of compliance with and response to behaviour therapy: results from a controlled trial. *Psychotherapy and Psychosomatics* (71): 255–62

Math SB, Janardhan ReddyYC (2007) Issues in the pharmacological treatment of obsessive-compulsive disorder. *International Journal of Clinical Practice* (61): 1188–97

McCracken JT, Suddath R, Chang S, Thakur S, Piacentini J (2008) Effectiveness and tolerability of open label olanzapine in children and adolescents with Tourette syndrome. *Journal of Child and Adolescent Psychopharmacology* (18): 501–8

McGuire JF, Kugler BB, Park JM, Horng B, Lewin AB, Murphy TK, Storch EA (2012) Evidence-based assessment of compulsive skin picking, chronic tic disorders and trichotillomania in children. *Child Psychiatry & Human Development* (43): 855–83

Mol Debes NM (2013) Co-morbid disorders in Tourette syndrome. *Behavioural Neurology* (27): 7–14

Muller-Vahl KR (2003) Cannabinoids reduce symptoms of Tourette's syndrome. *Expert Opinion on Pharmacotherapy* (4): 1717–25

Muller-Vahl KR (2013) Treatment of Tourette syndrome with cannabinoids. *Behavioural Neurology* (27):119–24

Muller-Vahl KR, Schneider U, Prevedel H, Theloe K, Kolbe H, Daldrup T, Emrich HM (2003) Delta 9-tetrahydrocannabinol (THC) is effective in the treatment of tics in Tourette syndrome: A 6-week randomized trial. *Journal of Clinical Psychiatry* (64): 459–65

Murray CJ, Lopez AD (1996) Evidence-based health policy – lessons from the Global Burden of Disease Study. *Science* (274): 740–3

Ninan PT, Knight B, Kirk L, Rothbaum BO, Kelsey J, Nemeroff CB (1998) A controlled trial of venlafaxine in trichotillomania: Interim phase I results. *Psychopharmacology bulletin* (34): 221–4

Ninan PT, Rothbaum BO, Marsteller FA, Knight BT, Eccard MB (2000) A placebo-controlled trial of cognitive-behavioral therapy and clomipramine in trichotillomania. *Journal of Clinical Psychiatry* (61): 47–50

Odlaug BL, Grant JE (2007a) Childhood-onset pathologic skin picking: Clinical characteristics and psychiatric comorbidity. *Comprehensive Psychiatry* (48): 388–93

Odlaug BL, Grant JE (2007b) N-acetyl cysteine in the treatment of grooming disorders. *Journal of Clinical Psychopharmacology* (27): 227–9

Odlaug BL, Grant JE (2008) Clinical characteristics and medical complications of pathologic skin picking. *General Hospital Psychiatry* 30: 61–66

Odlaug BL, Grant JE (2010) Pathologic skin picking *American Journal of Drug and Alcohol Abuse* (36): 296–303

Odlaug BL, Grant JE (2011) Phenomenology and epidemiology of pathological skin picking. In: Grant JE, Potenza MN (eds). *The Oxford Library of Psychology: Oxford Handbook of Impulse Control Disorders*. Oxford: Oxford University Press

Odlaug BL, Lust K, Schreiber LR, Christenson G, Derbyshire K, Grant JE (2013) Skin picking disorder in university students: Health correlates and gender differences. *General Hospital Psychiatry* (35):168–73

Pertusa A, Frost RO, Fullana MA, Samuels J, Steketee G, Tolin D, Saxena S, Leckman JF, Mataix-Cols D (2010) Refining the diagnostic boundaries of compulsive hoarding: A critical review. *Clinical Psychology Review* (30): 371–86

Pertusa A, Fullana MA, Singh S, Alonso P, Menchon JM, Mataix-Cols D (2008) Compulsive hoarding: OCD symptom, distinct clinical syndrome, or both? *American Journal of Psychiatry* (165): 1289–98

Perugi G, Akiskal HS, Gemignani A, Pfanner C, Presta S, Milanfranchi A, Lensi P, Ravagli S, Maremmani I, Cassano GB (1998) Episodic course in obsessive-compulsive disorder. *European Archives of Psychiatry and Clinical Neuroscience* (248): 240–4

Phillips KA (1996) *The Broken Mirror: Understanding and Treating Body Dysmorphic Disorder*. NewYork: Oxford University Press

Phillips KA (2005) Placebo-controlled study of pimozide augmentation of fluoxetine in body dysmorphic disorder. *American Journal of Psychiatry* (162): 377–9

Phillips KA Albertini RS Rasmussen SA (2002) A randomized placebo-controlled trial of fluoxetine in body dysmorphic disorder. *Archives of General Psychiatry* (59): 381–8

Phillips KA, Didie ER, Feusner J, Wilhelm S (2008) Body dysmorphic disorder: Treating an underrecognized disorder. *American Journal of Psychiatry* (165): 1111–8

Phillips KA, Hollander E, Rasmussen SA, Aronowitz BR, DeCaria C, Goodman WK (1997) A severity rating scale for body dysmorphic disorder: Development, reliability, and validity of a modified version of the Yale-Brown Obsessive Compulsive Scale. *Psychopharmacology Bulletin* (33): 17–22

Phillips KA, McElroy SL (2000) Personality disorders and traits in patients with body dysmorphic disorder. *Comprehensive Psychiatry* (41): 229–36

Phillips KA, Najjar F (2003) An open-label study of citalopram in body dysmorphic disorder. *Journal of Clinical Psychiatry* (64): 715–20

Phillips KA, Stein DJ, Rauch SL, Hollander E, Fallon BA, Barsky A, Fineberg N, Mataix-Cols D, Ferrao YA, Saxena S, Wilhelm S, Kelly MM, Clark LA, Pinto A, Bienvenu OJ, Farrow J, Leckman J (2010a) Should an obsessive-compulsive spectrum grouping of disorders be included in DSM-V? *Depression and Anxiety* (27): 528–55

Phillips KA, Wilhelm S, Koran LM, Didie ER, Fallon BA, Feusner J, Stein DJ (2010b) Body dysmorphic disorder: Some key issues for DSM-V *Depression and Anxiety* (27): 573–91

Pigott TA, L'Heureux F, Dubbert B, Bernstein S, Murphy DL (1994) Obsessive compulsive disorder: comorbid conditions. *Journal of Clinical Psychiatry* (55 Suppl): 15–27

Rapoport JL, Swedo SE, Leonard HL (1992) Childhood obsessive compulsive disorder. *Journal of Clinical Psychiatry* (53): 11–6

Rasmussen SA, Eisen JL (1992) The epidemiology and clinical features of obsessive compulsive disorder. *Psychiatric Clinics of North America* (15): 743–58

Rasmussen SA, Tsuang MT (1986) Clinical characteristics and family history in DSM-III obsessive-compulsive disorder. *American Journal of Psychiatry* (143): 317–22

Ravizza L, Maina G, Bogetto F (1997) Episodic and chronic obsessive-compulsive disorder. *Depression and Anxiety* (6): 154–8

Rettew DC, Swedo SE, Leonard HL, Lenane MC, Rapoport JL (1992) Obsessions and compulsions across time in 79 children and adolescents with obsessive-compulsive disorder. *Journal of the American Academy of Child & Adolescent Psychiatry* (31): 1050–6

Robertson MM, Eapen V, Cavanna AE (2009) The international prevalence, epidemiology, and clinical phenomenology of Tourette syndrome: A cross-cultural perspective. *Journal of Psychosomatic Research* (67): 475–83

Robertson MM, Schnieden V, Lees AJ (1990) Management of Gilles de la Tourette syndrome using sulpiride. *Clinical Neuropharmacology* (13): 229–35

Roessner V, Plessen KJ, Rothenberger A, Ludolph AG, Rizzo R, Skov L, Strand G, Stern JS, Termine C, Hoekstra PJ (2011) European clinical guidelines for Tourette syndrome and other tic disorders. Part II: pharmacological treatment. *European Child and Adolescent Psychiatry* (20): 173–96

Rosa-Alcázar AI, Sánchez-Meca J, Gómez-Conesa A, Marín-Martínez F (2008) Psychological treatment of obsessive-compulsive disorder: A meta-analysis. *Clinical Psychology Review* (28):1310–25

Rosen JC, Reiter J (1996) Development of the body dysmorphic disorder examination. *Behaviour Research and Therapy* (34): 755–66

Ruscio AM, Stein DJ, Chiu WT, Kessler RC (2010) The epidemiology of obsessive-compulsive disorder in the National Comorbidity Survey Replication. *Molecular Psychiatry* (15): 53–63

Sah DE, Koo J, Price VH (2008) Trichotillomania. *Dermatology and Therapy* (21): 13–21

Samuels J, Bienvenu OJ, Riddle MA, Cullen BA, Grados MA, Liang KY, Hoehn-Saric R, Nestadt G (2002) Hoarding in obsessive compulsive disorder: Results from a case-control study. *Behaviour Research and Therapy* (40): 517–28

Samuels JF, Bienvenu OJ, Grados MA, Cullen B, Riddle MA, Liang KY, Eaton WW, Nestadt G (2008) Prevalence and correlates of hoarding behavior in a community-based sample. *Behaviour Research and Therapy* (46): 836–44

Samuels JF, Bienvenu OJ, Pinto A, Fyer AJ, McCracken JT, Rauch SL, Murphy DL, Grados MA, Greenberg BD, Knowles JA, Piacentini J, Cannistraro PA, Cullen B, Riddle MA, Rasmussen SA, Pauls DL, Willour VL, Shugart YY, Liang KY, Hoehn-Saric R, Nestadt G (2007) Hoarding in obsessive-compulsive disorder: Results from the OCD Collaborative Genetics Study. *Behaviour Research and Therapy* (45): 673–86

Saxena S (2011) Pharmacotherapy of compulsive hoarding. *Journal of Clinical Psychology* (67): 477–84

Saxena S, Brody AL, Maidment KM, Baxter LR (Jr) (2007) Paroxetine treatment of compulsive hoarding. *Journal of Psychiatric Research* (41): 481–7

Saxena S, Maidment KM, Vapnik T, Golden G, Rishwain T, Rosen RM, Tarlow G, Bystritsky A (2002) Obsessive-compulsive hoarding: Symptom severity and response to multimodal treatment. *Journal of Clinical Psychiatry* (63): 21–27

Scahill L, Erenberg G, Berlin CM (Jr) Budman C, Coffey BJ, Jankovic J, Kiessling L, King RA, Kurlan R, Lang A, Mink J, Murphy T, Zinner S, Walkup J (2006) Contemporary assessment and pharmacotherapy of Tourette syndrome. *NeuroRX* (3): 192–206

Scahill L, Leckman JF, Schultz RT, Katsovich L, Peterson BS (2003) A placebo-controlled trial of risperidone in Tourette syndrome. *Neurology* (60): 1130–5

Scahill L, Riddle MA, Swiggin-Hardin M, Ort SI, King RA, Goodman WK, Cicchetti D, Leckman JF (1997) Children's Yale-Brown Obsessive Compulsive Scale: Reliability and validity. *Journal of the American Academy of Child & Adolescent Psychiatry* (36): 844–52

Schneider A, Storch EA, Geffken GR, Lack CW, Shytle RD (2008) Psychometric properties of the Hoarding Assessment Scale in college students. *Illness, Crisis & Loss* (16): 227–36

Shafran R, Tallis F (1996) Obsessive-compulsive hoarding: A cognitive-behavioral approach. *Behavioural and Cognitive Psychotherapy* (24): 209–21

Shapiro AK, Shapiro E (1981) Clonidine and haloperidol in Gilles de la Tourette syndrome. *Archives of General Psychiatry* (38): 1183–5

Shapiro AK, Shapiro E (1982) Clinical efficacy of haloperidol, pimozide, penfluridol, and clonidine in the treatment of Tourette syndrome. *Advances in neurology* (35): 383–6

Shytle RD, Silver AA, Sheehan KH, Wilkinson BJ, Newman M, Sanberg PR, Sheehan D (2003) The Tourette's Disorder Scale (TODS): Development, reliability, and validity. *Assessment* (10): 273–87

Simeon D, Stein DJ, Gross S, Islam N, Schmeidler J, Hollander E (1997) A double-blind trial of fluoxetine in pathologic skin picking. *Journal of Clinical Psychiatry* (58): 341–7

Skapinakis P, Papatheodorou T, Mavreas V (2007) Antipsychotic augmentation of serotonergic antidepressants in treatment-resistant obsessive-compulsive disorder: A meta-analysis of the randomized controlled trials. *European Neuropsychopharmacology* (17): 79–93

Skoog G Skoog I (1999) A 40-year follow-up of patients with obsessive-compulsive disorder [see comments]. *Archives of General Psychiatry* (56): 121–127

Snorrason I, Belleau EL, Woods DW (2012) How related are hair pulling disorder (trichotillomania) and skin picking disorder? A review of evidence for comorbidity, similarities and shared etiology. *Clinical Psychology Review* (32): 618–29

Stanley MA, Breckenridge JK, Sayder AG, Novy DM (1999) Clinician-rated measures of hairpulling: A preliminary psychometric evaluation. *Journal of Psychopathology and Behavioral Assessment* (21): 154–70

Stein DJ, Roberts M, Hollander E, Rowland C, Serebro P (1996) Quality of life and pharmaco-economic aspects of obsessive-compulsive disorder. A South African survey. *South African Medical Journal* (86): 79–1585

Steketee G, Frost RO (2007) *Compulsive hoarding and acquiring: Therapist guide*. New York: Oxford University Press

Steketee G, Frost RO, Tolin DF, Rasmussen J, Brown TA (2010) Waitlist-controlled trial of cognitive behavior therapy for hoarding disorder. *Depression and Anxiety* (27): 476–84

Steketee G, Frost RO, Wincze J, Greene K, Douglass H (2000) Group and individual treatment of compulsive hoarding: A pilot study. *Behavioural and Cognitive Psychotherapy* (28): 259–68

Stengler K, Olbrich S, Heider D, Dietrich S, Riedel-Heller S, Jahn I (2013) Mental health treatment seeking among patients with OCD: impact of age of onset. *Social Psychiatry and Psychiatric Epidemiology* (48): 813–9

Stewart RS, Nejtek VA (2003) An open-label, flexible-dose study of olanzapine in the treatment of trichotillomania. *Journal of Clinical Psychiatry* (64): 49–52

Storch EA, Lack CW, Simons LE, Goodman WK, Murphy TK, Geffken GR (2007) A measure of functional impairment in youth with Tourette's syndrome. *Journal of Pediatric Psychology* (32): 950–9

Storch EA, Muroff J, Lewin AB, Geller D, Ross A, McCarthy K, Morgan J, Murphy TK, Frost R, Steketee G (2011) Development and preliminary psychometric evaluation of the Children's Saving Inventory. *Child Psychiatry & Human Development* (42): 166–82

Storch EA, Murphy TK, Geffken GR, Sajid M, Allen P, Roberti JW, Goodman WK (2005) Reliability and validity of the Yale Global Tic Severity Scale. *Psychological Assessment* (17): 486–91

Streichenwein SM, Thornby JI (1995) A long-term, double-blind, placebo-controlled crossover trial of the efficacy of fluoxetine for trichotillomania. *American Journal of Psychiatry* (152): 1192–6

Sulkowski ML, Storch EA, Geffken GR, Ricketts E, Murphy TK, Goodman WK (2008) Concurrent validity of the Yale-Brown Obsessive-Compulsive Scale – Symptom Checklist. *Journal of Clinical Psychology* (64): 1338–51

Swedo SE, Leonard HL, Rapoport JL, Lenane MC, Goldberger EL, Cheslow DL (1989) A double-blind comparison of clomipramine and desipramine in the treatment of trichotillomania (hair pulling). *New England Journal of Medicine* (321): 497–501

Tay YK, Levy ML, Metry DW (2004) Trichotillomania in childhood: Case series and review. *Pediatrics* (113): e494-e498

Teng EJ, Woods DW, Twohig MP (2006) Habit reversal as a treatment for chronic skin picking: A pilot investigation. *Behavior Modification* (30): 411–22

Thomas R, Cavanna AE (2013) The pharmacology of Tourette syndrome. *Journal of Neural Transmission* 120: 689–94

Thomsen PH (2013) Obsessive-compulsive disorders. *European Child and Adolescent Psychiatry* (22 Suppl 1): S23-S28

Thomsen PH, Mikkelsen HU (1995) Course of obsessive-compulsive disorder in children and adolescents: A prospective follow-up study of 23 Danish cases. *Journal of the American Academy of Child & Adolescent Psychiatry* 34: 1432–1440

Tolin DF, Frost RO, Steketee G (2007) An open trial of cognitive-behavioral therapy for compulsive hoarding. *Behaviour Research and Therapy* 45 1461–70

Tolin DF, Frost RO, Steketee G (2010) A brief interview for assessing compulsive hoarding: The Hoarding Rating Scale-Interview. *Psychiatry Research* 178: 147–52

Torres AR, Moran P, Bebbington P, Brugha T, Bhugra D, Coid JW, Farrell M, Jenkins R, Lewis G, Meltzer H, Prince M (2006) Obsessive-compulsive disorder and personality disorder: Evidence from the British National Survey of Psychiatric Morbidity 2000. *Social Psychiatry and Psychiatric Epidemiology* 41: 862–7

Tucker BT, Woods DW, Flessner CA, Franklin SA, Franklin ME (2011) The Skin Picking Impact Project: Phenomenology, interference, and treatment utilization of pathological skin picking in a population-based sample. *Journal of Anxiety Disorders* 25: 88–95

Tukel R, Oflaz SB, Ozyildirim I, Aslantas B, Ertekin E, Sozen A, Alyanak F, Atli H (2007) Comparison of clinical characteristics in episodic and chronic obsessive-compulsive disorder. *Depression and Anxiety* 24: 251–5

Twohig MP, Hayes SC, Masuda A (2006) A preliminary investigation of acceptance and commitment therapy as a treatment for chronic skin picking. *Behaviour Research and Therapy* 44: 1513–1522

Twohig MP, Woods DW (2001) Habit reversal as a treatment for chronic skin picking in typically developing adult male siblings. *Journal of Applied Behavior Analysis* 34: 217–20

Uzun O, Ozdemir B (2010) Aripiprazole as an augmentation agent in treatment-resistant body dysmorphic disorder. *Clinical Drug Investigation* 30: 707–10

Van Ameringen M, Mancini C, Patterson B, Bennett M, Oakman J (2010) A randomized, double-blind, placebo-controlled trial of olanzapine in the treatment of trichotillomania. *Journal of Clinical Psychiatry* 71: 1336–43

Van Minnen A, Hoogduin KA, Keijsers GP, Hellenbrand I, Hendriks GJ, (2003) Treatment of trichotillomania with behavioral therapy or fluoxetine: A randomized, waiting-list controlled study. *Archives of General Psychiatry* 60: 517–22

Verdellen C, van de GJ Hartmann A Murphy T (2011) European clinical guidelines for Tourette syndrome and other tic disorders. Part III: Behavioural and psychosocial interventions. *European Child and Adolescent Psychiatry* 20: 197–207

Verdellen CW, Hoogduin CA, Kato BS, Keijsers GP, Cath DC, Hoijtink HB (2008) Habituation of premonitory sensations during exposure and response prevention treatment in Tourette's syndrome. *Behavior Modification* 32 215–227

Walther MR, Flessner CA, Conelea CA, Woods DW (2009) The Milwaukee Inventory for the Dimensions of Adult Skin Picking (MIDAS): Initial development and psychometric properties. *Journal of Behavior Therapy and Experimental Psychiatry* 40: 127–135

Weissman MM, Bland RC, Canino GJ, Greenwald S, Hwu HG, Lee CK, Newman SC, Oakley-Browne MA, Rubio-Stipec M, Wickramaratne PJ (1994) The Cross National epidemiology of obsessive compulsive disorder. The Cross National Collaborative Group. *Journal of Clinical Psychiatry* 55 (Suppl): 5–10

Wilhelm S, Keuthen NJ, Deckersbach T, Engelhard IM, Forker AE, Baer L, O'Sullivan RL, Jenike MA (1999)

Self-injurious skin picking: Clinical characteristics and comorbidity. *Journal of Clinical Psychiatry* (60): 454–9

Williams J, Hadjistavropoulos T, Sharpe D (2006) A meta-analysis of psychological and pharmacological treatments for Body Dysmorphic Disorder. *Behaviour Research and Therapy* 44: 99–111

Woods DW, Wetterneck CT, Flessner CA (2006) A controlled evaluation of acceptance and commitment therapy plus habit reversal for trichotillomania. *Behaviour Research and Therapy* 44: 639–56

Woody SR, Steketee G, Chambless DL (1995) Reliability and validity of the Yale-Brown Obsessive-Compulsive Scale. *Behaviour Research and Therapy* (33): 597–605

# Appendix: List of useful scales in the assessment of OCRDs

## A17.1 Obsessive-compulsive disorder (OCD)

- Children's Yale-Brown Obsessive Compulsive Scale (Scahill *et al.*, 1997): a semi-structured measure of obsessive-compulsive symptom severity in children and adolescents with obsessive-compulsive disorder
- Yale Brown Obsessive Compulsive (Symptoms) Checklist (Sulkowski *et al.*, 2008): a self-report version to help define the obsessions and compulsions prior to using the Yale Brown Obsessive Compulsive Scale (Y-BOCS – see below).
- Yale-Brown Obsessive Compulsive Scale (Goodman *et al.*, 1989a; Goodman, *et al.*, 1989b; Woody *et al.*, 1995): a standard observer-rated scale to rate severity of OCD symptoms.
- Obsessive Compulsive Inventory (OCI) (Foa *et al.*, 1998): a self-report measure of obsessive-compulsive symptoms.

## A 17.2 Body dysmorphic disorder (BDD)

- The BDD-Y-BOCS (Yale-Brown obsessive compulsive scale, modified for Body Dysmorphic Disorder) (Phillips *et al.*, 1997): a widely used measure to assess BDD symptom severity.
- The Body Dysmorphic Disorder Questionnaire (Brunhoeber and Maes, 2007; Kollei *et al.*, 2012): a measure to assess a wide range of BDD symptoms, containing two main scales and seven subscales with 42 items in total. It uses a 5-point rating scale for each item.
- The Body Shape Questionnaire (BSQ) (Cooper *et al.*, 1987; Evans and Dolan, 1993): one of the most widely used measures of body dissatisfaction, it consists of 34 items, each with a 6-point Likert-type scale.
- The Body Appreciation Scale (BAS) (Avalos *et al.*, 2005): a measure reflecting body appreciation (an aspect of positive body image).
- The Body Dysmorphic Disorder Examination (BDDE) (Rosen and Reiter, 1996): a measure designed to diagnose BDD and to measure symptoms of severely negative body image.

## A17.3 Hoarding disorder (HD)

- Saving Inventory-Revised (Frost *et al.*, 2004): a 23-item questionnaire that comprises three subscales designed to measure the main features of HD.
- Hoarding Rating Scale-Interview (Tolin *et al.*, 2010): a brief, 5-item semi-structured interview that assesses hoarding and its critical features.
- Hoarding Assessment Scale (Schneider *et al.*, 2008): a brief questionnaire with items focused on difficulties throwing away things, clutter, urges for acquisition and interferences or distress due to hoarding.
- Clutter Image Rating (Frost *et al.*, 2008): a novel assessment device designed to provide a measure of clutter; it is more objective and not dependent on beliefs about what constitutes clutter.
- Children's Saving Inventory (Storch *et al.*, 2011): a 21-item parent-rated scale of hoarding with four factors: difficulty discarding, clutter, excessive acquisition and distress or impairment.

## A17.4 Hair-pulling disorder (HPD or trichotillomania)

- Massachusetts General Hospital Hairpulling Scale (Keuthen *et al.*, 2007a): a brief, self-report instrument for assessing repetitive hair pulling.
- Milwaukee Inventory for Subtypes of Trichotillomania – Adult Version (MIST-A) (Flessner *et al.*, 2008b): assesses automatic and focused trichotillomania subtypes.

- Milwaukee Inventory for Styles of Trichotillomania – Child Version (MIST-C) (Flessner *et al.*, 2007): a 36-item self-report scale designed to assess the degree to which children and adolescents engage in focused and automatic hair pulling.
- NIMH Trichotillomania Severity Scale (NIMH-TSS) (Diefenbach *et al.*, 2005; Stanley *et al.*, 1999): a clinical interview modelled on the Y-BOCS, it consists of summative response scales assessing time, resistance, distress and interference.
- NIMH Trichotillomania Impairment Scale (NIMH-TIS) (Diefenbach *et al.*, 2005; Stanley *et al.*, 1999): a global measure of HPD impairment, based on hair loss, money spent on hair products and other hair treatments and time pulling or concealing hair loss, and the patient's sense of self-control over hair pulling.
- Psychiatric Institute Trichotillomania Scale (PITS) (Diefenbach *et al.*, 2005; Stanley *et al.*, 1999): a 6-item clinician-rated measure of hair-pulling symptoms that include pulling sites, duration, frequency, interference, distress and severity of hair loss.
- Trichotillomania Scale for Children–Child Report (TSC-C) (McGuire *et al.*, 2012): assesses severity, distress and impairment due to HPD symptoms.
- Yale-Brown Obsessive Compulsive-Scale-Trichotillomania (Y-BOCS-TM) (McGuire *et al.*, 2012): a 10-item measure modified from the Yale-Brown Obsessive Compulsive Scale (Y-BOCS). Items are rated on a scale from 0 to 5, and yield two subtotal scores – one for intrusive thoughts regarding hair pulling and the other for actual pulling behaviour.

## A17.5 Skin-picking disorder

- Milwaukee Inventory for the Dimensions of Adult Skin Picking (MIDAS) (Walther *et al.*, 2009): a measure to assess the degree to which individuals with skin-picking disorder engage in focused and/or automatic picking.
- Skin Picking Scale (SPS) (Keuthen *et al.*, 2001b): a 6-item self-report scale designed to assess the severity of skin picking.
- The Yale-Brown Obsessive Compulsive Scale modified for Neurotic Excoriation (Y-BOCS-NE) (Grant *et al.*, 2010): a semi-structured clinician-rated measure used to evaluate treatment efficacy in adults.
- The Skin Picking Impact Scale (SPIS) (Keuthen *et al.*, 2001a): focuses on the impact versus severity of skin-picking.

## A17.6 Tourette's disorder (TD)

- Child Tourette Syndrome Impairment Scale (CTIM) (Storch *et al.*, 2007): a 37-item parent-rated measure that assesses a child's tic-related impairment in school, home and social activities.
- Shapiro Tourette Syndrome Severity Scale (STSSS) (McGuire *et al.*, 2012): a clinician-rated scale that requires ordinal responses to each of its five items. The five questions focus on the number of tics (0–3 scale with anchor points), how noticeable they are to others (0–1), whether the tics elicit comments (0–2), if the patient is considered odd or bizarre (0–2) and if the tics interfere with functioning (0–2).
- Tourette Disorder Scale (TODS) (Shytle *et al.*, 2003): a 15-item scale to measure a broad range of common symptoms including tics, inattention, hyperactivity, obsessions, compulsions, aggression and emotional symptoms.
- Tourette Disorder Scale-Clinician Report (TODS-CR) (McGuire *et al.*, 2012): a clinician-administered measure that assesses the severity of tics and co-morbid conditions (e.g. hyperactivity, aggression and OCD).
- The Tourette Syndrome Symptom List (TSSL) (Cohen *et al.*, 1980; McGuire, *et al.*, 2012): a self-report or parent-report measure that contains a fairly comprehensive list of 35 symptoms covering the areas of motor tics, phonic tics and behaviour (e.g. touching, compulsions).
- Yale Global Tic Severity Scale (YGTSS) (Kircanski *et al.*, 2010; Leckman *et al.*, 1989; McGuire *et al.*, 2012; Storch *et al.*, 2005): a semi-structured interview that measures the number, frequency, intensity, interference and complexity of tics. It yields a total severity score and separate scores for motor and vocal tics, in addition to a clinician impairment rating.

CHAPTER

# 18 Somatic symptom and related disorders

Conrad Visser

## 18.1 Introduction

All bodily, or somatic, symptoms (including pain, weakness, tingling, chills and many more) are experienced psychically. Most of us are familiar with feelings of 'a lump in the throat', 'weakness at the knees' and 'butterflies in the stomach' in the face of psychological stress. These common experiences are examples of **somatising**, or the tendency to experience bodily distress in the face of psychological stress. We feel anxiety in our bodies. Somatising is also the central, defining feature of the somatic symptom disorders. In the DSM-5 (American Psychiatric Association, 2013), the characteristic feature of a somatic symptom disorder is the presence of somatic symptoms, suggesting a medical condition that cannot be fully explained by the presenting symptoms. (Somatic symptom disorders were classified as somatoform disorders in the DSM-IV-TR (American Psychiatric Association, 2000)). There must also be positive evidence or a strong presumption that links the observed bodily symptoms to psychological factors. We know that many patients who seek general medical services do not suffer from demonstrable physical ailments that require medical treatment. They also do not view themselves as psychiatrically ill and do not seek psychiatric help. Yet, many likely suffer from a somatic symptom condition (Epstein *et al.*, 1999).

Conceptualisations and attempts at categorical alignment have undergone repeated revision since the 19th century, yet the controversy continues. The controversy and debate stem from the diagnostic unwieldiness of some of the constructs on the one hand, and from our expanding understanding of the brain and behaviour emerging from modern neuroscience on the other. The DSM-5 recognises seven types of somatic symptom disorder (see Table 18.1) The approach adopted by the DSM-5 reflects the movement of clinical emphasis away from the medically unexplained quality of somatic symptoms to a greater recognition of psychological distress, functional impairment and poorer quality of life related to these symptoms. The International Classification of Diseases of the World Health Organisation (ICD-10) approaches these conditions quite differently. Conversion disorder, for example, is not classified as a somatoform disorder in the ICD-10 as it is conceptualised as a dissociative disorder.

**Table 18.1** List of somatic symptom disorders

- Somatic symptom disorder (DSM IV-TR Somatisation disorder)
- Illness anxiety disorder (DSM IV-TR Hypochondriasis)
- Conversion disorder (functional neurological symptom disorder)
- Psychological factors affecting other medical conditions
- Factitious disorder
- Other specified somatic symptom and related disorder
- Unspecified somatic symptom and related disorder

**Source:** Authors' own table

How does the DSM-5 account for entrenched DSM-IV-TR diagnoses like pain disorder? What is apparent in the leaner DSM-5 conceptualisation is the recognition of the similarities between the DSM-IV-TR somatisation, undifferentiated somatoform and pain disorder and their replacement with the single diagnostic construct 'somatic symptom disorder'. Within the DSM-5 individual differences, that reflect the predominant mode of presentation, are accommodated through type specifiers (e.g. 'pain disorder' becomes 'somatic symptom disorder with predominantly pain'). The classic hypochondriacal patient, where obsessive worry about health is prominent and somatic symptoms are in the background, is reconceptualised to have illness anxiety disorder. As bodily concerns are found in 'factitious disorder' and 'psychological factors affecting other medical conditions', these categories have been included in the renamed 'somatic symptom disorder' category. 'Body dysmorphic disorder' is reclassified as one of the obsessive-compulsive spectrum disorder category.

## 18.2 History

For millennia, the overlap of psychic and somatic experiences has been the focus of intellectual scrutiny. Strongly entrenched in the minds and vernacular of lay and professional people alike, 'hysteria' has been used synonymously with conversion and other instances of pathological somatising. The word itself is derived from the Greek hyster (uterus) and its use attributed to Hippocrates. The ancient Greeks and Egyptians understood hysteria to arise from a uterus wandering from its usual anatomical position into other parts of the body. The ancient Greeks also attributed certain maladies to disturbances in the viscera of the hypochondrium (abdomen below the ribcage). In the 1600s, hypochondriasis came to mean mental maladies arising from organs in the two hypochondria, leading to a preoccupation with bodily symptoms.

Thomas Sydenham (1624–1689) became aware of the importance of neurotic and hysterical symptoms and the frequency with which they occurred among his patients. He noted that psychosocial stress, or 'antecedent sorrows' was involved in causing hysterical symptoms. In the 1800s, more recognisably modern theories around hysteria and hypochondriasis emerged. Jean Martin Charcot, a French neurologist who worked at the Pitié-Salpêtrière Hospital in Paris, proposed that hysteria arose when patients, predisposed by heredity, were exposed to a traumatic event that produced a functional brain lesion. Charcot could evoke and manipulate hysteria through hypnosis and emphasised its role treating hysterical disorders.

Pierre Janet, who introduced the concept of dissociation, considered hysteria a disturbance in selective attention where, through dissociation, selected mental contents are removed from consciousness while continuing to produce motor and sensory deficits (Ford, 1985; Van der Hart and Rutger, 1989). Sigmund Freud studied at Charcot's clinic where he became interested in the problem of hysteria and considered it a genuine form of nervous system pathology. Freud came to suspect a connection between hysterical pathology and sexuality, providing one of the points of departure for psychoanalysis. Freud also introduced the term 'conversion' to medicine. Conversion was believed to be the defence mechanism responsible for converting mental stress and conflict into a somatic symptom.

In 1859 Paul Briquet described hysteria as an often chronic, poly-symptomatic condition that affected multiple organs. He argued that hysteria resulted from abnormal brain function when stressful events acted upon the 'affective part of the brain'. Regrettably, the term 'hysterical' came to be used loosely and pejoratively to describe any demanding patient with vague symptoms (Ford, 1985).

## 18.3 General notes on pathogenesis

The aetiologies of somatic symptom disorders are disparate and the pathogenic mechanisms are multiple and complex. Somatising conforms to the stressor-diathesis model with evidence of a hereditary predisposition (or diathesis). The universality of psychosocial trauma in the later development of somatising has been amply recognised. There is agreement that early occurrence of trauma, trauma of long duration and trauma that involves sexual or physical abuse are linked to an increased severity of conversion symptoms. Although the exact details of abuse may be debatable, abused patients probably experience significant problems with attachment, impaired-object relations and a dysfunctional family system (Krahn, 2008).

## 18.3.1 Neural information processing insights

The recent ascent of neuroscience, clinical experience, neuropsychological evidence, functional neuro-imaging and neurophysiological techniques have yielded insightful and practical pathogenic theories. Conversion and other somatising psychopathology appear to result from the dynamic restructuring of neural networks. This results in volition, sensory experience and motor behaviour to become functionally isolated, disconnected or dissociated. This disconnection occurs in the absence of an identifiable anatomical lesion and is thus considered functional. Dissociation is a common phenomenon experienced in health and disease and contributes to the presentation of somatising. Dissociation is conceptualised to involve two processes: compartmentalisation and detachment.

Compartmentalisation corresponds to Cardeña's (1984) concept of suspension of mental integration; it involves the inability to bring into conscious awareness information typically accessible to consciousness and susceptible to conscious influence. Despite their disconnection from consciousness, compartmentalised processes continue to function. Compartmentalisation can manifest as amnesia and other deficits such as blindness, anaesthesia and paralysis. Neurally, the process of compartmentalisation involves the top-down regulation of subordinate cortical functions by higher-order cortical regions. In the presence of a threat, for example, the prefrontal cortex may inhibit the primary motor cortex, thus preventing the final common pathway to initiate movement. In this instance, paralysis will result in the absence of any anatomically demonstrable lesion in the nervous system or muscle. The lesion thus is functional: it is as if the higher-order cortex had taken the subordinate cortex'offline'. Conversion paralysis, blindness or anaesthesia suggests compartmentalisation as a pathogenic mechanism. We have all heard of an animal rolling over and playing dead, or a hare frozen in a car's headlights on a rural road. In the animal kingdom, compartmentalised paralysis or tonic immobility is not uncommon and witnessed in, inter alia, sharks, snakes, cattle and hare.

Like compartmentalisation, detachment may also confer survival advantage on an animal under threat. By attenuation of the adverse emotional consequences of stress, detachment rations the brain's finite capacity for attention, thus freeing it to remain focused on the task at hand: to mitigate threat. Detachment results in traumatic amnesia, analgesia-anaesthesia, tunnel vision and visceral disturbances.

In light of these evolutionary theories, a question inevitably arises: how can an essentially adaptive system lead to disabling pathology? When exposed to serious threats, like abuse, a child may respond defensively through compartmentalisation or detachment. With repeated trauma, the dissociative response is strengthened through use-dependent conditioning. Over time, this dissociative response becomes the preferred response to threat. When faced with serious threats later in life, dissociation is activated and produces symptoms like blindness, paralysis, pain, dizziness and abdominal discomfort.

## 18.3.2 Psychodynamic understanding

Psychodynamic theory owes its origins to a need to understand hysteria, conversion and hypochondriasis. Psychodynamically, neurosis stems from unacceptable Id-impulses, which often are sexual or aggressive, attempting to break into consciousness and stamp their influence on behaviour. This gives rise to anxiety against which defences develop. Sometimes, intense anxiety spills into consciousness with debilitating effects. At other times, defences become overly rigid and neurotic behaviour results. In somatising, psychodynamic theory posits that regression is strongly exhibited. Patients defend themselves against the anxieties of adult life by regressing to the state of a sick child who wants attention, support and mollycoddling. In this situation the primary gain – relief from anxiety – is achieved. However, a secondary gain may also be achieved through comforting and release from responsibilities.

Conversion symptoms block awareness and expression of a forbidden impulse through incapacitating a body part related to that impulse: paralysis may arise as defence against murderous rage and glove anaesthesia against guilt over masturbation. Whatever the situation, the maintenance of elaborate defences monopolises and exhausts the Ego, thereby compromising the person's work and relationships.

### 18.3.3 Behavioural understanding

Behavioural theory interprets somatising as the product of a person's assumption of a social role reinforced by incidental consequences (Ullmann and Krasner, 1975). For a man conscripted into military service, conversion paralysis or conversion blindness is patently rewarding. Contingencies that continue to reward maladaptive behaviour or states may lead to a chronic maintenance of somatising. Learning plays a significant part in the modulation and experience of bodily sensations. Research data also suggest that parental interest in, and attention paid to, bodily symptoms in a patient's childhood, promote the likelihood of somatising in adulthood. Somatising could be considered a response to health care that emphasises care for physical afflictions (Kirmayer, 1984). With the common belief (partly reinforced by medicine's own biases) that physical disorders are respectable and mental illnesses shameful, somatising will likely continue to offer people a socially acceptable means of expressing psychic distress.

### 18.3.4 Humanistic-existential understanding

Like psychoanalysts, humanist-existential theorists view somatising to stem from anxiety due to intrapsychic conflicts. However, in humanist-existentialist theory, anxiety is understood not only as an individual problem but as a predictable outcome of conflict between the individual and society. Anxiety and psychological disturbance are inevitable as long as societies thwart the natural goodness of humans, oppose their innate drive for self-actualisation and frustrate their search for meaning. Humanist-existentialist theory posits that the root of anxiety is the discrepancy between our self-concept and our ideal self, which itself is regarded as the product of a hostile and rejecting upbringing.

## 18.4 General treatment considerations

Before embarking on an exploration of the individual disorders, let us pause to consider the principles of treatment. Since the somatic symptom disorders share many common features, a general treatment approach is feasible. The following points can be made (Allen *et al.*, 2001; Khouzam and Field, 1999; Mai, 2004; Kroenke and Swindle, 2000):

- Therapy is not a cure.
- The therapeutic aims are threefold:
  - improve patients' miserable experience and improve their quality of life
  - preserve and improve psychosocial functioning
  - minimise expensive health care use, unnecessary interventions and iatrogenic complications.
- Therapeutic aims are guided by a triad of principles:
  - to establish a solid therapeutic alliance from the outset
  - psycho-education that targets an understanding of symptoms and stress management
  - to offer consistent reassurance.
- Encourage relaxation, activity, employment and limit reliance on external support. Enhance awareness of emotions, decrease physical arousal and reframe distress.
- Achieving therapeutic aims yields reduced maladaptive health-seeking behaviour, regardless of the general mental or physical condition.
- Treat co-morbid medical and psychiatric conditions, especially depression and anxiety.
- Cognitive behavioural therapy (CBT) is able to achieve all aims and is considered the evidence-based treatment of choice.

- Pharmacotherapy has limited application and is used mainly to treat psychiatric co-morbidity.

## 18.5 Specific somatic symptom disorders

This discussion will present disorders using their DSM-5-nomenclature and order of listing.

### 18.5.1 Somatic symptom disorder

Paul Briquet (Pribor *et al.*, 1993) was the first to recognise this frequently chronic condition with its poly-symptomatic, multi-organ involvement. For this reason somatic symptom disorder (somatisation disorder in the DSM-IV-TR) is still sometimes referred to as Briquet's syndrome. In the mid-twentieth century, interest in Briquet's syndrome was reawakened, mainly through

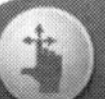

**Case study 18.1**

Jenny, 35, recently moved to Sasolburg following her boyfriend's appointment as a site manager at a petrochemical plant. She has been married twice and has three teenaged children from her first marriage.

As her boyfriend had loaded her as dependant on his medical aid, she decided to visit a local general practitioner instead of the state clinic, as she felt that private practitioners would better understand her 'dire state of health'. She complained to the attending doctor that she suffered from severe bloating, disabling and prolonged menstrual pain, frequent bouts of shortness of breath, sore muscles and joints and chronic headache. Her examination was unremarkable, except her slightly dishevelled appearance, onychomycosis, obesity and mild hypertension with no evidence of end-organ damage. He noted her sullen disposition. Appropriate bloodwork, chest and joint X-rays and abdominal ultrasound revealed no abnormalities. The doctor started treatment with a diuretic and provided dietary advice.

Over the ensuing weeks, Jenny repeatedly returned to the practice, preferring to see different doctors each time. She had complied with the anti-hypertensive treatment but had made no efforts to modify her diet or exercise. Her original symptoms were unchanged. Her treatment, now fragmented because of frequent changes of doctors resulted in investigations being repeated and illogical polypharmacy with various anti-inflammatory agents, analgesics, prokinetics, two benzodiazepines and three different antidepressants prescribed.

A few months later, she started attending another practice and also frequented the provincial hospital's clinic. At the provincial hospital, she complained to the nurse that nobody seemed capable, or willing, to understand her problems. She added that 'A doctor had dared to tell me it was all in my head.' Taking interest in the patient, the nurse inquired further, listening intently. Jenny was raised by a single mother. Her mother often moved house and had many relationships over the years. Although she stopped short of admitting abuse, she indicated that one of her mother's boyfriends had come 'too close for comfort' when she was eight years old. Jenny struggled academically, but managed to complete matric. She embarked on a secretarial course after matric, but never completed it as she fell pregnant with her firstborn and had to get married. She had two further babies, in rapid succession and said she felt used, 'like a mix between a prostitute and a baby machine'.

Tired of her husband's infidelity and verbal abuse, she filed for divorce and secured custody of her children. Then, aged 25, she started working for the first time. A relationship flared between her and the estate agent for whom she worked and the two were married within weeks. He, too, was unfaithful and divorce soon followed. Around this time, she started experiencing chronic headaches, shortness of breath and bloating. Her physical discomfort and frequent visits to doctors stymied her ability to sustain employment. She moved in with her sister, whose husband was a wealthy contractor. During this period, her physical condition improved somewhat. Around a year ago, she met her current boyfriend and moved in with him. Although he provided financial stability, his job was an itinerant one making severe demands on her. Shortly before their move to Sasolburg, she learnt that he too had been unfaithful and was obsessed with porn on his tablet. Not for the first time in her life, she took an overdose and tried to slit her wrists, spending a few days at a Johannesburg psychiatric clinic. 'I'm not psycho,' she protested, 'they all get it wrong, my body is packing up.'

the work of Purtell and Feighner (Hales, 2008). Feighner developed a comprehensive list of diagnostic criteria. However, Feighner's criteria were complicated and made diagnosis daunting and discouraging to practitioners. The term 'somatisation disorder' was first introduced in the DSM-III. Although abridged and simpler than Feighner's criteria, the DSM-III criteria remained complex (Hales, 2008). Subsequent editions of the DSM further pruned the criteria, but their operational complexity continued to hamper its recognition in primary care. The approach adopted by the ICD is also complicated.

The criteria have been much simplified in the DSM-5. The DSM-5 construct emphasises the psychological nature of symptoms such as cognitive distortions, high health-related anxiety, disproportionate and persistent concerns about the seriousness of symptoms, excessive time and energy devoted to the symptoms and somatic symptom disorder's chronic tendency. When pain is the predominant somatic symptom, it is coded as somatic symptom disorder with predominant pain. (Chronic pain is discussed briefly in Section 18.5.2.2.)

### 18.5.1.1 Diagnosis and clinical features

Patients present with complicated medical histories. Symptoms may be vaguely described or presented with dramatic exaggeration. Accounts of their symptom history are often contradictory and inconsistent: patients may even fail to distinguish between current, recent and past symptoms. Table 18.2 lists the DSM-5 diagnostic criteria for somatic symptom disorder.

Typical somatic complaints are pain and gastrointestinal, psychosexual, neurological, cardiological and pulmonological complaints. The nature and occurrence rates of symptoms vary across different cultures: tactile symptoms, for example, are more common in people of Afro-Caribbean than European descent. Concurrent anxiety and depressive symptoms are common: when a patient seeks psychiatric help it is usually because of these and not because the bodily symptoms are believed to have a psychological basis (Bagayogo *et al.*, 2013). Concurrent

**Table 18.2** DSM-5 Diagnostic Criteria for Somatic Symptom Disorder

| **Diagnostic Criteria** |
|---|
| A. One or more somatic symptoms that are distressing or result in significant disruption of daily life. |
| B. Excessive thoughts, feelings, or behaviors related to the somatic symptoms or associated health concerns as manifested by at least one of the following: |
| 1. Disproportionate and persistent thoughts about the seriousness of one's symptoms. |
| 2. Persistently high level of anxiety about health or symptoms. |
| 3. Excessive time and energy devoted to these symptoms or health concerns. |
| C. Although any one somatic symptom may not be continuously present, the state of being symptomatic is persistent (typically more than 6 months). |
| *Specify* if: |
| **With predominant pain** (previously pain disorder): This specifier is for individuals whose somatic symptoms predominantly involve pain. |
| *Specify* if: |
| **Persistent:** A persistent course is characterized by severe symptoms, marked impairment, and long duration (more than 6 months). |
| *Specify* current severity: |
| **Mild:** Only one of the symptoms specified in Criterion B is fulfilled. |
| **Moderate:** Two or more of the symptoms specified in Criterion B are fulfilled. |
| **Severe:** Two or more of the symptoms specified in Criterion B are fulfilled, plus there are multiple somatic complaints (or one very severe somatic symptom). |

**Source:** Reprinted with permission from the *Diagnostic and Statistical Manual of Mental Disorders*, Fifth Edition, (Copyright 2013). American Psychiatric Association.

occupational, interpersonal and marital difficulties abound. Patients may display histrionic and antisocial personality features. The presence of conversion and dissociative phenomena and strained interpersonal relationships further assist with recognition of the disorder (Hales, 2008). Suicide threats and acts of **deliberate self-harm** are not unusual. Female patients may dress seductively or appear demure, reminiscent of histrionic and borderline patients, as well as self-absorbed, manipulative, praise-seeking and dependent with an external locus of control. Patients have often seen many doctors, sometimes concurrently. In this regard it is helpful to access old medical records. Childhood trauma is common in patients' personal histories. The onset or exacerbation of symptoms also indicates trauma.

**Information box**

**Somatic symptom disorder essentials**

- Affects predominantly females
- Psychologically unsophisticated, lower socio-economic standing and education
- History of childhood trauma
- Symptom emergence tracks trauma
- Poly-symptomatic, multi-organ, chronic

### 18.5.1.2 Epidemiology

The prevalence rate varies between 0,5–2,8% (Escobar *et al.*, 1998). Women outnumber men by five to one, but cultural factors may modify the ratio (American Psychiatric Association, 2000). The disorder is believed common in primary care, with up to 10% of patients demonstrating features of it. However, because of the operational difficulties of diagnosis, many cases probably go unrecognised. The disorder is more common among rural and educationally deprived people.

### 18.5.1.3 Specific notes on pathogenesis

The pathogenesis of somatic symptom disorder is complex and multi-factorial. The occurrence of traumatic experiences in early development is a consistent finding in patients. The onset, exacerbation and maintenance of symptoms coincide with increased stress.

**Heredity, information processing and neuro-immunological factors**

Somatic symptom disorder occurs in about 20% of first-degree female relatives of patients with the disorder, and probably has a hereditary basis. Family studies also show a link between the disorder and either antisocial personality disorder or anxiety disorders. In women, the disorder probably shares its aetiological substrate with antisocial personality disorder; in men it may be more closely related to anxiety disorders (Hales, 2008). Monozygotic twin-studies demonstrating a 29% concordance for somatisation disorder coupled with evidence from adoption studies further support a genetic basis for the condition (Sadock BJ and Sadock VA, 2000).

Some biological evidence has implicated information processing in the pathogenesis of somatising; this involves aberrant cortical control of sensory afferents and motor efferents from and to the body. Functional imaging studies that point to abnormalities in blood flow and metabolism in the frontal parietal lobes, right parietal lobes, temporo-parietal regions, cerebellum and subcortical structures provide tentative support to this theory. Evoked potential studies also show abnormal sensory processing. Neuropsychological abnormalities like distractibility and circumstantial associations further support a neural substrate at play (Sadock BJ and Sadock VA, 2000).

The cytokines interleukin 1, 2 and 6 and tumour necrosis factor $\alpha$ are believed to be responsible for constitutional symptoms such as lethargy, depression, insomnia and anorexia, which is characteristic of infection and certain cancers. In somatic symptom disorder, cytokine dysregulation may evoke constitutional symptoms in the absence of infection or other causes. Cytokine-dysregulation has also been demonstrated in depression and schizophrenia (Rief *et al.*, 2001).

### 18.5.1.4 Differential diagnosis

The differential diagnosis of somatic symptom disorder includes chronic medical and neurological disorders with vague, transient and fluctuating symptoms referable to multiple organ systems. Multiple sclerosis and myasthenia gravis are prime candidates as are systemic lupus erythematosus, acute intermittent porphyria, porphyria variegata, inflammatory bowel disease and haemosiderosis. The sustained hypercalcaemia of hyperparathyroidism affects tissues in many organs, resulting in multiple symptoms including psychological ones. Syphilis, (known as the great mimicker) and its modern-day counterpart Acquired Immune Deficiency Syndrome (Aids) always warrant inclusion on a differentials list. As somatic symptom disorder typically begins before the age of 30, the onset of multiple physical symptoms later in life should raise the suspicion of a non-psychiatric condition.

Schizophrenia with multiple somatic delusions and tactile hallucinations as well as major depression with somatic symptoms may occasionally warrant differentiation from somatic symptom disorder (Bagayogo *et al.*, 2013). Although similar in many ways, conversion disorder can be distinguished from somatic symptom disorder by the occurrence of a single symptom or a set of symptoms of a neurological kind. In addition, conversion symptoms are typically short-lived. Other psychiatric diagnoses that must be considered are factitious disorder and malingering.

### 18.5.1.5 Course and outcome

Most often the pattern of multiple recurrent physical symptoms has its onset during adolescence. Somatic symptom disorder is a chronic illness and spontaneous remissions are rare, although fluctuations in the severity and number of symptoms do occur. The illness can have a significant impact on the lives of those who have the disorder, and symptoms may be severe and persistent enough to be incapacitating socially and occupationally. Doctors who fail to recognise the disorder may perform unnecessary surgical procedures or prescribe medication with avoidable adverse reactions. The prescription of analgesics or anxiolytics may well put the patient at risk of developing a substance use disorder. Major depressive disorder, personality disorder, substance related disorder and anxiety disorder are common psychiatric co-morbidities found among patients with somatic symptom disorder. Suicide attempts, completed suicide and other acts of deliberate self-harm are recognised complications of somatisation disorder.

### 18.5.1.6 Treatment

Somatic symptom disorder is therapeutically challenging. Whilst the presenting complaints may not involve a demonstrable medical disease, the suffering and dysfunction are very real and form the focus of treatment. The treatment schema set out in Section 18.4 applies. A solid therapeutic alliance is achievable when the patient's genuine suffering is recognised and authentic caring and interest is communicated. This must be followed by a thorough review of the patient's history and condition in order to rule out any underlying medical condition and to understand the patient's situation. Acceptance, mindful listening, patience and allowing the patient enough time to talk about his or her symptoms are indispensable elements of a good alliance.

Patients view their illness as physical and not psychiatric and are therefore often more comfortable seeking assistance from general practitioners. Secondly, patients often fail to recognise, or are reluctant to accept, the relationship between physical symptoms and psychological factors. In this regard psycho-education is an invaluable tool. Psycho-education must enlighten the patient about the nature of the diagnosis and frame it in a positive, yet realistic, way. Frank discussion about treatment, realistic goals and prognosis must follow. Without negating the morbid experience, reassure the patient that no ominous physical cause for the symptoms has been demonstrated. Emphasise the link between symptoms and stress and reassure the patient that his or her condition will continue to be monitored.

Other effective interventions include stress reduction, lifestyle modification and challenging and changing the sick role. CBT has evidence-based efficacy. With the exception of treating concurrent anxiety and depressive symptoms, the available evidence suggests that pharmacological treatment is not effective (Hales, 2008).

## 18.5.2 The special place of pain disorder, chronic pain or psychogenic pain

Pain is not just a sensation: it is an experience. Acute pain is a cardinal sign of, and adaptive response to, tissue damage that starts with nociception and elicits behaviour that limits tissue damage. In contrast, chronic pain is a dysfunctional remnant of a once adaptive response that involves layers of pain experience, suffering and behaviour. Pain behaviour involves a sufferer's efforts to avoid factors that trigger or exacerbate pain. Pain itself is maintained through different neural mechanisms and is exquisitely sensitive to emotional and motivational influences. The DSM-5 provides for the concept of chronic pain or a pain disorder by considering it under the rubric of somatic symptom disorder.

### 18.5.2.1 Diagnosis and clinical features

When the focus of clinical attention is pain and the patient's entire experience and behaviour are fashioned around it, pain becomes a disorder in its own right. Psychological factors are believed to play a role in its causation and maintenance. Involvement in litigation, notably personal injury suits, is recognised to exacerbate chronic pain and increases the risk of chronicity. The exact nature of the pain varies and can include headache, pelvic and joint pain. On closer scrutiny, the reported pain is grossly out of proportion to that suggested by other clinical findings.

Pain is rarely absent and is not alleviated through distraction. Analgesics provide little, if any relief. Patients become preoccupied with pain, lay all their sorrows and misfortunes at its door and imagine an idealised world without this pain. Patients may deny any other causes of distress. Evidence of depression, irritability, **alexithymia**, anhedonia, poor energy, limited libido, insomnia and weight loss are present in nearly all patients.

### 18.5.2.2 Specific notes on the pathogenesis of chronic pain

First-degree relatives of pain disorder probands are at increased risk of developing chronic pain. Other risks include childhood adversity, for example parental separation, alcohol abuse at home, quarrelling parents and lack of physical affection towards the child. An association between depression and chronic pain has long been acknowledged.

The conscious experience of pain is modulated by the cerebral cortex through descending inhibitory noradrenergic and serotonergic pathways. Substance P binding on neurokinin receptors enhances the experience of both pain and depression. Elevated cytokines may enhance pain experience, depression and possibly somatic symptom disorder. Endorphins modulate pain: decreased sensitivity of opioid receptors is demonstrable in both chronic pain and depression. It is feasible to question whether or not a primary lesion in one of these modulatory systems could cause a true, primary pain disorder, distinct from chronic pain that co-exists with another psychiatric disorder or following actual tissue damage. In chronic pain, kindling may be active in networks that relay pain-related information between the cortex and limbic system (Rome, 2000). Non-nociceptive fibres may be recruited in the spinal cord and peripheral nervous system to mediate pain. In the absence of tissue damage, sensitisation and amplification also maintain pain (Dworkin and Wilson, 1993; Shipton, 2008). Behavioural and interpersonal factors are also considered significant in the pathogenesis of chronic pain.

Psychodynamic theories of chronic pain relate to patients symbolically expressing intrapsychic conflicts through pain. Some patients may regard emotional suffering as weakness, thus displacing the problem to the body. Pain can also be used to obtain love and nurturance as well as averting responsibilities. These secondary gains reinforce pain and maintain pain behaviour.

Intractable pain has also been conceptualised as a means of manipulating others and gaining the upper hand in tense interpersonal situations, such as a strained marriage. Learning and conditioning mediate much of the persistence, experience and behaviours of chronic pain.

#### 18.5.2.3 Epidemiology

Pain is the most common complaint in all of medicine. In the developed world, estimates of the prevalence of some form of chronic pain range between 25–30% of the general population. Pain disorder is diagnosed twice as commonly in women as in men, with peak onset usually in the fourth or fifth decade of life. Demographically, chronic pain is associated with lower educational achievement and socioeconomic standing.

#### 18.5.2.4 Differential diagnosis

Medical conditions characterised by chronic pain are obvious candidates on a differentials' list. The following characteristics of nociceptive pain help differentiate it from the pain of pain disorder: the intensity of physical pain waxes and wanes and it is sensitive to emotional, cognitive, attentional and situational influences as well as analgesia. Although pain may be a complaint, hypochondriasis is characterised by a preoccupation with illness rather than a preoccupation with pain. Hypochondriacal symptoms are also more fluctuant than the pain of chronic pain. Conversion disorder is typically short-lived and symptoms are limited to a single pseudoneurological set. Factitious disorder can present as serious diagnostic challenges. Pain is commonly malingered, particularly in personal injury litigation. Here, so-called compensation neurosis, deceit and genuine chronic pain merge with menacing complexity. Pain without a physical basis occurs in other psychiatric disorders, like schizophrenia, major depression and anxiety disorders. Depression often accompanies chronic pain, although most pain patients do not display characteristic depressive vegetative disturbances.

#### 18.5.2.5 Course and outcome

Chronic pain generally has an abrupt onset and increases in severity over the next few weeks and months. The prognosis is variable, although it is typically chronic, distressing and disabling. If psychological factors are prominent, pain may subside once they are successfully treated or external reinforcements removed. With or without treatment, poor prognostic factors in chronic pain include premorbid maladjustment like **passivity**, litigation, the prospect of financial compensation, use of addictive pain medication and a long pain history.

#### 18.5.2.6 Treatment

The general treatment principles outlined in Section 18.4 apply. Pharmacological treatment has limited utility: sedative and anxiolytic agents should be avoided and opiates have no place in its management. A trial of tricyclic antidepressant medication is advised where medically possible. Selective serotonin and serotonin-noradrenaline reuptake inhibitors as well as anti-epileptic mood stabilisers show some promise in treatment. Psychotherapy has proven disappointing. However, behavioural treatments, such as biofeedback, may help in specific situations like chronic headache and myofacial pain. Acupuncture, transcutaneous nerve stimulation, bite blocks and hypnosis have shown some efficacy. Nerve blocks and surgical ablation are ineffective.

### 18.5.3 Illness anxiety disorder

Illness anxiety disorder is the DSM-5 reconceptualisation of hypochondriasis. Fundamentally, it is an over-concern about illness, a fearful attitude towards one's health and a faulty manner of thinking about one's body. Exaggerated awareness and inaccurate interpretation of bodily experiences fuel its erroneous beliefs and fears. Throughout its history, hypochondriasis has been subservient to other mental disorders (notably anxiety and depression) and its validity as a separate condition questioned. This has led to the reconceptualisation of hypochondriasis as a symptom dimension rather than a diagnostic category.

**Information box**

**Hypochondriasis essentials**

- Undue worry about having an illness
- Absence of demonstrable pathology
- Anxious disposition
- Reassurance not helpful
- Symptoms correlate with psychosocial stress

### 18.5.3.1 Diagnosis and clinical features

The DSM-5 diagnostic criteria for illness anxiety disorder are listed in Table 18.3. Whereas some patients display classical illness anxiety (or fear of having a serious medical condition without prominent somatic symptoms) others display a mixture of somatic symptoms and illness anxiety. Typically, the patient with illness anxiety disorder is preoccupied with bodily functions (e.g. heartbeat, bowel movements), troubled by minor physical abnormalities (e.g. a small mouth ulcer) or unsettled by vague and ambiguous physical sensations (e.g. aches). The patient views his or her symptoms as evidence of a dreaded disease and is overly concerned with their origin and meaning. Hypochondriacal symptoms also occur in depressive and anxiety disorders and delusional hypochondriacal beliefs in psychotic disorders. We must distinguish between illness anxiety disorder and the transient hypochondriacal experiences common to most people. We become sensitised when exposed to a friend who is ill, when learning about illness through the media or hearing a doctor discussing it. Thus sensitised, we may develop a fear for that illness, worry about having it and interpret neutral bodily sensations as indicative of its presence. This situation not infrequently affects medical students in their early days of clinical training, before they have integrated their knowledge and experienced real patients with real symptoms.

**Table 18.3** DSM-5 Diagnostic Criteria for Illness Anxiety Disorder

| Diagnostic Criteria |
|---|
| A. Preoccupation with having or acquiring a serious illness. |
| B. Somatic symptoms are not present or, if present, are only mild in intensity. If another medical condition is present or there is a high risk for developing a medical condition (e.g., strong family history is present), the preoccupation is clearly excessive or disproportionate. |
| C. There is a high level of anxiety about health, and the individual is easily alarmed about personal health status. |
| D. The individual performs excessive health-related behaviors (e.g., repeatedly checks his or her body for signs of illness) or exhibits maladaptive avoidance (e.g., avoids doctor appointments and hospitals). |
| E. Illness preoccupation has been present for at least 6 months, but the specific illness that is feared may change over that period of time. |
| F. The illness-related preoccupation is not better explained by another mental disorder, such as somatic symptom disorder, panic disorder, generalized anxiety disorder, body dysmorphic disorder, obsessive-compulsive disorder, or delusional disorder, somatic type. |
| *Specify* whether: |
| ▸ **Care-seeking type:** Medical care, including physician visits or undergoing tests and procedures, is frequently used. |
| ▸ **Care-avoidant type:** Medical care is rarely used. |

**Source:** Reprinted with permission from the *Diagnostic and Statistical Manual of Mental Disorders*, Fifth Edition, (Copyright 2013). American Psychiatric Association.

### 18.5.3.2 Epidemiology

In a general clinical population, hypochondriasis has a six-month prevalence of 4–6%, although wider ranges have been demonstrated by various studies (Escobar *et al.*, 1998). In Africa, its epidemiology is unknown. In contrast with conversion and somatic symptom disorder, the sexes are equally affected. Age of onset is typically in the twenties or thirties, but can start at any age. Social class, education and marital status do not appear to affect its expression.

### 18.5.3.3 Specific notes on pathogenesis

Psychodynamically, disturbed object relations with aggressive and hostile wishes towards others are posited to be transferred to the body through

**repression** and displacement. Hypochondriasis is also viewed as a defence against guilt – pain becomes a means of atonement and expiation. In learning theory, it may represent a defence against low self-esteem and inadequacy, with conditioned reinforcement of the sick role. Hypochondriasis is also considered a variant expression of other mental conditions, notably anxiety and depression. These conditions may establish a hyper-vigilant state in the body biased towards harm detection, like probable noxious signals originating from the person's own body.

#### 18.5.3.4 Differential diagnosis

Medical conditions with vague, transient and fluctuating symptoms require exclusion. Multiple sclerosis, systemic lupus erythematosus and occult neoplasms must also be excluded. Distinguishing between somatic symptom disorder and hypochondriasis hinges on the patient's focus of concern. The patient with hypochondriasis worries about developing a specific disease, while the patient with somatic symptom disorder complains of specific symptoms and not disease entities. Conversion disorder can be distinguished from illness anxiety disorder by the preponderance of younger, female patients with sudden and dramatic onset of pseudo-neurological symptoms. ***La belle indifférence*** (see Section 18.5.4) further assists in the differentiation of the two disorders. Pain and its attendant pain behaviour characterise pain disorder. Conceptualised as a variant of hypochondriacal disorder by the ICD-10, body dysmorphic disorder involves preoccupation with an anatomical abnormality, not anxiety about having an illness. If hypochondriacal concerns assume delusional qualities, a psychotic disorder must be considered. Anxiety and depressive disorders often co-exist with hypochondriasis; hypochondriacal complaints are not infrequent in these conditions. Identifying factitious patients and malingerers can be challenging.

#### 18.5.3.5 Course and outcome

Typically fluctuating, hypochondriacal concerns intensify during periods of heightened stress, notably the death or illness of a loved one. It also tends to have an episodic course with relapses and remissions, each lasting months to years. Significant long-term improvement is found in 30–50% of cases. Good outcomes are predicted by high socioeconomic status, sudden symptom onset following a distinct stressor, absence of significant personality pathology, no serious medical illness and treatment-responsive anxiety or depression.

#### 18.5.3.6 Treatment

The therapeutic approach outlined in Section 18.4 applies; early identification and treatment yield the best outcomes. Patients usually present to primary care but psychiatric treatment is helpful for those who acknowledge that their illnesses are stress related. Hypochondriacal symptoms associated with depression or anxiety resolve with effective treatment of the co-morbid conditions.

Kellner (1986) proposed a time-limited treatment for hypochondriasis uncomplicated by other psychiatric conditions. It relies on a strong therapeutic alliance, reassurance and psycho-education. It aims to shift the patient's preoccupation with a bodily condition towards understanding and handling psychosocial stressors. Whilst the patient's experience must not be negated, bodily concerns must not be overemphasised. To this end, regular, brief physical examinations must be scheduled, investigations used prudently and hospitalisation avoided. Some patients accept psychiatric treatment if it takes place in a medical setting and focuses on stress reduction and coping with chronic illness. Here, group therapy may be beneficial. CBT has shown promise and challenges a patient's beliefs, assumptions and interpretation of bodily experiences. Behavioural techniques target behaviours that maintain disease preoccupation. Relaxation and social skills training are further aids (Epstein *et al.*, 1999).

### 18.5.4 Conversion disorder

The hallmark of conversion disorder (also called functional neurological disorder) is its mono-symptomatic and pseudo-neurological nature. Mono-symptomatic refers to a single presenting symptom or a symptom-complex;

pseudo-neurological refers to symptoms suggesting a neurological nature that lack a conventional medical explanation. The ICD-10 considers conversion disorder under the rubric of dissociative conditions in deference to the presumed dissociative pathogenesis of conversion. By contrast, the DSM-5 retains its somatic symptom disorder categorisation by reason of its somatic mode of presentation and makes no claims to any specific pathogenesis, like dissociation, at play (American Psychiatric Association, 2013).

### 18.5.4.1 Diagnosis and clinical features

Conventionally, the diagnosis of conversion disorder has involved a process of exclusion. However, the DSM-5 recognises that the very nature of conversion symptoms suggests the presence of conversion. For instance, conversion symptoms disregard neurological constraints and anatomical boundaries and tend to demonstrate some degree of incongruence and inconsistency. The more patently fanciful the symptoms are, the more likely it is that the patient is of low intellect, poorly educated or psychologically unsophisticated. The patient may present as depressed, anxious or alexithymic (Grabe, 2000). *La belle indifférence* is observed in half of all patients and tends to occur alongside alexithymia. The utility of *la belle indifférence* in differentiating between conversion disorder and organic symptoms is doubtful (Stone *et al.*, 2006). Subtle cognitive impairments, notably concreteness and verbal expressive difficulty, are sometimes present. Conversion patients may display dependent, passive-aggressive, histrionic and anti-social traits. (Black, 2004; Ford, 1985; Krahn, 2008). Table 18.4 lists the DSM-5 diagnostic criteria for conversion disorder.

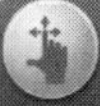

#### Case study 18.2

Justine, 19, lives outside Mosselbay on the Garden Route. She is a single mother of two toddlers, one of whom is mentally retarded. Following her father's unexpected death in a car accident two years earlier, she has been responsible for supporting her sickly mother and her children. She has part-time employment working as a teller at a local supermarket. Recently, she became involved with a civil servant seconded from Cape Town. The romance was soon spoiled by mistrust, resentment and physical abuse necessitating Justine to take out an interim protection order against the man. One weekend, the boyfriend appeared at her house and threatened her with a broken bottle. The following Monday morning at work, Justine collapsed and, unable to get up and walk was taken to the provincial hospital.

On admission, she was found to be fully conscious and provided an adequate, albeit superficial and somewhat emotionally detached, account of events. The general examination was unremarkable. She was unable to move her lower limbs against gravity. However, muscle tone was normal, deep tendon reflexes intact and plantar responses normal. **Hoover's sign** was present. She was transferred to Cape Town for specialist investigation. Detailed neurological examinations failed to demonstrate a neurological lesion. A psychiatrist was consulted who found her childlike, intellectually unsophisticated and emotionally unconcerned in the face of an apparently serious neurological problem. No evidence of major depression, anxiety disorder or psychosis was found.

Her developmental history revealed that she had grown up with her paternal uncle in Joubertina and saw her parents only during the festive season. Her uncle had abused alcohol and was often unemployed. The home environment was tense and disagreements settled violently. Justine admitted that she was frequently subjected to severe corporal punishment, but was never abused sexually. She recalled that she experienced a brief spell of blindness when she entered high school, aged 15. At the time, she had run away from her uncle's home and moved in with her parents after her father had finally settled down following his itinerant lifestyle as a member of the national defence force. She never returned to school and helped out at home after her mother's first stroke. She became very close to her father and was most distraught following his death.

During her hospital stay in Cape Town, she received regular supportive therapy. A week after her sudden collapse and paralysis, she regained control of her lower limbs, managed to stand and walk. She promptly discharged herself from hospital care.

## Case study 18.3

Dolly was admitted to a private hospital in Johannesburg following a suspected seizure. The paramedics remarked that her movements were severe and the episode prolonged. The convulsive movements eventually ceased after 4 mg intravenous lorazepam and she fell into a deep sleep. Now 48, Dolly has an unremarkable medical history, except recurrent but uncomplicated febrile convulsions as a child. She was assessed by a neurologist who found no clinical abnormalities. Bloodwork, analysis of her cerebrospinal fluid, neuro-imaging and halter-EEG were normal, as were echocardiography, ECG and Doppler studies of her neck arteries. She was not taking any medications, and neither smoked nor drank alcohol. During her stay on the neurology ward, she experienced a further two seizures. The seizures were atypical with notable flailing and sideways movement of the head. There were no injuries and incontinence. On both occasions, her daughter and grandchildren were present. The neurologist started anti-epileptic treatment and referred Dolly to a psychiatrist.

The psychiatrist elicited the following history: Dolly was brought up in a Christian home with very strict parents. Her father often used corporal punishment and locked her in a broom cupboard for hours on end when she had been naughty. During her matric year, she met a council worker and fell in love. To the horror of her parents, she fell pregnant. Her parents were most disapproving of the fact that she had married outside her religion – a man of the Hindu faith. She moved out of her parents' house and the couple settled in a small flat in Braamfontein. She found a job at a school for children with special needs, where she was tasked with looking after their play activities. She enjoyed her work as she had always dreamt of being a remedial teacher. When their child was three years old, her husband left her and her child. She was devastated by this and started doubting herself. She moved back with her parents. However, relations had become particularly strained. After witnessing her father striking her mother during a heated argument, she lost her voice and was unable to make a sound for about a week. Her mother arranged for her to live with a cousin in Empangeni where she met her second husband, a wealthy local trader. He wanted her to convert to Islam before the marriage and she did so. The couple had a good marriage from which one child was born. The day after their tenth wedding anniversary, her husband died unexpectedly of a heart attack. The day of the funeral, she started experiencing severe chest pain and panicky feelings. She was admitted to a local cardiac unit where myocardial ischaemia was ruled out.

She moved back to Johannesburg and returned to her old work at the special needs school. The demands of her work escalated: she was now also tasked to look after the children's hygiene and feeding and escorting them on field trips. Many of the children in her care are epileptic with poor seizure control. She often felt overwhelmed when having to deal with a child having a fit.

About a month before her presentation with a seizure, she was informed that the school would close and she would be retrenched. This was the second blow in short succession as earlier in the year, her elderly mother died. Her oldest child blamed her for causing religious confusion in the family and unfairly demanding her grandchildren to forsake their Hindu beliefs. This religious debate sparked an intense argument between the two. Her daughter left, angry. To her horror, when she arrived home, her mother's neighbour phoned to inform her of her mother's seizure.

On mental state examination, No cognitive impairments were apparent, but she appeared verbally unsophisticated. She was alexithymic with a dull affect. Mild anxiety was noted and she was not psychotic.

### Motor symptoms

Paralysis is the quintessential conversion disorder phenomenon. Other motor conversion symptoms are weakness, movement disorder and ataxia. Tell-tale features of conversion disorder weakness include normal deep tendon reflexes, muscle tone and bulk and absence of fasciculations. Hoover's sign, observed when the heel of an ostensibly paralysed limb pushes down onto the examiner's hand when the patient is instructed to raise the other leg, also raises suspicion of conversion disorder. Conversion hemiparesis may involve the impossibility of a patient's apparent inability to turn his or her head to the side of the weakness. Grotesque movement disturbances with swaying, bobbing, unusual tremor, blepharospasm, torticollis, oposthotonus, chorea and **athetosis** are suggestive of conversion disorder. **Astasia-abasia** is an outrageous gait disturbance with an uncharacteristic wildness with flailing, thrashing, and jerking movements. Movement and gait disturbances often worsen when attention is drawn to them.

**Information box**

**Conversion disorder – essentials**

- Affects females more than males
- Psychologically naïve, lower IQ
- History of childhood trauma
- Symptoms follow psychosocial stressor
- Mono-symptomatic and pseudo-neurological
- Symptoms: sensory, motor, seizure and mixed
- Usually brief course
- Co-existence of other neurological illness not uncommon

### Sensory symptoms

Anaesthesia and paraesthesia are common in conversion disorder, and tend to affect the extremities, assuming a glove-and-stocking distribution not typical of peripheral neuropathy, spinal cord lesions or brain lesions. Hemianaesthesia that strictly observes the midline demarcation between normal and anaesthetic skin is particularly suspicious. The organs of special sensation are also affected by blindness, monocular diplopia, tunnel vision, deafness and anosmia. Disequilibrium symptoms with unusual giddiness and feelings of lurching (referable to the vestibular apparatus) also occur.

### Pseudo-seizures

Pseudo-seizures are paroxysmal convulsive events in the absence of ictal electrical activity. Corneal and gag reflexes remain intact, extensor plantar responses are not elicited and, in the absence of neuroleptic treatment, serum prolactin concentration is not elevated. Other findings suggesting pseudo-seizures include the absence of injury, tongue biting and incontinence during falls. However, diagnosis is complicated because nearly a third of patients with pseudo-seizures have confirmed epilepsy. In fact, certain instances of pseudo-seizures may have their origin in true seizures and occur as a complex conditioned response. If a patient suffered a true seizure following stress, it is possible that the same neural networks recruited during the initial seizure can again be activated when faced with subsequent stress. The seizure thus becomes the preferential conditioned response: when stressed, the patient's brain behaves as it would during a true seizure, recruiting the same networks but without ictal electrical activity.

### Mixed symptoms

Mutism, hoarseness, bizarre affections of articulation and aphonia are examples of communication disturbances in conversion disorder. Conversion aphonia differs from true aphonia in that the ability to vocalise during a sneeze or snore is maintained. Globus hystericus (or lump in the throat) is common to many normal people and probably arises from mixed pharyngeal sensory-motor conversion phenomena. Psychogenic vomiting, diarrhoea, urinary retention and urinary frequency are visceral conversion symptoms. False memories, notably of physical or sexual abuse during childhood, are also considered conversion disorder phenomena (Krahn, 2008). Conversion pseudo-hallucinations are also recognised as conversion disorder symptoms but are not expressly included in the DSM-5. Pseudo-hallucinations are qualitatively different from psychotic or delirious hallucinations and may take on a utilitarian, supportive quality, as when a distressed girl hears the voice of her beloved comforting her. Magical and child-like imagery are more likely encountered in pseudo-hallucinations; patients typically retain insight into the unreality of pseudo-hallucinations (Hales, 2008).

Although conversion disorder is universal, the type of symptoms depends on sociocultural context. For example, falling down with loss of consciousness is a feature of a variety of culture-bound syndromes. This form of conversion reaction reflects local cultural idioms about acceptable ways to express distress. (See Chapter 26: Women's mental health, for further details.) In India, common pseudo-neurological complaints are feelings of heat, crawling sensations, numbness, burning hands and a hot peppery sensation in the head. Brain fag, a condition originally described in Nigerian university students, conforms to this presentation. *Ataque de nervios*, an affliction found in the Hispanic Caribbean, also involves heat rising to the head, numbness of extremities and pseudo-seizures (Escobar, 2004). So-called mass hysteria may represent conversion experiences shared by a collective and is socially communicated amongst members of a group.

### 18.5.4.2 Epidemiology

Transient conversion disorder symptoms insufficient to raise medical concern are common and encountered in nearly one-third of all people. Psychiatric patients have a 5–15% prevalence of conversion disorder symptoms. Conversion disorders are the most common of the somatic symptom disorders, particularly in the developing world. Conversion disorder occurs commonly in the youngest child in a family, lower socio-economic groups, rural areas and persons with sub-average intelligence and educational under-achievers. Psychological and medical naivety as well as exposure to war and combat further increase risk (Ford, 1985). Females outnumber males five to one, but a wide sex ratio range is noted. In males, conversion disorder symptoms often relate to occupational accidents, military service, trial and serving a sentence. Conversion disorder symptoms are rare in children younger than 10 and, if they do occur, typical involve gait problems and seizures. Conversion disorder more likely emerges in the teens through mid-thirties. Caution must be exercised in any person older than 40 who develops what appears to be a conversion disorder for the first time. In such cases, the presence of an underlying medical or neurological disorder must be strongly considered.

### 18.5.4.3 Specific notes on pathogenesis

Several theories have been put forward to explain the phenomenon of conversion disorder, but a unitary theory of conversion still eludes us. What is certain is that early trauma sets the scene for the emergence of conversion disorder symptoms in a genetically predisposed individual when that individual is faced with trauma

**Table 18.4** DSM-5 Diagnostic Criteria for Conversion Disorder (Functional Neurological Symptom Disorder)

| Diagnostic Criteria |
|---|
| A. One or more symptoms of altered voluntary motor or sensory function. |
| B. Clinical findings provide evidence of incompatibility between the symptom and recognized neurological or medical conditions. |
| C. The symptom or deficit is not better explained by another medical or mental disorder. |
| D. The symptom or deficit causes clinically significant distress or impairment in social, occupational, or other important areas of functioning or warrants medical evaluation. |
| *Specify* symptom type: |
| ▸ **(F44.4) With weakness or paralysis** |
| ▸ **(F44.4) With abnormal movement** (e.g., tremor, dystonic movement, myoclonus, gait disorder) |
| ▸ **(F44.4) With swallowing symptoms** |
| ▸ **(F44.4) With speech symptom** (e.g., dysphonia, slurred speech) |
| ▸ **(F44.5) With attacks or seizures** |
| ▸ **(F44.6) With anesthesia or sensory loss** |
| ▸ **(F44.6) With special sensory symptom** (e.g., visual, olfactory, or hearing disturbance) |
| ▸ **(F44.7) With mixed symptoms** |
| *Specify* if: |
| ▸ **Acute episode:** Symptoms present for less than 6 months. |
| ▸ **Persistent:** Symptoms occurring for 6 months or more. |
| *Specify* if: |
| ▸ **With psychological stressor** (*specify stressor*) |
| ▸ **Without psychological stressor** |

**Source:** Reprinted with permission from the *Diagnostic and Statistical Manual of Mental Disorders*, Fifth Edition, (Copyright 2013). American Psychiatric Association.

later in life. The argument that conversion disorder is a preferential dissociative response to threat was outlined earlier in this chapter.

Research findings are as confusing as they are plentiful. Do findings such as *la belle indifférence* and the preponderance of left-sided symptoms truly suggest dominant parietal dysfunction? *La belle indifférence* is curiously reminiscent of anosognosia, anosodiaphoria and neglect of non-dominant parietal cortical lesions. Lending credence to non-dominant, hemispheric involvement is the slight preponderance of left-sided symptoms, strangely more common in females. However, subtle impairments in vigilance, memory, verbal imprecision, affective incongruence and disordered processing of endogenous somatic percepts support left-dominant impairments instead. Impaired inter-hemispheric communication further compounds the picture (Stone *et al.*, 2006; Flor-Henry, 1965, cited in Black, 2004).

In neural information theory, conversion disorder is believed to follow on dynamic restructuring of neural networks, leading to a functional disconnection of volition, sensory experience and movement. Whilst primary perception and motor control are intact, integration of sensory percepts and motor planning are not. Paralysis ensues when disruption occurs at the level of preconscious motor planning. In support of this, functional neuro-imaging in conversion paralysis has demonstrated activation of the anterior cingulate gyrus and association motor cortices with contemporaneous inactivity of the primary motor strip. By contrast, when modality-specific attention is disrupted, sensory losses like blindness and anaesthesia follow (Black, 2004; Krahn, 2008; Mailis-Gagnon and Israelson, 2005; Sierra, 1998; Spence *et al.*, 2000). Unlike the homunculus of the primary somatosensory cortex, the body is not conformally mapped onto the inferior parietal association cortex. As a consequence, dysfunction in the inferior parietal cortex may explain the disregard for anatomical constraints so characteristic of sensory conversion symptoms. In support of this, decreased right inferior parietal functioning has been demonstrated. Further, right frontoparietal network disruptions may disturb self-recognition and appreciation of 'selfhood' (Black, 2004; Sierra, 1998).

Conversion disorder symptoms tend to reflect their cultural surroundings. Certain sick roles are sanctioned or tolerated in specific cultures. In different historical epochs and societies certain impulses and attitudes were either encouraged or deemed taboo. For example, during the Victorian era of repressed sexuality, orgasmic convulsions were common and tolerated. Fainting or swooning and languishing were also considered to be indicative of proper feminine demeanour. In contrast, such behaviours may now be minimised as vasovagal attacks or, perjoratively, deemed to be attention seeking.

### 18.5.4.4 Differential diagnosis

Many neurological diseases can be mistaken for conversion disorder and, where necessary, the appropriate investigations should be considered. Some of these disorders are:

- myasthenia gravis
- multiple sclerosis
- periodic paralysis
- optic neuritis
- Guillain-Barré syndrome
- other demyelinating encephalomyelopathy
- brain tumour
- Parkinson's disease
- subdural haematoma
- idiopathic and drug-induced dystonias
- Ménière's disease
- tardive dyskinesia.

Other conditions worth considering are malingering and factitious disorders, particularly in the presence of an identifiable external motivation, such as financial compensation. In conversion disorder, clinical diagnosis remains mainly one of exclusion, even if pseudo-neurological symptoms may be suggestive of conversion. Table 18.5 lists clues to conversion disorder.

**Table 18.5** Clues to conversion disorder

- Previous episodes of conversion (particularly if symptoms vary from episode to episode)
- Rapid onset of the symptoms
- Temporal relationship between onset and major psychosocial stressor. Suggestive symptoms, e.g. Hoover's sign, astasia-abasia, head bobbing
- Symbolic nature of symptoms, including pseudohallucinations
- *La belle indifférence*
- Suggestibility
- Inability to recall important pieces of historical information
- Psychological naivety, immaturity, low intellect
- Histrionic or dependent personality style
- Evidence of secondary gain

#### 18.5.4.5 Course and outcome

In 90–100% of cases, conversion symptoms resolve within a few days and rarely last longer than two weeks. Recurrence of conversion disorder during periods of psychosocial stress occurs in 25% of patients, often within a year of first diagnosis (Stonnington *et al.*, 2006). The longer the conversion symptoms last, the worse the outcome. Chronic conversion disorder can result in serious disability, with muscle atrophy, contractures and decubitus ulcers. The delayed emergence of a neurological condition always remains likely, necessitating meticulous examination and rigorous surveillance. Table 18.6 lists predictors of a favourable outcome.

#### 18.5.4.6 Treatment

The therapeutic principles outlined earlier in this chapter are applicable to conversion disorder. The primary goal of treatment is removal of the conversion symptom; the urgency to do so is dictated by the degree of distress and functional impairment. Confrontation must be avoided, since it usually serves to alienate the patient. It is possible that symptom resolution is not dependent on the specific technique employed but on the influence of suggestion. Suggestion will only succeed if the doctor elicits the patient's own understanding of the symptom. Suggestion can be effected by communicating to the patient that the symptom will improve (Cassem and Barsky, 1991). Further reassurance must follow, including good news about laboratory investigations and the certainty of recovery. Relaxation techniques and breathing exercises are handy adjuncts to suggestion. Since hypnotherapy works through suggestion, it may be effective. It must, however, be accompanied by exploring and treating the underlying psychological conflict. Medication is of little help. Most conversion disorders remit spontaneously.

### 18.5.5 Psychological factors affecting other medical conditions

Where psychological factors are judged to adversely affect the expression of a physical illness, a diagnosis of 'psychological factors affecting other medical conditions' is warranted. The DSM-5 diagnostic criteria are provided in Table 18.7. Psychological factors that adversely impact on medical conditions include poor stress-handling, maladaptive coping, interpersonal difficulties, denial and poor compliance with treatment. By contrast, when a medical condition evokes a strong psychological reaction it is best conceptualised as an adjustment disorder.

**Table 18.6** Predictors of a favourable prognosis in conversion disorder

- Sudden onset, following identifiable stressor
- Average to higher IQ, relatively stable personality structure and good premorbid adjustment
- No comorbid psychiatric condition
- Capacity for **introspection**
- Stable relationships: family and work
- Limited potential for secondary gain
- Able to relate to therapist; express and feel emotions without overwhelming affectivity. Symptom type: blindness and aphonia have better outcomes than **pseudoseizures**

**Source:** Binzer and Kullgren, 1998

### 18.5.6 Factitious disorder

Both factitious disorder and malingering involve the wilful and deceitful presentation of symptoms, illness, injury or impairment. The success of deceit rests on two pillars: familiarity with the subject of deceit and a communication style that avoids raising suspicion, notably through the suppression of anxiety. Deceitful communication that appears natural and targets the unsuspecting may prove sufficient for a successful dupe. Suspicion is more often raised by the nature of the communication than errors of fact contained in the deception. Factitious disorder concerns the intentional making of physical or psychological features of illness, injury or impairment in order to assume the sick role. Not only do patients deceive with their symptoms, they also misrepresent their medical histories and even their lives. Factitious disorder imposed on another person (colloquially known as Munchausen syndrome or factitious disorder by proxy) is the alarming situation where someone, usually a

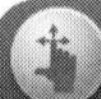

## Case study 18.4

Fanwell, a single man of 24, presented to a respected Johannesburg surgeon. Fanwell had a B.Tech-degree in medical chemistry and had been employed as a laboratory technician at a private pathology laboratory until his dismissal earlier in the year. He did not elaborate on the reasons for dismissal. Since his dismissal, he worked as a waiter at a pizzeria in Melville and was sharing accommodation nearby. He failed to provide details of next-of kin.

He explained to the surgeon that he had been experiencing repeated bouts of giddiness and fainting after meals. He first noticed the problem a year earlier and had been extensively investigated at various private hospitals. He produced a dossier of laboratory information suggesting that he experiences periods of sustained hypoglycaemia. In light of the presented laboratory findings, the surgeon immediately suspected the possibility of insulinoma. As an earlier dedicated arteriogram of the pancreas had failed to demonstrate a tumour, the surgeon arranged admission for a repeat arteriogram and other investigations.

His general examination and initial bloodwork failed to shed more light. However, the surgeon took note of obvious scars suggesting repeated laparotomies. Fanwell readily admitted to previous surgery and listed appendicectomy, cholecystectomy and several exploratory laparotomies. However, he was hesitant to provide further details. During his admission, he further revealed that he had been a sickly child and had spent months in hospital. His matric year was spent recuperating from a severe respiratory affliction that left him always out of breath. He also related how, in his gap year, he had been an honorary goodwill ambassador to Venezuela and had trekked the length of South America, stopping at various places to take in local culture. Whilst in Chile, he was employed as a disc jockey at a radio station and even took second place in the Cantare Panamericana talent competition in Santiago. Fanwell's very full life made the surgeon uneasy.

Shortly after admission, he experienced three episodes of severe hypoglycaemia resulting in two grand mal seizures. Acting on her intuition, an experienced nurse became suspicious. Following a fourth hypoglycaemic spell, she decided to inspect the drawer of his bedside locker. Shocked, but not surprised, she found several empty blister packs of metformin. With support from the surgeon, she gently enquired from Fanwell the reason for having the tablets. He became enraged, accused them of grossly unprofessional conduct and threatened litigation. The nurse and surgeon left the bedside, allowing Fanwell to regain his composure. Upon their return minutes later, he had disappeared from the hospital.

mother, intentionally simulates illness in another person entrusted to that person, usually a child.

Although Munchausen syndrome is used interchangeably with factitious disorder, its application is limited to a variant of factitious disorder characterised by feigned physical symptoms, migration from doctor to doctor and dramatic, but plausible-sounding, accounts of illness. The syndrome owes its name to Karl Friedrich Hieronymus Freiherr von Münchhausen. A retired 18th-century German cavalry officer and raconteur, he was renowned for his lavishly exaggerated stories: he recounted that he once extracted himself from a swamp by his own hair and had ridden a bisected horse into battle (Olry, 2002). Similarly, patients can present with *pseudologia phantastica*.

### 18.5.6.1 Clinical features and diagnosis

The DSM-5 lists two forms of factitious disorder: factitious disorder imposed on self and factitious disorder imposed on another. The diagnostic criteria are provided in Table 18.8.

Factitious disorder patients can present with a bewildering spectrum of symptoms. However, they tend to adopt one or more of the following strategies:

- fictitious histories consistent with a known diagnosis, without any supportive physical evidence; symptoms may consist of outright fabrications, exaggeration and distortion of existing symptoms, displacement and transformation of symptoms
- falsified evidence of an illness is presented (e.g. applying a flame to a thermometer)
- producing verifiable, true abnormal pathology (e.g. ingesting warfarin or metformin).

**Table 18.7** DSM-5 Diagnostic Criteria for Psychological Factors Affecting Other Medical Conditions

| Diagnostic Criteria |
|---|
| A. A medical symptom or condition (other than a mental disorder) is present. |
| B. Psychological or behavioral factors adversely affect the medical condition in one of the following ways: |
| 1. The factors have influenced the course of the medical condition as shown by a close temporal association between the psychological factors and the development or exacerbation of, or delayed recovery from, the medical condition. |
| 2. The factors interfere with the treatment of the medical condition (e.g., poor adherence). |
| 3. The factors constitute additional well-established health risks for the individual. |
| 4. The factors influence the underlying pathophysiology, precipitating or exacerbating symptoms or necessitating medical attention. |
| C. The psychological and behavioral factors in Criterion B are not better explained by another mental disorder (e.g., panic disorder, major depressive disorder, posttraumatic stress disorder). |
| *Specify* current severity: |
| ▸ **Mild:** Increases medical risk (e.g., inconsistent adherence with antihypertension treatment). |
| ▸ **Moderate:** Aggravates underlying medical condition (e.g., anxiety aggravating asthma). |
| ▸ **Severe:** Results in medical hospitalization or emergency room visit. |
| ▸ **Extreme:** Results in severe, life-threatening risk (e.g., ignoring heart attack symptoms). |

**Source:** Reprinted with permission from the *Diagnostic and Statistical Manual of Mental Disorders*, Fifth Edition, (Copyright 2013). American Psychiatric Association.

Patients may submit themselves to repeated dangerous procedures - the 'gridiron' or 'washboard' abdomen, feared on surgical firms, attests to repeated abdominal surgery. Factitious psychological symptoms are less common than physical ones. When simulating mental illness, patients may report depression, hallucinations or display bizarre behaviour.

Factitious disorder with psychological symptoms is more common in borderline patients and those with a close relative who is mentally ill. Factitious disorder patients are sick, distressed and functionally impaired. Factitious disorder does not confer immunity from other illnesses. Depression, anxiety and borderline traits are common co-morbid conditions.

**Table 18.8** DSM-5 Diagnostic Criteria for Factitious Disorder

| Diagnostic Criteria |
|---|
| **Factitious Disorder Imposed on Self** |
| A. Falsification of physical or psychological signs or symptoms, or induction of injury or disease, associated with identified deception. |
| B. The individual presents himself or herself to others as ill, impaired, or injured. |
| C. The deceptive behavior is evident even in the absence of obvious external rewards. |
| D. The behavior is not better explained by another mental disorder, such as delusional disorder or another psychotic disorder. |
| *Specify:* |
| ▸ **Single episode** |
| ▸ **Recurrent episodes** (two or more events of falsification of illness and/or induction of injury) |
| **Factitious Disorder Imposed on Another** |
| **(Previously Factitious Disorder by Proxy)** |
| A. Falsification of physical or psychological signs or symptoms, or induction of injury or disease, in another, associated with identified deception. |
| B. The individual presents another individual (victim) to others as ill, impaired, or injured. |
| C. The deceptive behavior is evident even in the absence of obvious external rewards. |
| D. The behavior is not better explained by another mental disorder, such as delusional disorder or another psychotic disorder. |
| **Note:** The perpetrator, not the victim, receives this diagnosis. |
| *Specify:* |
| ▸ **Single episode** |
| ▸ **Recurrent episodes** (two or more events of falsification of illness and/or induction of injury) |

**Source:** Reprinted with permission from the *Diagnostic and Statistical Manual of Mental Disorders*, Fifth Edition, (Copyright 2013). American Psychiatric Association.

### 18.5.6.2 Epidemiology

As the very nature of the disorder may result in failure to recognise the condition, the actual prevalence of factitious disorder has not been determined. Factitious disorder appears to occur more often in males and among hospital and health-care workers.

### 18.5.6.3 Aetiology

Adult factitious disorder probably stems from early childhood experience with emotional deprivation, absent parents and finding love and caring from doctors and nurses. By producing symptoms of an illness, patients may attempt to recreate this nurturing atmosphere that they experienced earlier. A similar pathogenesis is likely in Munchausen syndrome by proxy stemming from the caregiver's need to have a nurturing relationship with the doctor (Schreier and Libow, 1994).

### 18.5.6.4 Course and outcome

The onset of the disorder often follows a real illness or stressful event. This is followed by a path of maladaptive care-seeking as the condition traces its typically chronic course. Due to repeated or lengthy hospitalisation, the patient's functioning is seriously disrupted. Typically, the prognosis is poor: factitious disorder with psychological symptoms has a prognosis worse than schizophrenia or bipolar I disorder (Karukappadath *et al.*, 2013).

### 18.5.6.5 Differential diagnosis

The disorder has to be differentiated from other illness-affirming conditions such as somatic symptom disorder, illness anxiety and conversion disorder as well as medical and other psychiatric conditions and malingering.

Clues to factitious disorder are a long and involved medical, textbook-like presentation, sophisticated medical vocabulary, training or work in health care, demands for specific treatments or investigations and a history of multiple invasive procedures.

### 18.5.6.6 Treatment

Factitious disorder strains the therapeutic relationship. Sparked by apparent betrayal the temptation to strike back is ever present. But confrontation, exposure and blaming are not helpful and may precipitate personality disintegration, impulsive self-harm and frank psychosis. The general treatment guidelines outlined in Section 18.4 apply.

Safeguarding the victim is paramount in approaching factitious disorder imposed on another.

## 18.5.7 Malingering

Malingering is a behaviour, not an illness. It involves the wilful presentation of false symptoms, illness, injury or impairment in an attempt to avert threat or derive unjustified reward. Malingering occurs with full consciousness of both the fraudulent presentation and the motivation for it. Malingering is believed to occur, to some extent, among 60% of accused persons undergoing assessment. It is typically found in criminal prosecution, personal injury claims, drug-seeking and avoidance of military duty. Children can malinger to dodge school. Malingering is announced by factual errors in symptom presentation and a manner of communication suggestive of deceit. Context (such as prosecution or military duty) must always sound the siren that malingering is present (Du Plessis, 2003; Du Plessis and Visser, 2012).

## 18.5.8 Other somatic symptom disorders

The DSM-5 allows for the coding of two residual categories for conditions that fail to meet threshold criteria for any of the specified somatic symptom disorders. They are 'other specified somatic symptom and related disorders' and 'unspecified somatic symptoms and related disorders'. Their diagnostic criteria are listed in Tables 18.9 and 18.10, respectively. Only pseudocyesis, listed under 'other specified somatic symptom and related disorders' in the DSM-5, shall be considered here.

**Table 18.9** DSM-5 Diagnostic Criteria for Other Specified Somatic Symptom and Related Disorder

| |
|---|
| This category applies to presentations in which symptoms characteristic of a somatic symptom and related disorder that cause clinically significant distress or impairment in social, occupational, or other important areas of functioning predominate but do not meet the full criteria for any of the disorders in the somatic symptom and related disorders diagnostic class.<br>Examples of presentations that can be specified using the 'other specified' designation include the following:<br>1. **Brief somatic symptom disorder:** Duration of symptoms is less than 6 months.<br>2. **Brief illness anxiety disorder:** Duration of symptoms is less than 6 months.<br>3. **Illness anxiety disorder without excessive health-related behaviors:** Criterion D for illness anxiety disorder is not met.<br>4. **Pseudocyesis:** A false belief of being pregnant that is associated with objective signs and reported symptoms of pregnancy. |

**Source:** Reprinted with permission from the *Diagnostic and Statistical Manual of Mental Disorders*, Fifth Edition, (Copyright 2013). American Psychiatric Association.

#### 18.5.8.1 Pseudocyesis

Pseudcyesis involves a non-pregnant woman believing that she is pregnant. During the pseudo-pregnancy, she develops typical gravid features: oligomenorrhoea or amenorrhoea, abdominal distension, typical breast changes, lactation, nausea and vomiting, sensation of foetal movements and a duration of nine months. On examination, the abdomen feels firm with a tympanic ring, the umbilicus is not everted and a gravid uterus not palpated. However, negative test results may not convince the patient that she is not pregnant. It occurs from pre-teens to the seventies. Differential diagnoses are delusional pregnancy (notably in mania and schizophrenia), factitious disorder, malingering, pelvic neoplasia, endocrinopathy and hormonal manipulation in infertility treatment. Psuedocyesis also occurs in males. By contrast, Couvade syndrome (or sympathetic pregnancy) is a surprisingly common and widespread condition in which the husband or partner of a pregnant woman experiences symptoms of pregnancy or childbirth (Brennan *et al.*, 2007).

**Table 18.10** DSM-5 Diagnostic Criteria for Unspecified Somatic Symptom and Related Disorder

| |
|---|
| This category applies to presentations in which symptoms characteristic of a somatic symptom and related disorder that cause clinically significant distress or impairment in social, occupational, or other important areas of functioning predominate but do not meet the full criteria for any of the disorders in the somatic symptom and related disorders diagnostic class. The unspecified somatic symptom and related disorder category should not be used unless there are decidedly unusual situations where there is insufficient information to make a more specific diagnosis. |

**Source:** Reprinted with permission from the *Diagnostic and Statistical Manual of Mental Disorders*, Fifth Edition, (Copyright 2013). American Psychiatric Association.

### 18.5.9 Psychosomatic conditions

Controversial – and not included in the DSM-5 – psychosomatic conditions present with real clinical, diagnostic, treatment and ethical challenges. We shall consider four of these conditions: neurasthenia, chronic fatigue syndrome, irritable bowel syndrome and fibromyalgia.

#### 18.5.9.1 Neurasthenia

In the 1860s, American George M. Beard described a condition he believed was caused by 'nervous depletion' and came to be known as neurasthenia. Although it continues to be diagnosed in parts of Europe and Asia, neurasthenia has all but vanished from practice in the English-speaking world. DSM-I and DSM-II recognised it (Sadock BJ and Sadock VA, 2000), but its lack of distinctive features differentiating it from depression and anxiety contributed to its deletion since DSM-III. Neurasthenia is characterised by chronic weakness, fatigue, pains and nervousness. There are two types of neurasthenia: one dominated by mental fatigue and the other by physical fatigue and weakness. The mental syndrome features unpleasant intrusive, distracting recollections and associations, inattention and inefficient thinking. In the physical syndrome, bodily exhaustion occurs after minimal effort. Myalgia and inability to relax are prominent. Irritability, malaise, dizziness, headaches, poor sleep and anhedonia are common to both types (Sadock BJ and Sadock VA, 2000).

### 18.5.9.2 Chronic fatigue syndrome

Chronic fatigue syndrome, myalgic encephalomyalgia or "yuppie flu" is defined by disabling fatigue. Infection by the Epstein-Barr virus has been suggested as a cause. Other possible viruses have been identified. Autonomic dysfunction with orthostasis is a common finding and potential biomarker. Auto-immune factors similar to those in multiple sclerosis have been shown to be in its pathogenesis. Chronic fatigue syndrome is poly-symptomatic with pronounced mental and physical exhaustion, poor concentration and memory, anxiety, depression, insomnia, non-restorative sleep, sore throat, tender or enlarged lymph nodes, myalgia, arthralgia, headache, chills and flushes, night-sweats, palpitations, dyspnoea, diarrhoea, constipation, bloating, bitter taste, dysuria, sexual dysfunction, disequilibrium, eye pain, blurring, photophobia, alopecia, and post-exertion malaise. A physical examination is usually not helpful. Although it tends to be chronic, improvements do occur. It commonly co-exists with major depression, its primary differential diagnosis (Morris and Maes, 2013).

### 18.5.9.3 Irritable bowel syndrome

Irritable bowel syndrome (IBS) is the prototypical functional gastrointestinal disorder. Functional gastrointestinal disorders are so called because physiological bowel abnormalities are demonstrable in the absence of abnormal histological findings. Diverse abnormalities involving bowel muscle electrical and paracrine activity, bacterial flora, grey-matter density in the brain and cortical thickness are recognised. Certain food allergens may play a role. Altered hypothalamic-pituitary-adrenal axis modulation and sensitivity to visceral stimuli mediate symptom expression. Standardised diagnostic criteria were developed by the International Congress of Gastroenterology, comprising abdominal pain relieved by defecation, change in frequency or consistency of bowel movements, straining or urgency, feeling of incomplete evacuation and the passage of mucus per rectum. IBS is common and accounts for 50% of gastro-enterological outpatient visits. It often co-exists with major depression and anxiety (Fadgyas-Stanculete *et al.*, 2014).

### 18.5.9.4 Fibromyalgia

Fibromyalgia consists of multiple vague complaints of joint pain, stiffness, tender muscles, severe fatigue, distress and sleep disturbances. The American College of Rheumatology proposed a set of diagnostic criteria for fibromyalgia in 1990, identifying localised trigger points in muscles. Its differential diagnosis includes rheumatoid arthritis, osteoarthritis, systemic lupus erythematosus, metabolic and endocrine myopathies and psychiatric conditions such as depression, generalised anxiety and somatic symptom disorder. Whilst fibromyalgia is not regarded as a mental disorder it is well recognised that psychological factors play a role in its expression and maintenance. (Hawkins, 2013; Mease, 2005).

## Conclusion

Conditions characterised by somatising, or the physical expression of psychic distress, have taxed medicine for millennia. Whilst a physical presentation is central to the DSM-5 somatic symptom disorders, its nature and course suggest the presence of psychopathology. This psychopathology is cause for significant distress and psychosocial dysfunction, often much more so than the suggested physical condition. Somatic symptom disorders range from the pseudoneurological through multiple bodily complaints to the fear of illness. A common theme characterises the expression of somatic symptom disorders: early psychosocial adversity and the occurrence of a precipitant stressor. Apart from conversion disorder, that typically follows an acute course, somatic symptom disorders are usually chronic conditions characterised by periods of relapse and remission – often incomplete. Chronic fatigue syndrome, irritable bowel syndrome and fibromyalgia are related, but appreciably separate conditions that also involve substantial psychological factors. The ideal management approach to the somatic symptom and related disorders is multidisciplinary focusing on the recognition of psychosocial distress. Whilst the physical complaint should not be emphasised, thorough physical evaluation remains important to rule out, or in, serious physical disease.

# References


Allen LA, Woolfolk RL, Lehrer PM, Gara MA, Escobar JI (2001) Cognitive behavior therapy for somatization disorder: A preliminary investigation. *Journal of Behaviour Therapy and Experimental Psychiatry* 32(2): 53–62

American Psychiatric Association (2000) *Diagnostic and Statistical Manual of Mental Disorders* (4th edition). Text Revision. Arlington, VA: American Psychiatric Association

American Psychiatric Association (2013) *Diagnostic and Statistical Manual of Mental Disorders* (5th edition). Arlington, VA: American Psychiatric Association

Bagayogo IP, Interian A, Escobar JI (2013) Transcultural aspects of somatic symptoms in the context of depressive disorders. In: Iarcón RD (Ed). Cultural Psychiatry. *Advances in psychosomatic medicine* 33: 64–74

Binzer M, Kullgren D (1998) Motor Conversion Disorder: A Prospective 2- to 5-Year Follow-Up Study. *Psychosomatics* 39(6): 519–27

Black DS (2004) Conversion hysteria: lessons from functional imaging. *Journal of Neuropsychiatry and Clinical Neurosciences* 16(3): 245–51

Brennan A, Ayers S, Ahmed H, Marshall-Lucette S (2007) A critical review of the Couvade syndrome: the pregnant male. *Journal of Reproductive and Infant Psychology* 25(3): 173–89

Cardeña E (1984) The domain of disassociation. In: Rhue SJ. *Dissociation, Clinical and Theoretical Perspectives.* New York: Guilford Press

Cassem NH, Barsky AJ (1991) Functional somatic symptoms and somatoform disorder. In: Cassem NH (Ed). *Handbook of General Hospital Psychiatry.* St. Louis: Mosby

Du Plessis LM (2003) *An investigation into models for the assessment of malingering in criminal forensic evaluations.* Unpublished Master's dissertation. Unisa.

Du Plessis LM, Visser C (2012) Disorders with dissociative and somatic symptoms. In: Burke A (Ed). *Abnormal psychology* (2nd edition). Cape Town: Oxford University Press Southern Africa

Dworkin SF, Wilson L (1993) Somatoform pain disorder and its treatment. In: Dunner DD. *Current psychiatric therapy.* Philadelphia: WB Saunders

Epstein RM, Quill TE, McWhinney IR (1999) Somatization reconsidered: incorporating the patient's experience of illness. *Archives of Internal Medicine* 159(3): 215–22

Escobar J (2004) Transcultural aspects of dissociative and somatoform disorders. *Journal of Nervous and Mental Disease* (192): 324–7

Escobar JI, Gara M, Silver RC, Watzskin H, Holam A, Compton W (1998) Somatisation disorder in primary care. *British Journal of Psychiatry* (173): 262–6.

Fadgyas-Stanculete M, Buga A, Wagner AP, Dumitrascu DL (2014) The relationship between irritable bowel syndrome and psychiatric disorders: From molecular changes to clinical manifestations. *Journal of Molecular Psychiatry.* http://www.jmolecularpsychiatry.com/content/2/1/4 (Accessed 28 August 2014.)

Ford CV (1985) Conversion disorders: An overview. *Psychosomatics* (26): 371–85

Grabe HR (2000) The relationship between dimensions of alexithymia and dissociation. *Psychotherapy and Psychosomatics* (69): 128–31

Hales RY (2008) *American Psychiatric Publishing Textbook of Psychiatry* (8th edition). Washington, DC: American Psychiatric Publishing

Hawkins RA (2013) Fibromyalgia: A clinical update. *Journal of the American Osteopathic Association* 113(9): 680–9

Karukappadath RM, Russai R, Mohamed N, Kovari F (2013) Factitious disorder in intensive care unit – are we doing enough? *Journal of the Intensive Care Society* 14(4): 340–2

Kellner R (1986) *Somatization and hypochondriasis.* London: Greenwood Press

Khouzam HR, Field S (1999) Somatization disorder: Clinical presentation and treatment in primary care. *Hospital Physician* 45: 20–4

Kirmayer LJ (1984) Culture, affect and somatization. *Transcultural Psychiatry* (4): 159–8

Krahn, LB (2008) Looking toward DSM-V: should factitious disorder become a subtype of somatoform disorder? *Psychosomatics* 49: 277–82

Kroenke K, Swindle R (2000) Cognitive-behavioral therapy for somatization and symptom syndromes: A critical review of controlled clinical trials. *Psychotherapy and Psychosomatics* 69(4): 205–15

Mai F (2004) Somatization disorder: A practical review. Comment in *Canadian Journal of Psychiatry* 49(10): 649–51

Mailis-Gagnon A, Isrealson D (2005) *Beyond Pain: Making the Mind-Body Connection.* Toronto: Viking Canada/Penguin Books

Mease P (2005) Fibromyalgia syndrome: review of clinical presentation, pathogenesis, outcome measures, and treatment. *The Journal of Rheumatology* 75: 6–21

Morris, G, Maes, M (2013) Myalgic encephalomyelitis/chronic fatigue syndrome and encephalomyelitis disseminata/multiple sclerosis show remarkable levels of similarity in phenomenology and neuroimmune characteristics. *BMC Medicine.* http://www.biomedcentral.com/1741-7015/11/205 (Accessed 29 August 2014.)

Olry R (2002) Baron Munchhausen and the syndrome which bears his name: History of an endearing personage and of a strange mental disorder. *Vesalius* VIII(1): 53–7

Pribor EF, Yutzy SH, Dean JT, Wetzel RD (1993) Briquet's syndrome, dissociation, and abuse. *American Journal of Psychiatry* 150(10): 1507–11

Rief W, Pilger F, Ihle D, Bosmans E, Egyed B, Maes M (2001) Immunological differences between patients with major depression and somatization syndrome. *Psychiatry Research* 105(3): 165–74

Rome H.P (2000) Limbically augmented pain syndrome (LAPS): kindling, corticolimbic sensitization, and the convergence of affective an sensory symptoms in chronic pain disorders. *Pain medicine* 1(1): 7–23

Sadock BJ, Sadock VA (2000) *Kaplan & Sadock's Comprehensive Textbook of Psychiatry* (7th edition). Philadelphia: Lippincott, Williams & Wilkins

Sadock BJ, Sadock VA (2007) *Kaplan and Sadock's Synopsis of Psychiatry. Behavioural Sciences/Clinical* Psychiatry (10th edition). Philadelphia: Lippincott, Williams & Wilkins

Schreier HA, Libow JA (1994) Munchausen by proxy syndrome: A modern pediatric journal. *The Journal of Paediatrics* 125(6): 110–5

Shipton E (2008) The chronic pain experience. *New Zealand Medical Journal* 121(1270): 9–11

Sierra MB (1998) Depersonalization: neurobiological perspectives. *Biological Psychiatry* 44: 989–98

Spence CH, Crimlisk HL, Cope H, Ron RA, Grasby PM (2000) Discrete neuropsychological correlates in prefrontal cortex during hysterical and feigned disorder of movement. *The Lancet* 355(9211): 1234–43

Stone J, Smith ER, Carson A, Warlow C, Sharpe M (2006) La belle indifferénce in conversion symptoms and hysteria. Systematic review. *British Journal of Psychiatry* 188: 204–9

Stonnington CM, Barry J, Fisher RS (2006) Conversion disorder. *American Journal of Psychiatry* 163(9): 1510–7

Ullman LP, Krasner L (1975) A *Psychological Approach to Abnormal Behaviour* (2nd edition). Englewood Cliffs, N. J.: Prentice Hall

Van der Hart O, Rutger H (1989) The dissociation of Pierre Janet. *Journal of Traumatic Stress* 2(4): 1–11

CHAPTER

# 19 Dissociative disorders

*Christa Krüger*

## 19.1 Introduction

Dissociative disorders represent one of the biggest unresolved burning points in present-day psychiatry, where neurobiology and psychology – the 'hardware' and the 'software' of the brain – meet closely.

Dissociation may be defined from various angles. From a psychological perspective, dissociation is a protective psychological process to manage overwhelming emotions and experiences, usually of a traumatic or stressful nature (Brand and Loewenstein, 2010). Clusters of mental contents may be split off from conscious awareness, or ideas may be separated from their emotional significance and affect. Furthermore, dissociation may allow an individual to believe two contradictory truths while remaining unconscious of the contradiction (American Psychiatric Association, 2013).

See also Advanced reading block 19.1 for additional definitions of dissociation from neurobiological, cognitive, clinical, developmental and contextual perspectives.

Having considered the various definitions in Advanced reading block 19.1, it remains difficult to explain to a layperson, such as a colleague from another discipline, what dissociation is. Perhaps the following might be helpful: Dissociation is the brain's way of handling difficult information, for example, traumatic events or child abuse that is too painful to bear or information that is in conflict with one's experiences or expectations.

How much dissociation can occur before it becomes a disorder? 'Dissociative disorders (DDs) are characterised by a disruption of and/or discontinuity in the normal integration of consciousness, memory, identity, emotion, perception, body representation, motor control, and behaviour' (American Psychiatric Association, 2013). Dissociative disorders can be thought of as a cluster of clinical syndromes where dissociative processes, symptoms and **defence mechanisms** have become severe enough to be clinically significant, thereby affecting a person's functioning adversely to the extent that he or she is diagnosable as mentally ill. Dissociative disorders may also reflect an incredible ability to subdivide or compartmentalise one's mind to the point where it becomes dysfunctional rather than useful (Hunter, 2004).

Again, in lay language perhaps: Dissociative disorders mean there are significant problems with one's awareness, consciousness and sense of self. For example, a person blocks out traumatic memories or struggles to keep it all

### Case study 19.1

A patient presents to the emergency department with a bleeding laceration on the left forearm. The doctor finds the patient sitting in a dazed state, staring into space.

Doctor: 'What happened to your arm?'

Patient: 'I don't know, I only saw it this afternoon.'

## 19.1 Advanced reading block

**Definitions of dissociation (additional information)**

Psychologically speaking, dissociation is a protective psychological process to manage overwhelming emotions and experiences, usually of a traumatic or stressful nature (Brand and Loewenstein, 2010).

Neurobiologically speaking, dissociation is a regulatory strategy to cope with extreme arousal through hyper-inhibition of limbic regions – a strategy most active during the conscious processing of threat (Felmingham *et al.*, 2008).

Cognitively speaking, dissociation reflects an information processing style where multiple streams of information are processed simultaneously, but not integrated properly, in times of threat (Dorahy, 2006).

Clinically speaking, dissociation is an 'involuntary disruption of the normal integration of conscious awareness and control over one's mental processes' (Spiegel *et al.*, 2011). The manifestations include the loss of connections between memories, the emotions that go with memories, perception of one's self and one's environment, and hence confusion about one's identity and even alternating discordant behavioural states.

Developmentally speaking, dissociation represents a pattern of mental organisation where an integrated sense of self and the connections between mental processes never developed properly in the first place because of chronic complex traumatic experiences or chronic childhood abuse (Carlson *et al.*, 2009; Schore, 1996; Schore, 2009).

Contextually speaking, dissociation is a mostly normal information-processing tool to construct and maintain balanced, coherent selves-in-society, that is, individuals connected to each other in a world of conflicting messages, where the conflict is often interpersonal/cultural/societal in nature, rather than primarily intrapsychic (Krüger *et al.*, 2007).

together. When more severe, there might be 'breaks' in consciousness where a person may be unaware of behaving in contradictory ways, as if controlled by different forces at different times. The most severe example of a dissociative disorder – dissociative identity disorder (DID) – was previously called multiple personality disorder.

It is important that medical students and students of other health professions have an understanding of dissociation and dissociative disorders, since dissociative disorders are relatively common – much more common than schizophrenia or bipolar disorder – and cause at least as much suffering. Dissociative disorders are also difficult to diagnose; and when undiagnosed in general medical settings, present confusing clinical pictures and much frustration with unsuccessful treatment.

Dissociative disorders have a rich and interesting history in psychiatry and psychology. However, that history will not be covered here. In this chapter only the currently most widely accepted understanding of the field of dissociation is summarised.

### Critical thinking box

What would you think is the reason why a person with a given set of brain 'hardware' (genetic material, brain structure, neurotransmitters, etc.), may experience a certain mental state the one minute, and the very next second – with the exact same 'hardware' – the person switches into a completely different mental state with a different identity, different memories, different behaviour, different thoughts and emotions, and even different neurophysiological readings?

This chapter starts with an outline of the scope of dissociation and dissociative disorders, including recent changes in the diagnostic criteria of dissociative disorders, culture-specific presentations and how to recognise dissociative disorders. The second section covers the aetiology of dissociative disorders, with special reference to complex ongoing relational trauma, psychological and social theories of dissociation and neurobiological findings in dissociation. The third section concerns the relationship between dissociative disorders and other psychiatric disorders (e.g. post-traumatic stress disorder (PTSD), borderline personality disorder (BPD), depressive and anxiety disorders, psychotic disorders, and somatic symptom and related disorders) as well as the distinctions between them. The last section focuses on a trauma-informed approach to the management of dissociative disorders, and in particular the role of the general medical practitioner.

The most important areas for medical students to focus on are the clinical pictures of dissociative disorders, their traumatic aetiology, their relationships to other psychiatric disorders and the role of the GP in their management.

Note: this chapter has areas of overlap with several other chapters in this textbook: see Chapter 6: Culture and psychiatry, Chapter 11: Schizophrenia spectrum and other psychotic disorders, Chapter 12: Depressive disorders, Chapter 14: Anxiety, fear and panic, Chapter 15: Acute reactions to adverse life events, Chapter 16: Trauma, Chapter 18: Somatic symptom and related disorders, Chapter 24: Personality and personality disorder, Chapter 31: Psychiatry and medicine, Chapter 35: Legal and ethical aspects of mental health, Chapter 36: Pharmacological and other treatment in psychiatry and Chapter 37: Psychological interventions.

## 19.2 Scope of dissociation and the dissociative disorders

As with many other disorders, a certain degree of dissociation may be normal. It is only when dissociative symptoms become severe enough to cause clinically significant distress or disability in social, occupational or other important activities, that they are regarded as a disorder (American Psychiatric Association, 2013).

From the perspective of childhood development, dissociation has been considered a normal phase in healthy personality development. However, if the resolution of that phase is disrupted (e.g. by traumatic events such as childhood abuse) a dissociative disorder can be said to arise (see also Section 19.3).

### 19.2.1 Changes in the DSM-5 diagnostic criteria of the dissociative disorders

The main changes in the DSM-5 (American Psychiatric Association, 2013) to the diagnostic criteria of dissociative disorders are:

- the incorporation of possession trance with dissociative identity disorder
- the acceptance of self-reporting in the diagnosis of dissociative identity disorder
- the inclusion of amnesia for everyday events in the diagnosis of dissociative identity disorder (if excessive), in addition to amnesia for important personal information or traumatic events
- the addition of a functioning criterion in the diagnosis of dissociative identity disorder
- the incorporation of dissociative fugue as a specifier of dissociative amnesia (rather than as a separate disorder)
- the combination of depersonalisation and derealisation in depersonalisation/derealisation disorder
- the addition of a brief, transient 'acute dissociative reaction to stressful events' to the examples of other specified dissociative disorders (which lasts hours or days, typically less than one month, and consists of mixed dissociative symptoms)
- the broadening of the criteria for dissociative trance (another example of the other specified dissociative disorders) by removing the limitation that the trance experiences have to be indigenous to particular locations and cultures.

Most importantly, possession trance was incorporated in the main diagnostic criterion for dissociative identity disorder in the DSM-5, both as a cultural variant of dissociative identity disorder and as an alternative to 'distinct-personality-state dissociative identity disorder'. This incorporation means that a person does not necessarily have to have two or more distinct personality states/alter personalities, with accompanying switches, in order to be diagnosed with dissociative identity disorder, but might instead have possession experiences (reported by the person him- or herself or observed by others).

The inclusion of possession experiences might assist diagnosis of dissociative identity disorder in cultures where a disruption of identity might show itself as pathological possession states rather than as overtly multiple personality states. It is anticipated that the inclusion of possession would increase the global utility and cross-cultural applicability of the dissociative identity disorder diagnostic category. This inclusion might also lead to more frequent diagnoses of dissociative identity disorder in South Africa (see Case study 19.2). However, if the possession experience can be seen as a normal part of a broadly accepted cultural or religious practice, it is not regarded as a disorder and the person would not be diagnosed with dissociative identity disorder.

The disruption of identity that is the hallmark of dissociative identity disorder – whether manifesting as distinct personality states or as experiences of possession – involves marked discontinuity in the sense of self and the sense of agency, accompanied by related alterations in affect, behaviour, consciousness, memory, perception, cognition and/or sensory-motor functioning.

With regard to memory and amnesia in the DSM-5 definition of dissociative identity disorder, recurrent gaps in recall may occur for everyday events too and not just for traumatic events or important personal information. However, these memory gaps must be big enough to be inconsistent with ordinary (normal) forgetting.

A functioning criterion was also added to the criteria for dissociative identity disorder, which means that the symptoms of dissociative identity disorder only indicate a disorder if they cause clinically significant distress or impairment in functioning. Moreover, the disturbance is only a disorder when it falls outside of cultural norms. The addition of this functioning criterion implies that it is possible for healthy people to experience normal instances of multiplicity or discontinuities in identity and memory without suffering from dissociative identity disorder.

## 19.2.2 South African cultural idiom of distress: *Amafufunyana* and dissociative disorders

Although not listed in the DSM-5 (APA, 2013) glossary of cultural concepts of distress, *amafufunyana* – a local South African idiom of distress in which the angry spirits of ancestors are thought to enter the patient (Drennan, 2001) – may present as dissociative trance (one of the other specified dissociative disorders in the DSM-5) or even as dissociative identity disorder. In such cases, the syndrome usually starts with an emotional disturbance such as social withdrawal. This may be followed by somatic symptoms such as listlessness and loss of appetite, followed by behavioural disturbances such as grunting, falling down and aggressive behaviour. This phase of behavioural disturbance may resemble 'switching' behaviour. Subsequently, verbalisations may follow in which the *amafufunyana* (the evil spirits) speak. These voices may speak in a foreign language and may belong to someone of the opposite sex ('alter identity'). The patient is seen to undergo an altered state of consciousness and is amnesic regarding the event.

Case study 19.2 serves as an example of a pathological syndrome (dissociative identity disorder) where the patient presented with possession and an alter identity. The dissociative symptoms may have arisen from painful emotional experiences (the death of the young man). Furthermore, the dissociation may reflect a societal conflict around the practice of witchcraft. A community-based, spiritual-type intervention was employed to achieve healing on two levels: Nomthandazo stopped dissociating (individual healing) and the community managed to expel an undesirable witch from their midst (social healing).

## Case study 19.2

***Amafufunyana* as dissociative identity disorder**

Nomthandazo Grootboom (not her real name), a Xhosa girl in a rural village in the Eastern Cape, fell ill and became confused for a few days. There were no apparent acute precipitants or any ongoing stressors. Her family consulted a traditional healer but this did not help. Her symptoms of restlessness and confused speech worsened. Her behaviour became odd. She started walking on all fours. Her voice changed to that of a young man, and she called herself by this young man's name. Her family recognised the name and voice as those of a young man who had passed away two years earlier. Nomthandazo described the events that had led to his death. The voice of the deceased young man, through Nomthandazo, alleged that one of their neighbours had bewitched him and was using him as a slave. He said that he was not quite dead but could not come back to life as he had been bewitched.

As a means of healing and resolution the family decided to take Nomthandazo to the neighbour who had allegedly bewitched the young man. A crowd gathered in the house. The alleged witch was confronted with the information gathered and Nomthandazo, through the male voice, openly accused the neighbour of witchcraft. The alleged witch ran away. The girl and her family returned home, at which time her symptoms resolved and her voice returned to normal. She was, however, amnesic regarding these events. She was subsequently able to return to school and remained well.

**Source:** Adapted from Krüger *et al.*, 2007.

## 19.2.3 Recognising dissociative disorders

Patients who suffer from dissociative disorders may be identifiable provisionally in a general medical setting or in a casualty department by a confusing clinical presentation: many psychosomatic symptoms, unexplained injuries, self-harm or suicide attempts, incongruent affect (detachment from emotional pain), abrupt mood changes and a history or complaints of severe **acting-out** behaviour in a pleasant, compliant patient (Hunter, 2004). For the specific diagnosis of a dissociative disorder, the index of suspicion should be raised when there is a poly-symptomatic presentation, prominent co-morbidity, or an inconsistency in attendance, presentation and the patient's account.

However, in reality the road to a diagnosis of a dissociative disorder is often long and, in retrospect, often involved numerous hospital admissions and multiple medication trials that offered only limited benefit. It often happens that a patient with a dissociative disorder is not correctly diagnosed for many years.

'Switching' is the sudden transition from one identity state (**alter personality**) to another in dissociative identity disorder. Switching may be dramatic and obvious (e.g. associated with posturing and grunting by the patient) or subtle and barely noticeable by the clinician. Once switched, the new identity state or 'alter' may exhibit completely different characteristics from the previous state, including a different way of speaking, or difference in accent, posture, mannerisms and even adoption of the opposite gender.

It is possible to screen for the presence of a dissociative disorder with the Dissociative Experiences Scale (DES): a brief 28-item self-report questionnaire (Bernstein and Putnam, 1986; Carlson and Putnam, 1993). The items capture the percentage of the time that the patient experiences certain dissociative symptoms and experiences. An average score of ≥30 is highly suggestive that the patient might suffer from a severe dissociative disorder and should be followed up by a diagnostic interview by a psychiatrist or clinical psychologist (Carlson and Putnam, 1993).

Three subgroups of dissociative symptoms have been distinguished on the basis of recent neurobiological research: primary, secondary and tertiary dissociation (see Table 19.1). The neurobiological findings will be covered below under the aetiology of the dissociative disorders.

## 19.3 Aetiology of dissociative disorders

The aetiology of dissociative disorders can be understood according to a bio-psycho-social framework. Current psychological and neurobiological theories are starting to overlap in the sense that most of them link dissociation with a failure of normal developmental integration of parallel cognitive processes. This means that a child's mind does not develop the ability to handle conflicting types of information as it is supposed to. This developmental failure occurs when a child is traumatised (especially emotionally or sexually) because of chronic abuse or neglect.

Psychological trauma, and particularly complex, chronic and ongoing relational trauma (such as is found in abusive interpersonal relationships), leads to dissociative disorders. This link between trauma and dissociation (i.e. that trauma causes dissociation) is well-established and supported by substantial empirical evidence (Dalenberg *et al.*, 2012; Dorahy and Van der Hart, 2007; Dorahy *et al.*, 2014).

Dissociative identity disorder is currently understood as a chronic complex post-traumatic developmental disorder that usually begins before the age of five or six, usually as a result of chronic childhood abuse (physical, sexual or emotional abuse or emotional neglect). The alter identities result from the inability of many traumatised young children to develop a unified sense of self that is maintained across various discrete behavioural states (Howell and Blizard, 2009; Putnam, 2006).

Neurophysiological research on dissociation, including functional magnetic resonance imaging (fMRI), positron emission tomography (PET), single-photon emission computerised tomography (SPECT), electroencephalography (EEG) and quantitative electroencephalography (QEEG) studies show how intertwined is the psychological process of dissociation with cognitive and emotional processing (Dorahy *et al.*, 2014). (See also Table 19.1 and Advanced reading block 19.2.)

Current thinking includes that it is possible to distinguish between primary, secondary and tertiary dissociation in a so-called cortical processing model or cortico-limbic inhibition model of dissociation (Brand *et al.*, 2012). The cortico-limbic inhibition model involves down-regulation of neurotransmission in the infero-medial Papez circuit in the brain. This means that certain overactive deep limbic brain areas are dampened down or regulated by other more superficial cortical areas, to the extent that some areas are almost completely deactivated or numbed. (See also Table 19.1 and Advanced reading block 19.2.)

One might also call the above explanation a cognitive-emotional model of dissociation. The entire perceptual apparatus and cognition are affected because of emotional trauma.

## 19.4 Dissociative disorders in relation to other disorders: epidemiology, co-morbidity and differential diagnosis

Epidemiological studies have demonstrated the following prevalence figures in the general population: all dissociative disorders 8,6–18,3%, dissociative identity disorder 1,1–1,5%, depersonalisation disorder 0,8–2,8% and dissociative amnesia 1,8-3% (Johnson *et al.*, 2006; Martínez-Taboas *et al.*, 2013; Sar *et al.*, 2007a).

Co-morbidity with dissociative disorders is usually extensive and complicates the differential diagnosis. The most common co-morbid conditions – PTSD, BPD, depressive and anxiety disorders, psychotic disorders and somatic symptom and related disorders – can be difficult to distinguish from dissociative disorders.

### 19.4.1 Post-traumatic stress disorder (PTSD)

Much of the neurophysiological research on dissociation (see Advanced reading block 19.2) has been related to patients who suffer from

**Table 19.1** Dissociative symptom groups, symptoms, neurobiological findings, and corresponding DSM-5 disorders

| Symptom group | Dissociative symptom | Limited description | Neurobiological findings | Corresponding DSM-5 disorders |
|---|---|---|---|---|
| **Primary dissociation (hyper-aroused, hyperemotional)** | Flashbacks | Aspects of a traumatic event are re-experienced involuntarily as though they were reoccurring at that moment | Brain areas activated that represent under-controlled emotion, e.g., inhibition of activity in the anterior cingulate cortex, medial prefrontal cortex and thalamus, and at the same time, increased activity in the amygdala and insular regions. | PTSD |
| | Reliving experiences | As above, but more voluntary | | |
| | Intrusion | Unwanted thoughts or impulses enter one's mind, or unwanted emotions arise | | |
| | Autonomic hyper-arousal | Tachycardia, tachypnea, sweating, headache, diarrhoea, etc. | | |
| **Secondary dissociation (hypo-emotional)** | Distancing | Avoidance of socioemotional experience and interaction; restricted affectivity | Brain areas activated that may over-modulate emotion and alter one's sense of self (e.g. increased activity in the anterior cingulate cortex, medial prefrontal cortex and other regions, and at the same time, limbic inhibition). | PTSD with dissociative symptoms<br>Depersonalisation/ derealisation disorder<br>Dissociative amnesia |
| | Emotional numbing | Reduction in range and intensity of emotional expression | | |
| | Derealisation | Feeling detached from one's surroundings (as if an observer of unreal objects) | | |
| | Depersonalisation | Feeling detached from one's mental processes, body or actions (as if one's self is robotic or unreal) | | |
| | Amnesia | Inability to recall important autobiographical information, usually of a traumatic or stressful nature, that is inconsistent with ordinary forgetting | | |
| **Tertiary dissociation** | **Identity confusion** | A conscious feeling of uncertainty, puzzlement, or conflict about one's identity as a result of intrusions from a dissociated self-state | Different brain areas may be activated during different self-states. | Dissociative amnesia with dissociative fugue<br>Dissociative identity disorder |
| | **Identity alteration** | Discovering the fully-dissociated activities of another self-state (e.g. time loss, 'coming to', switches, being told of actions, finding evidence of one's recent behaviour) | | |
| | Conversion | Loss of or altered voluntary motor or sensory functioning, with or without impairment of consciousness or psychogenic non-epileptic seizures | | |

**Source:** This table is based on the theory of structural dissociation of the personality and the cortico-limbic inhibition model of dissociation (Frewen and Lanius, 2006; Lanius *et al.*, 2002, 2005, 2006; Nijenhuis and Den Boer, 2009; Nijenhuis *et al.*, 2010; Reinders *et al.*, 2003, 2006, 2012; Steele *et al.*, 2009; Van der Hart *et al.*, 2006; Dorahy and Van der Hart, 2007). The descriptions are based on the DSM-5 (American Psychiatric Association, 2013). This table gives only some examples of symptoms and is not exhaustive.

## 19.2 Advanced reading block

### Aetiology of the dissociative disorders (additional information)

### Psychological and social theories of dissociation

Various psychological theories help us understand dissociation and dissociative disorders, including theories relating to attachment, developmental psychopathology, structural dissociation of the personality, neural networks, conflict psychology and cognitive psychology.

According to the extensive recent research on attachment theory and developmental psychopathology, disorganised attachment of a child to its primary caretaker makes it impossible for normal instances of contradictory experiences (and their accompanying dissociated mental states) to be integrated into normal personality development. As a result, the child fails to mentalise normally and his or her sense of self remains fragmented (Carlson *et al.*, 2009; Sachs, 2013; Schore, 2009).

According to the theory of structural dissociation of the personality, there are 'apparently normal' and 'emotional' parts of the person's personality as a result of trauma (Nijenhuis *et al.*, 2010; Steele *et al.*, 2009; Van der Hart *et al.*, 2006). While the wounded emotional part of the personality remains in the background, the apparently normal part (or parts) of the personality help the person to get by in daily life.

According to neural network theory, dissociated mental states may be thought of as competition among groups of cortical neurons that excite one another but are unable to agree on a common frequency of oscillation (Bob, 2003; Bob and Faber, 2006).

According to socio-cognitive theories of dissociation, the processing of societal information may be problematic, for example when there is collective stimulus deprivation or stimulus overload in the individual's society, or when there are conflicting societal or ideological messages in the individual's context (Krüger *et al.*, 2007; Sar and Öztürk, 2007; Sar and Öztürk, 2013; Sar *et al.*, 2013; Sar *et al.*, 2014).

### Neurobiological findings in dissociation

Primary dissociation (see Table 19.1) refers to flashbacks, reliving, intrusion and hyper-arousal related dissociative symptoms, as is often found in PTSD. Emotions are under-modulated. Primary dissociation has been associated in fMRI, PET and SPECT studies with inhibition of activity in the anterior cingulate cortex, medial prefrontal cortex and thalamus with simultaneous increased activity in the amygdala and insular regions.

Secondary dissociation (see Table 19.1) refers to distancing and emotional numbing symptoms – more traditionally called 'dissociation' and also often found in PTSD. Emotions are over-modulated (Frewen and Lanius, 2006; Lanius *et al.*, 2002; Lanius *et al.*, 2005; Lanius *et al.*, 2006). Secondary dissociation has been associated in fMRI, PET and SPECT studies with the opposite to primary dissociation: increased activity in the anterior cingulate cortex, medial prefrontal cortex and other regions, and at the same time, limbic inhibition (Savoy *et al.*, 2012; Tsai *et al.*, 1999; Wolk *et al.*, 2012).

Tertiary dissociation (see Table 19.1) refers to the more differentiated dissociative symptoms of altered identity states as found in dissociative identity disorder. Several fMRI, PET and SPECT studies that have been done on patients with dissociative identity disorder show different patterns of activation during different identity states (Brand *et al.*, 2012; Nijenhuis and Den Boer, 2009; Reinders *et al.*, 2003; Reinders *et al.*, 2006; Reinders *et al.*, 2012; Sar *et al.*, 2001; Sar *et al.*, 2007b; Savoy *et al.*, 2012; Tsai *et al.*, 1999; Wolk *et al.*, 2012).

Interestingly, EEG and QEEG studies have demonstrated associations between dissociative symptoms and the temporal regions of the brain, rather than the cortico-limbic associations as found in fMRI, PET and SPECT studies (Coons *et al.*, 1988; Hopper *et al.*, 2002; Hughes *et al.*, 1990; Krüger *et al.*, 2013; Lapointe *et al.*, 2006; Mesulam, 1981; Spiegel and Vermetten, 1994).

In addition to the above cognitive-emotional model of dissociation, the somatoform dissociation model focuses on the involvement of somatosensory pathways (including the autonomic nervous system and other psychophysiological parameters) in dissociative processes (Nijenhuis, 2004).

There is currently limited evidence of a genetic basis to dissociative disorders. It appears that genetics might play a larger role in normal dissociation, whereas environmental factors – including ongoing relational trauma – might play a larger role in dissociative disorders (Becker-Blease *et al.*, 2004; Dalenberg *et al.*, 2012; Jang *et al.*, 1998; Lochner *et al.*, 2004). However, a recent genome-wide association study (Wolf *et al.*, 2014) in patients with the dissociative subtype of PTSD demonstrated two genes that are important in long-term potentiation, synaptic plasticity, synaptic integration and excitation.

PTSD, given the symptomatic overlap between these disorders. The DSM-5 includes a new subtype of PTSD – the dissociative subtype, specified as 'With dissociative symptoms' – which overlaps largely with dissociative disorders (American Psychiatric Association, 2013; see also Chapter 15: Acute reactions to adverse life events and Chapter 16: Trauma).

Unlike patients with PTSD, patients with dissociative identity disorder experience amnesia of many everyday, non-traumatic events, dissociative flashbacks that may be followed by amnesia of the content of the flashback, disruptive intrusions (unrelated to traumatic material) by dissociated identity states into the individual's sense of self and agency, and infrequent, full-blown changes among different identity states (American Psychiatric Association, 2013).

Unlike patients with PTSD, patients with dissociative amnesia may experience amnesia that extends beyond the immediate time of the trauma (American Psychiatric Association, 2013).

### 19.4.2 Borderline personality disorder (BPD)

Dissociative disorders are often confused with borderline personality disorder, since both are characterised by affect dysregulation, suicidality, self-harm and related symptoms (see also Chapter 24: Personality and personality disorder). Moreover, borderline personality disorder often occurs co-morbidly with the dissociative disorders, since the same trauma and disorganised attachment that lead to dissociative disorders may also contribute to borderline personality disorder.

Although it may be very difficult to distinguish between a dissociative disorder and borderline personality disorder, empirical research suggests that they are not the same disorder (Brand *et al.*, 2006; Brand *et al.*, 2009a; Korzekwa *et al.*, 2009a; Korzekwa *et al.*, 2009b; Ross, 2007; Ross *et al.*, 2014; Sar *et al.*, 2003; Sar *et al.*, 2006; Stiglmayr *et al.*, 2001; Stiglmayr *et al.*, 2008; Zanarini and Jager-Hyman, 2009). There appears to be consensus that BPD patients who dissociate are more impaired and require complex treatment. Furthermore, when compared psychometrically, patients with dissociative identity disorder show a greater capacity for self-reflection and introspection than BPD patients (Brand *et al.*, 2006; Brand *et al.*, 2009a).

Clinically, due to differences between identities, the longitudinal variability in personality style of patients with dissociative identity disorder differs from the pervasive and persistent dysfunction in affect management and interpersonal relationships typical of those with personality disorders (American Psychiatric Association, 2013).

### 19.4.3 Depressive and anxiety disorders

Depressive and anxiety disorders frequently occur co-morbidly in patients with dissociative disorders, and are often the presenting syndromes. With regard to the anxiety disorders, panic attacks are a frequent co-morbid occurrence.

In dissociative identity disorder sometimes only one or a few identity states suffer the depressive symptoms, in which case the depressed mood and cognitions fluctuate (American Psychiatric Association, 2013) and pharmacological treatment with antidepressants might not have the desired effect. Antidepressant treatment works best if the depressive or anxiety symptoms are experienced across the board by all alter identities (Loewenstein, 2005).

With regard to the close relationship of depersonalisation/derealisation with panic attacks, depersonalisation/derealisation disorder should only be diagnosed if the depersonalisation/derealisation symptoms exceed in duration and intensity the occurrence of the actual panic attacks, or continue after the panic disorder has remitted or been successfully treated (American Psychiatric Association, 2013).

### 19.4.4 Psychotic disorders

Not only is it sometimes difficult to distinguish between dissociative disorders and psychotic disorders, but also these disorders often occur co-morbidly. For example, patients with schizophrenia often also have dissociative symptoms. Patients with dissociative identity disorder very often experience hallucinations and Schneiderian first-rank symptoms, which include audible thoughts, voices arguing or commenting and **thought withdrawal** or broadcasting (Kluft, 1987; Moskowitz *et al.*, 2008; Ross *et al.*, 1990). In addition, the experience of interference by, or intrusions from, alternate identities into a patient's consciousness may be misdiagnosed as psychotic passive influence or first-rank symptoms (Brand and Loewenstein, 2010). In general however, patients with dissociative disorders do not report delusional explanations for hallucinations (American Psychiatric Association, 2013).

Patients with depersonalisation/derealisation disorder differ from psychotic patients in that the former's reality testing remains intact (American Psychiatric Association, 2013).

In the planning phases of the DSM-5, there was the possibility of including another new category under 'other specified dissociative disorder' – similar to the acute dissociative reactions to stressful events, of mixed dissociative symptoms, of less than 1 month's duration – but which would also include psychotic symptoms (a brief 'dissociative psychosis'). However, this was eventually not included in the DSM-5.

### 19.4.5 Somatic symptom and related disorders

Somatoform symptoms occur commonly in patients with dissociative disorders, and they have been considered a part of the construct of dissociation (somatoform dissociation as opposed to psychoform dissociation) (Nijenhuis, 2004). Examples of somatoform dissociative symptoms are pain while urinating, the whole body or a part of it being insensitive to pain, feeling that the body or part of it has disappeared, being unable to speak (or only with great effort) or only able to whisper.

At the disorder level, the ICD-10 classifies conversion disorder together with dissociative disorders (World Health Organization, 1992). Although thought was given to classifying conversion disorder with the dissociative disorders in the planning phases of the DSM-5, conversion disorder was eventually accommodated in the somatic symptom and related disorders section, as 'functional neurological symptom disorder' (American Psychiatric Association, 2013).

Clinically, dissociative identity disorder is differentiated from conversion disorder by its identity disruption or possession and more extensive amnesia (American Psychiatric Association, 2013).

## 19.5 Management of the dissociative disorders

The definitive treatment of dissociative disorders is most often and most appropriately carried out in a specialist context by psychiatrists, clinical psychologists and other clinical specialists. The mainstay of treatment is psychotherapy and the goal of therapy is more integrated functioning.

Psychiatric hospital admission may be necessary at times when patients are at risk of harming themselves or others, or when their dissociative or post-traumatic symptoms are overwhelming or out of control. Social support is also important in the journey to health. Dissociative disorders often have a chronic course. The longer the duration of symptoms, the more guarded the prognosis.

### 19.5.1 Psychotherapy

Psychotherapy for dissociative disorders often takes a number of years; it most often occurs on an out-patient basis, with an individual psychotherapist in a psychodynamically oriented framework (Brand *et al.*, 2009b; Brand *et al.*, 2009c; Brand *et al.*, 2013). Psychotherapy for dissociative identity disorder, for example, usually unfolds through three stages (International Society for the Study of Trauma and Dissociation, 2011): stabilisation, memory work and integration. The stabilisation phase focuses on establishing safety, teaching emotion regulation and reducing dissociative and other symptoms; this stage might take a number of years. The memory work phase involves confronting traumatic memories, working through them and integrating them. The integration phase involves helping the alter identities to be aware of one another as legitimate parts of the self, to negotiate and resolve their conflicts and to reach a workable form of integration, unification or harmony among the alter identities.

All of this happens in the context of a therapeutic relationship that provides a safe interpersonal space in which the patient can become aware of, learn and practise what was not learnt in early childhood or at the time of ongoing abuse: to develop a unified sense of self-in-relationship. Other techniques may be incorporated, such as hypnosis as a facilitator of psychotherapy and modified eye movement desensitisation and reprocessing therapy (EMDR) to aid the resolution of traumatic memories. Group therapy may also have an adjunctive role in the treatment of dissociative disorders.

**Critical thinking box**

If a person with dissociative identity disorder commits murder while in an alternate identity state or alter identity (of which the host identity has not been aware), should this person be held accountable for the crime? Should this person not be held accountable on the basis of mental illness?

### 19.5.2 Medication

The psychopharmacological treatment of dissociative disorders is mostly to assist with stabilisation and to treat co-morbid conditions, rather than being the primary treatment. Depending on the clinical presentation, antidepressants, mood stabilisers, antipsychotics and other medications may be used, for example to treat co-morbid disorders or to reduce intrusive symptoms. The use of medication in treating dissociative identity disorder should be to treat only the target symptoms that are found across all or most alternate identities (Brand and Loewenstein, 2010; Gentile *et al.*, 2013; Hunter, 2004; Loewenstein, 2005). Medication treatment is most appropriately done in a specialist psychiatric context.

### 19.5.3 Role of the general medical practitioner

The general practitioner's role is mainly diagnostic and supportive in nature.

Using a trauma-informed approach to patients in general medical settings will contribute to the assessment and appropriate management of patients with dissociative disorders. It should be routine to enquire about adverse childhood experiences and early childhood abuse. The general practitioner might include questions such as 'What has happened to you?' and 'How has it affected you later in life?', rather than 'What is the problem?' The ideal would be to foster a sense of safety, trust and openness by attending to trauma-related material non-judgementally and non-punitively with empathy, respect, dignity and a belief in recovery and resilience (in contrast to pity, condescension, and resignation) (Cook and Newman, 2014).

In addition to investing in physical, psychological and social safety, a trauma-informed approach should include an awareness of the patient's need to cope with difficult emotions, their grieving of multiple losses and their frequent sense of a foreshortened future (Corbin *et al.*, 2011).

Psycho-education and containment form important elements of the general practitioner's supportive role with regard to coping with trauma and the effects and side-effects of medication (Turkus and Kahler, 2006). It is helpful to explain procedures and treatment plans as thoroughly as possible.

Patients with a dissociative disorder may present to general practitioners with the same general medical conditions as patients without a dissociative disorder. One of the primary responsibilities of the general practitioner is to diagnose and manage such general medical conditions appropriately and sympathetically, despite any interfering psychiatric or psychological difficulties. Procedures might be adjusted to accommodate trauma-exposed patients, while maintaining appropriate boundaries (Cook and Newman, 2014).

It should also be borne in mind that a patient with a dissociative disorder may present with co-morbid psychiatric disorders, such as depressive disorders, anxiety disorders or PTSD, for which the general practitioner might have to provide the initial treatment. The index of suspicion of a dissociative disorder should be raised when treatment for a presenting psychiatric disorder fails. This treatment failure should be a sign to the general practitioner that something else might be the matter and that the patient might need to be referred to a psychiatrist.

The role of the general practitioner often focuses on referring the patient to psychiatrists and psychologists. In addition, the general practitioner might consider referring a patient with a dissociative disorder and who abuses substances to the relevant substance-abuse support groups.

The general practitioner's role also includes the careful evaluation of cultural factors in the patient's presentation. For this purpose, the Cultural Formulation Interview in the DSM-5 is useful (American Psychiatric Association, 2013). This cultural evaluation will help the general practitioner to assess whether the patient's problems reach pathological proportions, whether they go beyond the limits of what is considered culturally acceptable, whether there are signs of possession trance that might suggest a diagnosis of dissociative identity disorder and whether a referral to a psychiatrist or clinical psychologist is necessary.

## Conclusion

Dissociative disorders are relatively common and problematic; they warrant proper training of undergraduate medical students in the diagnosis, provisional supportive management and appropriate referral of patients with dissociative disorders.

Dissociative disorders are characterised by a lack of integration of consciousness, memory, identity, emotion, perception, body representation, motor control and behaviour that is severe enough to result in functional impairment. Patients with dissociative disorders will be more easily recognisable in a general medical setting if the general practitioner remains alert to a history of complex relational trauma and abuse, a poly-symptomatic presentation, prominent co-morbidity or an inconsistency in attendance, presentation and the patient's account.

Dissociative disorders may occur co-morbidly with, and be difficult to distinguish from, PTSD, borderline personality disorder, depressive disorders, anxiety disorders, psychotic disorders and somatic symptom and related disorders. Bearing in mind the new DSM-5 criteria for dissociative disorders, the general practitioner should pay increasing attention to cultural factors in the patient's presentation and to possible signs of possession trance that might suggest a diagnosis of dissociative identity disorder.

The established traumatic aetiology of dissociative disorders suggests that general practitioners should apply a trauma-informed, supportive approach to patients in a general medical setting. The mainstay of treatment of dissociative disorders remains psychotherapy.

# References


American Psychiatric Association (2013) *Diagnostic and Statistical Manual of Mental Disorders* (5th edition). Arlington, VA: American Psychiatric Association

Becker-Blease KA, Freyd JJ, Pears KC (2004) Preschoolers' memory for threatening information depends on trauma history and attentional context: Implications for the development of dissociation. *Journal of Trauma & Dissociation* 5(1): 113–31 (http://dx.doi.org/DOI: 10.1300/J229v05n01_07)

Bernstein EM, Putnam FW (1986) Development, reliability, and validity of a dissociation scale. *The Journal of Nervous and Mental Disease* 174(12): 727–35

Bob P (2003) Dissociation and neuroscience: history and new perspectives. *International Journal of Neuroscience* 113: 903–14 (DOI: 10.1080/00207450390220376)

Bob P, Faber J (2006) Dissociation in brain and mind as a consequence of competitive interactions. *Prague Medical Report* 107(3): 297–304

Brand B, Loewenstein RJ (2010) Dissociative disorders: An overview of assessment, phenomenology, and treatment. *Psychiatric Times* October: 62–9

Brand BL, Armstrong JA, Loewenstein RJ, McNary SW (2006) Psychological assessment of patients with Dissociative Identity Disorder. *Psychiatric Clinics of North America* 29(1): 145–68

Brand BL, Armstrong JA, Loewenstein RJ, McNary SW (2009a) Personality differences on the Rorschach of dissociative identity disorder, borderline personality disorder, and psychotic inpatients. *Psychological Trauma: Theory, Research, Practice, and Policy* 1(3): 188–205

Brand BL, Classen CC, Lanius RA, Loewenstein R, McNary S, Pain C, Putnam F. (2009c) A naturalistic study of dissociative identity disorder and dissociative disorder not otherwise specified patients treated by community clinicians. *Psychological Trauma: Theory, Research, Practice and Policy* 1(2): 153–71

Brand BL, Classen CC, McNary SW, Zaveri P (2009b) A review of dissociative disorders treatment studies. *The Journal of Nervous and Mental Disease* 197(9): 646–54

Brand BL, Lanius R, Vermetten E, Loewenstein RJ, Spiegel D (2012) Where are we going? An update on assessment, treatment, and neurobiological research in dissociative disorders as we move toward the DSM-5. *Journal of Trauma & Dissociation* 13(1): 9–31

Brand BL, McNary SW, Myrick AC, Classen CC, Lanius R, Loewenstein RJ, Pain C, Putnam FW (2013) A longitudinal, naturalistic study of dissociative disorder patients treated by community clinicians. *Psychological Trauma: Theory, Research, Practice & Policy* 5(4): 301–8

Carlson EA, Yates TM, Sroufe LA (2009) Dissociation and development of the self. In: Dell PF, O'Neil JA (Eds). *Dissociation and the dissociative disorders: DSM-V and beyond.* New York: Routledge

Carlson EB, Putnam FW (1993) An update on the Dissociative Experiences Scale. *Dissociation* VI(1): 16–27

Cook JM, Newman E, The New Haven Trauma Competency Group (2014) A consensus statement on trauma mental health: The New Haven Competency Conference process and major findings. *Psychological Trauma: Theory, Research, Practice, and Policy* 6(4): 300–307 (http://dx.doi.org/DOI: 10.1037/a0036747)

Coons PM, Bowman ES, Milstein V (1988) Multiple personality disorder: A clinical investigation of 50 cases. *The Journal of Nervous and Mental Disease* 176(9): 519–27

Corbin TJ, Rich JA, Bloom SL, Delgado D, Rich LJ, Wilson AS (2011) Developing a trauma-informed, emergency department-based intervention for victims of urban violence. *Journal of Trauma & Dissociation* 12(5): 510–25

Dalenberg CJ, Brand BL, Gleaves DH, Dorahy MJ, Loewenstein RJ, Cardeña E, Frewen PA, Carlson EB, Spiegel D (2012) Evaluation of the evidence for the trauma and fantasy models of dissociation. *Psychological Bulletin* (138): 550–88

Dorahy M (2006) The dissociative processing style: A cognitive organization activated by perceived or actual threat in clinical dissociators. *Journal of Trauma & Dissociation* 7(4): 29–53

Dorahy MJ, Brand BL, Šar V, Krüger C, Stavropoulos P, Martínez-Taboas A, Lewis-Fernández R, Middleton W (2014) Dissociative Identity Disorder: An empirical overview. *Australian and New Zealand Journal of Psychiatry* 48(5): 402–17 (DOI: 10.1177/0004867414527523)

Dorahy MJ, Van der Hart O (2007) Relationship between trauma and dissociation: A historical analysis. In: Vermetten E, Dorahy MJ, Spiegel D (Eds). *Traumatic Dissociation: Neurobiology and Treatment.* Washington, DC: American Psychiatric Publishing

Drennan G (2001) Cultural psychiatry. In: Robertson, B, Allwood, C, Gagiano, C (Eds.) *Textbook of psychiatry for Southern Africa* Cape Town: Oxford University Press Southern Africa

Felmingham K, Kemp AH, Williams L, Falconer E, Olivieri G, Peduto A, Bryant R (2008) Dissociative responses to conscious and non-conscious fear impact underlying brain function in post-traumatic stress disorder. *Psychological Medicine* 38: 1771–1780 (DOI:10.1017/S0033291708002742)

Frewen PA, Lanius RA (2006) Neurobiology of dissociation: Unity and disunity in mind-body-brain. *Psychiatric Clinics of North America* 29: 113–28

Gentile JP, Dillon KS, Gillig PM (2013) Psychotherapy and pharmacotherapy for patients with dissociative identity disorder. *Innovations in Clinical Neuroscience,* 10(2): 22–9

Hopper A, Ciorciari J, Johnson G, Spensley J, Sergejew A, Stough C (2002) EEG coherence and dissociative

identity disorder. *Journal of Trauma & Dissociation* 3(1): 75–88 (http://dx.doi.org/DOI: 10.1300/J229v03n01_06)
Howell EF, Blizard RA (2009) Chronic relational trauma disorder: A new diagnostic scheme for borderline personality and the spectrum of dissociative disorders. In: Dell PF, O'Neil JA (Eds). *Dissociation and the dissociative disorders: DSM-V and beyond*. New York: Routledge
Hughes JR, Kuhlman DT, Fichtner CG, Gruenfeld MJ (1990) Brain mapping in a case of multiple personality. *Clinical Electroencephalography* 21(4): 200–9
Hunter ME (2004) *Understanding dissociative disorders: A guide for family physicians and health care professionals.* Carmarthen, Wales, UK: Crown House Publishing
International Society for the Study of Trauma and Dissociation (ISSTD) (2011) Guidelines for treating dissociative identity disorder in adults, third revision. *Journal of Trauma & Dissociation*, 12(2): 115–187 (DOI: 10.1080/15299732.2011.537247)
Jang KL, Paris J, Zweig-Frank H, Livesley WJ (1998) Twin study of dissociative experience. *The Journal of Nervous and Mental* Disease 186(6): 345–51
Johnson JG, Cohen P, Kasen S, Brook JS (2006) Dissociative disorders among adults in the community, impaired functioning, and axis I and II comorbidity. *Journal of Psychiatric Research* 40: 131–40
Kluft RP (1987) First-rank symptoms as a diagnostic clue to multiple personality disorder. *American Journal of Psychiatry* 144: 293–8
Korzekwa MI, Dell PF, Links PS, Thabane L, Fougere P (2009b) Dissociation in borderline personality disorder: A detailed look. *Journal of Trauma & Dissociation* 10(3): 346–67 (DOI: 10.1080/15299730902956838)
Korzekwa MI, Dell PF, Pain C (2009a) Dissociation and borderline personality disorder: An update for clinicians. *Current Psychiatry Reports* 11(1): 82–8
Krüger C, Bartel P, Fletcher L (2013) Dissociative mental states are canonically associated with decreased temporal theta activity on spectral analysis of EEG. *Journal of Trauma and Dissociation* 14(4): 473–91 (DOI: 10.1080/15299732.2013.769480)
Krüger C, Sokudela BF, Motlana LM, Mataboge CK, Dikobe AM (2007) Dissociation: A preliminary contextual model. *South African Journal of Psychiatry* 13(1): 13–21 (http://repository.up.ac.za/handle/2263/4341)
Lanius RA, Bluhm R, Lanius U, Pain C (2006) A review of neuroimaging studies in PTSD: Heterogeneity of response to symptom provocation. *Journal of Psychiatric Research* 40: 709–29
Lanius RA, Williamson PC, Bluhm RL, Densmore M, Boksman K, Neufeld RWJ, Gati JS, Menon RS (2005) Functional connectivity of dissociative responses in posttraumatic stress disorder: A functional magnetic resonance imaging investigation. *Biological Psychiatry* 57: 873–84
Lanius RA, Williamson PC, Boksman K, Densmore M, Gupta M, Neufeld RWJ, Gati JS, Menon RS (2002) Brain activation during script-driven imagery induced dissociative responses in PTSD: A functional magnetic resonance imaging investigation. *Biological Psychiatry* 52: 305–11
Lapointe AR, Crayton JW, DeVito R, Fichtner CG, Konopka LM (2006) Similar or disparate brain patterns? The intra-personal EEG variability of three women with multiple personality disorder. *Clinical EEG and Neuroscience*, 37(3): 235–42
Lochner C, Seedat S, Hemmings SMJ, Kinnear CJ, Corfield VA, Niehaus DJH, Moolman-Smook JC, Stein DJ (2004) Dissociative experiences in obsessive-compulsive disorder and trichotillomania: Clinical and genetic findings. *Comprehensive Psychiatry* 45(5): 384–91
Loewenstein RJ (2005) Psychopharmacological treatments for dissociative identity disorder. *Psychiatric Annals* 35(8): 666–73
Martínez-Taboas A, Dorahy M, Sar V, Middleton W, Krüger C (2013) Growing not dwindling: International research on the world-wide phenomenon of dissociative disorders (Letter in response to Paris J. The rise and fall of dissociative identity disorder) (In: *The Journal of Nervous and Mental Disease* (2012) 200(12): 1076–1079.) *The Journal of Nervous and Mental Disease* 201(4): 353–4
Mesulam M-M (1981) Dissociative states with abnormal temporal lobe EEG: Multiple personality and the illusion of possession. *Archives of Neurology* 38: 176–81
Moskowitz A, Schäfer I, Dorahy MJ (Eds). (2008) *Psychosis, trauma and dissociation: Emerging perspectives on severe psychopathology*. Chichester, West Sussex, UK: Wiley-Blackwell
Nijenhuis ERS (2004) *Somatoform dissociation: Phenomena, measurement, and theoretical issues.* New York: WW Norton
Nijenhuis ERS, Den Boer JA (2009) Psychobiology of traumatization and trauma-related structural dissociation of the personality. In: Dell PF, O'Neil JA (Eds). *Dissociation and the dissociative disorders: DSM-V and beyond*. New York: Routledge
Nijenhuis ERS, Van der Hart O, Steele K (2010) Trauma-related structural dissociation of the personality. *Activitas Nervosa Superior* 52(1): 1–23
Putnam FW (2006) Dissociative disorders. In: Cicchetti D, Cohen DJ (Eds). *Developmental Psychopathology* (Vol. 2). New York: Wiley
Reinders AATS, Nijenhuis ERS, Paans AMJ, Korf J, Willemsen ATM, Den Boer JA (2003) One brain, two selves. *NeuroImage* 20: 2119–25
Reinders AATS, Nijenhuis ERS, Quak J, Korf J, Haaksma J, Paans AMJ, Willemsen ATM, Den Boer JA (2006) Psychobiological characteristics of dissociative identity disorder: A symptom provocation study. *Biological Psychiatry* 60: 730–40
Reinders AATS, Willemsen ATM, Vos HPJ, Den Boer JA, Nijenhuis ERS (2012) Fact or factitious? A psychobiological study of authentic and simulated dissociative identity states. *PLoS ONE* 7(6): e39279 (DOI:10.1371/journal.pone.0039279)
Ross CA (2007) Borderline personality disorder and dissociation. *Journal of Trauma & Dissociation* 8(1): 71–80
Ross CA, Ferrell L, Schroeder E (2014) Co-occurrence of dissociative identity disorder and borderline personality disorder. *Journal of Trauma & Dissociation* 15(1): 79–90 (DOI: 0.1080/15299732.2013.834861)
Ross CA, Miller SD, Reagor P, Bjornson L, Fraser GA, Anderson G (1990) Schneiderian symptoms in multiple personality disorder and schizophrenia. *Comprehensive Psychiatry* 31: 111–118
Sachs A (2013) Still being hurt: The vicious cycle of dissociative disorders, attachment, and ongoing abuse.

*Attachment: New directions in psychotherapy and relational psychoanalysis* 7: 90–100

Sar V, Akyüz G, Dogan O (2007a) Prevalence of dissociative disorders among women in the general population. *Psychiatry Research* 149: 169–76

Sar V, Akyuz G, Kugu N, Ozturk E, Ertem-Vehid H (2006) Axis I dissociative disorder comorbidity in borderline personality disorder and reports of childhood trauma. *Journal of Clinical Psychiatry* 67(10): 1583–90

Sar V, Krüger C, Martínez-Taboas A, Middleton W, Dorahy M (2013) Sociocognitive and posttraumatic models of dissociation are not opposed. (Letter in response to Boysen GA, vanBergen A: A review of published research on adult dissociative identity disorder 2000–2010. (In: *The Journal of Nervous and Mental Disease* (2013) 201(1): 5–11). *The Journal of Nervous and Mental Disease* 201(5): 439–40

Sar V, Kundakci T, Kiziltan E, Yargic IL, Tutkun H, Bakim B, Bozkurt O, Ozpulat T, Keser V, Ozdemir O (2003) The Axis-I dissociative disorder comorbidity of borderline personality disorder among psychiatric outpatients. *Journal of Trauma & Dissociation* 4(1): 119–36

Sar V, Middleton W, Dorahy M (Eds) (2014) *Global Perspectives on Dissociative Disorders: Individual and Societal Oppression*. Oxon, UK: Routledge

Šar V, Öztürk E (2007b) Functional dissociation of the self: A sociocognitive approach to trauma and dissociation. *Journal of Trauma & Dissociation* 8(4): 69–89

Sar V, Öztürk E (2013) Stimulus deprivation and overstimulation as dissociogenic agents in postmodern oppressive societies. *Journal of Trauma & Dissociation* 14(2): 198–212 (DOI: 10.1080/15299732.2013.724346)

Sar V, Unal SN, Kızıltan E, Kundakcı T, Öztürk E (2001) HMPAO SPECT study of cerebral perfusion in dissociative identity disorder. *Journal of Trauma & Dissociation* 2(2): 5–25

Sar V, Unal SN, Öztürk E (2007c) Frontal and occipital perfusion changes in dissociative identity disorder. *Psychiatry Research – Neuroimaging* 156: 217–23

Savoy RL, Frederick BB, Keuroghlian AS, Wolk PC (2012) Voluntary switching between identities in dissociative identity disorder: A functional MRI case study. *Cognitive Neuroscience* 3(2): 112–9

Schore AN (1996) The experience-dependent maturation of a regulatory system in the orbital prefrontal cortex and the origin of developmental psychopathology. *Development & Psychopathology* 8: 59–87

Schore AN (2009) Attachment trauma and the developing right brain: Origins of pathological dissociation. In: Dell PF, O'Neil JA (Eds). *Dissociation and the dissociative disorders: DSM-V and beyond.* New York: Routledge

Spiegel D, Loewenstein RJ, Lewis-Fernández R, Sar V, Simeon D, Vermetten E, Cardeña E, Dell PF (2011) Dissociative disorders in DSM-5. *Depression and Anxiety* 28: 824–52

Spiegel D, Vermetten E (1994) Physiological correlates of hypnosis and dissociation. In: Spiegel D (Ed.) *Dissociation: Culture, Mind, and Body*. Washington, DC: American Psychiatric Press

Steele K, Van der Hart O, Nijenhuis ERS (2009) The theory of trauma-related structural dissociation of the personality. In: Dell PF, O'Neil JA (Eds). *Dissociation and the dissociative disorders: DSM-V and beyond*. New York: Routledge

Stiglmayr CE, Ebner-Priemer UW, Bretz J, Behm R, Mohse M, Lammers CH, Anghelescu IG, Schmahl C, Schlotz W (2008) Dissociative symptoms are positively related to stress in borderline personality disorder. *Acta Psychiatrica Scandinavica* 117(2): 139–47

Stiglmayr CE, Shapiro DA, Stieglitz, RD, Limberger MF, Bohus M (2001) Experience of aversive tension and dissociation in female patients with borderline personality disorder – a controlled study. *Journal of Psychiatric Research* 35(2): 111–8

Tsai GE, Condie D, Wu MT, Chang IW (1999) Functional magnetic resonance imaging of personality switches in a woman with dissociative identity disorder. *Harvard Review of Psychiatry* 7: 119–22

Turkus JA, Kahler JA (2006) Therapeutic interventions in the treatment of dissociative disorders. *Psychiatric Clinics of North America* 29: 245–62

Van der Hart O, Nijenhuis ERS, Steele K (2006) *The Haunted Self: Structural Dissociation and the Treatment of Chronic Traumatization*. New York: Norton

Wolf EJ, Rasmusson AM, Mitchell KS, Logue MW, Baldwin CT, Miller MW (2014) A genome-wide association study of clinical symptoms of dissociation in a trauma-exposed sample. *Depression and Anxiety* 31: 352–60

Wolk PC, Savoy RL, Frederick BB (2012) The neural correlates of vertical splitting in a single case study. *Neuropsychoanalysis* 14(2): 157–63

World Health Organization (1992) *The ICD-10 classification of mental and behavioural disorders: Clinical descriptions and diagnostic guidelines*. Geneva: World Health Organization

Zanarini MC, Jager-Hyman S (2009) Dissociation in borderline personality disorder. In: Dell PF, O'Neil JA (Eds). *Dissociation and dissociative disorders: DSM-V and beyond.* New York: Routledge

CHAPTER

# 20 Alcohol-related disorders

Gerhard Grobler, Gerhard Jordaan

## 20.1 Introduction

Alcohol is probably the oldest psychoactive substance known to humankind. Fermented beverages containing ethyl alcohol have been traced back as far as 8000 BC. The distillation of alcohol dates from about 800 BC, when the process first began to be used in China, India and Arabia. Phenomenological descriptions of alcohol consumption, alcohol intoxication and its complications abound in ancient literature, including Egyptian hieroglyphics and Biblical writings.

The drinking of alcoholic beverages has become closely linked to the sociocultural customs of a particular society. Nowhere is this better demonstrated than in southern Africa, with its varied multicultural and multi-ethnic population. Historically, patterns of social drinking inherited from colonial migrants existed alongside traditional patterns of consuming slow-brewed or home-brewed beer at ceremonies and feasts that were an integral part of many religious and cultural rituals. In the colonial and apartheid eras, restrictive legislation prohibiting the consumption of'hard liquor' (i.e. spirits) by indigenous population groups gave rise to a phenomenon of illegal **shebeens** in urban and peri-urban communities. With the rapid growth of urbanisation and industrialisation, many of the traditional patterns of alcohol consumption are disappearing in communities throughout Africa, making populations increasingly vulnerable to the ravages of alcohol abuse.

## 20.2 Epidemiology

The World Health Organization's World Mental Health Survey studied 54 069 participants from 17 countries (USA, China, Colombia, Mexico, Belgium, France, Germany, Italy, the Netherlands, Spain, Ukraine, South Africa, Israel, Lebanon, Nigeria, Japan, and New Zealand) (Degenhardt *et al.*, 2008). Participants were asked if they had ever tried alcohol and/or tobacco and/or cannabis and/or cocaine (all in various forms). If they had used any of these drugs, their use was examined in further detail. The researchers found that alcohol was used by the vast majority of participants from the Americas, Europe, Japan and New Zealand and to a lesser extent in Africa, China and the Middle East. Males were more likely to have used any type of drug than females. The study found that drug use did not appear to correlate with drug policy, as countries with more stringent drug policies (such as the USA) did not have lower levels of substance use compared to countries with less stringent policies (such as the Netherlands). This study found between that 79–99% of young adults (by the age of 21 years) used alcohol in European countries, 78-93% in the Americas, 92% in Japan and 94% in New Zealand.

In the Middle East and Africa rates of alcohol use ranged between 40–63%. The threshold value of 60% of the population drinking by the age of 21 was crossed by all but three countries (South Africa, Nigeria and Lebanon). It was noted that the mid- to late-teenage years were a particularly risky time for the onset of alcohol use.

The South African Stress and Health Survey (SASH) (Stein *et al.*, 2008), undertaken between January 2002 and June 2004, found a lifetime prevalence of 11,4% for alcohol abuse in South Africa and a 12-month prevalence of 5,8%. Substance use disorders (with a prevalence of 13,3%) ranked the second-highest prevalent class of disorders following anxiety disorders (prevalence of 15,8%). A striking finding of this study was an earlier age of onset (mean age 24 years) for substance use disorders. Substance use disorders were also correlated with male gender, consistent with findings in other countries. According to the U.S. Center for Disease Control, about 17% of men and 8% of women meet criteria for alcohol dependence at some point in their lives. Alcohol was found to be the most commonly abused substance in the SASH study. Certain groups of individuals in South Africa (including farm workers in the Western Cape and migrant mine workers) have been shown to have particularly high prevalence rates of risky drinking.

The origins of all mental illnesses, including substance use disorders, are complex and multifactorial, but there is a correlation between poor mental health, poverty, deprivation (the so-called reduced access to social capital), low level of education, unemployment, lack of basic amenities, social exclusion and multiple stressors. Maternal use of alcohol is associated with foetal alcohol syndrome – of which South Africa has one of the highest incidences in the world (see Section 20.6). Maternal substance abuse is associated with increased risk of childhood mental illness, while alcohol use is highly associated with crime, violence and motor vehicle injuries. A study published in 1998 found in a random sample of drivers that 7% had blood alcohol levels above 0,08g/100ml – the legal limit for driving at the time (Parry and Bennetts, 1998). Alcohol contributes to more than half of all motor vehicle deaths each year in South Africa. Traumatic injuries are common in alcoholics. Minor household injuries are also frequent, as the alcoholic person may stumble and fall, sustaining bruises, fractures and lacerations. Subdural haematomas occur in many elderly alcoholics who fall and hit their head.

Other problems associated with alcoholism are largely social and occupational. People with alcohol problems commonly experience:

- marital problems leading to spousal abuse, separation and divorce
- frequent job problems, including absenteeism and job losses
- legal entanglements due to public intoxication, drunk driving, bar fights, etc.

## 20.3 Aetiology

The causes of alcohol-use disorder are multifactorial and include biological and psychosocial factors. The genetic basis of alcohol dependence is well recognised and heritability estimates range between 40–70% (Nieratschker *et al.*, 2013). Family studies of alcohol-use disorder (AUD) have consistently shown high rates of the disorder among first-degree relatives of persons with alcohol-use disorder. About 25% of fathers and brothers of patients with alcohol-use disorder also have alcohol-use disorder. Monozygotic twins have a higher concordance rate for alcohol-use disorder than dizygotic twins. Adoption studies have shown that the biological relatives of probands are significantly more likely to have alcohol-use disorder than the relatives of control adoptees. While it was previously believed that heritability differed between genders, recent large studies indicate equal heritability in men and women. The best classical candidate genes for alcohol dependence are alcohol dehydrogenase (ADH) and aldehyde dehydrogenase (ALDH) (Nieratschker *et al.*, 2013).

Early age of initiation of drinking significantly increases the risk of developing alcohol-use disorder. Approximately 50% of individuals drinking by the age of 14 develop alcohol-use disorder by the of age 21.

Social and environmental factors are also important factors in developing alcoholism. Risk factors include a history of childhood abuse and psychiatric disorders. Among the latter, mood and anxiety disorders are associated with greatest risk of developing alcohol-use disorder, especially social anxiety disorder and panic disorder.

Behavioural theory suggests that learning and gender socialisation may play a role in alcoholism. Children tend to follow their parents' drinking patterns. Boys are more likely to be encouraged to drink than girls, and binge-drinking rituals specifically intended to demonstrate masculinity and loyalty to an all-male peer group are common in Western culture.

The term '**co-dependency**' refers to the notion that an individual's drinking is enabled by his or her spouse, family or close friends. The co-dependent role is assumed when there is an (unconscious) denial of the alcohol dependence by family members or friends. By colluding with, rather than managing, the situation, they perpetuate the problem and also develop dysfunctional roles and behaviours themselves.

## 20.4 Pharmacology

Ethyl alcohol (ethanol) is a psychoactive substance that is classified as a central nervous system depressant. It is formed by either fermentation or distillation and is a drug of low molecular weight. It is readily absorbed from the intestines and metabolised by the liver. It distributes in total body water, being water soluble and fat insoluble. Alcohol is usually eliminated from the body by the Class I iso-enzymes of alcohol dehydrogenase (see Figure 20.1) (Jones, 2010).

Alcohol directly alters the activity of several ion channels, receptors and enzymes, which, when combined, leads to changes in synaptic function and plasticity. It has an effect on the glutamatergic and GABA-ergic system of the brain. Alcohol is shown to augment the functioning of GABA at certain $GABA_A$ receptors while inhibiting the effects of glutamate at the NDMA receptors.

## 20.5 Alcohol-induced disorders

The DSM-IV (American Psychiatric Asswociation,1994) specified the following disorders as alcohol-induced disorders, each with specified criteria:

- alcohol withdrawal/intoxication delirium
- alcohol-induced persisting dementia
- alcohol-induced persisting amnestic disorder
- alcohol-induced psychotic disorder
- alcohol-induced mood disorder
- alcohol-induced anxiety disorder
- alcohol-induced sexual disorder
- alcohol-induced sleep disorder.

The DSM-5 groups these disorders together (without specified criteria) as related disorders, where they 'are described in other chapters of

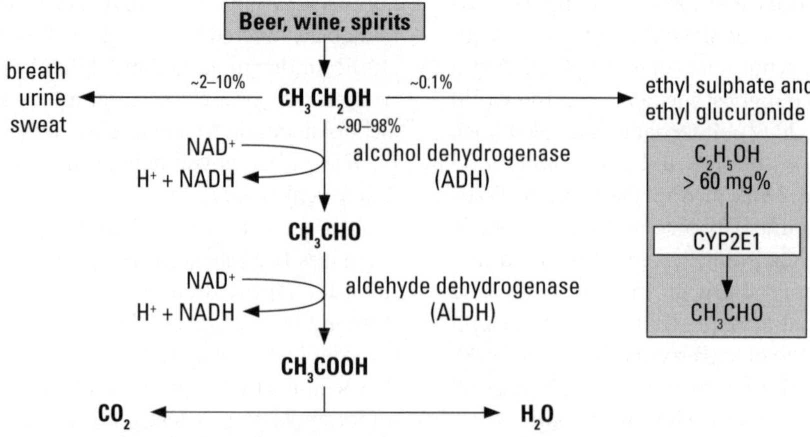


**Figure 20.1** Alcohol metabolism and elimination from the body

**Source:** Adapted from Jones, 2010. Reprinted with permission from Elsevier.

the manual with disorders with which they share phenomenology' (American Psychiatric Association, 2013). They include:

- alcohol-induced psychotic disorder ('schizophrenia spectrum and other psychotic disorders')
- alcohol-induced bipolar disorder ('bipolar and related disorders')
- alcohol-induced depressive disorder ('depressive disorders')
- alcohol-induced anxiety disorder ('anxiety disorders')
- alcohol-induced sleep disorder ('sleep-wake disorders')
- alcohol-induced sexual disorder ('sexual dysfunctions')
- alcohol-induced major or mild neurocognitive disorder ('neurocognitive disorders').

The symptom profiles for an alcohol-induced condition resemble independent mental disorders as described elsewhere in the DSM-5.

## 20.5.1 Alcohol intoxication

### 20.5.1.1 Diagnosis

The DSM-5 diagnostic criteria for alcohol intoxication are shown in Table 20.1.

### 20.5.1.2 Clinical picture

A person under the influence of alcohol displays the signs and symptoms of intoxication as described in Table 20.1 to a lesser or greater degree. The criteria require such a person to display emotional, cognitive or behaviour patterns not in keeping with the usual self. There is not a good correlation between a person's blood alcohol concentration (BAC) and the observable signs of intoxication (Sullivan *et al.*, 1987). A patient in the emergency room may therefore not appear intoxicated, while his or her blood alcohol level may exceed the legal limit for driving (see Text box Alcohol use and driving regulations).

The level of intoxication is dependent on characteristics of the drinker and the circumstances in which drinking occurs (Fisher *et al.*, 1987). Factors that influence the absorption and elimination of alcohol include:

- gender
- age
- physical wellness
- weight and body-fat composition
- level of fitness
- the absence or presence and content of food
- rate of alcohol intake and duration of consumption
- tolerance to alcohol
- fatigue.

**Table 20.1** DSM-5 Diagnostic Criteria for Alcohol Intoxication

| Diagnostic Criteria |
| --- |
| A. Recent ingestion of alcohol. |
| B. Clinically significant problematic behavioral or psychological changes (e.g., inappropriate sexual or aggressive behavior, mood lability, impaired judgment) that developed during, or shortly after, alcohol ingestion. |
| C. One (or more) of the following signs or symptoms developing during, or shortly after, alcohol use: |
| 1. Slurred speech. |
| 2. Incoordination. |
| 3. Unsteady gait. |
| 4. Nystagmus. |
| 5 Impairment in attention or memory. |
| 6 Stupor or coma. |
| D. The signs or symptoms are not attributable to another medical condition and are not better explained by another mental disorder, including intoxication with another substance. |

**Source:** Reprinted with permission from the *Diagnostic and Statistical Manual of Mental Disorders*, Fifth Edition, (Copyright 2013). American Psychiatric Association.

### Alcohol use and driving regulations

Section 15 of Chapter IV of the National Road Traffic Act (No. 93 of 1996) specifies that individuals with significant alcohol-use disorders may be disqualified from obtaining or holding a learner's or driver's license. It includes those 'addicted to the use of any drug having a narcotic effect or the excessive use of intoxicating liquor'. Chapter XI of the same Act also prohibits reckless or negligent driving or driving under the influence of intoxicating liquor or any drug having a narcotic effect. Section 65 of the Act rules that no person shall drive a vehicle on a public road or occupy the driver's seat of a motor vehicle with its engine running, while the concentration of alcohol in any specimen of blood taken from any part of his or her body is not less than 0,05 g/100 ml. The Act further stipulates that no person shall drive a motor vehicle on a public road or occupy the driver's seat of a motor vehicle with its engine running while the concentration of alcohol in any specimen of breath exhaled is not below 0,24 mg per 1 000 ml. These prohibitions apply regardless of whether or not that level causes clinical intoxication in the specific person.

### Alcohol content of common beverages

According to the South African Industry Association for Responsible Alcohol Use (ARA, *s.d.*):

- 340 ml malt beer (at a typical 5% alcohol by volume) contains 12 g of alcohol
- 340 ml cider (at a typical 6% alcohol by volume) contains 16 g of alcohol
- a 25 ml tot of brandy, whisky, gin, cane or vodka (at a typical 43% alcohol by volume) contains 11 g of alcohol
- a 120ml glass of wine (at a typical 12% alcohol by volume) contains 11 g of alcohol.

According to the same source a 'standard drink' in South Africa is considered to contain 12 g of alcohol.

Time is the only reliable factor in the metabolism of alcohol. Peak blood-alcohol levels are usually reached between 30 and 90 minutes after the last drink. The elimination rate varies between 0,01 g/dL/hour for moderate drinkers and 0,02 g/dL/hour for heavy drinkers. A moderate drinker who weighs 70 kg and drinks 10 standard tots (25 ml) of whiskey (40% alc/vol) will require 10 hours to be below the legal limit to drive.

## 20.5.2 Alcohol withdrawal

### 20.5.2.1 Diagnosis

The DSM-5 diagnostic criteria for alcohol withdrawal are shown in Table 20.2.

### 20.5.2.2 Clinical picture

In an alcohol-dependent patient the symptoms of withdrawal appear some 12 hours after his or her last drink. Symptoms peak in intensity after 48 to 72 hours, and usually disappear within seven days of the last drink. Studies show that between 5–20% of alcohol-dependent people admitted to a general hospital develop alcohol withdrawal symptoms severe enough to warrant treatment (Manasco *et al.*, 2012). Moderate to severe withdrawal is associated with increased in-hospital mortality and morbidity. It increases hospital stays, inflates costs and increases the burden on nursing and medical staff. Patients with alcohol withdrawal also suffer more medical co-morbidity and are at an increased risk of infections and sepsis. Alcohol withdrawal is detrimental to the central nervous system due to neuronal degeneration and neuronal death (Kalant, 1971). There is decreased memory performance with successive withdrawal episodes (Glenn *et al.*, 1988). Seizures may occur 18 to 48 hours after the last ingestion of alcohol. Occasionally, withdrawal symptoms may be delayed for three or more days after the last drink. Small proportions of patients in withdrawal develop delirium ('delirium tremens'). In such cases, an underlying general medical condition (such as Wernicke's encephalopathy/delirium) should be suspected.

**Table 20.2** DSM-5 Diagnostic Criteria for Alcohol Withdrawal

| **Diagnostic Criteria** |
|---|
| A. Cessation of (or reduction in) alcohol use that has been heavy and prolonged. |
| B. Two (or more) of the following, developing within several hours to a few days after the cessation of (or reduction in) alcohol use described in Criterion A: |
| 1. Autonomic hyperactivity (e.g., sweating or pulse rate greater than 100 bpm). |
| 2. Increased hand tremor. |
| 3. Insomnia. |
| 4. Nausea or vomiting. |
| 5. Transient visual, tactile, or auditory hallucinations or illusions. |
| 6. Psychomotor agitation. |
| 7. Anxiety. |
| 8. Generalized tonic-clonic seizures. |
| C. The signs or symptoms in Criterion B cause clinically significant distress or impairment in social, occupational, or other important areas of functioning. |
| D. The signs or symptoms are not attributable to another medical condition and are not better explained by another mental disorder, including intoxication or withdrawal from another substance. |
| *Specify* if: |
| ▸ **With perceptual disturbances:** This specifier applies in the rare instance when hallucinations (usually visual or tactile) occur with intact reality testing, or auditory, visual, or tactile illusions occur in the absence of a delirium. |

**Source:** Reprinted with permission from the *Diagnostic and Statistical Manual of Mental Disorders*, Fifth Edition, (Copyright 2013). American Psychiatric Association.

The recently developed Prediction of Alcohol Withdrawal Severity Scale (PAWSS) (Moldonado *et al.*, 2014) shows promise in predicting patients at risk of developing alcohol withdrawal with 100% sensitivity, specificity, positive predictive and negative predictive value. Schuckit (2009) found that approximately 50% of alcohol-dependent persons experience clinically significant withdrawal symptoms upon alcohol cessation.

A hangover is one way in which withdrawal presents. While 28% of drinkers reported never having a hangover, the majority of drinkers have experienced this phenomenon at least once (Howland *et al.*, 2008). Symptoms of hangover include drowsiness, cognitive problems, disturbed water balance, mood disturbance, balance problems, gastrointestinal problems, respiratory and cardiovascular problems, impulsivity and blunted affect, vomiting and feelings of guilt, headache and suicidal thoughts (Penning *et al.*, 2012).

### 20.5.2.3 Substance withdrawal delirium (delirium tremens)

Delirium tremens (alcohol withdrawal delirium) is arguably the most serious complication of alcohol withdrawal. The DSM-5 classifies this diagnosis in the neurocognitive disorders chapter under the general heading Delirium (see Chapter 10: Cognitive disorders).

The DSM-5 requires the clinician to specify whether the delirium develops during substance intoxication or substance withdrawal as follows: '**Substance withdrawal delirium:** This diagnosis should be made instead of substance withdrawal when the symptoms in Criteria A and C predominate in the clinical picture and when they are sufficiently severe to warrant clinical attention' (American Psychiatric Association, 2013).

#### Substance withdrawal delirium: General management

A thorough physical examination must exclude the following complications:

- cardiac arrhythmia or cardiac failure
- gastrointestinal bleeding (upper or lower)
- secondary infections (particularly pneumonia)
- liver failure
- head injuries
- neurological impairment, including peripheral neuropathies.

Many patients with mild withdrawal symptoms can be managed safely and effectively at home, or in non-medical **detoxification** centres.

## 20.1 Advanced reading block

**Neurochemistry of alcohol withdrawal**

Alterations in the glutamate and GABA balance in patients with alcohol withdrawal have been investigated (Brousse *et al.*, 2012). A markedly raised glutamate/GABA ratio has been demonstrated during acute withdrawal, indicating a hyper-glutamatergic state. Elevated plasma and brain glutamate levels are found in several conditions with neurological injury including stroke, motor neuron disease and preterm-birth asphyxia. Hyper-glutamatergic activity is a predictive factor in developing withdrawal symptoms; there also is a direct correlation between the plasma level of glutamate and the risk of immediate withdrawal. Elevated glutamate levels are neurotoxic and withdrawal symptoms are directly caused by disequilibrium between glutamate and GABA. It is suggested that anti-glutamatergic treatment (e.g. acamprosate) rather than GABA-reinforcement treatment (i.e. benzodiazepines) may be neuro-protective.

Some research suggests that homocysteine levels decline significantly during withdrawal (Heese *et al.*, 2012). Importantly, plasma folate and riboflavin levels influence homocysteine plasma levels in alcohol-dependent individuals. Increased homocysteine levels are associated with neurodegeneration, vascular disease, brain atrophy and short-term cognitive deficits during alcohol withdrawal. Homocysteine may play a role in alcohol withdrawal seizures. The recommendation of riboflavin and folate supplementation during alcohol withdrawal is supported by the fact that both these supplements influence the plasma level of homocysteine.

**Substance withdrawal delirium: Treatment (detoxification)**

Treat any of the above complications if present.

Benzodiazepines are universally accepted as the optimal medicinal treatment for alcohol withdrawal. Diazepam, being longer-acting, is the recommended drug, in a dosage that will make the patient calm and comfortable (5–15 mg every 6 to 8 hours, titrating against the response). Once the patient has settled, dosage can be reduced by 20% daily, and can be discontinued after five to seven days. A sensible safety precaution is to skip a dose if the patient appears over-drowsy. If the symptoms of withdrawal remain uncontrolled on diazepam, haloperidol (5–10 mg every 6 to 8 hours) can be added. It should subsequently be reduced in the same manner as described for diazepam.

Anticonvulsants such as phenytoin (100 mg three times daily) may be indicated, especially if there is a pre-existing history of seizures.

Fluids and electrolytes must be balanced, especially in cases of clinical dehydration. Glucose may be indicated. Supplement with vitamin B complex (especially thiamine and folic acid), and vitamin C.

Several regimens for the treatment of alcohol withdrawal syndrome exist.

### 20.5.3 Substance-induced or medication-induced neurocognitive disorder

Cognitive impairment is associated with a range of substances and medications. These include alcohol, methamphetamine (or tik), cocaine, inhalants (e.g. glue), benzodiazepines and opioids. The diagnostic criteria for substance/medication-induced major or mild neurocognitive disorder in the DSM-5 (American Psychiatric Association, 2013) are as follows:

A. The criteria are met for major or mild neurocognitive disorder.
B. The neurocognitive impairments do not occur exclusively during the course of a delirium and persist beyond the usual duration of intoxication and acute withdrawal.
C. The involved substance or medication and duration and extent of use are capable of producing the neurocognitive impairment.
D. The temporal course of the neurocognitive deficits is consistent with the timing of substance or medication use and abstinence (e.g., the deficits remain stable or improve after a period of abstinence).
E. The neurocognitive disorder is not attributable to another medical condition or is not better explained by another mental disorder

Specify if:
**Persistent:** Neurocognitive impairment continues to be significant after an extended period of abstinence.
(American Psychiatric Association, 2013).

Cognitive impairment tends to occur more frequently in individuals who have a longer history of heavy substance use, are older and have nutritional deficiencies. Nonetheless, the relationship between substance or medication use and cognitive impairment can be difficult to predict. A patient with a long history of alcohol use may describe considerable improvement in his or her memory after a period of abstinence and eating adequately, while a young occasional methamphetamine user may have severe cognitive deficits due to stimulant-related cerebrovascular disease.

Paramount are deep white-matter changes blurred with alcohol-induced vasculopathy, which is clinically often indistinguishable from vascular NCDs and with the same risk factors as precipitating and perpetuating causes. Note that both vascular and alcohol-induced NCD patients have relatively well-preserved personalities, compared with the degree of dementia present. Their excellent social skills or verbal ability may be misleading unless one screens for NCD using the Mini Mental State Examination (MMSE) (Folstein *et al.*, 1975).

## 20.5.4 Alcohol-induced persisting amnestic disorder

Alcohol-induced persisting amnestic disorder (Korsakoff's syndrome) is characterised by memory impairment associated with peripheral neuropathy, cerebellar ataxia and myopathy due to the thiamine deficiency associated with prolonged, heavy ingestion of alcohol. Patients with the disorder may fill the gaps in their memory with fictitious memories (or **confabulation**). The disorder often follows an episode of acute thiamine deficiency manifested by confusion, ataxia, nystagmus and cranial nerve III, IV and VI ophthalmoplegia (Wernicke's encephalopathy/delirium), but may have an insidious onset. Large doses of thiamine may prevent the full development of amnestic disorder in up to a third of patients. Thiamine deficiency may be precipitated by administering glucose in asymptomatic but thiamine-depleted patients who suffer from alcohol-use disorders (also from re-feeding after starvation such as with anorexia nervosa).

Parenteral thiamine in doses of at least 500 mg/day for three to five days should be given to all heavy drinkers with memory impairment, hypothermia, hypotension or delirium tremens. The Wernicke syndrome, characterised by a triad of confusion, ataxia and ophthalmoplegia, may result in permanent memory impairment if left untreated and may be precipitated by carbohydrate loading in the absence of thiamine.

## 20.5.5 Alcohol-induced psychotic disorder

Alcohol-induced psychotic disorder (AIPD) is a relatively rare disorder and should be distinguished from alcohol-withdrawal delirium (delirium tremens) and (paranoid) schizophrenia. Alcohol-induced psychotic disorder presents acutely (within a month of intoxication or withdrawal) with auditory hallucinations (often derogatory voices) and (often paranoid) delusions in a clear consciousness. Alcohol-withdrawal delirium may present with similar psychotic symptoms (often including visual hallucinations) in the presence of clouding of consciousness, disorientation and confusion. The distinction from schizophrenia in the presence of alcohol abuse may be difficult, yet is important because the management and prognosis differ. Alcohol-induced psychotic disorder usually presents at a later age (mid-thirties), typically without prodromal or residual negative symptoms and without thought-process disorder. Hospitalisation and treatment with antipsychotics are indicated in the acute phase. Depressive and suicidal symptoms and anxiety may coincide but are often transient. On-going antipsychotic treatment is usually not required once symptoms have cleared (within days or weeks), insight has been regained and provided abstinence can be maintained. Some patients have a recurrent or chronic course that may require indefinite use of antipsychotic treatment.

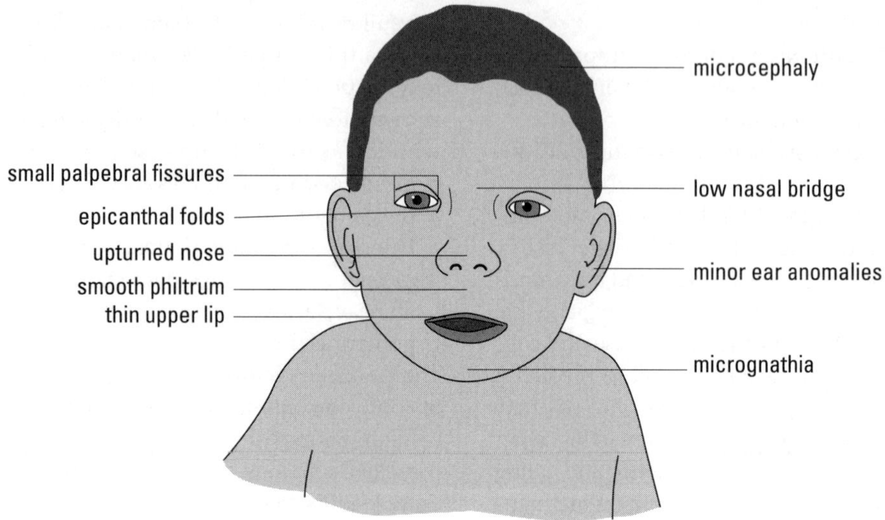


**Figure 20.2** Facial features of foetal alcohol syndrome

Parenteral thiamine in doses of at least 500 mg/day for three to five days should be given to all heavy drinkers with memory impairment, hypothermia, hypotension or delirium tremens. The Australian Government Department of Health and Aging advises an oral multivitamin preparation that contains vitamin B complex, vitamin C, zinc and magnesium for malnourished heavy drinkers (Haber *et al.*, 2009).

## 20.6 Foetal alcohol-spectrum disorder

Exposure to alcohol *in utero* is a leading preventable cause of birth defects and developmental impairment. Foetal alcohol-spectrum disorder (FASD) describes a range of physical, mental, cognitive and behavioural consequences in individuals with prenatal exposure to alcohol. Primary care providers should identify these features early and be cognisant of the educational, family support and treatment required by these individuals. Most individuals require a multidisciplinary approach.

A prevalence rate of 68,0 to 89,2 per 1 000 in the Western Cape province of South Africa (May *et al.*, 2007), gives this country the highest prevalence rate of foetal alcohol-spectrum disorder in the world. The authors found that severe episodic (binge) drinking on weekends by mothers of children with foetal alcohol syndrome and partial foetal alcohol syndrome accounted for 96% of all alcohol consumed in their cohort. An earlier study (Viljoen *et al.*, 2005) found the rates of foetal alcohol syndrome (at 65,2 to 74,2 per 1 000) was 33–148 times greater than the rates in the USA. Frequent, severe episodic (binge) drinking by both fathers and mothers of children with foetal alcohol syndrome was reported, leading to 'serious familial, social and economic challenges' (Viljoen *et al.*, 2005).

Some of the described risk factors for foetal alcohol syndrome (Kvigne *et al.*, 2003) include:

- low educational attainment
- higher maternal age
- higher gravidity and parity
- history of stillbirths and spontaneous abortions
- poor maternal nutrition during pregnancy
- history of foetal alcohol syndrome in previous children
- history of substance abuse, including nicotine
- history of mental health problems
- history of physical or sexual abuse of the mother

- social isolation during pregnancy, including living in a rural area
- history of violence inflicted by a intimate partner
- paternal alcohol and drug use during the pregnancy
- substance use by other maternal family members during the pregnancy
- poverty.

The clinical features required for the diagnosis of foetal alcohol syndrome (Bertrand *et al.*, 2004) include three facial dysmorphisms (short palpebral fissures, thin vermillion border and smooth philtrum) (Douzgou *et al.*, 2012), growth retardation and central nervous system impairment.

Other features include (May *et al.*, 2010; Jones *et al.*, 2010):

- epicanthal folds
- flat nasal bridge
- 'railroad track' ears
- upturned nose
- micrognathia
- clinodactyly, particularly of the fifth digit
- 'hockey stick' configuration of the upper palmar crease.

(See Chapter 29: Intellectual disability, for a further discussion on FASD.)

# 20.7 Alcohol-use disorder

## 20.7.1 Diagnosis

The DSM-5 diagnostic criteria for alcohol-use disorder are shown in Table 20.3.

## 20.7.2 Clinical picture

Alcohol-use disorder lies on a spectrum of severity from mild, occasional impairment to completely incapacitating. Denial is often a complicating factor in making the diagnosis but both the DSM-IV and DSM-5 require the person to have some degree of impairment before a diagnosis can be made. Collateral information is usually required to confirm the diagnosis.

Salience (or the relative value the person places on obtaining, using or recovering from alcohol) is often a key aspect of the clinical picture. Persons with an alcohol-use disorder tend to create opportunities to use alcohol and are willing to sacrifice social, occupational or relationship opportunities in favour of alcohol use. The behaviour is maintained even in the face of obvious self-defeating or negative consequences. Cravings can be seen in the person's longing for the effects of alcohol or seemingly irresistible urge to use alcohol. This often leads to cycles of alcohol use (in often increasing amounts on account of tolerance) followed by withdrawal, varying periods of sobriety before a relapse in use again. Earlier onset is usually associated with greater severity.

The process of developing an alcohol-use disorder is complex, involving an interaction of biogenetic, neurochemical and psychosocial factors. No general picture applies to the person with alcohol-use disorder and patterns of drinking and symptoms vary widely. In its earliest stages, alcohol-use disorder may be hard to identify. Symptoms may be minimal; denial of excessive drinking is common. Family members and co-workers are the most likely to identify early symptoms. These may include an insidious change in work habits or productivity, lateness or unexplained absences or minor personality disturbances, such as irritability or moodiness.

Co-morbidity, or **dual diagnosis**, is present in a large proportion of individuals with alcohol-use disorder. The most common forms of co-morbidity involve other substances of abuse, anxiety and depressive disorders and antisocial personality disorder. Co-morbidity influences choice of treatment, as well as response to treatment.

As the severity of alcohol-use disorder progresses, physical changes may occur, such as spider naevi on the face, trunk and hands, palmar erythema, painless enlargement of the liver consistent with fatty infiltration, an increasing number of minor respiratory or other infections, blackouts, minor accidents and bruises, complaints by others about the drinker's driving skills and perhaps an arrest or accident due to drunk-driving. Increasing signs of liver disease may develop, such as jaundice or

**Table 20.3** DSM-5 Diagnostic Criteria for Alcohol Use Disorder

| **Diagnostic Criteria** |
|---|
| A. A problematic pattern of alcohol use leading to clinically significant impairment or distress, as manifested by at least two of the following, occurring within a 12-month period:<br>1. Alcohol is often taken in larger amounts or over a longer period than was intended.<br>2. There is a persistent desire or unsuccessful efforts to cut down or control alcohol use.<br>3. A great deal of time is spent in activities necessary to obtain alcohol, use alcohol, or recover from its effects.<br>4. Craving, or a strong desire or urge to use alcohol.<br>5. Recurrent alcohol use resulting in a failure to fulfill major role obligations at work, school, or home.<br>6. Continued alcohol use despite having persistent or recurrent social or interpersonal problems caused or exacerbated by the effects of alcohol.<br>7. Important social, occupational, or recreational activities are given up or reduced because of alcohol use.<br>8. Recurrent alcohol use in situations in which it is physically hazardous.<br>9. Alcohol use is continued despite knowledge of having a persistent or recurrent physical or psychological problem that is likely to have been caused or exacerbated by alcohol.<br>10. Tolerance, as defined by either of the following:<br>a. A need for markedly increased amounts of alcohol to achieve intoxication or desired effect.<br>b. A markedly diminished effect with continued use of the same amount of alcohol.<br>11. Withdrawal, as manifested by either of the following:<br>a. The characteristic withdrawal syndrome for alcohol (refer to Criteria A and B of the criteria set for alcohol withdrawal, pp. 499–500).<br>b. Alcohol (or a closely related substance, such as a benzodiazepine) is taken to relieve or avoid withdrawal symptoms.<br>*Specify* if:<br>▶ **In early remission:** After full criteria for alcohol use disorder were previously met, none of the criteria for alcohol use disorder have been met for at least 3 months but for less than 12 months (with the exception that Criterion A4, 'Craving, or a strong desire or urge to use alcohol,' may be met).<br>▶ **In sustained remission:** After full criteria for alcohol use disorder were previously met, none of the criteria for alcohol use disorder have been met at any time during a period of 12 months or longer (with the exception that Criterion A4, 'Craving, or a strong desire or urge to use alcohol,' may be met).<br>*Specify* if:<br>▶ **In a controlled environment:** This additional specifier is used if the individual is in an environment where access to alcohol is restricted.<br>▶ *Specify* current severity:<br>▶ **305.00 (FI 0.10) Mild:** Presence of 2–3 symptoms.<br>▶ **303.90 (FI 0.20) Moderate:** Presence of 4–5 symptoms.<br>▶ **303.90 (FI 0.20) Severe:** Presence of 6 or more symptoms. |

**Source:** Reprinted with permission from the *Diagnostic and Statistical Manual of Mental Disorders*, Fifth Edition, (Copyright 2013). American Psychiatric Association.

ascites. Additional physical changes may occur, including testicular atrophy, gynaecomastia and the development of Dupuytren's contractures. At this stage, alcohol-use disorder may lead to job losses, broken marriages and estrangement from the family.

## 20.7.3 Medical complications

Alcohol-use disorders are associated with a variety of medical complications.

Alcohol has direct effects on the brain leading to cerebellar dysfunction with an unsteady gait, difficulty with standing steady and nystagmus. The amnestic syndromes (including **alcohol black-outs**) are also related to these effects. Wernicke's encephalopathy is characterised by palsy of the sixth cranial nerve, ataxia and amnesia. Korsakoff's syndrome is defined by an **anterograde** and **retrograde amnesia** with impairment in visuospatial and abstract learning. These deficits are often not in keeping with the global intellectual abilities of the person. Peripheral neuropathy is a risk for approximately 10% of persons with alcohol-use disorder.

Alcohol-use disorder is also associated with cardiovascular pathology (including a rise in blood pressure) and an increase in LDL cholesterol and triglycerides. Recent evidence, however, shows that moderate alcohol intake (one to two glasses of wine that contain flavonoids per day) may decrease cardiovascular risk. In high doses, alcohol is a striated-muscle toxin, which directly affects the heart muscle and sometimes results in cardiomyopathy.

Alcohol may also damage the gastrointestinal tract with inflammation of the oesophagus or stomach. Bleeds from oesophageal varices may be fatal. The liver and pancreas are also affected by alcohol. Excessive use of alcohol may initially lead to reversible swelling of the liver (known as fatty liver) on account of the accumulation of protein and fat in the liver cells. Continued use leads to hepatitis and ultimately to the destruction of the liver cells with cirrhosis (which the literature describes as a risk to approximately 15% of persons with alcohol-use disorder). Individuals may present with ascites, pancreatitis, diabetes, thrombocytopaenia or anaemia.

## 20.7.4 Management of alcohol-use disorder

### 20.7.4.1 Confirming the diagnosis of alcohol-use disorder

Confirming the diagnosis of alcohol-use disorder requires a high degree of clinical skill, a detailed history (including collateral information) and the ability to pursue an issue in the face of strong resistance. Ongoing physical complaints, anxiety or depression in a person who admits to heavy drinking, regular absenteeism from work and requests for medical certificates and conflicts with family members or work colleagues should alert the health worker to the possibility of alcohol abuse or dependence. Physical signs during a medical examination and confirmation of alcohol abuse from family members, work colleagues or the police will confirm the diagnosis. One useful self-administered screening questionnaire that has been validated in primary care settings is the CAGE questionnaire (Ewing, 1984). If one or more questions are positive, further screening for alcohol dependence should be done. One such instrument is the World Health Organization's Alcohol Use Disorders Identification Test (AUDIT)

**Assessment of the individual with alcohol-use disorder**

An assessment of a person with alcohol-use disorder should include:

1. establishing the lifetime pattern of alcohol consumption
2. establishing the current pattern of alcohol consumption
3. detecting signs of alcohol-use disorder and determining the level of severity
4. assessing physical health through examination and special investigations
5. assessing mental health
6. determining social, occupational and legal problems associated with alcohol-use disorder
7. describing previous treatment attempts and efforts to quit
8. describing the family history of alcohol use and alcohol-use disorder
9. determining the person's attitude to treatment
10. determining the person's goals.

for use by a suitably trained health care worker (Babor *et al.*, 2001).

Laboratory tests may be useful, but none are conclusive. People with alcohol-use disorder may develop increased high-density lipoprotein cholesterol, increased lactate dehydrogenase, decreased low-density lipoprotein cholesterol, decreased blood urea nitrogen, and increased uric acid levels. Mean corpuscular volume is increased in up to 10% of alcoholic patients. Liver enzymes are often abnormal. Gamma-glutamyl transferase (GGT) may be increased in 75% of individuals, and is often the earliest laboratory sign of alcohol-use disorder. Transaminases (serum glutamic-oxaloacetic transaminase (SGOT)) and serum glutamic pyruvic transaminase (SGPT)) are also increased.

### 20.7.4.2 Alcohol-use disorder and the health professional

Health-care workers are sometimes resistant to manage alcohol-related problems: they may feel that it is not their job to rehabilitate persons with alcohol-use disorder, that the problem is self-inflicted or that there is little likelihood of success. Professionals must understand that working in this area is often discouraging, frustrating and emotionally taxing, and that rewards may be few or even non-existent. However, the burden of alcoholism on the patient, family and society requires that health professionals tackle the problem with all available therapeutic approaches.

### 20.7.4.3 Planning treatment for alcohol-use disorder

Individuals with alcohol-use disorder often display marked ambivalence about whether they even have a problem, let alone about whether there is a need to change. In some individuals this may relate to memories of previous failed attempts to stop and a sense of hopelessness that recovery is not possible. The objectives of counselling are to help guide the individual with alcohol-use disorder towards making his or her own decision to change his or her drinking patterns or to quit altogether; and if change is not likely or possible, to guide him or her towards **harm reduction** and considering the possibility of future change. Motivational interviewing is a technique aimed at helping the individual move through the stages of change.

#### Motivational interviewing

Motivational interviewing (MI) is a process of steps that is driven by the person with AUD's motivation. In the first step, the health care worker communicates the diagnosis to the individual, describes the current and future effect of

#### Stages of change

A model for understanding motivation and action towards change in harmful patterns of alcohol-use was proposed by Prochaska and DiClemente (1983). Motivation is regarded as a prerequisite for, and a precursor of, action towards abstinence or more controlled alcohol (or drug) use. The stages of change are:

1. pre-contemplation: the person does not recognise that problem substance use exists, although this may be increasingly obvious to those around him/her
2. contemplation: the person may accept that there is a problem and begins to look at both the positive and negative aspects of continued substance use
3. decision: the point at which the person decides on whether to continue substance use or attempt change
4. action: the point of motivation where the person attempts change. A variety of routes exist by which change may be attempted, which may or may not include biomedical services
5. maintenance: a stage of maintaining gains made and attempting to improve those areas of life harmed by substance use
6. relapse: a return to previous behaviour but with the possibility of gaining useful strategies to extend the maintenance period on the next attempt.

alcohol-use disorder on health and life in general and encourages the individual to critically review his or her life. Together they establish consensus about the person's level of acceptance of his or her problem and its effects and his or her commitment to change. Freedom of choice is emphasised: the person takes responsibility for his or her own health and life. If there is no commitment to change, the person is encouraged to reconsider the issues and to return for further discussions. This is called the stage of pre-contemplation.

Subsequent stages may follow rapidly, slowly or not at all. When the person indicates concern and willingness to change (contemplation), the professional and the person can together explore possible options (decision), then initiate the change (action) and discuss maintenance of an alcohol-free lifestyle (including how to handle relapses).

**Deciding the goal of intervention**

Having diagnosed alcohol-use disorder and assessed the stage of change, one needs to then plan together with the individual the goal of intervention. Such goals may include:

- continue current drinking pattern: if the person is at the pre-contemplation stage and not able to cease drinking, it is preferable to give harm reduction advice and leave the door open to further assessment and help, rather than alienating the individual
- change to safer drinking pattern: if given appropriate advice, many individuals will be able to modify their harmful or risky drinking patterns (a 'drinking diary' may be a useful tool)
- attempt abstinence from alcohol: in some individuals the only safe course is to aim to abstain from alcohol completely.

The decision to stop drinking must be accompanied by considering whether detoxification treatment is indicated.

### 20.7.4.4 Psychosocial treatments for alcohol-use disorder

Comprehensive treatment programmes will incorporate elements of the following components:

**Psycho-education**

Psycho-education should focus on all aspects of alcohol use and abuse, and its effects on body, health, psychological, and social functioning. Provide the individual with information about local programmes and treatment facilities. The use of recovering addicts to reinforce the educational component can be useful.

**Individual therapy**

Individual therapy should include some or all of the following:

- social skills training
- problem-solving skills
- relaxation training
- anger management
- cognitive restructuring
- relapse prevention.

**Family therapy**

Families (including partners or spouses) should take part in psycho-education sessions and be included in the plan to manage the problem drinking. Co-dependency should be addressed to maximise the chances of successful treatment and staying abstinent.

**Group therapy**

Group therapy can be provided or accessed in various forms, both within and outside of the health services. Group therapy can help the individual to achieve proper self-management. This could include self-help groups (e.g. Alcoholics Anonymous (AA)), which is based on the premise that personal social-group support is necessary to maintain self-identification as a recovering person. Attendance at AA meetings was the best predictor of abstinence (Schuckit *et al.*, 1997). Other factors were female gender, older age at intervention, younger age of onset of alcoholism and being married. These programmes are often referred to as community support groups. In addition to self-monitoring, the teaching of coping skills and relapse prevention training play significant parts.

**Occupational therapy**

Occupational therapy plays an important part of the reconstruction process, given the loss of concentration, application and general skills in patients with long-standing alcohol-use disorder. Occupational therapy focuses on retraining in social skills, the constructive use of leisure time, appropriate relaxation exercises and coping mechanisms.

In summary, long-term support, advice, and positive reinforcement through periodic scheduled contacts with a counsellor or therapist are strongly recommended. It is often said that a treatment modality is only as good as its aftercare programme.

### 20.7.4.5 Pharmacotherapy of alcohol-use disorder

Pharmacotherapy will very often have to be used to treat co-morbid psychopathology (and which may be contributing to ongoing alcohol use). Antidepressant medication may be indicated to treat both anxiety and depression. Benzodiazepines should be avoided, except in the withdrawal stage or, occasionally, for very anxious patients. Medication for anxiety or depression is usually withheld until after detoxification, as these disorders may be bound up with the alcohol dependence itself. There is some evidence that lithium and serotonergic drugs have an ameliorating effect on alcohol craving by modulating impulse-control pathways in the brain.

The opioid system seems to play a role in the development and maintenance of alcohol-use disorders (Terenius, 1996; Del Arbol *et al.*, 1995). It is suggested that the rewarding effects of psychoactive drugs (including alcohol) is mediated by the release of dopamine in the nucleus accumbens, possibly by opioid-mediated mechanisms. The glutamate and endocannabinoid systems are also implicated in the development and maintenance of alcohol-use disorder (Heinz *et al.*, 2009).

Alcohol induces mesolimbic dopamine release, which is (at least partly) mediated by mu-opioid receptors within the cortico-mesolimbic system. Since endorphin levels decrease during stress, and alcohol induces the release of endogenous opioid, alcohol may be most rewarding at times when endorphins are low.

These findings support the potential role of opioid receptor blockers (naloxone and naltrexone) in decreasing alcohol intake. Naltrexone has been shown in animal studies and clinical trials to block opioid receptors. It also reverses alcohol-induced dopamine release in the nucleus accumbens.

An alternative to the opioid blockers for the long-term treatment of alcohol-use disorder is disulfiram (N,N′-diethylthiocarbamoyl disulphide). Disulfiram has been used in aversion therapy since the 1960s on account of the interaction between disulfiram and aldehyde dehydrogenase (Langeland and McKinley-McKee, 1996). Disulfiram causes drowsiness, forgetfulness and abdominal discomfort as toxic side effects with the risk of hepatotoxicity, peripheral neuropathy and cardiovascular abnormalities. There is evidence that adherence to disulfiram treatment lengthens the period of abstinence.

Acamprosate (N-acetyl homotaurine) is a N-methyl-D-aspartate receptor modulator which promotes a balance between the excitatory (glutamate) and inhibitory (GABA) neurotransmitters and may help individuals with alcohol dependence by reducing withdrawal-related distress (Witkiewitz *et al.*, 2012). Acamprosate may have neuromodulatory and neuro-protective effects, which is thought to modify the learned response to alcohol cues by reducing distress associated with alcohol withdrawal. Research suggests that acamprosate reduces the risk of returning to any drinking by 86% and improves the cumulative duration of abstinence by 11% compared to placebo. The same study showed that this benefit was retained for three to twelve months after discontinuation of treatment. The authors concluded that acamprosate is an efficacious treatment for alcohol dependence and is well-tolerated by patients. It also has no abuse potential and does not have significant drug interactions with many of the medications (including naltrexone, antidepressants, anxiolytics and hypnotics) that are commonly used to treat alcohol dependence and other psychiatric disorders. Feeney and

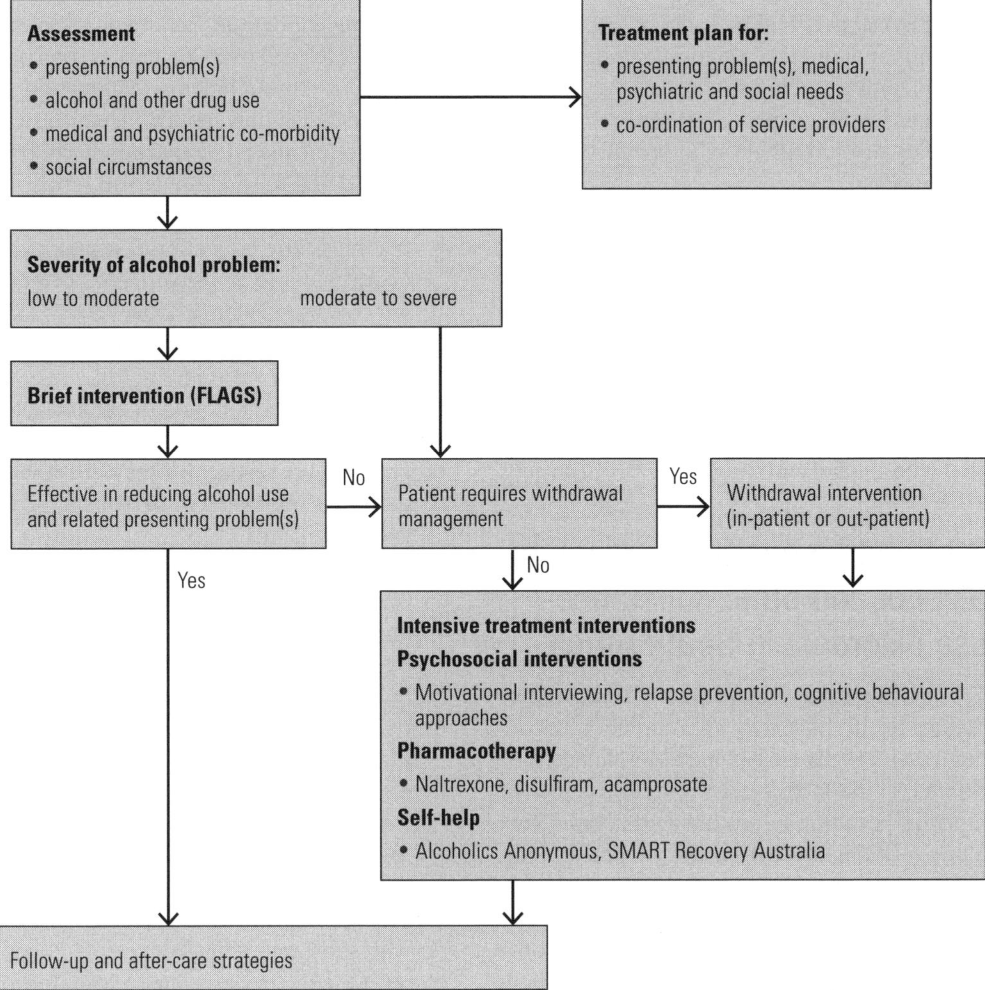


This is an example of a long-term treatment model from The Australian Government Department of Health and Aging, Canberra (Demirkol *et al.*, 2011). This model may be modified for use within the South African context, depending on the available treatment modalities.

**Figure 20.3** Model for management of problem drinking

**Source:** Reproduced with permission from The Royal College of General Practitioners from Dermirkol *et al.*, 2011

colleagues (2002) examined the effect of combining acamprosate with cognitive-behaviour therapy (CBT) in a mostly socially disadvantaged population and found that, even within an alcohol-dependent population characterised by poor prognostic indices, the addition of acamprosate to an established CBT outpatient programme significantly improved abstinence rates over a 12-week period.

## 20.7.5 Course and outcome of alcohol-use disorder

The unfortunate reality is that alcohol-use disorder is a condition with a high relapse rate and that usually requires long-term care.

Research shows a relapse rate of between 50-80% within six months following rehabilitation.

Factors associated with a poor outcome include:

- co-morbid use of other substances
- co-morbid mental disorders

- antisocial personality disorder
- emotional distress, relationship difficulties and family problems
- financial difficulties
- being around others who use alcohol and drugs.

Post-treatment difficulties are disproportionately higher among individuals who return to problematic alcohol use than among those who remain abstinent. Successful treatment can improve the quality of life in many areas for the individuals themselves, their families and their communities and also reduce the high economic costs associated with alcohol and drug abuse in our society.

## 20.8 Public-health approach to alcohol and other substance-use disorders in South Africa

The World Health Organization (WHO, 1946) defines health as 'a state of complete physical, mental and social well-being'. Mental health is defined as 'the successful performance of mental function, resulting in productive activities, fulfilling relationships with other people, and the ability to adapt to change and to cope with adversity; from early childhood until later life, mental health is the springboard of thinking and communication skills, learning, emotional growth, resilience and self-esteem' (US Department of Health and Human Services, 2003). In the South African National Mental Health Policy Framework and Strategic Plan 2013–2020 neuropsychiatric disorders (including substance use disorders) ranked third in contributing to the burden of disease in South Africa. Substance use disorders have a distinct role to play in the quadruple burden of disease. Traditionally, substance-abuse treatment programs in South Africa were the responsibility of both the Department of Social Development and the Department of Health and the policies defined by the National Drug Master Plan, drafted in 2006 and revised by the National Drug Master Plan 2013–2017 and the Prevention and Treatment of Substance Abuse Act (No. 70 of 2008).

The Prevention and Treatment of Substance Abuse Act (No. 70 of 2008) aims to combat substance abuse through demand reduction, harm reduction and supply reduction, which requires a multifaceted and integrated approach. The services rendered to service users in terms of this Act aim to:

- recognise the educational, social, cultural, economic and physical needs of persons affected by substance abuse
- promote access to information regarding prevention of substance abuse
- prevent the exploitation of persons affected by substance abuse
- promote the respect for the person, human dignity and privacy of persons affected by substance abuse
- prevent stigmatisation of persons affected by substance abuse
- promote the participation of persons affected by substance abuse in decision making processes
- recognise the special needs of people with disabilities
- ensure that services are made available without discrimination
- recognise persons affected by substance abuse as human beings in need of help
- coordinate the educational needs of children with substance abuse
- render effective, efficient, relevant, prompt and sustainable services
- respect the confidentiality of people affected by persons affected by substance abuse
- respect the right of persons affected by substance abuse to participate in research
- ensure age appropriate services for children and youths.

These interventions are expected to be community based and may be rendered by non-governmental organisations that must be registered with the provincial head of the Department of Social Development. At least one public treatment centre will be established in each province. The Act also makes provision for the establishment of aftercare and re-integration services.

## Conclusion

The complex relationship between humans and alcohol is an age-old phenomenon. While in many contexts alcohol use is a feature of acceptable social behaviour, it is also associated with a long list of problems that may be economic, social, criminal or health-related. Alcohol-use disorders are common in our society and frequently lead to co-morbid medical and psychiatric disorders. Any health practitioner working within the southern African context should have a sound understanding of these issues and be competent in adopting a truly bio-psycho-social approach in managing the array of problems associated with alcohol use.

# References


American Psychiatric Association (2013) *Diagnostic and Statistical Manual of Mental Disorders* (5th edition). Arlington, VA: American Psychiatric Association

Babor TF, Higgins-Biddle JC, Saunders JB, Monteiro MG (2001) *The alcohol use disorders identification test. Guidelines for use in primary care* (2nd ed.) (AUDIT). Geneva: World Health Organization http://whqlibdoc.who.int/hq/2001/who_msd_msb_01.6a.pdf (Accessed 19 February 2015)

Bertrand J, Floyd RL, Weber MK, O'Connor M, Riley EP, Johnson KA, Cohen DE, National Task Force on FAS/FAE (2004) *Fetal alcohol syndrome: Guidelines for referral and diagnosis*. Atlanta GA: Center for Disease Control and Prevention www.cdc.gov/ncbddd/fasd/documents/fas_guidelines_accessible.pdf (Accessed 24 February 2014)

Brousse G, Arnaud B, Vorspan F, Richard D, Dissard A, Dubois M, Pic D, Geneste J, Xavier L, Authier N, Sapin V, Llorca P-M, De Chazeron I, Minet-Quinard R, Schmidt J (2012) Glutamate/GABA balance during acute alcohol withdrawal in emergency department: A prospective analysis. *Alcohol and Alcoholism* 47(5): 501–8

Degenhardt L, Chiu W-T, Sampson N, Kessler RC, Anthony JC, Angermeyer M, Bruffaerts R, de Girolamo G, Gureje O, Huang Y, Karam A, Kostyuchenko S, Lepine JP, Mora ME, Neumark Y, Ormel JH, Pinto-Meza A, Posada-Villa J, Stein DJ, Takeshima T, Wells JE (2008) Towards a global view of alcohol, tobacco, cannabis and cocaine use: Findings from the WHO World Mental Health Surveys. Proceedings of the Library of Science and Medicine 5(7): e141 DOI:101371/journalpmed0050141

Del Arbol JL, Aguirre JC, Raya J, Rico J, Ruiz-Requena ME, Miranda MT (1995) Plasma concentrations of B-endorphin, adrenocorticotropic hormone, and cortisol in drinking and abstinent chronic alcoholics *Alcohol* 12(6): 525–9

Demirkol A, Conigrave K, Haber P (2011) Problem drinking: Management in general practice. *Australian Family Physician* 40(8): 576–82. Available at www.racgp.org.au/afp/2011/august/problem-drinking-management

Douzgou S, Breen C, Crow YJ, Chandler K, Metcalfe K, Jones E, Kerr B, Clayton-Smith J (2012) Diagnosing fetal alcohol syndrome: New insights from newer genetic technologies. *Archives of Disease in Childhood* 97(9): 812–7

Ewing JA (1984) Detecting alcoholism: the CAGE questionnaire. *The Journal of the American Medical Association* 252: 1905–7

Feeney GF, Young RM, Connor JP, Tucker J, McPherson A (2002) Cognitive behavioural therapy combined with the relapse-preventing medication acamprosate: Are short-term treatment outcomes for alcohol dependence improved? *Australian and New Zealand Journal of Psychiatry* 36(5): 622–8

Fisher HR, Simpson RI, Kapur BM (1987) Calculation of blood alcohol concentration (BAC) by sex, weight, number of drinks and time. *Canadian Journal of Public Health* 78(5): 300–4

Folstein MF, Folstein SE, McHugh PR (1975) 'Mini-mental state'. A practical method for grading the cognitive state of patients for the clinician. *Journal of Psychiatric Research* 12(3): 189–98

Glenn SW, Parsons OA, Sinha R, Stevens L (1988) The effects of repeated withdrawals from alcohol on the memory of male and female alcoholics. *Alcohol and Alcoholism* 23: 337–42

Haber P, Lintzeris N, Proude E, Lapotko O (2009) *Guidelines for the treatment of alcohol problems*. Canberra: The Australian Government Department of Health and Ageing. Available at: www.health.gov.au/internet/main//AustAlctreatguidelines%202009.pdf (Accessed 19/02/2015)

Heese P, Linnebank M, Semmler A, Muschler MAN, Heberlein A, Frieling H, Stoffel-Wagner B, Komhuber J, Banger M, Bleich S, Hillemacher T (2012) Alterations of homocysteine serum levels during alcohol withdrawal are influenced by folate and riboflavin: results from the German investigation on neurobiology in alcoholism (GINA). *Alcohol and Alcoholism* 47(5): 497–500

Heinz A, Beck A, Grüsser SM, Grace AA, Wrase J (2009) Identifying the neural circuitry of alcohol craving and relapse vulnerability. *Addiction Biology* 14(1): 108–18

Howland J, Rohsenow DJ, Edwards EM (2008) Are some drinkers resistant to hangover? A literature review. *Current Drug Abuse Reviews* 1: 42–6

Jones AW (2010) Evidence-based survey of the elimination rates of ethanol from blood with applications in forensic casework. *Forensic Science International* 200: 1–20

Jones KL, Hoyme HE, Robinson LK, Del Campo M, Manning MA, Prewitt LM, Chambers CD (2010) Fetal alcohol spectrum disorders: Extending the range of structural defects. *American Journal of Medical Genetics* 152A(11): 2731–5

Kalant H (1971) Absorption, diffusion, distribution and elimination of ethanol: Effects on biological membranes. In: Kissin B, Begleiter H (Eds) *Biology of Alcoholism* (Vol. 1). New York: Plenum Press

Kvigne VL, Leonardson GR, Borzelleca J, Brock E, Neff-Smith M, Welty TK (2003) Characteristics of mother who have children with fetal alcohol syndrome or some characteristics of fetal alcohol syndrome. *Journal of the American Board of Family Practice* 16(4): 296–303

Langeland BT, McKinley-McKee JS (1996) The effects of disulfiram on equine hepatic alcohol dehydrogenase and its efficiency against alcoholism: Vinegar effect. *Alcohol and Alcoholism* 31(1): 75–80

Manasco A, Chang S, Larriviere J, Hamm L, Glass M (2012) Alcohol withdrawal. *Southern Medical Journal* 105(11): 607–12

May PA, Gossage JP, Marais AS, Adnams CM, Hoyme HE, Jones KL, Robinson LK, Khaole NC, Snell C, Kalberg WO, Hendricks L, Brooke L, Stellavato C, Viljoen DL (2007) The epidemiology of fetal alcohol syndrome and partial FAS in a South African community. *Drug and Alcohol Dependence* 88(2–3): 259–71

May PA, Gossage JP, Smith M, Tabachnick BG, Robinson LK, Manning M, Cecanti M, Jones KL, Khaole N, Buckley D, Kalberg WO, Trujillo PM, Hoyme HE (2010) Population differences in dysmorphic features among children with fetal alcohol spectrum disorders. *Journal of Developmental and Behavioral Pediatrics* 31(4): 304–16

Maldonado JR, Sher Y, Ashouri JF, Hills-Evans K, Swendsen H, Lolak S, Miller AC (2014) The 'Prediction of Alcohol Withdrawal Severity Scale' (PAWSS): Systematic literature review and pilot study of a new scale for the prediction of complicated alcohol withdrawal syndrome. *Alcohol* 48: 375–390

Nieratschker V, Batra A, Fallgatter AJ (2013) Genetics and epigenetics of alcohol dependence. *Journal of Molecular Psychiatry* 1: 11

Parry CDH, Bennetts A (1998) *Alcohol Policy and Public Health in South Africa.* Cape Town: Oxford University Press, Southern Africa

Penning R, McKinney A, Verster JC (2012) Alcohol hangover symptoms and their contribution to the overall hangover severity. *Alcohol and Alcoholism* 47(3): 248–52

Prochaska J, DiClemente C (1983) Stages and processes of self-change in smoking: Toward an integrative model of change. *Journal of Consulting and Clinical Psychology* 5: 390–5

Schuckit MA (2009) Alcohol-use disorders. *The Lancet* 373: 492–501

Schuckit MA, Tipp JE, Smith TL, Bucholz KK (1997) Periods of abstinence following the onset of alcohol dependence in 1 853 men and women. *Journal for the Study of Alcoholism* 58(6): 581–9

South African Industry Association for Responsible Alcohol Use (sd) *Facts about alcohol and the effects it can have on the body*. Available at: http://www.ara.co.za/alcohol-facts (Accessed 26 September 2014)

Stein DJ, Seedat S, Herman A, Moomal H, Heeringa SG, Kessler RC, Williams DR (2008) Lifetime prevalence of psychiatric disorders in South Africa. *The British Journal of Psychiatry* 192: 112–7

Sullivan JB (Jr), Hauptman M, Bronstein AC (1987) Lack of observable intoxication in humans with high plasma alcohol concentration. *Journal of Forensic Science* 32(6): 1660–5

Terenius L (1996) Alcohol addiction (alcoholism) and the opioid system. *Alcohol* 13(1): 31–4

US Department of Health and Human Services. Mental Health: A Report of the Surgeon General. Rockville, MD: US Dept of Health and Human Services, 2003

Viljoen DL, Gossage JP, Brooke L, Adnams CM, Jones KL, Robinson LK, Hoyme HE, Snell C, Khaole NC, Kodituwakku P, Asante KO, Findlay R, Quinton B, Marais AS, Kalberg WO, May PA (2005) Fetal alcohol syndrome epidemiology in a South African community: A second study of a very high prevalence area. *Journal of Studies of Alcohol and Drugs* 66(5): 593–604

Witkiewitz K, Saville K, Hamreus K (2012) Acamprosate for treatment of alcohol dependence: Mechanism efficacy and clinical utility. *Therapeutics and Clinical Risk Management* 8: 45–53

World Health Organization (1946) *Preamble to the Constitution of the World Health Organization* as adopted by the International Health Conference, New York, 19–22 June, 1946; signed on 22 July 1946 by the representatives of 61 States (Official Records of the World Health Organization, no. 2, p. 100) and entered into force on 7 April 1948. The definition has not been amended since 1948. Available at http://www.who.int/about/definition/en/print.html

CHAPTER

# 21 Other substance-related and addictive disorders

*Jacobeth Mosidi Pooe, Kagisho Maaroganye*

## 21.1 Introduction

Substance-related disorders appear subsequent to substance use and are associated with serious medical, social and occupational consequences for the user. Knowledge of the aetiology of drug addiction and the clinical presentation of substance use disorders is essential for the correct management of these disorders. There is growing evidence of pathological brain changes due to substances even after first time use (Clay *et al.*, 2008). The DSM-5 cements this view by noting that, underlying substance use disorders, is a chronic change in the brain circuitry that leads to repeated relapses and intense drug cravings (American Psychiatric Association, 2013a). Being aware of the probable neurological changes and damage that can occur in the brain as a result of substance use, will enable physicians to rationalise their treatment of substance use disorders and to develop new treatments for drug dependence. It may also enable them to take the requisite longer term view of the management of these conditions, including referring patients for rehabilitation. Rehabilitation may assist in preventing the well-known phenomenon of frequent relapses by empowering users with prevention or remission strategies. Additionally it may be wise to set out a short-term and long-term plan with the patient's family through psycho-education or during family therapy sessions.

This chapter outlines our current knowledge about substance use disorders excluding alcohol-related disorders and discusses conditions related to specific substances, some of which may be more prevalent in southern Africa than others.

## 21.2 Classification and diagnosis of substance-related disorders

In the DSM-5, substance-related disorders are divided into 'substance use disorders' and 'substance induced disorders'. A substance use disorder is a constellation of cognitive, behavioural and physiological symptoms (including abuse and dependence) experienced by an individual who uses and continues to use a substance despite significant substance related problems. Substance use disorders are further refined into substance intoxication, substance withdrawal and other substance/medication-induced mental disorders such as psychotic disorders, bipolar and related disorders, depressive disorders, anxiety disorders, obsessive-compulsive and related disorders, sleep disorders, sexual dysfunctions, delirium and neurocognitive disorders. Intoxication is defined as the development of a reversible substance-specific syndrome due to the recent ingestion of a substance, whereas withdrawal is development of a substance-specific problematic behavioural change, with physiological and cognitive concomitants, that is due to the cessation of, or reduction in, heavy and prolonged substance use (American Psychiatric Association, 2013a).

The DSM-5 further categorises the severity of particular substance use disorders into mild (two to three symptoms), moderate (four to five symptoms) or severe (six or more symptoms). Further specifiers can be applied to substance use disorders and these are whether the remission is early or sustained and whether patient is in a controlled environment or on maintenance therapy (American Psychiatric Association, 2013a).

Whereas the DSM IV-TR denotes and clearly states the definition of abuse, dependency, intoxication and withdrawal syndromes, the term 'addiction' does not appear. Some authors define addiction as the incontrollable and continual urge to use a substance or drug despite negative consequences (Grant *et al.*, 2010; O'Brien *et al.*, 2006). DSM-5 introduces the term addiction and makes a distinction between dependence (with its associated withdrawal and tolerance characteristics) and addiction. It is reasoned that withdrawal symptoms and tolerance can emerge from the normal use of prescribed medication without the drug-seeking behaviour that is pertinent to addiction (American Psychiatric Association, 2013a). Therefore individuals whose substance-related symptoms occur as a result of the normal use of a prescription drug and without compulsive-drug seeking behaviour should not be regarded as being addicted. Whilst the term addiction is acknowledged by the DSM-5, it is not applied as a diagnostic criterion in the DSM-5 classification due to differences in opinion regarding its definition (O'Brien *et al.*, 2006). The DSM-5 also included the term 'craving' (a strong desire or urge for a substance or such a strong desire to use a substance that one can not think of anything else) as it was viewed as a potential biological treatment target (Hasin *et al.*, 2013). New to the DSM-5 are the following conditions: caffeine withdrawal, cannabis withdrawal, tobacco use disorder and gambling disorder, following peer consultation and research.

The criteria for recurrent substance-related legal problems or problems with law enforcement have been eliminated due to its difficulty applying it internationally and across cultures (American Psychiatric Association, 2013b).

DSM-5 refers to substance/medication induced disorders as those resembling the full criteria of an independent mental condition (Hasin *et al.*, 2013). Patients with substance/medication induced disorder are likely to have features associated with a specific drug but do not necessarily need to have symptoms that exceed the expected intoxication or withdrawal symptoms of that drug (American Psychiatric Association, 2013a).

### 21.2.1 Epidemiology

A review of epidemiological studies conducted in sub-Saharan Africa has revealed that cannabis and **khat** (an amphetamine-like stimulant) are widely used in the region and the use of cocaine, stimulants and heroin is increasing (Acuda *et al.*, 2011). Amongst the prescriptive drugs often abused in Africa by mostly the youth and women, are benzodiazepines, slimming tablets and simple analgesics.

A survey of the general South African population reveals that 8,4% abuse cannabis, 2% abuse other substances and 19,3% use psychoactive drugs for non-medicinal reasons (Van Heerden *et al.*, 2009). In the 2008 South African National Youth Risk Survey of students in Grade 8 to 11 in all nine provinces, 13% of participants admitted to having smoked cannabis, while 12% used inhalants, 7% used cocaine, 7% used 'tik' (crystal methamphetamine) and 7% used mandrax (Reddy *et al.*, 2010). It should be borne in mind that the use of substance may not necessarily be concentrated on school grounds. The most frequent location of drug use among high-risk adolescents may be in the adolescent's bedroom with friends (Valente *et al.*, 2004). A South African household survey conducted between 2002 and 2004 revealed that 13,3% of the respondents had a substance use disorder, which was more prevalent than mood disorders (Stein *et al.*, 2008). In other studies conducted in South Africa, the prevalence rate of alcohol and substance use disorders ranged from 15,3% in rural Limpopo Province of South Africa to 45% in a peri-urban township in Cape Town (Havenaar *et al.*, 2008).

Mentally ill patients can also abuse substances and end up having what is termed a 'dual diagnosis' of their primary mental illness and an additional substance use disorder (Kessler, 2004). This group of individuals tend to abuse alcohol, cannabis, cocaine, tranquillisers and hypnotics. In a Western Cape psychiatric hospital, 51% of the patients had co-morbid substance abuse and dependency (especially cannabis and methamphetamine) and in 8% of these in-patients, substances had led to substance-induced

**Table 21.1** Features for Substance/Medication-Induced Mental Disorders

A. The disorder represents a clinically significant symptomatic presentation of a relevant mental disorder.

B. There is evidence from the history, physical examination, or laboratory findings of both of the following:

1. The disorder developed during or within 1 month of a substance intoxication or withdrawal or taking a medication; and
2. The involved substance/medication is capable of producing the mental disorder.

C. The disorder is not better explained by an independent mental disorder (i.e., one that is not substance- or medication-induced). Such evidence of an independent mental disorder could include the following:

1. The disorder preceded the onset of severe intoxication or withdrawal or exposure to the medication; or
2. The full mental disorder persisted for a substantial period of time (e.g., at least 1 month) after the cessation of acute withdrawal or severe intoxication or taking the medication. This criterion does not apply to substance-induced neurocognitive disorders or hallucinogen persisting perception disorder, which persist beyond the cessation of acute intoxication or withdrawal.

D. The disorder does not occur exclusively during the course of a delirium.

E. The disorder causes clinically significant distress or impairment in social, occupational, or other important areas of functioning.

**Source:** Reprinted with permission from the *Diagnostic and Statistical Manual of Mental Disorders*, Fifth Edition, (Copyright 2013). American Psychiatric Association.

psychotic disorders (7%) and substance-induced mood disorders (1%) (Weich and Pienaar, 2009). Perhaps due to a difficulty in distinguishing between symptoms related to mental illness and substance abuse, relatives of both mentally ill patients and clinicians underestimate the extent of substance dependency among these patients. However, the high prevalence of substance abuse in psychiatric patients cannot be denied; it has a significant impact of the patient's recovery and prognosis (Hatfield, 2008).

The onset of substance use is usually early, specifically during the adolescent stage. In South Africa, it was found that that median age of onset for substance use disorders (21 years) was almost 10 years earlier than that of anxiety disorders or mood disorders (Stein *et al.*, 2008). Neurological and behavioural attributes of adolescents as well as the new era in which modern adolescents live (individualism and an incoherent family unit) may contribute to the early onset of substance abuse (Le Moal, 2009).The earlier the onset of substance use disorders, there more adverse are the outcomes including co-morbid psychiatric disorders (Larm *et al.*, 2010: Bakken *et al.*, 2004). Whilst it is commonly hypothesised that youth who start with more legal drugs tend to progress onto illicit drugs via cannabis use, very few youths progress as seamlessly as that (Odejide, 2006 ; Le Moal, 2009).

The greater use of substances amongst males is confirmed in South African studies (8–9 times more than females) and has perhaps led to the significant association between substance use disorders and male gender in the country (Stein *et al.*, 2008).

## 21.2.2 Aetiology

A combination of psychosocial and neurobiological factors may be responsible for the initial and continuous use of substance (Sadock BJ and Sadock VA, 2007).

### 21.2.2.1 Perinatal transmission

A mother's use of substances may influence the likelihood of her offspring using substances in future. Prenatal exposure to at least three substances (cocaine, tobacco, cannabis) has been linked to the child's use of these substances (Delaney-Black *et al.*, 2011; Cornelius, *et al.*, 2005; Day *et al.*, 2006; Porath and Fried, 2005).

### 21.2.2.2 Psychosocial dynamics

Stress can affect the developing brain, resulting in abnormalities that lead to substance use (Clay *et al.*, 2008). Although the mechanism behind this phenomenon is not clear, there is a strong association between child maltreatment (especially physical abuse) and substance dependence (Oshri *et al.*, 2011; Maniglio, 2011). Transitional periods of an individual's life may pose a heightened risk to the onset of substance use. Examples of such periods include entering puberty, starting high school, moving away from home and starting to work (National Institute on Drug Abuse, 2003). **Dynamics** within the family structure such as enabling and denial of the problem may also contribute to persistent substance use and subsequent substance use disorders (Sadock BJ and Sadock VA, 2007).

A large-scale Swedish study revealed that certain environmental factors that involve parents can strongly predict the risk for substance abuse in the offsprings. These include a history of divorce, death of a parent, criminal activity and parental alcohol problems. These factors become even more influential in offsprings with a high genetic risk for substance abuse (Kendler *et al.*, 2012). Epidemiological studies in South Africa also confirm that difficult family circumstances are associated with higher levels of substance use (Peltzer and Ramlagan, 2010). Risk factors for adolescent drug abuse also include peer substance use and early-onset sexual risk behaviours (Latimer and Zur, 2010). A study on adolescents in 6 African countries revealed that school attendance and parental supervision and connectedness protected against substance use, whereas school truancy, loneliness and poverty were associated with substance use (Peltzer, 2009). Violence towards the user and greater discrimination also led to higher levels of drug use amongst South African youth (Brook *et al.*, 2006).

### 21.2.2.3 Neurochemical or anatomical changes

Addiction has come to be regarded as a long-standing and relapsing 'disease of the brain' (Clay *et al* 2008; Vrecko, 2010; Kuhar, 2010). The brain-reward (and reinforcement) circuitry has been postulated to form the biological basis of addiction. Activation of this circuit leads to drug-seeking and drug-taking behaviours, whilst inhibition of this circuit is implicated in withdrawal dysphoria and dysphoria-mediated drug craving (Clay *et al.*, 2008). The circuit involves several major neuroanatomical areas including the ventral tegmental area (VTA), the medial forebrain bundle and the nucleus accumbens (Acb). Closely-related structures ventral to the nucleus accumbens (ventral pallidum and medial prefrontal cortex) and dorsal to the ventral tegmental area (locus coeruleus) also form part of this reward circuit. The major neurotransmitters probably involved in developing substance abuse and substance dependence are the opioid, norepinephrine, catecholamine (particularly dopamine), and gamma-aminobutyric acid (GABA) neurotransmitters. Other neurotransmitters, such as serotonergic and glutamatergic neurotransmitters, are also implicated. Addictive drugs primarily activate the dopaminegic neurons of the VTA-Acb axis, resulting in pleasurable or euphoric effects and uncontrollable cravings. Amphetamines, cocaine and phencyclidine activate these reward mechanisms directly, at the dopamine terminal loci in the Acb. Opiates and cannabinoids activate the VTA-Acb at both ends, whilst barbiturates, benzodiazepines and nicotine activate the reward circuitry at the VTA axis terminal. Opiates can also activate these reward mechanisms neurons indirectly via the locus coeruleus located close to the VTA. It is important to consider that the reward-enhancing power of addictive drugs is more powerful and immediate than the reward produced by natural reinforcers (Gardner, 2005).

### 21.2.2.4 Genetics

Genetic risk can be regarded as a strong risk factor for substance use. Genetic factors may account for as much as 50% of the variance in people with clinically defined alcohol or drug addiction (Uhl *et al.*, 1993). Specific control studies looking at probands with specific substance use disorders (opiates, cannabis, cannabis and alcohol) and their first-degree relatives show a eight-fold increased risk of drug disorders amongst first-degree relatives (Merikangas *et al.*,1998). Genetic effects may also underlie the transition from drug use to drug abuse

(Cadoret,1992). Not only are the levels of frequency or abuse of the substance under genetic control, but the subjective effects of cannabis (including its pleasant effects and negative effects) as well (Tsuang *et al.*, 1996; Lyons *et al.*, 1997). Genetic factors determine the individual's metabolism, sensitivity, tolerance and response to the emotional and psychological effects of the drug and hence sets their genetic vulnerability to the drug (Khantzian, 1985). It should also be borne in mind that other family, twin and adoption studies suggest that the risk of the vulnerable becoming addicted comes from both genetic factors (50%) and from environmental ones (50%) (Leyton, 2013).

#### 21.2.2.5 Other psychiatric disorders

Psychological distress has been frequently associated with substance use disorders. Higher levels of global psychological distress have been independently associated with more frequent use of both methamphetamine and heroin (Darke *et al.*, 2011). Certain personality trait disorders, such as antisocial (deceitfulness and lack of remorse), schizotypal (ideas of reference and social anxiety ) and borderline personality (identity disturbance and self-damaging impulsivity) traits have been linked to the persistence or chronicity of substance use disorders (Fenton *et al.*, 2012). A child's personality or temperament (withdrawn or aggressive) can eventually lead to substance abuse if it complicates into academic failure, peer rejection and subsequent association with deviant peers (National Institute on Drug Abuse, 2003).

The association between mental disorders and substance use disorders is significant (Lev-Ran, 2013). In the early years, Attention deficit/hyperactivity disorder (ADHD) has been implicated as leading to substance abuse and vice versa (Wilnes, 2004). In the later years, patients with psychotic disorders have also shown an increased use of substances, especially cannabis, compared with the general population (Kolliakou *et al.*, 2011). A small South African study (Brink *et al.*, 2003) has found that people with a vulnerability for psychosis started using cannabis at an earlier age than the general population. The self-medication theory used to explain the use of substances in patients with schizophrenia has not been convincingly proven (Kolliakou *et al.*, 2011), but it may be more pertinent in patients with anxiety disorders who are prone to abusing specific substances to ease their anxiety (Baigent, 2012). Cannabis use disorder, followed by cocaine use disorder and amphetamine use disorder, were the most common substance use disorders seen in patients with mood and anxiety disorders. Mania and panic disorders were more strongly related to sedative, tranquilliser and opioid use disorders than other mood and anxiety disorders (Conway *et al.*, 2006).

## 21.2.3 Assessment and management

### 21.2.3.1. Assessment and management approach

As substance use tends to be underreported due to its illegal nature, it is important that the clinician suspects it in any patient and assesses any patient for it; a treatment opportunity may otherwise be missed. It is important to recognise that these conditions can present subtly and may not be obvious until they are enquired about or noted by the keen physician. Assessment of substance use includes asking screening questions without discrimination, knowing the features of substance use disorders and being willing to test for substances through urine toxicology screen and blood tests. As the patient is being assessed, the multi-disciplinary team (MDT) can start considering recommending one of five levels of care to treat the individual's substance use disorder according to the American Society of Addiction Medicine (ASAM). These are: Level 0.5 (early intervention services), Level I (out-patient services), Level II (intensive out-patient services/partial hospitalisation services), Level III (low or high intensity residential and in-patient services), and Level IV (medically managed intensive in-patient services) (McCarty *et al.*, 2014).

There are a number of specialised medical and non-medical treatment approaches to treat substance use disorders. The longer the addicted individual remains in the programme, the better. Key to best treatment outcomes was high motivation within the addicted individual (Simpson, 2001). Age, criminal history, race or economic status did not influence the likelihood of staying longer in a rehabilitation program as much as motivation to change did (Ramlagan *et al.*, 2010).

When substance use disorders co-occur with another mental illness, an integrated, comprehensive and coordinated service, which provides substance abuse services within a community mental health service, may offer improved best results (Sterling *et al.*, 2011). The more severe the co-morbid conditions, the greater the need for more structured programmes that include intensive out-patient treatment, **case management** services and behavioural therapies such as Contingency Management (Kelly *et al.*, 2012). Integrated treatment for dual-diagnosis patients make use of many different treatment modalities, including intensive case management, motivational enhance therapy interviewing, 12-step programmes focused on dual diagnosis, cognitive-behavioral strategies for relapse prevention, 12-step facilitation, social skills training, contingency management and family psycho-education (Ziedonis *et al.*, 2005).

Obejide noted that in Africa there are few specialised drug treatment centres, and they were mostly located in South Africa, Nigeria and Kenya (Obejide, 2006). Experienced physicians at these centres may offer substitution treatment with methadone; but it was noted that in audited South African centres, detoxification services and substitution medications were less likely to be provided to individuals, perhaps due to the lack of experienced addiction clinicians (Medical Research Council, 2008). A study in historically disadvantaged communities in Cape Town revealed that stigma towards substance users and negative beliefs about treatment being ineffective and punitive from individuals involved in substance use treatment initiatives hinder treatment seeking for substance use disorders (Myers *et al.*, 2009).

### 21.2.3.2 General management of substance use disorders

**Pharmacotherapy**

The acute phase of the treatment of substance use disorders is usually dominated by the medical treatment of intoxication and withdrawal syndromes as well as substitute management for the addiction. There are medications to reduce the re-enforcing effects of substances and others that can assist to promote abstinence by inducing unpleasant consequences of substance use. Agonist treatment is used to contend against the drug of abuse. Medications to treat co-morbid psychiatric conditions are also available (American Psychiatric Association, 2010a). The possibility that the user may end up abusing some of the prescribed medications must be considered; but this should not dissuade the clinician from using medication where indicated. The primary focus of many studies has been the treatment of withdrawal syndromes of substance use disorders as well as substitute management of the addiction and these are alluded to under the various chapter sections below.

**Pharmacotherapy in dual diagnosis**

The treatment of patients with a dual diagnosis is challenging, partly due to the paucity of well-designed studies. Nevertheless, research does suggest that some psychotropic medication may be more effective than others in the treatment of various mental health disorders that co-morbid with substance use disorders (Murthy and Chand, 2012). There are also some key principles to help guide the clinician in managing patients with dual diagnosis. Clear symptom clusters should be elicited and treated and not vague complaints. The clinician should avoid medication with the potential to be addictive and should consider the safety of prescribed drugs for the patient. He or she should also be aware of drug-drug interactions with medication being specifically used for substance use disorder (American Psychiatric Association, 2010b).

### Mood and anxiety disorders

For depressed individuals with a nicotine dependence, bupropion has been proven to be able to treat both conditions (Wilkes, 2008). Valproate has been found to be effective in bipolar patients with a history of substance abuse in several randomised controlled studies. Not much is known about the effectiveness of other mood stabilisers such as lamotrigine, topiramate and gabapentin in dually diagnosed patients (Murthy and Chand, 2012). Individuals with substance use disorders are liable to abuse benzodiazepines that have been prescribed for their anxiety disorders. Therefore, consideration should first be given to whether the abused substance could have caused the anxiety and, second, whether detoxification should be the first action taken. If medication must be prescribed after detoxification, a combination of antidepressants (preferably selective serotonin reuptake inhibitors (SSRIs) because of their better side-effect profile and lack of addictive potential) and cognitive behavioural therapy (CBT) have good evidence-based support (Swinson, 2006).

### Psychotic disorders

Studies confirm that antipsychotics, especially atypical antipsychotics, are effective for a dual diagnosis of schizophrenia and substance use. Typical antipsychotic use is discouraged because patients who abuse substances are more likely to develop extra-pyramidal side effects (EPS), especially tardive dyskinesia (Bailey *et al.*,1997). Amongst the atypical antipsychotics, clozapine,

**Information box**

**Summary of psychosocial interventions for substance related disorders**

- Brief intervention: this intervention is meant to motivate a patient with a positive drug screen result to change his or her substance use habit because of the associated risks of the substance abuse (Henry-Edwards *et al.*, 2003).
- CBT encompasses motivational interventions, contingency management strategies and relapse prevention (McHugh *et al.*, 2010).
- Motivational interview: the therapist takes advantage of the individual's wish or motivation to reduce or stop his or her drug use whilst acknowledging their ambivalence about quitting substance abuse. This ambivalence is addressed with motivational interviewing as the uncertainty will make it difficult to remain in remission (Weich, 2006).
- Contingency management: a non-drug reinforcer (e.g. a money voucher) is used to encourage abstinence from substances after the patient has produced negative urine drug samples several times in a week (McHugh *et al*, 2010). There are also disincentives meant to punish specific targeted behaviour (Myers et al., 2008).
- Relapse prevention: the patient is taught about drug cue situations and how to avoid them in order to prevent a relapse into renewed substance abuse (Carrol and Onken, 2005).
- Family therapy: effective family-based therapies include behavioural couple's therapy, behavioural family therapies in adults (partner and family are taught to reinforce individual commitment to quit drugs and how to cope with cravings) and multiple systems-oriented treatments in adolescents (altering the multiple risk factors within the family that create and maintain adolescent substance abuse) (Rowe, 2012).
- Therapeutic communities: residents of rehabilitation centers undergo a number of psychotherapeutic programmes including the above-mentioned therapies; it may include detoxification in some cases. These communities are generally regarded as being effective but not all residents complete the programme and completion rates range from 9-56% (Malivert *et al*, 2012).
- Mutual-help group continuing care: examples of these include Narcotics Anonymous (NA). They follow the traditional 12-step principles. Participants should have a desire to stop their drug use by conceding that as an individual, without spiritual guidance, they are powerless to stop using substances (Alcoholics Anonymous, 2012).

olanzapine and risperidone are a better option and are commonly used for co-morbid schizophrenia and substance use disorders (Murthy and Chand, 2012; Drake *et al.*, 2007). Clozapine appears to be the most effective of the antipsychotics in reducing alcohol, cocaine and cannabis abuse among patients with schizophrenia (Kelly *et al.*, 2012).

**Attention deficit/hyperactivity disorder**

The efficacy of atomoxetine with respect to a decrease in substance abuse in patients with co-morbid adult ADHD is yet to be established (Murthy and Chand, 2012). There is concern that the use of stimulants for ADHD may lead to illicit substance abuse; a review of studies allays this fear (Faraone and Wilens, 2003).

**Psychosocial intervention**

There are a number of evidence-based psychotherapy treatments that can be used to treat substance use disorders. These include behavioural couple's therapy (CBT), (including relapse prevention, coping skills, contingency management, motivational enhancement/motivational interviewing), a community reinforcement approach and 12-step facilitation treatments (Manuel *et al.*, 2012). No single intervention can be regarded as the treatment of choice but, with all of these interventions, the clinician should aim to enhance the patient's motivation to stop or reduce substance use, improve the **self-efficacy** for change, strengthen coping skills and change reinforcement contingencies for recovery (Department of Veteran Affairs, Department of Defense, 2009). In patients with a dual diagnosis, the clinician should focus on motivational enhancement approaches during the initial phase and use both evidence-based pharmacological interventions and mental health psychosocial treatments. Community support through mutual help groups should also be encouraged (American Psychiatric Association, 2010b).

### 21.2.3.3 Harm reduction

Proponents of harm reduction take the view that the goal of establishing reduced use of substances with safer use practices or alternatives is also a desirable outcome en route to total abstinence from drugs. So, those who advocate harm reduction strategies have a lower threshold for patients to access support services that are not dependent on the patient changing their drug use behaviour. In the process they offer unconditional support to the patient. Traditional forms of harm reduction include needles exchange and the methadone maintenance program. These programs have been demonstrated to reduce rates of overdoses and transmission of infectious diseases (Mancini and Wyrick-Waugh, 2013). It has been noted that few centres in South Africa use the harm reduction approach (Parry, 2005).

Clinicians should strive to observe the following principles when managing drug abuse or are advocating for drug abuse management:

- early identification of at-risk consumption and harmful substance use, countered by psycho-education and advice
- facilitate the withdrawal phase through to detoxification and institute substitution treatment if concerned about continued use
- treat complications, including co-morbid mental disorders
- offer continuing care programmes to maintain remission and prevent relapse such as rehabilitation, as a substance use disorder should be viewed as a chronic disease
- recognise that no one intervention can be regarded as the treatment of choice for substance use disorders: substance use disorder is a chronic and relapsing brain disease and two or more interventions (including more than one visit to a rehabilitation facility) may be needed before the affected individual chooses abstinence. Each intervention increases the likelihood of success of other interventions: motivational interviewing, for example, increases the chances of retention in an in-patient rehabilitation programme (Weich, 2006; Hubbard, 1997).

# 21.3 Specific substance use disorders

## 21.3.1 Stimulant substances

The overarching term of stimulants includes amphetamine, methamphetamine, 3,4-methylenedioxymethamphetamine (MDMA, or 'ecstasy'), methcathinone ('meth cat' or 'cat'), ephedrine, methylphenidate and cocaine (the latter is discussed separately below). In the community, stimulants are also known as 'tik', 'speed', 'whizz', 'crystal meth' and 'ice'. Ephedrine is commonly found in appetite suppressants and bronchodilators, so these can be potential licit drugs of abuse. Amphetamines can be taken orally, snorted or injected. It gives users a sense of euphoria and energy through facilitating the release of dopamine, noradrenaline and adrenaline from the nucleus accumbens. In the long term, it results in early reduction of dopamine transporters in the caudate and putamen and changes in the levels of glucose metabolism in the thalamus and parietal cortex, which leads to emotional dysregulation (depression, negative symptoms of psychosis and anxiety) that is only partially improved with abstinence (Myers *et al.*, 2006). Its acute physiological effects include increases in pulse and blood pressure, pupil dilation and increases in temperature.

Tik is the street name for a potent form of methamphetamine used in South Africa by mostly poor communities because it is so cheap. Its effects are stronger and last longer than other forms of methamphetamine. In addition the 'crash' is worse. It is a white powder that can be smoked, snorted or injected. Its effects are instantaneous if injected or smoked. The initial affects are pleasurable and include euphoria, a heightened sense of contentment and satisfaction, confidence, energy and gratitude. Its after-effects are usually unpleasant and include anxiety, palpitations, panic attacks, sweating, hallucinations, itching (illusion that bugs are crawling on the skin), welts on the skin, involuntary body movements, headaches and aggression. In the long term it leads to malnutrition, depression, meth mouth (rotten and broken teeth), psychosis, insomnia, seizure and coma (False Bay Theurapeutic Community Centre, 2014).

Ecstacy is an example of a designer amphetamine-like substance. It contains a combination of amphetamines and hallucinogenic effects. It is often used at recreational gatherings with other drugs, including alcohol, LSD (lysergic acid diethylamide) , tobacco, opiods and cannabis (Robledo, 2010). Its harmful effects include hyperpyrexia and acute renal failure due to dehydration, as well as water intoxication in users who overcompensate. These adverse effects are usually responsible for ecstasy-related deaths (Gowing *et al.*, 2002).

The use of amphetamines is widespread throughout the world; after cannabis it is the most popular illicit substance in US and several parts of Western Europe (Sadock BJ and Sadock VA, 2007). Eight per cent of admissions to substance use treatment programs are due to amphetamine abuse (Brackins *et al.*, 2011). A SASH study (2002–2004) reported that the use of other drugs, including methamphetamine, stood at 2%, but this might be an underestimation: a survey conducted in 2005 revealed that methamphetamine was the primary drug of abuse in the Western Cape (Van Heerden, 2009). There has been a dramatic increase in admissions for amphetamine-related problems, especially of adolescents in the Western Cape, perhaps as a consequence of this (Kapp, 2008).

### 21.3.1.1 Stimulant use disorders

**Intoxication**

Amphetamines can lead to a myriad of symptoms and signs indicative of its psychostimulant and sympathomimetic effects. The affected individual may have nausea or vomiting, psychomotor agitation or retardation, chest pain, cardiac arrhythmia and respiratory depression. These effects usually last 48 hours but may resolve after 24 hours. Behaviourally, the individual may become euphoric, aggressive and hyper-vigilant. With chronic use or high doses, the individual may experience weight loss, muscular weakness, confusion, dyskinesia, dystonia, seizures, delirium or comas.

**Withdrawal**

After heavy or prolonged use, the individual may have the following symptoms and signs: dysphoric mood, fatigue, vivid and unpleasant dreams, insomnia or hypersomnia, increased appetite, psychomotor retardation or agitation. These symptoms occur from a few hours after cessation to a week thereafter. To meet the criteria for stimulant withdrawal disorder, two of these symptoms are required.

### 21.3.1.2 Stimulant-induced disorders

The DSM-5 (American Psychiatric Association, 2013a) recognises the following stimulant induced disorders:

- stimulant-induced psychotic disorders
- stimulant-induced bipolar disorder
- stimulant-induced depressive disorders
- stimulant-induced anxiety disorders
- stimulant-induced obsessive-compulsive disorders
- stimulant-induced sleep disorders
- stimulant-induced sexual dysfunction.

It is worth noting that, although rare, psychosis can occur at therapeutic doses of prescribed amphethamines such as methyphenidate. While stimulant-induced psychosis may be expected to last a few days or less than a month, it can continue for a much longer period than that, even after use has ceased (Hofmann, 1983). Paranoia can occur during intoxication, withdrawal, periods of sustained use and quickly after the individual resumes amphetamine use (Sato *et al.*, 1992). It can be difficult to distinguish between schizophrenia and amphetamine-induced psychotic disorder unless there is no prior history of psychotic symptoms, there is a positive urine toxicology result that indicates amphetamine use or resolution of psychotic symptoms after documented use. However, it has been noted that individuals with an amphetamine-induced psychotic disorder have more reactive affects and less formal thought disorder (Sweeting and Farrell, 2005).

Methamphetamine use has been associated with mental states or conditions such as suicide and depression (Darke *et al.*, 2008). Heavy use of methamphetamine can also lead to cognitive dysfunction, such as poorer performance on visuospatial memory and perceptual attention, but with individual variations possibly due to gene polymorphism and resultant reduced serotonin formation (Cuyas *et al.*, 2011).

### 21.3.1.3 Treatment and rehabilitation

There is no evidence-based pharmacological treatment for amphetamine withdrawal. Most of the withdrawal symptoms are short-lived; the clinician may treat insomnia with hypnotics. Pharmacologically, amphetamine intoxication or psychosis is treated with benzodiazepine and antipsychotics. Depending on their availability and the patient's tolerance to the side effects, olanzapine or haloperidol may be used to ameliorate the psychotic symptoms (Shoptaw *et al.*, 2009). Due to the limited knowledge of cellular and molecular mechanisms that lead to the development of amphetamine use disorders such as dependence, it is difficult to find treatment for stimulant dependence (Chen *et al.*, 2010). Various drugs such as sertraline, bupropion, mirtazapine, modafinil, risperidone, aripiprazole, topiramate and gabapentin have been used in clinical trials in an attempt to achieve abstinence from amphetamine use. None have been found to be consistently effective (Brackins *et al.*, 2011).

Still, it may be worthwhile to treat amphetamine-induced dependence with psychosocial interventions. These interventions include CBT and contingency management. CBT and contingency managements are moderately effective in reaching the stage of abstinence and are well tolerated (Vocci and Montoya, 2009). However, psychosocial interventions may not be highly effective in helping patients overcome mood, cognitive and motivation difficulties in the long term (Rose and Grant, 2008).

## 21.3.2 Cocaine

Although they produce a similar clinical picture, cocaine and amphetamine are two different drug forms, with varying specific mechanisms of action. Cocaine is derived from the coca plant, mainly in areas such as South America where it is of indigenous use to local inhabitants. It has medicinal use as in ENT surgery for its vasoconstrictive and analgesic properties. In addition to stimulating the brain, it can also suppress the appetite. It can be taken orally, by insufflation, intravenously or smoked ('crack' or 'freebase'). Neurochemically, cocaine leads to a rapid accumulation of catecholamine's and serotonin in the brain. It prevents the reuptake of these neurotransmitters; chronic use leads to relative dopaminergic deficiency. Cocaine has a much shorter half-life (1 hour) compared with amphetamine.

The use of cocaine is widespread throughout the world, leading to a variety of cocaine use disorders. The aetiology behind the use and abuse of cocaine is multifactorial and ranges from genetic influence, easy accessibility to cocaine, learned and conditioned behaviour (linked to its post-cocaine use 'rush') to environmental cues such as seeing white powder. Some people use cocaine for its pharmacological effects (including euphoria and belief that it enhances sexual performance). The development of mood disorders and alcohol-related disorders usually follows the onset of cocaine-related disorders, whereas anxiety disorders, antisocial personality disorder and ADHD are thought to precede the development of cocaine-related disorders (Sadock BJ and Sadock VA, 2007).

### 21.3.2.1 Cocaine use disorders

**Intoxication and withdrawal**

The clinical diagnosis of cocaine intoxication and withdrawal is similar to the diagnostic criteria of amphetamine intoxication and withdrawal. Treatment of cocaine-related intoxications is complicated by the uncommon knowledge that cocaine may be mixed with other drugs, such as atropine, when it is sold to users. The clinician should be aware that the clinical picture of cocaine intoxication may be influenced by the effects of other drugs (Vroegop *et al.*, 2009). Recovery from withdrawal usually takes one to two weeks (Sadock BJ and Sadock VA, 2007).

**Treatment and rehabilitation**

Most cocaine users do not seek treatment for their withdrawal experiences – in fact, in-patient or residential drug withdrawal treatment is not necessary when a person withdraws from cocaine. No drugs been proven effective in treating cocaine withdrawal symptoms, but short-acting benzodiazepine can be used to treat severe agitation or insomnia (Gorelick, 2014).

Without pre-existing psychiatric disorders such mood disorders, patients may not benefit from antidepressants, mood stabilisers or methylphenidate in the treatment of cocaine dependence. Dopamine agonists (bromocriptine and L-DOPA or carbidopa) have been investigated as treatment for cocaine abuse and dependence in clinical trials, but the effect sizes were not significant (Amato *et al.*, 2011).

Unless the impact of cocaine use on work and family responsibilities is emphasized by clinicians, abstinence from cocaine is difficult. There are no alternative drugs that can limit the craving for cocaine. The following interventions may be attempted: hospitalisation to limit access to the drug, frequent unscheduled urine tests, residential programmes, and cognitive and behavioural techniques.

## 21.3.3 Cannabis

Cannabis is the most commonly used illicit drug in the world; it is viewed as a gateway to harder drugs. It is also known as 'pot', 'dagga', 'marijuana', 'grass', 'weed', 'skunk' and 'dope', amongst others. Its source, the hemp plant (*Cannabis sativa*), has been cultivated for its psychoactive properties for more than 2000 years. Its main mind-altering ingredient is THC (delta-9-tetrahydrocannabinol). THC binds to endogenous cannabinoids receptors on cell membranes; this interaction between the endocannabinoid system and the dopaminergic and opioid systems may be responsible for cannabis dependence (Weinstein and Gorelick, 2011).

The amount of THC in the cannabis determines the strength of the drug, and is affected by factors like soil, weather, plant type and the time of harvest. In South Africa the most potent form of cannabis is called the Swazi. Cannabis can be smoked, sometimes in a pipe or water pipe, or as a loosely rolled cigarette known as a zol/joint. But it can also be brewed in tea or mixed in baked products (cookies and brownies), whereby unsuspecting individuals can suffer adverse effects of cannabis unknowingly. Cannabis is used by patients for a variety of conditions including anxiety, depression, GIT disorders, nausea due to chemotherapy, chronic pain, multiple sclerosis, AIDS, and glaucoma.

### 21.3.3.1 Cannabis use disorders

The development of the adverse effects of cannabis use depends on the weight and height of the user, the user's general health status, regularity of use, the person's mood, the manner in which the cannabis is used (whether ingested or smoked), the amount or concentration of the cannabis used and whether the cannabis is mixed with other drugs or not. Cannabis generally leads to an inability to learn and retain information, the inability to sustain attention and focus and to plan for as long as 24 hours ahead; the affected individual will also experience problems with mathematics and verbal skills.

**Intoxication**

The non-clinician may recognise cannabis intoxication by the user's reddish sclera and increased appetite ('the munchies'). The DSM-5 states that in order for cannabis intoxication to be diagnosed, there has to have been recent (within 2 hours) use of cannabis, clinically significant maladaptive behavioural or psychological changes (including impaired motor coordination, euphoria, anxiety, sensation of slowed time) and two (or more) of the following signs: conjunctival injection, increased appetite, dry mouth and tachycardia. A clinician may specify whether there are perceptual disturbances or not (American Psychiatric Association, 2013a).

**Withdrawal**

Previously cannabis withdrawal was not recognized, but the diagnosis has been included in the DSM-5, due to growing evidence of a 33–95% prevalence in cannabis users and use of cannabis to relieve withdrawal symptoms (Hasin *et al.* 2013). To define cannabis withdrawal syndrome the individual should have 'clinically significant distress or impairment in social, occupational or other important areas of functioning', characterised by at least three of the following symptoms irritability, anger or aggression, nervousness or anxiety, sleep difficulties, decreased appetite or weight loss, restlessness, depressed mood and physical symptoms like stomach pains, shakiness or tremors, sweating, fever, chills and headache (American Psychiatric Association, 2013a) Withdrawal symptoms often begin during the first week of abstinence and resolve after a few weeks (Weinstein and Gorelick, 2011).

### 21.3.3.2 Cannabis-induced disorders

Other cannabis-induced disorders include cannabis-induced psychotic disorder, cannabis-induced anxiety disorder and cannabis-induced sleep disorder. These cannabis-induced disorders are diagnosed instead of cannabis intoxication or cannabis withdrawal when the symptoms are sufficiently severe to warrant independent clinical attention.

Modest cannabis use can lead to delirium; at higher doses the level of consciousness of the user may become impaired as well. With delirium, it may then become difficult for a first-time user to give an account of what adverse effects they had after they had used cannabis and ended up in hospital. Psychotic disorder due to cannabis is rare; transient periods of psychosis are more common. In younger users, cannabis has been demonstrated to increase the risk of developing schizophrenia, although other risk factors are also important (Arseneault *et al.*, 2004). This suggests that the individual's vulnerability determines the outcome of schizophrenia or not in a cannabis user. Individuals with schizophrenia and who use cannabis may have a poorer outcome (Rathbone *et al.*, 2008).

#### 21.3.3.3 Treatment

There is no specific pharmacotherapeutics recommended for the treatment of marijuana intoxication, withdrawal or dependence. The following drugs have been investigated and hold some promise: cannabinoid 1 receptor antagonists (for intoxication), oral THC combined with an $\alpha$-adrenergic agonist such as lofexidine (for withdrawal) and buspirone (for dependence) (Weinstein and Gorelick, 2011). However, abstinence can still be attempted when premised on education about the adverse effects of cannabis and support programs.

### 21.3.4 Opioids

Opioid is a term given to natural occurring substance such as morphine, semi-synthetic drugs, such as heroin, or synthetic drugs, such as methadone or meperidine. Their pharmacologically active compounds are derived from the opium poppy, *Papaver somniferum* (Manchikanti *et al.*, 2010). Opioids are used as analgesics, cough suppressants, sedatives, pupil constrictors and anti-diarrhoea medication.

Opioid use disorders include opioid intoxication, opioid withdrawal, other opioid-induced disorders and unspecified opioid related disorders (American Psychiatric Association, 2013a). Opioid abuse and dependence have been grouped into a single opioid use disorder in the DSM-5 (American Psychiatric Association, 2013a).

Heroin is a morphine derivative and accounts for 70% of opiate abuse globally. It is estimated that South African has one of the highest prevalence rates of heroin use in Africa (Medical Research Council, 2004). Heroin is more potent and soluble than morphine. It crosses the blood-brain barrier faster and readily, leading to its propensity to cause addiction faster. Heroin can be combined with other drugs like cannabis, and is known as 'nyaope'. Nyaope first surfaced in the Pretoria region, South Africa, in the townships (Skosana, 2014). Since then it has spread far and wide throughout the country. In other areas, the heroin is mixed with cannabis and laced with bicarbonate of soda, rat poison and, allegedly, antiretroviral medication to give it volume. It is then called by different names in different regions. In KwaZulu-Natal, for example, it is known as '**whoonga**' (Chapman, 2013). In the Western Cape it is commonly used by tik addicts. '**Sugars**' is a mixture of heroin and cannabis that is laced with a residue of cocaine. To give it bulk, rat poison, bicarbonate of soda and teething powder are often used.

#### 21.3.4.1 Opioid use disorders

**Intoxication**

People who are intoxicated with opioids develop at least two symptoms that alter their normal mental function, change their behaviour or may impede their ability to carry out normal routine activities. The pupils may be dilated or constricted. Other symptoms of intoxication include slurred speech, drowsiness or coma, impairment in attention and memory. The diagnosis is made only after obtaining a history of recent use of an opioid drug or medication and lack of other psychological or physical conditions that could produce the same symptoms as that of opioid use.

**Withdrawal**

Opioid withdrawal occurs within minutes to days of reducing or stopping the drug or medication previously used. The severity of the withdrawal symptoms depends on the amount used and they may range from mild to severe. Mild symptoms may be anxiety, irritability and a desire to continue drug or medication use. If the withdrawal is moderate or severe, the patient may develop at least three of the following symptoms: dysphoric mood, nausea or vomiting, fever, muscle aches, lacrimation or rhinorrhoea, yawning, diarrhoea, pupillary dilation, piloerection or sweating and insomnia (Taylor *et al.*, 2012).

**Opioid-induced mood and anxiety disorders**

Anxiety, depression and insomnia may persist from the acute withdrawal stage and it should not be readily assumed to be a sign of an anxiety or depressive disorder. However, long-term use of opioids is commonly associated with moderate to severe depression (Substance Abuse and Mental Health Services Administration, 2005).

#### 21.3.4.2 Treatment and rehabilitation

A thorough assessment to determine the severity and nature of the addiction will determine the type of setting the patient will need. Medical conditions like HIV, tuberculosis, sexually transmitted infections, liver disease, pancreatitis and gastrointestinal and cardiovascular diseases are common in people with opioid addiction and may necessitate in-patient care. Patients with co-occurring psychiatric conditions must be admitted into a facility that can manage both disorders. Opioid withdrawal symptoms may be uncomfortable and painful but they are not life-threatening, especially in cases of mild use. Opioid withdrawal symptoms usually last for a week. The associated anxiety in relation to withdrawal may perpetuate the withdrawal symptoms that occur.

Treatment depends on the extent and nature of the patient opioid abuse problem. Concomitant factors like a medical or psychiatric disorder may influence the required setting for treatment. An opioid agonist like methadone and buprenorphine can be given as substitution treatment for the withdrawal symptoms by experienced clinicians. Clonidine, a $\alpha 2$ adrenergic agonist, can also be given to reduce the sympathetic nervous system response such as tachycardia and hypertension. The use of pharmacological agents like anxiolytics, opioid agonists, analgesics and sleep medication requires close monitoring and management to alleviate discomfort whilst reducing the potential for relapse.

Pregnant women should be stabilised and maintained on an opioid agonist for the duration of the pregnancy. Detoxification can lead to premature labour and poses the risk of relapse on other illicit drugs that are a risk to the fetus. Close monitoring by the obstetrician, social worker and psychiatric team should be sought. Special precautions should be taken for the young and old in the dose regime and appropriate treatment settings (Helmbrecht and Thiagarajah, 2008; Fajemirokun-Odudeyi *et al.*, 2006).

Successful treatment is dependent on other factors like the patient's readiness to stop the drug use, support from family members and others and the social environment. The involvement of support networks like Narcotics Anonymous should be encouraged.

### 21.3.5 Hallucinogens

Hallucinogens alter perception, producing psychedelic experiences. Examples of hallucinogens include lysergic acid diethylamide (LSD), phencyclidine (PCP or 'angel dust'), ketamine and 'magic mushrooms'. LSD is the main synthetic hallucinogen. They can be taken orally or intravenously. Agonistic action at 5-HT2 receptors is a likely common mechanism of action of these hallucinogens. PCP was initially used as an anaesthetic in humans but is now only used as a veterinary medicine. It can produce disorientation, agitation, delirium and unpleasant hallucinations in humans. Ketamine is still used as an anaesthetic; it has less adverse effects compared to PCP, but has the potential to be abused (Sadock BJ and Sadock VA, 2007). The LSD 'trip' starts about 3-6 hours after consumption, lasts for 8–12 hours, and consists of distorted sensory perception, alteration of the sense of time and scale, and changes in body image (e.g. out-of-body experiences). The effects can be very intense and occasionally terrifying (a 'bad trip').

PCP and related substances are sold as a crystalline powder, paste, liquid or drug soaked paper (blotter). It is often used with cannabis. The picture of PCP abuse can resemble those of schizophrenia. At least two of the following symptoms are necessary to make a diagnosis of PCP intoxication; nystagmus, tachycardia, hypertension, ataxia, dysarthria, hyperacusis, muscle rigidity, numbness or diminished responsiveness, seizures and coma. Other hallucinogens will produce pupillary dilation, tachycardia, sweating, blurred vision, tremors and incoordination.

Hallucinogens rarely cause physical addiction, although psychological addiction is common. Users are frequently addicted to the PCP-induced psychological state. These are associated with flashbacks in which the sensations of a trip are re-experienced long afterwards. Emergency psychiatric referral may be indicated because of the panic or agitation associated with a 'bad trip'. Reassurance, reorientation and 'talking down' the person are necessary, but may not be effective in people who are high on PCP. Sedation with benzodiazepines and dopamine receptor agonists like Haloperidol may be required so that use of physical restraints is avoided. The person may also come to harm from responding to the hallucinations. It is best to avoid excessive sensory stimuli from the environment: nurse the patient under supervision in a quiet, dark room. The symptoms, including psychotic features, usually resolve within 24–72 hours. In cases where there has been prolonged use, the symptoms can persist for 4–6 weeks. The symptoms will resolve despite antipsychotic medication.

## 21.3.6 Inhalant-related disorders

Inhalants are a group of volatile substances that have mind-altering effects when inhaled. The intoxicating effect renders the substances prone to abuse (Nayyer, 2001). Inhalants are cheap, legal and easily available: they are commonly found in households. They are classified into categories of inhalants: volatile solvents, aerosols, gases (including medical anaesthetics) and nitrites (used primarily as sexual enhancers) (Volkow, 2012). Volatile solvents, gases and aerosols are often the easiest and first options for abuse by young children. Solvent misuse (of glue, aerosols, petrol, etc.) is mainly an adolescent male group activity (MacLean *et al.*, 2012). The effects are rapid in onset and short-lived; manifesting as euphoria, disinhibitions, blurred vision and ataxia. Solvent users come to medical attention when complications arise, mainly cardiac dysrhythmias, inhalation of vomit or coma. Chronic damage to the central nervous system and other organs can also occur.

In South Africa, glue is the most commonly abused substance amongst street children and people in disadvantaged communities (Peltzer and Ramlagan, 2010). The abuse occurs in both urban and rural settings, mostly by young adolescents. These are usually adolescents from poor socioeconomic conditions, have poor grades, have a history of childhood abuse and/or are school dropouts. The inhalants are usually used in different forms, by either emptying the contents into a plastic bag and then inhaled through the mouth and nose ('bagging'), sniffing or snorting the fumes from containers, spraying the aerosol directly into the mouth, stuffing a soaked rag into the mouth ('huffing') or inhaling from balloons filled with nitrous oxide.

Inhaled chemicals are quickly absorbed into the blood stream through the lungs and distributed to the brain and other organs. Response is within seconds and the effects are similar to alcohol intoxication. Slurred speech, inability to coordinate movements, dizziness, euphoria, light-headedness, hallucinations, delusions, loss of consciousness and death are common symptoms associated with inhalant intoxication. The person abusing inhalants may have paint or other stains on the face, clothes or hands, a drunken or disorientated appearance, slurred speech, inattentiveness, irritability and depression. Hidden empty spray bottles or solvent containers and chemical stains on clothes may be evident.

Cognitive impairment, seizure, hallucinations, cranial and peripheral neuropathies have been associated with gasoline abuse and optic neuropathy associated with methanol. Multifocal disorder, dementia, encephalopathy, cognitive dysfunction, brainstem abnormalities and cranial neuropathies have been linked to **toluene** abuse. Peripheral neuropathy has been associated with methyl butyl ketone abuse and encephalopathy is associated with methylene chloride.

## 21.3.7 Sedatives, hypnotics and anxiolytics use disorder

Sedatives, hypnotics and anxiolytics are also known as tranquillisers. Benzodiazepines and barbiturates are common examples of this group of drugs. The primary uses of these drugs are to cause calmness (sedative or anxiolytic), or to produce sleep (sedative-anxiolytic), relax muscles or control seizures (Sadock BJ and Sadock VA, 2007). Sedatives, hypnotics and/or anxiolytics use disorder may emerge from a prolonged or inappropriate use of these drugs after being appropriately prescribed for psychiatric conditions. They may also be used to alleviate the unwanted effects of these other substances.

Withdrawal symptoms from benzodiazepines usually occur after abrupt cessation and the individual may present with rebound insomnia and anxiety. The gradual withdrawal of the drug may still lead to insomnia, loss of appetite, tension, apprehension and anxiety. Severe and prolonged dependence may lead to severe withdrawal symptoms such as muscle weakness, tremor, hyper analgesia, nausea, vomiting, weight loss and possibly convulsions.

Methaqualone is another sedative-hypnotic drug that can be abused. When combined with diphenhydramine, an antihistamine, it is known as Mandrax (Ewart and Priest, 1967). Methaqualone was initially marketed as a sedative but it started being used as a recreational drug in the late 1960s and early 1970s and became known as 'lupes' (US), 'mandies' (UK), buttons or whites (Inaba *et al.*,1973). A 'white pipe' is methaqualone mixed with cannabis. The use of Mandrax is popular in the Western Cape and Eastern Cape regions of South Africa where it is mostly used by young male Coloured adults (Bhana *et al.*, 2002). It is also used by sex workers to relax after sex or before the next work shift (Needle, 2008). Physiogically, it can cause drowsiness, bradycardia, bradyspnoea, aphrodisia and paresthesias. Behaviorally, it can lead to aggression, mental disorientation and confusion. An overdose of Mandrax can be recognized by the patient experiencing delirium, convulsions, hypertonia, hyperreflexia, vomiting, renal failure, coma and death through cardiac or respiratory arrest.

## 21.3.8 Nicotine addiction

*Nicotiniana tabacum* and *Nicotiana rustica* are two variants of a tobacco plant. The addictive component is nicotine. Leaves from the tobacco plant are dried and shredded, then rolled into cigarettes or cigars or packaged as pipe, chewing tobacco or snuff. During the 20th century, cigarette smoking caused about a million deaths a year worldwide. It is estimated that by the 21st century, about a billion deaths will be directly due to tobacco if the trend of smoking is not curbed (Pahl *et al.*, 2010).

The current international tobacco smoking control measures are focused on preventing people from starting to smoke, and to help smokers to quit. The South African government imposed tobacco control measures in the 1990s, which restrict and/or ban the use of cigarettes in public places, flights and legislated the provision of enclosed smoking areas in privately-owned businesses (Steyn *et al.*; Peer *et al.*,2009). According to the Cancer Association of South Africa, the rate of adult smokers decreased from 32–28%. Young people are, however, still continuously targeted to start smoking.

The trend of young women and girls smoking has steadily increased over the years after a decline in the early 2000s. Most started smoking for weight control purposes. Most Coloured women in the South Africa's Western Cape province continued to smoke during pregnancy, subjecting the fetus to potential harm like premature births and or low birth-weight babies (Peer *et al.*, 2009). The leading causes of death from cigarette smoking in South Africa are chronic obstructive pulmonary disease (COPD), tuberculosis, lung cancer and ischaemic heart disease (IHD). In high-income countries the causes are different, IHD and lung cancer being the two main causes of death due to smoking.

However, despite the decrease in cigarette consumption following the implementation of the tobacco control policies, South Africa remains the biggest tobacco consumer in comparison to other African countries. In 1998, South Africa became the first country in the world to include a history of smoking in the deceased and his or her next of kin in the death registration form. This enabled researchers to make an accurate and informed decision of the number of deaths due to tobacco smoking.

Most people with psychiatric disorders smoke. Those with anxiety disorders and depressive disorders fail more often to quit smoking than other people. Patients with schizophrenia tend to smoke more due to the ability of nicotine to reduce the extraordinary sensitivity to outside stimuli and to increase concentration (Ratschen *et al.*, 2011).

Exposure to environmental tobacco smoking can be from passive smoking, exhaled mainstream smoking and side stream smoking. Passive smoking is defined as inhalation of environmental tobacco smoke; it can lead to dangerous health risks for both children and adults like low birth weight, asthma, bronchitis, pneumonia, middle ear infections, sudden infant death syndrome, miscarriages and cancers. Exhaled mainstream smoking is when a person smoking a burning cigarette, cigar or pipe breathes out the smoke onto someone else. Side stream smoking is smoke that is released from a burning cigarette, cigar or pipe.

Smokeless tobacco products are thought to be less dangerous than smoked tobacco. Snuff, which is commonly used by women, contains carcinogens and may lead to cancers of the oral cavity and increases risk of cancers of the neck and head. Chewing tobacco may lead to early tooth decay, halitosis, gingivitis and disturbances in taste buds. ***Snus*** (snooze), which requires no spitting, has been linked to pancreatic carcinoma (Rantao and Olalekan, 2012).

Water pipes (**hookahs** or hubbly bubblies) may be more dangerous than cigarette smoking as the user inhales longer over a prolonged smoking session, which lasts up to 60 minutes (World Health Organization, 2005). Evidence shows that it contains toxic compounds including tar, carbon monoxide, heavy metals and carcinogens. It has been linked to oral cancers, lung disease and ischaemic heart disease.

Electronic nicotine delivery systems (e-cigarettes) were first introduced to the US market from China in 2007. They have become popular because smokers use them as a smoking cessation tool. They were marketed as a healthier and cheaper alternative to normal cigarettes (McAuley *et al.*, 2012). E-cigarettes are battery operated and may contain nicotine or not. They also contain a liquid that vaporises when heated and flavourants (Trimachi and Cassidy, 2011). As little is known about their safety and effect on an individual, they are not approved by the Food and Drug Authority.

#### 21.3.8.1 Management

Nicotine is an addiction and quitting may be a big challenge. Smokers often struggle to stay off nicotine: joining a support group is recommended. Nicotine supplements, such as gums, patches, nasal sprays, acupuncture, herbal therapy, inhalers and lozenges, are available over the counter, and their success depends on the individual's motivation and commitment to quit. Hypnosis works for some, but not for all, who intend to quit. Prescription medications like the antidepressants Wellbutrin SR®, Zyban® and Champix® have yielded some positive results. Patients with depression and emotional instability have been known to have their mood aggravated when on varenicline (Champix®). A thorough psychiatric history should be obtained, including previous attempts to quit, previous suicidal thoughts and suicide attempts. Suicidal behaviour and severe depression have been noted. Treatment of an underlying psychiatric problem should also be attended to simultaneously.

### 21.3.9 Caffeine-related disorders

Caffeine withdrawal is now included as a disorder in the DSM-5. Caffeine is described as a mild stimulant. It is commonly found in drinks, foods, prescription medication and over-the-counter medication (Sadock BJ and Sadock VA, 2007). Close to 85% of adults world-wide use caffeine. At low doses, caffeine functions as a mild reinforcer. Studies have shown that caffeine causes vasoconstriction of the cerebral blood flow, resulting in a decreased amount of blood flow to the brain.

Caffeine intoxication occurs after consumption of 250 g of brewed coffee or 2–3 cups at a time. The person may experience five or more symptoms, such as restlessness, nervousness, excitement, insomnia, flushed face, diuresis, gastrointestinal disturbances, twitching, rambling flow of thought and speech, psychomotor agitation and tachycardia or cardiac arrhythmias (American Psychiatric Association, 2013).

The symptoms associated with caffeine withdrawal are transitory. They usually appear 24 hours after reducing or stopping prolonged caffeine use.

The person may present with headache, marked fatigue, dysphoric irritable or depressed mood, difficulty concentrating and flu-like symptoms (American Psychiatric Association, 2013).

Analgesics are commonly sufficient for the treatment of caffeine withdrawal symptoms. The patient is advised to keep a diary of all consumed caffeine, including medication, chocolates and drinks. A gradual reduction in the daily caffeine amount will minimise the withdrawal symptoms that the person might experience.

## 21.4 Gambling disorder

Gambling is defined as placing something of value at risk in the hopes of gaining something of greater value. There are two types of gambling activities: casino games (blackjack, roulette and slot machines) and non-casino games gambling (bingo, lotteries, card games, coin/dice tossing and sports betting). Recent years have seen the emergence of Internet-based or online gambling, which should also be considered when investigating a patient for problematic gambling activities.

Gambling disorder is a term introduced in the DSM-5 to describe persistent and recurrent problematic gambling behaviour that leads to clinically significant impairment or distress (American Psychiatric Association, 2013a).

Previously, **pathological gambling** (gambling disorder) was classified as an impulse-control disorder. After a review of the research and contributions from experts, the DSM-5 authors concluded that gambling disorder was not only co-morbid with substance use disorder but similar to these disorders; hence it was re-classified under the 'Substance-related disorder and addictive disorders' category (Hasin *et al.*, 2013). For example, gambling disorder also presents with the phenomena of tolerance, withdrawal and craving, which are critical diagnostic features for substance-related disorders (Lupi *et al.*, 2014).

### 21.4.1 Epidemiology

A study conducted in 2005 by the National Gambling Board of South Africa involving 3 100 respondents nationally aged 18 years and older showed that just under half of the respondent's participated in legalised gambling activities: mostly the lottery, playing scratch cards, casino gambling, sports betting and online gambling (Lighthelm, 2005). While most people may gamble without problems, approximately 5% will develop gambling-related problems and those with more severe **gambling problems** may meet criteria for pathological gambling (Potenza, 2013). In the general population worldwide, the past-year prevalence rate of gambling disorder is 0,2–5,3%, while the lifetime prevalence rate is 0,4–1% (Lupi *et al.*, 2014). In South Africa, the National Prevalence Study of 2006 of 3 000 participants found that, using the Gamblers Anonymous 20 Questions, 0,9% were pathological gamblers and 4,8% were **problem gamblers** (Collins and Barr, 2006). More recently it was found that the prevalence of problem gambling amongst poor South Africans living in rural and peri-urban communities was 2% (Dellis *et al.*, 2013).

Gambling disorder can emerge at any age but it usually develops over the course of years with increases in frequency and size of wagers placed. It is important to note that the frequency of participation in a particular type of gambling may not be problematic or symbolic of a gambling disorder, but less frequent participation in other forms of gambling may lead to, or be part of, the individual's pathological gambling problem. Similarly the amount spent on a particular form of gambling does not mean there is a gambling disorder. Other individuals who spend small amounts on the same form of gambling may go on to have substantial gambling-related difficulties or meet the criteria for having a gambling disorder (American Psychiatric Association, 2013a). The individual may experience a varying intensity to his or her gambling disorder: from increases when stressed to total abstinence, only to return to problematic gambling again.

There is a higher prevalence rates amongst males compared to females (American Psychiatric Association, 2013a). Gambling disorders emerges late in females. If the disorder appears early, it appears to be associated with impulsivity and substance abuse. There is a low rate of treatment seeking, which is even lower in younger individuals and better in females (Schafffer and Martin, 2011).

## 21.4.2 Diagnosis and assessment

It is difficult to identify or recognise gambling disorder, unless the patient readily admits to it; patients will generally present with affective symptoms and/or substance use disorder problems. Patients also tend to deny or hide symptoms of pathological gambling that are central to its treatment (DeCaria *et al.*, 1996). Apart from using the DSM-5 criteria for the diagnosis of gambling disorder, screening tests may also be used to help make the diagnosis. Examples of screening tests include the Problem Gambling Severity Index (which uses the DSM-IV classification as criteria) as noted in the appendix (see A21.1).

There may be features present in the individual that support the diagnosis of gambling disorder. These include distortions in thinking, where the individual has overvalued ideas of having power and control over chance events or is superstitious. Other individuals are impulsive, competitive and energetic (American Psychiatric Association, 2013a). Studies have revealed cognitive deficits such as problems with working memory, planning and time management in individuals with pathological gambling (Hodgins *et al.*, 2011). Further probing may reveal complications of having a gambling disorder. The individual may have lost important relationships, been abstinent from work or performed poorly at work and they may have become financially indebted. (Sadock BJ and Sadock VA, 2007).

The following circumstances and clinical conditions should be considered in the differential diagnosis for sambling disorders:

- Non-disordered gambling such as professional and social gambling (American Psychiatric Association, 2013a)
- A manic episode, where the manic symptoms persist even when the individual is not gambling (Soberay *et al.*, 2014)
- Personality disorders, which may exist concurrently with a gambling disorder (Miller *et al.*, 2013)
- Gambling induced by certain drugs such as dopaminergic medications for a patient with Parkinson's disease (Schaffer and Martin, 2011).

Several conditions may occur concurrently with a gambling disorder. Depressive, bipolar and anxiety disorders can occur along with the gambling disorder especially in females (American Psychiatric Association, 2013a). Substance-related disorders, especially alcohol disorders, are common in individuals with gambling disorders: 30–40% of pathological gamblers have a substance use disorder (Bowden-Jones and Clark, 2011). Substance-related disorders usually appear subsequent to gambling disorder whereas mood and anxiety disorders usually precede the gambling disorder (Hodgins *et al.*, 2011).

## 21.4.3 Aetiology

There are a numbers of risk factors for gambling disorder. These are personal traumas such as experiencing death, separation, divorce, desertion of a child before the age of 15, harsh or inappropriate parental discipline, early exposure of teenagers to gambling environments, families that stressed materialism and poor family budgeting.

There are neurobiological, genetic and psychosocial factors that underlie the aetiology of gambling disorders. Once the gambling disorder has set in, certain environmental and economic factors can maintain it. These include close proximity to gambling centres and attraction of large prize monies on offer (Lighthelm, 2005).

## 21.4.4 Treatment

### 21.4.4.1 Psychopharmacological treatment

No drug has received regulatory approval in any jurisdiction as a treatment for gambling disorders. Better and longer studies are needed before specific treatment can be recommended for gambling disorder.

If pathological gambling is believed to be secondary to another **primary psychiatric** disorder (e.g. bipolar disorder, OCD) it may be beneficial

**Table 21.2** DSM-5 Diagnostic Criteria for Gambling Disorder

| **Diagnostic Criteria** |
|---|
| A. Persistent and recurrent problematic gambling behavior leading to clinically significant impairment or distress, as indicated by the individual exhibiting four (or more) of the following in a 12-month period:<br>1. Needs to gamble with increasing amounts of money in order to achieve the desired excitement.<br>2 Is restless or irritable when attempting to cut down or stop gambling.<br>3. Has made repeated unsuccessful efforts to control, cut back, or stop gambling.<br>4. Is often preoccupied with gambling (e.g., having persistent thoughts of reliving past gambling experiences, handicapping or planning the next venture, thinking of ways to get money with which to gamble).<br>5. Often gambles when feeling distressed (e.g., helpless, guilty, anxious, depressed).<br>6. After losing money gambling, often returns another day to get even ('chasing' one's losses).<br>7. Lies to conceal the extent of involvement with gambling.<br>8. Has jeopardized or lost a significant relationship, job, or educational or career opportunity because of gambling.<br>9. Relies on others to provide money to relieve desperate financial situations caused by gambling.<br>B. The gambling behavior is not better explained by a manic episode.<br>*Specify* if:<br>▶ **Episodic:** Meeting diagnostic criteria at more than one time point, with symptoms subsiding between periods of gambling disorder for at least several months.<br>▶ **Persistent:** Experiencing continuous symptoms, to meet diagnostic criteria for multiple years.<br>*Specify* if:<br>▶ **In early remission:** After full criteria for gambling disorder were previously met, none of the criteria for gambling disorder have been met for at least 3 months but for less than 12 months.<br>▶ **In sustained remission:** After full criteria for gambling disorder were previously met, none of the criteria for gambling disorder have been met during a period of 12 months or longer.<br>*Specify* current severity:<br>▶ **Mild:** 4-5 criteria met.<br>▶ **Moderate:** 6–7 criteria met.<br>▶ **Severe:** 8–9 criteria met. |

**Source:** Reprinted with permission from the *Diagnostic and Statistical Manual of Mental Disorders*, Fifth Edition, (Copyright 2013). American Psychiatric Association.

to treat the primary disorder in order to ameliorate the patient's gambling problem.

### 21.4.4.2 Psychosocial treatment

Various interventions have been tested for their efficacy in treating gambling disorders. A combination of cognitive and behavioural therapies has been thought to possibly produce better outcomes and have, indeed, largely produced favourable results (Lopez *et al.*, 1997).

Gamblers Anonymous (GA) is a self-help **advocacy** group that follow similar principles underlying Alcoholics Anonymous. These include accepting the individual's gambling problem and powerlessness over gambling and surrendering to a 'higher power'. GA may be helpful in making the individual abstain from gambling – especially if done in combination with other interventions – but there are few outcome studies evaluating the effectiveness of Gamblers Anonymous (Hodgins *et al.*, 2011).

### 21.4.4.3 Self-exclusion (banning)

Some gamblers may want to ban themselves from gambling by preoccupying their time with other activities incompatible with gambling or avoiding cues to gambling. In some countries, this self-exclusion can be legally enforced. Individuals can voluntarily ban themselves from gambling venues for six months to a lifetime and they can be fined or charged by the state with trespassing if they break the ban (Napolitano, 2003).

Although patients with gambling disorder usually do not seek treatment, a third of this population will recover without treatment (Slutske, 2006).

## Conclusion

The use of substances and its associated medical and psychosocial effects are a burden on the health-care system in southern Africa and globally. There are known risk factors for people with an established substance use disorder and these disorders in turn make users vulnerable to developing mental illness. Therefore any clinician with a special interest in mental illness needs to have knowledge of substance use disorders. Some psychiatrists may go on to become addiction specialists and this chapter is intended to provide background information in order to facilitate such academic development. Still, management of these patients requires a comprehensive and multidisciplinary team approach to deal with the underlying psychiatric disorder and/or substance-related conditions. In South Africa, such an approach is compromised or not possible due to the restricted budget allocated to mental health on the whole, never mind for specialist drug rehabilitation facilities. This constrained budget has led to a lack of appropriate facilities and shortage of personnel experienced to deal with problems of substance abuse. It is therefore important for medical health-care professionals to have a basic knowledge of substance abuse to identify those individuals at risk of abusing substances, to recognise the signs and symptoms of chronic use, to readily identify the intoxication and withdrawal states and manage these states and the chronic use of substances adequately.

New or emergent addiction disorders unrelated to substances or drugs have also become the focus of clinical attention because of their significant psychosocial presentations and impact on the social and occupational function of the affected individual. One such disorder is gambling disorder, and it is important for clinicians to be aware and conversant in how to assist patients on how to manage this form of addiction as well.

# References


Acuda W, Othieno CJ, Obondo A, Crome IB (2011) The epidemiology of addiction in Sub-Saharan Africa: A Synthesis of Reports, Reviews, and Original Articles. *American Journal on Addictions* 20(2): 87–99

Alcohol and Drug Abuse Research Group (2004) *The Nature and Extent of Heroin Use In Cape Town: Part 2 - A community survey*. Pretoria: Medical Research Council

Alcohol and Drug Abuse Research Unit (2006) *South African Community Epidemiology Network on Drug Use (SACENDU) Report Back Meetings* Tygerberg, Western Cape: Medical Research Council

Alcohol and Drug Abuse Research Unit (2008) Audit of Substance Abuse Treatment Facilities in Free State, Limpopo, Mpumalanga, North West and Northern Cape (2007 - 2008): Technical Report South Africa: Medical Research Council

Alcoholics Anonymous (2012) *The Twelve Steps of Alcoholics Anonymous*. Available at: http://wwwaaorg/assets/en_US/smf-121_enpdf (accessed 12 September 2014.)

Amato L, Minozzi S, Pani PP, Solimini R, Vecchi S, Zuccaro P, Davoli M (2011) Dopamine agonists for the treatment of cocaine dependence. *Cochrane Database of Systematic Reviews* Issue 12 Art No: CD003352 DOI: 101002/14651858CD003352pub3

American Psychiatric Association (2000) *Diagnostic and statistical manual of mental disorders DSM-IV-TR* Washington DC American Psychiatric Association

American Psychiatric Association (2010a) *Practice Guidelines for the Treatment of Patients with Substance Use Disorders* (2nd edition). Washington DC: American Psychiatric Association DOI: 101176/appibooks9780890423363141077

American Psychiatric Association (2010b) *Treating Substance Use Disorders: A Quick Reference Guide* (2nd edition). Washington DC: American Psychiatric Association DOI: 101176/appibooks9780890423370145633

American Psychiatric Association (2013a) *Diagnostic and Statistical Manual of Mental Disorders* (5th edition). Washington DC: American Psychiatric Assocation

American Psychiatric Association (2013b) *Substance-related and addictive disorders*. Available at: http://www.dsm5.org/Documents/Substance Use Disorder Fact Sheet (Accessed 27 March 2015)

Arseneault L, Cannon M, Witton J, Murray RM (2004) Causal association between cannabis and psychosis:

Examination of the evidence. *The British Journal of Psychiatry* 184: 110–7

Baigent M (2012) Managing patients with dual diagnosis in psychiatric practice. *Current Opinion in Psychiatry* 25(3): 201–5

Bailey LG, Maxwell S, Brandabur MM (1997) Substance abuse as a risk factor for tardive dyskinesia: A retrospective analysis of 1027 patients. *Psychopharmacology Bulletin* 33:177–181

Bakken K, Landheim AS, Vaglum P (2004) Early and late onset groups of substance misusers: Differences in primary and secondary psychiatric disorders. *Journal of Substance Use* 9(5): 224–34

Becker JB, Hu M (2008) Sex differences in drug abuse. *Frontiers in Neuroendocrinology* 29(1): 36–47

Bhana A, Parry CD, Myers B, Pliiddemann A, Morojele NK, Flisher AJ (2002) The South African Community Epidemiology Network on Drug Use(SACENDU) Project Phase 1–9 - Cannabis and Mandrax. *South African Medical Journal* 92: 542–547

Bjork JM, Grant SJ (2009) Does traumatic brain injury increase risk for substance abuse? *Journal of Neurotrauma* 26(7): 1077–82

Bowden-Jones H, Clark L 2011 Pathological gambling: a neurobiological and clinical update. *British Journal of Psychiatry* 199(2): 87–90

Brackins T, Brahm NC, Kissack JC (2011) Treatments for methamphetamine abuse: A literature review for the clinician. *Journal of Pharmacy Practice* 24(6): 541–50

Brink S, Oosthuizen P, Emsley R, Mbanga I, Keyter N (2003) Relationship between substance abuse and first-episode psychosis - a South African perspective. *South African Journal of Psychiatry* 9(1): 7–12

Brook JS, Pahl T, Morojele NK, Brook DW (2006) Predictors of drug use among South African adolescents. *Journal of Adolescent Health* 38(1): 26–34 DOI: 10.1016/j.jadohealth.2004.08.004.

Cadoret RJ (1992) Genetic and environmental factors in initiation of drug abuse and the transition to abuse. In: Glanz M, Pickens R (Eds). *Vulnerability to Drug Abuse.* Washington DC: American Psychological Association

Cancer Association of South Africa (CANSA) (2014) *Position statement on tobacco products.* http://www.cansa.org.za/files/2014/09/Position-Statement-Tobacco-Products-Sept-2014.pdf (Accessed 26 March 2015)

Carroll KM, Onken LS (2005) Behavioral therapies for drug abuse. *American Journal of Psychiatry* 162: 1452–60

Centre for Addiction and Mental Health (s.d.) *Problem Gambling Severity Index (PGSI).* Available at: http://www.problemgambling.ca/EN/ResourcesForProfessionals/pages/problemgamblingseverityindexpgsi.aspx. (Accessed 3 February 2015.)

Chapman S (2013) *Rat poison and heroin.* Available at: http://wwwmahalacoza/reality/rat poison and heroin (accessed 25 December 2013.)

Chen H, Wu J, Zhang J, Hashimoto K (2010) Recent topics on pharmacotherapy for amphetamine-type stimulants abuse and dependence. *Current Drug Abuse Reviews* 3(4): 222–38

Clay SW, Allen J, Parran T (2008) A Review of Addiction. *Postgraduate Medicine* 120(2): E01–7

Collins P, Barr G (2006) *The National Prevalence Study 2006: Gambling and problem gambling in South Africa.* Cape Town: National Centre for the Study of Gambling. Available from: http://www.responsiblegambling.co.za/media/user/documents/NRGP%20Prevalence%20Study%202006.pdf. (Accessed 5 September 2015)

Conway KP, Compton W, Stinson FS, Grant BF (2006) Lifetime comorbidity of DSM-IV mood and anxiety disorders and specific drug use disorders: Results from the National Epidemiologic Survey on Alcohol and Related Conditions. *Journal of Clinical Psychiatry* 67: 247–57

Cornelius MD, Leech SL, Goldschmidt L, Day NL (2005) Is prenatal tobacco exposure a risk factor for early adolescent smoking? A follow-up study. *Neurotoxicology and Teratology* 27(4):667–67

Cuyas E, Verdejo-Garcia A, Fagundo AB, Khymenets O, Rodriguez J, Cuenca A, de Sola Llopis S, Langohr K, Pena-Casanova J, Torrens M, Martin-Santos R, Farre M, de la Torre R (2011) The influence of genetic and environmental factors among MDMA users in cognitive performance. *PLoS ONE* 6(11): e27206

Darke S, Kaye S, McKetin R, Duflou J (2008) Major physical and psychological harms of methamphetamine use. *Drug and Alcohol Review* 27(3): 253–62

Darke S, Torok M, McKetin R, Kaye S, Ross J (2011) Patterns of psychological distress related to regular methamphetamine and opioid use. *Addiction Research and Theory* 19(2): 121–7

Day NL, Goldschmidt L, Thomas CA (2006) Prenatal marijuana exposure contributes to the prediction of marijuana use at age 14. *Addiction* 101(9): 1313–132

DeCaria CM, Hollander E, Grossman R, Wong CM, Mosovich SA, Cherkasky S (1996) Diagnosis, neurobiology and treatment of pathological gambling. *The Journal of Clinical Psychiatry* 57 (suppl 8): 80–4

Delaney-Black V, Chiodo LM, Hannigan JH, Greenwald MK, Janisse J, Patterson G, Huestis MA, Partridge RT, AgerJ, Sokol RJ (2011) Prenatal and postnatal cocaine exposure predict teen cocaine use. *Neurotoxicology and Teratology* 33(1): 110–9

Dellis A, Spurrett D, Hofmeyr A, Sharp C, Ross D (2013) Gambling participation and problem gambling severity among rural and peri-urban poor South African adults in KwaZulu-Natal. *Journal of Gambling Studies* 29(3): 417–33

Department of Veteran Affairs, Department of Defense (2009) *VA/DoD clinical practice guideline for management of substance use disorders (SUD).* Washington, DC: Department of Veteran Affairs, Department of Defense). Available at: http://wwwguidelinegov/contentaspx?id=15676 (Accessed 18 June 2014.)

Drake RE, Mueser KT, Brunette MF (2007) Management of persons with co-occurring severe mental illness and substance use disorder: Program Implication. *World Psychiatry* 6: 131–136

Evans DJ Pillay AL (2009) Mental health problems of men attending district-level clinical psychology services in South Africa. *Psychological Reports* 104(3): 773–83

Ewart RB, Priest RG (1967) Methaqualone addiction and delirium tremens. *British Medical Journal* 3: 92–93

Fajemirokun-Odudeyo O, Sinha C, Tutty S, Pairaudeau P, Armstrong D, Phillip T Lindow SW (2006) Pregnancy outcome in women who use opiates. *European Journal of Obstetrics and Gynecology and Reproductive Biology* 126(2): 170

False Bay Therapeutic Community Centre (2014) *Tik*. Available at: http://www.falsebaytc.co.za/drug-information/tik/ (Accessed 05 July 2014.)

Faraone SV, Wilens T (2003) Does stimulant treatment lead to substance use disorders? *Journal of Clinical Psychiatry* 64 (Suppl. 11): 9–13

Fenton MC, Keyes K, Geier T, Greenstein E, Skodol A, Krueger B, Grant BF, Hasin DS (2012) Psychiatric comorbidity and the persistence of drug use disorders in the United States. *Addiction* 107(3): 599–609

Ferris J, Wynne H J (2001a) *The Canadian Problem Gambling Index*. Ottawa: Canadian Centre on Substance Abuse

Gardner EL (2005) Endocannabinoid signaling system and brain reward: Emphasis on dopamine. *Pharmacology Biochemistry and Behavior* 81(2): 263–84

Gorelick DA (2014) *Treatment of cocaine use disorder in adults*. UpTodate Available at: http://wwwuptodatecom/contents/treatment-of-cocaine-use-disorder-in-adults (Accessed 23 June 2014.)

Gowing L, Henry-Edwards S, Irvine R, Ali R (2002) The health effects of ecstasy: A literature review. *Drug and Alcohol Review* 21: 53–63

Grant JE, Potenza MN, Weinstein A, Gorelick DA (2010) Introduction to behavioral addictions. American *Journal of Drug and Alcohol Abuse* 36(5): 233–41

Harvard Medical School (2010) *Addition in women*. http://www.health.harvard.edu/newsletter_article/addition-in-women (Accessed 27 March 2015)

Hasin DS, O'Brien CP, Auriacombe M, Borges G, Bucholz K, Budney A, Compton WM, Crowley T, Ling W, Petry NM, Schuckit M, Grant BF (2013) DSM-5 criteria for substance use disorders: Recommendations and rationale. *American Journal of Psychiatry* 170: 834–51

Hatfield AB (2008) *Dual diagnosis and mental illness. Schizophrenia and drug or alcohol dependence*. Available at: http://www.schizophrenia.com/family/dualdiaghtml (Accessed March 2014.)

Havenaar JM, Geerlings MI, Vivian L, Collinson M, Robertson B (2008) Common mental health problems in historically disadvantaged urban and rural communities in South Africa: Prevalence and risk factors. *Social Psychiatry and Psychiatric Epidemiology* 43(3): 209–15

Helmbrecht GD, Thiagarajah S (2008) Management of addiction disorders in pregnancy. *Journal of Addiction Medicine* 2(1): 1

Henry-Edwards S, Humeniuk R, Ali R, Monteiro M, Poznyak, V (2003) *Brief Intervention for Substance Use: A Manual for Use in Primary Care* (Draft Version 11 for Field Testing) Geneva: World Health Organization

Hodgins DC, Stea JN, Grant E (2011) Gambling disorders. *The Lancet* 378: 1874–84

Hofmann FG (1983) *A Handbook on Drug and Alcohol Abuse: The Biomedical Aspects* (2nd edition). New York: Oxford University Press

Hubbard RL, Craddock G, Rynn PM, Anderson J, Etheridge RM (1997) Overview of 1-year follow-up outcomes in the Drug Abuse Treatment Outcome Study (DATOS). *Psychology of Addictive Behaviors* 11(4): 261–278

Inaba DS, Gay GR, Newmeyer JA, Whitehead C (1973) Methaqualone abuse: 'Luding Out'. *JAMA* 224(11):1505–9

Kapp C (2008) Crystal meth boom adds to South Africa's health challenges. *The Lancet* 371(9608):193–4

Kelly TM, Daley DC, Douaihy AB (2012) Treatment of substance abusing patients with comorbid psychiatric disorders. *Addictive Behaviors* 37(1):11–24

Kendler KS, Sundquist K, Ohlsson H, Palmer K, Maes H, Winkleby MA, Sundquist J (2012) Genetic and familial environmental influences on the risk for drug abuse: A national Swedish adoption study. *Archives of General Psychiatry* 69(7): 690–697

Kessler RC (2004) The epidemiology of dual diagnosis. *Biological Psychiatry* 56:730–7

Khantzian EJ (1985) The self-medication thesis of addictive disorders: Focus on health and cocaine dependence. *American Journal of Psychiatry* 142: 1259–64

Kolliakou A, Joseph C, Ismail K, Atakan Z, Murray RM (2011) Why do patients with psychosis use cannabis and are they ready to change their use? *International Journal of Developmental Neuroscience* 29(3):335–46

Kuhar MJ (2010) Contributions of basic science to understanding addiction. *BioSocieties* 5(1 special issue): 25–35

Larm P, Hodgins S, Tengstrom A, Larsson A (2010) Trajectories of resilience over 25 years of individuals who as adolescents consulted for substance misuse and a matched comparison group. *Addiction* 105(7): 1216–25. DOI:10.1111/j.1360-0443. 2010.02914.x

Latimer W, Zur J (2010) Epidemiologic trends of adolescent use of alcohol tobacco and other drugs. *Child and Adolescent Psychiatric Clinics of North America* 19(3):451–64

Le Moal M (2009) Drug Abuse: Vulnerability and transition. *Pharmacopsychiatry* 42 (Suppl. 1): S42–S55)

Lev-Ran S, Imtiaz S, Rehm J, Le Foll B (2013) Exploring the association between lifetime prevalence of mental illness and transition from substance use to substance use disorders: Results from the National Epidemiologic Survey of Alcohol and Related Conditions (NESARC). *The American Journal on Addictions* 22: 93–98

Leyton M (2013) Are addictions diseases or choices? *Journal of Psychiatry and Neuroscience* 38(4):219–21

Lighthelm AA (2005) *Economic impact of legalised gambling in South Africa*. Pretoria: National Gambling Board

Lopez Viets VC, Miller WR (1997) Treatment approaches for pathological gamblers. *Clinical Psychology Review* 17(7): 689–702

Lupi M, Martinotti G, Acciavatti T, Pettorruso M, Brunetti M, Santacroce R, Cinosi E, Di Iorio G, Di Nicola M, Massimo Di Giannantonio M (2014) Pharmacological treatments in gambling disorder: A qualitative review. *Biomedical Research International*, 14. Article intellectual disability: 537306

Lyons MJ, Toomey R, Meyer JM, Green AI, Eisen SI, Goldberg J, True WR Tsuang MT (1997) How do genes influence marijuana use? The role of subjective effects. *Addiction* 92: 409–17

MacLean S, Cameron S, Harney A, Lee NK (2012) Psychosocial therapeutic interventions for volatile substance use: A systematic review. *Addiction* 107(2): 278–88

Malivert M, Fatseas M, Denis C, Langlois E, Auriacombe M (2012) Effectiveness of therapeutic communities: A systematic review. *European Addiction Research* 18(1): 1–11

Manchikanti L, Fellows B, Ailinani H, Pampati V (2010) Therapeutic use abuse and nonmedical use of opioids: A ten-year perspective. *Pain Physician* 13(5): 401–35

Mancini MA, Wyrick-Waugh W (2013) Consumer and practitioner perceptions of the harm reduction approach in a community mental health setting. *Community Mental Health Journal* 49: 14–24

Maniglio R (2011) The role of child sexual abuse in the etiology of substance-related disorders. *Journal of Addictive Diseases* 30(3): 216–28

McAuley TR, Hopke PK, Zhao J, Babaian S (2012) Comparison of the effects of e-cigarette vapour and cigarette smoke on indoor air quality. *Inhalation toxicology* 24(12): 850–7

McCarty D, BraudeL Russell LymanD, Dougherty RH, Daniels AS, Shoma Ghose S, Delphin-Rittmon ME (2014) Substance abuse intensive outpatient programs: Assessing the evidence. *Psychiatric Services* 65: 6. DOI: 10.1176/appi.ps.201300249

McHugh RK, Hearon BA, Otto MW (2010) Cognitive-behavioral therapy for substance use disorders. *Psychiatric Clinic of North America* 33(3): 511–25

Merikangas KR, McClair VL (2012) Epidemiology of substance use disorders. *Human Genetics* 131(6): 779–89

Merikangas KR, Stolar M, Stevens DE, Goulet J, Preisig MA, Fenton B, Zhang H, OMalley SS, Rounsaville BJ (1998) Familial transmission of substance use disorders. *Archives of General Psychiatry* 55:973–9

Miller JD, MacKillop J, Fortune EE, Maples J, Lance CE, Campbell WK Goodiet AS (2013) Personality correlates of pathological gambling derived from Big Three and Big Five personality models. *Psychiatry Research* 206: 50–55

Murthy P, Chand P (2012) Treatment of dual diagnosis disorders. *Current Opinion in Psychiatry* 25(3): 194–200

Myers B, Fakier N, Louw J (2009) Stigma, treatment beliefs, and substance abuse treatment use in historically disadvantaged communities. *African Journal of Psychiatry* 12: 218–22

Myers B, Harker N, Fakier N, Kader R, Mazok C (2008) *A review of evidence-based interventions for the prevention and treatment of substance use disorders.* (Draft report) Available at: http://www.sahealthinfo.org/admodule/evidencepdf (Accessed 3 March 2014.)

Myers B, Parry CDH, Karassellos C, Jardine G (2006) Methamphetamine abuse psychosis and your patient. *SA Family Practice* 48(2):56–7

Napolitano F (2003) The self-exclusion program: Legal and clinical considerations. *Journal of Gambling Studies* 19(3):303–15

National Institute on Drug Abuse (2003) *Preventing Drug Use among Children and Adolescents: A Research-Based Guide for Parents, Educators and Community Leaders* (2nd edition). Bethesda, MD: National Institute on Drug Abuse. Available at: http://wwwdrugabusegov/sites/default/files/preventingdruguse_2pdf (Accessed 5 March 2014.)

National Institute on Drug Abuse (2012) *DrugFacts: Inhalants.* Bethesda. MD: National Institute on Drug Abuse NIH DHHS Available at: http://www.drugabuse.gov/publications/drugfacts/inhalants Revised September 2012) (Accessed 15 December 2012.)

Nayyer I (2001) Neurotoxic effects of inhalants. *Annals of Saudi Medicine* 21(3–4): 216–8

Needle R, Kroeger K, Belani H, Achrekar A, Parry CD, Dewing S (2008) Sex, drugs, and HIV: Rapid assessment of HIV risk behaviors among street-based drug using sex workers in Durban, South Africa. *Social Science and Medicine* 67:1447–55

O'Brien CP, Volkow N, Li T-K (2006) What's in a word? Addiction versus dependence in DSM-V. *American Journal of Psychiatry* 163: 764–5

Odejide AO (2006) Status of drug use/abuse in Africa: A review. *International Journal of Mental Health Addict* 4: 87–102 DOI: 101007/s11469-006-9015

Oshri A, Rogosch FA, Burnette ML, Cicchetti D (2011) Developmental pathways to adolescent cannabis abuse and dependence: Child maltreatment, emerging personality, and internalizing versus externalizing psychopathology. *Psychology of Addictive Behaviors* 25(4):634–44

Pahl K, Brook DW, Morojele NK, Brook JS (2010) Nicotine dependence and problem behaviours among urban South African adolescents. *Journal of Behavioural Medicine* 33(2): 101–9

Pani PP, Trogu E, Vecchi S, Amato L (2011) Antidepressants for cocaine dependence and problematic cocaine use. *Cochrane Database of Systematic Reviews.* Issue 12, Art. No. CD002950. DOI: 101002/14651858CD002950pub3

Parry CDH (2005) Substance abuse intervention in South Africa. *World Psychiatry* 4(1): 34–5

Peer N, Bradshaw D, Laubscher R, Steyn K (2009) Trends in adult tobacco use from two South African demographic and health surveys conducted in 1998 and 2003. *South African Medical Journal* 99(10): 744–9

Peltzer K (2009) Prevalence and correlates of substance use among school children in six African countries. *International Journal of Psychology* 44(5): 378-386

Peltzer K, Ramlagan (2010) Illicit drug use in South Africa: Findings from a 2008 national population-based survey. *South African Journal of Psychiatry* 16(1): 8–15

Plüddemann A, Flisher AJ, McKetin R, Parry C, Lombard C (2010) Methamphetamine use, aggressive behaviour and other mental health issues among high school students in Cape Town, South Africa. *Drug and Alcohol Dependence* 109(1–3): 14–19

Porath AJ, Fried PA (2005) Effects of prenatal cigarette and marijuana exposure on drug use among offspring. *Neurotoxicology and Teratology* 27(2): 267–77

Potenza MN (2013) Neurobiology of gambling behaviours. *Current Opinion in Neurobiology* 23(4): 660–7

Ramlagan S, Peltzer K, Matseke G (2010) Epidemiology of drug abuse treatment in South Africa. *South African Journal of Psychiatry* 16(2): 40–9

Rantao M, Olalekan A (2012) Dual use of cigarettes and smokeless tobacco among South African adolescents. *American Journal of Health Behavior* 36(1):124–33

Rathbone J, Variend H, Mehta H (2008) Cannabis and schizophrenia. *Cochrane Database of Systematic Reviews.* Issue 3, Art. No. CD004837. DOI: 101002/14651858CD004837pub2

Ratschen E, Britton J, Mcnell A (2011) The smoking culture in psychiatry. *British Journal of Psychiatry* 198(1): 6–7

Reddy SP, James S, Sewpaul R, Koopman F, Funani NI, Sifunda S, Josie J, Masuka P, Kambaran NS, Omardien RG (2010) *Umthente Uhlaba Usamila – The South African Youth Risk Behaviour Survey 2008.* Cape Town: South African Medical Research Council Available at:

http://www.mrc.ac.za/pressreleases/2010/yrbs_2008_final_report.pdf (Accessed 15 November 2014)

Robledo P (2010) Cannabinoids, opioids and MDMA: neuropsychological interactions related to addiction. *Current Drug Targets* 11(4):429–39

Rose ME, Grant JE (2008) Pharmacotherapy for methamphetamine dependence: A review of the pathophysiology of methamphetamine addiction and the theoretical basis and efficacy of pharmacotherapeutic interventions. *Annals of Clinical Psychiatry* 20(3):145–55

Rowe CL (2012) Family therapy for drug abuse: Review and updates 2003 – 2010. *Journal of Marital and Family Therapy* 38(1):59–81

Rush CR, Stoops WW (2012) Agonist replacement therapy for cocaine dependence: A translational review. *Future Medicinal Chemistry* 4(2): 245–65

Sadock BJ, Sadock VA (2007) *Kaplan and Sadock's Synopsis of Psychiatry: Behavioral Sciences/Clinical Psychiatry* (10th edition). Philadelphia: Lippincott Williams and Wilkins

Sato M, Numachi Y, Hamamura T (1992) Relapse of paranoid psychotic state in methamphetamine model of schizophrenia. *Schizophrenia Bulletin* 18(1):115–22

Schafffer J, Martin R (2011) Disordered gambling: Etiology, trajectory and clinical considerations. *Annual Review of Clinical Psychology* 7:483–510

Shoptaw SJ, Kao U, Ling W (2009) Treatment for amphetamine psychosis. *Cochrane Database of Systematic Reviews*. Issue 1, Art. No. CD003026. DOI: 101002/14651858CD003026pub3

Simpson DD (2001) Modeling treatment process and outcomes. *Addiction* 96: 207–211

Skosana I (2014) We need to talk about caving in to nyaope. *The Mail and Guardian*. Available at: http://mgcoza/article/ (2014) -06-06-we-need-to-talk-about-caving-in-to-nyaope (Accessed 5 July 2014.)

Slutske WS (2006) Natural recovery and treatment-seeking in pathological gambling: Results of two US national surveys. *American Journal of Psychiatry* 163(2):297–302

Soberay A, Faragher JM, Barbash M, Brookover A, Grimsley P (2014) Pathological gambling, co-occurring disorders, clinical presentation and treatment outcomes at a university based counselling clinic. *Journal of Gambling Studies* 30:61–9

South African Community Epidemiology Network on Drug Use (2010) Monitoring alcohol and drug abuse trends in South Africa, July 1996 - June 2010. *SACENDU Research Brief* 13(2): 1–16

South African Medical Research Council (2003) *Umthenthe Uhlaba Usamila- The South African Youth Risk Behaviour Survey 2002.* Cape Town: South African Medical Research Council

Stein DJ, Seedat S, Herman A, Moomal H, Heeringa SG, Kessler RC, Williams DR (2008) Lifetime prevalence of psychiatric disorders in South Africa. *British Journal of Psychiatry* 192(2): 112–7

Sterling S, Felicia C, Hinman A (2011) Integrating care for people with co-occurring alcohol and other drug, medical, and mental health conditions. *Alcohol Research and Health* 33(4): 338–49

Substance Abuse and Mental Health Services Administration (2012) *Results from the 2011 National Survey on Drug Use and Health: Summary of National Findings.* Rockville MD: Substance Abuse and Mental Health Services Administration

Sweeting M, Farrell M (2005) Methamphetamine psychosis: How is it related to schizophrenia? A review of the literature. *Current Psychiatry Reviews* 1(2): 115–22

Swinson RP (2006) Clinical practice guidelines for the management of anxiety disorders. *Canadian Journal of Psychiatry* 51: 1S-92S

Taylor D, Paton C, Kapur S (2012) *Prescribing Guidelines in Psychiatry* (11th edition). Oxford: Wiley-Blackwell

Treatment Improvement Protocol (TIP) Series No 42 (2005) Center for Substance Abuse Treatment Rockville (MD): Substance Abuse and Mental Health Services Administration (US)

Trimachi M, Cassidy S (2011) *10 Little facts about e-cigarettes*. Available at: http://healthhowstuffworkscom/wellness/smoking cessation/10 facts (Accessed 19 September 2014.)

Tsuang MT, Lyons MJ, Eisen SA, Goldberg J, True W, Lin N, Meyer JM, Toomey R, Faraone SV, Eaves L (1996) Genetic influences on DSM-III-R drug abuse and dependence: A study of 3372 twin pairs. *American Journal of Medical Genetics* 67(5): 473–7

Valente TW, Gallaher P, Mouttapa M (2004) Using social networks to understand and prevent substance use: A transdisciplinary perspective. *Substance Use and Misuse* 39(10–12): 1685–712

Van Heerden MS, Grimsrud AT, Seedat S, Myer L, Williams DR, Stein DJ (2009) Patterns of substance use in South Africa: Results from the South African Stress and Health Study. *South African Medical Journal* 99(5 Pt 2): 358–66

Vocci FJ, Montoya ID (2009) Psychological treatments for stimulant misuse, comparing and contrasting those for amphetamine dependence and those for cocaine dependence. *Current Opinion in Psychiatry* 22(3):263–8

Volkow ND (2012) National institute of Drug Abuse Research report series Inhalant Abuse

Vrecko S (2010) Birth of a brain disease: Science, the state and addiction neuropolitics. *History of the Human Sciences* 23(4): 52–67

Vroegop MP, Franssen EJ, van der Voort PH, van den Berg TN, Langeweg RJ, Kramers C (2009) The emergency care of cocaine intoxications. *Netherlands Journal of Medicine* 67(4):122–6

Weich EW (2006) Substance use disorders. *Continuing Medical Education* 24(8): 436–40

Weich L, Perkel C, van Zyl N, Rataimane S, Naidoo L (2008) South African guidelines for the management of opioid dependence. *South African Medical Journal* 98(4): 280–3

Weich L, Pienaar W (2009) Occurrence of comorbid substance use disorders among acute psychiatric inpatients at Stikland Hospital in the Western Cape, South Africa. *African Journal of Psychiatry* 12(3):213–7

Weinstein AM, Gorelick DA (2011) pharmacological treatment of cannabis dependence. *Current Pharmaceutical Design* 17(14): 1351–8

Wilkes S (2008) The use of bupropion SR in cigarette smoking cessation. *International Journal of Chronic Obstructive Pulmonary Disease* Dis 3(1): 45–53. (Available at: http://www.ncb.inlm.nih.gov/pmc/articles/PMC2528204/

Wilnes MD (2004) Impact of ADHD and its treatment on substance abuse in adults. *Journal of Clinical Psychiatry* 65 (Suppl. 3):38–45

World Health Organisation Study Group on Tobacco Product Regulations (2005) *Water pipe tobacco smoking: Health effects, research needs by regulators*. Geneva: World Health Organization. Geneva Switzerland. Available at: http://webtoolsplace.com/doc/pdf/download/www__who__int--tobacco--global_interaction--tobreg--Waterpipe%20recommendation_Final.pdf . (Accessed 27 June 2014.)

Uhl G, Blum K, Noble E, Smith S (1993) Substance abuse vulnerability and $D_2$ receptor genes. *Trends in Neuroscience* 16(3):83–8

United States Department of Health and Human Services (2012) *Results from the 2011 National Survey on Drug Use and Health: Summary of national findings*. Rockville, MD: US Dept of Health and Human Services Available at: http://www.samhsa.gov/data/NSDUH/2k11MH_FindingsandDetTables/2K11MHFR/NSDUHmhfr2011.htm#1.1 (Accessed 14 March 2014.)

Ziedonis DM, Smelson D, Rosenthal RN, Batki SL, Green AI, Henry RJ, Montoya I, Parks J, Weiss RD (2005) Improving the care of individuals with schizophrenia and substance use disorders: consensus recommendations. *Journal of Psychiatric Practice* 11(5):315-39

# Appendix 21.1

**Table A21.3** Problem Gambling Severity Index (DSM-IV classification criteria)

Thinking about the last 12 months

1. Have you bet more than you could really afford to lose?

   Never=0 Sometimes=1 Most of the time=2 Almost always=3
2. Still thinking about the last 12 month, have you needed to gamble with larger amounts of money to get the same feeling of excitement?

   Never=0 Sometimes=1 Most of the time=2 Almost always=3
3. When you gambled, did you go back another day to try to win back the money you lost?

   Never=0 Sometimes=1 Most of the time=2 Almost always=3
4. Have you borrowed money or sold anything to get money to gamble?

   Never=0 Sometimes=1 Most of the time=2 Almost always=3
5. Have you felt that you might have a problem with gambling?

   Never=0 Sometimes=1 Most of the time=2 Almost always=3
6. Has gambling caused you any health problems, including stress or anxiety?

   Never=0 Sometimes=1 Most of the time=2 Almost always=3
7. Have people criticized your betting or told you that you had a gambling problem, regardless of whether or not you thought it was true?

   Never=0 Sometimes=1 Most of the time=2 Almost always=3
8. Has your gambling caused any financial problems for you or your household?

   Never=0 Sometimes=1 Most of the time=2 Almost always=3
9. Have you felt guilty about the way you gamble or what happens when you gamble?

   Never=0 Sometimes=1 Most of the time=2 Almost always=3

**Total Score**

Total your score. The higher your score, the greater the risk that your gambling is a problem.

Score of 0 = Non-problem gambling.

Score of 1 or 2 = Low level of problems with few or no identified negative consequences.

Score of 3 to 7 = Moderate level of problems leading to some negative consequences.

Score of 8 or more = Problem gambling with negative consequences and a possible loss of control.

**Source:** Ferris and Wynne, 2001

CHAPTER

# 22 Eating and sleep disorders

*Christopher Szabo, Chris Verster*

# Eating disorders

## 22.1 Introduction

The introduction of the Diagnostic and Statistical Manual for Mental Disorders (DSM-5) (American Psychiatric Association, 2013) has seen the conditions previously grouped as eating disorders in the DSM-IV (American Psychiatric Association, 1994) renamed 'Feeding and eating disorders'. This shift in focus consequently includes a range of diagnostic entities (e.g. **pica**, rumination disorder) that do not conform to those typically associated with eating disorders. For the purposes of this chapter the focus will be on those conditions most typically classified as eating disorders: anorexia nervosa (AN), bulimia nervosa (BN) and a newly recognised condition: binge-eating disorder (BED).

Eating disorders have typically constituted a group of diagnostic entities whose core pathology relates to an excessive and inappropriate concern with weight and shape. In essence, eating disorders operate on three levels: thinking, behaviour and consequences. Invariably the sufferer has made efforts to address his or her concerns about body weight and shape through dietary manipulation, thus leading to disturbances in physical and emotional well-being. Its impact on the sufferer's cognitive ability also impairs social, occupational and academic functioning.

These conditions affect predominantly young females, with 12-month prevalence rates of 0,4% for anorexia and 1%–1,5% for bulimia (American Psychiatric Association, 2013). Whilst this is generally understood as the group most at risk, eating disorders are not constrained by either age or gender. Specifically, they do occur in men, with South African research documenting their existence locally (Freeman and Szabo, 2005). Whilst the exact prevalence in men is not established, it has been noted that the ratio of women:men with these conditions is about 10:1 (American Psychiatric Association, 2013). In addition, the notion that race may also be a determinant of vulnerability (i.e. not occurring in black females) has certainly been dispelled both internationally and in South Africa (Szabo *et al.*, 1995). Members from all racial groups are at risk, specifically within urban settings. This has particular relevance to South Africa in terms of the emergence of eating disorders amongst black females. Aside from the impact of eating disorders on a range of domains of functioning, these conditions are also associated with mortality. Although most sufferers will recover to varying degrees, one should be mindful of the potential for fatal outcomes.

## 22.2 Diagnostic entities

According to the DSM-5 eating disorders are currently classified as 'feeding and eating disorders' with a range of diagnostic entities. These include:

- pica
- rumination disorder
- avoidant/restrictive food intake disorder
- anorexia nervosa
- bulimia nervosa
- binge-eating disorder

- other specified feeding or eating disorder
- unspecified feeding or eating disorder.

This chapter will focus on anorexia nervosa, bulimia nervosa and binge – eating disorder. Whilst each of these conditions has their own diagnostic criteria, there is some overlap with certain features being shared by the conditions.

## 22.2.1 Anorexia nervosa

Anorexia nervosa is characterised by restriction. In this regard, the eating behaviour is notable for a reduction in the quantity of food eaten, together with a reduction in the range of foods from which the sufferer selects his or her intake, as well as the frequency of intake. Eating behaviour is also influenced by the caloric value of foods. The sufferer not only has an intense preoccupation with packaging information in this regard but also develops a detailed knowledge of individual foods. The motivation for changes in eating behaviour often centre around health with a change to foods that have less fat and a preference for methods of food preparation that do not involve the use of oils or frying. Not infrequently one also sees a shift to vegetarianism: this is not to say that vegetarians constitute a group of individuals with an eating disorder, but rather that individuals with an eating disorder rationalise the change in their eating behaviour and do so in ways that ostensibly appear justifiable. However, the consequences of such choices are an indication that, rather than pursuing a healthier lifestyle, the individual has embarked on a process that will have an anything but a healthy outcome.

In terms of a diagnosis, a number of clinical features need to be assessed. These features include:

- weight: refusal to maintain body weight at or above a minimally normal weight for the person's age and height (< 85 % of that expected)
- fear: intense fear of gaining weight or becoming fat, even though the person is underweight
- perception: a disturbed experienced of the person's body weight or shape, influence of body weight or shape on self-evaluation or denial of the seriousness of the current low body weight.
- type: anorexia nervosa can either be of the restricting type or the binge-eating/**purging** type. Regarding the latter, here one sees the symptom overlap mentioned earlier; this will be echoed with regard to restriction when bulimia nervosa is discussed.

Specific diagnostic criteria, as per DSM-5, are noted in Chapter 28 (Table 28.8).

It should be noted that endocrine function in post-menarcheal females, with specific reference to amenorrhea, is no longer a diagnostic criterion in the DSM-5.

As with all psychiatric conditions, possible medical causes of any of the aforementioned criteria must be considered, not least of all because weight loss and ultimately the starvation process manifests in ways that might make anorexia nervosa the default diagnosis in a patient from a specific demographic (i.e. young and female). Earlier studies on starvation from the 1950s documented many forms of behaviour amongst physically and psychologically healthy individuals who were starved – and that are seen in anorexia nervosa sufferers - including a preoccupation with food, **ritualistic** approaches to food consumption, disturbed sleep, concentration problems, irritability, social withdrawal and isolation (Garner, 1997). From the aforementioned it is clear that the diagnostic criteria do not capture the range of clinical features that accompanies the illness.

## 22.2.2 Bulimia nervosa

Bulimia nervosa is characterised by excess in relation to food, in contrast with anorexia nervosa's generally restrictive and controlled presentation. This is not to say that bulimia nervosa sufferers do not restrict, it is simply that their restriction occurs as a secondary (rather than primary) phenomenon. As much as anorexia nervosa is about control, bulimia nervosa is about loss of control. Whilst anorexia nervosa and bulimia nervosa might be thought of as discrete conditions, they are not. A number of clinical scenarios illustrate this point:

- symptom overlap: restriction of food intake due to concerns with weight is a common feature
- features of one condition occurs simultaneously with another (e.g. anorexia nervosa, binge-eating/purging type)
- the possibility of the clinical presentation varying over time (e.g. a patient might at one time present with anorexia nervosa and at another with bulimia nervosa). Such diagnostic cross-over is well established and whilst generally this occurs over years, shorter periods (i.e. within months) have been described (Thomas *et al.*, 2010).

In this regard, some authors have suggested that the term 'eating disorders' with discrete conditions, be replaced by 'eating disorder' with a range of presentations that incorporate all the symptoms – thus acknowledging that symptoms are not all unique to either of the described conditions, that there is both symptom overlap and diagnostic shift.

In terms of a diagnosis, a number of clinical features need to be assessed. These features include:

- food intake: recurrent episodes of binge eating, with an episode of binge eating characterised by eating a quantity of food (that is definitely larger than what most people would eat in that time and under similar circumstances) within a discrete period of time (e.g. within a two-hour period) as well as a lack of control (related to quantity and type of food eaten) during the episode
- compensation: recurrent inappropriate compensatory behaviour in order to prevent weight gain, such as self-induced vomiting, misuse of laxatives, diuretics, enemas or other medications, fasting or excessive exercise
- frequency: the behaviour occurs, on average, at least once a week for three months
- perception: self-evaluation is unduly influenced by body shape and weight
- exclusion: the disturbance does not occur exclusively during episodes of anorexia nervosa
- type: bulimia nervosa can either be of the purging type or the non-purging type. If of the purging type, the person engages in vomiting or the use of laxatives, diuretics or enemas. If of the non-purging type, the person will use either fasting or excessive exercise to compensate for binge eating but seldom engages in purging behaviour.

Specific diagnostic criteria, as per DSM-5, are noted in Chapter 28 (Table 28.9).

When considering the diagnostic criteria for bulimia nervosa, the criterion overlap with anorexia nervosa in terms of self-evaluation should be noted, since this is a core criterion for an eating disorder. In addition, if a person meets the criteria for anorexia nervosa but also reports features of bulimia nervosa, then the diagnosis would be that of 'anorexia nervosa, binge-eating/purging subtype' (i.e. the diagnosis of anorexia is primary with the features of bulimia nervosa serving to type that diagnosis). The use of fasting, as compensation, is akin to the restrictive behaviour seen in anorexia nervosa; hence the context of such behaviour must be established for the purposes of diagnosis (together with other features). Food restriction is one of the causes of **bingeing** episodes amongst bulimia nervosa sufferers, and the means of compensation for a binge episode ultimately serves as the precipitant for the next binge episode, thus locking the sufferer into a destructive pattern of behaviour. Thus the significance of the shared criterion related to self-evaluation, whereby both anorexia nervosa and bulimia nervosa sufferers invariably commenced their progression to an eating disorder through dieting. In this regard, dieting is one of the major risk factors for the development of an eating disorder (see Section 22.3).

### 22.2.3 Other specified feeding or eating disorder/Unspecified feeding or eating disorder

As is the situation with all diagnostic entities in the DSM, provision is made for those patients whose clinical presentation does not meet the required criteria for a specific diagnosis, but whose presentation is characterised by features in keeping with a diagnosis from within a range of diagnoses that are grouped together. Whilst anorexia nervosa and bulimia nervosa are the two best described diagnoses within the 'feeding and eating disorders' category, it would appear that a significant number of sufferers (15-30%) are diagnosed from within the 'other specified feeding or eating disorder' or 'unspecified feeding or eating disorder' categories (Allen *et al.*, 2013). Any patient who presents with features of such conditions but who does not meet the full criteria would be so diagnosed. Whether patients diagnosed as such have discrete conditions or whether such presentations represent illness-in-evolution (i.e. either moving towards meeting full criteria as the disease progresses, or not meeting full criteria because the illness is improving), will be for the clinician to judge. Either way, subthreshold presentations do not diminish the seriousness of the presentation.

Two illustrative examples follow:

1. A presentation that does not meet the full criteria might be a preoccupation with weight and a fear of being overweight associated with restrictive intake but the weight loss does not meet the criterion for anorexia nervosa. Clearly anorexia nervosa is a consideration (all other possibilities having been excluded) but a diagnosis of 'Atypical anorexia nervosa' would be made.
2. Within the context of possible bulimia nervosa, one may be presented with a patient who engages in binge-eating episodes with purging, but the frequency is less than once per week while the duration is for longer than three months. In this instance a diagnosis of bulimia nervosa ('of low frequency and/or limited duration') will be made.

The current DSM iteration thus permits the clinician to note the predominant clinical features when making a diagnosis.

### 22.2.4 Binge-eating disorder

Essentially binge-eating disorder is bulimia nervosa without the purging or compensatory behaviour (i.e. binge eating with specific characteristics and frequency no different from bulimia nervosa). This condition occurs within the range of normal weight, overweight and obesity. While anorexia nervosa and bulimia nervosa occur predominantly amongst females, binge-eating disorder occurs more evenly amongst males and females (American Psychiatric Association, 2013).

## 22.3 Aetiology

Eating disorders are thought to be multifactorial in origin, with no single cause having been established. Thus it is probably more appropriate to consider the aetiology within the context of risk factors, whereby the emergence of a disorder most likely results from an interaction of individual vulnerability and environmental factors.

### 22.3.1 Individual vulnerability

Whilst the logical individual factor might be that of genetic predisposition, no such gene has been isolated and it is unlikely that a single gene will account for the heterogeneity of presentations within the diagnostic category of 'eating disorders'. The concept of individual vulnerability could relate to personality, and more specifically to aspects of personality that influence coping skills and communication. Poor coping skills are not uncommon, as is difficulty communicating, especially when communication may lead to conflict. Lack of self-esteem is commonly associated with eating disorders, as well as a sense of not being in control of one's life. All these individual aspects may characterise any eating disorder sufferer but none are specific to, or uniquely associated with, eating disorders. However, such individual characteristics may predispose an individual to what is arguably one of the most powerful risk factors, namely dieting (Szabo, 2002). Although dieting is highly prevalent amongst adolescent females (up to 85% in selected South African samples), and generally for aesthetic rather than health reasons, not all dieting leads to an eating disorder. It is not clear what unique factors may lead from one to the other, but a family history of an eating disorder, a mood disorder or substance abuse may confer elevated risk. In addition to dieting, gender appears to be a powerful factor, given that the vast majority of sufferers are female. A number of theories have been advanced, ranging from the influence of the media (with a focus on the idealisation of beauty being associated with slimness) to the relative percentage of body composition as fat during adolescence amongst girls relative to boys (i.e. greater amongst girls).

As most sufferers tend to be adolescent, and thus develop an eating disorder within the context of living with a family, both parent-child relationships and sibling relationships are relevant. Early researchers and theorists emphasised the role of the family in contributing to the emergence of eating disorders (e.g. parental over-involvement or inconsistent approaches to parenting). Such an understanding has changed over time. It is not a straightforward matter to establish cause versus effect (does the family dynamic contribute to the illness or does the sufferer contribute to the family dynamic?) The significance of such a shift in understanding is that it does not diminish the need to assess the family (for adolescent sufferers), but rather emphasises a need to understand the dynamics that exist within the family of a sufferer and within a therapeutic context. This is necessary in order to effect changes needed to restore health to the patient and harmony to the family. The latter statement highlights the fact that eating disorders contribute to significant disruption of family life and associated emotions.

## 22.3.2 Environmental factors

In recent times, eating disorders have emerged in settings not traditionally associated with eating disorders, namely non-Western countries. In South Africa the first cases of eating disorders amongst black females were described in 1995 (Szabo *et al.*, 1995). Eating disorders have been described amongst white females since the 1970s. Either these conditions were not recognised in the black community or they did not exist. And yet, case reports of eating disorders affecting black females from the rest of Africa had been published during the 1980s. The question arises as to what had changed in the environment that led to the emergence of eating disorders in settings other than urban and Western, with sufferers being predominantly white and relatively affluent? Such associations have led to the understanding that eating disorders are culture-bound. However, the emergence of eating disorders in settings and amongst people outside of those mentioned has led to a reconceptualisation of the term 'culture bound'. There is an understanding that 'modernity' appears to confer risk (Lee, 1996). In this regard a range of characteristics that constitute a modernising society have been highlighted:

- capitalism
- role choice for women
- decreased birth rates
- abundance of food
- increasing body weight
- body-orientated advertising
- urbanisation
- immigration
- the availability of information technology.

South African society post-1994 (the ending of Apartheid) is increasingly characterised by modernisation that may well have provided the impetus for the emergence of these conditions where previously they were unknown.

Aside from more general environmental changes, factors within the context of an individual's life, such as disappointment, changed circumstances and trauma, may also play a role. In this regard any such events must be established and documented in relation to the emergence of eating disorder symptoms.

# 22.4 Treatment

Eating disorders are complex both in terms of aetiology and in terms of treatment. Treatment follows consideration of the condition being treated as well as elements of a bio-psycho-social approach. In addition, depending on the age or marital status of the patient, the involvement of parents (and possibly siblings) or a spouse/partner should be considered. Family therapy has indeed been strongly recommended in the treatment of anorexia nervosa.

Regarding the individual, it is always important to be cognizant of the physical consequences of an eating disorder. In the DSM-IV (American Psychiatric Association, 1994) endocrine functioning in relation to anorexia nervosa was a diagnostic criterion, whereby the absence of three consecutive menstrual cycles was required to make the diagnosis. Although no longer incorporated in the diagnostic criteria, menstruation remains an important marker of health. In terms of physical complications these conditions impact on multiple organ systems. In anorexia nervosa such complications include hypotension and bradycardia, elevated liver enzymes, skin thinning and discolouration, scalp hair loss, osteopenia and osteoporosis and reduced brain volume. In bulimia nervosa such complications include electrolyte imbalances (hypokalaemia associated with purging), loss of dental enamel and dental abscesses, reflux gastritis (associated with vomiting) and cathartic colon (associated with laxative abuse). Aside from death due to either cardiac arrhythmia in bulimia nervosa or multiple organ failure in anorexia nervosa, suicide may occur. In this regard, it has been established that mortality rates among eating disorder sufferers, following hospitalisation for an eating disorder, are significantly higher than for age- and sex-matched individuals without an eating disorder (Hoang *et al.*, 2014).

Pharmacological interventions are not commonly used as a primary intervention, although the utility of serotonin specific reuptake inhibitors (SSRIs) – usually in doses higher than those used to typically treat major depression e.g. 40–60 mg/day of fluoxetine – as an antibulimic has been documented. No such intervention is indicated for the treatment of anorexia nervosa, although low doses of certain antidepressant agents (e.g. 100–150 mg trazadone at night) have been found to assist with the sleep disturbances associated with anorexia nervosa. Co-morbid psychiatric conditions, which are common (Treasure *et al.*, 2010), such as mood or anxiety disorders, may well require initiation or maintenance of pharmacological interventions. It should be noted that depressive symptoms are common in anorexia nervosa, but tend to respond to nutritional rehabilitation (Szabo and Terre Blanche, 1998).

The dominant intervention for either anorexia nervosa or bulimia nervosa is psychotherapy, and specifically, cognitive behavioural therapy (CBT). CBT targets both eating behaviour as well as ways of thinking and related issues that influence behaviour. With anorexia nervosa, weight restoration is critical, not only due to the risk of death but also due to the impact of the starvation process on emotional and cognitive functioning. With bulimia nervosa, stabilisation of eating is critical in terms of aiming for adequate consumption in a structured, predictable manner so as to eliminate binge eating and purging. Whilst such behavioural approaches are intuitively obvious – not only to the psychiatrist but sometimes to the patient too – implementation is difficult due to fear of change in terms of one specific consequence: weight gain. The art of psychotherapy lies in understanding how to connect with the patient, based on an appreciation of his or her preparedness for change, and guiding him or her towards such change. Aside from fear of change, lack of insight is a major obstacle. There are times when the clinician is obliged to intervene, which is generally easier with younger patients who are within the home environment and provided one can recruit and involve parents appropriately. In younger patients, specifically those who suffer from anorexia nervosa, involvement of the family (parents) is an important component of intervention insofar as equipping parents to implement the appropriate structures, supervise the necessary eating behaviour and deal with the emotional struggle that is inevitable in such situations. Whilst most sufferers are treated as out-patients, the need for hospitalisation does arise. This may result from physical complications that require medical intervention, while the severity and persistence of the eating disorder symptoms may necessitate an in-patient specialist eating disorder programme (Szabo and Terre Blanche, 1998).

The social aspects of intervention might be seen as those involving family, but within a broader context, societal value systems that promote eating disorder symptoms in a given individual must be addressed. In doing so, however, one should be careful not to adopt a rigid approach as to what is right and wrong but rather to facilitate individual awareness as to what is potentially better for their functioning and most likely to assist in fulfilling potential and aspirations.

## 22.5 Outcome

One of the major determinants of successful intervention is co-operation, from both patients and, where relevant, families. However, 'successful intervention' must be qualified. For example, moving from meeting all diagnostic criteria for either anorexia nervosa or bulimia nervosa to a diagnosis of 'other specified feeding or eating disorder' or 'unspecified feeding or eating disorder' may in fact be successful. Hence, success is relative and should be viewed within the context of the individual sufferer. Further, symptom resolution in terms of diagnostic criteria is a somewhat limited perspective by which to gauge success: the clinician should also consider emotional and cognitive functioning as well as meaningful participation in routine activities. Significant factors that have an impact on outcome include time (improvement will generally be slow) and trust (the patient must believe in the treating professional, which means that there is a need for honesty and sensitivity). With the appropriate intervention most sufferers will improve, usually as out-patients. Rather than a nihilistic attitude to eating disorder sufferers based on their apparent resistance, a realistic awareness of what is required and what is possible will be more conducive to positive outcomes.

# Sleep disorders

## 22.6 Introduction

Human beings spend about a third of their lives in a state of sleep. Although there is still much that is unknown about this phenomenon, there has been a dramatic increase in the knowledge about the evaluation and treatment of the various disorders that affect sleep.

## 22.7 Normal sleep

Subjective complaints of sleep as well as observed disturbances in sleep continuity and/or quality are common problems that face the psychiatrist. Although psychiatrists are seldom requested to evaluate patients with exclusively sleep-related problems, this is an area where psychiatry should become increasingly involved, especially when taking into consideration the fact that many of these problems are treated with psychotropic drugs and behavioural interventions.

Before a decision is made to intervene in the sleep habits or patterns, however, there must be an understanding as to what constitutes normal sleep.

### 22.7.1 Why do we sleep?

If normal sleep is a valid concept, we must consider the question of what function is served by this phenomenon. Various theories have been suggested, but the complete answer remains somewhat elusive. It is often suggested that the bodily systems and organs need time to shut down to rest or recover from the demands of daily activities. Whereas this theory has some merit, the reality is that physiological activities continue to be active and the body's metabolism continues to function and consume energy during sleep.

The next theory is the so-called learning theory. This implies that the brain needs a period of relative inactivity on a daily basis to consolidate the accumulation of facts and information obtained during the preceding day. This implies that late-night studying before exams or tests may even be counterproductive!

A final theory relates to evolutionary aspects and holds that the need for sleep is a remnant from ancient times when night-time was best spent in a shelter and in a state of inactivity. It is suggested that human eyes would have been no match for the night vision of dangerous predators, and that for the human species to survive, night-time inactivity (i.e. being asleep) was a necessity.

## 22.7.2 Sleep physiology

Sleep is recognised as a period of relative inactivity, but with ongoing physiological processes. Nevertheless, there are characteristic changes in various parameters during sleep (Vgontzas and Kales, 1999).

Normal sleep can broadly be divided into two types: rapid eye movement (REM) sleep and non-REM sleep. During REM sleep, there are observable movements of the eyes, visible even behind closed eyelids.

The use of EEG monitoring has led to significant advantages in the understanding of what happens during sleep. This has led to the description of different stages of sleep.

- **Stage 1**
  - transition between wakefulness and sleep
  - EEG changes (low amplitude theta activity with episodes of alpha activity)
  - normal sleep requires little time in this stage
- **Stage 2**
  - EEG changes (K-complexes and sleep spindles)
  - no discernible eye movements
  - decreased muscle tone
- **Stages 3 and 4**

  Stages 3 and 4 are similar in character, with somewhat more pronounced EEG changes in Stage 4.
  - EEG changes – slow-wave sleep (SWS); increased amounts of delta activity
  - considered to be the restorative phase
  - mostly during the first half of sleep
  - **REM sleep**
  - EEG reverts to a pattern similar to the waking state
  - muscle atonia
  - irregular respiratory and cardiovascular functions
  - penile erections
  - vivid dreams.

The sleep stages usually occur in succession, culminating in REM sleep. These recurring patterns are called sleep cycles and form the unique sleep architecture.

The first REM episode occurs after about 90 minutes and lasts for 5-10 minutes. The longer sleep persists, the more regular the REM episodes and the longer the duration. Slow-wave sleep mostly occurs during the first sleep cycles and decreases as the sleep progresses, whereas time spent in REM sleep increases as sleep progresses.

The phasic occurrence of sleep – usually on a 24 hour cycle – is determined by three interacting systems.

The homeostatic system regulates sleep drive and causes progressive drowsiness the longer sleep is postponed. This drive is dependent on the amount of sleep acquired during the preceding period. The system seeks to maintain a set amount of sleep and explains why sleep debt can be accumulated. This explains why students who do not spend enough time sleeping during the week, may easily sleep for 9-10 hours or even longer over a weekend.

The arousal system opposes the sleep drive, especially during daytime.

Circadian rhythms function independently of the other systems and help to ensure a 24-hour rhythmicity to sleep.

**Table 22.1** Physiological control of sleep

Sleep is governed by a complex set of biological factors:

- The suprachiasmatic nucleus (located in the hypothalamus) regulates the release of melatonin on a 25-hour cycle.
- The pineal gland secretes melatonin depending on environmental light or darkness.
- Multiple neurotransmitters are involved:
  - noradrenalin from cell bodies in the locus ceruleus
  - serotonin from the dorsal raphe nucleus
  - acetylcholine from the reticular formation.
  - dopamine – associated with wakefulness

**Source:** Saper *et al.*, 2001

#### 22.7.2.1 Circadian rhythms and chronobiology

Sleep cycles follow a circadian (*circa* = about; *dia* = day) rhythm and are usually maintained according to a pattern where sleep occurs during night-time. These rhythms are maintained by so-called *Zeitgebers* (literally, time-givers), of which light and darkness are the strongest influences. Other peripheral oscillators also influence circadian rhythmicity; these are in turn influenced by eating habits and social activities.

**Chronobiology** suggests that regular daily rhythms are essential for health. These various behavioural, physiological and hormonal rhythms are entrained with respect to sleep and the day-night cycle.

## 22.8 Sleep disorders

### 22.8.1 Classification

Various classification systems are used to describe the different sleep disorders. These include the DSM-5, the World Health Organization's ICD-10 and the International Classification of Sleep Disorders (ICSD).

Sleep disorders are broadly grouped under two subgroups. These are **dyssomnias** (conditions that cause insomnia or hypersomnia) and **parasomnias** (conditions that intrude into sleep).

Dyssomnias include conditions such as insomnia, narcolepsy, restless legs syndrome (RLS), obstructive sleep apnoea (OSA), periodic limb movement disorder (PLMD) and various circadian sleep disorders.

Various medical and psychiatric conditions may also influence sleep.

The latest versions of the ICSD-3 and the DSM-5 are now very similar and have been simplified from previous versions.

### 22.8.2 Diagnosis

Diagnosing the various sleep disorders requires an understanding of what happens during sleep, when it happens during the sleep cycle and what the consequences are.

The first step is to take a thorough clinical history as well as a specific sleep history. This includes questioning the bed-partner, obtaining a family history of sleep disorders and determining the nature, onset and impact of the sleep disturbance. The use of a sleep diary is also an important aid to determine sleep habits and patterns.

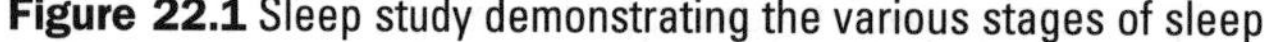

**Figure 22.1** Sleep study demonstrating the various stages of sleep

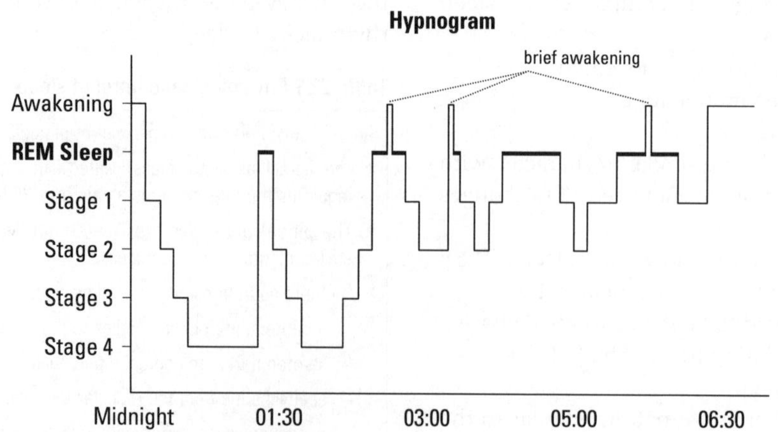

A physical and psychiatric evaluation is essential to further determine causative factors or comorbidities.

Technical diagnostic aids that may also be employed include Actigraphy, the Multiple Sleep Latency Test (MSLT) and polisomnography (PSG).

## 22.8.3 Dyssomnias

### 22.8.3.1 Insomnia

Of all the sleep disorders, insomnia is the most prevalent. It is estimated that 6–15% of adults meet the criteria for insomnia. The diagnosis of insomnia requires subjective (and/or objective) reports of a lack of sleep with daytime consequences such as feelings of irritability, fatigue or lack of concentration.

Short-term insomnia is often associated with situational stressors. Chronic insomnia is a much more serious problem and often persists independently of environmental factors. It also causes significant physical co-morbidities (increased risk of cardiovascular illness as well as cerebrovascular illness) and psychiatric co-morbidities (up to 40% risk of major depressive disorder (MDD) within the first year (Riemann, 2007)).

**Table 22.3** Causes of insomnia (according to ICSD-2)

| |
|---|
| Adjustment insomnia (acute insomnia, short-term insomnia) |
| Psychophysiological insomnia |
| Paradoxical insomnia (sleep-state misperception) |
| Idiopathic insomnia (primary insomnia) |
| Insomnia due to mental disorder |
| Inadequate sleep hygiene |
| Behavioural insomnia of childhood |
| Insomnia due to drug or substance |
| Insomnia due to a medical condition |
| Insomnia not due to a substance or a known physiological condition |
| Physiological (organic) insomnia, unspecified |

**Source:** International Classification of Sleep Disorders, 2014

### 22.8.3.2 Sleep-related breathing disorders

Sleep-related breathing disorders are characterised by sleep disruption due to problems related to breathing. Daytime sleepiness and symptoms such as headaches and impaired concentration may result.

Breathing through the nose may lead to excessive snoring in individuals with blocking of the nose or pharynx. The soft part of the pharynx

**Table 22.2** Classification of sleep according to different systems

| ICSD-3 | DSM-5 (sleep-wake disorders) | ICD-10 |
|---|---|---|
| insomnia | insomnia disorder | non-organic insomnia |
| sleep-related breathing disorders | breathing-related sleep disorders | |
| central disorders of hypersomnolence | hypersomnolence disorder | non-organic hypersomnia |
| | narcolepsy | |
| circadian rhythm sleep-wake disorders | circadian rhythm sleep-wake disorders | non-organic disorder of the sleep-wake schedule |
| parasomnias | parasomnias | ▶ sleepwalking<br>▶ sleep terrors<br>▶ nightmares |
| sleep-related movement disorders | | |
| | | other non-organic sleep disorders |
| | | unspecified |

may eventually collapse and obstructive sleep apnoea is the result.

#### 22.8.3.3 Circadian rhythm disorders

Circadian rhythm disorders include jet-lag, shift-work sleep disorder and sleep phase disorder (SPD).

Chronotypes refer to a person's preferred sleep period. Some people are morningness types and become drowsy relatively early at night (e.g. at 21h00). They tend to wake up early (e.g. at 05h00), but have no problems functioning well upon waking and do not experience impairment during the day because of sleepiness. The eveningness types prefer to stay awake later – their preferred bedtime is usually well after midnight. With a preferred waking time 08h00 and later, these individuals may experience substantial impairment due to sleep debt since social and occupational schedules usually do not accommodate such hours.

#### 22.8.3.4 Hypersomnia

Hypersomnia (or excessive daytime sleepiness) occurs in about 5% of the general population. These patients need a thorough clinical evaluation. The causes may vary from narcolepsy to drug abuse and various neurological causes. The Epworth Sleepiness Scale is a useful instrument for assessing daytime sleepiness.

#### 22.8.3.5 Narcolepsy

Narcolepsy is characterised by repeated irresistible sleep attacks and **cataplexy** (sudden loss of muscle tone, usually after an emotional response such as anger or joy). Sleep studies also demonstrate so-called REM-intrusions (REM sleep during the transition between sleep and wakefulness). This phenomenon may lead to the very distressing experience of sleep paralysis, due to the atonia of REM sleep persisting after wakening.

### 22.8.4 Parasomnias

#### 22.8.4.1 Non-REM sleep parasomnias

Non-REM sleep parasomnias occur during slow-wave sleep and include sleep-walking, sleep-eating and night terrors.

#### 22.8.4.2 REM sleep parasomnias

REM-sleep behavioural disorder occurs when dreams are acted out. Muscle atonia usually associated with REM sleep is absent. It mostly occurs in males over the age of 50. This condition could be an early predictor of neurodegenerative disease.

### 22.8.5 Sleep and psychiatric disorders

Sleep disturbances and psychiatric disorders often co-occur. Mood disorders have characteristic sleep problems, often used as part of the diagnostic criteria. Anxiety disorders and insomnia have a negative influence on each other: anxiety aggravates or maintains insomnia and insomnia (even short-term) worsens anxiety.

Depression can affect sleep in various ways, such as reduced total sleep time, reduced sleep efficiency, decrease in Stage 2 sleep and an increase in REM sleep (reduced latency and increased density).

Various psychiatric drugs have detrimental effects on sleep architecture as well as duration.

### 22.8.6 Treatment of sleep disorders

#### 22.8.6.1 Non-pharmacological measures

Behavioural sleep medicine is a rapidly expanding field and has clear evidence of efficacy in various sleep disorders, especially insomnia (Jacobs *et al.*, 2004).

The following interventions are employed in the management of insomnia:

- Stimulus control therapy (SCT) addresses the negative experience of, and associated anxiety related to, extended time spent in bed waiting to fall asleep. Awake time in bed is limited to a specified time (e.g. 15 minutes) after which the patient is advised to get up and to only return to bed when feeling drowsy or after a predetermined period of time has elapsed. This applies to sleep onset delays as well as waking during the night.

- Sleep restriction therapy (SRT) limits the actual time spent in bed to the total sleep time as determined by sleep diaries. The aim is to consolidate sleep and reduce the fragmentation of sleep. Small amounts of sleep time are then added as soon as good sleep-efficacy is achieved.
- CBT for insomnia addresses irrational assumptions and dysfunctional cognitions regarding sleep.
- Sleep hygiene emphasises good sleep habits and respect for a regular sleep routine.

These behavioural interventions have certain contraindications (Smith and Perlis, 2006):

- SCT instructions can be difficult and even potentially dangerous for frail patients or those with an increased risk of falls
- SRT may aggravate pre-existing conditions such as epilepsy, bipolar disorder, parasomnias or other illnesses
- SRT may increase daytime somnolence and reach a state where safety related to driving and operating machinery could be affected.

Treatment of circadian rhythm disorders may include bright-light therapy and chronotherapy. It is important to note that ordinary environmental illumination is usually not sufficient and that special light boxes may be needed.

Chronotherapy requires progressive delay of sleep onset for at least a week to eventually resynchronise circadian rhythms with the normal day/night rhythm. Clearly this will lead to major disruptions in lifestyle while the treatment is in progress (Wirz-Justice, 2003).

Other conditions such as sleep apnoea are treated with a combination of lifestyle interventions such as exercise and weight-loss programmes as well as specific interventions such as continuous positive airway pressure (CPAP) or nasal expiratory airway pressure (EPAP).

**Table 22.4** Psychotropic drugs that cause somnolence and insomnia

| | **Somnolence** | **Insomnia** |
|---|---|---|
| Antidepressants | amitryptiline | bupropion |
| | mianserin | fluoxetine |
| | trazodone | |
| | mirtazepine | |
| | trimipramine | |
| Antipsychotics | chlorpromazine | aripiprazole |
| | quetiapine | |
| | clozapine | |
| | olanzapine | |
| Other | antihistamines | methylphenidate |
| | benzodiazepines | modafanil |
| | zopiclone | |
| | zolpidem | |

#### 22.8.6.2 Pharmacological measures

The pharmacological management of insomnia has traditionally been employed more readily than the behavioural interventions, in spite of limited evidence for long-term efficacy. Benzodiazepines such as midazolam, nitrazepam, lormetazepam and others are still used and although they are effective in alleviating insomnia, the issues relating to tolerance, cognitive impairment, rebound insomnia after discontinuation as well as abuse and dependence remain real problems (Lavie *et al.*, 2002).

More recently, the so-called z-hypnotics such as zopiclone and zolpidem have been used widely (Nowell *et al.*, 1997), but as they also bind to the GABA receptor, cases of abuse and dependence have been reported.

Melatonin and melatonin agonists have been promoted, but remain more effective for circadian disorders rather than insomnia.

Antihistamines are also employed, but the evidence in insomnia is limited and problems related to tolerance and daytime drowsiness have been documented (Wilson *et al.*, 2010).

Sedating antidepressants (e.g. amitriptyline, trimipramine, mianserin, trazodone and mirtazapine) are also commonly used as hypnotics, but due to daytime sedation they are also not the ideal.

Intermittent use of hypnotics has been proposed and there is some evidence of longer term efficacy.

Dopaminergics such as pergolide, bromocriptine and pramipexole, benzodiazepines and opioids have been used in the treatment of RLS and PLMD (Richert and Baran, 2003).

Stimulants such as methylphenidate and modafanil are used in the treatment of narcolepsy (Richert and Baran, 2003).

### Case study 22.1

Mrs A is a 42-year-old divorced lady. She started to develop insomnia during difficult divorce procedures about 2 years ago. The insomnia persisted and 14 months later she was diagnosed with major depressive disorder. She was treated with a SSRI and some of her symptoms improved. The insomnia persisted and she continued to experience daytime impairment.

She was referred to a sleep behaviour therapist and with SCT and attention to sleep hygiene her sleep quality improved markedly; she is now in full remission of her mood disorder as well.

This case demonstrates the importance of considering chronic insomnia as a disorder to be managed by itself and not merely to be considered as a symptom of a mood disorder.

### Case study 22.2

Mr B is a 53-year-old businessman with a history of progressively poor sleep quality and marked impairment during the day because of poor concentration and headaches. He has a BMI of 35 and smokes 20 cigarettes per day. His work is also very stressful.

A course of benzodiazepine hypnotics was prescribed and although this improved his sleep latency (time to sleep onset) and subjective decrease in awareness of awakenings, his daytime functioning did not improve at all. Mrs B insisted on attending the follow-up visit and reported that his snoring had in fact worsened and that she was sure that he had stopped breathing on a number of occasions while sleeping.

Mr B was referred for a PSG and a diagnosis of obstructive sleep apnoea was made. He started using CPAP and together with ongoing weight loss, albeit slow, he experienced dramatic improvements in his quality of life. The hypnotics were also discontinued and smoking cessation is a work in progress.

This case demonstrates the importance of considering risk factors and getting a good collateral history from sleeping partners.

## Conclusion

Anorexia nervosa and bulimia nervosa are conditions predominantly affecting adolescent females, but not exclusively so. Further, these conditions have started to emerge in populations not previously thought to be affected. The impact on physical and psychological functioning and ultimately quality of life can be profound. Interventions need to be truly bio-psycho-social in approach, specifically taking into account both nutritional aspects as well as addressing dysfunctional beliefs and ways of thinking related to weight and shape. Resistance to intervention and change is common, and certainly with younger patients it is important to involve relevant family members in the management. Whilst recovery is often slow, both symptomatic improvement and improved quality of life are attainable.

A good understanding of sleep disorders, especially the more common conditions such as insomnia, is essential for any medical practitioner. Rational use of psychopharmacological interventions and the often neglected behavioural interventions, offer various treatment options in conditions with potentially significant morbidity.

# References


Allen KL, Byrne, SM, Oddy WH, Crosby RD (2013) DSM-IV-TR and DSM-5 eating disorders in adolescents: Prevalence, stability, and psychosocial correlates in a population-based sample of male and female adolescents. *Journal of Abnormal Psychology* 122(3): 720–32 (DOI: 10.1037/a0034004)

American Academy of Sleep Medicine (2014) *International Classification of Sleep Disorders* (3rd edition). Darien, IL: American Academy of Sleep Medicine

American Psychiatric Association (1994) *Diagnostic and Statistical Manual of Mental Disorders* (4th edition). Washington DC: American Psychiatric Association

American Psychiatric Association (2013) *Diagnostic and Statistical Manual of Mental Disorders* (5th edition). Arlington, VA: American Psychiatric Association

Freeman A, Szabo CP (2005) Eating disorders in South African males: A review of the clinical presentation of hospitalised patients. *South African Journal of Psychology* 35(4): 601–22

Garner DM (1997) Psychoeducational principles in treatment. In: Garner, DM, Garfinkel PE (Eds). *Handbook of Treatment of Eating Disorders* (2nd edition). London/New York: The Guilford Press

Hoang U, Goldacre M, James, A (2014) Mortality following hospital discharge with a diagnosis of eating disorder: National record linkage study, England 2001–2009. *International Journal of Eating Disorders* 47(5): 507–15

Jacobs GD, Pace-Schott EF, Stickgold R, Otto MW (2004) Cognitive behavior therapy for insomnia. *Archives of Internal Medicine* 164: 1888–96.

Lavie P, Pillar G, Malhotra A (2002) *Sleep Disorders: Diagnosis, Management and Treatment*. London: Martin Dunitz

Lee, S (1996) Reconsidering the status of anorexia nervosa as a western culture-bound syndrome. *Social Science & Medicine* 42(1): 21–34

Nowell PD, Mazumdar S, Buysse DJ, Dew MA, Reynolds CF, Kupfer DJ (1997) Benzodiazepines and zolpidem for chronic insomnia, *The Journal of the American Medical Association* 278: 2170–7

Richert AC, Baran AS (2003) A review of common sleep disorders. *CNS Spectrum*, 8(2): 102–9

Riemann D (2007) Insomnia and comorbid psychiatric disorders. *Sleep Medicine* 8 (Suppl. 4): S15–20

Saper CB, Chou TC, Scammell TE (2001) The sleep switch: Hypothalamic control of sleep and wakefulness. *Trends in Neurosciences* 24(12): 726–31

Smith MT, Perlis ML (2006) Who is a candidate for cognitive-behavioral therapy for insomnia? *Health Psychology* 25(1): 15–9

Szabo CP (2002) Youth at risk – dieting and eating disorders: A South African perspective. *South African Medical Journal* 92(4): 282–3

Szabo CP, Berk M, Tlou E, Allwood CW (1995) Eating disorders in black South African females: A series of cases. *South African Medical Journal* 85: 588–90

Szabo CP, Terre Blanche MJ (1998) Hospitalised anorexics: A preliminary evaluation of an inpatient programme. *South African Medical Journal* 88(3): 312–8

Thomas JJ, Delinsky SS, St Germain SA, Weigel TJ, Tangren CM, Levendusky PG, Becker AE (2010) How do eating disorder specialist clinicians apply DSM-IV diagnostic criteria in routine clinical practice? Implications for enhancing clinical utility in DSM-5. *Psychiatry Research* 178: 511–7

Treasure J, Claudino AM, Zucker N (2010) Eating disorders. *The Lancet* 375: 583–93

Vgontzas AN, Kales A (1999) Sleep and its disorders. *Annual Review of Medicine* 50: 387–400.

Wilson SJ, Nutt DJ, Alford C, Argyropoulos SV, Baldwin DS, Barteson AN, Britton TC, Crowe C, Dirk DJ, Espie CA, Gringas P, Hajak G, Idzikowski C, Krystal AD, Nash JR, Selsick H, Sharpley AL, Wade AG (2010) British Association for Psychopharmacology consensus statement on evidence-based treatment of insomnia, parasomnias and circadian rhythm disorders, *Journal of Psychopharmacy* 24(11): 1577–600

Wirz-Justice, A (2003) Chronobiology and mood disorders, *Dialogues in Clinical Neuroscience* 5(4): 315–25

# CHAPTER 23 Disorders of sexual function, preference and identity

*Carla Kotzé, Mo Nagdee, Hester Jordaan*

## Sexual dysfunction

### 23.1 Introduction

Disorders of sexual functioning are probably very common but due to the private nature of sexual problems, their full extent is unknown. This is a heterogeneous group of disorders that are typically characterised by a disturbance in a person's ability to respond sexually or to experience sexual pleasure.

Sexuality is determined by anatomy, physiology, psychology, the culture in which one lives, relationships with others and developmental experiences. It includes the perception of being male or female and all those thoughts, feelings and behaviours connected with sexual gratification. The sexual response is a psychophysiological experience. The normal sexual response cycle is summarised in Table 23.1.

**Table 23.1** DSM-IV-TR Phases of the Sexual Response Cycle and Associated Sexual Dysfunctions*

| Phases | Characteristics | Dysfunction |
|---|---|---|
| 1. Desire | Distinct from any identified solely through physiology and reflects the patient's motivations, drives, and personality; characterized by sexual fantasies and the desire to have sex. | Hypoactive sexual desire disorder; sexual aversion disorder; hypoactive sexual desire disorder due to a general medical condition (man or woman); substance-induced sexual dysfunction with impaired desire |
| 2. Excitement | Subjective sense of sexual pleasure and accompanying physiological changes; all physiological responses noted in Masters and Johnson's excitement and plateau phases are combined in this phase. | Female sexual arousal disorder; male erectile disorder (may also occur in stages 3 and 4); male erectile disorder due to a general medical condition; dyspareunia due to a general medical condition (man or woman); substance-induced sexual dysfunction with impaired arousal |
| 3. Orgasm | Peaking of sexual pleasure, with release of sexual tension and rhythmic contraction of the perineal muscles and pelvic reproductive organs. | Female orgasmic disorder; male orgasmic disorder; premature ejaculation; other sexual dysfunction due a general medical condition (man or woman); substance-induced sexual dysfunction with impaired orgasm |
| 4. Resolution | A sense of general relaxation, well-being, and muscle relaxation; men are refractory to orgasm for a period of time that increase with age, whereas women can have multiple orgasms without a refractory period. | Postcoital dysphoria; postcoital headache |

* DSM-IV-TR consolidates the Masters and Johnson excitement and plateau phases into a single excitement phase, which is preceded by the desire (appetitive) phase. The orgasm and resolution phases remain the same as originally described by Masters and Johnson.

**Source:** Sadock, 2000. Reprinted with permission from Wolters Kluwer Health.

In the DSM-5 changes were made in the chapter on sexual dysfunctions in an attempt to correct, expand and clarify the different diagnoses and their respective criteria and to improve the validity. Some noteworthy changes include diagnostic classifications made separately according to gender and the elimination of classifications based on simple linear sexual response (Sungur and Gunduz, 2014). Many of the diagnostic criteria were updated for increased precision and most now require a minimum duration of six months as well as a frequency of 75–100%. Substance-induced and medication-induced sexual dysfunction have been excluded.

Table 23.2 lists the sexual dysfunctions included in DSM-5 (IsHak and Tobia, 2013).

**Table 23.2** List of sexual dysfunctions

| **Male dysfunctions:** |
|---|
| ▶ delayed ejaculation<br>▶ erectile disorder<br>▶ male hypoactive sexual desire disorder<br>▶ premature (early) ejaculation |
| **Female dysfunctions:** |
| ▶ female orgasmic disorder<br>▶ female sexual interest/arousal disorder<br>▶ genito-pelvic pain/penetration disorder |
| **Other:** |
| ▶ substance/medication-induced sexual dysfunction<br>▶ other specified sexual dysfunction<br>▶ unspecified sexual dysfunction |

**Source:** Authors' own Table

The time of onset may indicate different aetiologies and interventions, and thus subtypes are classified according to the onset of the difficulty. 'Lifelong' refers to a sexual problem that has been present from first sexual experiences, while 'acquired' applies to sexual disorders that develop after a period of relatively normal sexual function. 'Situational' refers to sexual difficulties that only occur with certain types of stimulation, situations or partners; when it is not limited by these factors it is referred to as 'generalised'.

Several factors should be considered during the evaluation, because they can be relevant to the aetiology, prognosis, course and treatment. These factors include (American Psychiatric Association, 2013):

- partner factors (e.g. the partner's sexual or health problems)
- relationship factors (e.g. poor communication, discrepancies in sexual desire)
- individual vulnerability factors (e.g. poor body image, history of abuse), psychiatric co-morbidity or stressors (e.g. job loss or bereavement)
- cultural or religious factors (e.g. inhibitions related to prohibitions against sexual pleasure, attitudes toward sexuality)
- medical factors.

**Information box**

Sexuality depends on four interrelated psychosexual factors:

- sexual identity (pattern of biological sexual characteristics)
- gender identity (a person's sense of maleness or femaleness)
- sexual orientation (describes the object of a person's sexual impulses)
- sexual behaviour (includes desire, fantasies, pursuit of partners, auto-eroticism and all activities engaged in to express and gratify sexual needs).

These factors affect personality, development and functioning (Sadock, 2000).

Sexual function involves a complex interaction of biological, sociocultural and psychological factors that should all be taken into consideration. Because of the enormous individual variation in sexual preferences, expectations and needs, as well as transcultural variations in sexual practices, a disorder should only be diagnosed if it is judged to cause marked distress or interpersonal difficulty.

Making the diagnosis of a sexual disorder also requires that other problems should be ruled out.

This includes other psychiatric conditions, the effects of substances or medications and other medical conditions or relationship problems, partner violence or other stressors. If the sexual dysfunction is better explained by another non-sexual psychiatric disorder (e.g. mood or anxiety disorder), then a separate diagnosis of sexual dysfunction should not be made. If sexual difficulties are the result of inadequate sexual stimulation, there might be a need for care without diagnosing a sexual dysfunction (Sadock, 2000).

## 23.2 Male sexual dysfunctions

### 23.2.1 Delayed ejaculation

The distinguishing feature of delayed ejaculation is a marked delay or inability to achieve ejaculation despite adequate stimulation and the desire to ejaculate. There is no consensus as to what constitutes a reasonable time to reach orgasm. Because of this lack of precise definition the prevalence is unclear, but it is the least common male sexual complaint.

Delayed ejaculation must be differentiated from retrograde ejaculation, where the seminal fluid passes backwards into the bladder. Retrograde ejaculation always has an organic cause, for example after genito-urinary surgery or anticholinergic side effects of medication (American Psychiatric Association, 2013).

### 23.2.2 Erectile disorder

Between 35% and 50% of all men treated for sexual disorders have erectile dysfunction as the main complaint. Repeated failure to obtain or maintain erections during partnered sexual activities is the main feature of erectile disorder. This may be associated with low self-esteem; avoidance of future sexual encounters may occur. Few men pass through life without experiencing erectile dysfunction on at least one occasion. A disorder is diagnosed if the problem persists for six months on almost all occasions (75–100%) of sexual activity (American Psychiatric Association, 2013).

The incidence of erectile disorder increases with age, when it is often associated with biological factors. Statistics indicate that 50–80% of men with erectile dysfunction have a medical basis for their problem. Common causes include: diabetes mellitus, endocrine disease, vascular disease, multiple sclerosis, pelvic fractures, spinal cord injuries and pelvic surgery.

The most difficult aspect of the differential diagnosis of erectile disorder is ruling out erectile problems that are fully explained by medical

#### 23.1 Advanced reading block

**Brain areas, hormones and neurotransmitters involved with sexual behaviour**

- Chemical and electrical stimulation of various sites of the limbic system have elicited penile erection.
- The hippocampus is believed to influence genital tumescence and regulation of gonadotropin release.
- Substances that increase dopamine levels can increase libido, while an increase in serotonin in the upper pons and midbrain can have an inhibitory effect on sexual desire. Many other neurotransmitters can also influence sexual behaviour.
- Testosterone is believed to increase libido in men and women.
- In men, stress is inversely correlated with testosterone blood concentration.
- Factors such as sleep and mood also affect the circulating levels of testosterone.
- Oestrogen is a key factor for lubrication involved in female arousal and may increase sensitivity to stimulation.
- Progesterone, excessive prolactin and cortisol mildly depress desire in men and women.
- Oxytocin is involved in pleasurable sensations during sex and is increased after orgasm (Sadock, 2000).

factors. Such cases will not receive a diagnosis of a mental disorder, but the distinction is often unclear and many cases will have complex combinations of biological and psychiatric aetiologies. The presence of an organic disease known to cause erectile problems does not confirm a causal relationship. A history of acute onset after a stressful life event, spontaneous erections, morning erections or satisfactory erections during masturbation, suggest a psychological basis for the problem (Sadock, 2000).

### 23.2.3 Male hypoactive sexual desire disorder

Both a low or an absent desire for sex and deficient or absent sexual thoughts or fantasies are required for a diagnosis of male hypoactive sexual desire disorder. Interpersonal context must be taken into account when making the diagnosis; a discrepancy between the man's level of desire for sex and that of his partner is not sufficient to make the diagnosis. A low sexual desire may represent an adaptive response to adverse life conditions, and for this reason the time period of six months with persistent symptoms is included. The prevalence of this disorder varies greatly among different age groups and increases with age (American Psychiatric Association, 2013).

### 23.2.4 Premature (early) ejaculation

To make a diagnosis of premature ejaculation there must be a persistent or recurrent pattern of ejaculation that occurs during partnered sexual activity within approximately one minute following vaginal penetration and before the male wishes it. No specific duration criteria have been established for situations of non-vaginal sexual activities. There is often an accompanying sense of lack of control over ejaculation and apprehension about the inability to delay ejaculation. 20–30% of men between the ages of 18–70 report concern about how rapidly they ejaculate. With the time period of ejaculation within one minute after penetration added, only 1–3% of men would be diagnosed with the disorder. Difficulty in ejaculatory control may be associated with anxiety regarding the sex act. Both anxiety and ejaculation are mediated by the sympathetic nervous system. Other psychological factors include sexual guilt, interpersonal hypersensitivity and perfectionism (American Psychiatric Association, 2013).

## 23.3 Female sexual dysfunctions

### 23.3.1 Female orgasmic disorder

Female orgasmic disorder is characterised by difficulty in experiencing orgasm and/or a markedly reduced intensity of orgasmic sensations. Subjective descriptions of orgasm vary greatly; to make the diagnosis it must be accompanied by clinically significant distress. The causes are usually multifactorial or cannot be determined. Reported prevalence rates for orgasmic problems vary widely (10–42%) and do not take into account the presence of distress. Approximately 10% of women do not experience orgasm throughout their lifetime. Numerous psychological factors are associated with female sexual inhibition, including fears of impregnation, rejection by a partner, hostility towards men and guilt feelings about sexual impulses (American Psychiatric Association, 2013).

### 23.3.2 Female sexual interest/arousal disorder

To make a diagnosis of female sexual interest/arousal disorder, the interpersonal context must be taken into account. A situation where the woman has a lower desire for sexual activity than her partner is not sufficient to diagnose female sexual interest/arousal disorder. There must be an absence or a reduced frequency or intensity of at least three of the six indicators (sexual activity, erotic thoughts, initiation of sexual activity, sexual excitement or pleasure, sexual interest or arousal, genital or non-genital sensations during sexual activity) for at least six months. Short-term changes in sexual interest or arousal are common and may be adaptive responses to events or stressors and do not represent a

## Case study 23.1

A couple presented with a complaint of lack of desire on the wife's part. Mr and Mrs B. were in their 40s and were both professionals. They sustained a satisfactory sex life up to the year before they came for the consultation. Mrs B felt sufficiently attracted to her husband before this time, but now agreed to seek help because of his increasing complaints about their lack of sexual interaction. Mrs B was physically healthy and all her blood results, including hormone levels, were within normal limits. She reported that juggling all her obligations at home and work had been very demanding. She had to put off certain projects at work because her husband was working long hours and she had to take on more of the responsibility at home. Mr B has been attending conferences, networking and writing articles. He made it clear that he could not put his career on hold and felt that his wife's demands on his time were unreasonable. Mrs B's current lack of desire was associated with anger at her husband whom she perceived as no longer willing to support her career. She felt that he was being selfish. Mrs B was diagnosed with female sexual interest/arousal disorder, because her symptoms have been present for approximately 12 months.

sexual dysfunction. In clinical practice, relationship problems are the most commonly given reason for decreased sexual activity (American Psychiatric Association, 2013).

### 23.3.3 Genito-pelvic pain/ penetration disorder

Genito-pelvic pain/penetration disorder refers to four commonly co-morbid symptom dimensions. It presents with persistent or recurrent difficulties with one or more of the following symptoms:

- vaginal penetration during intercourse
- genito-pelvic pain
- fear of, or anxiety over, pain or vaginal penetration
- tension of the pelvic floor muscles during attempted vaginal penetration.

Note: In the DSM-5, this disorder represents both vaginismus and dyspareunia, which were terms previously used in DSM-IV.

The diagnosis can be made on the basis of marked difficulty in only one symptom dimension if it causes clinically significant distress. Although the prevalence of genito-pelvic pain/ penetration disorder is unknown, it is frequently associated with other sexual dysfunctions and relationship problems (American Psychiatric Association, 2013).

## 23.4 Other sexual dysfunctions

### 23.4.1 Substance-induced or medication-induced sexual dysfunction

This diagnosis is made when there is clinically significant disturbance in sexual function that is associated with substance intoxication or withdrawal or after exposure to medication capable of producing the sexual dysfunction. The diagnosis of substance-induced sexual dysfunction is made instead of a diagnosis of substance intoxication or substance withdrawal only when the sexual symptoms predominate in the clinical picture. The onset of antidepressant-induced sexual dysfunction may be as early as eight days after the initiation of the medication. There is some evidence that sexual dysfunction related to substances or medication increases with age (American Psychiatric Association, 2013).

**Table 23.3** Substances and medications commonly associated with sexual dysfunction

| | |
|---|---|
| **Intoxication or withdrawal** | alcohol<br>opioids<br>sedative<br>hypnotics or anxiolytics<br>stimulants |
| **Medications** | antidepressants<br>antipsychotics<br>anticonvulsants (excluding lamotrigine)<br>benzodiazepines<br>cytotoxic agents<br>centrally-acting antihypertensives<br>hormonal contraceptives |

**Source:** Sadock, 2000

## 23.4.2 Other specified sexual dysfunction and unspecified sexual dysfunction

These classifications are used when the symptoms of the sexual dysfunction does not meet the full criteria for any of the specific disorders. With 'other specified sexual dysfunction' the clinician must communicate the specific reason that the presentation does not meet the criteria for a specific sexual dysfunction. With 'unspecified sexual dysfunction' the clinician does not specify this reason; this includes presentations where there is not enough information available to confirm a diagnosis (American Psychiatric Association, 2013).

## 23.2 Advanced reading block

**Antipsychotic drugs**

Most antipsychotic drugs are dopamine-receptor antagonists that also block adrenergic and cholinergic receptors, which accounts for their adverse sex effects. Agents with potent anticholinergic effects impair erection and ejaculation in men and inhibit vaginal lubrication and orgasm in women.

**Antidepressant drugs**

Sexual dysfunction, including changes in libido, impaired erectile capacity and delayed or inhibited ejaculation or orgasm, has been reported with almost all antidepressants. With selective serotonin reuptake inhibitors (SSRIs) the increased serotonin concentration can cause a decreased libido and difficulty in reaching orgasm in both genders. Of the SSRIs, the most frequent sexual adverse effects are seen with paroxetine, then with fluoxetine and the least with sertraline. Reversal of negative effects has been achieved with cyproheptadine (antihistamine with antiserotonergic effects), amantadine (dopamine agonist), yohimbine (central alpha$_2$ adrenergic receptor antagonist), methylphenidate (dopaminergic and adrenergic effects), buspirone and sildenafil. The tricyclic and tetracyclic antidepressants have anticholinergic effects that interfere with erection and delay ejaculation.

Antidepressants that can be considered for use in patients with sexual side effects are bupropion, reboxetine or mirtazapine.

Note: Since depression is associated with a decreased libido and sexual dysfunction, the evaluation of possible sexual side effects from medication is very difficult and should be monitored carefully.

**Alcohol**

Alcohol suppresses central nervous system (CNS) activity and can produce erectile disorders in males. Alcohol has a direct gonadal effect that decreases testosterone concentrations in men. Paradoxically, it can produce a slight increase in testosterone in women. Long-term use of alcohol reduces the ability of the liver to metabolise oestrogenic compounds, which can lead to testicular atrophy and gynecomastia in men (Sadock, 2000).

## 23.5 Taking a sexual history

Most patients with sexual problems present to primary care doctors with other complaints, such as gynaecological problems, disturbed sleep or mood problems. It is important to develop a positive doctor-patient relationship and to be non-judgemental, because patients often feel embarrassed to talk about their sexual difficulties. Learn to take a sexual history without shame or embarrassment. The specifics of the current sexual complaint should be obtained, as well as usual patterns of sexual practice, fantasies, masturbatory history, relationship issues and the degree of commitment. The onset and frequency of the problem and the patient's perception of the partner's contribution to the present problem should be described. Early sexual development and education should also be discussed. All interviews should review high-risk sexual behaviour (regardless of sexual orientation) since transmission of HIV is a major problem among all groups. Additionally, the issue of sexual abuse must be explored, since a history of abuse predisposes to the development of sexual dysfunction. During the assessment it is important to screen for co-morbid psychiatric conditions, such as depression and anxiety. The doctor should supply information and offer reassurance (Sadock, 2000).

## 23.6 Management of sexual dysfunction

When faced with an individual or a couple with a sexual problem, the first priority is to consider the possibility of medical causes. A thorough medical evaluation, including a medical and psychiatric history, physical examination and appropriate laboratory investigations, should be done. If a medical cause is found it should be treated appropriately (e.g. antibiotics for genital infections, change of causal medication or initiating antidepressant treatment if depression is diagnosed). When a medical condition is not reversible (e.g. peripheral vascular disease or neuropathies) patients should be reassured and educated about their condition and different management options. In most cases the patient will have to be referred to the appropriate specialist for further investigation and treatment.

In cases of erectile disorder, nocturnal penile tumescence monitoring or an ultrasound flow meter can be performed. Angiography may identify vascular causes of erectile dysfunction and cases that may be suitable for vascular reconstructive surgery. Other laboratory tests that may be indicated include a glucose tolerance test, thyroid and liver function tests, prolactin, luteinising hormone and follicle-stimulating hormone levels.

Sexual dysfunction, especially in men, may be associated with many modifiable risk factors that should be addressed. All patients should be provided with general advice to modify these risk factors, including losing weight, lowering alcohol intake, addressing sleeping problems (e.g. obstructive sleep apnoea) and managing depression and diabetes. (Martin *et al.*, 2014).

Once all medical factors have been addressed or excluded and the diagnosis of a sexual dysfunction is confirmed, the individual or couple should be referred for psychotherapy. The clinician should not label one individual in a couple as having the problem and should rather make the couple the focus of attention. Relationship issues should be addressed as well as the different therapy methods (e.g. dual sex therapy, assertiveness training, behavioural therapy, group therapy and integrated sex therapy) that are available.

Principles of sex therapy are relatively simple to learn, and emphasise education about sexual functioning, assisting couples to improve communication and correcting dysfunctional attitudes about sex that one or both partners may hold. Therapy involves assignments that help the couple in learning how to increase sensory awareness; these assignments can be completed at home. Techniques may include self-masturbation, sensate focus exercises, special coital techniques and learning to separate pleasure from physiological response (e.g. erection) (Sadock, 2000).

### 23.6.1 Biological management

Biological treatment, including pharmacotherapy and surgery, have application in specific cases of sexual dysfunction. Some medications used in the treatment of erectile disorder include sildenafil, vardenafil, tadalafil, oral prostaglandin, alprostadil (Caverject), injectable phentolamine and a transurethral alprostadil. The drugs should be used in conjunction with, not as a replacement for, sex therapy.

Sildenafil is a nitric oxide enhancer that facilitates blood flow to the penis; it has no effect in the absence of sexual stimulation. Common adverse effects include headaches, flushing and dyspepsia. Other drugs that work with a similar mechanism include tadalafil and vardenafil. The difference between the drugs are for how long they are effective and how quickly they work. Vardenafil are effective for approximately five hours and sildenafil for approximately four hours. They both take effect in about 30 minutes. Tadalafil works a bit faster (within approximately 15 minutes) and the effect lasts up to 36 hours.

This group of medications is contraindicated for people using nitrates or alpha-blockers and should be used with caution in men with a recent history of myocardial infarction, stroke, arrhythmia, cardiac failure, angina pectoris and extreme hypotension or hypertension (Sadock, 2000).

In contrast to oral medication, injectable and transurethral prostadil act locally on the penis and can produce erections in the absence of sexual stimulation. Alprostadil contains a naturally occurring form of prostaglandin E1, which is a powerful vasodilating agent.

### 23.6.2 Other pharmacological agents

Anti-anxiety agents may have some application in tense patients, although they can also interfere with the sexual response. The side effects of SSRIs have been used to prolong the sexual response in patients with premature ejaculation that do not respond to behavioural interventions. Some substances, like ginseng and yohimbine, have popular standing as aphrodisiacs, but this has not been confirmed by any studies. The antidepressant bupropion has dopaminergic effects and has increased sex drive in some patients, but should be used with caution if the patient has not been diagnosed with depression. All biological treatments should only be used in combination with therapy or when a patient does not respond to therapy alone (Sadock, 2000).

**23.3 Advanced reading block**

The physiological mechanism of penile erection involves the release of nitric oxide in the corpus cavernosum during sexual stimulation. Nitric oxide activates guanylate cyclase, which increases cyclic guanosine monophosphate, which then produces smooth muscle relaxation in the corpus cavernosum. This process allows the penile blood vessel to dilate and admit blood. Sildenafil, tadalafil and vardenafil augment this natural process by inhibiting the enzyme that degrades cyclic guanosine monophosphate (Sadock, 2000).

# Paraphilic disorders

## 23.7 Introduction and context

The term 'paraphilia' is derived from the Greek *para* (to the side of or beyond the usual) and *philia* (love)). The DSM-5 defines a paraphilia as 'any intense and persistent sexual interest other than sexual interest in genital stimulation or preparatory fondling with phenotypically normal, physically mature, consenting human partners' (American Psychiatric Association, 2013). A paraphilic disorder (the term used in the DSM-5, and which will be used in this chapter) or disorder of sexual preference (the term used by ICD-10 (World Health Organization, 1992) may be diagnosed in individuals in whom a paraphilia causes significant distress or functional impairment in the individual concerned, or whose satisfaction has entailed risk of harm or actual harm to others. A paraphilia is a necessary, but insufficient, condition for the diagnosis of a paraphilic disorder: a paraphilia by itself does not necessarily justify or require clinical attention or intervention.

Other terms that have been used for paraphilic disorders include sexual deviance or sexual perversion. There is much overlap between paraphilic disorders, sexual offending and inappropriate sexual behaviour. They all involve a range of sexual behaviours that cause offence and/or harm to others. They may, and often do, involve activities that are criminal or illegal (depending on many factors such as the nature of the paraphilic disorder in question and its specific attributes in the individual concerned, whether coercion was used, the nature and degree of a human rights violation or harm to others, and the specific legislation of the country concerned). This notwithstanding, they remain separate concepts. A man who commits a sexual offence against a child may or may not have paedophilic disorder. A 15-year-old adolescent boy who has sexual intercourse with his 14-year-old girlfriend is committing a sexual offence, but will not necessarily be displaying inappropriate or unusual sexual behaviour, nor be sexually deviant or perverted.

This section of the chapter will initially outline the clinical features, classification, epidemiology, aetiology and clinical assessment principles of paraphilic disorders. This will be followed by a brief overview of specific paraphilic disorders, and summary of the course, clinical management and prognosis of paraphilic disorders.

## 23.7.1 Clinical features

People with paraphilic disorder experience recurrent and intense sexually arousing fantasies, urges, impulses and/or behaviour that involve inappropriate and/or unusual objects or activities. Such individuals either act on their fantasies, urges and impulses, are markedly distressed by them and/or are functionally impaired (in social, occupational or other important spheres of life) as a result (see Table 23.4).

The specialised sexual paraphilic fantasies or urges, and their behavioural manifestations, are usually considered the pathognomonic component of paraphilic disorders, with sexual arousal and/or orgasm being associated phenomena. The sexual behaviour of people with paraphilic disorder diverges from normal sexual behaviour and is unconventional in not conforming to generally accepted social norms (though this differs significantly in each society and at different periods in history). The consequences of paraphilic disorders extend beyond the sexual sphere to negatively influence and pervade people's lives (both the person with paraphilic disorder and those of others). People with paraphilic disorder usually conceal their paraphilic fantasies, impulses and urges. The associated behaviour often involves the degradation, coercion, humiliation or dehumanisation of people who are either unable or unwilling to consent (although this is not necessarily always the case) and are often significantly harmful and/or illegal. While many people with paraphilic disorder may make numerous resolutions to stop, they seem generally unable to abstain for too long. Whilst paraphilic arousal and behaviour may occur only during periods of stress, conflict, anxiety or even depression, people with paraphilic disorders usually have more pervasive and lifelong problems, with paraphilic imagery and interests starting before or during puberty. Acting on paraphilic urges is often followed by marked distress in people with paraphilic disorder. The distress may be the result of many factors, including attitudes of society, conflict between paraphilic urges and the individual's moral standards, feelings of guilt or remorse at causing harm to others and fear of social, interpersonal, occupational or legal consequences of disclosure. The validity of the DSM-5 and ICD-10 diagnostic requirement that significant distress or functional impairment must always be present has been questioned, as many people with paraphilias experience distress only upon disclosure of their paraphilic activity, and not necessarily as a result of their condition.

**Table 23.4** The core features of a paraphilic disorder

| Feature | Description |
|---|---|
| Sexual fantasies, urges or impulses | ▸ involves inappropriate, unusual or specialised objects or activities<br>▸ recurrent, intense and persistent<br>▸ experienced for at least six months |
| Sexual arousal | ▸ depends on mental or behavioural elaboration of such fantasies, urges or impulses |
| Sexual behaviour | ▸ does not conform to generally accepted social norms<br>▸ is ritualised, stereotyped and/or compulsive in nature |
| Consequences to self and others | ▸ causes distress and/or functional impairment to the individual<br>▸ often involves coercion of people who are unable or unwilling to consent<br>▸ usually causes personal harm or harm to others |

The general diagnostic criteria common to all paraphilic disorders specified in the DSM-5 are outlined in Table 23.5. Diagnostic criteria for specific paraphilic disorders are provided later in the chapter.

In the light of the distinction between paraphilia and paraphilic disorders, the diagnosis of a paraphilic disorder is reserved for individuals who meet both criterion A and B. An individual who meets criterion A only denotes a particular paraphilia (which may be discovered during the course of the clinical assessment for some other mental disorder).

**Table 23.5** General diagnostic criteria for paraphilic disorder

| Criterion | Description |
|---|---|
| A | Specifies the qualitative nature of the paraphilia (i.e. disturbed or anomalous sexual activity or target preferences) for at least 6 months |
| B | Specifies the negative consequences of the paraphilia, for example acting on these urges with a non-consenting person, or clinically significant distress or functional impairment to self |

**Source:** Authors' own Table

## 23.7.2 Classification

The specific paraphilic disorders listed in the ICD-10 and the DSM-5 are similar, as shown in Table 23.6.

The rationale for selecting the specific paraphilic disorders traditionally included in the ICD-10 and the DSM-5 classification systems is based on two observations:

- the listed paraphilic disorders are relatively common (in relation to the dozens of other distinct but rare paraphilic disorders, which are placed in the residual categories
- many of the listed paraphilic disorders entail behavioural manifestations that are classified as criminal offences (due to their noxious nature and potential to violate and/or harm others).

The order of listing in the DSM-5 system is based on the system outlined in Figure 23.1, in which paraphilic preferences are grouped according to anomalous activity and target preferences respectively.

## 23.7.3 Epidemiology

Since many individuals with paraphilic disorders do not present to mental health services for help or are unlikely to disclose sexually anomalous preferences and behaviour in surveys because of social and legal stigma, it is difficult to obtain accurate prevalence and other epidemiological data. People with paraphilic disorders often come to the attention of mental health professionals only when their paraphilic behaviour has brought them into conflict with their families,

**Table 23.6** Specific paraphilic disorders included in the ICD-10 and the DSM-5

| ICD-10 | DSM-5 | Paraphilic focus or preference |
|---|---|---|
| voyeurism | voyeuristic disorder | Observing others engaged in private activities |
| exhibitionism | exhibitionistic disorder | Exposing genitals to strangers |
| - | frotteuristic disorder | Touching or rubbing against strangers |
| sadomasochism | sexual masochism disorder | Undergoing humiliation, bondage, pain or suffering |
| | sexual sadism disorder | Inflicting humiliation, bondage, pain or suffering |
| paedophilia | paedophilic disorder | Sexual focus on children |
| fetishism | fetishistic disorder | Sexual focus on inanimate objects or on specific non-genital body parts |
| fetishistic transvestitism | transvestic disorder | Sexual focus on cross-dressing |
| multiple, other and unspecified disorders of sexual preference | other specified and unspecified paraphilic disorders | Residual categories for other paraphilic disorders (e.g. necrophilia, zoophilia, coprophilia, urophilia, etc.) |

sexual partners or the law. Prevalence rates from such legally identified cases of sexual offending are unlikely to be accurate approximations of rates of paraphilic disorders in clinical samples or the general population. This notwithstanding, a number of general conclusions can be drawn from the available evidence in respect of the epidemiology of paraphilic disorders (Abel *et al.*, 1987; Abel and Osborn, 2006). It is estimated that

- paraphilic disorders are far more common in males than females (estimated male:female ratio is approximately 30:1)
- the age of onset is usually from mid-adolescence to early adulthood

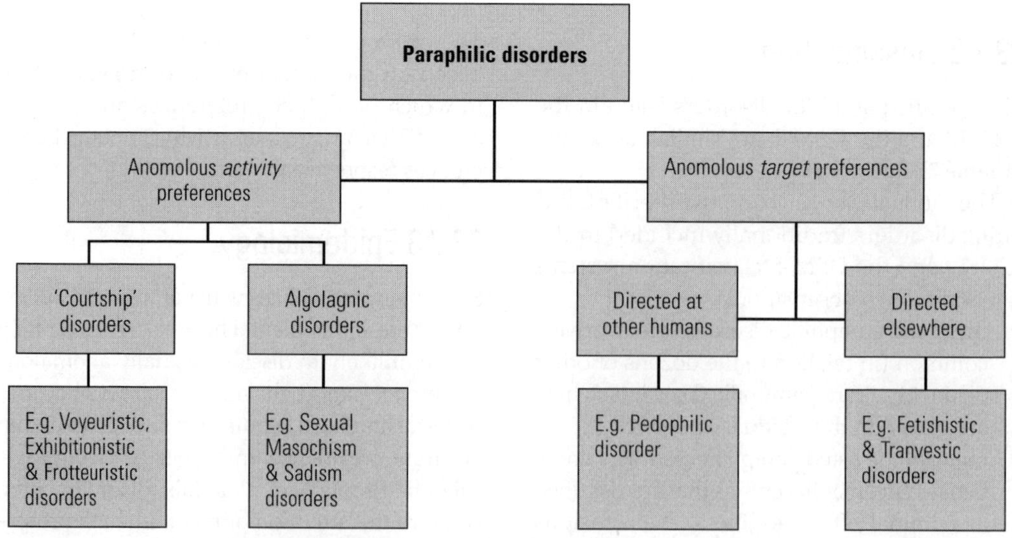


**Figure 23.1** Paraphilic disorders grouped by anomalous preference

**Source:** Author's own diagram

- many individuals have multiple paraphilic disorders and/or co-morbidity with other psychiatric disorders
- a large survey of over 561 participants seeking assessment and/or treatment for their sexual interests within a psychiatric setting reported the most common paraphilic disorders to be paedophilia (approximately 50% of cases), followed by exhibitionism (12%), voyeurism (5%) and frotteurism (5%).

## 23.7.4 Aetiology

Paraphilic disorders are complex behavioural and psychiatric syndromes of which the cause remains largely unknown. While numerous aetiological theories have been proposed, there remains insufficient evidence to draw specific conclusions about causality. The main theories relate to biological and psychosocial factors.

### 23.7.4.1 Biological theories

The main biological theories advanced paraphilic disorders are:

- genetic: chromosomal abnormalities have been implicated but there is insufficient data available to draw specific conclusions
- physiological: intra-uterine hormonal influences have been suggested to contribute to the nature and intensity of sexual drive and preferences later in life; early CNS insults at critical stages of growth may also impair control mechanisms that govern sexual behaviour
- neurological: reportedly a disproportionate number of people with paraphilic disorder have soft neurological signs, abnormal EEGs and co-morbid neuropsychiatric disorders (e.g. epilepsy, intellectual impairment, autism-spectrum disorders and traumatic brain injury).

### 23.7.4.2 Psychosocial theories

The main psychosocial theories advanced for paraphilic disorder are:

- psychodynamic: failure to complete normal psychosexual development is postulated to manifest in paraphilic behaviours as an outlet for anomalous or deviant sexual and aggressive drives
- cognitive-behavioural learning models stress the importance of early experience, learning and conditioning in the development of paraphilic preferences. The earliest choice or use of inappropriate objects or behaviour for sexual gratification (viewed as random, idiosyncratic occurrences) may predispose people to develop paraphilic choices in later life. The expression of early paraphilic interests results from the extent to which the child anticipates the consequences of acting on those interests
- social learning models suggest that the sociocultural environment of people with paraphilic disorders is an important factor. Lack of parental care, harsh and erratic discipline, poor role models, violence and sexual and non-sexual abuse in the family may predispose children to paraphilic disorders, via deficient attachment bonds, lowering of self-esteem, and maladaptive identification with aggression and social deviance
- addiction models view deviant sexual behaviour as addictive in nature, and fulfilling some unspecified need, much as many substances of abuse do.

## 23.7.5 Assessment and diagnostic principles

A focused and comprehensive clinical interview, mental state examination, physical examination, and special investigations (as indicated) are necessary in every case presenting with suspected paraphilic disorder. The goals of the interview, context of clinical assessment (e.g. forensic versus clinical), potential limits on confidentiality (e.g. in cases which may involve criminal processes or identified potential victims) and informed consent are important considerations in all cases. The clinician must attend to the following questions and issues during the course of assessment:

- **Why is the individual presenting now?** People with paraphilic disorders may present themselves directly or upon request of another party (e.g. partner, legal agency, social worker) when the paraphilic behaviour is discovered, causing problems in relationships or during the course of legal proceedings following the commission of an offence. Patients may present with another sexual dysfunction or mental disorder (see below), with the paraphilic disorder coming to light upon further assessment.

- **Is there another co-morbid medical or mental disorder present, and is there more than one paraphilic disorder present in the same individual?** Various co-morbid medical and psychiatric disorders may lead to unusual, inappropriate or anomalous sexual behaviour e.g. traumatic brain injury and other neurological conditions (e.g. seizure disorders, frontal lobe syndromes, post-encephalitic syndromes, multiple sclerosis, mood disorders (bipolar and depressive disorders), psychotic spectrum disorders, anxiety disorders, substance-related disorders, intellectual impairment, neurocognitive disorders or personality disorders). Suicide risk may be high if individuals are charged with sexual offences or are exposed in their community or family. Co-morbidity is more common in patients who present with paraphilic disorders in middle age or later. It is also relatively common for individuals to manifest two or more paraphilic disorders, with the paraphilic foci of each paraphilic disorder being closely related (e.g. foot fetishism in addition to shoe fetishism) or multiple paraphilic foci occurring without obvious inter-connectedness (e.g. transvestic and sexual sadism disorder). Any co-morbid disorders (including adjustment responses, such as depression, anxiety or guilt over the paraphilic disorder itself) will require further clinical assessment and management as indicated.
- **Comprehensive psychosexual assessment** is clearly essential for anyone who presents with a paraphilic disorder. Clinicians should make an effort to put patients at ease and adopt an empathic and open approach to facilitate discussion and disclosure of sexual matters. The involvement of partners and significant others may be helpful (either by obtaining collateral information or inclusion in the interview process). Psychosexual themes to be covered should include a relationship history (e.g. partner details, nature of relationships, interpersonal conflict, sexual issues), sexual history (e.g. development of sexual interest, age and nature of first sexual encounter, masturbation, intercourse, libido, sexual experience, sexual dysfunction), sexual knowledge, sexual attitudes to self and others, sexual fantasies, urges and impulses (e.g. onset, development, content, and intensity of fantasies, urges and impulses as well as emotional responses to them), specific paraphilic sexual behaviours (range, context, frequency and duration, materials and paraphernalia used, conditions for arousal, associated sexual offending or legal issues and details), associated distress, thoughts, attitudes or feelings and degree and nature of any functional impairment. In some circumstances, the 'intense and persistent' criterion may be difficult to apply (e.g. people who are severely medically ill or very old who may not have sexual interests of any kind). In such cases, a paraphilia may be present when the sexual interest is greater than or equal to normophilic sexual interest.
- **Risk assessment:** The risk of sexual offending should be assessed using clinical judgement, actuarial and structured risk assessment tools.
- **What does the individual seek from clinical assessment or management?** The context of the assessment, whether the person wants professional clinical help or has presented by socio-legal coercion, and their motivation for change (e.g. do they wish to change the focus of their paraphilic sexual arousal, desist from overt paraphilic sexual behaviour or adapt better without necessarily changing such behaviour?) are all important considerations.
- **Are any further investigations required?** A number of specialised investigations that attempt to assess sexual interest (e.g. penile plethysmography, polygraphy, visual reaction times) are available but their clinical availability, utility and value are limited.

The issues outlined above vary considerably amongst individuals presenting to mental health services. Each person being assessed is unique and there is a large degree of heterogeneity of presentation. The clinical approach (and hence management plan) must therefore be individualised.

## 23.7.6 Specific paraphilic disorders

### 23.7.6.1 Voyeuristic disorder

The act of voyeurism is usually secretive, and individuals may not come to clinical or criminal attention. Individuals with voyeuristic disorder often return to the same environment repeatedly to fulfil their voyeuristic fantasies and urges. Opportunistic observation without distress or impairment (e.g. an adolescent male who watches his female neighbour sunbathing in her back yard without her top on) should not be labelled as voyeuristic disorder. When people with voyeuristic disorder are arrested it is commonly for acts such as trespassing or housebreaking, with voyeurism often not identified as the main offence.

### 23.7.6.2 Exhibitionistic disorder

Exhibitionists are usually males exposing themselves to females. Their aim is not to frighten the victim. Cognitive distortions involving the reaction of victims are common (e.g.'They screamed like they would if I were a rock star','They laugh because they like it'. They often find it difficult to grasp the distress victims may experience (e.g.'There was no physical attack, and I did not touch her'). Masturbation and fantasy involving the victim(s) in a sexual role before, during or after the event often take place. Co-morbid paedophilic disorder is common and should not be overlooked.

**Table 23.7** DSM-5 Diagnostic Criteria for Voyeuristic Disorder

| Diagnostic Criteria |
|---|
| A. Over a period of at least 6 months, recurrent and intense sexual arousal from observing an unsuspecting person who is naked, in the process of disrobing, or engaging in sexual activity, as manifested by fantasies, urges, or behaviors. |
| B. The individual has acted on these sexual urges with a nonconsenting person, or the sexual urges or fantasies cause clinically significant distress or impairment in social, occupational, or other important areas of functioning. |
| C. The individual experiencing the arousal and/or acting on the urges is at least 18 years of age. |
| *Specify* if: |
| ▸ **In a controlled environment:** This specifier is primarily applicable to individuals living in institutional or other settings where opportunities to engage in voyeuristic behaviour are restricted. |
| ▸ **In full remission:** The individual has not acted on the urges with a nonconsenting person, and there has been no distress or impairment in social, occupational, or other areas of functioning, for at least 5 years while in an uncontrolled environment. |

**Source:** Reprinted with permission from the *Diagnostic and Statistical Manual of Mental Disorders*, Fifth Edition, (Copyright 2013). American Psychiatric Association.

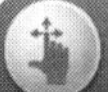

**Case study 23.2**

**Voyeuristic disorder**

A 33 year old male is found in the garden of a girl's hostel and is arrested for trespassing. Residents report that he is frequently seen in the area although he lives about 12 km away. He denies spying on the girls and claims he was looking for his cat. His mother reports that he does not own a cat and a check of his criminal record reveals that he was previously arrested for trespassing on two occasions dating back to his late teens. On both occasions he received a warning only. His cellphone has several video recordings and photographs of girls in various states of undress in front of windows.

**Table 23.8** DSM-5 Diagnostic Criteria for Exhibitionistic Disorder

| Diagnostic Criteria |
|---|
| A. Over a period of at least 6 months, recurrent and intense sexual arousal from the exposure of one's genitals to an unsuspecting person, as manifested by fantasies, urges, or behaviors.<br>B. The individual has acted on these sexual urges with a nonconsenting person, or the sexual urges or fantasies cause clinically significant distress or impairment in social, occupational, or other important areas of functioning.<br>*Specify* whether:<br>▸ **Sexually aroused by exposing genitals to prepubertal children**<br>▸ **Sexually aroused by exposing genitals to physically mature individuals**<br>▸ **Sexually aroused by exposing genitals to prepubertal children and to physically mature individuals**<br>*Specify* if:<br>▸ **In a controlled environment:** This specifier is primarily applicable to individuals living in institutional or other settings where opportunities to expose one's genitals are restricted.<br>▸ **In full remission:** The individual has not acted on the urges with a nonconsenting person, and there has been no distress or impairment in social, occupational, or other areas of functioning, for at least 5 years while in an uncontrolled environment. |

**Source:** Reprinted with permission from the *Diagnostic and Statistical Manual of Mental Disorders*, Fifth Edition, (Copyright 2013). American Psychiatric Association.

## 23.7.6.3 Frotteuristic disorder

People with frotteuristic disorder usually choose crowded areas (e.g. trains, sporting events or bars) to touch and rub against victims. It is a criminal offence but seldom has serious legal consequences. The act is often carefully planned, with the location and victim pre-selected, and movements can be very well rehearsed. Such individuals may wear a condom or extra clothing to prevent ejaculate from showing on clothes. Cognitive distortions are frequently noted (e.g. 'I did not actually harm her... she did not even know it was happening... it is not like I tried to rape her').

**Table 23.9** DSM-5 Diagnostic Criteria for Frotteuristic Disorder

| Diagnostic Criteria |
|---|
| A. Over a period of at least 6 months, recurrent and intense sexual arousal from touching or rubbing against a nonconsenting person, as manifested by fantasies, urges, or behaviors.<br>B. The individual has acted on these sexual urges with a nonconsenting person, or the sexual urges or fantasies cause clinically significant distress or impairment in social, occupational, or other important areas of functioning.<br>*Specify* if:<br>▸ **In a controlled environment:** This specifier is primarily applicable to individuals living in institutional or other settings where opportunities to touch or rub against a nonconsenting person are restricted.<br>▸ **In full remission:** The individual has not acted on the urges with a nonconsenting person, and there has been no distress or impairment in social, occupational, or other areas of functioning, for at least 5 years while in an uncontrolled environment. |

**Source:** Reprinted with permission from the D*iagnostic and Statistical Manual of Mental Disorders*, Fifth Edition, (Copyright 2013). American Psychiatric Association.

### Case study 23.3

**Exhibitionistic disorder**

A 25-year-old male is arrested for exposing himself to two teenage girls. They started running away but decided to follow the man from a distance after he left the scene. They contacted the police and the man was apprehended in the student residence where he lived. He reported that the startled reaction and screams from the girls were delight and amazement and when they glanced back at him whilst running away it was because they had to have a second look. Local residents report a young male known as 'the flasher' exposing himself regularly to teenagers in the area for the past year.

### 23.7.6.4 Sexual masochism disorder

Masochists seldom seek psychiatric help and are not likely to present to the criminal justice system as the behaviour is not illegal. They are sometimes seen in medical settings due to injuries sustained as a result of masochistic behaviour e.g. bruises, foreign objects in orifices, burns and cut wounds. There is a risk of accidental death while practicing asphyxiophilia or other auto-erotic procedures, such as suffocation, hanging or other complicated procedures to cut off oxygen supply whilst masturbating.

**Table 23.10** DSM-5 Diagnostic Criteria for Sexual Masochism Disorder

| Diagnostic Criteria |
|---|
| A. Over a period of at least 6 months, recurrent and intense sexual arousal from the act of being humiliated, beaten, bound, or otherwise made to suffer, as manifested by fantasies, urges, or behaviors. |
| B. The fantasies, sexual urges, or behaviors cause clinically significant distress or impairment in social, occupational, or other important areas of functioning. |
| *Specify* if: |
| ▸ **With asphyxiophilia:** If the individual engages in the practice of achieving sexual arousal related to restriction of breathing. |
| *Specify* if: |
| ▸ **In a controlled environment:** This specifier is primarily applicable to individuals living in institutional or other settings where opportunities to engage in masochistic sexual behaviors are restricted. |
| ▸ **In full remission:** There has been no distress or impairment in social, occupational, or other areas of functioning for at last 5 years while in an uncontrolled environment. |

**Source:** Reprinted with permission from the *Diagnostic and Statistical Manual of Mental Disorders*, Fifth Edition, (Copyright 2013). American Psychiatric Association.

### 23.7.6.5 Sexual sadism disorder

Sexual sadists are not only interested in subduing victims but inflict excessive pain and torture to satisfy their sexual urges. Partners often start out as willing masochistic participants. The disorder is more common in males. There are multiple problems related to the definition, application of the diagnostic criteria and the reliability of the diagnosis. It has a significant impact on how the individual will be managed in the legal system. Most research relates to aggressive behaviour associated with sexual crimes but this is not necessarily motivated by sexual sadism disorder. Indicators of sexual sadism associated with crimes include torture, ritualistic elements, humiliation, victim confinement, bondage, post-death mutilation and careful planning of the offence.

**Table 23.11** DSM-5 Diagnostic Criteria for Sexual Sadism Disorder

| Diagnostic Criteria |
|---|
| A Over a period of at least 6 months, recurrent and intense sexual arousal from the physical or psychological suffering of another person, as manifested by fantasies, urges, or behaviors. |
| B. The individual has acted on these sexual urges with a nonconsenting person, or the sexual urges or fantasies cause clinically significant distress or impairment in social, occupational, or other important areas of functioning. |
| *Specify* if: |
| ▸ **In a controlled environment:** This specifier is primarily applicable to individuals living in institutional or other settings where opportunities to engage in sadistic sexual behaviours are restricted. |
| ▸ **In full remission:** The individual has not acted on the urges with a nonconsenting person, and there has been no distress or impairment in social, occupational, or other areas of functioning, for at least 5 years while in an uncontrolled environment. |

**Source:** Reprinted with permission from the *Diagnostic and Statistical Manual of Mental Disorders*, Fifth Edition, (Copyright 2013). American Psychiatric Association.

### 23.7.6.6 Paedophilic disorder

The diagnostic criteria for paedophilic disorder are intended to apply to both individuals who freely disclose this paraphilia as well as those individuals who deny any sexual attraction to prepubescent children, despite substantial objective evidence to the contrary. Extensive use of pornography depicting prepubescent children is a useful diagnostic indicator. Paedophiles with antisocial personality disorder are more likely to act out sexually. Higher rates of **recidivism** are also found in paedophiles with male

**Table 23.12** DSM-5 Diagnostic Criteria for Pedophilic Disorder

| **Diagnostic Criteria** |
|---|
| A. Over a period of at least 6 months, recurrent, intense sexually arousing fantasies, sexual urges, or behaviors involving sexual activity with a prepubescent child or children (generally age 13 years or younger). |
| B. The individual has acted on these sexual urges, or the sexual urges or fantasies cause marked distress or interpersonal difficulty. |
| C. The individual is at least age 16 years and at least 5 years older than the child or children in Criterion A. |
| Note: Do not include an individual in late adolescence involved in an ongoing sexual relationship with a 12- or 13-year-old. |
| *Specify* whether: |
| ▶ **Exclusive type** (attracted only to children) |
| ▶ **Nonexclusive type** |
| *Specify* if: |
| ▶ **Sexually attracted to males** |
| ▶ **Sexually attracted to females** |
| ▶ **Sexually attracted to both** |
| *Specify* if: |
| ▶ **Limited to incest** |

**Source:** Reprinted with permission from the *Diagnostic and Statistical Manual of Mental Disorders*, Fifth Edition, (Copyright 2013). American Psychiatric Association.

victims, multiple previous victims and unrelated victims. Paedophilia is not synonymous with sexual abuse of children. Not all child molesters have paedophilic disorder (in fact, the majority do not), as behaviour may be motivated by other factors such as opportunistic sexual offending when an appropriate and consenting adult partner is unavailable, opportunistic and impulsive sexual behaviour in people with intellectual impairment, poor impulse control in the context of traumatic brain injury or substance intoxication or criminal sexual contact with children to avoid contracting HIV (since children are less likely to carry the virus). Child molesters are more likely to abuse children of varying ages, genders and familial relationship to them. Individuals with paedophilic disorder tend to be more preferential in choosing potential victims. Such individuals often seek occupational roles that place them in close proximity to children (e.g. teachers, youth counsellors, volunteers at youth organisations). Cognitive distortions often involve some form of misdirected sex education (e.g.'I was showing the child what to expect in future and what people are not allowed to do to them') or **rationalisation** (e.g.'The child did not cry or ask me to stop so I was not upsetting them').

### 23.7.6.7 Fetishistic disorder

Many individuals with fetishistic interests are not distressed or impaired by them, and do not meet the diagnostic criteria for fetishistic disorder. It is common for sexualised fetishes to combine inanimate objects (e.g. shoes) with a body part (e.g. feet). The exclusive focus of sexual interest on a specific body part is called partialism. Fetishism does not necessarily require the participation of a partner as sexual activity may be with the object itself (e.g. masturbating whilst fondling a shoe). Individuals may find it difficult

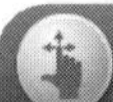

## Case study 23.4

**Paedophilic disorder**

A 38-year-old male was arrested after approaching an 11-year-old boy outside a primary school and offering him money to accompany him. He had previously been noticed outside the school talking to young boys. His computer contained multiple images of child pornography. There was email correspondence with four different boys between the ages of 10 and 14 years where he posed as a 15 year old boy wanting to meet new friends. He has a history of three previous arrests for exposing himself outside primary schools and an arrest for sexual assault of a 10 year old boy when he was 19 years old. He has never been involved in a long-term relationship and denied any sexual arousal from exposing himself or looking at images of children. He was adamant that he was just friendly towards the boy and refused to co-operate any further.

**Table 23.13** DSM-5 Diagnostic Criteria for Fetishistic Disorder

| Diagnostic Criteria |
|---|
| A. Over a period of at least 6 months, recurrent and intense sexual arousal from either the use of nonliving objects or a highly specific focus on nongenital body part(s), as manifested by fantasies, urges, or behaviors. |
| B. The fantasies, sexual urges, or behaviors cause clinically significant distress or impairment in social, occupational, or other important areas of functioning. |
| C. The fetish objects are not limited to articles of clothing used in cross-dressing (as in transvestic disorder) or devices specifically designed for the purpose of tactile genital stimulation (e.g., vibrator). |
| *Specify*: |
| ▸ **Body part(s)** |
| ▸ **Nonliving object(s)** |
| ▸ **Other** |
| *Specify* if: |
| ▸ **In a controlled environment:** This specifier is primarily applicable to individuals living in institutional or other settings where opportunities to engage in fetishistic behaviours are restricted. |
| ▸ **In full remission:** There has been no distress or impairment in social, occupational, or other areas of functioning for at least 5 years while in an uncontrolled environment. |

**Source:** Reprinted with permission from the *Diagnostic and Statistical Manual of Mental Disorders*, Fifth Edition, (Copyright 2013). American Psychiatric Association.

to relate sexually without the presence of the object and they may also try to incorporate it into sexual activity with a partner. When people with fetishistic disorder come to the attention of the legal system it is usually for shoplifting, theft or housebreaking (in an attempt to obtain fetishistic objects) or as a result of co-morbid paraphilias.

### 23.7.6.8 Transvestic disorder

The majority of individuals involved in transvestic behaviour do not experience distress or impairment due to their sexual interests and

**Table 23.14** DSM-5 Diagnostic Criteria for Transvestic Disorder

| Diagnostic Criteria |
|---|
| A. Over a period of at least 6 months, recurrent and intense sexual arousal from crossdressing, as manifested by fantasies, urges, or behaviors. |
| B. The fantasies, sexual urges, or behaviors cause clinically significant distress or impairment in social, occupational, or other important areas of functioning. |
| *Specify* if: |
| ▸ **With fetishism:** If sexually aroused by fabrics, materials, or garments. |
| ▸ **With autogynephilia:** If sexually aroused by thoughts or images of self as female. |
| *Specify* if: |
| ▸ **In a controlled environment:** This specifier is primarily applicable to individuals living in institutional or other settings where opportunities to cross-dress are restricted. |
| ▸ **In full remission:** There has been no distress or impairment in social, occupational, or other areas of functioning for at least 5 years while in an uncontrolled environment. |

**Source:** Reprinted with permission from the *Diagnostic and Statistical Manual of Mental Disorders*, Fifth Edition, (Copyright 2013). American Psychiatric Association.

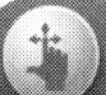

## Case study 23.5

**Fetishistic disorder**

Mr and Mrs G are in their 40's and present to a therapist with marital problems. Their sexual relationship has become a source of conflict. They met four years ago and Mrs G found it exciting when her husband asked her to keep her high-heeled shoes on during intercourse. He would spend an inordinate amount of time touching, rubbing and licking her feet. As time went, by the attention he showed her feet made her very uncomfortable but he persisted despite her objections. When she refused he would abruptly stop any sexual activity. She feels he is being unreasonable and that she has accommodated him enough; if he really loved her he would stop his behaviour. She found the situation unbearable: after he had ignored her for five weeks, she found him masturbating in her shoe cupboard. Mr G was very reluctant to engage with the therapist and appeared angry and humiliated.

would not meet the criteria for a disorder. Associated fetishism decreases the likelihood of gender dysphoria (persistent discomfort with one's gender role or identity). The presence of autogynaephilia increases the likelihood of gender dysphoria.

The DSM-5 diagnostic system includes two other categories of paraphilic disorder: 'other specified paraphilic disorder' (see Table 23.15) and 'unspecified paraphilic disorder' (see Table 23.16).

## 23.7.7 Principles of management

Intervention in paraphilic disorders should be individualised. Factors that should guide management are:

- the nature and severity of the paraphilia
- co-morbid paraphilias
- co-morbid psychiatric diagnoses
- criminal charges
- readiness for intervention
- intellectual functioning
- future risk of offending.

Three main areas that should be addressed are psychotherapy, pharmacotherapy and legal aspects.

### 23.7.7.1 Psychotherapy

Psychotherapeutic intervention is considered the mainstay of clinical management, and may involve various modalities.

#### a) Cognitive-behavioural therapy (group and individual)

Cognitive-behavioural therapy (CBT) is currently the treatment of choice in paraphilias and sexual offenders. The focus should be on aspects such as cognitive distortions used to rationalise the behaviour, victim empathy, social skills training, sex education, identifying triggers and high risk situations for paraphilic behaviour, anger management and co-morbid substance abuse.

**Table 23.15** DSM-5 Diagnostic Criteria for Other Specified Paraphilic Disorder

| |
|---|
| This category applies to presentations in which symptoms characteristic of a paraphilic disorder that cause clinically significant distress or impairment in social, occupational, or other important areas of functioning predominate but do not meet the full criteria for any of the disorders in the paraphilic disorders diagnostic class. The other specified paraphilic disorder category is used in situations in which the clinician chooses to communicate the specific reason that the presentation does not meet the criteria for any specific paraphilic disorder. This is done by recording 'other specified paraphilic disorder' followed by the specific reason (e.g., 'zoophilia'). |
| Examples of presentations that can be specified using the 'other specified' designation include, but are not limited to, recurrent and intense sexual arousal involving telephone scatologia (obscene phone calls), necrophilia (corpses), zoophilia (animals), coprophilia (feces), klismaphilia (enemas), or urophilia (urine) that has been present for at least 6 months and causes marked distress or impairment in social, occupational, or other important areas of functioning. Other specified paraphilic disorder can be specified as in remission and/or as occurring in a controlled environment. |

**Source:** Reprinted with permission from the *Diagnostic and Statistical Manual of Mental Disorders*, Fifth Edition, (Copyright 2013). American Psychiatric Association.

#### b) Individual psychotherapy

Insight-orientated longer term intervention aims at understanding how the paraphilic interest developed, how it impacts on functioning in multiple spheres, matters regarding self-esteem and developing alternative, pro-social and appropriate coping mechanisms.

#### c) Couples, marital and family therapy

It is important that people with paraphilic disorder learn to relate more appropriately with significant others and develop personal relationships that are meaningful, supportive and rewarding.

#### d) Maintenance therapy and relapse prevention

Paraphilic disorders are chronic conditions. A treatment program should incorporate support groups, regular visits to treating clinicians, community supervision and support (e.g. from parole officers, family members, work colleagues and friends). Avoiding high-risk situations and

**Table 23.16** DSM-5 Diagnostic Criteria for Unspecified Paraphilic Disorder

| This category applies to presentations in which symptoms characteristic of a paraphilic disorder that cause clinically significant distress or impairment in social, occupational, or other important areas of functioning predominate but do not meet the full criteria for any of the disorders in the paraphilic disorders diagnostic class. The unspecified paraphilic disorder category is used in situations in which the clinician chooses *not* to specify the reason that the criteria are not met for a specific paraphilic disorder, and includes presentations in which there is insufficient information to make a more specific diagnosis. |
|---|

**Source:** Reprinted with permission from the *Diagnostic and Statistical Manual of Mental Disorders*, Fifth Edition, (Copyright 2013). American Psychiatric Association.

recognising stressors that lead to paraphilic behaviour should be a focus of attention in an effort to prevent relapse and/or criminal conviction.

### 23.7.7.2 Pharmacotherapy

Pharmacotherapy may assist in reducing sex drive but has little effect on the paraphilic interest. A reduced sexual desire to commit paraphilic behaviour may make the individual more amenable to psychological and behavioural intervention. Medication should not be initiated without psychological intervention. A number of pharmacotherapeutic strategies are available.

**a) Reduction of testosterone**

There are many medical and ethical concerns regarding the initiation of these drugs. Close monitoring of possible side effects (e.g. hypertension, hyperglycaemia, obesity, gynaecomastia, decreased bone mineral density, depression) is essential.

- Anti-androgens reduce testosterone by competitive inhibition of testosterone and dihydrotestosterone at androgen receptors throughout the body. The most commonly used agent is cyproterone acetate, for which oral and long-acting depot formulations are available.
- Gonadotropin-releasing hormone agonists or analogues (GnRH analogues) stimulate the hypothalamic-pituitary axis leading to an increase in GRH secretion, followed by a dramatic reduction (and the eventual elimination) of testosterone secretion.

**b) Serotonergic drugs**

Antidepressant medications, such as SSRIs, can reduce the sexual drive as part of their side-effect profile. Some paraphilic disorders have a strong compulsive element, and SSRIs may be effective in these cases.

**c) Pharmacotherapy of co-morbid psychiatric conditions, as clinically appropriate.**

### 23.7.7.3 Legal aspects

Individuals with paraphilia sometimes break the law in response to sexual urges. Mental health professionals are frequently involved in the clinical evaluation, forensic assessment and the legal outcome of these offences. The findings may have significant impact on the individual (and on society) and be scrutinised in a legal setting. Clinical assessment of people with paraphilic disorder should, as detailed earlier in this chapter, therefore be:

- **Comprehensive**: including clinical interviews, collateral, medical and criminal records, medical and behavioural evaluation, appropriate risk assessment instruments where indicated
- **Individualised**
- In line with **recognised diagnostic criteria and classification systems** (e.g. DSM, ICD)
- Sensitive to addressing relevant legal aspects.

In addition, the following guidelines should be employed in cases which involve legal processes:

- **Treating clinicians**
  - Patients should be informed that it is the clinician's ethical, professional and legal duty to break confidentiality if a crime is brought to their attention or the identity of a victim of a sexual offence is revealed (past, present or even potential future victims).

- **Risk assessment and management**
  - Clinicians may be required by the court to assess the future risk of sexual offending using their clinical judgement or actuarial or structured risk assessment tools. This may impact on factors such as sentencing, community supervision and future treatment options.
- **Forensic assessment**
  - Paraphilic disorders alone do not cause cognitive impairment, impairment in reality testing or volitional impairment. Whilst paraphilic disorders are included in diagnostic classification systems such as the DSM and the ICD, they have little or no impact on competence to stand trial or on criminal responsibility (i.e. an appreciation of wrongfulness and capacity to act accordingly). They are not usually considered by the court as mitigating factors; on the contrary, they are often viewed as an aggravating factor leading to harsher sentencing outcomes.

### 23.7.8 Course

Paraphilic disorders are pervasive, chronic disorders that usually commence in adolescence. Most paraphilic thoughts and fantasies increase in frequency during the course of adolescence, with increased sex drive eventually resulting in paraphilic behaviour. The course tends to fluctuate, with paraphilic behaviour increasing during times of stress and decreasing with age and or ill-health.

### 23.7.9 Prognostic factors

Poor prognostic indicators include early age of onset, high frequency of acts, no guilt or shame associated with paraphilic acts, and co-morbidity (e.g. antisocial-personality disorder, substance abuse, additional paraphilic diagnoses). Favourable prognostic indicators are a history of successful adult attachment and healthy interpersonal relationships, normal intellectual functioning, self-referral to mental health services (as opposed to referral via the legal system), and absence of co-morbid psychiatric disorders.

# Gender dysphoria

## 23.8 Introduction

Gender dysphoria refers to the distress that may accompany the incongruence between one's experienced or expressed gender and the gender one has been assigned. Many individuals will only be distressed if the desired physical interventions by means of hormones and/or surgery are not available. The prevalence rates range from 0,005–0,014% for natal males and from 0,002–0,003% for natal females, but are likely to be modest underestimates. A diagnosis should not be made before a specialist assessment has been carried out. Although parents may seek reassurance if their children do not fit their own or the cultural stereotypes of masculinity or femininity, a diagnosis of gender dysphoria is only appropriate in cases where there is a profound distress on the part of the individual regarding his or her assigned gender. Adults with gender dysphoria are preoccupied with their wish to live as a member of the other gender. They are uncomfortable functioning as members of their assigned gender and may wish to acquire the physical appearance of the other gender through hormonal or surgical manipulation (American Psychiatric Association, 2013).

Most individuals with gender dysphoria in association with a disorder of sex development have come to medical attention at an early age. Issues of gender assignment and infertility are usually addressed from a young age. In the majority of cases of sex-development disorder, the individual may experience uncertainty about his or her gender, as opposed to developing a firm conviction that one is another gender.

**Table 23.17** DSM-5 Diagnostic Criteria for Gender Dysphoria

| Diagnostic Criteria |
|---|
| **Gender Dysphoria in Children** |
| A. A marked incongruence between one's experienced/expressed gender and assigned gender, of at least 6 months' duration, as manifested by at least six of the following (one of which must be Criterion A1): |
| 1. A strong desire to be of the other gender or an insistence that one is the other gender (or some alternative gender different from one's assigned gender). |
| 2. In boys (assigned gender), a strong preference for cross-dressing or simulating female attire: or in girls (assigned gender), a strong preference for wearing only typical masculine clothing and a strong resistance to the wearing of typical feminine clothing. |
| 3. A strong preference for cross-gender roles in make-believe play or fantasy play. |
| 4. A strong preference for the toys, games, or activities stereotypically used or engaged in by the other gender. |
| 5. A strong preference for playmates of the other gender. |
| 6. In boys (assigned gender), a strong rejection of typically masculine toys, games, and activities and a strong avoidance of rough-and-tumble play; or in girls (assigned gender), a strong rejection of typically feminine toys, games, and activities. |
| 7. A strong dislike of one's sexual anatomy. |
| 8 A strong desire for the primary and/or secondary sex characteristics that match one's experienced gender. |
| B The condition is associated with clinically significant distress or impairment in social, school, or other important areas of functioning. |
| *Specify* if: |
| ▸ **With a disorder of sex development** (e.g., a congenital adrenogenital disorder such as 255.2 [E25.0] congenital adrenal hyperplasia or 259.50 [E34.50] androgen insensitivity syndrome). |
| **Gender Dysphoria in Adolescents and Adults** |
| A. A marked incongruence between one's experienced/expressed gender and assigned gender, of at least 6 months' duration, as manifested by at least two of the following: |
| 1. A marked incongruence between one's experienced/expressed gender and primary and/or secondary sex characteristics (or in young adolescents, the anticipated secondary sex characteristics). |
| 2. A strong desire to be rid of one's primary and/or secondary sex characteristics because of a marked incongruence with one's experienced/expressed gender (or in young adolescents, a desire to prevent the development of the anticipated secondary sex characteristics). |
| 3. A strong desire for the primary and/or secondary sex characteristics of the other gender. |
| 4. A strong desire to be of the other gender (or some alternative gender different from one's assigned gender). |
| 5 A strong desire to be treated as the other gender (or some alternative gender different from one's assigned gender). |
| 6 A strong conviction that one has the typical feelings and reactions of the other gender (or some alternative gender different from one's assigned gender). |
| B. The condition is associated with clinically significant distress or impairment in social, occupational, or other important areas of functioning. |
| *Specify* if: |
| ▸ **With a disorder of sex development** (e.g., a congenital adrenogenital disorder such as 255.2 [E25.0] congenital adrenal hyperplasia or 259.50 [E34.50] androgen insensitivity syndrome). |
| *Specify* if: |
| ▸ **Posttranstion:** The individual has transitioned to full-time living in the desired gender (with or without legalization of gender change) and has undergone (or is preparing to have) at least one cross-sex medical procedure or treatment regimen—namely, regular cross-sex hormone treatment or gender reassignment surgery confirming the desired gender (e.g., penectomy, vaginoplasty in a natal male; mastectomy or phalloplasty in a natal female). |

**Source:** Reprinted with permission from the *Diagnostic and Statistical Manual of Mental Disorders*, Fifth Edition, (Copyright 2013). American Psychiatric Association.

As regards terminology:

- '**gender**' is used to denote the public lived role as boy or girl, man or woman
- '**transgender**' refers to the broad spectrum of individuals who transiently or persistently identify with a gender different from their natal gender
- '**transsexual**' denotes an individual who seeks, or has undergone, a social transition from male to female or from female to male, which in many cases also involves a somatic transition by cross-sex hormone treatment and sex reassignment surgery
- '**transvestism**' refers to cross-dressing behaviour used by men for the purpose of sexual excitement (Sadock, 2000).

Monitoring over an extended period of time is usually necessary to clarify the diagnosis in children and young adolescents. The treatment of gender dysphoria is highly specialised and possible cases should be referred at the outset. Therapy is aimed at helping the individual to be comfortable with the gender identity he or she desires; in some cases, it also involves complex assessments for possible sex-reassignment surgery.

## 23.4 Advanced reading block

**Intersex conditions**

Intersex conditions are syndromes in which a person has gross anatomical or physiological aspects of the opposite sex.

**Congenital virilising adrenal hyperplasia**

Congenital virilising adrenal hyperplasia is a disorder characterised by an enzymatic defect in the production of cortisol by the adrenal gland. The resultant excessive androgenic adrenal hormone production begins prenatally. At birth, affected females show varying degrees of genital virilisation. After birth, excessive androgen production can be controlled by cortisone. Male or female patients diagnosed neonatally appear to develop a gender identity consistent with their chromosomal and gonadal sex and sex of rearing.

**Turner's syndrome**

In Turner's syndrome one sex chromosome – sexual karyotype XO – is missing. The genitals are female at birth, but have poorly developed ovaries. They require oestrogen replacement for female secondary sex characteristics to develop.

**Klinefelter's syndrome**

In Klinefelter's syndrome an additional X chromosome is present together with the typical XY male pattern. Infants appear normal males at birth, but the testes are small and they may develop gynaecomastia in adolescence. Testosterone levels are low and a higher rate of gender dysphoria has been suggested.

**5-$\alpha$-reductase deficiency**

In 5-$\alpha$-reductase deficiency an enzymatic defect prevents the conversion of testosterone to dihydrotestosterone. An XY-affected individual is born with female-appearing genitalia because prenatal virilisation did not occur. At puberty testosterone causes extensive virilisation, with phallic growth. When an individual is raised as a male, with androgen supplementation, they function as relatively normal men.

**Androgen-insensitivity syndrome**

Androgen-insensitivity syndrome is a metabolism disorder in the XY individual. Tissue cells are unable to use testosterone or other androgens. The person appears to be a normal female at birth. Testes are undescended and no internal female reproductive structures are present. During puberty, testosterone converts to estradiol and brings female-type breast development. A vagina has to be constructed. Gender identity usually evolves as female, with a sexual interest in males (Sadock, 2000).

## 23.8.1 Other specified gender dysphoria

'Other specified gender dysphoria' applies to presentations in which symptoms characteristic of gender dysphoria do not meet the full criteria. The clinician must communicate the specific reason the individual does not meet the criteria for gender dysphoria (American Psychiatric Association, 2013).

## 23.8.2 Unspecified gender dysphoria

'Unspecified gender dysphoria' applies to presentations in which symptoms characteristic of gender dysphoria do not meet the full criteria and the clinician chooses not to specify the reason that the criteria for gender dysphoria are not met (American Psychiatric Association, 2013).

## Conclusion

In this chapter we have covered three distinct phenomena/groups of phenomena that are related only because they pertain to human sexuality. Sexual dysfunctions are disorders of sexual functioning, while paraphilias are disorders of sexual preference. Gender dysphoria represents a disorder of sexual identity only when the incongruence between experienced/expressed gender and assigned gender gives rise to significant distress or impairment in the individual. We wish to be clear that grouping the three categories in a single chapter in no way suggests that they coexist or overlap – this was simply an editorial decision for the purposes of structuring the book.

Issues of human sexuality are frequently overlooked, often owing to discomfort on the part of both clinicians and patients with addressing intimate topics. It is critical that health practitioners familiarise themselves with the range of sexuality-problems people experience and live with. In providing holistic health care to our patients, the onus very often lies on us to raise the issue of sexuality with patients in an informed, open and non-judgemental manner that provides them the freedom to seek help.

# References


Abel GG, Becker JV, Mittelman MS, Cunningham-Rathner J, Rouleau JL, Murphy WD (1987). Self-reported sex crimes of non-incarcerated paraphiliacs. *Journal of Interpersonal Violence* 2: 3–25

Abel GG, Osborn CA. (2006) The paraphilia's. In: Gelder MG, Lopez-Ibor JJ (Jr), Andreasen NC (Eds). *New Oxford Textbook of Psychiatry*. Oxford: Oxford University Press

American Psychiatric Association (2013) *Diagnostic and statistical manual of mental disorders* (5th edition). Washington: American Psychiatric Association

IsHak WW, Tobia G (2013) *DSM-5 Changes in Diagnostic Criteria of Sexual Dysfunctions* [Online] Available at: http://dx.doi.org/10.4172/2161-038X.1000122 (Accessed 3 April 2014.)

Martin SA, Atlantis, E, Lange K, Taylor AW, O'Loughlin P, Wittert GA, *et al.* (2014) Predictors of sexual dysfunction incidence and remission in men. *Journal of Sexual Medicine* (abstract) [Online] Available at: http://onlinelibrary.wiley.com/doi/10.1111/jsm.12483/abstract (Accessed 30 April 2014)

Sadock BT, Sadock VA (2000) *Kaplan and Sadock's Comprehensive Textbook of Psychiatry* (7th edition). Philadelphia: Lippincott Williams and Wilkins

Sungur MZ, Gunduz A. (2014) *A Comparison of DSM-IV-TR and DSM-5 definitions for sexual dysfunctions: Critiques and challenges* [Online] Available at: http://www.ncbi.nim.nih.gov/pubmed/24251514 (Accessed 3 April 2014)

World Health Organization (1992) *International classification of diseases and related health problems* (10th revision). Geneva: World Health Organization

CHAPTER

# 24 Personality and personality disorder

*Mo Nagdee, Stoffel Grobler, Zukiswa Zingela*

## 24.1 Introduction

Personality exerts important influences on mental health. It can predispose a person to mental ill-health, determine how patients react when they are ill and is often mistaken for (or co-morbid with) other mental disorders. People with personality disorder (PD) are commonly encountered and may present significant diagnostic and management challenges. This chapter will discuss the concepts of normal personality and personality disorder (including definitions, classification systems, aetiology, epidemiology, assessment and diagnostic principles), as well as outline specific personality disorders using contemporary classification systems (the DSM-5 and the ICD-10). The relationship between a personality disorder and other mental disorders, an overview of clinical management principles, and the natural evolution of personality disorder (outcome, course and prognosis) will be discussed. Lastly, we will address personality disorder within the South African context.

## 24.2 Normal personality

We all recognise, in people we know well, attributes and qualities that describe the characteristic way in which they think, feel and behave in response to situations encountered in daily life. People may describe these qualities or traits in various ways: introverted, confident, shy, angry, entitled, withdrawn, moody, sensitive, callous, labile, obsessive, odd, anxious, energetic, flexible, hostile, impulsive or suspicious, to name a few. Every individual has a unique combination of personality traits, which may vary between and within individuals over context and time. Whilst these traits are fairly stable over time, they may transiently be exaggerated at times of stress. It is both the personality traits and the nature of stressors that determine, or even predict, an individual's unique behavioural responses.

Personality therefore describes a person's totality of innate, enduring and recognisable patterns of perceiving, relating to and thinking about themselves, others and the environment. It has a strong genetic basis, but is also influenced by developmental and environmental factors. In most cases, an individual's unique personality is fully formed by adolescence (or earlier) and remains relatively stable and predictable throughout adulthood. Personality forms a significant component of the contextual understanding of each patient, and interacts with, and is influenced by, ill-health of any nature.

## 24.3 Concept of personality disorder

Some individuals exhibit personality traits that are either excessive or deficient in comparison to the range of variation found within that person's culture. Such people tend to exhibit limited, stereotyped and rigid responses (e.g. aggression, seduction, avoidance, mood instability) in diverse social and interpersonal situations. These individuals repeatedly and predictably apply these limited responses particularly in situations they find stressful or difficult, even when such strategies have proved unsuccessful or inappropriate in the past. If this leads to significant subjective distress, difficulties in relationships with others, and/or functional impairment, this may indicate the presence of a personality disorder.

The study of personality disorder has been beset by problems with respect to definitions, conceptualisation and classification.

Whilst there are many definitions of personality disorder in clinical use, the DSM-5 (American Psychiatric Association, 2013) and the ICD-10 (World Health Organization,1992) classification systems include a number of common elements in their respective descriptions (see Table 24.1).

**Table 24.1** Defining features of personality disorder

| | |
|---|---|
| **Characteristic patterns of...** | ▶ **cognition** (ways of thinking, perceiving and interpreting oneself, others and events)<br>▶ **emotion** (range, intensity and appropriateness of affect, and emotional responses)<br>▶ **behaviour** (in various interpersonal, social and occupational settings) |
| **which are...** | ▶ evident from early life (adolescence/ early adulthood)<br>▶ enduring and persistent into adulthood<br>▶ pervasive and stable over time<br>▶ inflexible and rigid<br>▶ maladaptive<br>▶ deviant from sociocultural norms and expectations |
| **and lead to...** | ▶ distress to self, others or society<br>▶ impairment in interpersonal, social and/or occupational relationships and performance |
| **but are not due to...** | ▶ other major psychiatric disorders (e.g. schizophrenia, mood disorders)<br>▶ substance abuse or medications<br>▶ medical conditions (e.g. traumatic brain injury, epilepsy, HIV) |

Patients with personality disorder present to health services in various ways. They may be concerned about themselves, or others are concerned or affected by their behaviour. Personality disorder may also be detected during the course of assessment or treatment of another psychiatric or medical disorder. A patient's self-description, attitudes and behavioural responses may also be influenced by co-morbid mental disorders, giving a misleading impression of their baseline personality (baseline being when they are not mentally ill).

Many patients with a personality disorder perceive and experience their personality traits as natural and acceptable attributes that do not require change or therapeutic attention. This is referred to as ego-syntonic. They believe that other people misunderstand or mistreat them. Such patients may respond to stress or difficulties by attempting to modify the environment, rather than their own response to it. This is referred to as using alloplastic defences. They are also more likely to deny or minimise their problems and resist help from health professionals. They may seem disinterested or even obstructive in treatment settings, and impervious to recovery.

A smaller proportion of patients with a personality disorder find their own personality traits objectionable and distressing, and in need of change (ego-dystonic). They respond to stress by attempting to alter their own internal thoughts, feelings and behavioural responses (autoplastic defences). Such patients may appear to be more troubled or anxious about their problems and maladaptive behaviour. They often seek help from professionals, albeit most commonly for associated problems (e.g. marital or occupational dysfunction, substance-related problems, co-morbid mental disorders).

Despite attempts to clarify the concept of a personality disorder, there remain significant controversies, such as:

- **Is a personality disorder a mental illness?** Some may consider individual differences in personality as normal variation rather than pathological; they argue that a personality disorder is not a clinical entity and should not be treated by health professionals.
- **Is the diagnosis of a personality disorder reliable?** The clinical validity of diagnostic criteria have been questioned as they are not based on solid empirical evidence and use confusing terminology derived from different theoretical perspectives.

- **Is there a distinction between a personality disorder and other psychiatric disorders?** There is significant overlap and co-morbidity with other psychiatric disorders, and it is often difficult to make clear distinctions.
- **Is the term 'personality disorder' pejorative, dismissive or stigmatising?** Some health professionals use the term 'personality disorder' to describe individuals they may not like or as a justification to avoid patients whose problems they find difficult to manage.

## 24.4 Classification

There are three main approaches to the classification of a personality disorder: ideographic, nomothetic, and hybrid models (Cooke and Hart, 2004; Lopez-Ibor, 2009; Reich and De Girolamo, 2009).

### 24.4.1 Ideographic approaches

Ideographic approaches emphasise individuality and seek to understand personality and its disorders by relating to individual uniqueness rather than by reference to common factors. Examples are:

- psycho-analytic models in which thoughts, feelings and behaviours are explained by influences of early development, unconscious drives, inner conflicts, and various defence mechanisms
- cognitive-behavioural models in which maladaptive cognitive schemata and the behavioural responses are seen to contribute to personality traits
- situationist models which consider the most important determinants of personality, affect and behaviour to be the unique situations people find themselves in.

Critics of ideographic approaches point out their poor scientific validity.

**Table 24.2** DSM-5 and ICD-10 categorical classification of personality disorder

| DSM-5 | | ICD-10 |
|---|---|---|
| **Cluster** | **Personality disorder** | **Personality disorder** |
| **A** | paranoid | paranoid |
| | schizoid | schizoid |
| | schizotypal | schizotypal |
| **B** | antisocial | dissocial |
| | borderline | emotionally unstable – borderline type |
| | - | emotionally unstable – impulsive type |
| | histrionic | histrionic |
| | narcissistic | - |
| **C** | avoidant | anxious (avoidant) |
| | dependent | dependent |
| | obsessive-compulsive | anankastic |
| **Other** | personality change due to another medical condition<br>other specified personality disorders and unspecified personality disorders | mixed and other personality disorders |

**Source:** Authors' own Table

### 24.4.2 Nomothetic approaches

Nomothetic approaches are derived from population studies and view personality and personality disorders in terms of the attributes shared by individuals. There are two subdivisions within this category:

#### 24.4.2.1 Type or categorical models

Type or categorical models distinguish individual personality disorders according to pre-defined archetypes or categories. Personality traits are viewed on a continuum from absent to severe. Those that reach a specific threshold of severity are regarded as disordered. In order to diagnose a specific personality disorder, it is necessary to have a distinct collection of traits that are sufficiently above or below the threshold. This approach formed the basis of the DSM-5 and the ICD-10 classification systems. These describe ten categories of a personality disorder, with DSM-5 further grouping certain categories into three clusters (A, B and C) according to their apparent clinical similarities (see Table 24.2). Whilst both the DSM-5 and the ICD-10 approaches are similar, there are personality disorders that appear in one but not the other and different terms are used for the same categories.

Personality disorders were previously encoded in the DSM-IV-TR multi-axial system on Axis II (together with 'mental retardation/intellectual disability'), in an attempt to separate them from the major mental disorders (previously encoded on Axis I) and to highlight them as a focus of clinical attention (American Psychiatric Association, 2000). DSM-5 has moved to a non-axial documentation of diagnoses (formerly encoded on Axes I, II and III), with separate notations for important psychosocial and contextual factors (formerly on Axis IV) and functional impairment (formerly Axis V) respectively. Patients may, however, have another psychiatric diagnosis co-morbid with a personality disorder (e.g. major depressive disorder in a patient with avoidant personality disorder), but with certain exceptions (e.g. a personality disorder cannot be diagnosed in people with schizophrenia). In addition, many patients may meet the diagnostic criteria for more than one personality disorder. This does not imply that they suffer from more than one actual personality disorder: each person has only one personality, which may or may not be disordered. If it is disordered, the clinical features may simply be inadequately described by a single category. Clinically it is more important to understand and describe the unique features of each patient than to assign them to a single category.

The advantages of categorical approaches are their relative simplicity, wide use in clinical and research settings and ability to facilitate professional communication in a way that dimensional approaches cannot. A significant disadvantage is the questionable clinical reliability and validity. Many people with abnormal personalities do not fit into any single diagnostic category, or may meet the criteria of several categories, or of none of them. The DSM-5 and the ICD-10 systems deal with this problem by having residual categories (see Table 24.2) for patients whose predominant features do not conform to any specific personality category, and also allow for more than one personality disorder diagnosis to be made.

#### 24.4.2.2 Trait or dimensional models

Trait or dimensional models are more modern approaches that assume that a limited number of universal traits apply to everyone. Each trait is on a continuous scale. A person's positioning on each trait continuum, as well as their overall trait combinations, describe their personality. People with a personality disorder have sufficiently maladaptive traits to cause distress or dysfunction. Some of the more prominent dimensional models and their respective traits include (Cooke and Hart, 2004; Lopez-Ibor, 2009):

- Eysenck's three-factor model: neuroticism, extraversion, psychoticism
- Costa and McCrae's five-factor model: neuroticism, extraversion, openness to experience, agreeableness, conscientiousness
- Cloninger's seven-factor model: novelty seeking, harm avoidance, reward

dependence, persistence, self-directedness, cooperativeness, self-transcendence

Advantages of the dimensional approach include its versatility, its ability to describe unique combinations of personality traits more accurately and its avoidance of the simplistic distinction between a personality disorder and its absence (which characterises categorical approaches). Disadvantages include its complexity and the fact that it may be less helpful in certain clinical and research settings where distinct categories are more valuable.

### 24.4.3 Categorical-dimensional approach

An alternative hybrid categorical-dimensional approach has recently been included in the DSM-5, consisting of ratings of both trait constructs and specific personality disorder categories (see Section 24.8). This system has a better supported evidence base in predicting antecedent variables (e.g. family history, history of childhood abuse), concurrent variables (e.g. functional impairment, medication use) and predictive variables (e.g. hospitalisation, suicide risk). The clinical utility of such hybrid, multidimensional personality trait models lie in their ability to focus attention on multiple areas of personality variation in each individual patient. This assists the clinician in formulating more comprehensive and individualised diagnostic descriptions, treatment plans and prognostic forecasts.

## 24.5 Aetiology

Little is known about the aetiology of personality disorders, partly because little is understood about the determinants of 'normal' personality. Whilst there is no single, convincing evidence-based theory that explains the genesis of a personality disorder, there are a number of contributory factors. The complex interaction of biological and psychosocial variables is likely to lead to problematic personality development, and if severe enough, the emergence of a personality disorder by adolescence or early adulthood. A relative paucity of robust research has allowed the proliferation of theories with much influence and appeal, but little scientific merit. This notwithstanding, genetic, neurobiological, childhood and development, psychological and sociocultural factors may contribute to the development of PD (Cloninger and Svrakic, 2009; Tobena, 2009).

### 24.5.1 Genetic factors

Studies demonstrate that normal personality traits are at least moderately heritable.

Twin studies show heritability of personality traits to be approximately 30–50%. Pairs of twins raised apart are as similar on several measures of personality as pairs raised together, and monozygotic twins display greater concordance for many personality traits than dizygotic twins.

Family studies demonstrate important relationships between various personality disorders and other mental disorders in first-degree relatives (e.g. between cluster A personality disorders and psychotic disorders, cluster B personality disorders and mood disorders, and cluster C personality disorders and anxiety disorders).

Linkage studies are inconclusive, but suggest associations between loci on chromosome 11 with novelty-seeking behaviour, chromosome 17 with harm-avoidance behaviour and chromosome 1 with emotional reactivity.

### 24.5.2 Neurobiological factors

Neurophysiological and neurochemical abnormalities have been associated with certain personality traits and disorders:

- electroencephalogram (EEG) changes in antisocial/dissocial personality disorder
- neurotransmitter (especially serotonin) and hormonal (especially testosterone) dysfunction associated with impulsivity, aggression and mood instability
- abnormal dexamethasone suppression tests, reduced thyroid-releasing hormone response and reduced rapid eye movement (REM) latency associated with vulnerability to stressful events.

Neurological factors may be influential:

- functional neuro-imaging abnormalities have been demonstrated in psychopathy (a severe variant of antisocial/dissocial personality disorder)
- approximately 50% of patients with a personality disorder have some form of neurological dysfunction (e.g. 'soft' neurological signs, a history of traumatic brain injury or attention-deficit hyperactivity disorder (ADHD), or co-morbid neurological disorders such as epilepsy).

## 24.5.3 Childhood and developmental factors

The influence of early life experience on personality development is difficult to determine, mainly because of the long interval between childhood experiences and the mature adult personality. Early childhood experience may influence adaptive and coping skills, rather than personality structure itself. Examples of some associations between childhood experiences and personality disorder include:

- a high prevalence of early abuse in patients with borderline personality disorder
- early-onset conduct disorder and the later development of antisocial personality disorder
- children who are temperamentally fearful may develop avoidant personality disorder
- insecure, ambivalent or disorganised attachments to parental figures may also predict personality disorder (especially those in cluster B).
- certain child-rearing practices (especially where there is a mismatch between the child's temperament and parenting style) have been associated with some personality disorders. Harsh and inconsistent parenting, for example, is associated with conduct disorder and antisocial personality disorder, while authoritarian and enmeshed parenting is associated with histrionic personality disorder.

## 24.5.4 Psychological factors

### 24.5.4.1 Psychoanalytic model

Psychoanalytic models stress the important influence of early childhood experiences in personality development. Traumatic or distressing experiences may predispose individuals to develop lifelong patterns of pathological adaptation (Millon and Davis, 1996). Such early events are proposed to lead to a cluster of defence mechanisms (unconscious mental processes used by the ego to resolve internal conflicts). When such defences are ineffective or abandoned, this increases distress and dysfunctionality. Progressive maladaptation then leads to personality disorder.

### 24.5.4.2 Cognitive-behavioural model

Maladaptive schemata (core beliefs derived from interactions between childhood experiences and innate patterns of behaviour) contribute to the development of a personality disorder. Such schemata are said to form in early childhood and are rigid and unconditional (e.g. 'Nobody loves me') in comparison to affective disorders (e.g. 'If someone important criticises me, then they don't love me').

### 24.5.4.3 Dialectical-behavioural model

This is a hybrid model that synthesises cognitive-behavioural and psychodynamic themes. Innate temperamental traits and vulnerabilities interact with dysfunctional environments, leading to emotional dysregulation. This manifests as instability of affect and behaviour, maladaptive problem-solving, and poor coping strategies seen in personality disorder.

## 24.5.5 Sociocultural factors

Whilst there is little scientific evidence to support this, it is widely believed that sociocultural factors play some role in the development of personality and personality disorder. Certain personality disorders may be more influenced than others: cultures that encourage aggression, for example, may unwittingly contribute to the development of antisocial personality disorder. Similarly, cultures that emphasise subservience or submission to authority may contribute to dependent personality disorder.

## 24.6 Epidemiology

Studies investigating the epidemiology of personality disorder have been hampered by methodological problems. The following broad conclusions can nonetheless be drawn from available evidence (Casey, 2000; Guzetta and De Girolamo, 2009; Suliman *et al.*, 2008):

- The overall prevalence of personality disorder in the community is between 2–22%, with the most widely accepted median prevalence estimate being 12,5%. The prevalence in South Africa is estimated to be about 7%.
- There is a gradient of increasing prevalence from community to institutional settings:
  - primary care or general practice: 5–8%
  - psychiatric outpatients: 30–40%
  - psychiatric inpatients: 40–50%
  - prison populations: 25–75%.
- There are high rates of co-morbidity with other mental disorders in all settings.
- Overall, personality disorder seems to be equally prevalent in males and females, though this may not apply to certain personality disorders: antisocial, schizoid and obsessive-compulsive personality disorders are seen more often in men and avoidant, dependant and borderline personality disorder may be more common in women.
- The prevalence of personality disorder appears higher in younger than older adults, and possibly higher in urban than rural settings.
- Specific types of personality disorder have different prevalence rates (see Table 24.3).

**Table 24.3** Median prevalence rates of specific personality disorders in the community (using DSM-5 PD categories)

| Cluster | Personality disorder | Median prevalence rate (%) |
|---|---|---|
| A | paranoid | 1,6 |
| | schizoid | 0,8 |
| | schizotypal | 0,7 |
| B | antisocial | 1,5 |
| | borderline | 1,6 |
| | histrionic | 1,8 |
| | narcissistic | 0,2 |
| C | avoidant | 1,3 |
| | dependent | 0,9 |
| | obsessive-compulsive | 2,0 |

**Source:** Guzetta and De Girolamo, 2009

## 24.7 Assessment and diagnostic principles

Assessing personality and personality disorder is often challenging, especially to the inexperienced clinician. Some difficulties include negative counter-transference, relying on diagnoses made by others without conducting an independent assessment, not recognising co-morbid psychiatric conditions or diagnosing personality disorder with inadequate information. The diagnosis of a personality disorder should be based on a thorough and accurate assessment of the patient's enduring and pervasive patterns of cognition, emotion and behavioural responses. Obtaining reliable collateral information from as many sources as possible is essential. Repeated interviews over time are usually necessary to confirm the diagnosis. Once the diagnosis is made, clinicians should be aware of the potential for patients to be stigmatised or discriminated against.

A number of structured instruments are available for assessing personality disorder. Examples include:

- self-report questionnaires, for example the Millon Clinical Multi-axial Inventory (MCMI) (Millon *et al.*, 2009) or the Minnesota Multiphasic Personal Inventory (MMPI) (Butcher, 1989)
- structured clinical interviews with the patient, for example the Structured Clinical Interview for DSM-IV Personality Disorder (SCID II) (First *et al.*, 1997)
- structured clinical interviews with informants, for example the Standardised Assessment of Personality (SAP) (Moran *et al.*, 2003)
- instruments to assess specific personality disorders, for example the Diagnostic Interview for Borderline Patients (DIB) (Kolb and Gunderson, 1980) or the Psychopathy Check List – Screening Version (PCL-SV) (Hare and Neumann, 2009)

The DSM remains the most widely used classification system for mental disorders in South Africa. An alternative hybrid dimensional-categorical model for personality disorders was initially considered for the DSM-5 but, due to widespread criticism and controversy, this was dropped only weeks prior to publication of the DSM-5 in favour of the same system used in DSM-IV-TR. In contrast to the categorical approach, the dimensional perspective holds that personality disorders represent maladaptive variants of personality traits that merge imperceptibly into normality and into one another. This model is now included in Section III of the DSM-5 to stimulate further research on this modified classification system.

The personality disorders described in the DSM-5 are as follows:

- Cluster A personality disorders
  - paranoid personality disorder is a pattern of distrust and suspiciousness such that others' motives are interpreted as malevolent
  - schizoid personality disorder is a pattern of detachment from social relationships and a restricted range of emotional expression
  - schizotypal personality disorder is a pattern of acute discomfort in close relationships, cognitive or perceptual distortions and eccentricities of behaviour.
- Cluster B personality disorders
  - antisocial personality disorder is a pattern of disregard for, and violation of, the rights of others
  - borderline personality disorder is a pattern of instability in interpersonal relationships, self-image and affects and marked impulsivity
  - histrionic personality disorder is a pattern of excessive emotionality and attention seeking
  - narcissistic personality disorder is a pattern of grandiosity, need for admiration and lack of empathy.
- Cluster C personality disorders
  - avoidant personality disorder is a pattern of social inhibition, feelings of inadequacy, and hypersensitivity to negative evaluation
  - dependent personality disorder is a pattern of submissive and clinging behaviour related to an excessive need to be taken care of
  - obsessive-compulsive personality disorder is a pattern of preoccupation with orderliness, perfectionism and control.
- Other personality disorders
  - personality change due to another medical condition is a persistent personality disturbance that is judged to be due to the direct physiological effects of another medical condition (e.g. frontal lobe lesion)
  - 'other specified personality disorder' and 'unspecified personality disorder' is a category provided for two situations: 1) the individual's personality pattern meets the general criteria for a personality disorder, and traits of several different personality disorders are present, but the criteria for any specific personality disorder are not met; or 2) the individual's personality pattern meets the general criteria for a personality disorder, but the individual is considered to have a

personality disorder that is not included in the DSM-5 classification (e.g., passive-aggressive personality disorder) (American Psychiatric Association, 2013).

A personality disorder is an enduring pattern of inner experience and behaviour that deviates markedly from the expectations of the individual's culture, is pervasive and inflexible, has an onset in adolescence or early adulthood, is stable over time, and leads to distress or impairment (American Psychiatric Association, 2013). Table 24.4. provides an overview of the general criteria for personality disorder as described in the DSM-5.

## 24.8 Personality disorder types in the DSM-5

Based on their descriptive similarities, the personality disorders are grouped in the DSM-5 into three clusters. DSM-5 cautions though that this clustering system, although useful in research and educational situations, has serious limitations and has not been consistently validated (American Psychiatric Association, 2013). Cluster A includes paranoid, schizoid, and schizotypal personality disorders. Individuals with these disorders may appear unusual or eccentric. Cluster B includes antisocial, borderline, histrionic, and narcissistic personality disorders. Individuals with these disorders may appear

**Table 24.4** DSM-5 General Personality Disorder Criteria

| Criteria |
| --- |
| A. An enduring pattern of inner experience and behavior that deviates markedly from the expectations of the individual's culture. This pattern is manifested in two (or more) of the following areas:<br>1. Cognition (i.e., ways of perceiving and interpreting self, other people, and events).<br>2. Affectivity (i.e., the range, intensity, lability, and appropriateness of emotional response).<br>3. Interpersonal functioning.<br>4. Impulse control. |
| B. The enduring pattern is inflexible and pervasive across a broad range of personal and social situations. |
| C. The enduring pattern leads to clinically significant distress or impairment in social, occupational, or other important areas of functioning. |
| D. The pattern is stable and of long duration, and its onset can be traced back at least to adolescence or early adulthood. |
| E. The enduring pattern is not better explained as a manifestation or consequence of another mental disorder. |
| F. The enduring pattern is not attributable to the physiological effects of a substance (e.g., a drug of abuse, a medication) or another medical condition (e.g., head trauma). |

**Source:** Reprinted with permission from the *Diagnostic and Statistical Manual of Mental Disorders*, Fifth Edition, (Copyright 2013). American Psychiatric Association.

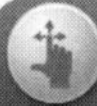

### Case study 24.1

**Paranoid personality disorder**

Mr A is a 67-year-old widower who is taken by his sister to see her GP. She reports that living with him has become increasingly difficult. He often rants about the whole family for maltreating him when he was in his teens, is hypersensitive to being wronged and has at least six civil suits pending against his ex-employer and co-workers for various injurious acts dating back ten years. These range from being passed over for promotions to co-workers excluding him from office parties and meetings. Lately he has been frequenting the local police station to complain about the nursery next to his house because 'they deliberately make the children cry to cause him mental suffering'.

**Key features:** persistent suspiciousness, sensitive to slights, bears grudges, litigious, hostile.

melodramatic, emotional, or erratic and unpredictable. Cluster C includes avoidant, dependent, and obsessive-compulsive personality disorders. Individuals with these disorders may seem anxious or fearful.

## 24.8.1 Cluster A personality disorders

### 24.8.1.1 Paranoid personality disorder

The basic capacity for trusting other human beings appears to be deficient in people with paranoid personality disorder. Other people are perceived as the enemy, waiting to strip them of their already questionable safety and expose their vulnerabilities. From the perspective of others they are often perceived as guarded, hostile, rigid and self-righteous, unwilling to consider the objective evidence and draw rational conclusions. Instead they attribute hidden motives to others and often accuse lifelong friends of betrayal. They envelop themselves with righteous indignation and self-pity, further fuelling their anger. Individuals with paranoid personality disorder are reluctant to confide in or become close to others because they fear

**Table 24.5** DSM-5 Diagnostic Criteria for Paranoid Personality Disorder

| **Diagnostic Criteria** |
|---|
| A. A pervasive distrust and suspiciousness of others such that their motives are interpreted as malevolent, beginning by early adulthood and present in a variety of contexts, as indicated by four (or more) of the following: |
| 1. Suspects, without sufficient basis, that others are exploiting, harming, or deceiving him or her. |
| 2. Is preoccupied with unjustified doubts about the loyalty or trustworthiness of friends or associates. |
| 3. Is reluctant to confide in others because of unwarranted fear that the information will be used maliciously against him or her. |
| 4. Reads hidden demeaning or threatening meanings into benign remarks or events. |
| 5. Persistently bears grudges (i.e., is unforgiving of insults, injuries, or slights). |
| 6. Perceives attacks on his or her character or reputation that are not apparent to others and is quick to react angrily or to counterattack. |
| 7. Has recurrent suspicions, without justification, regarding fidelity of spouse or sexual partner. |
| B. Does not occur exclusively during the course of schizophrenia, a bipolar disorder or depressive disorder with psychotic features, or another psychotic disorder and is not attributable to the physiological effects of another medical condition. |
| **Note:** If criteria are met prior to the onset of schizophrenia, add 'premorbid,' i.e., 'paranoid personality disorder (premorbid).' |

**Source:** Reprinted with permission from the *Diagnostic and Statistical Manual of Mental Disorders*, Fifth Edition, (Copyright 2013). American Psychiatric Association.

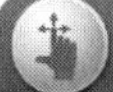

## Case study 24.2

**Schizoid personality disorder**

Mr B, a 39-year-old male, has applied to work as a gardener at the local clinic after being retrenched. The clinic manager contacts his previous employer for a character reference and gets the following report. 'Mr B is a hard worker who is of even temperament and generally keeps to himself. He lives alone and does not seem interested in mixing with other staff members in or outside of work. He seems happier in his own company and although he has been with us for more than 12 years, he is the only employee who has never once attended our annual Christmas party. He is always punctual at work and is often seen walking around the company grounds by himself during his lunch hour. He interacts so little with his co-workers that he is often excluded in invitations to office parties because one simply forgets about him unless he is in front of you.'

**Key features:** detached, solitary existence, quiet, restricted emotional expression.

that the information they share will be used against them. They persistently bear grudges and are unwilling to forgive the insults, injuries or slights that they think they have received. They are extremely insecure – which stems from a feeling of inferiority – but they then tend to blame others instead of themselves for these perceived shortcomings.

### 24.8.1.2 Schizoid personality disorder

Individuals with schizoid personality disorder exhibit a pattern of detachment from social relationships and a restricted range of emotional expression. Typically distant and viewed as introverted, these individuals keep to themselves and appear to have no need for relationships, whether platonic or sexual. Seemingly immune to either criticism or praise, they also seem almost incapable of experiencing emotional extremes of anger or pleasure. Preferring a solitary life, they are rarely noticed by others because they are so quiet and unobtrusive. They are often described by others as detached and emotionally flat. (See Table 24.6.)

### 24.8.1.3 Schizotypal personality disorder

People with schizotypal personality disorder are viewed by others as odd and eccentric in their appearance, beliefs and behaviour. They display restricted emotional responses and appear to

**Table 24.6** DSM-5 Diagnostic Criteria for Schizoid Personality Disorder

| **Diagnostic Criteria** |
|---|
| A. A pervasive pattern of detachment from social relationships and a restricted range of expression of emotions in interpersonal settings, beginning by early adulthood and present in a variety of contexts, as indicated by four (or more) of the following:<br>1. Neither desires nor enjoys close relationships, including being part of a family.<br>2. Almost always chooses solitary activities.<br>3. Has little, if any, interest in having sexual experiences with another person.<br>4. Takes pleasure in few, if any, activities.<br>5. Lacks close friends or confidants other than first-degree relatives.<br>6. Appears indifferent to the praise or criticism of others.<br>7. Shows emotional coldness, detachment, or flattened affectivity. |
| B. Does not occur exclusively during the course of schizophrenia, a bipolar disorder or depressive disorder with psychotic features, another psychotic disorder, or autism spectrum disorder and is not attributable to the physiological effects of another medical condition. |
| **Note:** If criteria are met prior to the onset of schizophrenia, add 'premorbid,' i.e., 'schizoid personality disorder (premorbid).' |

**Source:** Reprinted with permission from the *Diagnostic and Statistical Manual of Mental Disorders*, Fifth Edition, (Copyright 2013). American Psychiatric Association.

## Case study 24.3

**Schizotypal personality disorder**

Ms P, a 28-year-old female primary school teacher, agrees to see a psychologist after several parents complained to the head mistress that she read their children's palms and 'predicted their future'. Otherwise the school had no complaints about her work but admitted that she was seen as eccentric by the rest of the staff. At the interview she was colourfully and oddly dressed with a purple bandana on her head. She states that she has few close friends and studies reincarnation, astrology and astral projection at home. She believes she has had special powers of clairvoyance since childhood.

**Key features:** confused boundaries between self and others, eccentricity, unusual thought processes, preference for being alone.

be aloof and isolated. They tend to be socially withdrawn and have difficulty forming close and lasting relationships. They tend to be suspicious of others and harbour doubts about the loyalty or fidelity of people around them. Whilst they often express unusual or idiosyncratic ideas or beliefs, frank thought disorder or delusional thinking is absent. Under stress, however, they are vulnerable to psychotic, depressive or dissociative symptoms. (See Table 24.7.)

## 24.8.2 Cluster B personality disorders

### 24.8.2.1 Antisocial personality disorder

Individuals with antisocial personality disorder often seem to be high-functioning, but upon scrutiny their personal life reveals many areas of dysfunction. A number of behavioural problems are described in childhood, such as deceitfulness, truancy, running away from home, theft, fighting with peers, substance abuse and criminality. They have a low tolerance for frustration, act impetuously and cannot delay gratification.

**Table 24.7** DSM-5 Diagnostic Criteria for Schizotypal Personality Disorder

| Diagnostic Criteria |
|---|
| A A pervasive pattern of social and interpersonal deficits marked by acute discomfort with, and reduced capacity for, close relationships as well as by cognitive or perceptual distortions and eccentricities of behavior, beginning by early adulthood and present in a variety of contexts, as indicated by five (or more) of the following: |
| 1. Ideas of reference (excluding delusions of reference). |
| 2. Odd beliefs or magical thinking that influences behavior and is inconsistent with subcultural norms (e.g., superstitiousness, belief in clairvoyance, telepathy, or 'sixth sense': in children and adolescents, bizarre fantasies or preoccupations). |
| 3. Unusual perceptual experiences, including bodily illusions. |
| 4. Odd thinking and speech (e.g., vague, circumstantial, metaphorical, overelaborate, or stereotyped). |
| 5. Suspiciousness or paranoid ideation. |
| 6. Inappropriate or constricted affect. |
| 7. Behavior or appearance that is odd, eccentric, or peculiar. |
| 8. Lack of close friends or confidants other than first-degree relatives. |
| 9. Excessive social anxiety that does not diminish with familiarity and tends to be associated with paranoid fears rather than negative judgments about self. |
| B. Does not occur exclusively during the course of schizophrenia, a bipolar disorder or depressive disorder with psychotic features, another psychotic disorder, or autism spectrum disorder. |
| **Note:** If criteria are met prior to the onset of schizophrenia, add 'premorbid,' e.g., 'schizotypal personality disorder (premorbid).' |

**Source:** Reprinted with permission from the *Diagnostic and Statistical Manual of Mental Disorders*, Fifth Edition, (Copyright 2013). American Psychiatric Association.

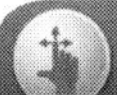

## Case study 24.4

**Antisocial personality disorder**

Mr Z is a 24-year-old inmate in prison who was referred to the psychiatrist for assaulting a fellow inmate. He was jailed for armed robbery. When asked about the assault, he responded 'I didn't like his face and I felt like it'. He showed no remorse about severely injuring his fellow inmate. He then angrily demanded sleeping tablets from the psychiatrist and threatened further violence should he not receive them. In spite of his urine testing positive for cannabis, he vehemently denies use and claimed it was the wardens who 'wanted to get him into trouble'.

**Key features:** lack of remorse, manipulation, intimidation, dishonesty, impulsivity.

They rarely consider the consequences of their behaviour, disregard authority and rules and often engage in criminal activities. They tend to be brash, arrogant and resentful. Others regard them as untrustworthy and unreliable. People with antisocial personality disorder seldom appear anxious or depressed, although suicidal threats and somatic preoccupations may be present. They may attempt to impress clinicians with seductive aspects of their personalities, though they are usually regarded as manipulative and demanding.

Note: not all criminals have antisocial personality disorder though, and not all people with antisocial personality disorder are criminals. (See Table 24.8.)

### 24.8.2.2 Borderline personality disorder

The core features of borderline personality disorder are instability of self-image, affect and interpersonal interactions. Emotional responses tend to be intense and unpredictable. Although individuals with borderline personality disorder seek attention and affection from others, they often behave in ways that are unpredictable, manipulative and volatile. They dislike being alone, and may easily accept strangers as friends

**Table 24.8** DSM-5 Diagnostic Criteria for Antisocial Personality Disorder

| Diagnostic Criteria |
| --- |
| A. A pervasive pattern of disregard for and violation of the rights of others, occurring since age 15 years, as indicated by three (or more) of the following: |
| 1. Failure to conform to social norms with respect to lawful behaviors, as indicated by repeatedly performing acts that are grounds for arrest. |
| 2. Deceitfulness, as indicated by repeated lying, use of aliases, or conning others for personal profit or pleasure. |
| 3. Impulsivity or failure to plan ahead. |
| 4. Irritability and aggressiveness, as indicated by repeated physical fights or assaults. |
| 5. Reckless disregard for safety of self or others. |
| 6. Consistent irresponsibility, as indicated by repeated failure to sustain consistent work behavior or honor financial obligations. |
| 7. Lack of remorse, as indicated by being indifferent to or rationalizing having hurt, mistreated, or stolen from another. |
| B. The individual is at least age 18 years. |
| C. There is evidence of conduct disorder with onset before age 15 years. |
| D. The occurrence of antisocial behavior is not exclusively during the course of schizophrenia or bipolar disorder. |

**Source:** Reprinted with permission from the *Diagnostic and Statistical Manual of Mental Disorders*, Fifth Edition, (Copyright 2013). American Psychiatric Association.

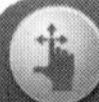

## Case study 24.5

**Borderline personality disorder**

Ms M is a 22-year-old waitress, brought in to the emergency department by her boyfriend of six weeks. She insisted that he cancel a planned business trip and stay with her to prove he loves her. She cut her wrists and took an overdose when he refused. She tells the doctor on call that her boyfriend is her soul mate and the best thing that ever happened to her. She cannot survive without him because he saved her from her ex-boyfriend who is 'the son of Satan'. The boyfriend describes Miss M as unpredictable and emotional and mentions that she has violent outbursts if she doesn't get her way. She has cut off contact with her family and has recently fallen out with her best friend. This is her fourth overdose in four weeks.

**Key features:** impulsivity, self-harming behaviour, fear of abandonment, over-idealisation and **devaluation**, instability of mood, instability of relationships.

or act promiscuously. They often display repetitive and deliberate acts of self-harm, commonly in the form of superficial cutting. This self-injurious behaviour may be an attempt to elicit help from others, express anger, or may occur in response to overwhelming affect. They may report intermittent, fleeting psychotic-like symptoms (e.g. isolated and transient hallucinations) at times of distress. Individuals with borderline personality disorder appear to be in a near-constant state of crisis. They are reliant on those around them and are fearful of rejection or separation.

Psychodynamic theory suggests that individuals with borderline personality disorder use complex defence mechanisms to deal with their distress. An example of a defence mechanism commonly cited is projective identification: when the patient's own unacknowledged or unacceptable feelings are attributed to others. Splitting is another immature defence mechanism that is used: this is the tendency to appraise others in extreme terms (as either all good or all bad. For example, as in-patients they may idealise some staff members and disparage others. These defence behaviours can be highly disruptive to the therapeutic process and to the functioning of the multi-disciplinary team. (See Table 24.9.)

**Table 24.9** DSM-5 Diagnostic Criteria for Borderline Personality Disorder

| **Diagnostic Criteria** |
|---|
| A pervasive pattern of instability of interpersonal relationships, self-image, and affects, and marked impulsivity, beginning by early adulthood and present in a variety of contexts, as indicated by five (or more) of the following: |
| 1. Frantic efforts to avoid real or imagined abandonment. (**Note:** Do not include suicidal or self-mutilating behavior covered in Criterion 5.) |
| 2. A pattern of unstable and intense interpersonal relationships characterized by alternating between extremes of idealization and devaluation. |
| 3. Identity disturbance: markedly and persistently unstable self-image or sense of self. |
| 4. Impulsivity in at least two areas that are potentially self-damaging (e.g., spending, sex, substance abuse, reckless driving, binge eating). (**Note:** Do not include suicidal or self-mutilating behavior covered in Criterion 5.) |
| 5. Recurrent suicidal behavior, gestures, or threats, or self-mutilating behavior. |
| 6. Affective instability due to a marked reactivity of mood (e.g., intense episodic dysphoria, irritability, or anxiety usually lasting a few hours and only rarely more than a few days). |
| 7. Chronic feelings of emptiness. |
| 8 Inappropriate, intense anger or difficulty controlling anger (e.g., frequent displays of temper, constant anger, recurrent physical fights). |
| 9. Transient, stress-related paranoid ideation or severe dissociative symptoms. |

**Source:** Reprinted with permission from the *Diagnostic and Statistical Manual of Mental Disorders*, Fifth Edition, (Copyright 2013). American Psychiatric Association.

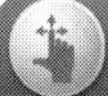

## Case study 24.6

**Histrionic personality disorder**

Mrs M is a 35 year old bank teller brought in to see her GP by her husband. She has streaks of orange in her ash-blonde hair, is dressed in a pink mini-skirt, a low-cut orange tank top with her midriff showing and high-heeled red shoes. She is complaining of a terrible headache which she describes as the worst pain she has ever had. She says she is blind in one eye because of the pain and declares tearfully and loudly that she has been blinded forever. Her husband has often had to rush her to their GP after a disagreement at home with similar symptoms; these usually pass after a few hours or when he gives in to her demands. The precipitant now is that his mother is due to arrive for a week's visit with them.

**Key features:** excessively emotional, dramatic, attention seeking, seductive.

### 24.8.2.3 Histrionic personality disorder

Frequently described as 'the life of the party', these individuals are typically dramatic and often seductive. They make every effort to remain the centre of attention and feel unappreciated when they are not. Their behaviour and opinions conform to suit whomever they are interacting with. Often lively and dramatic, they tend to draw attention to themselves and may initially charm new acquaintances by their enthusiasm, apparent openness or flirtatiousness. These qualities wear thin, however, as these individuals continually demand to be the centre of attention. They may do something dramatic (e.g. make up stories, create a scene) to draw the focus of attention to themselves. This need is often apparent in their behaviour with a clinician (e.g. being flattering, bringing gifts, providing dramatic descriptions of physical and psychological symptoms). The appearance and behaviour of individuals with this disorder are often inappropriately sexually provocative or seductive.

**Table 24.10** DSM-5 Diagnostic Criteria for Histrionic Personality Disorder

| Diagnostic Criteria |
|---|
| A pervasive pattern of excessive emotionality and attention seeking, beginning by early adulthood and present in a variety of contexts, as indicated by five (or more) of the following: |
| 1. Is uncomfortable in situations in which he or she is not the center of attention. |
| 2. Interaction with others is often characterized by inappropriate sexually seductive or provocative behavior. |
| 3. Displays rapidly shifting and shallow expression of emotions. |
| 4. Consistently uses physical appearance to draw attention to self. |
| 5. Has a style of speech that is excessively impressionistic and lacking in detail. |
| 6. Shows self-dramatization, theatricality, and exaggerated expression of emotion. |
| 7. Is suggestible (i.e., easily influenced by others or circumstances). |
| 8. Considers relationships to be more intimate than they actually are. |

**Source:** Reprinted with permission from the *Diagnostic and Statistical Manual of Mental Disorders*, Fifth Edition, (Copyright 2013). American Psychiatric Association.

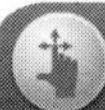

## Case study 24.7

**Narcissistic personality disorder**

Captain A is a defence force member who attended the sick-bay with complaints of nausea. His wife had left him in the previous week. On questioning he becomes agitated and exclaims: 'After all I have done for her, how dare she... she is nothing without me... someone of my rank and importance doesn't deserve to be treated this way!' He then looks at the young attending doctor and asks, 'But what would you know about life, you're still wet behind the ears?'

**Key features:** Self-centredness, exaggerated self-appraisal, sense of entitlement, admiration seeking, condescending

## Case study 24.8

**Avoidant personality disorder**

Ms Q is an attractive and intelligent 21-year -old female university student brought by her mother to a psychiatrist after failing her first semester at university and complaining of feeling depressed. She seldom attended classes for fear of being asked a question in front of everybody and saying 'something stupid'. She believed she was 'ugly' and that men were therefore not interested in her. She avoided social functions as a result.

**Key features:** Low self-esteem, sensitivity to rejection, avoidance of social contact.

They consistently use their physical appearance to draw attention to themselves and are overly concerned with impressing others by their appearance. They may spend an excessive amount of time, energy and money on clothes and grooming. They may search for compliments regarding appearance. These individuals have a style of speech that is extremely impressionistic, however lacking in detail. (See Table 24.10.)

### 24.8.2.4 Narcissistic personality disorder

People with narcissistic personality disorder have exaggerated self-appraisal, are attention-seeking and self-serving. They appear entitled and grandiose. They constantly seek approval and expect special treatment from others. Such individuals tend to handle criticism or confrontation poorly, and may become irritable, enraged or withdrawn as a result. Their disregard for the needs of others leads to superficial and fragile interpersonal relationships. (See Table 24.11.)

## 24.8.3 Cluster C personality disorders

### 24.8.3.1 Avoidant personality disorder

Patients with avoidant personality disorder are commonly described by lay people as having an inferiority complex. They show extreme sensitivity to rejection by others. They are apt to

**Table 24.11** DSM-5 Diagnostic Criteria for Narcissistic Personality Disorder

| **Diagnostic Criteria** |
|---|
| A pervasive pattern of grandiosity (in fantasy or behavior), need for admiration, and lack of empathy, beginning by early adulthood and present in a variety of contexts, as indicated by five (or more) of the following: |
| 1 Has a grandiose sense of self-importance (e.g., exaggerates achievements and talents, expects to be recognized as superior without commensurate achievements). |
| 2. Is preoccupied with fantasies of unlimited success, power, brilliance, beauty, or ideal love. |
| 3. Believes that he or she is 'special' and unique and can only be understood by, or should associate with, other special or high-status people (or institutions). |
| 4. Requires excessive admiration. |
| 5. Has a sense of entitlement (i.e., unreasonable expectations of especially favourable treatment or automatic compliance with his or her expectations). |
| 6. Is interpersonally exploitative (i.e., takes advantage of others to achieve his or her own ends). |
| 7. Lacks empathy: is unwilling to recognize or identify with the feelings and needs of others. |
| 8. Is often envious of others or believes that others are envious of him or her. |
| 9. Shows arrogant, haughty behaviors or attitudes. |

**Source:** Reprinted with permission from the *Diagnostic and Statistical Manual of Mental Disorders*, Fifth Edition, (Copyright 2013). American Psychiatric Association.

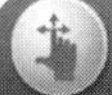

**Case study 24.9**

**Dependent personality disorder**

Mrs V is a 45-year-old housewife who presents with a low mood and suicidal ideation after her fourth husband had left her for a younger woman. She is terrified of being alone and feels distressed that her husband has filed for a divorce, even though he was very controlling and overbearing. She relied on him to make most decisions and does not know what to do now that he is gone. Since he left she has been increasingly relying on her recently widowed neighbour to help her make decisions and is thinking of asking the neighbour to move in with her even though she is still awaiting finalisation of the divorce. She married her first husband when she was 18 years old and has never been alone since.

**Key features:** needy, exaggerated fear of being unable to care for himself or herself, difficulty making everyday decisions.

misinterpret the comments of others as derogatory or ridiculing. They are timid and shy and their feelings are easily hurt. Despite their perpetual social unease, they do desire companionship. They lack self-confidence and are tentative, uncertain and anxious in their relationships. Instead of confronting their anxieties, they tend to escape social encounters whenever possible. This serves only to perpetuate their problems, leaving them socially withdrawn. (See Table 24.12.)

### 24.8.3.2 Dependent personality disorder

People with dependent personality disorder are caring to a fault, allowing others' well-being to come first no matter the cost to themselves. In a way they live their lives through others and for others. They prefer harmony in their relationships and tend to be apologetic even when others should take the greater part of responsibility for a disagreement. On the surface they are warm and affectionate but underneath they see themselves as helpless and fear doing things on

**Table 24.12** DSM-5 Diagnostic Criteria for Avoidant Personality Disorder

| Diagnostic Criteria |
|---|
| A pervasive pattern of social inhibition, feelings of inadequacy, and hypersensitivity to negative evaluation, beginning by early adulthood and present in a variety of contexts, as indicated by four (or more) of the following: |
| 1. Avoids occupational activities that involve significant interpersonal contact because of fears of criticism, disapproval, or rejection. |
| 2. Is unwilling to get involved with people unless certain of being liked. |
| 3. Shows restraint within intimate relationships because of the fear of being shamed or ridiculed. |
| 4. Is preoccupied with being criticized or rejected in social situations. |
| 5. Is inhibited in new interpersonal situations because of feelings of inadequacy. |
| 6. Views self as socially inept, personally unappealing, or inferior to others. |
| 7. Is unusually reluctant to take personal risks or to engage in any new activities because they may prove embarrassing. |

**Source:** Reprinted with permission from the *Diagnostic and Statistical Manual of Mental Disorders*, Fifth Edition, (Copyright 2013). American Psychiatric Association.

**Table 24.13** DSM-5 Diagnostic Criteria for Dependent Personality Disorder

| Diagnostic Criteria |
|---|
| A pervasive and excessive need to be taken care of that leads to submissive and clinging behavior and fears of separation, beginning by early adulthood and present in a variety of contexts, as indicated by five (or more) of the following: |
| 1. Has difficulty making everyday decisions without an excessive amount of advice and reassurance from others. |
| 2. Needs others to assume responsibility for most major areas of his or her life. |
| 3. Has difficulty expressing disagreement with others because of fear of loss of support or approval. (**Note:** Do not include realistic fears of retribution.) |
| 4. Has difficulty initiating projects or doing things on his or her own (because of a lack of self-confidence in judgment or abilities rather than a lack of motivation or energy). |
| 5. Goes to excessive lengths to obtain nurturance and support from others, to the point of volunteering to do things that are unpleasant. |
| 6. Feels uncomfortable or helpless when alone because of exaggerated fears of being unable to care for himself or herself. |
| 7. Urgently seeks another relationship as a source of care and support when a close relationship ends. |
| 8. Is unrealistically preoccupied with fears of being left to take care of himself or herself. |

**Source:** Reprinted with permission from the *Diagnostic and Statistical Manual of Mental Disorders*, Fifth Edition, (Copyright 2013). American Psychiatric Association.

their own. By putting their lives in the control of others, they suffocate their partners with clinginess and in turn leave themselves vulnerable to abandonment. When a relationship dissolves, their self-esteem is devastated. (See Table 24.13.)

### 24.8.3.3 Obsessive-compulsive personality disorder

People with obsessive-compulsive personality disorder are overly conscientious and rigidly perfectionistic. They are extraordinarily concerned with rules, details, organisation and order. As a result they lack flexibility and are intolerant of mistakes or changes in routine. Novel ideas and unfamiliar circumstances tend to upset them. They appear incapable of spontaneity. They display an unusual adherence to social convention, preferring to maintain formal and polite personal relationships. Whilst they see themselves as productive and efficient, they often have difficulty completing tasks as a result of their rigidity.

People with obsessive-compulsive personality disorder use defence mechanisms such as **reaction-formation**. This is when an unacceptable

## Case study 24.10

**Obsessive-compulsive personality disorder**

Mr O is a 36-year-old man referred by the Employee Assistance Programme for assessment after he screamed at a co-worker for accidentally spilling some tea on the table in the staff tea-room. He admits that he 'hates slobs' and 'people who always leave the tea-room in a mess'. He goes on to boast that his office is always perfectly neat and he knows exactly where everything is. He believes others are jealous of him because he is so devoted to his work that 'I make others look bad'. He had been married twice and said both divorces were the result of him 'being married to his job'.

**Key features:** rigid perfectionism, sense of self derived from work, relationships seen as secondary to work.

**Table 24.14** DSM-5 Diagnostic Criteria for Obsessive-Compulsive Personality Disorder

| Diagnostic Criteria |
|---|
| A pervasive pattern of preoccupation with orderliness, perfectionism, and mental and interpersonal control, at the expense of flexibility, openness, and efficiency, beginning by early adulthood and present in a variety of contexts, as indicated by four (or more) of the following:<br>1. Is preoccupied with details, rules, lists, order, organization, or schedules to the extent that the major point of the activity is lost.<br>2. Shows perfectionism that interferes with task completion (e.g., is unable to complete a project because his or her own overly strict standards are not met).<br>3. Is excessively devoted to work and productivity to the exclusion of leisure activities and friendships (not accounted for by obvious economic necessity).<br>4. Is overconscientious, scrupulous, and inflexible about matters of morality, ethics, or values (not accounted for by cultural or religious identification).<br>5. Is unable to discard worn-out or worthless objects even when they have no sentimental value.<br>6. Is reluctant to delegate tasks or to work with others unless they submit to exactly his or her way of doing things.<br>7. Adopts a miserly spending style toward both self and others; money is viewed as something to be hoarded for future catastrophes.<br>8. Shows rigidity and stubbornness. |

**Source:** Reprinted with permission from the *Diagnostic and Statistical Manual of Mental Disorders*, Fifth Edition, (Copyright 2013). American Psychiatric Association.

impulse is transformed into its opposite, such as engaging in socially commendable actions that are, in fact, diametrically opposite their own feelings. (See Table 24.14.)

## Case study 24.11

**Personality change due to another medical condition**

Mr PG is a 59-year-old male who suffered an anoxic brain injury following a myocardial infarction. In the subsequent months his wife complained to their GP that Mr. PG was 'not the same person he was before'. Before the heart attack he used to be a highly intelligent, driven, perfectionistic man; the CEO of a small company who was known for his sense of humour. In the subsequent months, she has noticed that he had become unpredictably irritable, labile and prone to bouts of unprovoked anger and that he paid less attention to his appearance. He would justify his behaviour by saying, 'Well, I yell at you because you deserve it', seemingly oblivious to the fact that he had hurt her feelings. He also seemed to have lost his sense of humour and seemed to have lost all interest in his hobby of making wooden children's toys. Whilst previously being a regular church-goer, he now preferred reading his Bible on his own for hours, making copious notes in the process. He also seemed to have become suspicious of her and would frequently ask her where she had been after she had gone out, insinuating that she was seeing another man.

**Key features:** change in temperament following another medical condition e.g. increased irritability, mood lability, behavioural disinhibition, apathy, social withdrawal, suspiciousness, reduced empathy.

**Table 24.15** DSM-5 Diagnostic Criteria for Personality Change Due to Another Medical Condition

| Diagnostic Criteria |
|---|
| A. A persistent personality disturbance that represents a change from the individual's previous characteristic personality pattern.<br>**Note:** In children, the disturbance involves a marked deviation from normal development or a significant change in the child's usual behavior patterns, lasting at least 1 year.<br>B. There is evidence from the history, physical examination, or laboratory findings that the disturbance is the direct pathophysiological consequence of another medical condition.<br>C. The disturbance is not better explained by another mental disorder (including another mental disorder due to another medical condition).<br>D. The disturbance does not occur exclusively during the course of a delirium.<br>E. The disturbance causes clinically significant distress or impairment in social, occupational, or other important areas of functioning.<br>*Specify* whether:<br>▸ **Labile type:** If the predominant feature is affective lability.<br>▸ **Disinhibited type:** If the predominant feature is poor impulse control as evidenced by sexual indiscretions, etc.<br>▸ **Aggressive type:** If the predominant feature is aggressive behavior.<br>▸ **Apathetic type:** If the predominant feature is marked apathy and indifference.<br>▸ **Paranoid type:** If the predominant feature is suspiciousness or paranoid ideation.<br>▸ **Other type:** If the presentation is not characterized by any of the above subtypes.<br>▸ **Combined type:** If more than one feature predominates in the clinical picture.<br>▸ **Unspecified type** |

**Source:** Reprinted with permission from the *Diagnostic and Statistical Manual of Mental Disorders*, Fifth Edition, (Copyright 2013). American Psychiatric Association.

### 24.8.4 Other personality disorders

#### 24.8.4.1 Personality change due to another medical condition

Personality change due to another medical condition is a persistent personality disturbance that is judged to be due to the direct physiological effects of a medical condition (e.g. frontal lobe lesion) (see Table 24.15).

#### 24.8.4.2 Other specified personality disorder and unspecified personality disorder

This category provides for two situations:

- the individual's personality pattern meets the general criteria for a personality disorder, and traits of several different personality disorders are present, but the criteria for any specific personality disorder are not met
- the individual's personality pattern meets the general criteria for a personality disorder, but the individual is considered to have a personality disorder that is not included in the DSM-5 classification (e.g. passive-aggressive personality disorder).

## 24.9 Personality disorders and mental illness

The definitions of a mental illness and disorder in the ICD-10 and the DSM-5 are similar (see Table 24.16) and emphasise the resultant distress and functional impairment caused by the disorder (Kendell, 2002).

Personality disorders are considered to be mental disorders because they:

- present with cognitive, emotional and behavioural symptoms
- cause distress
- lead to an impairment in functioning (World Health Organization, 1992; Kendell, 2002).

The interaction between personality disorder and other mental disorders is important and manifold (Harrison *et al.*, 2010).

Personality and personality disorders may:

- predispose to another mental disorder (Harrison *et al.*, 2010) for example schizotypal personality disorder and schizophrenia
- co-exist with other mental disorders (co-morbidity) (Harrison *et al.*, 2010) for example antisocial personality disorder and substance-related disorders
- be misdiagnosed as other mental disorders, and vice versa, for example borderline personality disorder and bipolar disorders
- be affected by other mental disorders (Harrison *et al.*, 2010), for example personality change following neurocognitive disorders
- affect other mental disorders (e.g. a depressive disorder exaggerated by obsessive-compulsive traits).

Genetic, biological, environmental and psychological factors interact to influence temperament and personality. These influences apply similarly to the genesis of other mental disorders. Associations between PDs and other mental disorders are therefore unsurprising. In the World Health Organization's Mental Health Surveys, 51,2% of people with personality disorder also met the criteria for at least one mental disorder (Huang, 2009). Examples of associations between personality disorder and other mental disorders include:

- schizotypal personality disorder is found more commonly in first-degree relatives of patients with schizophrenia
- mood, anxiety and substance-related disorders are commonly co-morbid in patients with borderline personality disorder and narcissistic personality disorder and in their first-degree relatives
- patients with avoidant personality disorder and obsessive-compulsive personality disorder are prone to anxiety and depressive disorders.

The co-existence of personality disorders and other mental disorders affects treatment outcomes, often in unpredictable ways (Tyrer *et al.*, 1997). Psychopathology in both personality disorder and other mental disorders may influence

**Table 24.16** Definitions of mental illness and disorder

| Mental illness | Mental disorder: ICD-10 | Mental disorder: DSM-5 |
|---|---|---|
| A disease of the mind characterised by impairment of an individual's normal cognitive, emotional or behavioural functioning | A clinically recognisable set of symptoms or behaviours associated in most cases with distress and with interference with personal functions | A mental disorder is a syndrome characterized by clinically significant disturbance in an individual's cognition, emotion regulation, or behavior that reflects a dysfunction in the psychological, biological, or developmental processes underlying mental functioning. Mental disorders are usually associated with significant distress or disability in social, occupational, or other important activities. |

the motivation to, and capacity of, patients for seeking help. Co-morbidity may complicate the clinical presentation, leading to delays in diagnosis and appropriate treatment. Patients may have difficulty in sustaining contact with mental health services and adhering to treatment programmes. This may have significant effects on treatment outcomes and prognosis.

## 24.10 Personality disorders in the South African context

In South Africa, a large survey found that almost 7% of South African people age 20 or older have a personality disorder (Suliman *et al.*, 2008). This rate is similar to other low- and middle-income countries and slightly lower compared to the United States. In the same study, less than one-fifth of the people with PD received mental health treatment in the year before the study. Male gender was the only independent variable significantly associated with personality disorder. Other psychiatric disorders found to occur co-morbidly with personality disorders in the South African survey were substance-related disorders, anxiety disorders, mood disorders and impulse-control disorders. In the population sampled, there was a higher prevalence of cluster A disorder compared with cluster B and C disorders, but the reasons for this were unclear.

## 24.11 Principles of management

Intervention in personality-disordered individuals is aimed at alleviating distress and improving level of functioning. Principles of management are:

- thorough clinical assessment and diagnosis
- multiple clinical interviews
- adequate and reliable collateral information
- assessment for co-morbidity
- risk assessment
- identifying and targeting acute psychosocial stressor(s)
- a multidisciplinary bio-psycho-social approach to clinical management

### 24.11.1 Biological intervention

Some personality disorder symptoms that may respond to medication include:

- anxiety
- agitation
- mood dysregulation
- hypersensitivity to rejection
- anger or hostility
- acting-out behaviour
- depression
- escalation in impulsive or risky behaviour
- self-harming
- suicide attempts (Taylor *et al.*, 2012).

Symptoms responsive to medication may also be related to co-morbid mental disorders. Rational prescribing principles, namely defining the indications and goals for medication and prescribing minimum effective dose for the minimum duration required, should be followed. Certain psychotropic medication may have the potential for abuse and may influence the psychotherapeutic process. The prescribing clinician must therefore monitor for the abuse of, or dependence on, prescription medication. In order to minimise side effects, abuse and inappropriate use of medication (e.g. deliberate overdose) polypharmacy should be the exception rather than the rule. Short-duration prescriptions are useful in patients with an increased suicide risk. The following medications may be useful (see Table 24.17):

- Antidepressants (e.g. SSRIs) may be useful to reduce impulsivity and aggression. Antidepressants may also be used to treat other co-morbid psychiatric disorders (e.g. depressive and anxiety disorders).
- Mood stabilisers (e.g. lithium, sodium valproate) may help to reduce impulsivity, anger, hostility and affect dysregulation (e.g. in borderline personality disorder). Lithium may be beneficial in patients with deliberate self-harm or aggression. The potential benefits should be weighed against the potential risks of medication, for example the potential efficacy of lithium versus its potential toxicity and lethality in overdose.
- Antipsychotics (both first- and second-generation antipsychotics) may be beneficial for a wide range of symptoms, including affect dysregulation, impulsivity, cognitive-perceptual symptoms, aggression and impulsivity. The prescription of antipsychotics in patients with a personality disorder should similarly be balanced against the burden of extrapyramidal and metabolic side effects. Clozapine may decrease aggression in some patients with a personality disorder.
- Sedative hypnotics (e.g. zopiclone, zolpidem, zaleplon, benzodiazepines) may be useful in acute crisis management or as short-term adjuvants to other interventions (e.g. psychotherapy or whilst commencing SSRI, mood stabiliser or antipsychotic medication). The long-term use of sedative hypnotic medication should be avoided in patients with a personality disorder who are prone to substance-related disorders. Benzodiazepines may cause paradoxical disinhibition (e.g. in patients with personality disorder who have co-morbid intellectual disability or neuropsychiatric disorders).
- Other medications (e.g. beta-blockers, anti-histamines) may be useful in, for example, patients with avoidant personality disorder prior to social interaction or sedating antihistamines (which have a lower risk of being habit-forming) in patients with borderline personality disorder.

Psychological and social interventions are discussed in Section 24.11.2 and Section 24.11.3. Also see Chapter 37: Psychological interventions, and Chapter 38: Social interventions in psychiatry, for more detailed discussion of these treatment modalities.

## 24.11.2 Psychological intervention

Both individual and group psychotherapy may be useful in the management of people with personality disorder. Psychotherapy with patients with personality disorders may present many challenges, including:

- excessive dependence on the therapist
- fear of intimacy
- difficulty in establishing rapport and trust
- fear of rejection
- acting out or self-destructive behaviour
- failure to sustain therapy
- interpersonal conflict between the patient and therapist
- boundary violations.

### 24.11.2.1 Individual psychotherapy

**Cognitive-behavioural therapy**

Cognitive-behavioural therapy (CBT) focuses on cognition (thoughts, beliefs and attitudes) and how these impact on behaviour and emotions. Negative patterns of thinking and their behavioural responses are identified. The therapist helps the patient challenge cognitive and behavioural patterns that lead to distress and dysfunction.

**Dialectical behaviour therapy**

Dialectical behaviour therapy (DBT) is based on CBT principles and adapted to meet the emotional needs of people with borderline personality disorder. DBT facilitates change by focusing on the patient's acceptance of who they are. At the same time, harmful behaviours are identified as a focus of change. DBT balances acceptance techniques with change techniques.

**Insight-orientated (psychodynamic) therapy**

Insight-orientated (psychodynamic) therapy examines conflicts and symptoms that arise from past dysfunctional relationships and that are thought to influence present behaviour. The therapist helps the patient to explore past events, and the feelings or meaning attached to them. Awareness of the connection between such events and the person's maladaptive coping styles is encouraged.

**Supportive psychotherapy**

Supportive psychotherapy uses reassurance, direction, suggestion and persuasion to relieve symptoms. This strengthens the patient's defences, problem-solving skills and adaptation to psychosocial stressors.

**Crisis intervention**

Crisis intervention is an immediate, short-term intervention for individuals who present with psychological, physical and behavioural distress. Patients in crisis present with a sudden inability to use effective problem-solving and coping skills. The therapist offers empathetic, practical, problem-solving intervention aimed at reducing distress and restoring function. Short-term admission, whilst providing practical assistance with modifying psychosocial stressors, may be a form of crisis intervention

### 24.11.2.2 Group psychotherapy

In group psychotherapy a group of people with personality disorder are guided by a therapist who facilitates group interaction. Such interactions facilitate desired changes in cognition, emotional expression and behaviour. Group therapy may employ a range of psychotherapeutic approaches (e.g. supportive psychotherapy, CBT). Some patients with personality disorder may react negatively or anxiously when placed in a group setting. Therapeutic communities similarly use a group therapy approach. These are supported residential units for people with personality disorder and/or other mental disorders. Residents are encouraged and guided by the clinical team to provide mutual support to each other, behave in a pro-social manner and take responsibility for running of the unit (Schimmel, 1997; Campling, 2001). Intensive, longer-term therapeutic community treatment for PDs can achieve a significant reduction in symptomatic distress, and improve functionality.

## 24.11.3 Social intervention

Social problems may be the main reason why some people with personality disorder seek help. Social workers may assist with a range of problems, such as breaking free from an abusive environment, assistance with alternative accommodation, child access and custody issues and accessing community-based resources (e.g. substance-abuse rehabilitation centres and other social support networks). Quick access to assistance from a social worker may also be a form of crisis intervention.

## 24.11.4 Other interventions

Helping the patient with a personality disorder to re-establish optimal function is always a priority in management. Many other health professionals and agencies may contribute to this:

- an occupational therapist may conduct a functional assessment and assist with a structured program of daily activities, which may help reduce rumination about stressors or negative experiences and help optimise functionality
- local support groups or 24-hour help lines may be contacted in times of crisis or distress
- short-term hospital admissions may be necessary at times of acute crisis (e.g. admitting an acutely suicidal patient with borderline personality disorder)

- somatic symptoms (e.g. chronic pain) may require management by a general practitioner or referral to a physiotherapist.

## 24.12 Course, outcome and prognosis

Effects of enduring personality disorder symptoms include lower levels of educational or occupational achievement, on-going interpersonal conflict, social withdrawal, substance-related problems and persistence of co-morbid mental disorders.

Personality disorders were previously regarded as stable over time. Whilst maladaptive personality traits are more stable than personality disorder diagnoses, more recent evidence suggests that personality disorders may improve over time (Skodol, 2008). Even when personality disorder symptoms improve, residual effects may persist in the form of functional impairment, continuing behavioural problems, reduced future quality of life, and on-going other psychopathology. These residual effects have a negative effect on treatment outcome and prognosis (see Table 24.17).

**Table 24.17** Summary of personality disorder management, course and prognosis

| Personality disorder | Examples of symptoms and traits | Examples of biological intervention | Examples of psychological therapies | Course & prognosis |
|---|---|---|---|---|
| **CLUSTER A ('odd and eccentric')** | | | | |
| Paranoid | sensitive to slights<br>distrustfulness<br>suspiciousness<br>bears grudges | ▶ antipsychotics | ▶ supportive therapy<br>▶ crisis intervention<br>▶ not amenable to group therapy due to high levels of mistrust | chronic course<br>may herald schizophrenia<br>symptoms may wax and wane throughout lifetime<br>persistent functional and social impairment |
| Schizoid | detached<br>solitary existence<br>quiet<br>restricted emotional expression | ▶ antipsychotics<br>▶ antidepressants | ▶ supportive therapy<br>▶ group therapy | chronic course<br>persistent isolation results in poor social interaction and reduced quality of life |
| Schizotypal | magical thinking<br>eccentricity<br>peculiar ideas | ▶ antipsychotics<br>▶ antidepressants | ▶ CBT<br>▶ group therapy | chronic course<br>may develop schizophrenia<br>risk of suicide<br>reduced quality of life |
| **CLUSTER B ('dramatic and erratic')** | | | | |
| Antisocial | impulsivity<br>self-centredness<br>low frustration tolerance<br>aggression<br>criminality | ▶ antipsychotics<br>▶ antidepressants | ▶ group therapy<br>▶ psychodynamic therapy | variable course<br>may improve in adulthood<br>legal problems<br>substance use problems<br>depression<br>risk of death by violence or suicide<br>reduced quality of life |

| Personality disorder | Examples of symptoms and traits | Examples of biological intervention | Examples of psychological therapies | Course & prognosis |
|---|---|---|---|---|
| Borderline | instability of mood<br>identity and relationships<br>suicide attempts<br>self-harming<br>anxiety symptoms | ▶ antidepressants<br>▶ mood stabilizers<br>▶ antipsychotics | ▶ CBT<br>▶ DBT<br>▶ therapeutic community | variable course<br>ageing may lead to stability<br>risk of suicide<br>mood disorders<br>substance abuse<br>poorer function socially and vocationally<br>reduced quality of life |
| Histrionic | excessively emotional<br>dramatic<br>attention seeking<br>seductive | ▶ antidepressants<br>▶ antipsychotics | ▶ group therapy<br>▶ psychodynamic | may wax and wane with advancing age<br>may be at risk of substance abuse or somatisation disorder<br>prone to dissociation |
| Narcissistic | grandiosity<br>sensitivity to criticism<br>narcissistic rage | ▶ antidepressants | ▶ group therapy<br>▶ psychodynamic therapy | chronic course<br>difficult to treat<br>may develop depression and substance abuse |
| **CLUSTER C ('anxious and fearful')** | | | | |
| Avoidant | intense sensitivity to rejection<br>need for reassurance<br>anxious in social interaction | ▶ anxiolytics<br>▶ antidepressants<br>▶ beta blockers | ▶ CBT<br>▶ group therapy<br>▶ social skills training<br>▶ psychodynamic therapy | chronic course<br>risk of depression and social phobia<br>phobic avoidance may lead to isolation |
| Dependent | needy<br>exaggerated fear of being unable to care for oneself<br>difficulty making everyday decisions | ▶ antidepressants | ▶ CBT<br>▶ assertiveness training<br>▶ psychodynamic therapy<br>▶ group therapy | persistent occupational function impairment<br>prone to physical/ psychological abuse due to lack of assertiveness<br>prone to depressive disorders |
| Obsessive-compulsive | inflexible<br>perfectionistic<br>pre-occupied with rules<br>unable to compromise | ▶ antidepressants<br>▶ antipsychotics<br>▶ anxiolytics | ▶ CBT<br>▶ psychodynamic therapy | variable<br>isolated personal life<br>may develop anxiety/ depressive disorders |

## Conclusion

People with a personality disorder display characteristic patterns of cognition, emotion and behaviour that are pervasive and maladaptive, lead to significant distress to self and others and are associated with functional impairment.

The conceptualisation and classification of personality disorders remains controversial and the subject of ongoing debate. The aetiology is likely to be multifactorial, involving biological, psychological and socio-environmental factors. People with personality disorder often present significant diagnostic and management challenges. A thorough, longitudinal psychiatric assessment, including adequate collateral information, is important.

Co-morbidity (especially with other mental disorders) is common, and often complicates clinical presentation and management. Clinical intervention requires an individualised and holistic care plan within a multidisciplinary team context, and is aimed at relieving distress, treating co-morbidity and improving functionality. Psychotherapeutic interventions are the mainstay of clinical management, with various modalities being useful.

Medication that targets specific symptoms and/or treat co-morbid conditions may be useful in some individuals. Course, outcome and prognosis are variable, although many people experience residual symptoms and a chronic course.

# References


American Psychiatric Association (2000) *Diagnostic and statistical manual of mental disorders* (4th edition). (Text Revision). Washington DC: American Psychiatric Association

American Psychiatric Association (2013) *Diagnostic and statistical manual of mental disorders* (5th edition). Washington DC: American Psychiatric Association

Butcher JN (1989) *Minnesota Multiphasic Personality Inventory*. John Wiley & Sons

Campling P (2001) Therapeutic communities. *Advances in Psychiatric Treatment* 7: 365–72

Casey, P (2000) The epidemiology of personality disorder. In: Tyrer P (Ed). *Personality disorders: Diagnosis, Management and Cause.* Oxford: Butterworth Heinemann

Cloninger CR, Svrakic DM (2009) Personality disorders. In: Sadock BJ, Sadock VA, Ruiz P (Eds.) *Kaplan & Sadock's Comprehensive Textbook of Psychiatry* (9th edition) Philadelphia: Lippincott Williams & Wilkins

Cooke DJ, Hart SD (2004) Personality disorders. In: Johnstone EC, Cunnigham Owens DG, Lawrie SM, Sharpe M, Freeman CPL (Eds). *Companion to Psychiatric Studies* (7th edition). Edinburgh: Churchill Livingstone

First MB, Gibbon M, Spitzer RL, Williams, JBW, Benjamin LS (1997) *Structured Clinical Interview for DSM-IV Axis II Personality Disorders (SCID-II)*. Washington DC: American Psychiatric Press

Guzetta F, De Girolamo G (2009) Epidemiology of personality disorders. In: Gelder MG, Andreasen NC, Lopez-Ibor JJ (Jr), Geddes JR (Eds). *New Oxford Textbook of Psychiatry* (2nd edition). Oxford: Oxford University Press

Hare RD, Neumann CS (2009) *Psychopathy*. Chicago: Oxford University Press

Harrison P, Geddes J, Sharpe M (2010) *Psychiatry* (10th edition). Chichester: Wiley-Blackwell

Huang Y (2009) DSM–IV personality disorders in the WHO World Mental Health Surveys. *British Journal of Psychiatry* 195: 46–53

Kendell RE (2002) The distinction between personality disorder and mental illness. *British Journal of Psychiatry* 181: 76–7

Kolb JE, Gunderson JG (1980) Diagnosing borderline patients with a semistructured interview. *Archives of General Psychiatry* 37(1): 37–41

Lopez-Ibor JJ (Jr) (2009) Personality disorders: An introductory perspective. In: Gelder MG, Andreasen NC, Lopez-Ibor JJ (Jr), Geddes JR (Eds). *New Oxford Textbook of Psychiatry* (2nd edition). Oxford: Oxford University Press

Millon T, Davis R (1996) *Disorders of Personality: DSM-IV and Beyond*. New York: John Wiley & Sons

Millon T, Millon C, Davis R, Grossman S (2009) *MCMI-III Manual* (4th edition). Minneapolis: Pearson Education

Moran P, Leese M, Lee T, Walters P, Thornicroft G, Mann A (2003) Standardised Assessment of Personality – Abbreviated Scale (SAPAS): Preliminary validation of a brief screen for personality disorder. *British Journal of Psychiatry* 183(3): 228–32

Reich R, de Girolamo G (2009) Diagnosis and classification of personality disorders. In: Gelder MG, Andreasen NC, Lopez-Ibor JJ (Jr), Geddes JR (Eds). *New Oxford Textbook of Psychiatry* (2nd edition). Oxford: Oxford University Press Sadock BJ, Sadock VA (2010) *Pocket Handbook of Clinical Psychiatry* (5th edition). Philadelphia: Lipincott Williams and Wilkins

Schimmel P (1997) Swimming against the tide? A review of the therapeutic community. *Australian and New Zealand Journal of Psychiatry* 31(1): 120–7

Skodol E (2008) Longitudinal course and outcome. *Psychiatric Clinics of North America* 31(3): 495–503, viii. DOI: 10.1016/j.psc.2008.03.010

Suliman S, Stein DJ, Williams DR, Seedat S (2008) DSM-IV Personality Disorders and their Axis I correlates in the South African population. *Psychopathology* 41(6): 356–64

Taylor D, Paton C, Kapur S (2012) *Prescribing Guidelines in Psychiatry* (11th edition). London: Wiley Blackwell

Tobena, A (2009) Neuropsychological templates for abnormal personalities: From genes to biodevelopmental pathways. In: Gelder MG, Andreasen NC, Lopez-Ibor JJ (Jr), Geddes JR (Eds). *New Oxford Textbook of Psychiatry* (2nd edition). Oxford: Oxford University Press

Tyrer P, Gunderson J, Lyons M, Tohen M (1997) Extent of comorbidity between mental state and personality disorders. *Journal of Personality Disorders* 11(3): 242–59

World Health Organization (1992) *International Classification of Diseases and related Health Problems* (10th revision). Geneva: World Health Organization

CHAPTER

# 25 Impulse-control disorders

*Mo Nagdee, Heidi Loffstadt, Willem Esterhuysen*

## 25.1 Introduction and context

The group of conditions called the impulse-control disorders are broadly defined by a range of harmful behaviours performed in response to irresistible impulses. The ICD-10 classification system defines them as 'repeated acts that have no clear rational motivation and that generally harm the patient's own interests and those of other people' (World Health Organization, 1992). The DSM-IV-TR refers to 'failure to resist an impulse, drive or temptation to perform an act that is harmful to the person or others' (American Psychiatric Association, 2000). The DSM-5, on the other hand, describes the impulse-control disorders as involving 'problems in the self-control of emotions and behaviours', that 'bring the individual into significant conflict with societal norms or authority figures' (American Psychiatric Association, 2013). The specific impulse-control disorders listed in the ICD and DSM systems are generally similar, but with a few key differences in approach and categorisation, as indicated by the comparative summary in Table 25.1.

The chapter focuses on intermittent explosive disorder, pyromania, kleptomania, and other/unspecified impulse control disorders. See Chapter 21: Other substance-related and addiction disorders, for pathological gambling (gambling disorder), Chapter 17: Obsessive-compulsive and related disorders, for trichotillomania (hair pulling disorder), and Chapter 27: Child and adolescent psychiatry 1: Assessment and the young child, for oppositional defiant and conduct disorder.

## 25.2 Clinical features

There are many psychological conditions and mental disorders, in addition to impulse-control disorders, that often involve significant problems in emotional or behavioural regulation or poor impulse control and that may result in harm to self or others. These include (but are not limited to) neurodevelopmental disorders (e.g. intellectual impairment, autism spectrum disorders, ADHD), psychotic disorders (schizophrenia and others), mood disorders (especially mania), substance-related and addictive disorders, obsessive-compulsive and related disorders, neurocognitive disorders (e.g. delirium and dementia involving the frontal lobe) and many personality disorders, paraphilic disorders, mental disorders due to medical conditions (e.g. complex partial epilepsy, frontal lobe syndromes). The underlying causes of impulsivity and its behavioural manifestations also vary considerably between different disorders and individuals. In addition, many of the symptoms and behaviours associated with impulse-control disorders can occur to some degree as part of normal development. It is therefore important to consider the clinical context, frequency, persistence, pattern and associated impairments or consequences when conducting a diagnostic assessment.

Impulse-control disorders are a complex, heterogeneous group of conditions. This notwithstanding, there are a number of core clinical features that are common to the impulse-control disorders, as outlined in Table 25.2.

**Table 25.1** Specific impulse-control disorders included (or not) in ICD-10, DSM-IV-TR and DSM-5

| | ICD-10 (in Habit & Impulse-Disorder category) | DSM-IV-TR (in Impulse- control disorders Not Elsewhere Classified category) | DSM-5 (in Disruptive, Impulse-control Disorders & Conduct Disorders category) |
|---|---|---|---|
| Intermittent explosive disorder | no[1] | yes | yes |
| Kleptomania | yes | yes | yes |
| Pyromania | yes | yes | yes |
| Pathological gambling | yes | yes | no[4] |
| Trichotillomania | yes | yes | no[5] |
| Oppositional defiant disorder | no[2] | no[3] | yes[6] |
| Conduct disorder | no[2] | no[3] | yes[6] |
| Other/Unspecified impulse-control disorders | yes | yes | yes |

[1] Subsumed into 'Other habit and impulse disorders' category of the ICD-10
[2] Included in 'Behavioural & Emotional Disorders with onset occurring in childhood and adolescence' category
[3] Included in 'Disorders usually diagnosed in infancy, childhood or adolescence' category (under the section 'Attention-deficit & disruptive behavior disorders')
[4] Included in 'Substance-related and addictive disorders' chapter (in both the DSM-5 and this textbook)
[5] Included in 'Obsessive-compulsive and related disorders' (in both the DSM-5 and this textbook)
[6] See Chapter 27: Child and adolescent psychiatry 1: Assessment and the young child

# 25.3 Aetiology

Impulse-control disorders are complex behavioural and psychiatric syndromes whose cause remains largely unknown. Whilst numerous aetiological theories have been proposed, there remains insufficient evidence to draw specific conclusions about primary causality. As with many other mental disorders, the underlying mechanisms that result in the characteristic impulsivity and emotional or behavioural dyscontrol of impulse-control disorders, is likely to be multi-factorial. The main theories proposed include:

## 25.3.1 Biological theories

- Genetic: there is insufficient data available to draw specific conclusions on genetic factors.
- Neurotransmitter dysfunction: disturbances in central serotonergic function have been consistently implicated as the neurobiological substrate of impulsive aggression and completed suicide. Reduced concentrations of certain serotonin metabolites have been demonstrated in the suicidal behaviour of violent offenders and impulsive fire-setters (Virkunnen *et al.*, 1989). Noradrenaline and dopamine have also been implicated.
- Frontal and limbic network dysfunction: functional neuro-imaging studies suggest a role for impaired frontal-limbic control or inhibition of behavioural response sets. Exaggerated amygdala reactivity and reduced orbito-frontal cortical activation in response to perceived social threats in individuals with impulsive aggression have also been demonstrated (Coccaro *et al.*, 2007).
- Endocrine: certain hormones (e.g. elevated testosterone levels) are associated with impulsive aggression.
- Other biological associations: there are reportedly a disproportionate number

**Table 25.2** Core clinical features of impulse-control disorders

| Feature | Description |
|---|---|
| Impulsivity | ▶ Long-standing, recurrent, intense inability to control impulses or resist temptations to behave in specific manner or perform a specific act<br>▶ Magnitude of dyscontrol of emotions and/or behaviour disproportionate to context, provocation or psychosocial stressors |
| Compulsivity | ▶ Underlying force, motivation or drive compels individual to carry out specific behavioural responses (e.g. impulsive, aggressive outbursts) or specific activities (e.g. fire-setting or stealing)<br>▶ Behaviour does not entail obvious external gain |
| Arousal or tension prior to the behaviour or act | ▶ Increasing or mounting arousal or tension (which may be mixed with anticipatory pleasure) prior to engaging in the behaviour or committing the act |
| Pleasure, gratification and/or relief during or upon completion of the behaviour or act | ▶ Release of tension and pleasurable gratification experienced whilst acting out or upon completion of the behaviour or act |
| Regret, remorse, guilt, self-reproach and/or dysphoria following the behaviour or act | ▶ For variable periods following the behaviour or act<br>▶ Individuals usually harbour shameful secrecy about repetitive impulsive behaviour or activities |
| Harmful consequences to self and/or others | ▶ Behavioural and emotional dyscontrol cause distress and/or impairment to the individual<br>▶ Impulsive behaviour and activities violate the rights of others and bring the individual into conflict with societal norms, authority figures and the law<br>▶ Typically brought to attention of mental health services due to harmful consequences (e.g. criminal, interpersonal or financial) of impulsivity |
| Other shared features | ▶ Onset during childhood or early adolescence<br>▶ Tend to be more common in males (with possible exception of kleptomania)<br>▶ Not due to or better accounted for by other medical conditions (e.g. frontal lobe pathology) or other mental disorders (e.g. substance-related or personality disorders)<br>▶ High degree of co-morbidity with other mental disorders (especially substance-related disorders)<br>▶ Many shared personality dimensions (e.g. trait impulsivity or compulsivity, disinhibition, mood dysregulation and negative emotionality) |

of people with impulse-control disorders who have a history of perinatal insults (e.g. encephalitis), soft neurological signs, abnormal electroencephalogram's, mixed cerebral dominance and co-morbid neuropsychiatric disorders (e.g. complex partial epilepsy).

## 25.3.2 Psychosocial theories

- Psychodynamic theory hypotheses that acting out on impulses may represent a defence against perceived threats, anxiety, tension, guilt or emotional distress. Impulsive acts may also relate to the need to express sexual or aggressive drives or a sub-conscious need to experience punishment.
- Social learning models suggest that the socio-cultural environment in which people with impulse-control disorders grow up and live is an important factor. Exposure to domestic violence, antisocial or disinhibited parental or family role models, emotional deprivation, neglect and abuse, deficient attachment bonds and early and persistent psychosocial stressors all may contribute to the clinical manifestation of impulse-control disorders.

- Addiction models view impulsive behaviour and activities as addictive in nature, fulfilling some unspecified need as many substances of abuse do.

## 25.4 Epidemiology

Most individuals with impulse-control disorders only come to the attention of mental health-care professionals when their behaviour has brought them into conflict with their families, partners or the law. There are very few epidemiological studies available on this topic, but the DSM-5 draws the following broad conclusions (American Psychiatric Association, 2013):

- intermittent explosive disorder is more prevalent among younger individuals, and one-year prevalence data in the United States is about 2,7%
- kleptomania occurs in about 4–24% of individuals arrested for shoplifting. Prevalence in the general population is very rare, at approximately 0,3–0,6%. Females outnumber males at a ratio of 3:1
- pyromania as a primary diagnosis appears to be very rare. Among a sample of persons reaching the criminal system with reported fire setting, only 3,3% had symptoms that met the full criteria for pyromania. This disorder is more prevalent in men.

## 25.5 Specific impulse-control disorders

### 25.5.1 Intermittent explosive disorder

The impulsive and aggressive outbursts in intermittent explosive disorder have a rapid onset and a short or no prodromal period. Outbursts typically last for less than 30 minutes and commonly occur in response to a minor provocation. After the episode, patients usually show genuine regret. These patients usually do not seek help spontaneously and are brought to the attention of mental health care professionals by others who have to bear the brunt of their outbursts or are referred by law enforcement agencies.

Aggressive behaviour secondary to a another medical condition (especially delirium and intracranial pathology), dementia, personality change due to a another medical condition, substance withdrawal or intoxication, antisocial and borderline personality disorder, bipolar disorder, schizophrenia, conduct disorder and malingering should be considered in the differential diagnosis of intermittent explosive disorder.

### 25.5.2 Kleptomania

The defining symptom of kleptomania is the repetitive theft of items that are usually of little monetary value and are not realistically needed. Patients usually report increasing tension before stealing, feelings of relief and gratification during the act, and feelings of remorse, guilt and self-loathing after the incident. Kleptomania is usually repugnant to many sufferers, and inconsistent with their otherwise ethical behaviour and beliefs.

Ordinary theft, malingering, antisocial personality disorder, conduct disorder, manic episodes, psychotic episodes and neurocognitive disorders should be considered in the differential diagnosis.

### 25.5.3 Pyromania

Pyromania is the recurrent, deliberate and purposeful setting of fires. A typical episode begins with rising tension linked to thoughts of fire setting. These thoughts may possess a distinctly erotic quality and may be accompanied by restlessness, headaches, palpitations and tinnitus. Persons with pyromania regularly watch fires in their neighbourhood, frequently set off false alarms and show interest in fire-fighting paraphernalia. Their curiosity is evident but they typically show little or no remorse, and may be indifferent to the consequences for life or property. Commonly associated features include alcohol intoxication, sexual dysfunction, below-average intelligence, chronic personal frustration and resentment towards authority figures. Some patients may become sexually aroused by fire.

**Table 25.3** DSM-5 Diagnostic Criteria for Intermittent Explosive Disorder

| Diagnostic Criteria |
|---|
| A. Recurrent behavioral outbursts representing a failure to control aggressive impulses as manifested by either of the following: |
| 1. Verbal aggression (e.g., temper tantrums, tirades, verbal arguments or fights) or physical aggression toward property, animals, or other individuals, occurring twice weekly, on average, for a period of 3 months. The physical aggression does not result in damage or destruction of property and does not result in physical injury to animals or other individuals. |
| 2. Three behavioral outbursts involving damage or destruction of property and/or physical assault involving physical injury against animals or other individuals occurring within a 12-month period. |
| B. The magnitude of aggressiveness expressed during the recurrent outbursts is grossly out of proportion to the provocation or to any precipitating psychosocial stressors. |
| C. The recurrent aggressive outbursts are not premeditated (i.e., they are impulsive and/or anger-based) and are not committed to achieve some tangible objective (e.g., money, power, intimidation). |
| D. The recurrent aggressive outbursts cause either marked distress in the individual or impairment in occupational or interpersonal functioning, or are associated with financial or legal consequences. |
| E. Chronological age is at least 6 years (or equivalent developmental level). |
| F. The recurrent aggressive outbursts are not better explained by another mental disorder (e.g., major depressive disorder, bipolar disorder, disruptive mood dysregulation disorder, a psychotic disorder, antisocial personality disorder, borderline personality disorder) and are not attributable to another medical condition (e.g., head trauma, Alzheimer's disease) or to the physiological effects of a substance (e.g., a drug of abuse, a medication). For children ages 6–18 years, aggressive behavior that occurs as part of an adjustment disorder should not be considered for this diagnosis. |
| **Note:** This diagnosis can be made in addition to the diagnosis of attention-deficit/hyperactivity disorder, conduct disorder, oppositional defiant disorder, or autism spectrum disorder when recurrent impulsive aggressive outbursts are in excess of those usually seen in these disorders and warrant independent clinical attention. |

**Source:** Reprinted with permission from the *Diagnostic and Statistical Manual of Mental Disorders*, Fifth Edition, (Copyright 2013). American Psychiatric Association.

## Case study 25.1

### Intermittent explosive disorder

A 42-year-old car salesman sought assistance for difficulties with his anger. He had been verbally abusive towards clients on a number of occasions and also had sudden outbursts of anger towards his girlfriend. This occurred in the absence of clear conflict. Between the episodes he was a kind and patient individual.

Mental state examination revealed a generally cooperative patient. He had no history of substance abuse or medical conditions, and has never received psychiatric care prior to this evaluation.

**Table 25.4** DSM-5 Diagnostic Criteria for Kleptomania

| Diagnostic Criteria |
|---|
| A. Recurrent failure to resist impulses to steal objects that are not needed for personal use or for their monetary value. |
| B. Increasing sense of tension immediately before committing the theft. |
| C. Pleasure, gratification, or relief at the time of committing the theft. |
| D. The stealing is not committed to express anger or vengeance and is not in response to a delusion or a hallucination. |
| E. The stealing is not better explained by conduct disorder, a manic episode, or antisocial personality disorder. |

**Source:** Reprinted with permission from the *Diagnostic and Statistical Manual of Mental Disorders*, Fifth Edition, (Copyright 2013). American Psychiatric Association.

Dementia, intellectual disability, substance intoxication, schizophrenia, conduct disorder and antisocial personality disorder should always be excluded.

## 25.5.4 Other specified disruptive, impulse-control and conduct disorders

This includes presentations in which symptoms characteristic of these disorders do not meet the full criteria for any of the disorders in the separate classes. This category is used in situations where the clinician chooses to communicate the specific reason why the presentation does not meet the criteria for a specific disorder.

## 25.5.5 Unspecified disruptive, impulse-control and conduct disorders

This category includes situations in which the clinician chooses not to specify the reason that the criteria for disruptive, impulse-control and conduct disorders are not met, and/or in situations where there is insufficient information to make a more specific diagnosis.

**Table 25.5** DSM-5 Diagnostic Criteria for Pyromania

| Diagnostic Criteria |
|---|
| A. Deliberate and purposeful fire setting on more than one occasion. |
| B. Tension or affective arousal before the act. |
| C. Fascination with, interest in, curiosity about, or attraction to fire and its situational contexts (e.g., paraphernalia, uses, consequences). |
| D. Pleasure, gratification, or relief when setting fires or when witnessing or participating in their aftermath. |
| E. The fire setting is not done for monetary gain, as an expression of sociopolitical ideology, to conceal criminal activity, to express anger or vengeance, to improve one's living circumstances, in response to a delusion or hallucination, or as a result of impaired judgment (e.g., in major neurocognitive disorder, intellectual disability [intellectual developmental disorder], substance intoxication). |
| F. The fire setting is not better explained by conduct disorder, a manic episode, or antisocial personality disorder. |

**Source:** Reprinted with permission from the *Diagnostic and Statistical Manual of Mental Disorders*, Fifth Edition, (Copyright 2013). American Psychiatric Association.

### Case study 25.2

**Kleptomania**

A 19-year-old lady is referred by the court for psychiatric evaluation after she has been caught stealing toiletries from the local supermarket. This is the third time that she has been caught doing this. She is a college student who performs very well academically; she also has never been convicted of any other offence. She is part of a stable family and has no financial difficulties. She claims that she cannot suppress the urge to take these objects, and only feels relief if she steals them. On mental state examination she is clearly distressed about her behaviour, and expresses genuine remorse.

### Case study 25.3

**Pyromania**

A 23-year-old fire setter reported that he felt intensely sexually aroused by the sight of the fire after he set his sister's bedroom alight. He also reported that he has been fascinated with fires since an early age, and cannot resist his impulses to set fires.

# 25.6 Principles of management

## 25.6.1 General principles

Although literature and research into impulse-control disorders are growing, most of what is known and recommended on the treatment of these disorders are based on case studies, case series and small clinical trials. To further complicate the matter, most patients who present for treatment do so via the legal system, which may influence the patient's willingness to cooperate with a proposed treatment regime. Despite the lack of clear evidence based treatments, the following general guidelines should be considered:

- assessment of patients with impulse-control disorder should include a comprehensive psychiatric and medical history, mental state examination and physical examination, with particular emphasis on the patient's legal or criminal history (patients with impulse-control disorder often have previous convictions and pending charges)
- due to significant co-morbidity, clinicians should actively screen and manage co-morbid psychiatric disorders, which include amongst others:
  - substance-use disorders
  - mood disorders
  - anxiety disorders
  - eating disorders
  - personality disorders
  - obsessive-compulsive disorders
  - other disruptive, impulse-control and conduct disorders
- due to the covert nature of impulse-control disorders and the embarrassment patients often experience when arrested, the clinician should assess carefully for adjustment reactions, depressed mood and suicidality
- a thorough risk assessment should be conducted, particularly in patients with intermittent explosive disorder and pyromania, in respect of risk to others and risk to property.

As with all other psychiatric disorders, building and maintaining a therapeutic relationship with the patient will improve treatment outcomes.

**Table 25.6** DSM-5 Diagnostic Criteria for Other Specified Disruptive, Impulse-Control, and Conduct Disorder

| This category applies to presentations in which symptoms characteristic of a disruptive, impulse-control, and conduct disorder that cause clinically significant distress or impairment in social, occupational, or other important areas of functioning predominate but do not meet the full criteria for any of the disorders in the disruptive, impulse-control, and conduct disorders diagnostic class. The other specified disruptive, impulse-control, and conduct disorder category is used in situations in which the clinician chooses to communicate the specific reason that the presentation does not meet the criteria for any specific disruptive, impulse-control, and conduct disorder. This is done by recording 'other specified disruptive, impulse-control, and conduct disorder' followed by the specific reason (e.g., 'recurrent behavioral outbursts of insufficient frequency'). |
|---|

**Source:** Reprinted with permission from the *Diagnostic and Statistical Manual of Mental Disorders*, Fifth Edition, (Copyright 2013). American Psychiatric Association.

**Table 25.7** DSM-5 Diagnostic Criteria for Unspecified Disruptive, Impulse-Control, and Conduct Disorder

| This category applies to presentations in which symptoms characteristic of a disruptive, impulse-control, and conduct disorder that cause clinically significant distress or impairment in social, occupational, or other important areas of functioning predominate but do not meet the full criteria for any of the disorders in the disruptive, impulse-control, and conduct disorders diagnostic class. The unspecified disruptive, impulse-control, and conduct disorder category is used in situations in which the clinician chooses *not* to specify the reason that the criteria are not met for a specific disruptive, impulse-control, and conduct disorder, and includes presentations in which there is insufficient information to make a more specific diagnosis (e.g., in emergency room settings). |
|---|

**Source:** Reprinted with permission from the *Diagnostic and Statistical Manual of Mental Disorders*, Fifth Edition, (Copyright 2013). American Psychiatric Association.

## 25.6.2 Psychological management

### 25.6.2.1 Intermittent explosive disorder

The recommendation for using psychological treatment in intermittent explosive disorder is based on the success of this approach in managing impulsive-aggression in the broader context of psychiatric disorders. Cognitive behavioural therapy (CBT), group therapy, family therapy and social skills training have all been shown to be effective in reducing aggressive behaviour. An important therapeutic goal would be to help the patient recognise and appropriately express thoughts and feelings that precede explosive behavioural outbursts (as opposed to simply acting out impulsively).

### 25.6.2.2 Kleptomania

Several case studies have shown promising results for using CBT in patients with kleptomania. The techniques used include systematic desensitisation, aversion therapy, relaxation training and alternative sources of gratification. Insight-oriented psychotherapy and psychoanalysis have also been used but these techniques are more dependent on a patients' motivation to change than CBT approaches are.

### 25.6.2.3 Pyromania

There is little evidence-based literature available on effective treatment of pyromania. Despite this, the mainstay of treatment at present is psychological intervention, with an emphasis on behavioural techniques (such as behaviour modification programmes, specific fire-setting offender treatment programmes, social supervision and support). Early intervention programmes and addressing problematic fire-setting behaviour in children and adolescents have been implemented in some developed countries, with mixed success. This approach cannot be generalised to all patients with pyromania.

## 25.6.3 Pharmacological management

### 25.6.3.1 Intermittent explosive disorder

Several classes of medication have shown some efficacy in reducing impulsive aggression in a range of clinical populations. These include lithium carbonate, anticonvulsants, antidepressants, antipsychotics and beta-blockers. Clinical experience suggests that the anticonvulsants (e.g. sodium valproate, carbamazepine) are commonly prescribed in the symptomatic treatment of impulsive aggression, despite mixed results from clinical trials. Lithium carbonate is possibly more effective in reducing impulsivity but arguably lacks the better safety and tolerability profile of sodium valproate and carbamazepine. The SSRI fluoxetine has been evaluated in the treatment of intermittent explosive disorder and demonstrated some efficacy in reducing aggressive outbursts in these patients, but only a small percentage of patients who respond to treatment sustain full remission. Since there is no approved medication for the treatment of intermittent explosive disorder, it is recommended that the pharmacological treatment for such patients be individualised and guided by the clinical setting and additional management of co-morbid conditions.

### 25.6.3.2 Kleptomania

Several case studies have reported the effective treatment of kleptomania with several different classes of medication. These include antidepressants, mood stabilizers, electroconvulsive therapy, opioid antagonists and glutamatergic agents. Promising results have been demonstrated with the opioid antagonists (e.g. naltrexone). One clinical trial with a SSRI failed to show improvement in the symptoms of kleptomania, but the high co-morbidity of this condition with mood and anxiety disorders suggests possible benefits (Schreiber *et al.*, 2011).

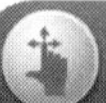

**Case study 25.4**

**Kleptomania**

Heidi is a 34-year-old married woman with three children who is referred by a social worker for assessment and treatment, following her second arrest for shoplifting. Heidi gives a clear history of kleptomania and reports that she steals mainly G-strings (which she never wears) from lingerie stores every time she goes to the mall for groceries (at least ten times a month). As part of her treatment regime aversive therapy techniques are used where Heidi has to visualise going into the lingerie store stealing an item, being caught by the store manager, being driven in the back of a police van to the holding cells and appearing before a judge for a charge of shoplifting. Heidi is then further helped to visualise having to phone her husband from the cells and the subsequent breakdown of her marriage and the children being placed with their father. Following 12 sessions Heidi reported no relapses over a 12-month follow-up period.

### 25.6.3.3 Pyromania

There are no clear evidence-based guidelines for the pharmacological treatment of pyromania but, as with the other impulse-control disorders, co-morbid conditions should be actively treated.

## 25.7 Course and prognosis

As a general rule, the impulse-control disorders are considered chronic disorders with a waxing and waning course and a guarded prognosis.

Intermittent explosive disorder most often has its onset during late childhood or early adolescence and rarely presents after the age of 40 years. The course is typically persistent and chronic.

Kleptomania tends to start in adolescence but has a variable age of onset. It may continue for years despite multiple convictions for shoplifting. Three patterns in the evolution of the disorder have been suggested:

- sporadic with brief episodes and long periods of remission.
- episodic with protracted periods of stealing and periods of remission.
- chronic with some degree of fluctuation.

Pyromania probably also has its onset in childhood or early adolescence but there is insufficient data to establish a typical age of onset. It seems to have a chronic course, with episodic fire-setting incidents.

## Conclusion

Impulse-control disorders are complex behavioural and psychiatric syndromes whose cause remains largely unknown. Despite evidence that these disorders are common they tend to be under-diagnosed in clinical populations. Optimal treatment and early detection of patients with impulse-control disorders are important due to their strong association with other psychiatric co-morbidity and the potential risk these patients pose to themselves and others. The mainstay of treatment includes a combination of pharmacological interventions, psychotherapy, and detection and management of potential risks.

# References

American Psychiatric Association. (2000) *Diagnostic and statistical manual of mental disorders* (4th edition). Text Revision) Washington DC: American Psychiatric Association

American Psychiatric Association (2013) *Diagnostic and statistical manual of mental disorders* (5th edition). Washington DC: American Psychiatric Association

Coccaro EF, McCloskey MS, Fitzgerald DA, Phan KL (2007) Amygdala and orbitofrontal reactivity to social threats in individuals with impulsive aggression. *Biological Psychiatry* 62: 168–78

Schreiber L, Odlaug BL, Grant JE (2011) Impulse control disorders: Updated review of clinical characteristics and pharmacological management. *Frontiers in Psychiatry* 2: 1–11

Virkkunen M, de Jong J, Bartko J, Linnoila M (1989) Psychobiological concomitants of history of suicide attempts among violent offenders and impulsive fire-setters. *Archives of General Psychiatry* 46: 604–6

World Health Organization (1992) *International classification of diseases and related health problems* (10th revision). Geneva: World Health Organization

# PART 5

# Special topics in psychiatry

CHAPTER

# 26 Women's mental health

Nadira Khamker

## 26.1 Introduction

Gender differences in the prevalence, expression and risk of developing illness is becoming an area of increased interest. This requires familiarity with psychobiological factors unique to both men and women. Revisions to the DSM-5 included a review of the potential differences in the expression of mental illness in men and women (American Psychiatric Association, 2013). There are gender differences in cognitive function and in the prevalence of many other neuropsychiatric disorders. The biological basis for these differences is still an area of research, but has been attributed to the effects of oestrogen on brain function in regions that are implicated in neuropsychiatric disorders.

## 26.2 Cellular actions of oestrogen

The role of oestrogen, in particular, along with that of other hormones has profound implications for the aetiology and treatment of women's psychiatric illness (Steiner *et al.*, 2003.) The stress of specific life events, such as puberty, miscarriage, abortion and menopause, can also affect women's mental health from both a biological and psychosocial perspective with the potential for the development of **secondary psychiatric disorders** (Freeman *et al.*, 2002; Lolak *et al.*, 2005; Steiner *et al.*, 2003).

Ovarian oestrogen, especially 17β oestradiol, regulates reproductive function and that of reproductive-associated tissue of the breast and uterus. Long-term positive effects of oestrogen on other target organs include bone mineralisation and decreasing serum cholesterol.

Oestrogens have trophic actions in the brain and these trigger expression by binding to oestrogen receptors. These receptors do not only differ from tissue to tissue but in different brain regions as well. Apart from oestrogen receptors, there are receptors for progesterone, androgens and other steroids such as gluco- and mineral corticoids.

Gonadal steroid receptors are located in different areas of the brain including the amygdala, hippocampus, basal forebrain, cortex, cerebellum, locus coeruleus, midbrain raphe nuclei, pituitary gland and hypothalamus. It has been suggested that steroid hormone receptors function as transcription factors to achieve integration of neural information in the central nervous system (CNS). Oestrogen exerts its trophic influence through low levels of glutamate activation leading to spine formation and synaptogenesis; this may be one of the hypotheses to explain the mechanism of cyclical formation and removal of synapses. Other cellular actions of oestrogen include its ability to act as an anti-oxidant and therefore provide neuro-protection against free radicals (Craig and Cutter 2004; Sherwin 2003).

Steroid hormones modulate neuronal transmission by a variety of mechanisms:

- they may affect the synthesis and/or release of neurotransmitters
- they may modulate the expression of receptors
- they may modulate membrane plasticity and permeability.

## 26.3 Effects of oestrogen on neurotransmitter systems

### 26.3.1 The cholinergic system

In rat studies, oestradiol has been reported to:

- enhance cholinergic muscarinic receptor density
- enhance choline uptake and the activity of choline acetyltransferase in the basal forebrain and two of its projection areas, namely the hippocampus and frontal cortex
- modulate acetylcholine release, thus exerting an effect on the cholinergic system and diminishing cognitive function with time following loss of ovarian function.

### 26.3.2 The serotonergic system

- There is increasing evidence that oestrogen interacts with the 5-HT system at multiple levels. The serotonergic system is in close reciprocal relationship with gonadal hormones. In the hypothalamus, oestrogen induces a fluctuation in 5-HT whereas progesterone increases the turnover rate of 5-HT.
- The suggestion that oestrogen modulates expression of 5-HT receptors is supported by recent positron emission tomography (PET) findings of increased $5\text{-HT}_{2A}$ receptor density in women on hormone replacement therapy.
- It has also been demonstrated that oestrogen replacement therapy significantly modulates age-related reduction in serotonergic responsivity.
- The $5\text{-HT}_{2A}$ receptor is important in many neuropsychiatric disorders, including depression, schizophrenia and Alzheimer's disease.

The density of $5\text{-HT}_{2A}$ receptors in the frontal and cingulate cortex increases significantly during the high-oestrogen phase. Oestrogen treatment causes an increase in central $5\text{-HT}_2$ receptors and a decrease in $5\text{-HT}_1$ receptors (Craig and Murphy, 2006; Steiner *et al.*, 2003; Stahl, 2000; Sherwin, 2003).

### 26.3.3 The dopaminergic system

Gender differences in maturation of the dopaminergic system have been reported and may also be influenced by oestrogen. Earlier studies on humans and animals indicate that oestrogen modulates many aspects of dopaminergic function. These studies suggest that:

- dopaminergic neurons start to develop earlier in females and then exhibit a steeper pattern of decline in mid-life
- oestrogen deprivation for a period of time has been reported to lead to loss of dopaminergic cells in brain regions
- the duration of oestrogen therapy administration may affect dopaminergic responsivity because acute therapy has been reported to convert high $D_2$ dopamine binding sites to low affinity sites
- in humans, dopamine $D_2$ receptor concentration reduces significantly with increasing age, especially in frontal and basal ganglia regions. A more pronounced decline in women than in men is observed (Craig and Murphy, 2006; Sherwin, 2003; Stahl, 2000; McEwen and Alves, 1999).

## 26.4 Hormones and mood

### 26.4.1 Epidemiology

Epidemiological studies have consistently demonstrated higher rates of mood disorders (especially depressive illness) in women than in men. The lifetime prevalence of mood disorders in women is approximately twice that of men (Wu and Anthony, 2000). With the exception of an increased incidence during the peri-menopause, this higher incidence is less marked in the years after menopause.

Potential links have been identified between changes in oestrogen levels across the female life cycle with the observation that depression is more common in women than men during certain stages of the life cycle. In women, the incidence of depression mirrors the oestrogen levels changing across the life cycle: as oestrogen levels increase during puberty, the incidence of depression increases and then decreases again after menopause. Thus, females have the same frequency of depression as males before puberty and after menopause. In males the incidence of depression rises in puberty and then remains constant throughout life, despite a slowly declining level of testosterone from the age of 25. The underlying cause of this gender difference is not clear, but it is hypothesised that a dysregulation in the hypothalamic-pituitary-gonadal axis could play a role (Deecher *et al.*, 2008, Steiner *et al.*, 2003; Craig and Cutter 2004; Lolak *et al.*, 2005).

### 26.4.2 Aetiology

The underlying causality of this gender difference in mood-related disorders is unclear. However, there are multiple factors associated with the aetiology of these disorders. They include a genetic predisposition and an increased vulnerability or exposure to stressful life events that can cause biochemical changes in the neuro-endocrine systems and neuro-anatomical areas in the brain. Alterations in the neurotransmitter systems (e.g. serotonin, noradrenalin and dopamine systems) are also implicated in the aetiology of depressive disorders (Deecher *et al.*, 2008; Steiner 2006). Several psychosocial and environmental factors have been linked with depression, including life stress, relational difficulties, trauma, violence and poverty. Childhood abuse and a history of previous mood disorders during the early reproductive years are associated with a greater risk of a depressive disorder developing in women than in men (Steiner, 2006; Steiner, 2008).

Oestrogen levels vary across the female life cycle in relation to various reproductive events. Oestrogen levels begin to rise and cycle during puberty, and this cycling persists during childbearing years. The oestrogen levels are very high during pregnancy and decrease drastically postpartum. Another fluctuation in oestrogen levels occurs around the time of the menopause, prior to complete cessation of menstrual cycles, and hormonal levels are thus unpredictable during these years. Menopause is the final stage of transition of oestrogen in the female life cycle (Deecher *et al.* 2008; Steiner, 2006; Sherwin, 2003; McEwen and Alves 1999).

It has been suggested that oestrogen may provide protection against depression and this is supported by reports of an increased incidence of depressive symptoms during periods associated with low oestrogen concentrations, for example the premenstrual and postpartum periods. A study conducted in a peri-urban setting in South Africa found the rate of postpartum depression to be three times that found in British postpartum samples (Cooper *et al.*, 1999). However, it has also been reported that depression may be equally high at times of high oestrogen concentration such as the antenatal period. Although pregnancy is traditionally viewed as a period of emotional well-being, studies show that the prevalence of antenatal depression is higher than that of postnatal depression (Mannikam and Burns, 2012). The cause for these varying expressions remains to be elucidated (Craig and Murphy 2006; Deecher *et al.*, 2008).

## 26.5 Phases of life and psychiatric disorders

### 26.5.1 Menarche and mood disorders

Epidemiological studies consistently show that, beginning at menarche, mood disorders are twice as common in women as men. Significant changes occur in the hormonal milieu during adolescence and with this come social, psychological and physiological changes (Boyd and Amsterdam, 2004; Steiner *et al.*, 2003).

The newly fluctuating levels of gonadal hormones and gonadotropins, which mark the onset of menarche and the establishment of menstrual cycles, introduce a major change in the hormonal milieu to which the rest of the systems have to adjust. This is the period during which the hypothalamic-pituitary-adrenal (HPA) axis matures and becomes sensitised to a variety of new feedback mechanisms. It is also during this time that the HPA axis may be particularly vulnerable to external psychosocial stressors, sleep deprivation and other influences, resulting in a higher incidence of HPA dysregulation and mood instability (Steiner, 2006; Miller *et al.*, 2009).

There is both direct and indirect evidence of involvement of the serotonergic system in the aetiology of depressive disorders in child and adolescent depression. Gonadal hormones effect the production of serotonin receptors; an altered distribution or function of serotonin receptor subtypes brought on by changes in the hormonal milieu at menarche may increase vulnerability to developing mood disorders. It is thus important that pubertal and other hormonal changes be monitored prospectively along with individual, genetic, constitutional and psychological characteristics in order to predict the development of negative affect during puberty (Steiner *et al.*, 2003; Cohen, 2003).

## 26.5.2 Premenstrual dysphoric disorder

Many women may experience physical, psychological and behavioural changes related to their menstrual cycles. Menstruation-related mood disorders are amongst the earliest recorded biologically linked behavioural disturbances. The inclusion of pre-menstrual dysphoric disorder (PMDD) in the DSM-5 recognises the fact that some women have extremely distressing premenstrual emotional and behavioural symptoms. There is a growing database in the literature that reports a link between premenstrual dysphoric disorder and mood disorders (American Psychiatric Association, 2013).

### 26.5.2.1 Epidemiology

Epidemiological surveys have estimated that as many as 75% of women with regular menstrual cycles experience some symptoms of premenstrual syndrome. Premenstrual dysphoric disorder, however, is much less common, affecting 3–8% of women. It is found to be more severe and exerts a greater psychological toll than does premenstrual syndrome. These women report premenstrual symptoms that significantly interfere with their lifestyle and relationships.

The twelve-month prevalence of premenstrual dysphoric disorder is between 1,8–5,8% of menstruating women (Gehlert *et al.*, 2009; Witchen *et al.*, 2002). The most rigorous estimate of premenstrual dysphoric disorder is 1,8% for women whose symptoms meet the full criteria without functional impairment and 1,3% for women whose symptoms meet the current criteria with functional impairment and without co-occurring symptoms from another mental disorder (Gehlert *et al.*, 2009). Onset of premenstrual dysphoric disorder can occur at any point after menarche. Incidence of new cases over a 40-month follow-up period is 2,5%.

### 26.5.2.2 Aetiology

The aetiology of premenstrual dysphoric disorder is largely unknown, but that it may have a biological component is underscored by recent evidence of the heritability of premenstrual symptoms and the elimination of premenstrual complaints with suppression of ovarian activity or surgical menopause. The current consensus is that normal ovarian function (rather than hormonal imbalance) is the cyclic trigger for biochemical events within the CNS and other target tissues, which results in premenstrual symptoms in vulnerable women. The current literature suggests that thyroid dysfunction may also be found in a small group of women with premenstrual symptoms, but premenstrual dysphoric disorder is not considered to be a masked form of hypothyroidism.

Environmental factors associated with the expression of premenstrual dysphoric disorder include stress, history of interpersonal trauma, seasonal changes and sociocultural aspects of female sexual behaviour (Deuster *et al.*, 1999; Girdler *et al.*, 2004, Maskall *et al.*, 1997).

**Genetic factors**

Heritability of premenstrual dysphoric disorder is unknown. However, estimates for heritability of premenstrual symptoms range between 30–80%. One study found that 70% of daughters of mothers with premenstrual stress (PMS) also have premenstrual dysphoric disorder symptoms, compared with only 37% of daughters of unaffected mothers (Parry and Berga, 2003; Miller *et al.*, 2009; Cohen *et al.*, 2002).

**Physiological factors**

*Gonadal steroids and gonadotropins*

The role of female sex hormones in premenstrual symptomatology has been considered to be of central importance. An area of increasing attention in the manifestation of premenstrual symptomatology is the metabolite of progesterone namely allopregnanolone. Treatment studies have suggested that progesterone and progestogens may provoke, rather than ameliorate, the cyclical symptom changes of premenstrual dysphoric disorder.

Early investigations of androgens have suggested that women with PMS or premenstrual dysphoric disorder have elevated levels of testosterone in the luteal phase compared with controls; this may contribute primarily to the symptom of irritability. (Androgens promote sexual drive in humans and have been tentatively linked with mood and impulsive behaviour.)

A relationship between serotonin and androgens and their effects on human behaviour has been proposed; the behavioural effects of androgens may therefore partly be mediated by a reduction in serotonin activity (Miller at al., 2009; Steiner, 2006; Deuster *et al.*, 1999).

*Beta endorphin*

A decreased level of B endorphin is found in patients with pre-menstrual dysphoric disorder.

*Neurotransmitters*

Of the neurotransmitters studied to date, evidence increasingly suggests that serotonin may be important in the pathogenesis of premenstrual dysphoric disorder. Premenstrual dysphoric disorder shares many features of other mood and anxiety disorders linked to serotonergic dysfunction. In addition, reduction in serotonin neurotransmission is thought to lead to poor impulse control, depressed mood, irritability and increased carbohydrate craving: all mood and behavioural symptoms associated with premenstrual dysphoric disorder.

Additional evidence suggesting the involvement of the serotonergic system has emerged from treatment studies indicating that drugs that facilitate serotonergic transmission (e.g. SSRIs) are effective in reducing premenstrual symptoms. These studies imply a possible change in $5HT_{1A}$ receptor sensitivity in women with premenstrual dysphoria. The current consensus is that women with premenstrual dysphoria may be behaviourally or biochemically sub- or supersensitive to the serotonergic system (Miller *et al.*, 2009; Boyd and Amsterdam, 2004).

### 26.5.2.3 Diagnosis and clinical features

**Diagnostic criteria**

*Recording procedures*

If symptoms have not been confirmed by prospective daily ratings of at least two symptomatic cycles, 'provisional' should be noted after the name of the diagnosis (i.e. 'premenstrual dysphoric disorder, provisional') (American Psychiatric Association, 2013).

**Diagnostic features**

More than 150 symptoms have been reported during the latter half of the menstrual cycle, which can cause problems in women's ability to function. Typically, symptoms peak around the time of the onset of menses (Hartlage *et al.*, 2012) and, although it is not uncommon for symptoms to linger into the first few days of menses, the individual must have a symptom-free period in the follicular phase after the menstrual period begins.

Mood and behavioural symptoms constitute a major component among the various symptoms associated with a premenstrual syndrome. Irritability, depression, anxiety and mood lability are among the most common. Physical complaints include changes in sleep, temperature, appetite, reduced energy and difficulty concentrating. Joint or muscle pain, breast tenderness or swelling and abdominal bloating can also occur. Diagnosis can be complicated by the fact that specific symptom patterns vary among women. Syndromes such as epilepsy, migraine and various psychiatric disorders may show a

**Table 26.1** DSM-5 Diagnostic Criteria for Premenstrual Dysphoric Disorder

| **Diagnostic Criteria** |
|---|
| A. In the majority of menstrual cycles, at least five symptoms must be present in the final week before the onset of menses, start to *improve* within a few days after the onset of menses, and become *minimal* or absent in the week postmenses. |
| B. One (or more) of the following symptoms must be present: |
| 1. Marked affective lability (e.g., mood swings: feeling suddenly sad or tearful, or increased sensitivity to rejection). |
| 2. Marked irritability or anger or increased interpersonal conflicts. |
| 3. Marked depressed mood, feelings of hopelessness, or self-deprecating thoughts. |
| 4. Marked anxiety, tension, and/or feelings of being keyed up or on edge. |
| C. One (or more) of the following symptoms must additionally be present, to reach a total of five symptoms when combined with symptoms from Criterion B above. |
| 1. Decreased interest in usual activities (e.g., work, school, friends, hobbies). |
| 2. Subjective difficulty in concentration. |
| 3. Lethargy, easy fatigability, or marked lack of energy. |
| 4. Marked change in appetite; overeating; or specific food cravings. |
| 5. Hypersomnia or insomnia. |
| 6. A sense of being overwhelmed or out of control. |
| 7. Physical symptoms such as breast tenderness or swelling, joint or muscle pain, a sensation of 'bloating,' or weight gain. |
| **Note:** The symptoms in Criteria A–C must have been met for most menstrual cycles that occurred in the preceding year. |
| D. The symptoms are associated with clinically significant distress or interference with work, school, usual social activities, or relationships with others (e.g., avoidance of social activities; decreased productivity and efficiency at work, school, or home). |
| E. The disturbance is not merely an exacerbation of the symptoms of another disorder, such as major depressive disorder, panic disorder, persistent depressive disorder (dysthymia), or a personality disorder (although it may co-occur with any of these disorders). |
| F. Criterion A should be confirmed by prospective daily ratings during at least two symptomatic cycles. (Note: The diagnosis may be made provisionally prior to this confirmation.) |
| G. The symptoms are not attributable to the physiological effects of a substance (e.g., a drug of abuse, a medication, other treatment) or another medical condition (e.g., hyperthyroidism). |

**Source:** Reprinted with permission from the *Diagnostic and Statistical Manual of Mental Disorders*, Fifth Edition, (Copyright 2013). American Psychiatric Association.

pattern of premenstrual exacerbations distinct from the syndrome of premenstrual dysphoric disorder (Boyd and Amsterdam, 2004; Miller *et al.*, 2009; Steiner, 2008).

These symptoms may be accompanied by behavioural and physical symptoms. Symptoms must have occurred in most of the menstrual cycles during the past year and must have an adverse effect on work or social functioning. The intensity and/or expressivity of the accompanying symptoms may be closely related to social and cultural background characteristics, family perspectives, religious beliefs, social tolerance and female gender role issues (American Psychiatric Association, 2013).

### 26.5.2.4 Differential diagnosis

- **Premenstrual syndrome**
  Premenstrual syndrome differs from premenstrual dysphoric disorder in that the minimum of five symptoms is not required to make the diagnosis and that the symptom expression is less severe in nature. There is also no stipulation of affective symptoms (American Psychiatric Association, 2013).
- **Dysmenorrhea**
  Dysmenorrhea is a syndrome of painful menses and begins with the onset of menses. This syndrome is distinct from premenstrual dysphoric disorder, where symptoms begin before the onset of menses, and can linger into the first few days of menses.

- **Bipolar disorder, major depressive disorder, and persistent depressive disorder (dysthymia)**
  Many women with bipolar disorder, major depressive disorder or persistent depressive disorder believe that they have premenstrual dysphoric disorder. However, when the symptoms are charted, they are not found to follow a premenstrual pattern. Women with other mental disorders may experience chronic or intermittent symptoms that may be unrelated to a menstrual cycle phase, but may report that symptoms occur only or worsen premenstrually. The overlap between the symptoms of premenstrual dysphoric disorder and some other diagnoses makes a differential diagnosis very difficult.
- **Use of hormonal treatments**
  Some women who present with moderate to severe premenstrual symptoms may be using hormonal treatments, including hormonal contraceptives. If such symptoms occur after initiation of exogenous hormone use, the symptoms may be due to the use of hormones rather than to the underlying condition of premenstrual dysphoric disorder. If the woman stops the hormonal treatment and the symptoms disappear, this is consistent with substance-induced or medication-induced depressive disorder.

### 26.5.2.5 Co-morbid conditions

A range of medical disorders (e.g. migraine, asthma, allergies, seizure disorders) or other mental disorders (e.g. depressive disorder, bipolar disorder, anxiety disorder, bulimia nervosa, substance use disorders) may worsen during the premenstrual phase but the absence of a symptom-free period during the post-menstrual interval excludes a diagnosis of premenstrual dysphoric disorder. The range of medical and psychiatric conditions are thus considered to be premenstrual exacerbation of a current mental or medical disorder (Hartlage *et al.*, 2004).

The diagnosis of premenstrual dysphoric disorder is not usually made in situations in which an individual only experiences a premenstrual exacerbation of another mental or physical disorder. However, it can be considered in addition to the diagnosis of another mental or physical disorder if the individual experiences symptoms and changes in level of functioning that are characteristic of premenstrual dysphoric disorder and are markedly different from the symptoms experienced as part of the ongoing disorder.

### 26.5.2.6 Course and prognosis

Several authors believe that premenstrual symptoms tend to worsen over time and increase in duration if left untreated. Women who seek treatment for the disorder are usually in their thirties. It is reported that women who use oral contraceptives may have fewer premenstrual complaints than women who do not use oral contraceptives. Many women who approach menopause report that symptoms worsen during this time and cease after menopause, although cyclical hormone replacement can trigger the re-expression of symptoms.

### 26.5.2.7 Management

**Pharmacological treatment**

Since women may present with a variety of premenstrual symptoms, it is important to chart these variations for at least two menstrual cycles to determine if the symptoms are linked to the menstrual cycles.

More than fifty treatment options for treating and managing PMDD have been proposed. The number of treatment options reflects the lack of a single effective cure.

Biological treatment includes treatment with SSRIs, given either continuously or during the luteal phase when premenstrual symptoms occur and stopping them after the onset of the menses. Recently, several studies have indicated the intermittent (premenstrually only) treatment with SSRIs is equally effective in these women.

SSRIs show greater efficacy when compared with noradrenergic agents, for example maprotiline and desipramine or dopaminergic agents such as bupropion.

Other treatment options include regimens to alleviate various symptoms experienced during this period. These include diuretics, bromocriptine, clonidine, anxiolytics, atenolol, prostaglandin and antiprostaglandin treatment. As far as hormonal treatment is concerned, studies have not found progesterone to be more effective than placebo. Oral contraceptives suppress ovulation but may cause psychological side effects and are capable of inducing depression. Studies using oral contraceptives as treatment for premenstrual dysphoric disorder have shown inconsistent results. Oestradiol percutaneous patches or subcutaneous implants at adequate doses can be used. Conservative treatment includes psychotherapy, exercise and dietary changes (Steiner, 2008; Boyd and Amsterdam, 2004; Miller *et al.*, 2009; Cohen, 2003; Lolak *et al.*, 2005).

## 26.5.3 The impact of reproductive events on the course of bipolar disorders

As mentioned, sex hormones play an important role in mood disorders and although bipolar disorder is equally prevalent in men and women, women experience rapid cycling, mixed episodes and depressive episodes more frequently. Women with bipolar disorder are at a high risk for relapse (25–40%) during the postpartum period. Some studies indicate that 18% of female patients with bipolar disorder have onset of the disorder within one year of the menarche (Joffe, 2007; Freeman *et al.*, 2002).

Little is known about the impact of female reproductive hormones on the course of bipolar disorder and its implications for treatment. Treatment considerations in bipolar disorder differ between men and women. One important difference arises because of factors specific to the reproductive system. Some psychotropic medications that are used to treat bipolar disorder can affect the hypothalamic-pituitary-gonadal (HPG) axis. When psychiatric medications affect the HPG axis, menstrual cycle patterns may change. Disruption of the menstrual cycle can have important effects, including reduced fertility. Hormonal changes associated with menstrual irregularities may also increase the risk of specific chronic medical conditions, such as osteoporosis in the case of prolactin disorder or endometrial hyperplasia and diabetes mellitus in patients with polycystic ovarian syndrome (Joffe, 2007; Freeman *et al.*, 2002).

Women with bipolar disorder may be more likely to have menstrual cycle irregularities than women with depression and healthy individuals. In a study of menstrual cycle dysfunction prior to initiation of psychiatric medication, 34% of women with bipolar disorder reported a history of menstrual cycle abnormalities, which was significantly higher than that found in healthy control subjects (20%) and patients with depression (24%). This study suggests that approximately one-third of patients with bipolar disorder have irregular cycles before they start treatment.

The data from the study support the hypothesis that times of hormonal fluctuation are associated with increased risk of affective dysregulation or mood episodes in women with bipolar disorder (Joffe, 2007; Lolak *et al.*, 2005; O'Donovan, 2002).

### 26.5.3.1 Treatment of bipolar disorder

Treatment of bipolar disorder in women of reproductive age requires attention to the potential effects of psychotropic drugs and reproductive biology. When specific medications are selected, reproductive side effects should be considered together with concerns about health risks, such as weight gain, insulin resistance and thyroid and renal dysfunction. Management of bipolar disorder in premenopausal women involves complicated decision making about benefits and risks of medication.

Valproate is often used as a mood stabiliser in treating patients with bipolar disorders. Valproate has been reported to be associated with features of polycystic ovarian syndrome (PCOS) in patients taking this treatment for epilepsy and bipolar disorders (Ernst and Goldberg, 2002; Cohen *et al.*, 2010; Cohen, 2003; Joffe, 2007; Lolak *et al.*, 2005).

## 26.5.4 Polycystic ovarian syndrome

Polycystic ovarian syndrome is a chronic reproductive-endocrine disorder that occurs in 4–10% of women of reproductive age.

### 26.5.4.1 Aetiology

The aetiology of polycystic ovarian syndrome remains unknown, although the available data suggest a number of factors, including genetic predisposition, ovarian defects, epilepsy and insulin resistance. These may interact with environmental or iatrogenic factors, such as psychotropic medications and obesity.

### 26.5.4.2 Clinical features

Clinical features associated with polycystic ovarian syndrome include hirsutism, alopecia, acne, menstrual irregularity and obesity. Hormonally, women with polycystic ovarian syndrome manifest increased levels of total and free serum testosterone, decreased follicle-stimulating hormone (FSH), increased serum prolactin, and increased serum-luteinising hormone (LH). Insulin resistance, hyperlipidaemia, impaired glucose tolerance and hyperinsulinaemia are other endocrinological complications of polycystic ovarian syndrome. Corresponding morbidities associated with polycystic ovarian syndrome may include non-insulin dependent diabetes mellitus (NIDDM), infertility, endometrial hyperplasia or malignancy, hypertension, coronary artery disease and adverse lipid profiles.

### 26.5.4.3 Polycystic ovarian syndrome and bipolar disorder

Some authors have begun to raise the possibility of a direct association between polycystic ovarian syndrome and affective disorders. Hormonal abnormalities in a significant percentage of bipolar women compared with those who have other psychiatric diagnoses have been reported. More recently, 27% of women with a primary diagnosis of polycystic ovarian syndrome were found to screen positively for features of bipolar spectrum disorder. It has been hypothesised that a common neuro-endocrine defect may be responsible for the pathogenesis of polycystic ovarian syndrome and affective illness.

Three theories have been described to account for why valproate might confer an increased risk for polycystic ovarian syndrome.

- The potential for hyperandrogenism and menstrual abnormalities that may result from weight gain or obesity during valproate therapy.
- Increased levels of GABA resulting from valproate use may contribute to the development of polycystic ovarian syndrome by affecting gonadotropin-releasing-hormone (GnRH) release from the hypothalamus, which could in turn affect the secretion of the gonadotropins LH and FSH.
- Valproate could have a direct effect on the formation of androgens in the ovary, by inhibiting the conversion of testosterone to oestradiol or by stimulating the production of more androgens.

### 26.5.4.4 Management of polycystic ovarian syndrome

Management of polycystic ovarian syndrome involves:

- correcting hyperandrogenaemia, long-acting gonadotropin releasing hormones and anti-androgens
- promoting induction of ovulation
- managing metabolic abnormalities, for example diet modification, weight loss, exercise and oral hypoglycaemics (Joffe, 2003; Freeman *et al.*, 2002; Ernst *et al.*, 2002; O'Donovan *et al.*, 2002).

# 26.6 Pregnancy and psychiatric disorders

## 26.6.1 Postpartum mood disorders

### 26.6.1.1 Postpartum blues

This condition, also commonly known as the baby blues or maternity blues, is a condition that affects 20–85% of women after delivery and is distinct from postpartum depression (see Section 26.6.1.2). This is a transient condition and usually begins three to four days postpartum and can last between one day and a week. Women may present with intermittent tearfulness, despondency, anxiety and poor concentration. The anxiety symptoms usually relate to situational difficulties, such as problems with breast feeding. Symptoms usually remit within two weeks postpartum. This period could be considered a time of postpartum reactivity, including heightened lability of mood in reaction to stimuli possibly resulting from hormonal withdrawal (Pearlstein *et al.*, 2009; Cohen *et al.*, 2010; Miller and LaRusso, 2011).

### 26.6.1.2 Postpartum depression

Postpartum depression is a complex mix of physical, emotional and behavioural changes that occur after giving birth and are attributed to the genetic, social, and psychological changes associated with having a baby. Postpartum depression is classified as a major depressive disorder with a postpartum onset specifier. The symptoms should occur within four weeks post-delivery. Symptoms of major depressive disorder tend to overlap with what is considered to be normal changes that occur in the postpartum period, for example weight changes, sleep disturbances, fatigue and occasional crying. These symptoms are not uncommon in new mothers but can pose a challenge and complicate the accurate assessment of postpartum depression. Women may not discuss these symptoms with the health care providers, either due to poor symptom recognition, stigma attached to the diagnosis or perhaps as a result of the symptoms that they are experiencing (e.g. lack of energy or motivation, hopelessness). Identifying these symptoms is important and prompt treatment is required as postpartum depression can lead to chronic depression, suicide, maternal-infant interaction disturbances and, in rare cases, infanticide (Pearlstein *et al.*, 2009; Cohen *et al.*, 2010; Miller and LaRusso, 2011).

The strongest predictors for developing postpartum depression include depression, anxiety during pregnancy, stressful life events (either during pregnancy or postpartum), low levels of social support, premenstrual dysphoric disorder, adolescence, being from a low socioeconomic group and recent diagnosis of an eating disorder (Boyd and Amsterdam, 2004).

The primary goal in the assessment process is to identify women at risk for postpartum depression, those who are already in the depths of depression and those women who are at immediate risk to themself and others. It is important for health care providers who provide perinatal care to screen for postpartum depression, educate women and refer them for complete psychiatric evaluation. The Edinburgh Postnatal Depression Scale is a useful tool to screening for postpartum depression (Miller and LaRusso, 2011; Pearlstein *et al.*, 2009; Kornstein, 2001; Mian, 2005).

#### Treatment options

Many women with postpartum depression remain untreated, possibly from lack of information about treatment effectiveness and the residual effects of antidepressants on nursing infants. SSRIs are considered the drug class of choice; sertraline and paroxetine offer the best safety profile. The benefits of taking antidepressants will have to be weighed against the risk of infant exposure to psychotropics. Benefits will probably outweigh the risks when moderate to severe symptoms with significant functional deterioration or a progressive worsening of the condition are present. Psychotherapy has a place in the treatment armamentarium and may be a good indication as a combined treatment or as monotherapy in milder cases in women who breastfeed and/or are opposed to medication. Electroconvulsive therapy (ECT) is another safe and effective alternative in postpartum depression and should be considered in severely suicidal patients (Pearlstein *et al.*, 2009; Cohen *et al.*, 2010; Mian, 2005; Boyd and Amsterdam, 2004).

## 26.6.2 Postpartum psychotic disorders

### 26.6.2.1 Postpartum psychosis

Postpartum psychosis is a severe but rare psychiatric disorder that may or may not co-exist with postpartum depression. One to three in 1 000 women without a previous psychiatric diagnosis will experience postpartum psychosis and about 4,5–9% of women who have a previous psychiatric diagnosis will develop postpartum psychosis. Women who have a bipolar disorder or a family history of postpartum psychosis are at an increased risk of experiencing future episodes of psychosis during their lifetime. The differential diagnosis for postpartum psychosis can include major depression with psychotic features, bipolar disorder I and II, schizophrenia, schizo-affective disorder and brief psychotic disorder.

The onset of psychosis tends to be rapid, occurring three to five days after delivery and can last between one week and several months in the absence of treatment. Symptoms may include severe agitation, confusion, delusions or hallucinations, paranoia, feelings of hopelessness and shame, hyperactivity, rapid speech or frank mania. The delusions frequently focus on denying the baby's existence or the need to kill self or the infant.

Risk factors of developing postpartum psychosis include living in a poor socioeconomic environment, having a female child, delivery by caesarean section, complications during delivery, low birth-weight infants and perinatal death. Evidence to support these risk factors is, however, inconclusive.

Research indicates that prevention of postpartum psychosis consists of pharmacotherapy and, given the association of postpartum psychosis with bipolar disorders, mood stabilisers (e.g. lithium) are commonly used as prophylactic measures and to decrease the risk of postnatal relapse. Treatment for postpartum psychosis includes antipsychotic drugs, counselling and hospital admission if the woman is a danger to herself or others. ECT is also effective in treating severe and treatment-resistant cases of postpartum psychosis (Pearlstein *et al.*, 2009; Lolak *et al.*, 2005).

## 26.6.3 Postpartum anxiety disorders

### 26.6.3.1 Obsessive-compulsive disorder

Fluctuations in gonadal steroids during the various phases in the life cycle seem to increase the risk of emotional disturbances in women. Although most studies are focused on mood disorders, some authors have described a worsening of panic disorder, trichotillomania and obsessive-compulsive disorder (OCD). The perinatal period is associated with an increase in the incidence of obsessive-compulsive disorder. Exacerbations of obsessive-compulsive disorder occurs in up to 50% of women in the postpartum period; patients with an onset or worsening of obsessive-compulsive disorder during this time report a history of previous depressive disorder, including postpartum depression and premenstrual mood symptoms. Aggressive obsessions appear to be common in postpartum obsessive-compulsive disorder and include disturbing intrusive thoughts about harming newborns.

Apart from fluctuations in gonadal hormones that may play a role in the onset and course of obsessive-compulsive disorder in certain women, preliminary data show that the presence of the hormone oxytocin may also contribute to the high incidence of obsessive-compulsive disorder during this period. Prospective studies are, however, required to confirm these findings (Lolak *et al.*, 2005; Labad and Menchon, 2005).

## 26.7 Oestrogen and schizophrenia

The cause of schizophrenia remains unclear, but evidence suggests both genetic and environmental causes for the disease. Early studies identified schizophrenia as a predominantly male neuropsychiatric illness, in contrast with depression that was considered to be a predominantly female neuropsychiatric illness. However, careful analysis of the pattern of onset has led to the following conclusions:

- there are gender differences in pre-morbid functioning, age of onset, symptomatology and outcome of schizophrenia
- oestrogen is hypothesised to protect women against early onset of severe symptoms of schizophrenia. The 'oestrogen hypothesis' was derived from epidemiological, clinical and animal studies (Huber and Borsutzky, 2004; Kulkarni and Riedel, 2001; Huttner, 2003; Lolak *et al.*, 2005).

## 26.7.1 Epidemiology

Earlier studies reported the incidence of schizophrenia in men and women to be equal. However, recent epidemiological studies show unequal incidences of schizophrenia for men and women (Longnecker *et al.*, 2010). These gender differences in the incidence and course of schizophrenia have been ascribed to the neuroprotective effects of oestrogen in women. In early adulthood the incidence rate of schizophrenia is lower in women than in men and the age of onset of schizophrenia occurs three to four years later in women (Huttner, 2003). On average, men are hospitalised for psychotic episodes in their late teens and early twenties, whereas women seek psychiatric care for psychosis in their late twenties and early thirties (Kulkarni and Riedel, 2001).

Additionally, a second peak incidence occurs when women develop psychotic or delusional manifestations around the time of the menopause (between 45–55 years). Clinical studies also reveal greater differences in the symptoms suffered, with men tending to have more negative symptoms of schizophrenia and women experiencing more affective and paranoid symptoms. Life-cycle studies show that women are more vulnerable to either a first episode of psychosis or relapse of an existing illness at two major periods of hormonal change: during the postpartum period and during menopause (Smith, 2001; Ernst and Goldberg, 2002; Craig and Murphy 2006).

There have been case reports of women whose schizophrenia symptoms exacerbated at low-oestrogen phases of the menstrual cycle.

When women with schizophrenia are given adjunctive treatment with exogenous oestrogen there is a slight increase in speed of recovery, but no improvement overall compared with antipsychotic medication alone.

## 26.7.2 Neurobiology

- Oestrogen may in itself have a direct neuroleptic effect through rapid membrane effects on the $D_2$ receptor presynaptically. In this way oestrogen may mimic the action of typical antipsychotics.
- Oestrogen has also been shown to affect the $5\text{-}HT_{2A}$ receptor density in animal studies, thus mimicking the effect of atypical antipsychotic drugs.
- Oestrogen may potentiate the effect of antipsychotic drugs by enhancing the uptake through increased activation of liver microsomal drug metabolism enzymes or by affecting antipsychotic drug absorption.
- Oestrogen may impact on psychotic symptoms via interaction with prolactin, which has been shown to modulate the biphasic effect of oestrogen administration on $D_2$ receptors.
- Patients on classic antipsychotic drugs often have altered HPG axis function with resultant hypo-oestrogenism and menstrual irregularities. It has been suggested that young women with schizophrenia who may have to take antipsychotic medication for many years are at particular risk of artificially induced premature menopause with its attendant cardiovascular, osteoporosis and other general health problems.

### 26.7.3 Managing women taking prolactin-elevating antipsychotics

Serum levels of prolactin increase during pregnancy and lactation but can also be increased by specific medical conditions and medications. Antipsychotic agents are a common cause of hyperprolactinaemia. Prolactin is a hormone produced and secreted by the anterior pituitary. Its secretion is tonically inhibited by dopaminergic neurons from the hypothalamus acting on dopamine $D_2$ receptors. Antipsychotics that have a strong affinity for $D_2$ receptors block these receptors in the anterior pituitary, thus increasing prolactin secretion.

The antipsychotics most strongly associated with hyperprolactinaemia are the typical agents as well as risperidone amongst the atypical antipsychotics. The other atypical antipsychotic agents (clozapine, olanzapine, quetiapine, ziprasidone, aripiprazole) have a low affinity for $D_2$ receptors and are thus prolactin sparing.

A common symptom of hyperprolactinaemia is infrequent menstrual cycles or amenorrhea, which occurs in at least 25% of women who take typical antipsychotics and 50% of women who take risperidone. Infrequent menses reflect infrequent ovulation and reduced production of ovarian oestrogen, which can lead to infertility and osteoporosis if left untreated for a prolonged period. Other symptoms of hyperprolactinaemia include galactorrhoea and symptoms of sexual dysfunction.

A small increase in the risk of breast cancer has been observed in a large study of women who use long-term typical antipsychotics. The association between use of prolactin-elevating medication and breast cancer is difficult to reconcile with the oestrogen-deficient state that result from hyperprolactinaemia, because an oestrogen deficiency should provide relative protection against breast cancer.

Treatment options for symptomatic hyperprolactinaemia induced by antipsychotics include:

- adding a hormonal contraceptive to reduce the risk of osteoporosis
- changing the antipsychotic to a prolactin-sparing antipsychotic or mood stabiliser
- reducing the dose of the antipsychotic
- adding a dopamine agonist to directly lower the prolactin level (Ernst, 2002; Joffe, 2007; Cohen, 2003; Gentile, 2011); Maguire, 2002.

## 26.8 Menopause and psychiatric disorders

### 26.8.1 Peri-menopause and menopause

The transition into menopause is a major hormonal event associated in many women with both physical and psychological changes. The term peri-menopause describes the period immediately before the menopause (from the time when the hormonal and clinical features of approaching menopause commence until the end of the first year after the menopause) (Sherman, 2005).

The physiological hallmark of transition into menopause is gradual oestrogen depletion. Changes most commonly associated with oestrogen depletion include vasomotor symptoms, such as hot flushes and night sweats, as well as urogenital changes that cause dyspareunia. There is also an increased risk for osteoporosis and cardiovascular disease over time (Steiner *et al.*, 2003; Parry, 2008; Soares and Frey, 2010; Soares and Taylor, 2007).

According to epidemiological data, the majority of post-menopausal women do not experience prominent symptoms of depression. There is, however, a higher than expected prevalence of depressive-like symptoms observed in peri-menopausal and post-menopausal women. These include irritability, tearfulness, anxiety, depressed or labile mood, lack of motivation and energy, poor concentration and interrupted sleep. These symptoms have been linked to predictable fluctuations in oestradiol levels, especially abrupt withdrawal from very high erratic levels (Parry, 2008; Steiner *et al.*, 2003; Soares and Frey, 2010; Cohen, 2003; Robinson, 2001).

#### 26.8.1.1 Management of menopause symptoms and depression

A critical window of opportunity may exist when interventions for different systems, including cognition and mood, are effective in patients who are getting older, suffering from depression and making the transition to menopause (Deecher *et al.*, 2008; Steiner, 2006; Soares, 2007; Boyd and Amsterdam, 2004; Parry, 2008).

**Hormonal therapies**

Menopause-related hormone therapy has been a subject of controversy, given a recent study questioning their long-term safety and efficacy. Oestrogen plus progesterone used in post-menopausal women aged 45-80 years did not prevent cardiovascular disease as previously thought but increased the risk of stroke and breast cancer (Parry, 2008; Rapp *et al.*, 2003).

Furthermore, oestrogen alone was effective for the short-term treatment of depression when given to women going through peri-menopause, but was ineffective for the treatment of depression or mood in post-menopausal women who have been deprived of oestrogen for many years. The evidence suggests that peri-menopausal women with first-onset depression and vasomotor symptoms are more likely to respond to oestrogen alone, or in combination with antidepressants, than are post-menopausal women with a history of multiple depressive episodes and no vasomotor symptoms.

Preliminary studies seem to indicate the beneficial effects of combining oestrogen replacement therapy (ORT) with SSRIs in the treatment of depressed post-menopausal women.

**Psychological treatment**

Psychological treatment may be of help to women who are distressed at this time of life. Psycho-education is important in addressing and alleviating anxiety, distress and fears during this transitional phase. Supportive psychotherapy and group therapy have also been suggested as therapeutic options (Steiner, 2006; Parry, 2008; Rapp *et al.*, 2003; Soares and Taylor, 2007; Soares and Frey, 2010; Cohen, 2003; Stahl, 2000; Kornstein, 2001; Spinelli, 2004).

### 26.8.2 Oestrogen and cognitive functioning in women

Declining cognitive function is a growing public health concern for older adults, given the well-documented pattern of age-associated changes in many areas of cognitive performance. The prevalence of age-associated memory impairment in the general older population is estimated at 17–34%. In post-menopausal women, the effect of reduced sex hormones, especially oestrogen and progesterone, on cognitive decline is of particular interest because of their modulating effects on neurotransmitters, neuroconnectivity and neuroprotection (Steiner, 2006; Freeman and Sammel, 2004; Sherwin, 2003).

Accumulated data are beginning to suggest that there may be a critical period during the immediate post-menopausal years for the protective effect of ORT on cognition. For example, elderly women who initiate ORT at the time of the menopause have less cognitive decline than non-users, whereas the incidence of cognitive decline is not different in women with more recent exposures.

Studies conclude that oestrogen plus progestin therapy:

- are associated with significantly greater age-related cognitive decline
- do not prevent mild cognitive impairment and significantly increases the risk for dementia of all causes.

Currently, the available evidence suggests that if ORT is started at a crucial time (at or around the menopause) it may have beneficial effects on cognition and reduce the risk of developing Alzheimer's disease. In contrast, if ORT is started when women are older than 65, this may have no beneficial effect on the brain and may increase the risk for all-cause dementia (Rapp *et al.*, 2003; Shumaker *et al.*, 2003; Geerlings *et al.*, 2001; LeBlanc at al., 2001).

## Conclusion

Basic research indicates that oestrogen may affect brain maturation and subsequent modulation of brain function in regions that are implicated in neuropsychiatric disorders. The findings of a number of studies do not indicate the use of oestrogen as a first-line treatment in clinical practice. Current evidence suggests that oestrogen alone has no role in the treatment of established Alzheimer's disease but may delay its onset. The evidence base for the use of oestrogen as an adjunct to antipsychotics in schizophrenia or in the treatment of postnatal and peri-menopausal depression is currently too weak to merit its use in clinical practice. Larger prospective studies are required to establish whether oestrogen has a role in the prophylaxis and treatment of numerous psychiatric disorders.

When specific medications are selected, reproductive side effects should be considered together with concerns about health risks. Management of psychiatric disorders in women involves complicated decision-making about the benefits and risks of medications. The risk of side effects should be weighed against the risk of under-treating or destabilising a woman with severe mental illness when medications are withheld or discontinued. Collaboration with gynaecologists, endocrinologists and primary-care physicians during consideration of reproductive effects or reproductive side effects and drug interactions can help optimise care in these complicated conditions.

# References


American Psychiatric Association (2013) *Diagnostic and statistical manual of mental disorders* (5th edition). Washington DC: American Psychiatric Publishing

Boyd RC, Amsterdam JD (2004) Mood disorders in women from adolescence to late life: An overview. *Clinical Obstetrics and Gynaecology* 47(3): 515–26

Cohen LS (2003) Gender specific considerations in the treatment of mood disorders in women across the life cycle. *Journal of Clinical Psychiatry* 64:5 (Suppl.): S18-S29

Cohen LS, Soares CN, Otto MW, Sweeney BH, Liberman RF, Harlow BL (2002) Prevalence and predictors of premenstrual dysphoric disorder in older premenopausal women: The Harvard Study of moods and cycles. *Journal of Affective Disorders* 70(2): 125–32

Cohen LS, Wang, B, Nonacs, R, Viguera, A.C, Lemon, E.L, Freeman, M.P (2010) Treatment of mood disorders during pregnancy and postpartum. *Psychiatric Clinics of North America* 33: 273–93

Cooper, PJ, Mark T, Swartz L, Woolgar M, Murray L, Molteno C (1999) Post-partum depression and the mother-infant relationship in a South African peri-urban settlement. *British Journal of Psychiatry* 175: 554–8

Craig M, Cutter W (2004) Estrogens, brain function and neuropsychiatric disorders. *Current Opinion in Psychiatry* 17(3): 209–14

Craig MC, Murphy DG (2006) Estrogen, cognition and maturing female brain. *Journal of Neuroendocrinology* 19: 1–6

Deecher D, Andree T, Sloan D, Schechter LE (2008) From menarche to menopause: Exploring the underlying biology of depression in women experiencing hormonal changes. *Psychoneuroendocrinology* 33: 3–17

Deuster PA, Adera T, South-Paul J (1999) Biological, social, and behavioural factors associated with premenstrual syndrome. *Archives of Family Medicine* 8(2): 122–8

Ernst CL, Goldberg JF (2002) The reproductive safety profile of mood stabilizers, atypical antipsychotics and broad spectrum psychotropics. *Journal of Clinical Psychiatry* 63(4): 42–55

Freeman EW, Sammel MD (2004) Hormones and menopausal status as predictors of depression in women in transition to menopause. *Archives of General Psychiatry* 61: 62–70

Freeman MP, Smith KW, Freeman SA, McElroy SL, Kmetz GE, Wright R, Keck PE (Jr) (2002) The impact of reproductive events on the course of bipolar disorder in women. *Journal of Clinical Psychiatry* 63(4): 284–7

Geerlings MI, Ruitenberg A, Witteman JCM, Van Swieten JC, Hofman A, Van Duijn CM, Breteler MM, Launer LJ (2001) Reproductive period and risk of dementia in postmenopausal women, *Journal of the American Medical Association* 285(11): 1475–81

Gehlert S, Sang IH, Chang CH, Hartlage DA (2009) The prevalence of premenstrual dysphoric disorder in a randomly selected group of urban and rural women. *Psychological Medicine* 39(1): 129–36

Gentile S (2011) Drug treatment for mood disorders in pregnancy. *Current Opinion in Psychiatry* 24(1): 34–40

Girdler SS, Thompson KK, Light KC, Leserman J, Pedersen CA, Prange AJ (Jr) (2004) Historical sexual abuse and current thyroid axis profiles in women with premenstrual dysphoria. *Psychosomatic Medicine* 66(3): 403–10

Hartlage SA, Brandeburg DL, Kravitz HM (2004) Premenstrual exacerbation of depressive disorders in a community-based sample in the United States, *Psychosomatic Medicine* 66(5),698–706

Hartlage SA, Freels SA, Gotman N, Yonkers K (2012) Criteria for premenstrual dysphoric disorder (PMDD): Secondary analyses of relevant data sets. *Archives of General Psychiatry* 69(3): 300–5

Huber TJ, Borsutzky M (2004) Psychotic disorders and gonadal function: Evidence supporting the estrogen hypothesis. *Acta Psychiatrica Scandinavica* 109(4): 269–74

Huttner RP, Shepherd JE (2003) Gonadal steroids, selective serotonin reuptake inhibitors and mood disorders in women. *Medical Clinics of North America* 87(5): 1065–76

Joffe H (2007) Reproductive biology and psychotropic treatments in premenopausal women with bipolar disorder. *Journal of Clinical Psychiatry* 68(9): 10–5

Kornstein SG (2001) The evaluation and management of depression in women across the life span. *Journal of Clinical Psychiatry* 62(24) (suppl.): S11-S7

Kulkarni J, Riedel A (2001) Estrogen – a potential treatment for schizophrenia. *Schizophrenia Research* 48: 137–4

Labad J, Menchon JM (2005) Female reproductive cycle and obsessive-compulsive disorder. *Journal of Clinical Psychiatry* 66(4): 428–35

LeBlanc ES, Janowsky J, Chan BKS, Nelson HD (2001) Hormone replacement therapy and cognition, systematic review and meta-analysis. *Journal of the American Medical Association* 285(11): 1489–99

Lolak S, Rashid N, Wise TN (2005) Interface of women's reproductive health. *Current Psychiatry Reports* 7(3): 220–7

Longnecker J, Genderson J, Dickneson D, Malley J, Elvevåg B, Weinberger DR, Gold J (2010) Where have all the women gone? Participant gender in epidemiological and non-epidemiological research in schizophrenia. *Schizophrenia Research* 119: 240–5

Maguire GA (2002) Prolactin elevation with antipsychotic medications: Mechanisms of action and clinical consequences. *Journal of Clinical Psychiatry* 63(4) (Suppl.): S56-S62

Mannikam L, Burns JK (2012) Antenatal depression and its risk-factors: An urban prevalence study in KwaZulu-Natal. *South African Medical Journal* 102(12): 940–4

Maskall DD, Lam RW, Misri S, Carter D, Kuan AJ, Yatham LN, Zis AP (1997) Seasonality of symptoms in women with late luteal phase dysphoric disorder. *American Journal of Psychiatry* 154(10): 1436–41

McEwen BS, Alves SE (1999) Estrogen action in the central nervous system. *Endocrine Reviews* 20: 279–307

Mian AI (2005) Depression in pregnancy and the postpartum period: Balancing adverse effects of untreated illness with treatment risks. *Journal of Psychiatric Practice* 11(6): 389–96

Miller LG, Girgis C, Gupta R (2009) Depression and related disorders during the female reproductive cycle. *Women's Health* 5(5): 577–87

Miller LJ, La Russo EM (2011) Preventing postpartum depression. *Psychiatric Clinics of North America* 34: 53–65

O'Donovan C, Kusumakar V, Graves GR, Bird DC (2002) Menstrual abnormalities and polycystic ovarian syndrome in women taking valproate for bipolar mood disorder. *Journal of Clinical Psychiatry* 63(4): 322–30

Parry BL (2008) Perimenopausal depression. *American Journal of Psychiatry* 165(1): 23–7

Parry BL, Berga SL (2003) Premenstrual dysphoric disorder. In: Sadock BJ, Sadock VA (Eds). *Kaplan and Sadock's Comprehensive Textbook of Psychiatry* (Vol. 2, 8th edition). Philadelphia: Lippincott, Williams and Wilkins

Pearlstein T, Howard M, Salisbury A, Zlotnick C (2009) Postpartum depression. *American Journal of Obstetrics and Gynaecology* 200(4): 357–64

Rapp RS, Espeland MA, Shumaker SA, Henderson VW, Brunner RL, Manson JE, Gass MLS, Stefanick ML, Lane DS, Hays J, Johnson KC, Coker LH, Dailey M, Bowen D (2003) Effects of estrogen plus progestin on global cognitive function in postmenopausal women. The Women's Health Initiative Memory Study: A randomised controlled trial. *Journal of American Medical Association* 289(20): 2663–72

Robinson GE (2001) Psychotic and mood disorders associated with the peri-menopausal period. *CNS Drugs* 15(3): 175–184

Sherman S (2005) Defining the menopausal transition. *American Journal of Medicine* 118(2) (Suppl): S3-S7

Sherwin BB (2003) Estrogen and cognitive functioning. *Endocrine Reviews* 24(2): 133–51

Shumaker SA, Legault C, Rapp SR, Thal L, Wallace RB, Ockene JK *et al.*, (2003) Estrogen plus progestin and the incidence of dementia and mild cognitive impairment in postmenopausal women. The Women's Health Initiative Memory Study: A randomised controlled trial. *Journal of the American Medical Association* 289(20): 2651–62

Smith YR (2001) Effects of long term hormone therapy on cholinergic synaptic concentrations in healthy postmenopausal women. *Journal of Clinical Endocrinology and Metabolism* 86(2): 679–84

Soares CN, Frey BN (2010) Challenges and opportunities to manage depression during the menopausal transition and beyond. *Psychiatric Clinics of North America* 33: 295–308

Soares CN, Taylor V (2007) Effects and management of the menopausal transition in women with depression and bipolar disorder. *Journal of Clinical Psychiatry* 68(9) (Suppl.): S16-S21

Spinelli MG (2004) Depression and hormone therapy. *Clinical Obstetrics and Gynaecology* 47(2): 428–36

Stahl S (2000) *Essential Psychopharmacology – Neuroscientific Basis and Practical Applications* (2nd edition). New York: Cambridge University Press

Steiner M, (2006) Female-specific mood disorders. *Psychiatry* 5(4): 131–4

Steiner M (2008) Female-specific mood disorders. *Psychiatry* 8(2): 61–6

Steiner M, Dunn E, Born L (2003) Hormones and mood: From menarche to menopause and beyond. *Journal of Affective Disorders* 74: 67–83

Witchen H, Becker E, Lieb R, Kramer P (2002) Prevalence, incidence and stability of premenstrual dysphoric disorder in the community. *Psychological Medicine* 32(1): 119–132

Wu L, Anthony JC (2000) Estimated rate of depressed mood in US adults: Recent evidence for a peak in later life. *Journal of Affective Disorders* 60: 157–71

CHAPTER 27

# Child and adolescent psychiatry 1: Assessment and the young child

*Khatija Jhazbhay, Enver Karim*

## 27.1 Introduction

Behavioural and emotional disorders are common in childhood. Southern Africa, with its diversity of people, cultures and socioeconomic status, presents many risk factors for the development of severe emotional and behavioural difficulties in children from all communities. These difficulties impact negatively on the developmental trajectory of children and may result in psychopathology in adulthood. Identifying and intervening early may contribute towards a healthy society.

When a child has symptoms, it is usually the parent who seeks help, and therefore whether a child's difficulty comes to the attention of a clinician or not depends not only on the nature and severity of the problem but also on the attitude of, and resources accessible to, the parent. Some healthy children are brought to the doctor by overanxious parents for advice on behaviour that is usual for the child's age, whilst other children with serious problems are not brought to the doctor.

Health care workers, especially at primary care level, have an important role in identifying children who are experiencing difficulties and intervening appropriately. Child psychiatry services are a priority to help children who are vulnerable to developing mental health problems.

This chapter will focus on assessing and managing young children (younger than 10 years) who present with mental health problems.

## 27.2 Aetiology of child psychiatry disorders

The causes of childhood psychiatric disorders may be complex and often involve multiple interacting factors that are included in the following broad domains:

- *biological*: genetic, another medical condition (e.g. HIV, malnutrition, brain injury, metabolic, endocrine), substances
- *psychological*: poor early attachment, abuse and neglect, discordant relationships, family dysfunction, traumatic events
- *social*: school functioning and circumstances, environment, cultural factors, socioeconomic status.

All domains must be assessed, which means that a bio-psycho-social approach and all contributing factors, strengths and difficulties should be integrated in a diagnostic formulation to help the child and family.

## 27.3 Special considerations when assessing a child

Children are not just little adults; therefore there are important differences in emphasis and approach when you assess a child. You will have to operate like a 'detective' to gather 'clues' that lead to an understanding of the difficulties the child and family are experiencing and for implementation of effective interventions.

- A developmental approach is emphasised, rather than the cross-sectional approaches that are typically used in assessing adults. This developmental and longitudinal approach must take into account where the child is at in his or her natural trajectory of growth and maturation processes, and assess his or her strengths and difficulties in the light of each particular child's life situation. All evaluation and intervention in child psychiatry takes place in this context. The stage of development of the child is important: some behaviour may be normal for a child at a particular age (e.g. repeated bedwetting is normal in an 18-month-old child but not in a six-year-old child). A basic understanding of child development is fundamental to child assessment. Keeping in mind the variability in development in children will help in identifying and intervening in developmental areas of concern and minimise the risk of over-diagnosis and over-pathologising. A developmental approach to a child's assessment helps to identify competencies or strengths as well as areas of need or difficulty. In the case of children, treatment is not focused on a specific diagnostic disorder, but rather on intervening to help the child in areas of developmental concern with the aim of developing him or her to his or her full potential.
- The context in which problems arise is important: a child may be distressed because of frequent family quarrels at home, for example, or an older child may present with truancy because of being bullied at school. It is also important to understand whether the child is having difficulties in all contexts, or only specific ones, such as behaving well at home but having behavioural difficulties at school. This may help clarify the nature of the difficulty and point to specific areas of intervention.
- A comprehensive assessment is essential to understand the child's difficulties and to plan effective therapeutic interventions; this involves gathering information from multiple sources (e.g. parents, guardians or caregivers, other family members, school, the child and others). Previous assessments and school reports must be taken into consideration. The evaluation of family functioning is integral to the assessment.
- Interviewing children of different ages with the goal of understanding the child's inner world and perspectives demands creativity and the use of different techniques to fit the developmental needs of the child. Techniques may range from observation to play to developmentally appropriate conversation. Requesting a drawing may be a useful additional tool for assessments at all ages.
- Diagnoses are more complicated in children. Although children may technically be diagnosed with almost any DSM-5 diagnosis, there are many controversial issues, such as in interpretation of symptoms, lack of diagnostic and aetiological specificity of many symptoms, issues of over-diagnosis, misdiagnosis or under-diagnosis, long-term effects of diagnostic **labelling**, validity or cultural factors that may cast a cloud over a diagnosis. Furthermore, it is imperative not to ignore psychosocial issues that may be prominent in the genesis of presentations in children.

## 27.4 Assessment of the child

The assessment of the child in primary care requires an understanding of the problem, the situational context in which it occurs, the child and family functioning, and an assessment of severity and planning appropriate interventions.

To achieve this, the following steps must to be taken:

- history taking
- examination (observation and interview or mental state examination)
- investigations (collateral information, rating scales, referrals or further assessments)
- diagnostic formulation
- management planning.

## 27.4.1 History taking

To elicit enough information to gain an in-depth understanding of the child's internal and external life requires a trusting, empathic and non-judgemental clinical space in which the parent feels comfortable with giving information.

The interview begins with the parent(s) and child seen together. The child may be occupied with drawing or play in a child-friendly area in the consulting room.

The components of information needed in the primary care situation are outlined below.

### 27.4.1.1 Presenting problem

This is a critical part of gathering information as it sets the scene for careful further enquiry and active exploration of concerns and expectations. At this stage you are already considering and exploring various diagnostic and aetiological possibilities, such as:

- reason for referral
- onset, duration, frequency and intensity
- precipitants and context
- degree of distress
- how the family members have handled the situation
- impact on family members
- social and school functioning.

### 27.4.1.2 Past psychiatric history

Past psychiatric history should include:

- previous assessments
- previous diagnoses
- previous hospitalisation and treatments
- previous response
- current treatment.

### 27.4.1.3 Medical history

Medical history should contain information regarding:

- hospitalisations, operations, serious injuries
- physical disabilities
- chronic and acute illnesses
- allergies
- seizure-like episodes
- visual or hearing impairment
- toxin exposure
- medication
- substance use.

### 27.4.1.4 Developmental history

The developmental history should take into account such aspects as:

- conception
- pregnancy and perinatal history
- infancy
- milestones
- school functioning
- emotional development and behaviour
- relationships with family and peers
- interests
- traumatic or unusual circumstances.

### 27.4.1.5 Family assessment

A family assessment should supply information regarding:

- genogram (useful)
- composition of family
- family medical history
- family functioning including relationships, roles and cultural beliefs
- parenting methods and discipline
- income means
- areas of conflict.

## 27.4.2 Examination

### 27.4.2.1 Physical examination of the child

Look for biological factors that may be associated with mental health difficulties, for example, HIV and depression, anaemia and poor school performance.

### 27.4.2.2 Psychiatric examination of child

Use interview and observation methods to assess developmental functioning and the presence and severity of psychopathology.

- Direct observation of general activity level, attention span, posture, mannerisms, dress and grooming, motor skills, eye contact, anxiety, confidence, child-caregiver interaction, separation, quality of rapport, affect, over-familiarity, verbal expression and vocabulary assist in the assessment.
- Adapt assessment procedures to developmentally appropriate techniques and language.
- Imaginative play, speech, draw-a-person, three wishes/sad/happy/fears questions can elicit valuable information.
- An interview with the child covers general and neutral topics to build rapport, after which structured and specific questions may be asked.

### 27.4.3 Collateral information

Collateral information may be gathered from other family members, the school, social welfare agencies and previous medical records.

### 27.4.4 Physical investigations

Where appropriate blood, EEG and imaging investigations should be performed.

### 27.4.5 Further assessment

Further investigation should include:

- psychological assessment and testing
- occupational therapy assessment
- speech, language and hearing assessment
- assessment by a social worker, where deemed necessary).

### 27.4.6 Diagnostic formulation

The diagnostic formulation will encompass the biological, psychological and sociocultural domains to highlight predisposing, precipitating and perpetuating factors and strengths and difficulties that are identified. The purpose of a diagnostic formulation is to provide an integrated synthesis of the possible diagnosis and aetiology. The severity of the difficulties, which is usually assessed on the basis of degree of impairment of the child's functioning, will indicate whether there is a need for referral to the next level of care.

### 27.4.7 Management planning

Psycho-education, giving feedback to parents and involving parents in planning are important. Planning interventions should be goal orientated, holistic and built on strengths that are present. It may be necessary to work together with other involved agencies like schools, social and justice departments. As psychiatric problems in children may sometimes be complicated, consultation with, and referral to, higher levels of care is encouraged to benefit the child.

## 27.5 Neurodevelopmental disorders

### 27.5.1 Intellectual disability in children

(See also Chapter 29: Intellectual disability.)
A child with intellectual disability has limitations in intellectual functioning and adaptive behaviours, evident by not achieving expected milestones along the childhood developmental trajectory.

There are many different signs of intellectual disability in children. Depending on the severity of the disability, signs may appear during infancy or they may not be noticeable until a child reaches school-going age. Some of the most common signs of intellectual disability are:

- late in rolling over, sitting up, crawling or walking
- late in talking or having trouble with talking
- slow to master things like potty training, dressing, and feeding himself or herself
- difficulty in remembering things
- inability to connect actions with consequences
- behavioural problems, such as explosive tantrums
- difficulty with problem-solving or logical thinking.

In children with severe or profound intellectual disability, there may be other health problems as well. These problems may include seizures, mental disorders, motor **handicaps**, vision problems or hearing problems.

Early detection and developmentally sensitive multimodal intervention is required for best outcomes. Early intervention may include speech therapy, occupational therapy, physical therapy, psychological counselling, family counselling and social worker services. It is important that services are well coordinated and that there is an effective multidisciplinary collaboration in the care of children with complex and multiple disabilities.

The prognosis is variable, depending on the severity of intellectual disability. In general, children with a mild intellectual disability can anticipate gaining academic skills at about Grade 8 level, with the ability to hold a job and function with minimal support in the community. The prognosis is markedly improved with early intervention and education, appropriate skills development, good medical care and a supportive environment

(Also see Chapter 29: Intellectual disability, for a further discussion.)

## 27.5.2 Communication disorders

Communication disorders affect learning, language and/or speech. The DSM-5 communication disorders include language disorder (which combines DSM-IV expressive and mixed receptive-expressive language disorders), speech sound disorder (a phonological disorder), and childhood-onset fluency disorder (stuttering). Also included is social (pragmatic) communication disorder, a new condition for persistent difficulties in the social uses of verbal and nonverbal communication. Because social communication deficits are one component of autism-spectrum disorder (ASD), it is important to note that social (pragmatic) communication disorder cannot be diagnosed in the presence of restricted repetitive behaviours, interests and activities (the other component of ASD). The symptoms of some patients diagnosed with the DSM-IV's 'Pervasive developmental disorder not otherwise specified' may meet the DSM-5 criteria for social communication disorder.

Certain characteristics are common to all communication disorders:

- the disorder is not a consequence of intellectual disability
- the child's communication ability resembles that of a much younger child, which creates problems at school, at home and with peers (particularly in school)
- these disorders may run in families (e.g. there may be a genetic component to some communication disorders)
- they are more frequently diagnosed in boys than in girls and are more common among younger children than in older children
- there is a wide range of subtypes and varying levels of severity among these disorders.

### 27.5.2.1 Management

Children with communication disorders are usually referred to speech therapists, who conduct an assessment that generates a treatment plan. Parents are expected to participate actively in the treatment and are given speech exercises for the child to practise with supervision at home.

## 27.5.3 Autism-spectrum disorder

Autism-spectrum disorder was classified as pervasive developmental disorders in the DSM-IV (American Pychiatric Association, 2000). In the DSM-5 (American Pychiatric Association, 2013) it is now classified under the neurodevelopmental disorders. Furthermore, the individual disorders such as autistic disorder, Asperger's disorder and childhood disintegrative disorder have been collapsed into an all-encompassing autism-spectrum disorder; Rett's syndrome has been removed from the DSM-5.

### 27.5.3.1 Epidemiology

Autism-spectrum disorder has in the past been considered very uncommon. In recent years, increasing prevalence rates have been reported

**Table 27.1** DSM-5 Diagnostic Criteria for Autism Spectrum Disorder

| **Diagnostic Criteria** |
|---|
| A. Persistent deficits in social communication and social interaction across multiple contexts, as manifested by the following, currently or by history (examples are illustrative, not exhaustive; see text):<br>1. Deficits in social-emotional reciprocity, ranging, for example, from abnormal social approach and failure of normal back-and-forth conversation; to reduced sharing of interests, emotions, or affect; to failure to initiate or respond to social interactions.<br>2. Deficits in nonverbal communicative behaviors used for social interaction, ranging, for example, from poorly integrated verbal and nonverbal communication; to abnormalities in eye contact and body language or deficits in understanding and use of gestures: to a total lack of facial expressions and nonverbal communication.<br>3. Deficits in developing, maintaining, and understanding relationships, ranging, for example, from difficulties adjusting behavior to suit various social contexts; to difficulties in sharing imaginative play or in making friends; to absence of interest in peers. |
| *Specify* current severity: |
| ▸ **Severity is based on social communication impairments and restricted, repetitive patterns of behavior** (see Table 2). |
| B. Restricted, repetitive patterns of behavior, interests, or activities, as manifested by at least two of the following, currently or by history (examples are illustrative, not exhaustive; see text):<br>1. Stereotyped or repetitive motor movements, use of objects, or speech (e.g., simple motor stereotypies, lining up toys or flipping objects, echolalia, idiosyncratic phrases).<br>2. Insistence on sameness, inflexible adherence to routines, or ritualized patterns of verbal or nonverbal behavior (e.g., extreme distress at small changes, difficulties with transitions, rigid thinking patterns, greeting rituals, need to take same route or eat same food every day).<br>3. Highly restricted, fixated interests that are abnormal in intensity or focus (e.g., strong attachment to or preoccupation with unusual objects, excessively circumscribed or perseverative interests).<br>4. Hyper- or hyporeactivity to sensory input or unusual interest in sensory aspects of the environment (e.g., apparent indifference to pain/temperature, adverse response to specific sounds or textures, excessive smelling or touching of objects, visual fascination with lights or movement). |
| *Specify* current severity: |
| ▸ **Severity is based on social communication impairments and restricted, repetitive patterns of behavior** (see Table 2). |
| C. Symptoms must be present in the early developmental period (but may not become fully manifest until social demands exceed limited capacities, or may be masked by learned strategies in later life). |
| D. Symptoms cause clinically significant impairment in social, occupational, or other important areas of current functioning. |
| E. These disturbances are not better explained by intellectual disability (intellectual developmental disorder) or global developmental delay. Intellectual disability and autism spectrum disorder frequently co-occur; to make comorbid diagnoses of autism spectrum disorder and intellectual disability, social communication should be below that expected for general developmental level. |
| **Note:** Individuals with a well-established DSM-IV diagnosis of autistic disorder, Asperger's disorder, or pervasive developmental disorder not otherwise specified should be given the diagnosis of autism spectrum disorder. Individuals who have marked deficits in social communication, but whose symptoms do not otherwise meet criteria for autism spectrum disorder, should be evaluated for social (pragmatic) communication disorder. |
| Specify if: |
| ▸ **With or without accompanying intellectual impairment** |
| ▸ **With or without accompanying language impairment** |
| ▸ **Associated with a known medical or genetic condition or environmental factor** |
| ▸ **Associated with another neurodevelopmental, mental, or behavioral disorder** |
| ▸ **With catatonia** (refer to the criteria for catatonia associated with another mental disorder, pp. 119–120, for definition) |

**Source:** Reprinted with permission from the *Diagnostic and Statistical Manual of Mental Disorders*, Fifth Edition, (Copyright 2013). American Psychiatric Association.

in many countries. Currently prevalence rates of 1% and sometimes even more have been reported in North America, Europe and parts of Asia. There is, unfortunately, limited data on the incidence of these disorders in Africa, although anecdotal evidence suggests that there is an increasing prevalence in keeping with that seen in other parts of the world.

The disorder shows a male predominance, with boys affected four to five times more frequently than girls (Center for Disease Control and Prevention, 2015).

### 27.5.3.2 Aetiology

There is a strong genetic underpinning for autism spectrum disorders. It has been estimated that the heritability of autism spectrum disorders is 90% (Freitag, 2007). The relatives of persons diagnosed with autism spectrum disorders are at increased risk of the same condition. Even people who do not meet the criteria for the diagnosis of the condition often display attenuated features of the condition. Its strong biological underpinnings are highlighted by an increased incidence of the disorder in association with other neurodevelopmental disorders, such as fragile X syndrome and tuberose sclerosis. Children with autism spectrum disorders also display an increased incidence of epilepsy and developmental delays. While many environmental factors have been proposed in the aetiology of autism spectrum disorders, the evidence in support of these factors remains unconvincing (Lai *et al.*, 2014).

### 27.5.3.3 Symptoms

The disorder is characterised by two main symptom domains. The social-communication domain is characterised by persistent qualitative impairments in social interaction and reciprocal emotional engagement. Deficits in non-verbal communication, such as failure to use gestures or facial expression to facilitate communication, may be present. Language delays, although a prominent feature in the DSM-IV, is no longer a requirement for the diagnosis. This reflects its lack of specificity and the marked variation of language ability seen in the disorder.

The behavioural domain is characterised by restricted, repetitive and often stereotyped interests, activities and behaviours. Abnormal patterns of reaction to sensory stimuli may also occur.

The disorder is present early in life, although it may only come to attention at a later stage, generally when social demands have increased. The disorder must cause significant distress and dysfunction.

### 27.5.3.4 Diagnosis

In most patients the diagnosis can be made on the basis of a comprehensive history and observation of the child's behaviour. A variety of screening instruments are available to facilitate the evaluation process, but they are not essential for the diagnosis. There are no special investigations necessary to diagnose autism spectrum disorders, but investigations may be useful to exclude other conditions such as fragile X syndrome and co-morbid epilepsy.

**Childhood disintegrative disorder**

Childhood disintegrative disorder (CDD) is part of the autism spectrum disorders. In this condition, normal development proceeds uneventfully for at least two years (but not beyond the age of ten). This is followed by marked regression in language skills, social skills, bowel and bladder control and motor skills.

### 27.5.3.5 Differential diagnosis

Differential diagnoses to consider include mixed receptive-expressive language disorder, acquired aphasia with convulsions, congenital deafness, intellectual impairment, severe psychosocial deprivation and childhood schizophrenia.

### 27.5.3.6 Treatment

There is no definitive treatment available for autism spectrum disorder. The treatment aims at enhancing the child's development in terms of cognitive functioning, communication and social skills. Since individuals with the disorder display such diversity in terms of symptoms and symptom severity, treatment has to be individualised. Intensive interventions using principles of behaviour therapy are generally used. Multidisciplinary approaches from psychology, occupational therapy, speech therapy and specialised educational services may be useful. Greater improvements are associated with earlier commencement of interventions and the intensity of interventions. Caregivers play an important role in ensuring that the ASD patient receives the structure and stimulation that he or she requires in the home setting. Caregivers should receive appropriate psycho-education about the disorder and can be taught to implement basic home-based interventions (American Academy of Child and Adolescent Psychiatry, 2014). Autism support groups may be a valuable resource in ensuring that caregivers receive ongoing support and encouragement.

There are no specific pharmacotherapeutic interventions. Medication may be used to treat co-morbid disorders such as ADHD, as well as to target severe behavioural problems such as self-harming or aggressive behaviour. Medication includes antipsychotics (e.g. risperidone), stimulant medication (e.g. methylphenidate) and selective serotonin reuptake inhibitors (e.g. fluoxetine) (McPheeters *et al.*, 2011).

## 27.5.4 Reactive attachment disorder and disinhibited social engagement disorder

These conditions are believed to be the consequences of severe early childhood psychosocial deprivation. Children with these conditions were generally exposed to an early environment that prevented them from forming secure attachments to a caregiver, such as children exposed to severe childhood neglect or to multiple foster care placements. These children display a pervasive pattern of behaviour that reflects their inability to engage with adults in a socially appropriate manner. Their pattern of engagement is characterised by two extremes. In reactive attachment disorder, the child is inhibited, withdrawn, fails to engage socially and displays a lack of emotional responsiveness to others. Children with disinhibited social engagement disorder show a pattern of indiscriminate engagement with adults, which is clearly developmentally and socially inappropriate. It is important to distinguish these conditions from others in which social engagement may be inappropriate, such as autism-spectrum disorder.

## 27.5.5 Attention deficit hyperactivity disorder (ADHD)

Attention deficit hyperactivity disorder (ADHD) is the most commonly diagnosed disorder in children. ADHD is characterised by a combination of problems, such as difficulty sustaining attention, hyperactivity and impulsive behaviour; presents in multiple settings (e.g. school and home) and gives rise to social and educational difficulties. Children with ADHD also may struggle with low self-esteem, troubled relationships and poor performance in school. ADHD is a clinical diagnosis based on a comprehensive assessment. Treatment typically involves medication and behavioural interventions. Early diagnosis and treatment can make a big difference in outcome.

### 27.5.5.1 Epidemiology

Various studies show that the prevalence of the disorder ranges from 3%–12% of preschool and primary school children. It appears to be diagnosed less often in African children in sub-Saharan Africa. It is far more common in boys than in girls, with a ratio of approximately 3:1.

### 27.5.5.2 Aetiology

Multiple factors have been implicated in the development of ADHD. A common feature is relative dysfunction of the prefrontal cortex, with deficits in executive functioning, such as planning, organisation and impulse control. ADHD often runs in families, and studies indicate that genes play a role, with heritability estimated at 75%. Certain environmental factors also may increase risk at critical periods in development.

Risk factors for ADHD may include:

- family history of ADHD
- maternal drug use, alcohol use or smoking during pregnancy, exposure to environmental poisons, poor maternal health and viral infections during pregnancy
- perinatal factors, such as premature birth, hypoxia, foetal distress, central nervous system infection
- environmental, such as severe abuse and neglect during infancy.

### 27.5.5.3 Clinical features

The DSM-5 divides symptoms into two categories of inattention as well as hyperactivity and impulsivity. Children must have at least six symptoms from either (or both) the inattention group of criteria and the hyperactivity and impulsivity criteria. These symptoms must be present in two or more settings (e.g. home and school) and give rise to school or social difficulties. The symptoms must not be better accounted for by another mental disorder such as a specific learning disorder, dissociative disorder, depression or anxiety. The core symptoms of ADHD are grouped as follows:

- Inattention
  - careless mistakes in schoolwork or other activities
  - attention difficulties in tasks or play activities
  - listening problems
  - loses items (e.g. pencil, books) needed for tasks or activities
  - organisational skills lacking (e.g. difficulty managing sequential tasks, difficulty in keeping materials and belongings in order, messy)
  - forgets daily activities (e.g. brushing teeth, routine school activity)
  - fails to follow through instructions and fails to finish schoolwork or chores
  - reluctant to engage in tasks that require sustained mental effort (e.g. schoolwork or chores at home homework)
  - easily distracted by extraneous stimuli (e.g. a bird outside the classroom).
- Hyperactivity and impulsivity
  - restless (e.g. runs about or climbs in situations where it is inappropriate)
  - unable to await his or her turn (e.g. while in a queue)
  - unable to play quietly
  - on the go or often acts as if driven by a motor (e.g. unable or uncomfortable keeping still for an extended time, as in restaurants)
  - fidgets with hands or feet or squirms in a chair
  - blurts out answers, completes people's sentences for them and cannot wait for their turn in conversation
  - staying seated is difficult (e.g. repeatedly leaves his or her place in the classroom)
  - talks excessively
  - tends to interrupt or intrudes on others (e.g. butts into conversations, games or activities, use other people's things without asking or receiving permission).

ADHD may be specified based on the current presentation.

- Combined presentation: if both inattention and hyperactivity-impulsivity criteria are met for the past six months.
- Predominantly inattentive presentation: if criteria for inattention are met but criteria for hyperactivity-impulsivity are not met, and three or more of the latter have been present for the past six months.
- Inattentive presentation (restrictive): if criteria for inattention are met but no more than two symptoms for hyperactivity-impulsivity have been present for the past six months.
- Predominantly hyperactive/impulsive presentation: if criteria for hyperactivity-impulsivity are met and criteria for inattention are not met for the past six months.

ADHD not elsewhere classified may be coded in cases where the child's symptoms are below the threshold for ADHD or for whom there is insufficient opportunity to verify all criteria. However,

ADHD-related symptoms should be associated with impairment, and they are not better explained by any other mental disorder.

#### 27.5.5.4 Normal behaviour vs. ADHD

Most healthy children are inattentive, hyperactive or impulsive at one time or another. It's normal for pre-schoolers to have short attention spans and be unable to stick with one activity for long. Even in older children and teenagers, attention span often depends on the level of interest.

The same is true of hyperactivity. Young children are naturally energetic – they often wear their parents out long before they themselves are tired. In addition, some children just naturally have a higher activity level than others do. Children should never be classified as having ADHD just because they're different from their friends or siblings.

Children who have problems in school but get along well at home or with friends are likely struggling with something other than ADHD. The same is true of children who are hyperactive or inattentive at home, but whose schoolwork and friendships remain unaffected.

#### 27.5.5.5 Clinical assessment

The diagnosis of ADHD is made clinically, based on careful history taking, clinical examination and information from multiple sources and multiple settings like school, home and community.

The assessment of the child is the same as for any other mental health difficulty. A comprehensive assessment is not only essential in making an accurate diagnosis and to understand the child's difficulties but also to rule out other primary or co-morbid psychiatric disorders, medical problems or side effects of other medications. Reports from school and assessing functional disability in multiple domains are also important. Laboratory investigations may be done as clinically indicated. Psychology testing is useful in assessing intellectual ability and possible specific learning disorders. ADHD rating scales (parent and teacher forms) may be useful to document a baseline and as a follow-up of treatment effectiveness. It is important to note that all tests are useful only in the context of a comprehensive assessment.

#### 27.5.5.6 Co-morbidity

The risk of having other psychiatric disorders is increased in children with ADHD and thus co-morbidity is common. Co-existing disorders that may be present include learning disorders, disruptive behaviour, depression, anxiety, and an adjustment reaction to a pathological or abusive home environment.

ADHD can make life difficult for children and they:

- often struggle in the classroom, which can lead to academic failure and judgement by other children and adults
- tend to have more accidents and injuries of all kinds than children who do not have the disorder
- often have poor self-esteem
- are more likely to have trouble interacting with, and being accepted by, peers and adults
- are at increased risk of alcohol and drug abuse and other delinquent behaviour.

#### 27.5.5.7 Differential diagnosis

It is essential to differentiate between ADHD from developmentally age-appropriate over-activity and other disorders that are listed in Table 27.2.

#### 27.5.5.8 Treatment

The treatment of ADHD is multimodal and includes biological (medication) and psycho-social interventions. Once the diagnosis has been communicated and psycho-education given, it is important to assess the impact of the condition and to provide support by addressing parental concerns, providing written information and referral to support groups. Treatment usually involves a combination of medication and behavioural management. Extensive research has shown that medication is the most effective treatment for the core symptoms (hyperactivity, impulsivity and inattention)

**Table 27.2** Disorders that may present similar to ADHD

- Biological or other medical conditions
  - hearing or vision impairment
  - epilepsy
  - genetic abnormalities
  - thyroid disorders
  - medications
  - heavy metal poisoning
  - fetal alcohol syndrome
- Psychosocial conditions
  - poor nutrition
  - abuse/neglect
  - chaotic family functioning
  - community conflict
  - school situation
- Psychiatric disorders
  - neurodevelopmental disorders
  - disruptive behaviours
  - mood disorders
  - anxiety disorders
  - tic disorders
  - substance use disorders
  - sleep disorders

of ADHD, as well as effects on cognition and social function.

The most widely studied and used medication is the psychostimulant methylphenidate, which is available in a short-acting, a long-acting and an extended-release form. The usual starting dose is 5 mg, increasing weekly until either marked behavioural improvement or significant side effects occur. The usual maximum dose is 0,5 mg/kg per day, although higher doses may occasionally be needed. The right dose varies from child to child, so it may take some time to find the correct dose. The dose may have to be adjusted if significant side effects occur or as the child matures. Unless symptoms are extreme, the medication is usually restricted to school days, and reviewed after six months. Besides inhibition of appetite, growth suppression and insomnia, side effects include headaches, irritability and dysphoria. (See Chapter 36: Pharmacological and other treatments in psychiatry for further information on methylphenidate).

Other medication that may be used include atomoxetine, and tricyclic antidepressants like imipramine. Clonidine (alpha agonist) is used as a first-line treatment in children with both ADHD and tic disorder. Atypical antipsychotics like risperidone are considered when most other medications are ineffective.

Psychosocial interventions may include

- *Behaviour therapy*. Teachers and parents can learn behaviour-changing strategies for dealing with difficult situations. These strategies may include token reward systems and time-outs.
- *Psychotherapy*. This allows older children with ADHD to talk about issues that bother them, explore negative behavioural patterns and learn ways to deal with their symptoms.
- *Parenting skills training*. This can help parents develop ways to understand and guide their child's behaviour (consistency, routines, organisation, reducing stimulation, decreasing frustration, anticipating difficulties, behaviour modification).
- *Family therapy*. To reduce conflict and improve communication and problem solving within the family.
- *Social skills training*. This can help children learn appropriate social behaviours. The best results usually occur when a team approach is used, with teachers, parents, and therapists or physicians working together.
- *Schooling*. Classroom modification strategies and teacher understanding. Remedial learning provides additional support where necessary.

### 27.5.5.9 Prognosis

Approximately 50% of children with this disorder have a satisfactory outcome. A significant percentage of the remaining half will continue to have problems with attention and impulsivity throughout adolescence and, in some cases, into adulthood. Approximately 25% will go on to have personality problems in adulthood. Those with a co-morbid conduct disorder are more

**Table 27.3** DSM-5 Diagnostic Criteria for Attention-Deficit/Hyperactivity Disorder

| Diagnostic Criteria |
|---|
| A. A persistent pattern of inattention and/or hyperactivity-impulsivity that interferes with functioning or development, as characterized by (1) and/or (2): |
| 1. **Inattention:** Six (or more) of the following symptoms have persisted for at least 6 months to a degree that is inconsistent with developmental level and that negatively impacts directly on social and academic/occupational activities: |
| **Note:** The symptoms are not solely a manifestation of oppositional behavior, defiance, hostility, or failure to understand tasks or instructions. For older adolescents and adults (age 17 and older), at least five symptoms are required. |
| a. Often fails to give close attention to details or makes careless mistakes in schoolwork, at work, or during other activities (e.g., overlooks or misses details, work is inaccurate). |
| b. Often has difficulty sustaining attention in tasks or play activities (e.g., has difficulty remaining focused during lectures, conversations, or lengthy reading). |
| c. Often does not seem to listen when spoken to directly (e.g., mind seems elsewhere, even in the absence of any obvious distraction). |
| d. Often does not follow through on instructions and fails to finish schoolwork, chores, or duties in the workplace (e.g., starts tasks but quickly loses focus and is easily sidetracked). |
| e. Often has difficulty organizing tasks and activities (e.g., difficulty managing sequential tasks; difficulty keeping materials and belongings in order; messy, disorganized work; has poor time management; fails to meet deadlines). |
| f. Often avoids, dislikes, or is reluctant to engage in tasks that require sustained mental effort (e.g., schoolwork or homework; for older adolescents and adults, preparing reports, completing forms, reviewing lengthy papers). |
| g. Often loses things necessary for tasks or activities (e.g., school materials, pencils, books, tools, wallets, keys, paperwork, eyeglasses, mobile telephones). |
| h. Is often easily distracted by extraneous stimuli (for older adolescents and adults, may include unrelated thoughts). |
| i. Is often forgetful in daily activities (e.g., doing chores, running errands; for older adolescents and adults, returning calls, paying bills, keeping appointments). |
| 2. **Hyperactivity and impulsivity:** Six (or more) of the following symptoms have persisted for at least 6 months to a degree that is inconsistent with developmental level and that negatively impacts directly on social and academic/occupational activities: **Note:** The symptoms are not solely a manifestation of oppositional behavior, defiance, hostility, or a failure to understand tasks or instructions. For older adolescents and adults (age 17 and older), at least five symptoms are required. |
| a. Often fidgets with or taps hands or feet or squirms in seat. |
| b. Often leaves seat in situations when remaining seated is expected (e.g., leaves his or her place in the classroom, in the office or other workplace, or in other situations that require remaining in place). |
| c. Often runs about or climbs in situations where it is inappropriate. (**Note:** In adolescents or adults, may be limited to feeling restless.) |
| d. Often unable to play or engage in leisure activities quietly. |
| e. Is often 'on the go,' acting as if 'driven by a motor' (e.g., is unable to be or uncomfortable being still for extended time, as in restaurants, meetings; may be experienced by others as being restless or difficult to keep up with). |
| f. Often talks excessively. |
| g. Often blurts out an answer before a question has been completed (e.g., completes people's sentences; cannot wait for turn in conversation). |
| h. Often has difficulty waiting his or her turn (e.g., while waiting in line). |
| i. Often interrupts or intrudes on others (e.g., butts into conversations, games, or activities; may start using other people's things without asking or receiving permission; for adolescents and adults, may intrude into or take over what others are doing). |
| B. Several inattentive or hyperactive-impulsive symptoms were present prior to age 12 years. |
| C. Several inattentive or hyperactive-impulsive symptoms are present in two or more settings (e.g., at home, school, or work; with friends or relatives; in other activities). |
| D. There is clear evidence that the symptoms interfere with, or reduce the quality of, social, academic, or occupational functioning. |

E. The symptoms do not occur exclusively during the course of schizophrenia or another psychotic disorder and are not better explained by another mental disorder (e.g., mood disorder, anxiety disorder, dissociative disorder, personality disorder, substance intoxication or withdrawal).

*Specify* whether:

- **314.01 (F90.2) Combined presentation:** If both Criterion A1 (inattention) and Criterion A2 (hyperactivity-impulsivity) are met for the past 6 months.
- **314.00 (F90.0) Predominantly inattentive presentation:** If Criterion A1 (inattention) is met but Criterion A2 (hyperactivity-impulsivity) is not met for the past 6 months.
- **314.01 (F90.1) Predominantly hyperactive/impulsive presentation:** If Criterion A2 (hyperactivity-impulsivity) is met and Criterion A1 (inattention) is not met for the past 6 months.

*Specify* if:

- **In partial remission:** When full criteria were previously met, fewer than the full criteria have been met for the past 6 months, and the symptoms still result in impairment in social, academic, or occupational functioning.

*Specify* current severity:

- **Mild:** Few, if any, symptoms in excess of those required to make the diagnosis are present, and symptoms result in no more than minor impairments in social or occupational functioning.
- **Moderate:** Symptoms or functional impairment between 'mild' and 'severe' are present.
- **Severe:** Many symptoms in excess of those required to make the diagnosis, or several symptoms that are particularly severe, are present, or the symptoms result in marked impairment in social or occupational functioning.

**Source:** Reprinted with permission from the *Diagnostic and Statistical Manual of Mental Disorders*, Fifth Edition, (Copyright 2013). American Psychiatric Association.

likely to show antisocial personality traits in adulthood.

It is also important to consider the effects secondary to having ADHD, such as academic failure, loss of interest in education, low self-esteem, and depressed mood.

The long-term outcome is improved with effective treatment, psychosocial interventions and support.

## 27.5.6 Specific learning disorders

These disorders are characterised by an inability to achieve in a specific area of learning (reading, written language or mathematics) at a level consistent with the child's overall IQ, age and education. Typically, individuals with these disorders have intelligence that falls within the normal range (although it may be low or high), but have a specific inability to learn at least one and sometimes several of these academic skills.

Specific learning disorder in the DSM-5 is now a single, overall diagnosis, incorporating deficits that impact academic achievement. Rather than limiting learning disorders to diagnoses particular to reading, mathematics and written expression, the criteria describe shortcomings in general academic skills and provide detailed specifiers for the areas of reading, mathematics, and written expression.

### 27.5.6.1 Epidemiology

Twenty per cent of most school populations have difficulties in performing academically. Apart from learning disorders, overall below-average intelligence and emotional problems can cause poor school achievement. The incidence of learning disorders in children is 5%–10%, with a far greater frequency in boys. Many children with these disorders have no other sign of psychopathology, and are usually detected and treated within the educational system rather than the mental health system.

### 27.5.6.2 Aetiology

Learning disorders result from varying degrees and types of neurological anomaly, and are often inherited. They represent a specific difficulty with information processing.

#### 27.5.6.3 Diagnosis

The diagnoses is made through a clinical review of the individual's developmental, medical, educational, and family history, reports of test grades and teacher observations, and response to academic interventions. The diagnosis requires persistent difficulties in reading, writing, arithmetic or mathematical reasoning skills during formal years of schooling. Symptoms may include inaccurate or slow and effortful reading, poor written expression that lacks clarity, difficulties remembering number facts or inaccurate mathematical reasoning. Current academic skills must be well below the average range of scores in culturally and linguistically appropriate tests of reading, writing or mathematics. The individual's difficulties must not be better explained by developmental, neurological, and sensory (vision or hearing), or motor disorders and must significantly interfere with academic achievement, occupational performance, or activities of daily living.

Because of the changes in the DSM-5, clinicians will be able to make this diagnosis by identifying whether patients are unable to perform academically at a level appropriate to their intelligence and age. After a diagnosis, clinicians can provide greater detail into the type of deficit(s) that an individual has through the designated specifiers.

#### 27.5.6.4 Management

These problems can have long-term impact on a person's ability to function because so many activities of daily living require a mastery of number facts, written words, and written expression.

Early identification and intervention are particularly important. The broader DSM-5 category of specific learning disorder ensures that fewer affected individuals will go unidentified; while the detailed specifiers will help clinicians effectively target services and treatment.

Intervention is educational, the earlier the better. A full psychometric and educational evaluation is necessary wherever possible. Remedial teaching is undertaken to shore up the skill deficits. This may need to be intensive if the learning disorder is severe. It should always be supportive, sympathetic and aimed at raising the learner's self-esteem and confidence. This is often sufficient to alleviate any secondary emotional or behavioural problems.

### 27.5.7 Motor disorders

The following motor disorders are included in the DSM-5: developmental coordination disorder, stereotypic movement disorder, Tourette's disorder, persistent (chronic) motor or vocal tic disorder, provisional tic disorder, other specified tic disorder, and unspecified tic disorder. The tic criteria have been standardised across all of these disorders. Stereotypic movement disorder has been more clearly differentiated from body-focused repetitive behaviour disorders that are in the DSM-5 chapter on obsessive-compulsive disorder.

Tics are defined as sudden, rapid, recurrent, non-rhythmic stereotyped motor movements or vocalisations. They are repetitive involuntary movements of discrete muscle groups and can be suppressed for varying lengths of time, usually when the patient is concentrating, but eventually become uncontrollable. For example, they may be less evident during school hours, but very prominent when the child or adolescent is at home in the evenings. Tics are exacerbated by stress, fatigue, anxiety and boredom, and occur less often or are absent during sleep or absorbing enjoyable activities.

Motor tics include eye-blinking, neck-jerking, shoulder-shrugging, and facial movements. The head and neck are more involved than the trunk and the lower limbs are seldom involved. Complex motor tics include facial gestures, jumping, compulsive touching, smelling objects, grooming behaviours and repetitive sequences (such as complex jumps or stepping in a particular pattern). These tics may be semi-purposeful, and therefore are sometimes construed as a form of bad behaviour.

Simple vocal tics include grunting, coughing, throat-clearing, animal-like noises, humming, snorting, screaming, and shouting. Complex vocal tics include repeating certain words or phrases, the use of socially unacceptable words, echolalia, or nonsensical verbal patterns.

There may be a strong aggressive or sexual component to complex tics, with sexual touching, obscene gestures, or coprolalia (uttering obscenities) occurring. **Coprolalia** is present in less than 15% of children with Tourette's disorder.

### 27.5.7.1 Tourette's disorder in children

Children with Tourette's disorder have both multiple motor tics and vocal tics that are temporarily suppressible and proceeded by a premonitory urge. Characteristically, the tics in Tourette's disorder wax and wane and high emotions typically exacerbate tics. The tics usually begin in early childhood, with motor tics that typically fluctuate and change over time. Vocal tics begin in the early school-going years.

#### Epidemiology

The highest incidence is in children from 7–11 years, and the condition is much more common in boys. Many cases remain mild and most settle by the time adulthood is reached, having been at their worst in adolescence. A minority of patients retain severe symptoms.

Co-morbidity with other disorders is frequent. ADHD is present in as many as 40% of patients, and may in fact precede the onset of the tics. It can be severe and hard to treat. Obsessive-compulsive disorder occurs in nearly 50% of those with Tourette's disorder.

There is also a higher incidence of learning disorders. These children can be very problematic in the school setting, and many develop secondary emotional and behavioural problems, especially when their behaviour is labelled as voluntary misbehaviour and they are punished.

#### Aetiology

Tourette's disorder is considered to be hereditary, with a probable polygenetic inheritance and variable penetration. The abnormality is thought to occur in the corticostriatothalamocortical circuits and to involve dopamine, adrenalin and serotonin neurotransmitters. Other factors that have been implicated include perinatal events, such as low birth weight, maternal stress and obstetric complications. Auto-immune processes may affect the tic onset and exacerbation in some cases. Current research focuses on role of paediatric auto-immune neuropsychiatric disorders associated with streptococcal infections (PANDAS), in the onset of tic disorders and OCD.

#### Diagnosis

The diagnosis is based on the clinical findings, including the family history. In the differential diagnosis, neurological disorders, such as hyperkinetic movement disorders, stereotypic behaviour, dystonias, choreiform disorders and myoclonus may be confused with tics and should be ruled out. Co-morbidities include OCD and ADHD. Learning disorders, sleep disorders, disruptive behaviour disorders and mood disorders may also complicate the clinical condition of children with Tourette's disorder.

#### Management of tic disorders

Treatment involves a careful assessment of the impact of the condition, any co-morbid disorders, and problems within the family or at school. Psycho-education and explanation of the condition to parents and teachers often facilitate better management and understanding of the child. Information brochures and support groups may be available. Behavioural interventions (habit reversal training) and supportive psychotherapy may be helpful. In many cases, these steps are sufficient to bring relief and improvement. If the tics are sufficiently troublesome to warrant medication, referral to a specialist is advised.

Medication used include atypical antipsychotics, alpha-2a agonists or antidepressants, depending on the clinical situation. In patients with co-morbid ADHD that is significant and impairing, the cautious use of stimulants is recommended. Atomoxetine may be useful if alpha agonists and stimulant medication do not appropriately treat a severe tic disorder with ADHD.

## 27.6 Conduct disorder

Conduct disorder refers to a condition wherein the child persistently displays a range of behaviours that is deemed inappropriate in that he or she violates the rights of others or accepted standards of behaviour. The disorder presents major challenges for the caregivers, schooling, welfare and justice authorities and indeed for society in general.

### 27.6.1 Epidemiology

Prevalence rates of conduct disorder are estimated to be 2%–8%. There is a male predominance, with ratios of 4–10:1. There have been concerns about increasing rates of conduct disorder in females (Scott, 2012).

### 27.6.2 Aetiology

The condition is presumed to have a multi-factorial aetiology. Factors implicated include genetics, parental and environmental factors, child abuse and neglect.

### 27.6.3 Clinical features

According to the DSM-5, the child must, in the preceding 12 months, have displayed at least three behaviour symptoms from the following categories:

- aggressive behaviour directed towards people and animals
- behaviour involving the destruction of property
- deceitfulness and stealing
- major violations of rules.

At least one of these behaviours must have occurred in the previous six months; and these behaviours must be responsible for functional impairment.

A distinction is made between childhood-onset and adolescent-onset types, based on the presence or absence respectively, of at least one criterion before the age of 10 years. The DSM-5 also makes provision for recording the presence of a specifier, 'limited prosocial emotions', characterised by at least two of the following over at least 12 months and in multiple relationships and settings:

- lack of remorse or guilt
- callous – lack of empathy
- unconcerned about performance
- shallow or deficient affect.

### 27.6.4 Investigations

There are no specific investigations for conduct disorder. Commonly used rating scales such as the Connors (Connors, 1997), Child Behaviour Checklist (CBL) (Achenbach and Edelbrock, 1991) and the Strengths and Difficulties Questionnaire (SDQ) (Goodman, 1997) have components that can be used to assess conduct disorder symptoms.

### 27.6.5 Differential diagnosis

Since a diagnosis of conduct disorder often carries very negative connotations, it is imperative that other conditions that may resemble it are actively sought and excluded. Children with ADHD may sometimes display behaviour usually associated with conduct disorder. In ADHD these behaviours are often as a result of impulsivity and hyperactivity, however, and not necessarily seen as a deliberate intent to break the rules. Unfortunately ADHD and conduct disorder commonly co-exist. Adjustment disorders may present with disturbances of conduct. Depression in children is also sometimes associated with externalising behaviour, including conduct symptoms. In some situations childhood bipolar disorder could resemble conduct disorder.

### 27.6.6 Course and prognosis

The earlier the onset of the disorder and increased frequency and severity of the behavioural symptoms, the worse the longer-term prognosis. The disorder is associated with an increased vulnerability to develop substance-related and anti-social personality disorders.

### 27.6.7 Treatment

The disorder is often difficult to treat and demands a multi-modal approach. Parents and caregivers must receive psycho-education about the disorder from the start as their involvement is critical. The psychological treatments generally use principles of behaviour therapy (National Center for Health and Care Excellence, 2013). Parent Management Training is one such approach. This treatment trains parents to modify their child's behaviour by reinforcing prosocial behaviour while providing consistent but non-punitive consequences for aberrant behaviour. Medication has a role to play, especially in the treatment of comorbid disorders. Since ADHD and conduct disorder commonly overlap, the use of stimulant medication such as methylphenidate may be useful. Other medication that has shown effectiveness, especially in controlling aggressive behaviour, include risperidone and mood stabilisers, such as lithium, sodium valproate and carbamazepine (Pappadopulos *et al.*, 2006).

## 27.7 Oppositional defiant disorder

Oppositional defiant disorder (ODD) describes a condition where the child displays symptoms of angry or irritable mood, argumentative or defiant behaviour and vindictiveness. (American Psychiatric Association, 2013). While these symptoms may occur in normally developing children, in the case of ODD they are deemed to be excessive due to their frequency and persistence. Children with the condition do not, however, display the severe symptoms involving violation of the rights of others or major societal norms as seen in conduct disorder. It is sometimes seen as a less severe variant of conduct disorder, with which it shows many similarities.

### 2.7.1 Epidemiology

The prevalence of the disorder is 2-10%. As with conduct disorder, there is a male predominance (Costello *et al.*, 2003). The first symptoms are generally present in the preschool period. Peak age is between 5-10 years with rates declining thereafter.

### 27.7.2 Clinical features

According to the DSM-5 the child must have in the preceding six months, displayed at least four symptoms from the following categories:

- angry or irritable mood
- argumentative or defiant behaviour
- vindictiveness.

This behaviour must be more frequent and intense from what is generally encountered within the range of normative development. Symptoms must be associated with distress in the patient or those around him or her, or must cause functional impairment. It is important to exclude other psychiatric conditions such as sepression and disruptive mood dysregulation disorder (American Psychiatric Association, 2013).

### 27.7.3 Investigations

A comprehensive clinical interview, with information on the child obtained from multiple informants, is generally sufficient to make a diagnosis. Commonly used rating scales such as the Connors, Child Behaviour checklist (CBL) and the Strengths and Difficulties Questionnaire (SDQ) include components to evaluate the presence of ODD (Steiner and Remsing, 2007).

### 27.7.4 Differential diagnosis

Some degree of oppositional symptoms may be considered to be normative and it is important to reserve the diagnosis for those displaying severe symptoms only. In addition, oppositional behaviour may occur in the context of other disorders such as depression, anxiety disorders, ADHD and conduct disorder.

## 27.7.5 Treatment

The main focus of treatment is psychosocial. Parents Management Training can be used to teach parents to modify their behaviour towards their child in order to ultimately bring about changes in the child's behaviour. Parents are taught how to reinforce their child's positive behaviours, while responding appropriately to their disruptive behaviours. Some children may also benefit from social-skills training. Except for the treatment of co-morbid conditions (Steiner and Remsing, 2007) such as ADHD, there is little role for medication in the management of oppositional defiant disorder.

# 27.8 Separation anxiety disorder

The DSM-5 characterises separation anxiety disorder as a disorder in which an individual displays a disproportionate degree of anxiety or fear in response to separation or anticipation of separation from a significant attachment figure.

A degree of separation anxiety is considered to be developmentally appropriate in younger children; however this tends to diminish by the age of 3-4 years in most children. In children with the disorder, the anxiety or fear may persist and is in excess of what is normally expected. The DSM-5 requires that the symptoms must persist for at least six months..

Children with the disorder commonly display excessive and unreasonable worry about harm befalling their loved ones. They may manifest their distress in clinging behaviour, nightmares and sleep disturbance and multiple vague somatic complaints. Efforts to avoid separation may cause them to avoid social functions like parties or sleepovers; in some cases it may even lead to school refusal.

# 27.9 Social anxiety disorder

The DSM-5 describes social anxiety disorder as one in which the individual's anxiety or fear revolves around fear of being negatively evaluated by others: they fear being embarrassed or humiliated. This can happen when required to perform tasks in front of, interact with others or be observed by them. Symptoms must persist for at least six months and must cause distress and functional impairment.

A subtype of this condition is selective mutism. In selective mutism, the child consistently fails to speak in certain situations, for example at school. The child is, however, capable of speaking normally in other situations, such as at home. This failure to speak impacts negatively on academic, occupational and social functioning.

# 27.10 School refusal

While school refusal is not a psychiatric diagnosis, it does represent a problem that commonly presents to child psychiatric services. School refusal can have serious consequences in terms of disruption of a child's education, as well as creating stress and conflict within the family setting. School refusal may occur in a variety of contexts. In conduct disorder and oppositional defiant disorder, the child may wilfully refuse to attend school. Children with major depressive disorder, bipolar disorder or schizophrenia may refuse to attend school due to lack of drive or presence of psychotic symptoms.

Anxiety disorders are a common reason for school refusal. Specific phobias involving the school may render the child too fearful to attend. Similarly, children who develop post-traumatic stress disorder as a result of school-based violence may seek to avoid school-based reminders of the trauma. Children with social anxiety disorder may refuse to attend school, since it represents a situation where they will be evaluated by others. School refusal occurs frequently as a consequence of separation anxiety disorder, especially in younger children.

School refusal can be an emergency, and requires urgent intervention. It is important to return the child to school as soon as possible to limit the risk of the behaviour being reinforced by secondary gains. Obtaining the co-operation of both the parents and the school is essential. A graded re-introduction to school can be considered. In the initial stages this may entail allowing the child to remain in school even if the child is not able to participate meaningfully in the school programme. Parents could also be allowed to accompany the child to school, with a gradual decrease in the time spent as the child's anxiety improves. The underlying anxiety disorder must be treated (Figueroa *et al.*, 2012).

## 27.11 Disruptive mood dysregulation disorder

Disruptive mood dysregulation disorder (DMDD) is a new concept introduced by the DSM-5. Its inclusion arose mainly in response to concerns that increasing numbers of children were being diagnosed as having bipolar disorder. While many children do display features typically associated with mania in adults, others may display symptoms of severe irritability that is chronic and not episodic (Mikita and Stringaris, 2012). The belief that this represented a childhood presentation of mania has been widely challenged. These children have been found to differ significantly from bipolar adult patients, hence the need to classify them separately (Leibenluft, 2011).

### 27.11.1 Symptoms

Disruptive mood dysregulation disorder refers to a disorder in which children display severe recurrent temper outbursts. Between these episodes the child will continue to experience negative mood states. Symptoms have to be present for at least 12 months and must occur in at least two settings. The condition can only be diagnosed in children from the age of six, and onset must be before the age of 10.

### 27.11.2 Treatment

Treatment options include psychotherapy, in particular behavioural approaches, skills training and parenting programmes. Pharmacological options that have been used include antidepressants, mood stabilisers and the typical antipsychotics (Zeft and Holtman, 2012). This is a new condition and further research is needed to clarify the optimum treatment modalities.

## 27.12 Elimination disorders

The development of continence for urine and faeces represents an important task for the developing child. Failure to successfully achieve this task may have an adverse impact on the child, including poor self-esteem, ostracisation, impaired peer relationships and conflictual family relationships.

There is considerable variation in the age at which continence is achieved; however children tend to follow a similar sequence in the development of continence. Nocturnal faecal continence is often the first to develop, followed closely by diurnal faecal continence. Diurnal urinary continence then develops, followed lastly by

**Case study 27.1**

**Disruptive mood dysregulation disorder**

G is an 8-year-old boy who was referred for evaluation. His parents and his teachers expressed concern about his behaviour, as G had been displaying severe temper tantrums of increasing frequency. These temper outbursts are now happening on an almost daily basis and are usually precipitated by minor issues such as his brother touching his possessions or minor reprimands by parents and or teachers. He has on several occasions become physically aggressive during these tantrums, and has even been suspended from school for attacking a schoolmate. His mood is generally quite low, as he feels that he is the one who is being unfairly treated. Examination failed to demonstrate any convincing evidence of depression, oppositional-defiant or conduct disorder. A provisional diagnosis of disruptive mood dysregulation disorder was made.

nocturnal urinary continence. Alterations in this pattern may indicate potential problems.

### 27.12.1 Enuresis

Enuresis is characterised by the repeated voiding of urine into inappropriate places (clothes, bed, etc.) This inappropriate voiding may be deliberate or not and may be diurnal or nocturnal. Diagnosis of the condition according to the DSM-5's guidelines requires that the problem occurs at least twice a week for three months, and the child must be at least five years old. The disorder can only be diagnosed if general medical conditions such as urinary tract infections, diabetes mellitus and structural problems such as posterior urethral valve have been excluded as causes.

A diurnal pattern is less common and may be associated with greater psychopathology in the child. Nocturnal enuresis is the commoner clinical presentation. The disorder is commoner in males. Children with enuresis often have relatives who have experienced the same disorder. Children may develop enuresis after having attained a period of continence, often in response to stressful life events. Rates of enuresis tend to fall as children mature.

Diagnosis is made on the basis of a comprehensive history and examination. Medical conditions that can cause incontinence must be excluded. The treatment of the condition requires a holistic approach. Treatment should commence with psycho-education of parents and child. General measures include addressing issues of embarrassment by ensuring a change of clothes and dealing with harsh parental responses to bedwetting. Parents are advised to limit giving fluids in the evenings and to ensure that the child goes to the toilet at night. Behavioural treatment has proven effective (Caldwell *et al.*, 2013). These include 'star charts' (which seek to provide positive reinforcement for dry nights) via the principle of **operant conditioning**. The 'bell and pad' method, using classical conditioning, is also effective (Glazener *et al.*, 2005). In this method, the child sleeps on an alarm pad that triggers if he or she wets the bed. Medication used includes anticholinergic medication such as the tricycle antidepressants and antidiuretic hormone analogues such as desmopressin. Medication is most useful when used in conjunction with behavioural treatment. Prognosis for enuresis is generally good with high rates of remission in most cases.

### 27.12.2 Encopresis

The DSM-5 characterises encopresis as the passage of faeces into inappropriate places. This can be under voluntary control or not. Soiling should occur at least once a week for a period of three months, in a child of at least four years old. In order for the disorder to be diagnosed, a medical condition must be excluded.

A distinction is made between children with constipation and associated overflow incontinence and those without. Many children with encopresis have constipation. This may occur as a result of poor sphincter tone or psychological factors. Psychological factors could include, for example, phobias involving the toilet, oppositional-defiant behaviour and even anxiety related to harsh toilet training. With constipation, the faeces accumulate in the bowel. The faeces liquefy and may leak out causing overflow incontinence.

In some cases encopresis may occur after a period of normal functioning. This is often in response to stressful life events.

General treatment measures include psycho-education of the parents. Harsh toilet training methods are to be avoided. Issues of embarrassment and stigmatisation must be addressed by ensuring that the child has multiple changes of clothes in the event of an accident. Behavioural methods have proven effective in most cases. These include toilet training (e.g. ensuring that the child sits on the toilet at regular and planned intervals). When the child successfully passes faeces in the toilet, this behaviour is then reinforced by the parent. Laxatives, preferably osmotic or mineral oil laxatives, may be prescribed for patients with constipation. The prognosis of the condition depends largely on the cause. Many children will continue to have a lifelong disturbed bowel function (Von Gontard, 2012).

## 27.13 Feeding and eating disorders of infancy and early childhood

In feeding and eating disorders of infancy and early childhood the infant or child fails to eat appropriately, to the extent that he or she loses weight or fails to gain weight. These disorders are only diagnosed if medical conditions that could account for the symptoms have been excluded. There are three conditions described: pica, rumination disorder and a revised category of avoidant/restrictive food intake disorder.

### 27.13.1 Pica

Pica is a condition where the child or infant persistently eats non-food substances for at least one month. The condition is fairly common, occurring in 15% of children aged 2–3 year, with both sexes being equally affected. It occurs more commonly in individuals with intellectual disability. Complications of the disorder include lead poisoning, gastrointestinal parasite infestation and (rarely) intestinal obstruction. In many cases, the disorder is transient in nature and most remit. The condition is sometimes associated with deficiencies of iron or zinc and levels of these minerals should be investigated.

### 27.13.2 Rumination disorder

Infants with rumination disorder induce regurgitation of food by sucking their tongue, arching their back or even putting their hand into their mouth. The regurgitated food may be expelled or reswallowed. The infant appears to derive pleasure and comfort from the act of rechewing and reswallowing the food. The condition is rare, but should be considered in a child that fails to thrive.

### 27.13.3 Avoidant or restrictive food intake disorder

Children with avoidant or restrictive food intake disorder fail to feed or eat appropriately. This may result from factors such as lack of interest in eating, consuming a severely limited diet (by only choosing foods that share certain sensory characteristics) and displaying aversion to eating or feeding. These abnormal eating or feeding patterns are not caused by other general medical conditions or other psychiatric illnesses, such as depression. Whatever the cause, the behaviours are severe enough to cause weight loss or disturbed growth, nutritional deficiencies and sometimes dependence on nutritional supplements. The condition also impacts negatively on psychosocial functioning. The condition can be differentiated from eating disorders such as anorexia nervosa and bulimia nervosa by the fact that body image concerns are usually not present.

### 27.13.4 Treatment of feeding and eating disorders of infancy and early childhood

The child's parents or caregivers play an important role in the treatment of these conditions. Parent education and ongoing support should be considered a critical part of treatment. In general, treatment involves behavioural techniques, including negative reinforcement and aversive therapy. Environmental manipulation may also be required. There is little justification for pharmacotherapy (Sadock BJ and Sadock VA, 2009).

## 27.14 Special areas involving children

### 27.14.1 Poor school performance

Learning and education are important aspects of a child's development and every child should have the opportunity to reach his or her academic potential. Poor school performance should be viewed as a symptom that reflects an underlying difficulty that must be identified and managed. Neglecting to address the symptom of poor school performance has significant negative consequences for the child, such as low self-esteem, stress and fewer opportunities.

A comprehensive evaluation is required to find the cause of the poor school performance: a wide variety of biological, psychological and social factors may give rise to this symptom. A careful history obtained from multiple informants (including the child, parents or caregivers, teacher and school counsellor) and a physical examination assist in making a provisional diagnosis. This will inform further investigations and appropriate referral to a psychologist, paediatrician, child psychiatrist, ENT specialist, optometrist etc. as necessary for further management.

It is important to find the reason(s) for a child's poor school performance and come up with a treatment plan early so that the child can reach his or her full potential.

#### 27.14.1.1 Causes of poor school performance

- Medical conditions that may have an independent effect on school performance include:
  - preterm birth and low birth weight
  - malnutrition and nutritional deficiencies
  - worm infestations
  - hearing impairment
  - visual impairment
  - habitual snoring
  - asthma and allergic rhinitis
  - epilepsy
  - other chronic diseases (e.g. HIV, cancer).
- Psychiatric disorders include:
  - intellectual disability
  - specific learning disability
  - ADHD
  - autism
  - mood and anxiety disorders.
- Psychological or emotional factors such as:
  - abuse and neglect
  - bullying and fears
  - adjustment difficulties
  - relationship problems.
- Social factors such as:
  - poor socioeconomic status
  - environmental factors
  - cultural influences.

#### 27.14.1.2 Management of poor school performance

Poor school performance can be managed by:

- taking a careful history from multiple informants
- a complete examination
- being on the look out for reversible medical conditions
- doing appropriate investigations to find a cause
- making relevant referrals, if necessary, for further evaluation and management.

### 27.14.2 HIV and child mental health

An estimated 3,4 million children globally were living with HIV at the end of 2011; 91% of them were from sub-Saharan Africa. HIV-infection has had a major impact on the mental health of affected children in southern Africa. Children are affected by the medical and psychosocial consequences of having the disease themselves and by the psychosocial sequelae of caregivers having the disease.

Most HIV infections in children are passed from mother to child during pregnancy, labour and delivery or breastfeeding. Blood transfusions using infected blood or injections with unsterilised needles can lead to HIV infection in children. Although sexual transmission is not a main cause of HIV/Aids among children, it does occur in countries where children become sexually active at an early age. Children may also become infected through sexual abuse.

Many babies and children living with HIV are known or suspected to have the infection because their mothers are known to be infected. However, sometimes infection is not suspected until a child develops symptoms. Symptoms of HIV infection varies by age and individual child. Some of the more common symptoms are given below.

- failure to thrive and to reach developmental milestones during the expected time frame
- as HIV infection becomes more advanced, children start to develop opportunistic infections

- neurological problems like seizures, difficulty with walking or poor performance in school
- psychiatric manifestations that may range from psychosis, depression and anxiety to cognitive deterioration. HIV infection must be excluded when a child presents with mental health difficulties.

#### 27.14.2.1 Psychiatric relevance in HIV infection

The relationship between HIV and mental health may be best understood from the bio-psycho-social perspective that explains the genesis of psychiatric illnesses. There are various factors associated with HIV/Aids that can predispose an HIV-infected child to develop psychiatric symptoms or disorders. These factors may be classified into biological, psychological and societal factors. This classification is, however, arbitrary as one factor (e.g. biological) can lead to the occurrence of other factors (psychological or social) which may, in turn, predispose a child for psychiatric illness.

**Biological**

- The predilection of HIV to affect the central nervous system, thus developing a risk to develop psychiatric illness.
- Effects of having a chronic illness.
- Body infirmity because of physical effects of HIV infection leading to body image disturbance.
- Neuropsychiatric adverse effects of antiretroviral treatment as well as other medication used in HIV infection.

**Psychosocial**

- History of repeated hospitalisation and isolation from peers are known to have an adverse effect on a child's social, cognitive and communicative development.
- The effect of stigma and discrimination.
- Fear of death and suffering.
- Family conflict and stress because of the illness.
- Grief with loss of family member due to HIV/Aids.
- Lack of provision of care and support of child, poor socioeconomic environment.

#### 27.14.2.2 Psychiatric manifestation in HIV-infected children

A number of factors make the task of diagnosing psychiatric disorders in HIV infection difficult. First, there are a number of non-pathological states, such as grief and mourning in relation to personal loss, which must be differentiated from major psychiatric illness such as depression and anxiety. Second, many children who present with symptoms that resemble depression or anxiety may have these symptoms because of organic conditions ranging from central nervous system (CNS) infections and encephalopathy to malnutrition and growth stunting. Finally, signs or symptoms that resemble psychiatric illness may be the side effects of medication used to treat HIV and related conditions. Thus one must take a number of factors into account before making a diagnosis of psychiatric illness.

#### 27.14.2.3 Psychosocial aspects of HIV in children

Psychosocial aspects are the major concern in the case of children in southern Africa. In many instances, HIV infection co-exists with social adversity. Families in which HIV infection occurs may have any or all of the following problems:

- where parent(s) are ill and cannot work (with resulting poverty) or cannot cope adequately with the demands of parenting, emotions often run high, with anger, guilt, anxiety and fear of death being experienced
- loss of one or both parents places the burden of child-rearing on members of the extended family, who may or may not be willing or able to cope with these demands
- when there is no suitable adult available to care for surviving children, children have to assume adult responsibilities in a child-headed family
- for the children involved, there are the traumas of parental illness and death. In

southern Africa, the social structures needed to assist single parents (especially those who are ill) and to care for children when their parents are in hospital or when they become orphaned, are grossly inadequate.

#### 27.14.2.4 Management

- A multidisciplinary case management is important to provide holistic care and support.
- Improved antiretroviral treatment adherence is associated with improved neurocognitive outcomes in children with HIV.
- Consider a psychiatric illness when any behavioural or psychological symptoms that are not fully explained by medical illness are encountered.
- Pharmacological management of psychiatric illness in children with HIV must be carefully considered. Initiate with low doses to avoid the side effects to which these children are susceptible.

### 27.14.3 Child abuse and neglect

Child abuse and child neglect include all types of physical and/or emotional ill-treatment, sexual abuse, neglect, negligence and commercial or other exploitation, which result in actual or potential harm to the child's health, survival, development or dignity in the context of a relationship of responsibility, trust or power.

In South Africa, the statistics for child abuse and neglect are high; however, the statistics do not accurately reflect the real extent, as many cases go unreported. Given the high estimates of unreported cases, one must be vigilant in recognising abuse when a child presents with behavioural changes. Children who have been abused may display a range of emotional and behavioural reactions, many of which are characteristic of children who have experienced other types of trauma.

The following behaviours are some of the indicators that may suggest abuse:

- being nervous of physical contact with adults
- crying when it is time to leave a protected environment
- an increase in nightmares and/or other sleeping difficulties
- withdrawn behaviour
- angry outbursts
- anxiety
- depression
- regression
- not wanting to be left alone with a particular individual(s)
- lying and stealing
- a drop in scholastic performance
- sexual knowledge, language, and/or behaviour that are inappropriate for the child's age
- absence from school.

#### 27.14.3.1 Management of child abuse or neglect

- Compulsory reporting to South African Police Services, to a commissioner of child welfare or to a social worker for investigation, is required if there is a legitimate suspicion of abuse and neglect.
- Ensure the immediate safety of the child and the prevention of further abuse.
- Provide counselling for child and family, if needed.
- Provide monitoring to detect development of psychiatric symptoms, which may require treatment.

## 27.15 General principles of management

- Co-morbidity is common: assess for other disorders that may co-occur.
- Although most behavioural and emotional difficulties respond to psychosocial interventions, pharmacotherapy may at times be indicated in addition to psychosocial methods. The judicious use of medication is essential; weigh up the benefits of medication use against the potential risk. Children have a higher metabolic rate of breakdown of medication than adults; therefore they may need higher and more frequent doses of medication

than expected for their weight. Keep in mind that there is considerable variation between children in their response to the same dose of medication. Children also differ from adults with regard to their sensitivity to certain medication and their vulnerability to side effects. Since negative perceptions may affect compliance, address all concerns raised regarding the use of medication by clear explanations.

- Psychosocial treatment includes a variety of modalities, including psycho-educational counselling, supportive counselling, crisis intervention counselling, parent counselling, family counselling, education support services, individual and group therapy and family therapy.
- Hospital admission is indicated as a last resort as, in accordance with the MHCA (No. 17 of 2002) one is obliged to provide treatment in the least restrictive environment. However, in situations where the difficulties are serious, where there is impairment in functioning in more than one area of the child's life, in cases where the safety of the child and those around him or her are compromised or where outpatient treatments have failed, it may be in the child's best interests to be admitted in a unit that provides a multidisciplinary team approach to assessment and care. Young children are usually managed in a paediatric ward.
- Ethical considerations are particularly pertinent to children, being a doubly vulnerable population. The doctor is obliged to assume an advocacy role for the child and to make decisions that are in the best interests of the child as stipulated by the The Children's Act (No. 38 of 2005). There is a duty to report suspected cases of abuse and neglect of a child. Parental informed consent is required as most children may not be of sufficient maturity to make informed decisions regarding their treatment options.

## Conclusion

Children are a particularly vulnerable population as they depend on adults for their basic physical and emotional needs. Therefore it is an imperative to be ethically mindful in their care. As the biopsychosocial development of children can be affected adversely by unmet needs or adverse circumstances, and their rates of development vary greatly across ages, it is important to assess children from this developmental perspective and in a comprehensive biopsychosocial context. Information is best gained from multiple informants such as parents, caregivers, and teachers as views may be biased. Assessing a child clinically calls upon the clinician to be flexible in approach according to the child's age and capabilities. Behavioural and emotional difficulties are common in the young child, and psychological interventions are often the most effective. Pharmacotherapy use in the young child has to be cautious, as long-term effects on the developing brain are unknown. There is a responsibility to advocate for the opportunity of each child to flourish and reach its best potential.

## 27.1 Advanced reading block

**Current legislation and policy guidelines relevant to relevant to the mental health care of children**

**1. The Constitution of the Republic of South Africa, 1996**

Section 28 of the Constitution provides for children's rights in terms of the rights to basic care.

**2. The Reconstruction and Development Program (RDP) of South Africa**

The RDP contains a series of national goals for children that serve as a means to entrench the rights of children, such as providing improved protection of children in difficult circumstances.

**3. The United Nations Convention on the Rights of the Child (CRC)**

In June 1995, the South African government ratified this convention, and by so doing, the government pledged itself to enhance the survival, protection and development of the children of South Africa. This was encapsulated in the principle of the First Call for Children in South Africa.

**4. The National Program of Action for Children in South Africa, 1996**

The National Program of Action for Children in South Africa (NPA) is the instrument by which South Africa's commitments to children in terms of the UN's Convention is expressed.

**5. The Mental Health Care Act (No. 17 of 2002)**

The Mental Health Care Act does not specifically emphasise the mental health needs of children and adolescents, but their inclusion is implicit in the definition of a mental health care user in the Act. Of particular relevance in this regard are the emphasis on holistic, integrated and community-based care at primary, secondary and tertiary levels of care and the promotion of mental health in the population as whole.

**6. Child and Adolescent Mental Health Policy Guidelines, 2003**

These policy guidelines serve as framework for establishing mental health services for children and adolescents at national, provincial and local levels of health care within the primary health care approach and by using an intersectoral approach. They have been developed in relation to other South African policies, legislation and treaties that address the enhancement of survival as well as well the protection and development of children and adolescents.

**7. The Children's Act (No. 38 of 2005)**

This is the foremost statute for the protection of children and pertains to matters regarding the best interest of the child, informed consent, abuse and neglect. It compels health care professionals, social workers, teachers and managers and staff of children's homes, places of care and shelters to report suspected ill treatment of children attended by them.

**8. The National Health Policy Guidelines for Improved Mental Health in South Africa**

One of the key priority areas identified in the intervention framework is the mental health service for children. It is indicated that the priority for mental health services for children should be prevention and that the services need to be integrated into general primary health care. Areas of special focus are prevention of delays in emotional and intellectual development, introduction of life skills education and prevention of substance-related problems such as foetal alcohol syndrome.

# References


Achenbach TM, Edelbrock C (1991) *The Child Behavior Checklist and Revised Child Behavior Profile*. Burlington, VT: University Associates in Psychiatry

American Academy of Child and Adolescent Psychiatry. (2014). Practise parameters for the assessment and treatment of children and adolescents with Autism Spectrum Disorder. *Journal of the American Academy of Child and Adolescent Psychiatry* 53(2): 237–257

American Psychiatric Association (2000) *Diagnostic and Statistical Manual of Mental Disorders* (4th edition). Washington, DC: American Psychiatric Association

American Psychiatric Association (2013) *Diagnostic and Statistical Manual of Mental Disorders* (5th edition). Washington, DC: American Psychiatric Association

Caldwell PHY, Nankivell G, Sureshkumar P (2013) Simple behavioural interventions for nocturnal enuresis in children. *Cochrane Database of Systematic Reviews* Issue 7. Article No. CD003637. DOI: 10.1002/14651858. CD003637.pub3

Center for Disease Control and Prevention (*s.d.*) *Austism*. www.http://www.cdc.gov/ncddd/autism/data.html (Accessed 30 October 2015)

Conners CK (1997) *Conners' Rating Scales — Revised*. Toronto, ON: Multi-Health Systems

Costello EJ, Mustillo S, Erkanli A, Keeler G, Angold A. (2003) Prevalence and development of psychiatric disorders in childhood and adolescence. *Archives of General Psychiatry* 60(8): 837–44

Department of Health, Republic of South Africa (1997) *The National Health Policy Guidelines for Improved Mental Health in South Africa*. Pretoria: Department of Health, Republic of South Africa

Department of Health, Republic of South Africa (2003) *National Policy Guidelines for Child and Adolescent Mental Health*. Pretoria: Department of Health, Republic of South Africa

Department of Women, Children and People with Disabilities, Republic of south Africa (1996) *The National Plan of Action for Children in South Africa*. Pretoria: Department of Women, Children and People with Disabilities, Republic of South Africa))

Figueroa A, Soutullo C, Ono Y, Saito K (2012) Separation anxiety. In: Rey JM. *IACAPAP Textbook of Child and Adolescent Mental Health* Available at: htpp: //iacapap-textbook-of-child-and-adolescent-mental-health) Geneva: International Association for Child and Adolescent Psychiatry and Allied Profession

Freitag C (2007) The genetics of autistic disorders and its clinical relevance: A review of the literature. *Molecular Psychiatry* 12: 2–22

Glazener CMA, Evans JHC, Peto RE (2005) Alarm interventions for nocturnal enuresis in children. *Cochrane Database of Systematic Reviews*, Issue 2. Article No. CD002911 DOI:10.1002/14651858.CD002911.pub2

Goodman R (1997) The Strengths and Difficulties Questionnaire: A research note. *Journal of Child Psychology and Psychiatry* 38: 581–6

Lai MC, Lombardo MV, Baron-Cohen S (2014) Autism. *The Lancet* 383: 896–910

Leibenluft E (2011) Severe mood dysregulation, irritability, and the diagnostic boundaries of bipolar disorder. *American Journal of Psychiatry* 168: 129–42

McPheeters M, Warren Z, Sathe N, Bruzek J, Krishnaswami S, Jerome RE (2011) A systematic review of medical treatments for children with autism spectrum disorders. *Pediatrics* 127(5): 1312–21

Mikita N, Stringaris A (2012) Mood dysregulation. *European Child and Adolescent Psychiatry* 22 (Suppl 1): S11–S6

National Institute for Health and Care Excellence (NICE) (2013). *Antisocial behaviour and conduct disorders in children and young people: recognition, intervention and management.*

Pappadopulos E, Woolston S, Chait AE (2006) Pharmacotherapy of aggression in children and adolescents: Efficacy and effect size. *Journal of the Canadian Academy of Child and Adolescent Psychiatry* 15(1): 27–39

Republic of South Africa (1994) *The Reconstruction and Development Programme* Republic of South Africa

Sadock BJ and Sadock VA (2009) *Feeding and eating disorders of infancy and childhood. Concise textbook of child and adolescent psychiatry*. Philadelphia: Lippincott, Williams and Wilkins

Scott S (2012) Conduct disorders. In Rey JM (Ed.) *IACAPAP e-Textbook of Child and Adolescent Mental Health*. Geneva: International Association for Child and Adolescent Psychiatry and Allied Professions

Steiner H, Remsing L (2007) Practice parameter for the assessment and treatment of children and adolescents with oppositional defiant disorder. *Journal of the American Academy of Child and Adolescent Psychiatry* 46(1): 126–41

United Nations (1989) *The United Nations Convention on the Rights of the Child*. Available at: http://www.refworld.org/docid/3ae6b38f0.html (Accessed 19 January 2015)

Von Gontard A (2012) Encopresis. In: Rey JM (Ed.) *IACAPAP e-Textbook of Child and Adolescent Mental Health*. Geneva: International Association for Child and Adolescent Psychiatry and Allied Professions http://iacapap.org/iacapap-textbook-of-child-and-adolescent-mental-health (Accessed 29 January 2015)

Von Gontard A (2012). Enuresis. In: Rey JM (Ed.) *IACAPAP e-Textbook of Child and Adolescent Mental Health*. Geneva: International Association for Child and Adolescent Psychiatry and Allied Professions (Accessed 29 January 2015)

Zepf FD, Holtmann M (2012) Disruptive mood dysregulation disorder. In: Rey JM (Ed.) *IACAPAP e-Textbook of Child and Adolescent Mental Health*. Geneva: International Association for Child and Adolescent Psychiatry and Allied Professions http://iacapap.org/iacapap-textbook-of-child-and-adolescent-mental-health (Accessed 29 January 2015)

# CHAPTER 28 Child and adolescent psychiatry 2: The older child and adolescent

*Saeeda Paruk, Debbie van der Westhuizen, Angelo Lasich*

## 28.1 Introduction

Adolescence is a unique period of maturation; a creative transitional period between childhood and adulthood (Goodman and Scott, 2012). Adolescence is marked by its own bio-psycho-social growth features. Physical changes include the development of primary and secondary sexual characteristics, the surging of sexual hormones of puberty and marked growth in stature and muscle mass (Pataki, 2005). Cognitive and social developmental changes in adolescence include a dramatic growth in cognitive abilities, deepening of peer relationships, growth of autonomy in decision making, seeking intellectual recreation and social belonging. Likewise, adolescence is a period of paradoxes: sexual maturity is reached well before that of cognitive and emotional maturity, resulting in a confusing legal status comprising a mixture of privileges and reprimands (Martin and Volkmar, 2007; Arnett, 2000; Scott and Woolard, 2004).

The 'stress and storm debate' regarding the frequency and severity of adolescent turmoil has been decided: most normal adolescents go through this developmental period with hopefulness, good-self-esteem, maintaining good peer relationships and sustaining a satisfying relationship with their families (Robins and Trzesniewski, 2005; Martin and Volkmar, 2007; Arnett 1999).

Additionally, adolescents are trying to work towards a sense of identity that bridges internal inspirations and external realities of modern world challenges such as globalisation, smaller families, longer lifespans and urbanisation. Although society offers adolescents a puzzling variety of possible adult roles, in practice, the options are limited and unspectacular (Goodman and Scott, 2012).

A substantial proportion of adolescents may experience an increase in conflict with their parents, suffer from mood difficulties and engage in high-risk behaviour. The commonest causes of arguments with parents are about issues concerning autonomy and rules. However, only 20% of adolescents have diagnosable clinical disorders. Psychiatric disorders diagnosed in adolescence are either the continuation of childhood disorders or early manifestations of adult disorders (Goodman and Scott, 2012).

Adolescent sexual behaviour usually starts off with healthy sexual experimentation such as fantasy and masturbation. A number of factors may prevent physically safe sexual practices, giving rise to major challenges for society. Adolescent mothers may be vulnerable to an accumulation of health risks including difficulties in caring for the child, inability to attend antenatal care, issues related to abortions with her parents' consent, prostitution, sexually transmitted diseases such as HIV/Aids and drug use (e.g. alcohol, nicotine, cannabis, cocaine, opioids, heroin). High-risk sexual behaviour has been associated with personality traits, gender, cultural and religious background, racial factors, family attitudes towards prevention and sex-education programs (Sadock BJ and Sadock VA, 2007).

Violence in adolescence includes violent crimes and homicides. School violence (murder and suicides) is associated with male gender, growing up with guns and knives or an absent father or a father substitute, bullying, gang violence, impulsivity, learning difficulties, low IQ and fearlessness (Dishion *et al.*, 2005; Harris, 2005; Ozer, 2005).

Consequently, adolescent development is secured in the child's capacity to develop independence and autonomy from the parents, grow the ability to develop interdependence and form and sustain mutually supportive relationships outside the family. Following the ecological perspective, individual adolescent's relationships are seen as rooted in the interrelated contexts of family, school, neighbourhood and culture (Collins and Steinberg, 2006).

## 28.2 Psychiatric assessment of the adolescent

It is far better to start a thorough psychiatric assessment of an adolescent with a clear idea of the goals of the interview and then to pursue them flexibly (Goodman and Scott, 2012).

One of the goals of the clinical psychiatric assessment is to identify the presence of psychopathology; this is based on detecting any developmental deviations and maladaptive psychodynamic patterns. Listing of target symptoms should then follow.

The next step is to guide the planning of appropriate interventions and/or treatment, such as addressing co-morbidities and multiple problems that may influence adherence to treatment efforts (e.g. relevant environmental variables such as family or school factors, as well as protective and resilience factors (Goodman and Scott, 2012).

A comprehensive psychiatric assessment consists of multiple interviews with the parent, the adolescent, family members and gathering information regarding current school functioning (see Table 28.1). If available, details regarding standardised assessment of the adolescent's intellectual level and academic achievement should be acquired. In some cases, standardised measures of developmental level and neuropsychological development are valuable. Psychiatric assessments should include information obtained about the parents, the family and the school, as well as information from social and legal agencies to appreciate the reasons behind the evaluation (see Table 28.2) (Dulcan, 2010).

The psychiatric assessment of adolescents is more similar to the psychiatric assessment of adults than that of younger children (see Table 28.3, Table 28.4, Table 28.5) (Dulcan, 2010).

**Table 28.1** Elements of a comprehensive assessment

| |
|---|
| ▶ Adolescent interview |
| ▶ Parent interview |
| ▶ Interview with teachers (could be by phone after obtaining consent from parents) |
| ▶ Family interview as appropriate |
| ▶ Interviews with other family members (siblings, grandparents, other caretakers) |
| ▶ Medical records from primary care physician |
| ▶ Prior mental health treatment records |
| ▶ School records |
| ▶ Records from other involved agencies (e.g. social services, juvenile justice) |
| ▶ Standardised measures (rating scales, symptom checklists, diagnostic interviews) as needed to assess problem behaviour or symptoms |
| ▶ Psychological testing |

**Source:** Reprinted with permission from *Dulcan's Textbook of Child and Adolescent Psychiatry*, First Edition, (Copyright ©2010). American Psychiatric Association. All Rights Reserved.

There are typical differences between adolescent psychiatric assessments and adult assessments.

- Adolescents rarely initiate psychiatric assessment or treatment themselves; in most cases it is the parent or caregiver who seeks treatment for the adolescent.
- The adolescent's behaviour usually may cause greater distress to the parents or adults than to themselves.
- Sometimes, the parents may expect too much of the adolescent and seek ways to change the adolescent to suit their own needs; an adult's expectations for the adolescent might exceed the adolescent's abilities, for example, or the adult's parenting or teaching style may be a poor fit with that of the adolescent.
- Adolescents may not recognise their behaviour as problematic for others (Dulcan, 2010).

## 28.2.1 Start of the assessment

The first decision is to decide whom to invite to the initial interview: autonomy issues and struggles for separation are important to take into consideration. The way the initial interview is handled can have a significant positive or negative effect. Seeing the parent(s) first may result in resistance and oppositional behaviour, as the adolescent may place the clinician in the role of an agent of the parent.

In most cases, starting the initial assessment with parent(s) and adolescent together may be productive. It also allows the clinician to assess the relationship between the adolescent and the parent(s). Both parent and adolescent should understand the structure and process of the evaluation.

For the adolescent to feel comfortable providing details about his or her life and feelings, confidentiality issues must be explained to both the parent and the adolescent. Both parties must know how much will be communicated to the parent. Coming to an understanding of how confidentiality will be handled will avoid some uncomfortable situations and allows for an easier first interview (Dulcan, 2010).

## 28.2.2 Detailed psychiatric assessment of an adolescent

Performing a detailed psychiatric assessment of an adolescent involves appropriate engagement between interviewer and the family in order to start laying the foundations for treatment while focusing on five key questions discussed below (Goodman and Scott, 2012; Le Couteur and Gardner, 2008; Taylor and Rutter, 2008).

A. Symptom identification to clarify what sort of problem it is. Most psychiatric syndromes that affect adolescents involve combinations of symptoms and signs from more than one domain:
   1. Emotional symptoms: enquire about anxiety, fears, any subsequent avoidance, discontent and associated depressive features; worthlessness, hopelessness, self-harm, inability to take pleasure in activities usually enjoyable (anhedonia), poor appetite, sleep disturbance and lack of energy. Obtain parental reports and self-reports in older children. Where there are disagreements on emotional symptoms between parent and child, accept that there are multiple perspectives rather than one single truth.
   2. Behavioural symptoms or problems usually dominate adolescent and child practice. Focus enquiries on three domains of behaviour: defiant behaviour (irritability and temper outbursts), aggression and destructiveness and anti-social behaviour (stealing, fire-setting, substance abuse). Adolescents find it hard to recognise their own unreasonable and defiant behaviour.
   3. Developmental symptoms delay: a background in child and adolescent health will assist the clinician in the identification of age and developmental delays; growth charts are useful to spot very small or tall adolescents. Observing family interactions in the

waiting or consulting room may be helpful:

- Particular relevant areas of delay for adolescents include attention and activity regulation, speech and language, play, motor skills, bladder and bowel control, and scholastic attainments in reading, spelling and mathematics. Current levels of functioning may be judged through direct observation and interview of the adolescent and parents as well as reports from parents and teachers.
- Gathering information from parents about the adolescent's developmental milestones can tell us about previous developmental course.
- Another taxing task is assessing the adolescent's difficulties in social relatedness. Autistic individuals seem to have an aloof indifference to other people as people, a passive acceptance of interactions when others take the initiative and an awkward and un-empathetic social interest. This tends to put others off.
- Attachment may be insecure with the main caregiver but secure with other caregivers (attachment may be secure, resistant, aloof, disorganised). See how the adolescent relates to you during the physical and mental state examination (shy, monosyllabic or welcomes you as a best friend trying to hug or kiss you).

4. Relationship difficulties both at home (sibling, parents) and/or at school (peer group, teachers).

B. Impact of these symptoms on functioning: elicit how much distress or impairment the symptoms cause. Impact criteria are judged on social impairment (family life, classroom learning, friendships, leisure activities), distress for the adolescent himself or herself and disruption for others.

C. Risk factors identification: establish what factors have initiated and maintained the problem. Most of the causes in adolescent and child psychiatry are best thought of as risk factors. The presence of a disorder can be explained by predisposing, precipitating and perpetuating factors in the absence of protective factors.

D. Strengths identification: elicit what resources there are to work with. The treatment plan must build on the strengths of the individual and the family and also on the strengths of the school and wider social network. Focusing exclusively on the negatives may leave the family feeling emotionally mistreated. When seeing parents who seem to have particularly obvious weaknesses, put more effort into identify their strengths.

E. Explanatory model of the family: understand what expectations and beliefs the family brings with them. After asking the family about the presenting complaint, enquire about how they see the problem, what they think it is due to, and how they think it might be investigated and treated. Knowing about families' explanatory models gives the clinician a chance to present the bio-psycho-social views of the doctor in a way that will be most relevant to them. It will also allow them to update their explanatory model if you take time to explain the facts (i.e. psycho-education).

**Table 28.2** Elements of data collection from the parents

| **Parental history** | **Developmental history of identified adolescent** |
|---|---|
| ▸ How they met<br>▸ History of the relationship<br>▸ Problems in the relationship<br>▸ Decision to marry<br>▸ Having children: planned?<br>▸ Response to pregnancy: happy/anxious?<br>▸ Relationship after children<br>▸ Style of discipline<br>▸ Marital problems<br>▸ Their expectations for the child?<br>▸ What were their childhoods like?<br>▸ Do they agree on rules and discipline application?<br>▸ Circumstances: housing, debt, contact with social services?<br>▸ Family assessment: family's structure, relationships and boundaries, communication, belief systems and regulatory processes | ▸ Problems during pregnancy<br>▸ Perinatal problems<br>▸ Birth and delivery<br>▸ What sort of baby? Easy/difficult?<br>▸ Developmental milestones:<br>– feeding problems<br>– motor development<br>– language problem<br>– play<br>– peer relationships<br>– educational history: schools' names, grades and dates?<br>– difficulties in classroom?<br>– learning disabilities<br>▸ Physical health: fits and faints, illnesses, special investigations, hospital or psychiatric contact? |
| **Sibling relationship** | **Family history of mental illness** |
| ▸ Birth order<br>▸ Relationship with siblings<br>▸ Physical or emotional problems with siblings | ▸ Examination of each parent may be needed<br>▸ Draw a family tree (a genogram)<br>▸ Ask a few details about the relatives, medical and psychiatric problems |
| **Presenting complaint** | **Current functioning** |
| ▸ When did it begin? When last was he or she completely well?<br>▸ How does the presenting complaint show itself? Give specific examples<br>▸ What happens before, after and what is your response? Effect on rest of family?<br>▸ Review symptoms: behaviour, attention, activity, emotions, eating, sleeping, bladder, bowels, pains and tics | ▸ Typical day's activities: dressing, eating, playing and leisure, going to bed, sleeping; how involved are the parents?<br>▸ Social relationships: any friends? Sleepovers? How often? Leader? Sexuality?<br>▸ Adults: How does child get on with each parent? Other carers? How do they feel about the child?<br>▸ Spend time with siblings? Like/dislike/jealous? |

**Source:** Reprinted with permission from *Dulcan's Textbook of Child and Adolescent Psychiatry*, First Edition, (Copyright ©2010). American Psychiatric Association. 

**Table 28.3** How to see the adolescent alone: elements of data collection during the adolescent interview

| |
|---|
| ▶ Do not rush into difficult topics; engage first by focusing initially on pleasant or neutral topics<br>▶ Some parents have used referrals to clinic as a threat: ensure a positive experience |
| ▶ Observe: activity and attention: fidgeting, distracted? Quality of social interaction: too much or too little anxiety about coming to you? Good eye contact? Inappropriate, friendly, over-familiar, cheeky? Developmental level: complexity of language, ideas, drawings, play?<br>▶ Find out where the adolescent would measure his or her current life situation on a scale (bad (0%), good and bad (50/50), good (100%)?<br>▶ Address undisclosed abuse: sometimes nasty things happen to people; has anything like that ever happened to you? |
| ▶ Chief complaint |
| ▶ History of present illness |
| ▶ Screening for psychiatric disorders |
| ▶ Substance use |
| ▶ Educational history |
| ▶ Family relationships |
| ▶ Peer relationships |
| ▶ Hobbies, interests, sports, music |
| ▶ Sexual history |
| ▶ Religious, spiritual, cultural history |

**Source:** Dulcan, 2010; Goodman and Scott, 2012

**Table 28.4** Elements of the mental status evaluation

| **Mental status of the adolescent** |
|---|
| ▶ Attitude and behaviour |
| ▶ Eye contact |
| ▶ Hygiene and style of dress |
| ▶ Speech: fluency, rate, rhythm, prosody |
| ▶ Motor: gait, co-ordination, abnormal movements |
| ▶ Orientation (person, place, time, circumstances) |
| ▶ Affect (perceived by interviewer) |
| ▶ Mood (reported by adolescent) |
| ▶ Suicidal or homicidal ideation, plan, intent |
| ▶ Thought process and form of thinking (logical or looseness of associations, flight of ideas or poverty of thinking, thought blocking, preservation?) |
| ▶ Thought content and thinking about (ideas, beliefs, pre-occupations, obsessions, suicide, delusions) |
| ▶ Perceptions: auditory, visual, tactile or olfactory hallucinations |
| ▶ Memory: immediate, recent, remote or long term |
| ▶ Intellectual functioning: calculations, geography, presidents |

| ▶ Abstraction: proverbs, similarities |
|---|
| ▶ Insight |
| ▶ Judgement |
| ▶ Reliability |

**Source:** Reprinted with permission from *Dulcan's Textbook of Child and Adolescent Psychiatry*, First Edition, (Copyright ©2010). American Psychiatric Association. All Rights Reserved.

**Table 28.5** Other important information to be obtained

| Obtain information from teachers: school report or teacher feedback |
|---|
| Physical examination: especially vital signs, weight, height |
| Basic neurological evaluation:<br>▶ measure head circumference and plot it<br>▶ walk, run, hop and walk on a line on the floor<br>▶ observe the adolescent standing with feet together, arms outstretched, eyes closed<br>▶ check eye, face and tongue movements<br>▶ move and shake all four limbs<br>▶ test strengths<br>▶ test reflexes<br>▶ test co-ordination<br>▶ check visual or hearing problems. |
| Ideally all presenting adolescents need neurological examinations, especially if there is a history of seizures or regression, developmental delay or intellectual disability, abnormal gait, not using both hands well (e.g. when playing), **dysmorphic features**, skin signs of neuro-cutaneous disorder, speech difficulties, history of fever fits or head injuries with loss of consciousness |

**Source:** Goodman and Scott, 2012

All assessments should be seen as provisional and generating working hypotheses that have to be updated and corrected over the entire course of your contact with the family.

The final formulation (see Table 28.6) is based on inputs from all team members, not only to inform feedback to the family but also to be used as a guide for subsequent management. Consider the need for reassessment if treatment does not work (Goodman and Scott, 2012).

**Table 28.6** The adolescent formulation should include the following elements

| ▶ Socio-demographic summary |
|---|
| ▶ Clinical presentation |
| ▶ Diagnosis |
| ▶ Causation |
| ▶ Management plan |
| ▶ Predicted outcome |

**Source:** Goodman and Scott, 2012

### 28.2.3 Motivational interviewing

Dealing with resistant and high-risk taking adolescents can pose a special challenge for the mental health care practitioner (Dulcan, 2010).

Motivational interviewing (MI) is an effective approach for raising problem awareness and facilitating change with youth who may be stuck or not yet ready to modify their high-risk behaviour, such as substance abuse, sexual risk taking or driving at speed.

Motivational interviewing is now being used with adolescents and children seen in a variety of settings including paediatric practice, schools, justice settings and emergency rooms (Friedman, 2006).

Motivational interviewing is a client-centred, directive method to improve intrinsic motivation for change by exploring and resolving indecision. This is accomplished through showing adolescent patients respect and by applying a certain set of skills. Once they experience a safe and comfortable therapeutic environment, they will be more likely to engage in an open examination of their lives to determine how to resolve their problems.

Motivational interviewing seems to be a particular good match with adolescents as it is brief, personalised and focused on normal development attractions towards identity formation, independence, acceptance and connection. It has shown to improve the adolescent's engagement and self-efficiency (Friedman, 2006).

**Information box**

**Motivational interviewing skills**

- Express empathy: this refers to the ability of the mental health care practitioner to view the world through the eyes of the adolescent, by seeing, feeling and understanding things as if living the same life experiences (i.e. put yourself in their shoes) and reassuring the adolescent that he or she is understood and not crazy.
- Develop discrepancy by using motivational change. This occurs when the adolescent recognises that there is a faulty connection between his or her behaviour, self-image, desires and goals. MI encourages adolescents to examine whether they are living with full integrity and, if not, to consider making changes.
- As resistance is common when working with adolescents, it is helpful to accept resistance by using a friendly and co-operative style and by not by arguing with or provoking the adolescent.
- Support self-efficacy: a troubled adolescent may be used to critical judgements and negative attention and may have lost hope. The mental health care practitioner should assist adolescents to identify their strengths by guiding them to recall past victories and achievements; this might enlighten positive abilities to confront new challenges.

## 28.3 Mood disorders in children and adolescents

The clinical presentation of mood disorders varies with age and developmental level. The recognition of mood disorders in children and adolescents is important as untreated mood disorders may have negative implications for growth and development, family and peer relationships, school performance, substance abuse and increased risk of suicide (Cook *et al.*, 2009; Keenan-Miller *et al.*, 2007; Thapar *et al.*, 2012).

### 28.3.1 Depression

#### 28.3.1.1 Prevalence

Mood disorders increase with age and prevalence ranges from 2% in younger children to 4–8% in adolescents (Jane Costello *et al.*, 2006). There is a marked increase in prevalence of depression in females after puberty (Thapar *et al.*, 2012).

#### 28.3.1.2 Aetiology

The risk factors for depression in children are similar to those in adults but genetic vulnerability to mood disorders is associated with an earlier age of onset in each successive generation. Having a parent with a mood disorder increases

**Information box**

**Motivational interviewing strategies to be used when working with adolescents and children**

- Be prepared and be a good host as the adolescent often arrives to an initial appointment angry.
- Conduct the initial interview with care, with a detailed discussion of the legal and professional limits of confidentiality as well as an overview of the possible range and scope of services offered.
- Establish rapport to construct a therapeutic patient-doctor relationship. This can be achieved through enquiring about less threatening topics first, followed by discussion of more threatening topics.
- Talk about the change process by discussing change. This is to provide a frame for discussions about goal-setting and measuring progress.
- Consider and validate the adolescent's worldview to ensure that he or she feels heard and understood.
- When providing personal feedback, stick to the facts and inform the adolescent fully and honestly about your decisions. First ask permission of the adolescent before offering any feedback advice.
- Carefully look for and acknowledge successes by recognising the patient's strengths and achievements.
- Be a good role model, as the power of a positive role model will inspire the adolescent (e.g. through motivating a healthy lifestyle.)
- Work enthusiastically to help make change worthwhile: help the adolescent to see the benefit of change.
- Ask for, and respond to, feedback.
- Avoid traps that will interfere with efforts to establish a meaningful relationship with the adolescent. When an adolescent is resistant, it usually is a signal that the mental health care practitioner's approach may be a problem. Examples of a problematic approach include asking too many questions, giving advice without permission, focusing prematurely on topics that the adolescent would prefer to avoid and using labels to describe problem behaviour.

**Source:** Friedman, 2006

the risk two- to threefold (Beardslee *et al.*, 1998; Weissman *et al.*, 1997). Psychosocial risk factors include abuse, neglect, family conflict and peer victimisation. General stressful life events often precipitate a depressive episode in biologically vulnerable adolescents (Goodyer *et al.*, 2000).

### 28.3.1.3 Clinical features

The DSM-5 diagnostic criteria for depression in children and adolescents are the same as for adults, except in children a failure to make expected weight gains may be noted instead of significant weight gain or loss as in adults (American Psychiatric Association, 2013).

Children often present with somatic complaints, temper tantrums, behavioural problems and poor school performance. Adolescents tend to present with apathy, psychomotor retardation, a sense of hopelessness, suicidal ideation, depressed mood (or, more commonly, irritable mood), insomnia and impaired concentration. They often describe themselves as 'useless' or life as 'no fun, boring and a waste'. The diagnosis of depression may be missed as older adolescents may present with oppositional or antisocial behaviour, use of substances, withdrawal and school difficulties. Less commonly, children and adolescents with severe depression may have hallucinations and delusions, which are generally mood congruent. It is also important to identify youth with subsyndromal depressive symptoms as they are at increased risk of later depressive disorders (Thapar *et al.*, 2012).

In the South African context, detecting underlying depressive disorders in children and adolescents living with chronic medical conditions such as HIV is important to promote optimal mental and physical development and treatment adherence (see Chapter 27: Child and adolescent psychiatry 1: Assessment and the young child, for the psychiatric complications of HIV in children). In chronically medically ill children, depression may be missed, as the **vegetative symptoms** from the medical disorder or complications of treatment (e.g. appetite and energy changes) overlap with the symptoms of depression.

### 28.3.1.4 Differential diagnosis

General medical conditions, substance-related disorders, anxiety and bereavement and disruptive behaviour disorders may have similar presentations.

### 28.3.1.5 Co-morbidity

Two-thirds of children and adolescents with depression have co-morbid psychiatric conditions. Common co-morbid disorders are anxiety disorders, attention-deficit hyperactivity disorder (ADHD), disruptive behaviour disorders, obsessive-compulsive disorder, eating disorders or substance-related disorders (Birmaher *et al.*, 1996).

### 28.3.1.6 Management

A suicide-risk assessment must always be a routine part of the assessment at every visit.

Hospitalisation is indicated if patient is a danger to themselves or others.

Treatment of depression is multimodal with combination treatment of psychotherapy and antidepressants.

Psychotherapy, including psycho-education of the patient and his or her family and cognitive behavioural therapy (CBT) is generally the first-line treatment in mild depression (Thapar *et al.*, 2012).

Treatment with antidepressants for six months to a year may be indicated for moderate to severe depression, recurrent depression, poor response to psychotherapy and in the presence of psychosocial stressors. Tricyclic antidepressants are not effective in children (National Institute for Health Care and Excellence, 2012; Taylor *et al.*, 2009). Selective serotonin reuptake inhibitors (SSRIs) are considered a first-line intervention for adolescents with depression; fluoxetine currently has the greatest evidence in child and adolescent depression (Rey, 2012; National Institute for Health Care and Excellence, 2012).

The risk of suicide with SSRI antidepressant initiation in children and adolescents is controversial (Hetrick *et al.*, 2007). The potential risk of treatment-emergent agitation and suicidal ideation can be managed with close monitoring of the patient for self-harm and informed consent from the caregiver for the use of psychotropic medication in children. Treatment should be tapered off over 6–12 weeks at the end of treatment.

### 28.3.1.7 Prognosis

Prognosis for a single episode is generally good but the risk of recurrence is estimated to increase to 70% after 5 years (Cook *et al.*, 2009). Age of onset, severity of symptoms and co-morbid disorders also influence outcome.

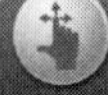

## Case study 28.1

**Case JJ**

J, a 15-year-old boy presents with a problem of chronic headache for the past six months. His parents report that he has become increasingly withdrawn and irritable, his grades have dropped this year and he has stopped playing sport, which he had previously enjoyed.

On enquiry, JJ admits to feeling hopeless for the past six months after discovering his 21-year-old sister is HIV positive. He calls himself a retard and feels guilty for not being able to help her. He denied suicidal ideation and psychotic symptoms. He was assessed as having moderate depression.

JJ and his parents chose to begin with psychotherapy.

## 28.3.2 Bipolar mood disorder

Bipolar I disorder is rare in pre-pubertal children and is more common in older adolescents with an estimated lifetime prevalence of 1% (Lewinsohn *et al.*, 1996).

### 28.3.2.1 Aetiology

Early onset of bipolar disorder is more common with a family history of bipolar disorder (Baldessarini, 2000). Twenty to forty per cent of children who present with psychotic depression will later develop bipolar disorder (Geller *et al.*, 1994).

Neurophysiological risk factors are similar to those in adults.

### 28.3.2.2 Clinical features

The DSM-5 criteria are as for adults. Adolescents with mania present with irritability, increased energy, increased self-esteem, unrealistic ambitions and, if challenged, they may have an aggressive outburst. Excessive spending, sexual disinhibition and an increase in risk-taking behaviour may also be features of mania. Children and adolescents may be more prone to rapid cycling (more frequent episodes of rapid mood fluctuations) or even ultra-rapid cycling (in contrast to the more discrete mood episodes experienced by adults) (Faedda *et al.*, 2004), making diagnosis more challenging in this age group.

Mixed episodes with mood fluctuating between mania/hypomania and depression may also occur.

### 28.3.2.3 Differential diagnosis

ADHD may be difficult to distinguish from bipolar disorders as the hyperactivity, talkativeness and impulsivity overlap, but adolescents with bipolar disorder tend to be more grandiose, sexually disinhibited and have a decreased need for sleep. ADHD may also be co-morbid in some children (Geller *et al.*, 1994).

Mood swings, aggressive outbursts and irritability may also be associated with severe depression or dysphoric mood dysregulation disorder (see Chapter 27: Child and adolescent psychiatry 1: Assessment and the young child).

Disruptive behaviour disorders, anxiety disorders, substance-related disorders, general medical conditions, psychosis and post-traumatic stress disorder (PTSD), which all have overlapping presentations, must be excluded.

### 28.3.2.4 Co-morbidity

Common co-morbid disorders include ADHD, disruptive-behaviour disorders and anxiety disorders. Case study 28.2 illustrates the co-morbid presentation of ADHD and bipolar mood disorder.

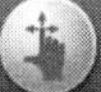

**Case study 28.2**

**Case SN**

SN, who is 15 years old, was diagnosed with ADHD at the age of 8 and has always had behavioural problems. He has been on methylphenidate for several years, with some improvement.

In the past six months, SN's grades have dropped and he has become increasingly irritable and stayed out overnight twice without explanation. He is constantly giggling in class, stays up late at night listening to loud music, wants to drop out of school and start his own music band.

His parents are concerned about possible substance use. There is a strong family history of mood disorders.

On assessment he was very talkative, hyperactive, and had an irritable mood.

SN was commenced on a mood stabiliser and responded well to treatment.

#### 28.3.2.5 Management

The adolescent may require hospitalisation in the acute phase of mania or if severely depressed.

First-line treatment in the acute manic episode is a mood stabiliser such as lithium, sodium valproate and/or an atypical antipsychotic with mood stabilising properties such as risperidone or clothiapine, depending on the clinical picture.

In the depressed phase, mood stabilisers such as lithium, sodium valproate or lamotrigine may be useful. There is little evidence for the use of antidepressants in children with bipolar depression; they should only be used in conjunction with a mood stabiliser.

Maintenance treatment with a mood stabiliser and psychotherapy is indicated. Patients should be monitored for side effects.

Psychosocial management includes psychoeducation, supportive psychotherapy, educational and vocational counselling and family intervention.

#### 28.3.2.6 Prognosis

Prognosis is generally good for an individual episode but guarded to poor in the long term with early-onset symptoms (Baldessarini, 2012).

## 28.4 Anxiety disorders in children and adolescents

Anxiety disorders are said to be among the most common ailments that affect children and adolescents, with a prevalence ranging from 4–20%.

These conditions have an adverse effect on the young person's self-esteem, social relationships and academic performance.

The recognition, understanding and treatment of anxiety disorders in childhood are extremely important as they represent strong predictors of anxiety disorders in adulthood. They also confer a greater risk for other forms of psychopathology either concurrently or later in life. Prospective studies show that temperamentally shy, inhibited infants and toddlers are at an increased risk of developing anxiety disorders later on (Goodman *et al.*, 2012).

Anxiety disorders run in families: affected parents are more likely to have affected children, and vice versa.

Most anxiety disorders of childhood are diagnosed using criteria applicable to adults (see Chapter 14: Anxiety, fear and panic) with separation-anxiety disorder (see Chapter 27: Child and adolescent psychiatry 1: Assessment and the young child) no longer regarded as an exception by the DSM-5.

### 28.4.1 Clinical features of anxiety in children and adolescents

Adolescents who present with anxiety disorders may not directly express their worries, but behaviour patterns may often reflect either separation anxiety or another anxiety disorder: they exhibit discomfort about leaving home, engage in solitary activities due to fears of performance situations involving their peers or feel distress when away from their families. Children with anxiety disorders may retreat from social or group activities and express feelings of loneliness because of their self-imposed isolation. When a family relocates, a child may cling intensely to a mother figure as the result of separation anxiety. Sleep difficulties are common in children and adolescents with an anxiety disorder. It is not unusual for an anxious child to go to a parent's bed or sleep at the parents' bedroom door when woken by anxiety, a morbid fear or a nightmare. Fear of the dark and imaginary or bizarre concerns may be associated with anxiety disorders.

Such children are inclined to be more sensitive than their peers and more easily brought to tears. Somatic complaints are frequent and include gastrointestinal symptoms, unexplained pain in various sites of the body, sore throats and flu-like symptoms. Older children usually complain of somatic experiences classically reported by adults with anxiety.

### 28.4.2 Special investigations in anxiety disorders

No specific laboratory measures aid in the diagnosis of separation anxiety disorder or other anxiety disorders.

### 28.4.3 Differential diagnosis

In the very young child, clinical judgement is necessary to distinguish between normal anxiety and separation-anxiety disorder in this age group, as some degree of separation anxiety is a normal phenomenon.

In school-age children, the refusal to attend school on a regular basis is an indicator that the child is experiencing more than normal distress. It is necessary to distinguish whether fear of separation, general worry about their performance or more specific fears of humiliation in front of their peers or teachers are responsible for the reluctance to attend school. The anxiety in generalised anxiety disorder is not based on separation. Anxiety over separation, which might occur in pervasive developmental disorders and schizophrenia, is the product of the disorder itself. Depressive disorders and separation anxiety disorder often co-exist; criteria for both disorders must be met to confirm the diagnosis.

Truancy is common in conduct disorder; staying away from school is not the result of separation from key figures.

Panic disorder with agoraphobia tends to be uncommon prior to the age of 18.

Children with conditions such as simple phobias, social phobia or fear of failure because of a learning disorder may also refuse to attend school.

### 28.4.4 Course and prognosis of childhood anxiety disorders

The course and prognosis of separation anxiety disorders, generalised anxiety disorder and social phobia are varied and are determined by factors such as the age of onset, duration of symptoms and the development of co-morbid anxiety and depressive disorders. Those children who can maintain school attendance, after-school activities and peer relationships generally enjoy a better prognosis than children or adolescents who refuse to attend school and/or drop out of social activities. There appears to be a significant overlap of separation anxiety disorders and depressive disorders; the prognosis is guarded in these complicated cases. A follow-up study of children and adolescents over a three-year period reported that up to 82% no longer met criteria for anxiety disorders at follow-up (Sadock BJ and Sadock VA, 2009).

In this group, 96% of children with separation anxiety disorder had a remission at follow-up. Most children who recovered did so within the first year. Predicted slower recovery was determined by early age of onset and later age at diagnosis. Nearly one third of the group studied, however, had developed another psychiatric disorder within the follow-up period and 50% of these children developed another anxiety disorder. Reports indicate that children with severe school phobia continue to resist attending school for many years.

### 28.4.5 Treatment of anxiety disorders in children and adolescents

Cognitive behavioural therapy (CBT) is widely accepted as a first-line treatment for a range of anxiety disorders that occur in children and include separation anxiety disorder, social phobia and selective mutism. It is usually necessary to adopt a comprehensive treatment approach utilising CBT, family education, family psychosocial intervention and pharmacological intervention. As regards medication, SSRIs have been shown to be both safe and efficacious in the treatment of childhood anxiety disorders. Other options include tricyclic agents such as imipramine or amitriptyline.

# 28.5 Trauma and stressor-related disorders in children and adolescents

## 28.5.1 Post-traumatic stress disorder

Post-traumatic stress disorder (PTSD) is now listed in the DSM-5 under'trauma and stressor-related disorders'. Characteristic symptoms that occur in PTSD include re-experiencing symptoms, distressing recollections, persistent avoidance and hyper-arousal in response to exposure to one or more traumatic events. Many children and adolescents are exposed to traumatic events such as physical or sexual abuse, domestic violence, being in war-torn areas, natural and other disasters or may experience severe medical illnesses directly (witnessed) or indirectly (un-witnessed). Such experiences may lead to PTSD or milder forms with at least some symptoms in many others (Hamblen and Barnett, 2012).

The manifestation of symptoms is influenced by developmental factors and the age of the child and reflects internal states that are identified by what the child articulates verbally. In children and adolescents the re-experiencing of a traumatic event is often observed through play activity, recurrent nightmares (that may or may not reflect aspects of trauma) and behaviour characterised by disorganisation, regression, agitation and re-enactment of the traumatic event (Sadock BJ and Sadock VA, 2009).

### 28.5.1.1 Epidemiology of post-traumatic stress disorder

A survey of pre-school children (4–5 years) found a prevalence rate of 1,3 per cent of PTSD, whereas children aged 2 to 3 did not meet the full criteria for PTSD. Other studies of children aged 9–17 have found three-month prevalence rates of PTSD ranging from 0,5–4% percent. Those children who experience trauma on a long-term basis are at the greatest risk of developing PTSD (National Collaborating Centre for Mental Health, 2005a).

### 28.5.1.2 Aetiology

**Biological factors**

Research indicates that the risk factors of children developing PTSD include pre-existing anxiety disorders, which suggest that a genetic predisposition for anxiety disorders as well as a family history with increased risk of depressive disorders may predispose a child exposed to trauma to develop PTSD. An increased secretion of adrenergic and dopaminergic metabolites, smaller intracranial volume and corpus callosum, memory deficits and lower intelligence quotients have been found in children with PTSD when compared to age-matched controls (Kelleher *et al.*, 2008; Yehuda, 2001).

**Psychological factors**

Although exposure to trauma is the primary causative factor in the development of PTSD, the enduring symptoms characteristic of PTSD, such as avoidance of stimuli (places, people, activities), can be ascribed in part to the result of both classic and operant conditioning. A site (neutral cue) where the traumatic event occurred may become paired with an intensely fearful past event caused by persons or factors linked to the site. Operant conditioning occurs when a child learns to avoid traumatic reminders to prevent the emergence of distressing feelings. The mechanism of modelling may be implicated in the development and maintenance of PTSD symptoms as a form of learning (Sadock BJ and Sadock VA, 2009).

**Social factors**

The support and reactions of the family to a child's traumatic experience may play a significant role in the development of PTSD. Adverse parental emotional responses to a child's trauma may increase the risk of developing PTSD. In addition, the lack of parental support and psychopathology among parents has been identified as risk factors in the development of PTSD in traumatised children (True *et al.*, 1993).

### 28.5.1.3 Diagnosis and clinical features

Key to the development of PTSD is exposure to a traumatic event, which involves either a direct personal experience or witnessing or learning of a traumatic event that involves a close family member or friend. Such an event includes the threat of death, serious injury or serious harm. The most common traumatic events for children and adolescents include physical or sexual abuse, being kidnapped, violence encountered at school, the community or home, motor vehicle or household accidents, car-hijacking, living in a war zone and natural disasters such as floods, earthquakes and fires. To make a diagnosis, the child must respond with intense fear, terror, helplessness, horror or disorganised or agitated behaviour (McCloskey and Walker, 2000).

### 28.5.1.4 Critical clinical features of PTSD

- Re-experiencing the traumatic event in at least one of the following ways: recurring, intrusive thoughts perceived as entering their head, memories, images or bodily sensations that remind them of the event. In the very young it is common to observe play that includes aspects of the traumatic event or behaviour not developmentally appropriate. Flashbacks as described by adults may also be experienced by children.
- Avoidance and numbing: children with PTSD display avoidance by physically avoiding the places which would present traumatic reminders of the event or being unable to recall important aspects of the traumatic event. Children may, after a traumatic event, experience a sense of detachment from their customary play activities or a decreased capacity to feel emotions (psychological numbness). A sense of a foreshortened future may be found in older adolescents, expressed as a fear of dying.
- Symptoms of hyper-arousal: children may have difficulty falling asleep or staying asleep. Hyper-vigilance as regards safety and increased checking that doors or windows are locked and exaggerated startle reactions are characteristic. Increased irritability, outbursts, general inability to relax and an impaired ability to concentrate may reflect hyper-arousal in some children.

To meet the diagnostic criteria for PTSD, the symptoms must be present for at least one month and cause distress or impaired functioning socially and scholastically. Should symptoms resolve within three months, acute PTSD is diagnosed. When symptoms persist for more than three months, chronic PTSD is diagnosed. Should the entire syndrome occur more than six months after the exposure to trauma, a diagnosis of PTSD with delayed expression is made. (See Chapter 16: Trauma, for the DSM-5 diagnostic criteria for PTSD.)

The DSM-5 includes a subtype 'With dissociative symptoms' characterised by either depersonalisation or derealisation. Should the full diagnostic criteria not be met six months after the event, the term 'delayed expression' is used. An age criterion for children six years and younger has been introduced.

Children and adolescents with PTSD not uncommonly experience survival guilt – especially if others people died in the particular event. They may blame themselves for the death of others and may develop co-morbid depression. Childhood PTSD tends to be associated with increased rates of other anxiety disorders in addition to depressive episodes, substance use disorders and inattentiveness.

### 28.5.1.5 Differential diagnosis

Anxiety disorders in childhood feature a number of overlapping symptoms such as recurrent intrusive thoughts in obsessive-compulsive disorder and avoidance in social phobia. Children with depressive disorders often display withdrawal and feel isolated from their peers, as well as feeling (unrealistic) guilt about life events. Irritability, insomnia, poor concentration and decreased interest in usual activities can also be observed in both PTSD and major depressive disorder. Children with PTSD may be misdiagnosed with disruptive behaviour disorders because of the presence of poor concentration, inattention and irritability. The loss of a loved one in a traumatic event may cause a child to experience both PTSD and a major depressive disorder when bereavement persists beyond its expected course (Sadock BJ and Sadock VA, 2009).

### 28.5.1.6 Course and prognosis

The outcome of PTSD depends on the severity and intensity of the trauma as well as pre-existing emotional and psychiatric states of the child. Symptoms may persist for one to two years in children and adolescents with a milder form of PTSD, after which they diminish. PTSD symptoms in more severe instances may persist for many years with spontaneous remission occurring in only a number of children and adolescents.

A poor prognosis is associated with untreated PTSD and the presence of serious co-morbidities and psycho-biological abnormalities associated with PTSD. A good prognosis is predicted by a rapid onset of symptoms (less than six months), healthy pre-morbid functioning, strong social support and the absence of co-morbid psychiatric disorders, medical disorders or serious injury. In general, the very young and the very old have more difficulty in coping with traumatic events (Sadock BJ and Sadock VA, 2009).

### 28.5.1.7 Treatment

There is clinical evidence for the efficacy of trauma-focused CBT in the treatment of PTSD. Components of CBT include psycho-education, stress inoculation, gradual exposure and cognitive processing. These are carried out in sequence. A parental treatment component is added to provide the parent with management strategies to assist the child (National Collaborating Centre for Mental Health, 2005b; Cahill and Foa, 2004).

A variant of trauma-focused CBT for PTSD is eye movement desensitisation and reprocessing (EMDR), in which exposure and cognitive reprocessing interventions are paired with directed eye movements (Shapiro and Maxfield, 2002).

Crisis intervention (or psychological debriefing), which consists of providing several sessions immediately after exposure to a traumatic event, has also been used as a treatment approach (Gillies *et al.* 2012).

Psychopharmacological treatment involves the use of SSRIs as a first- line treatment in children with PTSD. Most of the SSRI efficacy data have been obtained through open trials with adults that suggest they are beneficial.

Citalopram in a dose of 20–40mg daily has been reported to be helpful with the management of PTSD in children and adolescents based on results of an eight-week open trial.

Propanolol has been used for the management of agitation and hyper-arousal. Transdermal clonidine treatment of pre-school children with PTSD in an open study has indicated possible efficacy in decreasing activation and hyper-arousal. Other studies have involved the use of imipramine and guanfacine (Cooper *et al.*, 2005; Berger *et al.*, 2009; Khoshhu, 2006).

## 28.6 Obsessive-compulsive disorder

A significant number of patients with obsessive-compulsive disorder (OCD) have onset of symptoms in childhood or adolescence, although presentation is often delayed for several years. The DSM-5 criteria are the same for children and adolescents except that children may not have the insight that their thoughts or behaviours are unreasonable or unusual. The hallmark of the disorder is the presence of obsession and/or compulsions (American Psychiatric Association, 2013).

### 28.6.1 Aetiology

A genetic vulnerability for the development of OCD is supported by family studies that suggest a fourfold increase risk in first-degree relatives of early- onset OCD (Black *et al.*, 2003). The association with group A beta haemolytic streptococcal exposure in some children has also suggested an auto-immune process; these cases are called paediatric auto-immune neuropsychiatric disorders (PANDAS) (Murphy *et al.*, 2010). An acute onset of OCD symptoms with neuropsychiatric symptoms not associated with an infectious cause is referred to as paediatric acute neuropsychiatric syndrome (PANS) (Swedo *et al.*, 2012).

As is the case with adults, serotonin and dopamine dysregulation are implicated in the development of OCD in children.

### 28.6.2 Clinical features

Children may present with ritualistic and repetitive behaviour regarding contamination, counting or checking and worries about accidents or disease. The Children's Yale-Brown Obsessive Compulsive scale (CY-BOCS) is a comprehensive tool to aid diagnosis (Scahill *et al.*, 1997).

### 28.6.3 Differential diagnosis

Anxiety disorders, tic disorders, psychosis and the ritualistic stereotypical behaviour of autistic spectrum disorders may all have overlapping symptoms.

### 28.6.4 Treatment

Treatment follows similar principles as with managing OCD in adults, but younger patients often have a poorer response to treatment (Lack, 2012).

## 28.7 Psychosis in children and adolescents

Psychosis in children is very rare (1%) (American Psychiatric Association, 2013) and children and adolescents with psychotic symptoms need careful assessment; they generally warrant specialist referral. The onset of schizophrenia is generally in late adolescence to mid-30s. Onset of psychosis before the age of 18 is referred to as early-onset psychosis and before the age of 10, as very-early-onset psychosis.

Whilst the DSM-5 diagnostic criteria are the same for children and adults, diagnosis may be more complex. Symptomatology differs based on the developmental level.

### 28.7.1 Aetiology

Genetic predisposition, high incidence of pregnancy and birth complications, early cannabis use (before the age of 15) and sexual abuse are risk factors in early-onset schizophrenia (Brown, 2011). The precise mechanisms of biological vulnerabilities and environmental triggers that result in early-onset psychosis require further study. An increasing body of evidence suggests that schizophrenia is a neurodevelopmental disorder, since prospective studies of individuals who later develop schizophrenia often have impaired neurocognitive functioning in childhood (Kolvin and Berney, 1990; Owen *et al.*, 2011).

### 28.7.2 Clinical features

Onset is often insidious and varied. Children may have a history of delayed motor and language milestones and limited social skills. Children and adolescents commonly present with auditory hallucinations (often commentatory or commanding in nature), visual hallucinations, delusions and a blunted or inappropriate affect. Formal thought disorder and illogical thinking may be present.

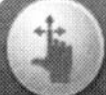

**Case study 28.3**

**Case BB**

BB, a 10-year-old boy, presented with a six-month history of persistent concern that he may have said a vulgar word; he kept checking with his parents for reassurance that he had not been rude. He threw temper tantrums if his mother was not willing to reassure him. He also insisted on wearing something red every day and spent hours washing, as he felt contaminated whenever he left the house. BB was assessed as having OCD and was treated with CBT and anxiolytics, which helped relieve his concerns.

### 28.7.3 Differential diagnosis

A comprehensive assessment is most valuable; focus on longitudinal presentation is important in psychotic illnesses. Psychotic phenomena are also common in mood disorders in children. Pervasive developmental disorders and schizotypal personality disorder also share similarities with schizophrenia. General medical conditions and substance-related disorders must be comprehensively excluded before considering a diagnosis of schizophrenia.

### 28.7.4 Management

The treatment of psychosis is multi-modal and follows similar principles as in adults. Antipsychotic medication is the mainstay of treatment, with most guidelines advocating the use of atypical antipsychotics as first-line treatment in children and adolescents. Patients on antipsychotics must be closely monitored for potential side effects, especially extrapyramidal side effects and complications associated with weight gain.

Psychosocial treatment includes ongoing supportive care, family education and support and addressing psychosocial morbidity and vocational difficulties.

### 28.7.5 Prognosis

Early-onset psychosis has a guarded to poor long-term outcome as the psychosis can be very disruptive in a critical development period.

**Information box**

**Principles of prescribing psychotropic medication in children**

- Treat target symptoms, not diagnosis.
- Technical aspects of paediatric prescribing: start low and go slow.
- More than one type of medication may be required.
- Allow time for medication to work.
- Change one drug at a time where possible.
- Monitor outcome.
- Provide patient and family psycho-education (Taylor *et al.*, 2009).

## 28.8 Suicide in adolescents

### 28.8.1 Introduction

With teen suicide the third most common cause of death among adolescents in the USA, the rise in youth suicidal behaviour remains an important clinical problem. Advancing our understanding of the underlying social factors, cultural issues and sociological issues may help clinicians to achieve more efficient prediction, prevention and treatment strategies (Amitai and Apter, 2012).

**Information box**

**Summary of findings regarding suicidal behaviour and suicide prevention in adolescents**

1. The risk of suicide attempts, suicide ideation and deliberate self-harm is high amongst young people; with an annual rate of deliberate self-harm reported as 7,3% and lifetime prevalence of 12–13% (Harkavy-Friedman *et al.*,1987).
2. Although suicide thoughts and behaviours can occur in the context of a depressive disorder, most youth who contemplate, attempt or complete suicide are not in the midst of a major depressive disorder (Sadock BJ and Sadock VA, 2007). However, the primary risk factor for teen suicide is the presence of a mental illness (Friedman, 2006; Beautrais, 2000).
3. While suicide ideation occurs in all age groups (children and adolescents), it is more common in adolescents, with as many as 60% reporting having experienced suicide ideation on at least one occasion; it is seen with greater frequency in children and adolescents with severe mood disorders (Harkavy-Friedman *et al.*,1987).
4. In the last 15 years, rates of both completed suicide and suicide ideations have decreased among adolescents. This decrease coincides with the increase in SSRIs prescribed to adolescents with mood and behaviour disturbance (Sadock BJ and Sadock VA, 2007).

In order to correct a history of inconsistent and unclear terminology regarding suicide-related behaviour, O'Caroll *et al.*, (1996) developed a defined set of terms (see Table 28.7).

**Table 28.7** Suicide terminology

| Term | Definition |
|---|---|
| ▸ Suicide | Fatal, self-inflicted, destructive act with explicit or implicit intent to die. |
| ▸ Suicide attempt | Non-fatal, destructive act (not necessarily resulting in injury) with explicit or implicit intent to die. |
| ▸ Suicide ideation | Thoughts of harming or killing oneself. |
| ▸ Suicidality | All suicide-related behaviour or thoughts. |
| ▸ Non-suicidal self-injurious behaviour | Any self-inflicted, destructive act without intent to die but with full intent of inflicting physical harm to oneself (viewed as distinct from suicide). |

**Source:** O'Carroll *et al.*, 1996. This material is reproduced with permission from John Wiley and Sons Inc.

## 28.8.2 Protective factors

A positive parent-child connection, with active parental supervision as well as clear behavioural and academic expectations, has been associated with lower levels of suicidal behaviour (Borowsky *et al.*, 2001).

## 28.2.3 Risk factors for adolescent suicidal behaviour

- A previous suicide attempt is the strongest predictor of future suicide (Brent *et al.*, 1999).
- Suicidal ideation: frequent high levels of suicide intent or suicide planning in youth are associated with a 60% chance of making a suicide attempt within one year of ideation onset (Hagedom and Omar, 2002).
- Availability of lethal means: firearms are much more common in the homes of suicide completers (Goldston *et al.*, 1997).
- Precipitant: assessing physicians should explore the history: the most common triggers include a fight with the parents, the end of a relationship, other disappointments, important losses, financial difficulties, rejection, humiliation and disgrace.
- Impulsivity: completed suicide is more likely among teens who act impulsively on suicidal thoughts (Links, 2007).
- Age: the rates of attempted and completed suicide increase dramatically with age throughout childhood into adolescence. This could be due to decreased supervision with an elevated risk of psychopathology in adolescence. The cognitive maturity of pre-pubertal children limits their ability to plan and execute lethal suicide attempts.
- Gender: in Western countries, the rates of suicide across ethnicities are higher in adolescent boys than adolescent girls (ratio of 5:1). However, the rates of suicidal ideation and attempted suicide are higher in girls (ratio 3:1) (Amitai and Apter, 2012). Explanations for higher suicide rates in boys include higher suicide intent, use of more violent methods, a higher prevalence of antisocial disorder and substance abuse and a greater vulnerability to stressors such as legal difficulties, financial problems and interpersonal loss. Boys may also have more difficulties in asking for help and communicating their distress (Amitai and Apter, 2012). Girls tend towards suicidal behaviour as a language that commands attention and respect and as a desire for a relationship, while boys turn to violence as an alternative to feeling helpless and powerless (Gilligan, 2004).
- Race and socioeconomic status: some studies show that adolescents who engage in deliberate self-harming behaviour tend to be from the lower socioeconomic strata, with an increased suicide risk conveyed by a lower socioeconomic status (Kokkevi *et al.*, 2012). The rate of completed suicide among young African-American males has been growing disproportionately in recent years (Joe and

Kaplan, 2002). Children who frequently moved residence were more likely to make suicide attempts during adolescence (Qin *et al.*, 2009).

- Mental illness: mental illness is the most important risk factor for adolescent suicide (Friedman, 2006; Beautrais, 2000). Most serious psychiatric illnesses, including depression, anxiety and substance abuse, start in the early teens to early twenties. There is a typical delay of 10 to 20 years before a diagnosis is made, delaying important life-saving treatment (Friedman, 2006). More than 90% of suicide victims had psychiatric illnesses at the time of their deaths (Fleischmann *et al.*, 2005).
- Medical disorders: chronic medical conditions, including diabetes and epilepsy, have been associated with suicidality in paediatric populations (Goldston, 1997). There is a prospective association between suicide attempts and functionally impairing physical illness or injury (Lewinsohn *et al.*, 1996).
- Family factors: the parents of teens who attempt suicide or complete suicide have higher-than-expected rates of mood disorder, substance abuse and antisocial behaviour (Lewinsohn *et al.*, 1996). Research has pointed to the importance of the family environment as a predictor of suicidal behaviour among adolescents. The relevant family-related risk factors are parental psychopathology, family history of suicidal behaviour, family discord, loss of a parent to death or divorce, poor quality of parent-child relationship and maltreatment (Bridge *et al.*, 2006).
- Physical and sexual abuse: a history of physical, sexual or emotional abuse is common among teens who present with suicidal thoughts and behaviours (Fergusson, 2008; Hagedom and Omar, 2002). (This type of information should be elicited in a respectful and compassionate manner by, for example, asking 'Has anything really awful ever happened to you?')
- Other risk factors: teens who attempt suicide are more likely to be in trouble with the police, be involved in physical fights, have difficulties at school, function badly at school and to lack academic motivation (Flouri and Buchanan, 2002).

## 28.8.4 Assessment: the role of the family physician

Taking into consideration that parents are unaware of 90% of suicide attempts made by their teenagers, prevention and screening are important (Friedman, 2006). Physicians should be aware of warning signs for adolescent suicide and use chance patient encounters or periodic health examination visits as opportunities to screen for mental illness, hopelessness and suicidal thoughts (Links, 2007; Canadian Mental Health Association, 2010).

**Information box**

**Common warning signs for adolescent suicide**

- Sudden change in behaviour
- Apathy
- Withdrawal
- Change in eating patterns
- Unusual preoccupation with death or dying
- The giving away of valued personal possessions
- Signs of depression
- Moodiness
- Hopelessness

**Source:** Adapted from the Canadian Mental Health Association (2010)

## 28.8.5 Clinical management

Suicidal ideation should be assessed according to both severity (intent) and pervasiveness (frequency and intensity). Suicidal ideation characterised by a high degree of severity and pervasiveness is associated with a greater likelihood of suicide attempts in adolescents (Lewinsohn, 1996).

- Screen for mental illness: periodic health assessments are ideal opportunities for physicians to use adolescent questionnaires (e.g. Reach Institute, 2014) to identify at-risk youth. It is important for physicians to realise that the incidence of mental illness is substantial, even though teens are unlikely to present with psychological issues as their chief complaint.

- Treatment: data from psychosocial and pharmacological studies suggest that the treatment of depression may not be sufficient to reduce the risk of suicide risk and that specific treatment targeting suicidality may be required (Levinkron, 1998). These include clinical interventions such as safety planning, hospitalisation and psychosocial treatment that include cognitive, emotion regulation and interpersonal approaches.
- The development of a safety plan is considered to be one of the most critical parts of the assessment and treatment of suicidal youth. It involves the collaboration of the clinician, the patient and the family. A safety plan consists of a hierarchical list of strategies that the patient agrees to use in the event of a suicidal crisis.
- Discuss confidentiality: studies indicate that teens believe that the disclosure of suicidal thoughts could result in a breach of confidentiality. The clinician should explain that the visit between teen and physician is confidential, but that the clinician also has to act responsibly.
- Address self-harming behaviour: self-mutilation is associated with serious mental illness and converts to a high risk of eventual completed suicide. It is not reasonable to dismiss self-mutilating behaviour as manipulative or attention-seeking behaviour, as it is associated with serious mental pathology and a considerable lifetime risk of eventual completed suicide (Links, 2007).
- Assess level of intent: acts of self-harm might or might not be associated with a true intent to commit suicide (Levenkron, 1998). Physicians must ask whether the self-harm was intended to relieve psychological pain or whether there was an intention to commit suicide. Ultimately, the physician should exercise good judgement based on the patient's situation, symptoms and risk factors.
- Assess reasons for living: the belief that it is acceptable to end one's life confers a 14-fold increased likelihood of making a suicide plan (Martin and Wait, 1994). The clinician should access reasons for living such as family responsibility, moral objections to suicide, and fear of disapproval.
- Identify and mobilise protective factors: the most important protective factors are social support, a sense of family cohesion, connectedness at school, involvement in sports and academic achievement (Chiqueta and Stiles, 2007).
- Reduce access to lethal means: parents or other caregivers should be counselled regarding the reduction of access to lethal means for youth suicide.
- Consider hospitalisation if necessary: the risk of suicide is highest after discharge from hospital, thus making the transition particularly important (Kjelsberg *et al.*, 1994). All adolescents who come to medical attention because of suicide attempts must be evaluated before determining whether hospitalisation is necessary. Adolescents who fall into the high-risk group should be hospitalised until the acute suicidality is no longer present. High-risk groups include previous suicide attempts, boys older than 12 with a history of aggressive behaviour and substance abuse, those who have made a lethal suicide attempt, those with major depressive disorder characterised by social withdrawal, hopelessness and a lack of energy, girls who have run away from home, are pregnant or have made an attempt with a method other than ingesting a toxic substance and any person who exhibits persistent suicidal ideation.
  - Diagnostic criteria: family physicians should refer to the DSM-5 to review symptoms of paediatric and adolescent mental illnesses, including depressive and bipolar mood disorders. Physicians should be aware of impulsivity, poor coping skills and a history of self-harm

  as signs of potentially serious mental pathology (American Psychiatric Association, 2013).
  - Psychotherapeutical approaches should include CBT, skills-based therapy and school-based prevention plans.
- Pharmacological approaches: SSRIs, lithium
  - No studies have expressly examined the effect of fluoxetine or any other SSRI on impulsive aggression on youth. A study that evaluated the effectiveness of fluoxetine hydrochloride therapy, CBT and their combination in adolescents with major depressive disorder found that suicidal events were more common in patients receiving fluoxetine therapy than combination therapy or CBT. Adding CBT to medication enhances the safety of medication. It is important to note that all SSRIs exhibit a significant decrease in suicidal ideation (March *et al.*, 2004). Most commonly, suicidality occurred early in treatment and consisted of increased or new-onset suicidal ideation, with very few suicide attempts and no suicide completions. A recent meta-analysis supports the assertion that many more youth will show a good clinical response to SSRIs than will become suicidal (Bridge *et al.*, 2007).
  - Data support the use of lithium for the treatment of aggression in adolescents and children (Malone *et al.*, 2000). Examination of the use of lithium for the treatment of suicidality in youth appears warranted.
  - Divalproex has demonstrated efficacy in the treatment of impulsive aggression, mood lability and behavioural symptoms in studies of children, adolescents, and adults (Hollander *et al.*, 2003).
  - Although the use of neuroleptics for the treatment of youth suicidality has not been evaluated, atypical neuroleptics have been shown to be efficacious in the treatment of aggressive behaviour in children and adolescents (Findling *et al.*, 2000).

**Information box**

**Tips for prescribing antidepressant medication in youth**

- Inform the patient and the family about the risks and benefits of SSRIs and discuss the black box warning.
- Be sure to inform family members specifically about the risk of suicide behaviour.
- Therapy should be started at a low dose (equivalent of 5–10 mg of fluoxetine).
- If needed, dose increases should be considered every two weeks.
- The Food and Drug Administration recommends weekly monitoring for the first four weeks of antidepressant therapy and thereafter dose adjustment.

**Source:** Adapted from Canadian Mental Health Association (2010).

### 28.8.6 Concluding comments on adolescent suicide

The public-health implications of youth suicide are serious, although progress has been made in improving our understanding of risk and protective factors for suicidality in youth. A great deal remains to be known about the effective prevention for those at highest risk, as well as the neurobiology associated with suicidality in youth. (For further information on suicide, see Chapter 34: Suicide and the aggressive patient.)

## 28.9 Eating disorders in adolescents

Overeating related to tension, poor nutritional habits and food fads are relatively common problems for youngsters. In addition, two psychiatric eating disorders, anorexia nervosa and bulimia nervosa, are on the increase among teenage girls and young women and often run in families. These two eating disorders also occur in boys, but less often.

Parents frequently wonder how to identify symptoms of anorexia nervosa and bulimia nervosa. These disorders are characterised by a pre-occupation with food and a distortion of body image. Unfortunately, many teenagers hide these serious – and sometimes fatal – disorders from their families and friends.

### 28.9.1 Symptoms and signs of anorexia nervosa and bulimia nervosa in adolescents

Symptoms and warning signs of anorexia nervosa and bulimia nervosa in adolescents include the following:

- Teenagers with anorexia nervosa are typically perfectionists and high achievers in school. At the same time, they suffer from low self-esteem, irrationally believing they fat regardless of how thin they become. Desperately needing a feeling of mastery over their life, teenagers with anorexia nervosa experience a sense of control only when they say'no'to the normal food demands of their body. In a relentless pursuit to be thin, they starve themselves. This often reaches the point of serious damage to the body and, in a small number of cases, may lead to death.
- The symptoms of bulimia nervosa are usually different from those of anorexia nervosa. The patients binge on huge quantities of

**Table 28.8** DSM-5 Diagnostic Criteria for Anorexia Nervosa

| **Diagnostic Criteria** |
|---|
| A. Restriction of energy intake relative to requirements, leading to a significantly low body weight in the context of age, sex, developmental trajectory, and physical health. *Significantly low weight* is defined as a weight that is less than minimally normal or, for children and adolescents, less than that minimally expected. |
| B. Intense fear of gaining weight or of becoming fat, or persistent behavior that interferes with weight gain, even though at a significantly low weight. |
| C. Disturbance in the way in which one's body weight or shape is experienced, undue influence of body weight or shape on self-evaluation, or persistent lack of recognition of the seriousness of the current low body weight. |
| *Specify* whether: |
| ▸ **(F50.01) Restricting type:** During the last 3 months, the individual has not engaged in recurrent episodes of binge eating or purging behavior (i.e., self-induced vomiting or the misuse of laxatives, diuretics, or enemas). This subtype describes presentations in which weight loss is accomplished primarily through dieting, fasting, and/or excessive exercise. |
| ▸ **(F50.02) Binge-eating/purging type:** During the last 3 months, the individual has engaged in recurrent episodes of binge eating or purging behavior (i.e., self-induced vomiting or the misuse of laxatives, diuretics, or enemas). |
| *Specify* if: |
| ▸ **In partial remission:** After full criteria for anorexia nervosa were previously met. Criterion A (low body weight) has not been met for a sustained period, but either Criterion B (intense fear of gaining weight or becoming fat or behavior that interferes with weight gain) or Criterion C (disturbances in self-perception of weight and shape) is still met. |
| ▸ **In full remission:** After full criteria for anorexia nervosa were previously met, none of the criteria have been met for a sustained period of time. |
| *Specify* current severity: |
| The minimum level of severity is based, for adults, on current body mass index (BMI) (see below) or, for children and adolescents, on BMI percentile. The ranges below are derived from World Health Organization categories for thinness in adults; for children and adolescents, corresponding BMI percentiles should be used. The level of severity may be increased to reflect clinical symptoms, the degree of functional disability, and the need for supervision. |
| ▸ **Mild:** BMI $\geq$ 17kg/m$^2$ |
| ▸ **Moderate:** BM1 16–16.99 kg/m$^2$ |
| ▸ **Severe:** BM1 15–15.99 kg/m$^2$ |
| ▸ **Extreme:** BMI < 15 kg/m$^2$ |

**Source:** Reprinted with permission from the *Diagnostic and Statistical Manual of Mental Disorders*, Fifth Edition, (Copyright 2013). American Psychiatric Association.

high-caloric food and/or purges their body of dreaded calories by self-induced vomiting and often by using laxatives. These binges may alternate with severe diets, resulting in dramatic weight fluctuations. Teenagers may try to hide the signs of throwing up by running a tap while spending long periods of time in the bathroom. Purging presents a serious threat to the patient's physical health, including dehydration, hormonal imbalance, the depletion of important minerals and damage to vital organs.

## 28.9.2 Management of anorexia nervosa and bulimia nervosa in adolescents

With comprehensive treatment, most teenagers can be relieved of the symptoms or helped to control eating disorders. The psychiatrist is trained to evaluate, diagnose, and treat these psychiatric disorders. Treatment of eating disorders usually requires a team approach, including individual therapy, family therapy, working with a primary care physician and a nutritionist and

**Table 28.9** DSM-5 Diagnostic Criteria for Bulimia Nervosa

| **Diagnostic Criteria** |
|---|
| A. Recurrent episodes of binge eating. An episode of binge eating is characterized by both of the following:<br>1. Eating, in a discrete period of time (e.g., within any 2-hour period), an amount of food that is definitely larger than what most individuals would eat in a similar period of time under similar circumstances.<br>2. A sense of lack of control over eating during the episode (e.g., a feeling that one cannot stop eating or control what or how much one is eating).<br>B. Recurrent inappropriate compensatory behaviors in order to prevent weight gain, such as self-induced vomiting; misuse of laxatives, diuretics, or other medications; fasting; or excessive exercise.<br>C. The binge eating and inappropriate compensatory behaviors both occur, on average, at least once a week for 3 months.<br>D. Self-evaluation is unduly influenced by body shape and weight.<br>E. The disturbance does not occur exclusively during episodes of anorexia nervosa.<br>*Specify* if:<br>▶ **In partial remission:** After full criteria for bulimia nervosa were previously met, some, but not all, of the criteria have been met for a sustained period of time.<br>▶ **In full remission:** After full criteria for bulimia nervosa were previously met, none of the criteria have been met for a sustained period of time.<br>*Specify* current severity:<br>The minimum level of severity is based on the frequency of inappropriate compensatory behaviors (see below). The level of severity may be increased to reflect other symptoms and the degree of functional disability.<br>▶ **Mild:** An average of 1–3 episodes of inappropriate compensatory behaviors per week.<br>▶ **Moderate:** An average of 4–7 episodes of inappropriate compensatory behaviors per week.<br>▶ **Severe:** An average of 8–13 episodes of inappropriate compensatory behaviors per week.<br>▶ **Extreme:** An average of 14 or more episodes of inappropriate compensatory behaviours per week. |

**Source:** Reprinted with permission from the *Diagnostic and Statistical Manual of Mental Disorders*, Fifth Edition, (Copyright 2013). American Psychiatric Association.

medication. Many adolescents also suffer from other problems including depression, anxiety, and substance abuse. It is important to recognise and get appropriate treatment for these problems as well.

(See Chapter 22: Eating and sleep disorders, for further information on eating disorders.)

## Conclusion

A number of challenges have been identified: a growing body of empirical research supports the view that young people over the past fifty years have become increasingly prone to problems known to be sensitive to psychosocial circumstances-behavioural problems, crime, substance abuse, depression and suicide. Many traumatised children and adolescents have never had the opportunity to talk freely to an informed adult about their normal experiences. Furthermore, parents only insist on referral once a child's problems are a substantial burden to them. So, most child and adolescent psychiatric disorders go untreated.

Assessment of the child with multifaceted mental problems requires careful assessment to identify all relevant adverse circumstances, where correcting only one of these factors could break the vicious circle. Assisting the child to develop problem solution- and social skills competencies would lessen the impact of psychiatric disorders and improve self-confidence.

Future cross-cultural studies are needed to show whether our current ideas on classification, treatment, prognosis and prevention apply equally to children and adolescents from all backgrounds, taking our multicultural society into account.

# References

American Psychiatric Association (2013) *Diagnostic and Statistical Manual of Mental Disorders* (5th edition). Washington DC: American Psychiatric Association

Amitai M, Apter A (2012) Social aspects of suicidal behaviour and prevention in early life: A review. *International Journal of Environmental Research and Public Health* 9: 985–94

Arnett JJ (1999) Adolescent storm and stress, reconsidered. *American Psychologist* 54: 317–26

Arnett JJ (2000) Emerging adulthood: A theory of development from the late teens through the twenties. *American Psychologist* 55:469–80

Baldessarini RJ (2000) A plea for integrity of the bipolar disorder concept. *Bipolar Disorders* 2: 3–7

Baldessarini RJ (2012) Comparing tolerability of olanzapine in schizophrenia and affective disorders: A meta-analysis. *Drug Safety* 35(12): 1183–4

Beardslee WR, Versage EM, Gladstone T (1998) Children of affectively ill parents: A review of the past 10 years. *Journal of the American Academy of Child and Adolescent Psychiatry* 37: 1134–41

Beautrais AL (2000) Risk factors for suicide and attempted suicide among young people. *Australian and New Zealand Journal of Psychiatry* 34(3): 420–36

Berger W, Mendlowicz MV, Marques-Portella C, Kinrys G, Fontenelle LF, Marmar CR, Figueira I (2009) Pharmacologic alternatives to antidepressants in posttraumatic stress disorder: A systematic review. *Progress in Neuro-Psychopharmacology and Biological Psychiatry* 17: 33(2): 169–80

Birmaher B, Ryan ND, Williamson DE, Brent DA, Kaufman J, Dahl RE, Perel J, Nelson B (1996) Childhood and adolescent depression: A review of the past 10 years. Part I. *Journal of the American Academy of Child and Adolescent Psychiatry* 35(11): 1427–39

Black DW, Gaffney GR, Schlosser S, Gabel J (2003) Children of parents with obsessive-compulsive disorder - a 2-year follow-up study. *Acta Psychiatrica Scandinavica* 107: 305–13

Borowsky IW, Ireland MA, Resnick MD (2001) Adolescent suicide attempts: Risks and protectors. *Pediatrics* 107: 485–93

Brent DA, Baugher M, Bridge M, Chen J, Chiapetta L (1999) Age- and sex-related risk factors for adolescent suicide. *Journal of the American Academy of Child and Adolescent Psychiatry* 38: 1497–1505

Bridge J, Iyengar S, Salary CB, Barbe RP, Birmaher B, Pincus HA, Ren L, Brent DA (2007) Clinical response and risk for reported suicidal ideation and suicide attempts in pediatric antidepressant treatment: A meta-analysis of randomized controlled trails. *The Journal of the American Medical Association* 297: 1683–96

Bridge JA, Goldstein TR, Brent D.A (2006) Adolescent suicide and suicidal behaviour. *Journal of Child Psychology and Psychiatry* 47: 372–94

Brown AS (2011) The environment and susceptibility to schizophrenia. *Progress in Neurobiology* 93: 23–58

Cahill SP and Foa EB (2004) A glass half empty or half full? Where we are and directions for future research in the treatment of post-traumatic stress disorder. In Taylor S (Ed). *Advances in the treatment of post-traumatic stress disorder. Cognitive behavioral perspectives* New York: Springer 267–313

Canadian Mental Health Association (2010) Available at: http://www.cmha.ca/?s=suicide&submit=Search&lang=en (Accessed 16 Jun 2010) http://www.cmha.ca

Chiqueta AP, Stiles TC (2007) The relationship between psychological buffers, hopelessness, and suicidal ideation: Identification of protective factors. *Crises* 28(2): 67–73

Collins WA, Steinberg L (2006) Adolescent development in interpersonal context. In: Damon W, Lerner RM (Eds). *Handbook of child psychology* (Vol 3, 6th edition). Hoboken, NJ: Wiley

Cook M, Peterson J, Sheldon C (2009) Adolescent depression: An update and guide to clinical decision making. *Psychiatry* 6 (9): 17–31

Cooper J, Carty J, Creamer M (2005) Pharmacotherapy for posttraumatic stress disorder: Empirical review and clinical recommendations. *Australian and New Zealand Journal of Psychiatry 39*(8): 674–82

Dishion TJ, Nelson SE, Yasui M (2005) Predicting early adolescent gang involvement from middle school adaptation. *Journal of Clinical Child and Adolescent Psychology* 34(1): 62–73

Dulcan MK (2010) Assessing adolescents. In: Dulcan MK (Ed). *Dulcan's Textbook of Child and Adolescent Psychiatry.* Washington DC: American Psychiatric Publishers

Faedda GL, Baldessarini RJ, Glovinsky IP, Austin NB. (2004) Pediatric bipolar disorder: Phenomenology and course of illness. *Bipolar Disorders* 6: 305–13

Fergusson DM, Boden JM, Horwood LJ (2008) Exposure to childhood sexual and physical abuse and adjustment in early adulthood. *Child Abuse and Neglect* 32: 607–19

Findling Rl, McNamara NK, Branicky LA, Schluchter MD, Lemon E, Blumer JL. (2000) A double-blind pilot study of risperidone in the treatment of conduct disorder. *Journal of the American Academy of Child Psychiatry* 4:509–16

Fleischmann A, Bertolote JM, Belfer M, Beautrais AL (2005) Completed suicide and psychiatric diagnosis in young people: A critical examination of the evidence. *American Journal of Orthopsychiatry* 75(4): 676–83

Flouri E, Buchanan A (2002) The protective role of parental involvement in adolescent suicide. *Crises* 23(1): 17–22

Friedman RA (2006) Uncovering an epidemic-screening for mental illness in teens. *New England Journal of Medicine* 355: 2717–9

Geller B, Fox LW, Clark KA (1994) Rate and predictors of prepubertal bipolarity during follow-up of 6- to 12-year-old depressed children. *Journal of the American Academy of Child and Adolescent Psychiatry* 33: 461–8

Gillies D, Taylor F, Gray C, O'Brien L, d'Abrew N (2012) Psychological therapies for the treatment of posttraumatic stress disorder in children and adolescents. *Cochrane Database of Systematic Reviews* 12.

Gilligan C (2004) Strengthening healthy resistance and courage in children: A gender–based strategy for preventing youth violence. *Annals of the New York Academy of Science* 1036: 128–40

Goldston DB, Kelley AE, Reboussin DM, Daniel SS, Smith JA, Lorentz W, Hill C (1997). Suicidal ideation and behaviour and noncompliance with the medical regimen among diabetic adolescents. *Journal of the American Academy of Child and Adolescent Psychiatry* 36: 1528–36

Goodman R, Scott S (2012) *Child and Adolescent Psychiatry* (3rd edition). London: Wiley-Blackwell

Goodyer IM, Herbert J, Tamplin A, Altham PM (2000) Recent life events, cortisol, dehydroepiandrosterone and the onset of major depression in high-risk adolescents. *British Journal of Psychiatry* 177: 499–504

Hagedom J, Omar H (2002) Retrospective analysis of youth evaluated for suicide attempt or suicidal ideation in an emergency room setting. *International Journal of Adolescent Medicine and Health* 14(1): 55–60

Hamblen J, Barnett E (2012) *PTSD in children and adolescents.* VA National Center for Posttraumatic Stress Disorder. Available at: http://www. ttsd.va.gov/professional/pages/ptsd-in- children-and-adolescents-overview-for-professionals.asp (Accessed June 2013.)

Harkavy-Friedman JM, Asnis GM, Boeck M, Di Fiore J (1987) Prevalence of specific suicidal behaviours in a high school sample. *American Journal of Psychiatry* 144: 1203–6

Harris S (2005) Bullying at school among older adolescents. *School Nurse News* 22(3): 18–21

Hetrick S, Merry S, McKenzie J, Sindahl P, Proctor M (2007) Selective serotonin reuptake inhibitors (SSRIs) for depressive disorders in children and adolescents. *Cochrane Database Systematic Review* 18(3):CD004851

Hollander E, Tracy KA, Swann AC, Coccaro EF, McElroy SL, Wozniak P (2003) Divalproex in the treatment of impulsive aggression: Efficacy in Cluster B personality disorders. *Neuropsychopharmacology* 28: 1186–97

Jane Costello E, Erkanli A, Angold A (2006) Is there an epidemic of child or adolescent depression? *Journal of Child Psychology and Psychiatry* 47: 1263–71

Joe S, Kaplan MS (2002) Firearm-related suicide among African-American males. *Psychiatric Service* 53: 332–4

Keenan-Miller D, Hammen C, Brennan P (2007) Health outcomes related to early adolescent depression. *Journal of Adolescent Health* 41: 256–62

Kelleher I, Harley M, Lynch F, Arseneault L, Fitzpatrick C, Cannon M (2008) Association between childhood trauma, bullying and psychotic symptoms among a school-based adolescent sample. *British Journal of Psychiatry* 193(5): 378–82

Khoshnu E (2006) Clonidine for treatment of PTSD. *Clinical Psychiatry News* 34(10): 22

Kjelsberg E, Neegaard E, Dahl AA (1994) Suicide in adolescent psychiatric inpatients: Incidence and predictive factors. *Acta Psychiatrica Scandinavica* 89: 235–41

Kokkevi A, Rotsika V, Arapaki A, Richardson C (2012) Adolescent's self-reported suicide attempts, self-harm thoughts and their correlates across 17 European countries. *Journal of Child Psychology and Psychiatry* 53: 381–9

Kolvin I, Berney TP (1990) Childhood schizophrenia. In: Tonge BJ, Burrows GD, Werr JS (Eds). *Handbook of Studies on Child Psychiatry*. New York: Elsevier

Lack CW (2012) Obsessive-compulsive disorder: Evidence-based treatments and future directions for research. *World Journal of Psychiatry* 2(6): 86–90

Le Couteur A, Gardner F (2008) Use of structured interviews and observational methods in clinical settings. In: Rutter M, Bishop D, Pine D, Scott S, Stevenson JS, Taylor EA, Thapar A (Eds). *Rutter's Child and Adolescent Psychiatry* (5th edition). Chichester: Wiley-Blackwell

Levenkron S (1998) *Cutting: Understanding and Overcoming Self-mutilation.* New York, NY: Lion's Crown

Lewinsohn P M, Rohde P, Seeley JR (1996), Adolescent suicidal ideation and attempts: Prevalence, risk factors, and clinical implications. *Clinical Psychology: Science and Practice* 3: 25–46

Links P (2007) Arthur Sommer Rottenberg Chair in Suicide Studies; Professor of Psychiatry Lecture. *Assessing and managing suicide risk in psychiatric patients*. Toronto, ON: University of Toronto

Malone R, Delaney MA, Luebbert JF, Cater J, Campbell M (2000) A double-blind placebo-controlled study of lithium in hospitalized aggressive children and adolescents with conduct disorder. *Archives of General Psychiatry* 57: 649–54

March JS, Silva S, Petrycki S, Curry J, Wells K, Fairbank J, Burns B, Domino M, McNulty S, Vitiello B, Severe J (2004) Treatment for Adolescents With Depression Study (TADS) Team (2004) Fluoxetine, cognitive behavioral therapy, and their combination for adolescents with depression: Treatment for adolescent depression study (TADS) randomized controlled trail. *Journal of the American Medical Association* 292: 807–20

Martin A, Volkmar FR (2007) Adolescence. In: Martin A, Volkmar FR (Eds). *Lewis's Child and Adolescent Psychiatry: A Comprehensive Text* (4th edition). Philadelphia: Lippincott Williams & Wilkins

Martin G, Wait S (1994) Parental bonding and vulnerability to adolescent suicide. *Acta Psychiatrica Scandinavica* 89(4): 246–54

McCloskey LA, Walker M (2000) Posttraumatic stress in children exposed to family violence and single-event trauma. *Journal of the American Academy of Child and Adolescent Psychiatry* 39(1): 108–15

Murphy TK, Kurlan R, Leckman J (2010) The immunobiology of Tourette's disorder, pediatric autoimmune neuropsychiatric disorders associated with streptococcus, and related disorders: A way forward. *Journal of Child and Adolescent Psychopharmacology* 20: 317–31

National Collaborating Centre for Mental Health (UK) (2005) *Post-traumatic stress disorder, section 2: Incidence and prevalence.* NICE Clinical Guidelines, No. 26. Gaskell: Royal College of Psychiatrists

National Collaborating Centre for Mental Health (UK) (2005) *Post-traumatic stress disorder: The management of PTSD in adults and children in primary and secondary care.* NICE Clinical Guidelines, No.26. Gaskell: Royal College of Psychiatrists

National Institute for Health Care and Excellence (NICE) (2012) *Social and emotional wellbeing: early years.* Available at: https://www.nice.org.uk/Guidance/PH40/Documents

O'Carroll PW, Berman AI, Maris RW, Moscicki EK, Tanney BL, Silverman MM (1996) Beyond the Tower of Babel: A nomenclature for suicidology. *Suicide and Life Threatening Behavior* 26: 237–52

Owen MJ, O Donovan MC, Thaper A, Craddock N (2011) Neurodevelopmental hypothesis of schizophrenia. *British Journal of Psychiatry* 198(3): 173–175

Ozer EJ (2005) The impact of violence on urban adolescents: Longitudinal effects of perceived school connection and family support. *Journal of Adolescent Research* 20(2): 167–92

Pataki CS (2005) Normal adolescence. In: Sadock BJ, Sadock VA (Eds). *Kaplan & Sadock's Comprehensive Textbook of Psychiatry* (Vol. 2, 8th edition). Baltimore: Lippincot Williams & Wilkins

Qin P, Mortensen PB, Pedersen CB (2009) Frequent change of residence and risk of attempted and completed suicide among children and adolescents. *Archives of General Psychiatry* 66: 628–32

Reach Institute (2014) *Guidelines for adolescent depression in primary care (GLAD-PC) toolkit.* New York: The Reach Institute. Available at: http://www.glad-pc.org/

Rey JM (Ed). (2012) IACAPAP *Textbook of Child and Adolescent Mental Health.* Geneva: International Association for Child and Adolescent Psychiatry and Allied Professions.

Robins RW, Trzesniewski KH (2005) Self-esteem development across the lifespan. *Current Directions in Psychological Science* 14(3): 158–62

Rosenberg ML, Smith JC, Davidson LE, Conn JM (1987) The emergence of youth suicide: An epidemiologic analysis and public health perspective. *Annual Review of Public Health* 8: 417–40

Sadock BJ, Sadock VA (2007) *Kaplan & Sadock's Synopsis of Psychiatry: Behavioral Sciences /Clinical Psychiatry* (10th edition). Philadelphia: Lippincott Williams & Wilkins

Sadock BJ, Sadock VA (2009) *Concise Textbook of Child and Adolescent Psychiatry*. Philadelphia PA: Lippincott Williams and Wilkins

Scahill L, Riddle MA, McSwiggin-Hardin M, Ort SI, King RA, Goodman WK, Cicchetti D, Leckman JF (1997) Children's Yale-Brown Obsessive Compulsive Scale: Reliability and validity. *Journal of the American Academy of Child and Adolescent Psychiatry* 36: 844–52

Scott E, Woolard J (2004) The legal regulation of adolescence. In: Lerner R, Steinberg L (Eds). *Handbook of Adolescent Psychology* (2nd edition). Hoboken, NJ: Wiley

Shapiro F, Maxfield L (2002) Eye movement desensitization and reprocessing (EMDR): Information processing in the treatment of trauma. *Journal of clinical psychology* 58(8): 933–46

Swedo SE, Leckman JF, Rose NR (2012) From Research Subgroup to clinical syndrome: modifying the PANDAS criteria to describe PANS (Pediatric Acute-Onset Neuropsychiatric syndrome). *Pediatrics and Therapeutics* 2(2) http:// dx.doi/10. 4172/2161-0665.1000113

TADS Team (2007) The Treatment for Adolescents with Depression Study (TADS): Long-term effectiveness and safety outcomes. *Archives of General Psychiatry* 64(10): 1132–43

Taylor D, Paton C, Kapur S (2009) *The Maudsley prescribing guidelines* (10th edition). London: Informa

Taylor E, Rutter M (2008) Clinical assessment and diagnostic formulation. In: Rutter M, Bishop D, Pine D, Scott S, Stevenson JS, Taylor EA, Thapar A (Eds). *Rutter's Child and Adolescent Psychiatry* (5th edition). Chichester: Wiley-Blackwell

Taylor S (Ed) (2004) *Advances in the Treatment of Posttraumatic Stress Disorder: Cognitive-Behavioral Perspectives.* New York: Springer

Thapar A, Collishaw S, Pine DS, Thapar AK (2012) Depression in adolescence. *The Lancet* 379: 1056–67

True WR, Rice J, Eisen SA (1993) A twin study of genetic and environmental contributions to liability for posttraumatic stress symptoms. *Archives of General Psychiatry* 50(4): 257–64

Weissman M, Warner V, Wickramaratne P, Moreau D, Olfson M (1997) Offspring of depressed parents: 10 years later. *Archives of General Psychiatry* 54: 932–939

Yehuda R (2001) Biology of posttraumatic stress disorder. *Journal of Clinical Psychiatry* 62 (Suppl. 17): 41–6

CHAPTER

# 29 Intellectual disability

*Richard Nichol, Colleen Adnams*

## 29.1 Introduction

Historically, people with an intellectual disability (ID) have been both severely stigmatised and marginalised. This has occurred on a worldwide scale, not only societally, but also through discriminatory laws, policies, actions and inactions by decision makers in all community spheres.

During the past two decades a new era has emerged for people with disabilities in which their human rights and needs have been recognised resulting in improvements in the lives of those with disabilities in many countries.

This chapter aims to provide the reader with an understanding of the complex, multidimensional nature of IDs and to present practical aspects of identification and assessment, health management and related care of people with ID. The basic epidemiology and known aetiologies of ID are presented, including prevention of the condition where possible. Anyone caring for people with ID will know there are distinct challenges to management and care. Both behavioural and psychopharmacological management strategies and special considerations in ID are suggested.

Specific medico-legal and ethical issues are also discussed in the chapter.

## 29.2 Definitions

Intellectual disability is described in the DSM-5 (American Psychiatric Association, 2013) as a developmental disorder, referring to a neurodevelopmental disorder with its onset during the developmental period. These disorders are characterised by intellectual and adaptive functioning deficits in conceptual, social and practical domains.

**Adaptive functioning** refers to the ability to adapt to the needs of everyday living and requires conceptual, social and practical skills. With an intellectual disability, a person's lower intellectual functioning leads to a reduced adaptive functioning.

The DSM-5 aligns the conceptualisation and terminology of intellectual disability with that of other currently accepted approaches to disability. Historically there has been uncertainty about whether intellectual disability should be regarded as a disability or a health condition (Salvador-Carulla *et al.*, 2011). However it can be regarded as both. The bio-psycho-social model builds upon biological, individual and social experiences of disability and provides a comprehensive basis for understanding disability and focusing on the function of the whole person in a social context. By combining the best of previously disparate disability models, it allows intellectual disability to be regarded as a health condition (the medical model), thus providing for appropriate health support approaches that allow a framework to minimise the negative impact caused by environmental and societal circumstances that impair the person with a disability (the social model). The social model is based on a human rights framework.

The International Classification of Diseases, version 10 (ICD10) (World Health Organization, 2010) is the classification system most widely used across all member countries of the World Health Organization. The Working Group for the ICD version 11 revision proposed the term 'intellectual developmental disorder' and defines the disorder as 'a group of developmental conditions characterised by significant impairment of cognitive functions, which are associated with limitations of learning, adaptive behaviour and skills' (Salvador-Carulla *et al.*, 2011).

There is congruence between the DSM-5 and the proposed ICD-11 definitions: both classification systems recognise impairment of adaptive functioning in addition to intelligence. The International Classification of Functioning, Disability and Health (ICF) (WHO, 2001) complements the definition of the ICD10 and incorporates the concepts disability and functional adaptation to disability. Other international organisations such as the American Association on Intellectual and Developmental Disabilities (AAIDD) have developed similar definitions (American Association on Intellectual and Developmental Disabilities, 2010).

## 29.3 Classification and functional impairments

At present there is much uncertainty as to whether intellectual disability should be regarded as a disability or a health condition (Salvador-Carulla *et al.*, 2011). However it can be regarded as both.

Although many organisations have called for a discontinuation of specific categories based solely on IQ (intelligence quotient), in practice these categories are important due to their diagnostic and clinical utility (Salvador-Carulla *et al.*, 2011).

According to the DSM-5, criteria in three domains must be met to make a diagnosis of intellectual disability: deficits in intellectual functioning, deficits in adaptive functioning and onset of intellectual and adaptive deficits during the developmental period. These criteria are detailed in Table 29.1.

In the DSM-5, the use of specifiers enables a description of the course and symptomatology of the developmental disability, for example age of onset (e.g. the perinatal period), association with a medical condition (e.g. epilepsy) or a genetic condition (e.g. Down syndrome).

For intellectual disability in the DSM-5, levels of severity are included as specifiers, and 'the various levels of severity are defined on the basis of adaptive functioning, and not IQ scores, because it is adaptive functioning that determines the level of support required'. (American Psychiatric Association, 2013). Refer to Table 1 Severity Levels for intellectual disability (intellectual development disorder) in the DSM-5.

The ICD10-defined levels of severity are mild (IQ 50–69), moderate (IQ 35–49), severe (IQ 20–34), and profound (IQ <20). Deficits in functioning across a number of domains and levels of disability can be assessed in detail using the ICF.

## 29.4 Epidemiology

Intellectual disability is the most common developmental disorder and affects a large number of individuals. Intellectual disabilities are a broad group of heterogeneous conditions. Because of the complex nature of the condition and the fact that it is usually life-long, ID has an impact on individuals, on families, communities and societies. The impact of health needs constitutes a major public-health problem.

### Understanding intelligence quotient (IQ)

The term intelligence quotient or IQ, describes a score on a test that rates the person's intellectual function, or cognitive ability, as compared to the general population. IQ tests, for example the Wechsler Intelligence Scale for Children or the Wechsler Adult Intelligence Scales, use a standardised scale normed for particular populations, with a mean score of 100. On most tests, a score between 85 and 115 (or the mean plus or minus 15) indicates average intelligence. An intellectual disability may be diagnosed when the IQ score is 2 or more standard deviations below the population mean, including a margin of error of measurement of 5 points (an IQ score of ≤ 65–75 or ≤ 70 ± 5). An exceptional intelligence would be an IQ ≥ 130 ± 5.

**Table 29.1** DSM-5 Diagnostic Criteria for Intellectual Disability (Intellectual Developmental Disorder)

| **Diagnostic Criteria** |
|---|
| Intellectual disability (intellectual developmental disorder) is a disorder with onset during the developmental period that includes both intellectual and adaptive functioning deficits in conceptual, social, and practical domains. The following three criteria must be met:<br>A. Deficits in intellectual functions, such as reasoning, problem solving, planning, abstract thinking, judgment, academic learning, and learning from experience, confirmed by both clinical assessment and individualized, standardized intelligence testing.<br>B. Deficits in adaptive functioning that result in failure to meet developmental and sociocultural standards for personal independence and social responsibility. Without ongoing support, the adaptive deficits limit functioning in one or more activities of daily life, such as communication, social participation, and independent living, across multiple environments, such as home, school, work, and community.<br>C. Onset of intellectual and adaptive deficits during the developmental period.<br>**Note:** The diagnostic term intellectual disability is the equivalent term for the ICD-11 diagnosis of intellectual developmental disorders. Although the term intellectual disability is used throughout this manual, both terms are used in the title to clarify relationships with other classification systems. Moreover, a federal statute in the United States (Public Law 111–256, Rosa's Law) replaces the term mental retardation with intellectual disability, and research journals use the term intellectual disability. Thus, intellectual disability is the term in common use by medical, educational, and other professions and by the lay public and advocacy groups.<br>*Specify* current severity (see Table 1):<br>**(F70) Mild**<br>**(F71) Moderate**<br>**(F72) Severe**<br>**(F73) Profound** |

**Source:** Reprinted with permission from the *Diagnostic and Statistical Manual of Mental Disorders*, Fifth Edition, (Copyright 2013). American Psychiatric Association.

## 29.4.1 Prevalence

Globally, wide variations in ascertainment methods and use of terminology have contributed to a lack of comparable epidemiological data for intellectual disability. Many factors can affect the estimates of intellectual disability, such as the definitions and classification system used, severity of the disorder, co-existing disabilities and health conditions, gender, age, study population and design, geographical area and socioeconomic status (Maulik and Harbour, 2010). Many large population studies involve household surveys about the existence and experience of disabilities. Some studies have focussed on cognitive function while excluding adaptive functioning. Simple validated questionnaires, such as the Ten Questions Screen (Durkin *et al.*, 1994), have been used for epidemiological studies in developing countries.

Environmental risk factors are more commonly associated with mild intellectual disability, whereas biological and genetic risk factors are more commonly found in the severe condition. Hence, there is a higher prevalence of mild intellectual disability in lower socioeconomic populations compared with higher socioeconomic populations. Notwithstanding, a poor environment will further negatively influence the developmental potential of an individual with a severe intellectual disability.

The global prevalence of intellectual disability is reported to vary according to region and ascertainment methods. In terms of severity, mild intellectual disability is more common. Of the population with an intellectual disability, the relative occurrence of mild, moderate, severe, and profound severity is about 85%, 10%, 4%, and 2%, respectively. In a meta-analysis of 52 worldwide studies, the global prevalence of intellectual disability was estimated to be 10,37 per 1 000 of the population (Maulik *et al.*, 2011). The highest rates were reported in low- and middle-income countries and amongst children and adolescents.

There is evidence of an association between poverty and intellectual disability (including in the world's richer countries) (Emerson, 2004; Emerson, 2007). However, as in other developing countries, in South Africa there is little data on the mechanisms through which poverty and disability affect each other.

Studies in South Africa that have attempted to describe the epidemiology of intellectual disability report prevalence rates of 1–2% for all intellectual disabilities to 17% for mild intellectual disability (Adnams, 2010). In a study that confirmed survey-reported data through clinical assessments, the prevalence of mild and severe intellectual disability in children was 2,9% and 0,64% respectively, with a male predominance of all intellectual disabilities (ratio 3:2) (Kromberg *et al.*, 2008).

## 29.4.2 Aetiology

A range of factors is associated with intellectual disability, and the multifactorial aetiology of intellectual disability is now well recognised. The American Association on Intellectual and Developmental Disabilities (2010) describes four categories of risk factors (biomedical, social, behavioural and educational) that interact across time, including the lifespan of the individual and across generations from parent to child. The multiple risk factors are not distinct and frequently interact.

Biomedical risk factors (see Table 29.2) usually relate to genetic or acquired conditions such as prenatal conditions (genetic disorders, syndromes, metabolic disorders, congenital cerebral malformations, exposure to toxins, maternal illness), perinatal conditions (prematurity, birth injuries, birth asphyxia, neonatal disorders) and postnatal conditions (head injury, childhood infections including meningitis, seizure disorders, malnutrition, neurodegenerative disorders). Biomedical factors interfere with neurological function and are influenced by environmental factors, including psychosocial influences such as poverty, social deprivation, lack of environmental stimulation and lack of opportunity to learn or practise skills. In the last decade, with rapid advances in knowledge and diagnostic capacity in the field of genetics, the recognised contribution of genetic disorders to the aetiology of intellectual disability has increased significantly. Many specific genes have been now implicated in learning, behavioural and psychiatric syndromes. More than 1 000 genetic disorders are known to be associated with intellectual disability. These include chromosome abnormalities such as Trisomy 21 (Down syndrome), single-gene abnormalities (such as fragile-X syndrome) and microdeletion abnormalities

**Table 29.2** Summary of biomedical risk factors in the development of intellectual disability

- **Pre-natal factors**
  - genetic disorders
  - metabolic disorders
  - congenital cerebral malformations
  - exposure to toxins
  - maternal illness (e.g. retroviral disease)
  - fetal alcohol spectrum disorders.
- **Peri-natal factors**
  - prematurity
  - birth injuries
  - birth asphyxia
  - neonatal disorders.
- **Post-natal factors**
  - head injury
  - childhood infections
  - seizure disorders
  - malnutrition
  - neurodegenerative disorders.
- **Biomedical factors are influenced by environmental factors (e.g. psychosocial influences)**
  - poverty
  - social deprivation
  - lack of environmental stimulation
  - lack of opportunities to learn or practise skills.

**Source:** American Association on Intellectual and Developmental Disabilities, 2010 (adapted). Republished with permission from the American Association on Intellectual and Developmental Disabilities. Permission conveyed through the Copyright Clearance Centre.

(such as Prader-Willi syndrome). The most common genetic syndrome associated with ID is Down syndrome, a trisomy abnormality of chromosome 21, with an incidence of 1 per 700 births. In a significant number of individuals (30–50%) the aetiology remains unknown (Maulik *et al.*, 2010).

No reliable data exist on the aetiology of intellectual disability in South Africa. Clinic-derived reports suggest that a number of causes of intellectual disability in South Africa have a similar a prevalence to that of developed countries. A few studies have examined aetiology in small population samples. In a study of a rural population, Kromberg *et al.*, (2008), reported a congenital aetiology in 20,6% of affected children, an acquired aetiology in 6,3%, and an undetermined aetiology in 73,1%. In the Western Cape Province the prevalence of intellectual disability was estimated at 3% (Kleintjes *et al.*, 2006).

High prevalence rates in South Africa for conditions that are associated with the onset of an intellectual disability in the pre-natal and developmental period suggest a higher total prevalence of intellectual disability than in high-income countries. Many of these conditions are preventable and, in themselves, contribute significantly to overall burden of disease and care. This has implications for addressing effective prevention and interventions to reduce the prevalence of conditions that contribute to intellectual disabilities in South Africa. Preventable conditions that impact on the burden of disability, either through a high prevalence or severity, include nutritional deficiencies and growth stunting (which are strong predictors for poor educational outcomes) (Grantham-McGregor *et al.*, 2005), tuberculous meningitis, fetal alcohol spectrum disorder (FASD) and trauma and violence.

### 29.4.2.1 Fetal alcohol spectrum disorder

The burden of mental and physical disease associated with high levels of alcohol abuse in South Africa has major implications for intellectual disabilities. FASD results from pre-natal alcohol exposure due to excessive maternal drinking. In high-risk regions in South Africa, the prevalence rates of FASD, of which fetal alcohol syndrome (FAS) is the most severe expression of the spectrum, are the highest in the Western world at 6,7%–11% (Urban *et al.*, 2008; May *et al.*, 2013). The majority of children and adults with FASD in South Africa function in the mild intellectual disability range and demonstrate associated social and behavioural difficulties. (See Chapter 20: Addictions 1: Alcohol-related disorders, for further discussion on FASD).

### 29.4.2.2 Violence and injury

In South Africa, violence and injury carry a high burden of morbidity and mortality (Lalloo and Van As, 2004). Traumatic brain injury (TBI) contributes significantly to this burden. TBI is an important preventable cause of intellectual disability in children across the developmental span and also of cognitive impairment in older adolescents and adults. Especially in children, there is a high burden of disablement due to TBI resulting from traffic accidents and physical assault. Alcohol plays a significant role in the epidemiology of traumatic brain injury, both in children and adults who may be victims of violence and motor vehicle accidents.

### 29.4.2.3 Retroviral disease (neuro-Aids)

South Africa is severely affected by the HIV/Aids epidemic, with both the highest reported prevalence of HIV/Aids per capita and the world's largest population. More than 15% of the population aged 15–49 years and 280 000 children aged 0–14 years, are living with HIV. Ninety-five per cent of children infected with HIV in sub-Saharan Africa (SSA) acquire infections from their mothers. HIV/Aids is the leading cause of death in South African children under younger than five. Those children who manage to survive without early treatment have a high prevalence of cognitive disability, visual-spatial and motor deficits, neurological impairment, seizures and encephalopathy. (See Chapter 33:

HIV and mental health, for further information on HIV and cognition.)

#### 29.4.2.4 Nutritional deficiencies

Nutritional deficiencies and growth stunting represent multiple biological and psychosocial risks and are indicators of poor development (Grantham-McGregor *et al.*, 2005). Childhood under-nutrition is generally associated with concurrent and long-term global deficiencies in cognition, behaviour and motor skills (although the relationship is often confounded by socioeconomic factors). In South Africa, the prevalence of protein-energy malnutrition (PEM) has increased and is regarded as a complication of HIV/Aids epidemic.

## 29.5 Assessment and diagnosis of a person with an intellectual disability

Assessment and diagnosis of children and adults with an intellectual disability should be made in the context of their developmental delay and intellectual impairment (Hurley *et al.*, 2007).

The goal of the diagnostic assessment is to:

- determine the nature of the problem
- identify the aetiology
- suggest potential interventions
- address issues of prognosis.

The general health assessment of a person with an intellectual disability should always precede a mental health or psychometric assessment and should begin with a thorough history, usually provided by the parent or carer. The history or interview includes developmental, medical and family information and informs the physical examination and subsequent evaluations and special investigations. Many individuals with an intellectual disability have limitations in participating in a health or educational evaluation process and the interview and assessment procedures should be conducted with special consideration for the person's abilities, for example, by communicating using simple, understandable language and short sentences (Hurley *et al.*, 2007).

### 29.5.1 Medical and neurodevelopmental history

The medical history includes an enquiry of the mother's pregnancy, birth, key developmental milestones, educational progress, early, previous and current health problems (including seizures and other physical problems such as visual and hearing disabilities). Biomedical and other risk factors for intellectual disability should be identified. Record information about medications interventions and any previous assessments such as intelligence testing and educational or occupational evaluations.

### 29.5.2 Family and social history

A detailed three-generation family history is ideal: ask for information about the family's general health conditions, genetic disorders and syndromes, intellectual disability and mental illness. Knowledge of a person's social circumstances is important because individuals with an intellectual disability are generally dependent on family members for care and support and the family will be closely involved with health-care provision.

### 29.5.3 Clinical examination

The clinical examination should include observation of the person to assess social interaction, behaviour, physical disabilities and dysmorphic facial and other features characteristic of genetic syndromes. Growth and head circumference should be measured, especially in children, since individuals with an intellectual disability frequently present with growth abnormalities. The physical examination should include all systems, including the central nervous system. Include an assessment or enquiry about hearing and vision as part of the neurological examination.

### 29.5.4 Psychometric and adaptive functioning assessment

A good history will provide a gauge of the level of intellectual and adaptive functioning of the individual with an intellectual disability. In South Africa most suspected cases of intellectual disability are diagnosed after a clinical evaluation of the patient's delays in intellectual functioning abilities and social adaptive functioning.

Diagnosis of intellectual disability can be confirmed by administering standardised tests, such as IQ tests or other tests that have been especially developed to assess domains of cognitive and adaptive function in people with more severe levels of intellectual disability. In South Africa, psychometric tests that are commonly used in specialist intellectual disability services include the Grover Counter Test to measure level of intellectual functioning and the Vineland Adaptive Behavior Scales to measure personal and social skills of individuals from birth through adulthood.

### 29.5.5 Levels of intellectual disability

Psychiatric classifications describe four levels of severity of intellectual disability: mild, moderate, severe and profound. The most accurate diagnosis of intellectual ability is determined using input from members of the multi-disciplinary team.

#### 29.5.5.1 Mild

IQ is generally between 50 and 69 and accounts for about 80% of cases. Development during early life is slower than in typically developing children and developmental milestones are delayed. These children and adults are able to communicate and learn basic skills. Their ability to learn to read and master computing skills is on par with school children in Grades 3–6.

#### 29.5.5.2 Moderate

IQ is usually between 35 and 49 and accounts for about 12% of cases. These children and adults are slow in meeting intellectual developmental milestones. Their ability to learn and think logically is impaired but they are able to communicate and look after themselves with some assistance. With supervision they can perform unskilled or semi-skilled work.

#### 29.5.5.3 Severe

IQ is usually between 20 and 34 and accounts for 3–4% of all cases. Every aspect of their development in the early years is distinctly delayed. They have difficulty pronouncing words and have a restricted vocabulary. Through considerable practise and time, they may gain basic self-help skills but still need support at school, home and in the community.

#### 29.5.5.4 Profound

IQ is usually below 20 and accounts for 1–2% of all cases. These children and adults cannot take care of themselves and have little or no verbal language. Their capacity to express emotions may be poorly understood. Seizures, physical disabilities and reduced life expectancy are common.

### 29.5.6 Mental health evaluation

The mental health assessment includes obtaining a detailed history about behaviour, possible psychosocial or environmental stressors and symptoms of mental illness. (See Chapter 7: Clinical assessment in psychiatry, for more information on mental health evaluation.) The standard evaluation procedure may have to be flexibly adapted in order to optimise the interview and observations. Individuals with an intellectual disability may not display typical features of mental illness. In addition, the relationship between medical conditions and a mental health disorder in individuals with an intellectual disability is not always understood by the patient, his or her family or health-care providers. It is important to be aware that medical problems may be the source of the person's presenting complaints. For example, chronic pain may be the source of depressed mood or of a behavioural disturbance such as irritability or aggression. Medication and side effects should be asked about. In higher functioning individuals substance abuse should not be overlooked as a cause of behaviour and mood disturbances. Diagnosis of a suspected psychiatric illness may have to be confirmed or re-evaluated after further assessment and observation.

## 29.6 Associated health conditions and co-morbidities

### 29.6.1 Associated health conditions

People with an intellectual disability are at an increased risk of a number of congenital physical malformations and neurodevelopmental disabilities. They may develop chronic primary and secondary medical problems that occur more commonly than in the general population (see Table 29.3). Those with a severe and profound intellectual disability and who are not ambulant are at a particular risk of health problems and shortened life expectancy. People with an intellectual disability have a significantly increased lifetime risk of developing epilepsy. There is an association with higher prevalence of epilepsy and increasing disability. It is important for health-care providers to be aware that any illness may markedly reduce cognitive and adaptive functioning in people with an intellectual disability. Common medical or emotional disorders may provoke symptoms that mimic psychiatric illness.

Certain genetic syndromes may also have clinical features or health conditions as part of the phenotype. Table 29.4 lists a few examples.

### 29.6.2 Health care needs of people with intellectual disability

The health needs of people with an intellectual disability should be integrated into general health services and should be met through comprehensive approaches at a primary-health care level. Those with an intellectual disability have

**Table 29.3** Chronic health system conditions associated with intellectual disability

| | |
|---|---|
| **Central nervous system or neurological** | ▸ epilepsy |
| **Oro-dental** | ▸ dental caries<br>▸ dental malocclusion<br>▸ gum disease<br>▸ bony, facial and palate abnormalities<br>▸ swallowing inco-ordination |
| **Sensory** | ▸ visual problems<br>▸ hearing problems |
| **Cardiovascular** | ▸ congenital heart disease<br>▸ ischaemic heart disease |
| **Musculo-skeletal** | ▸ skeletal (especially spine) and joint deformities<br>▸ postural abnormalities<br>▸ muscle tone and power abnormalities<br>▸ osteoporosis |
| **Gastrointestinal** | ▸ constipation<br>▸ gastro-oesophageal reflux disease<br>▸ upper gastrointestinal cancer |
| **Urinary tract** | ▸ enuresis<br>▸ urinary retention<br>▸ urinary tract infections |
| **Respiratory** | ▸ upper and lower respiratory tract infections |
| **Endocrine** | ▸ type I and type II diabetes mellitus<br>▸ obesity<br>▸ hypothyroidism<br>▸ metabolic syndrome |
| **Multiple system disorders** | ▸ cerebral palsy<br>▸ ageing problems |
| **Mental health** | ▸ behavioural problems<br>▸ mental health problems |

**Source:** Van Schrojenstein Lantman-de Valk and Walsh, 2008. Adapted with permission from the BMJ Publishing Group Ltd.

**Table 29.4** Physical manifestations and clinical features of specific genetic syndromes

| Syndrome | Physical manifestations |
|---|---|
| **Cornelia de Lange** | ▸ gastrointestinal disturbances – painful reflux<br>▸ hearing impairments |
| **Prader-Willi** | ▸ hyperphagia (presents in childhood)<br>▸ childhood and adulthood obesity<br>▸ diabetes mellitus |
| **Tuberous sclerosis complex** | ▸ epilepsy<br>▸ abnormal growths in multiple organs (e.g. brain tumours with headaches, double vision, dizziness) |
| **Down** | ▸ congenital cardiac defects (childhood and adulthood)<br>▸ hypothyroidism (childhood and adulthood)<br>▸ premature menopause<br>▸ Alzheimer's-type dementia in adults |
| **Williams** | ▸ congenital cardiac defects (mostly present in childhood)<br>▸ heightened response to auditory stimuli |
| **Angelman** | ▸ epilepsy |
| **Smith-Magenis** | ▸ hearing impairments |

**Source:** Waite *et al.*, 2014 (adapted)

important health care support needs, including early identification and intervention of at-risk conditions, access to health services, lifelong **health promotion**, screening for at-risk conditions to encourage healthy lifestyles and rehabilitation of co-morbid disabilities. In recent years, there has been an increase in the quality of life and life expectancy of the population with intellectual disability, largely due to improved intervention of health disorders driven by increased recognition of the rights of people with disabilities to health care. Survival of individuals has increased dramatically over past decades due to advances in cardiac surgery in childhood, general health management and increased social inclusion. The average life expectancy of a person with Down Syndrome is now 55-60 years. In addition, increased longevity in people with ID has been accompanied by a significant increase in mid-life health problems that are common to the general ageing population. This has resulted in a large ageing population of people with an intellectual disability who experience health disorders such as ischaemic heart disease and Alzheimer's-type dementia (Sheehan *et al.*, 2014).

In spite of increased longevity, there is ongoing evidence that although the population with an intellectual disability has more health needs than does the general population, they still face many barriers to health care and their needs are inadequately met (Bouras, 2010), especially in middle- and low-income countries. In order to address their health needs, health programmes are required that can provide both surveillance for at-risk conditions and rehabilitation. Medical interventions aim to prevent or treat health conditions that may cause increased morbidity and mortality if neglected. It is therefore important to know about or monitor the health course or trajectory of a particular intellectual disability (especially if associated with a known aetiology), the medical complications that may occur and their relative prevalence in different age-groups.

## 29.6.3 Multidisciplinary health management

Because persons with an intellectual disability have a range of needs that impact on their health, and to ensure that they receive optimum comprehensive care, a team consisting of more than one health professional is essential. Multidisciplinary teams often include psychiatrists, paediatricians, neurologists, psychologists, medical officers, nurses, occupational therapists, social workers, physiotherapists and speech therapists. In most instances the team is much smaller. Where different members of the professional team are able to work together and meet regularly, patient care is enhanced.

## 29.7 Associated behavioural and psychiatric symptoms and psychiatric disorders

### 29.7.1 Diagnostic overshadowing

Diagnostic overshadowing refers to the tendency of clinicians to attribute symptoms or behaviour in learning-disabled individuals to their underlying cognitive deficits. This means that co-morbid psychopathology is often under-diagnosed (Jones *et al.*, 2008). People with an intellectual disability must be evaluated comprehensively to ensure co-morbid conditions are not missed.

### 29.7.2 Challenging behaviour

Challenging behaviour, also referred to as problem behaviour, comprises the most common form of mental disorder in children and adults with an intellectual disability and is often the reason for presenting to mental health and related services. These behaviour, which may be directed at themselves or at significant others, represent a wide range of behaviour that may pose a risk to the person with an intellectual disability, to others or to property. Although the behaviour serve a function for the individual with an intellectual disability, they may make care-giving difficult and stressful and also affect the person's well-being. The behaviour is often maintained or reinforced if the person is successful in altering his or her internal or external environment through the behaviour, which may be an attempt to communicate, gain attention or control of their life, avoid duties or demands or achieve access to preferred activities or objects.

The causes of challenging behaviour are complex and multifactorial and include medical, other co-morbid psychiatric conditions and environmental factors.

- Medical factors
  - unrecognised pain or discomfort
  - side effects of medication
  - substance abuse
  - physical illness (e.g. epilepsy)
  - **behavioural phenotypes** – specific to a syndrome.
- Other co-morbid psychiatric conditions (discussed later in this chapter)
- Environmental factors
  - problems in the living and working environment
  - life events (e.g. change of school, death, separation or returning to a residential facility after being home for a short period)
  - communication problems (e.g. inability to communicate needs or emotions effectively, carers maladjusted to needs of the person with an intellectual disability, inappropriate responses and management that reinforces challenging behaviour)
  - life stages (e.g. puberty)
  - behaviour serves a function or purpose for the person with an intellectual disability: challenging behaviour is maintained if the person is successful in altering their internal or external environment through their behaviour.

Three of these behaviours – aggression, self-mutilation or self-harm and inappropriate sexual behaviour – will now be discussed.

Aggressive behaviour may be unpredictable and unprovoked. Patients may display aggression towards family members, peers, carers or health workers. Reduced frustration tolerance and disinhibited behaviour is common. Sometimes patients can become destructive, breaking windows or damaging personal objects. As the person displaying the aggressive behaviour may often not able to verbalise his or her pain, care should be taken to examine the person physically to exclude fractures, infections or other lesions before administering sedating medication.

Individuals may direct aggression towards themselves in the form of self-injury, such as head banging, continuous scratching of a painful self-induced physical wound, self-biting or even ingestion of objects or chemicals.

Adolescents and adults may exhibit sexualised behaviour such as masturbation in public, imitating or performing acts of coitus, or inappropriate sexual fondling of peers or carers. A distinction should be made between hyper-sexuality and simple excessiveness (Walsh, 2000). Where possible, the conditions relating to hypersexual behaviour should be identified and managed (e.g. exclude possible side effects of risperidone or carbamazepine that may cause increased sexual behaviour) (El-Gabalawi *et al.*, 2007). When a child or adult with an intellectual disability presents with inappropriate sexual behaviour, the possibility of sexual abuse of that person should always be excluded.

## 29.7.3 Comorbid psychiatric conditions

People with an intellectual disability manifest with the entire spectrum of psychiatric disorders described in the general population, but are more susceptible to developing co-morbid psychiatric conditions than those with a normal intelligence. In children and adolescents with an intellectual disability, emotional and behavioural problems are 3–7 times more frequent than in typically developing youth. Symptoms of psychiatric disorders are often attributed to the intellectual disability rather than recognised as co-morbid psychiatric symptomatology (diagnostic over-shadowing). Additionally, some mental conditions may manifest differently in individuals with an intellectual disability, compared with individuals in the general population (e.g. psychotic features may represent symptoms of depression in individuals with an intellectual disability). These symptoms may be exacerbated in those with a severe form of intellectual disability due to restricted communication skills and bland symptomatology known as psychosocial masking.

The correct psychiatric diagnosis is not always made with certainty in persons with severe and profound intellectual disability. Because of all factors, and despite high levels of mental-health conditions, psychiatric illness often remains undiagnosed.

Co-morbid psychiatric conditions (or dual diagnosis) occur in about 40–50% of ID individuals including:

- attention deficit hyperactivity disorder (ADHD)
- depressive disorders and suicidal behaviour
- autism spectrum disorders (ASD)
- oppositional defiant disorder (ODD)
- conduct disorder (CD)
- anxiety disorders.

## 29.7.4 Behavioural phenotypes

O'Brien (2006) describes behavioural phenotypes as patterns of behaviour that present in syndromes caused by chromosomal or genetic abnormalities. They may also occur when there is an etiological factor such as a neurotoxin. They have both physiological and behavioural manifestations with distinctive social, linguistic, cognitive and motor profiles. Knowledge of behavioural phenotypes can assist carers to understand how a person with an intellectual disability interacts with the environment and adapts it to suit his or her needs.

Specific examples of behavioural phenotypes in genetic syndromes include attachment to a preferred adult in Smith-Magenis syndrome and attachment to objects in cri-du-chat syndrome. Self-injurious behaviour occurs in almost all people with Lesch-Nyhan syndrome. Children and adults with Angelman syndrome and Smith-Magenis syndrome have been shown to be more than three times more likely to show aggression than those without these syndromes (Waite *et al.*, 2014).

## 29.7.5 Psychopharmacology

Individuals with an intellectual disability have vulnerable neurological and other biological systems. They have an increased sensitivity to dose effects at normal prescribed levels and are at risk of adverse or paradoxical responses to sedatives, stimulants and anticonvulsants and other pharmacological treatment of behavioural problems or psychiatric illness. Due caution should

**Table 29.5** Summary of psychotropic medications by class used for people with intellectual disability

| |
|---|
| **Antipsychotic drugs**<br>Risperidone is often the most commonly prescribed antipsychotic drug for people with an intellectual disability with behavioural disturbances and aggression. There is evidence that risperidone may reduce the total symptom burden in ADHD in children with moderate intellectual disability. It should only be used where stimulants have proved to be ineffective. Care should be taken to monitor patients for early signs of metabolic syndrome. |
| **Anticonvulsants**<br>Anticonvulsants are commonly used for co-morbid seizure disorders. They may be useful to stabilise mood or behaviour. |
| **Antidepressants**<br>Selective serotonin reuptake inhibitors (SSRIs) are useful for major depression, especially for those individuals with ID who have repetitive movement disorders. Behavioural activation is more common in children and other persons with an intellectual disability compared to the general population. Treatment should be commenced with low doses of SSRIs and increased gradually.<br>Tricyclic antidepressants (TADs) may be useful for insomnia. |
| **Psychostimulants (methylphenidate)**<br>Stimulant drugs are among the most commonly prescribed psychotropic medications used for ADHD. |
| **Adrenergics**<br>Clonidine may be prescribed as an alternate medication for ADHD. |
| **Other drugs**<br>Cyproterone may be used in males displaying unacceptable levels of sexual and aggressive behaviour where comprehensive behaviour therapy has not proved to be effective. |

**Source:** Dulcan, 2010

be taken when prescribing medication and individuals with ID should be monitored carefully. A sound pharmacological rule is to 'start low and go slow' when prescribing psychotropic medications in people with an intellectual disability.

More than one-third of all persons with an intellectual disability receive at least one psychotropic drug (Dulcan, 2010). The type of medication used depends on which co-morbid conditions are present (e.g. an antidepressant for major depression or a stimulant for ADHD) (see Table 29.5). Doses of medication should be calculated according to the patient's weight and age.

Polypharmacy and inadequate medication review are acknowledged problems in this population (International Association for Scientific Study of Intellectual and Developmental Disabilities, 2001). Care should be taken to avoid polypharmacy unless there are clear indications for combining drugs. Prescription charts should be reviewed at least once a year to avoid chronic use of unnecessary drugs.

## 29.7.6 Management of challenging behaviour

Challenging behaviour interferes with the daily life of individuals with an intellectual disability and their caregivers and reduces their quality of life and survival. The starting point is to ascertain whether the behaviour is linked to treatable physical causes, including pain, which often necessitate the use of medication.

A clinical psychologist may conduct a behaviour analysis that includes:

- a detailed description of the behaviour being targeted
- the context in which it takes place (time, place, who, what, why, etc.)
- the sequence of events and interactions with others, including possible triggers and responses, and whether these responses reinforce the target behaviour
- potential needs met by the challenging behaviour.

The psychologist then devises means of extinguishing negative behaviour and reinforcing positive behaviour (behaviour therapy). Clinical staff and/or the patient's family are often also involved in this process

Medication may be prescribed, especially if the behaviour therapy has proved to be ineffective. Risperidone, haloperidol, clozapine or other antipsychotic medication may help to prevent aggressive behaviour. Although its use has been considered controversial, hormonal manipulation using medications such as cyproterone may be effective in cases of inappropriate sexual behaviour or hyper-sexuality where behavioural interventions failed.

# 29.8 Special considerations in intellectual disability

## 29.8.1 Early detection and intervention

Prenatal screening (sonography and amniocentesis) plays an important role in identifying certain conditions *in utero,* such as Down syndrome.

When a specific genetic disorder is detected in a child with an intellectual disability, the parents should be included in a genetic counselling programme. Parents often have many questions to ask the paediatrician concerning the well-being of future offspring and the chances of the condition recurring. Advice and information concerning the nature and implication of the specific condition are very important.

Psychological support is vital to help parents work through their own response and grief processes concerning the impact their child's condition will have on their lives, but also to assist them with decisions about subsequent pregnancies.

## 29.8.2 Normalisation and de-institutionalisation

Due to ignorance and stigmatisation many people believe that people with an intellectual disability should live in government or other residential institutions away from their families and communities. Over the past 20 or more years there has been a strong move to de-institutionalise psychiatric patients (except where the person has a compromised social support system and/or continuous and extensive health-care support needs).

In South Africa the rights of all people with disabilities are protected by international charters and treaties and national laws and policies to ensure recognition of their human rights, including the right to be regarded with humanity and respect. South African people with an intellectual disability have the right to be equal citizens of their local communities and country according to the South African Constitution. Examples of international charters are the human rights based United Nations Convention on the Rights of Persons with Disabilities (www.un.org/disability/documents/convention/convopt.prot-e.pdf) and the United Nations Convention on the Rights of the Child (www.childrights.ie/sites/default/files/UNCRCEEnglish.pdf), to both of which South Africa is a signatory.

Within the relevant sectors, policies make provision for social security (disability) grants for children and adults, health security in the form of free primary health care for disability grant recipients and fiscal or tax benefits.

Within the education system, policies provide for inclusion of learners with an intellectual

### Why people with an intellectual disability need an administrator

Although most people with an intellectual disability have limited financial resources, there are some individuals who may accumulate financial resources through an inheritance or other reasons. The person with an intellectual disability is at high risk of exploitation by others wanting to have their money. On the other hand, should someone with an intellectual disability sign a contract, unless he or she has fully understood the contract, his or her signature may not be valid and the contract may be considered null and void.

Where possible all people with an intellectual disability should have an **administrator** to protect themselves and their interests. In the case of institutionalised individuals, the chief executive officer of the institution fulfils this role. Parents or an designated adult family member of a person with an intellectual disability are regarded as the person's guardian, or a formal curator may be appointed in a court of law.

If the administrators feel that their charges have need of some article or service and finances are available, they may purchase the item on that person's behalf. However, should there be a formal inquiry into the person with an intellectual disability's affairs, the administrator may have to explain to the Master of the High Court why the expenses were in the best interest of their charge.

disability in the mainstream system and for specialised education support. Unfortunately, according to the official policy, learners may need to fail three or more academic years before the Inclusive Education section of the Department of Education is prepared to intervene. The educational needs of many learners are frequently not met in the mainstream education system.

Although people with an intellectual disability have difficulty in competing in the open market labour system, those with less severe degrees of impairment are able to work with supervision in the open labour market and in facilities that provide supervised occupational activities.

Where possible, adults with an intellectual disability should be able to live as autonomously as possible. People with an intellectual disability have a right to consensual intimate relationships and should have access to health and other community services, such as health promotion and HIV testing and counselling.

## 29.9 Medico-legal and ethical issues in intellectual disability

### 29.9.1 Legal rights of people with an intellectual disability

People with an intellectual disability have human rights protection under international disability conventions and national laws and policies, including the Mental Health Care Act of 2002.

Individuals with an intellectual disability should be evaluated to determine their ability to care for themselves and to manage their own affairs. Most require support from others to do this and therefore need an administrator to assist them. Mostly this role is undertaken informally by a parent, adult sibling or a family member, but any other independent person may fulfil this role as the need arises. Applications are made to a Master of the High Court.

This process is described in Chapter VIII of the Mental Health Care Act of 2002 (The care and administration of property of mentally ill person or person with severe or profound intellectual disability).

The affairs of people with a severe or profound intellectual disability, who are permanently institutionalised, are administered by the administrative head of that institution.

### 29.9.2 Sterilisation of persons with an intellectual disability

Families and carers of people with an intellectual disability may request that surgical procedures for permanent contraception be undertaken to ensure lifelong infertility. There is little literature to guide health care providers on how to respond ethically (Van Schrojenstein Lantman-de Valk, 2008). Sexuality education and reversible contraception should always be the first option offered to individuals with ID. Permanent sterilisation for the purpose of infertility should be undertaken on the basis of full, free and informed consent. According to the World Health Organization (OHCHR *et al.*, 2014), persons with an intellectual disability should not be coerced or unwillingly undergo sterilisation procedures.

The South African Constitution protects the rights and human dignity of persons, in particular those who are incapable of giving their consent or who are mentally disabled, by ensuring that any decisions about sterilisation are made in a manner that is ethical, responsible and considerate and in the best interests of the person.

Should surgical sterilisation be considered for any reason, including for medical reasons, this should be decided by a multi-disciplinary professional panel that includes a disability rights advocate and the guardian representing the person with an intellectual disability, if the person is not cognitively capable of understanding the consent or surgical procedure.

### 29.9.3 Involvement in criminal activity

People with an intellectual disability may be implicated in criminal activity. Where mental illness or intellectual disability is suspected the person is referred to a forensic psychiatric team in order to determine whether or not a formal

30-day forensic evaluation is warranted. (See Chapter 35: Legal and ethical aspects of mental health, concerning the Criminal Procedures Act).

The 30-day evaluation will determine whether the alleged perpetrator should be considered:

- fit to stand trial (understands the nature of the charge against him or her, is able to follow the court proceedings and is able to give instructions to his or her defence lawyers)
- criminally accountable for his/her deeds (the person was able to distinguish between right and wrong at the time of the alleged crime(s) and had the ability to stop him/herself doing it.)

By and large most people with an intellectual disability are not found to be fit for trial or criminally accountable for their deeds. Each case should be considered separately, especially where the accused person has a borderline or mild degree of intellectual disability.

## 29.9.4 Ability to give evidence in court

There have been incidents where people with an intellectual disability may have been the victim of crime, or witnessed criminal activities. The court may request that they be evaluated to determine whether they are capable of giving evidence in a trial. Each person with ID should be assessed individually rather than an assumption made that they are incapable of assisting the court. In some centres in South Africa, trained facilitators provide support to people with an intellectual disability to give evidence as witnesses in court.

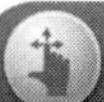

### Case study 29.1

Jamie is a 26-year-old man whose parents have noticed a change is his behaviour. He has never attended mainstream education (IQ = 60), but coped well in a school for children with specialised needs and completed his education there.

Jamie has an amiable nature and is usually able to relate to others in his own way. He spends most days in a supervised occupational facility where he undertakes uncomplicated activities. His younger brother, who also has an intellectual disability, works in a different section of the facility. Every evening the brothers return to the family home.

**Early history**

Jamie's mother states that her pregnancy and subsequent delivery were uneventful, but she soon realised that he had physical and mental handicaps.

Jamie's muscle strength in his right arm and leg muscles was weaker than his left side. His developmental milestones were delayed, but he was eventually able to walk (with assistance) by the age of two and spoke by the age of four. Although he has adequate bladder sphincter control during the day, he uses an adult nappy at night.

He is very friendly to people around him but he has a restricted vocabulary, with many words being spoken indistinctly. His parents (both professional workers) are knowledgeable of their sons' conditions. Their home environment is stable.

Recently Jamie has had repeated bouts of irrational fretting regarding the future. During these episodes, he shares his concerns with anyone who is prepared to listen, but becomes verbally and sometimes even physically aggressive when they don't agree with him.

Jamie's parents now feel incapable of managing his behaviour.

**Suggested questions for discussion**

1. Broadly speaking, what do you think are the most likely cause of the brothers' conditions?
2. How would you rate Jamie's level of functioning?
3. Which co-morbid conditions are present?
4. Do you think medication would be of value?
5. What other treatment modalities should be utilised?

| Information to aid the discussion | |
|---|---|
| Classification and functional impairment | mild ID degree<br>primary nocturnal enuresis<br>decreased muscle strength (unilaterally)<br>inability to walk unassisted<br>dysarthria |
| Epidemiology | Jamie is one of the 1–2% of the population with ID<br>as both brothers have ID, there is a strong possibility of a genetic aetiology, but no chromosomal tests have been performed |
| Assessment and diagnosis | he was evaluated by a paediatrician and a neurologist in his early years |
| Associated conditions | cerebral palsy |
| Associated behavioural and psychiatric symptoms | OCD-like symptoms and general anxiety disorder; the condition responded well to a SSRI<br>aggression well managed with risperidone (low doses) |
| Special considerations | Jamie lives with his parents in the family home. He looks forward to work and is accepted in the community |
| Medico-legal and ethical issues | Internal arrangements have been made for a younger member of the extended family to become Jamie and his brother's guardian when the parents are no longer able to manage the sons' affairs |

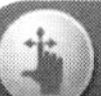

## Case study 29.2

Denzel is an 8-year-old boy whose parents had misused alcohol for many years and who were caught up in their own problems. Even from an early age he was different from other children. He isolated himself from the other children in the home, preferring to rock on his haunches for many hours each day. He never learnt to talk but eventually communicated some of his needs to his grandmother using gestures in a manner she could understand.

Both Denzel's parents died the previous year due to chronic medical conditions. Apparently these tragedies had little noticeable effect on Denzel.

During the evaluation, Denzel's grandmother stated that he was a very busy child who found it difficult to sit without fidgeting or moving about. She had tried to teach him how to recognise numbers and colours, but without success. When given crayons and paper he would sometimes scrawl a few lines before losing interest. He needed constant supervision at home and was unable to comprehend or complete the basic tasks of daily living. He was not fully toilet trained.

During examination the doctor felt she was unable to connect with Denzel. He spent most of the interview playing in a non-constructive way with parts of toys.

**Suggested questions for discussion**

1. What would be the most likely cause of Denzel's intellectual disability?
2. Name two other co-morbid conditions.
3. How would you rate Denzel's level of intellectual disability compared to Jamie's?
4. What treatment modalities should be considered when managing Denzel's condition?

| Information to aid the discussion | |
|---|---|
| Classification and functional impairment | ID moderate degree<br>primary nocturnal enuresis<br>primary encopresis receptive and expressive communication disorder |
| Epidemiology | Denzel is one of the 1–2% of the population with an intellectual disability<br>FASD |
| Assessment and diagnosis | he was recently evaluated by a paediatrician and a child psychiatrist |
| Associated conditions | facial features FASD, microcephaly |
| Associated behavioural and psychiatric symptoms | autism spectrum disorder (ASD) and ADHD |
| Special considerations | Denzel should be referred for educational support for children with specialised learning needs. This may be to a special school or mainstream school with a special unit that are able to facilitate support for learners with ASD and ID |
| Medico-legal and ethical Issues | arrangements have been made for the CEO of the school hostel to act as Denzel's guardian and for future foster or children's home placement (Denzel's grandmother passed away soon after the social workers became aware of his condition) |

## Conclusion

This chapter provided an overview of aspects of intellectual disability that are pertinent to general and mental health care. People with an intellectual disability are at higher risk of general health problems, behavioural problems and mental illness than the general population. All health workers should have knowledge of the determinants of intellectual disabilities and should be able to respond to the mental health management and care needs of individuals with an intellectual disability.

# References

Adnams CM (2010) Perspectives of intellectual disability in South Africa: Epidemiology, policy, services for children and adults. *Current Opinion in Psychiatry* 23: 436–40

American Association on Intellectual and Developmental Disabilities (AAIDD) (2010) *Intellectual Disability: Definition, Classification and Systems of Supports* (11th edition). Washington, DC. AAIDD Publishing

American Psychiatric Association (2013) *Diagnostic and Statistical Manual of Mental Disorders* (5th edition). Washington DC: American Psychiatric Publishing

Bouras N (2010) Unmet needs of people with developmental and intellectual disability. *Current Opinion in Psychiatry* 23(5): 405–6

Dulcan MK (2010) *Dulcan's Textbook of Child and Adolescent Psychiatry*. Washington DC: American Psychiatric Publishing

Durkin MS, Davidson LL, Desai P, Hasan ZM, Khan N, Thorburn MJ, Shrout PE, Wang W (1994). Validity of the ten-question screen for childhood disability: Results from population based studies in Bangladesh, Jamaica and Pakistan. *Epidemiology* 5: 283–9

El-Gabalawi F, Johnson RJ (2007) Hypersexuality in inpatient children and adolescents: Recognition, differential diagnosis, and evaluation. *CNS Spectrum* 12(11): 821–7

Emerson E (2004) Poverty and children with intellectual disabilities in the world's richer countries. *Journal of Intellectual and Developmental Disabilities* 29(4): 319–38

Emerson E (2007) Poverty and people with intellectual disabilities. *Mental Retardation Developmental Disabilities Research Reviews* 13(2): 107–13

Fletcher R, Loschen E, Stavrakaki C, First M (2007) Intellectual Disabilities. In: *Diagnostic Manual – Intellectual Disability (DM-ID): A Textbook of Diagnosis of Mental Disorders on Persons with Intellectual Disability*. New York: NADD Press/National Association for the Dually Diagnosed: 63–8

Grantham-McGregor S, Baker-Henningham H (2005) Review of the evidence linking protein and energy to mental development. *Public Health Nutrition* 8(7A): 1191–201

Hurley AD, Levitas A, Lecavalier L, Parry RJ (2007). Assessment and Diagnostic Procedures. In: *Diagnostic Manual – Intellectual Disability (DM-ID): A Textbook of Diagnosis of Mental Disorders in Persons with Intellectual Disability*. New York: NADD Press

International Association for Scientific Study of Intellectual and Developmental Disabilities (2001) *Health Guidelines for Adults with an Intellectual Disability*. Available at: http://iassid.org/pdf/healthguidelines.pdf (Accessed 03 February 2014.)

Jones S, Howard L, Thornicroft G (2008) 'Diagnostic overshadowing': worse physical health care for people with mental illness. *Acta Psychiatry Scandinavia* 118(3):169–71

Kleintjes S, Flisher A, Fick M, Raioun A, Lund C, Molteno C, Robertson BA (2006) The prevalence of mental disorders among children, adolescents and adults in the Western Cape, South Africa. *South Africa Psychiatry Review* 9: 157–60

Kromberg J, Zwane E, Manga P, Venter A, Rosen E, Christianson A (2008) Intellectual disability in the context of a South African population. *Journal of Policy and Practice in Intellectual Disabilities* 5(2): 9–95

Lalloo R, van As AB (2004) Profile of children with head injuries treated at the trauma unit of Red Cross War Memorial Children's Hospital, 1991–2001. *South African Medical Journal* 94: 544–546

Maulik PK, Harbour, CK (2010) Epidemiology of intellectual disability. In: Stone JH, Blouin M (Eds). *International Encyclopedia of Rehabilitation*. Buffalo. Available at: http://cirrie.buffalo.edu/encyclopedia/en/article/144/ (Accessed 15 July 2014.)

Maulik PK, Mascarenhas MN, Mathers CD, Dua T, Saxena S (2011) Prevalence of intellectual disability: A meta-analysis of population-based studies. *Research in Developmental Disabilities* 32(2): 419–436

May PA, Blankenship J, Marais AS, Gossage JP, Kalberg WO, Barnard R, de Vries M, Robinson LK, Adnams CM, Buckley D, Manning M, Jones KL, Parry C, Hoyme HE, Seedat S (2013) Approaching the prevalence of the full spectrum of fetal alcohol spectrum disorders in a South African population-based study. *Alcoholism Clinical and Experimental Research* 37(5): 818–30

O'Brien G (2006) Behavioural phenotypes: Causes and clinical implications. *Advances in Psychiatric Treatment* 12: 338–48

OHHCHR, UN Women, UNAIDS, UNDP, UNFPA, UNICEF, WHO (2014) *Eliminating forced, coercive and otherwise involuntary sterilization: An interagency statement*. World Health Organization. Available at: http://www.who.int/reproductivehealth/publications/gender_rights/eliminating-forced-sterilization/en/ (Accessed 17 June 2014.)

Salvador-Carulla L, Reed GM, Vaez-Assisi LM, Cooper S, Martinez-Leal R, Bertelli M, Adnams C, Cooray, S Shoumitro, D Akoury-Dirani, L Girimaji, SC Katz G, Kwok H, Luckasson R, Simeonsson R, Walsh C, Munir K, Saxena S (2011) Intellectual developmental disorders: Towards a new name, definition and framework for 'mental retardation/ intellectual disability' in ICD 11. *World Psychiatry* 10: 175–80

Sheehan R, Ali A, Hassiotis A (2014) Dementia in intellectual disability. *Current Opinion in Psychiatry* 27(2): 143–8

Urban MF, Chersich MF, Fourie L-A, Chetty C, Olivier L, Viljoen D (2008) Fetal alcohol syndrome among grade-one children in the Northern Cape Province: Prevalence and risk factors. *South African Medical Journal* 98(11): 887–2

Van Schrojenstein Lantman-de Valk HM, Walsh PN (2008) Managing health problems in people with intellectual disabilities. *British Medical Journal* 337: a2507

Waite J, Heald M, Wilde L, Woodcock K, Welham A, Adams D, Oliver C (2014) The importance of understanding the behavioural phenotypes of genetic syndromes associated with intellectual disability. *Paediatrics and Child Health* 24(10): 468–72

Walsh, A (2000) Improve and care: Responding to inappropriate masturbation in people with severe intellectual disabilities. *Sexuality and Disability* 18(1): 27–30

World Health Organization (2001) *International Classification of Functioning, Disability and Health*. Geneva: World Health Organization

World Health Organization (2010) *International statistical classification of diseases and related health problems* (10th revision). Geneva: World Health Organization

CHAPTER

# 30 Psychogeriatrics

Felix Potocnik

'A medical revolution has extended the life of our elder citizens without providing the dignity and security those later years deserve.'

*John F. Kennedy (1917–1963) US Statesman. Acceptance Speech, Democratic National Convention, Los Angeles, 15 July 1960.*

## 30.1 Introduction

From an evolutionary point of view there must be some advantage for the continued survival of humankind following the end of reproductive life. Since humans are unique in both the richness and complexity of their memories and experiences and have the ability to share this knowledge with others, one presumes this to be a major reason (Pitt, 1974). While each generation adds to the gifts it has received from its ancestors, the lessons taught are unfortunately not always fully integrated. Hence, history repeats itself unnecessarily and painfully, the elderly often being perceived (at a very primitive level) as a problem rather than being acknowledged for the contributions that they could make. Going by the dictum that 'in the old days parents had many children, and now children have lots of parents' this problem has uniquely become our problem. The challenge, therefore, is to change this paradigm, allowing the elderly to continue to contribute to society within the social model of the extended family, in spite of the increasing number of nuclear families. One of the first steps in this direction is to ensure their psychological and physical health and the promotion of a sense of well-being so that they continue to be an asset and not a burden to society.

## 30.2 Ageing

### 30.2.1 Definitions

Ageing is the progressive decline in function and performance, which accompanies advancing years. It is multifactorial in origin, partly inborn (primary ageing) involving concepts such as apoptosis or programmed cell death, the biological clock and other genetic factors, and partly environmental (secondary ageing) due to a wearing out by stress and strain and the accumulation of toxins. Gerontology covers all knowledge pertaining to the ageing process; geriatrics deals mainly with the care and treatment of physical illness in the elderly; while psychogeriatrics involves the socio-psychiatric and cognitive disorders and their management in the elderly. It is the fastest growing field in psychiatry.

### 30.2.2 Demographic effects

The World Health Organization predicts a world population of 9 billion for the year 2050, which is due to decrease to 8.4 billion by the end of this century owing to complex medical and social reasons. By 2100, 34% of the world's population will be 60 years or older. The international trend is to describe as 'elderly' people aged 65 and over, while lesser developed countries would include those aged 60 years and older in order to highlight the current needs of the aged. South Africa's Rainbow Nation reflects a demographic diversity, in that elderly blacks constitute 6,5% of their population group, compared to whites at 16%, with Indians and coloureds in between. The current 4,5 million (8,4%) elderly people (those

60 years and older) will more than double within the next 25 years (Statistics South Africa, 2014). In general, this increase has been due to reduced fertility rates and decreased mortality rates in the young, rather than any marked extension in life expectancy. Thus, future demographic trends are dependent on measures of population control and improved health services. Under normal circumstances, 2,1 children per family unit are required to maintain steady population numbers.

With the passing decades the population 'pyramid' will change shape, forming a 'bulge' and finally becoming a 'kite' (see Figure 30.1). The potential impact of HIV/Aids on the population demographic is also shown.

From a variety of data a theoretical human lifespan of about 120 years has been calculated (Hayflick, 1985). Owing to mental and physical factors, however, we not only die at an earlier age but also live a portion of our lives disabled. This amounts to 18% of our given life-years in lesser developed countries as opposed to 8% in the more developed countries. At present, in lesser developed countries in the poorer socioeconomic sectors, the life expectancy of a woman is around 64 years while that of a man is approximately 60 years, in contrast with 79 and 74 years respectively in the more affluent sectors (United Nations, 2013). Though Aids in South Africa is steadily reducing the life expectancy of certain population groups, it should be noted that persons of any population group currently approaching the 60-year mark can look forward to an average of another 18 years of life. The causes of death in those over the age of 65 years in developed countries are generally cardiovascular disease (53%), neoplasms (17%) and respiratory disease (14%). In fourth place are the neurodegenerative disorders (such as Alzheimer's disease), which are becoming notably more prevalent as other causes are brought under control (Fries, 1990). There is a mutual relationship between old age and disease: disease hastens ageing and age renders the old person more vulnerable to diseases, especially of the degenerative kind (Pitt, 1974).

### 30.2.3 Psychosocial implications

The increase of elderly in the upper age brackets has enormous financial implications. Approximately 30% of the elderly suffer from psychiatric symptoms while 80% suffer from some physical illness, and many from both (Pitt, 1974; Fries, 1990). Individuals in this group are on at least one medication, thus the need for setting up effective services for the elderly becomes quite clear. A common psychiatric illness in the elderly is depression, at a prevalence of about 18% in women and 12% in men. Major neurocognitive disorder (NCD), depending on age category, has a much lower prevalence rate of 5–10%, frequently complicated by bouts of delirium. Anxiety disorder (often co-morbid with depression) is present in some 15% of the elderly, while 34% complain of sleep disturbance (Katona and Robertson, 1995). Prior to the mid-1980s there was a tendency to keep psychiatrically disturbed elderly patients in hospital. Following a change in policy, mainly because of more effective medication, these patients are now increasingly being placed back in the community, resulting in an ever-increasing burden on out-patient health services, non-governmental organisations and individual caregivers.

With regard to community care, one has to remember that in the last 50 years the proportion of middle-aged people (35–65 years) to elderly has dwindled from 10 to 1 to roughly 4 to 1 in more developed countries. This means that fewer people are supporting pension funds and providing financial aid towards their health requirements (Pitt, 1974; Statistics South Africa, 2013). Over the same period the proportion of middle-aged women (traditionally the caregivers of the elderly) going out to work has risen from some 10% to 60%. Lesser developed countries are now pursuing this trend. In lesser developed countries up to 50% of the population is younger than 25 years (Adamchak, 1996). These young people, in turn, compete with the elderly for support from the high-income 25–45-year group. The latter group, though, is contending

**Figure 30.1** Population pyramids demonstrating population trends

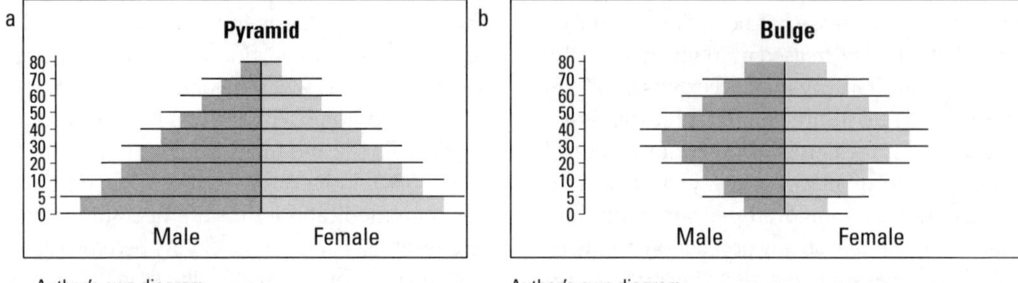


Author's own diagram

Author's own diagram

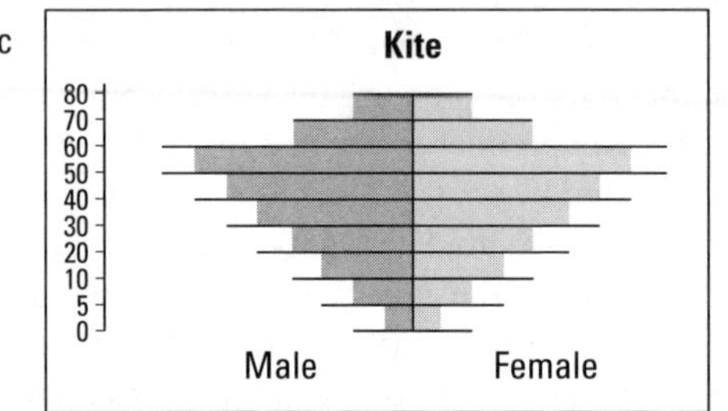


Author's own diagram

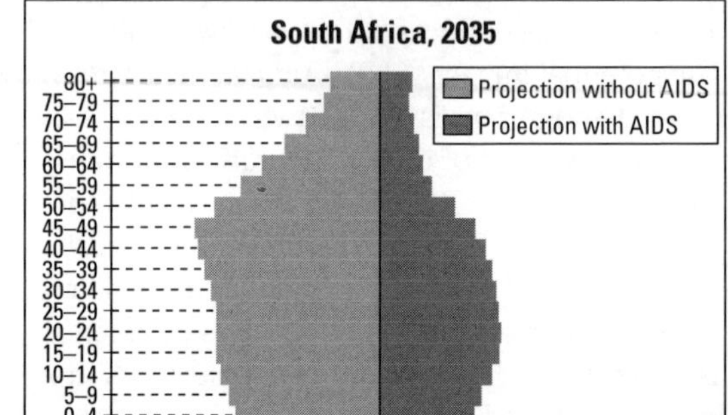


with problems of its own. They have a very high HIV-infection rate (due to reach a projected steady state of 32% within a decade). Other problems include dwindling natural and economic resources, competition with the more advanced nations on an industrial and technological level, the high rate of unemployment and the effects of migration (Adamchak, 1996). Some 25% of potential workers in South Africa are unemployed, and most of these originate from the poorer socioeconomic groups. In these instances a caregiver is available for the elderly, but the latter's pension is often now the chief source of income for that particular family. In addition, the care required for a mental illness is often beyond the scope of most families. All these factors must be taken into account by policy-makers.

Generally, the elderly fall victim to poor housing and poverty, pensions that cannot keep pace with the daily cost of living and a decreasing intellect that gives rise to an inability to use financial resources to best advantage. All this requires an increase in the number of services for the elderly, such as primary health care, home visits, day centres, liaison services, day hospitals, hospital-based services, residential and old age homes, council houses and villages (Pitt, 1974).

## 30.2.4 Physical changes

Height decreases by some 8 cm by the age of 80 years owing to a decrease in bone mass and an increased curvature of the spine. Body weight steadily decreases, while joints stiffen and osteoarthritis becomes more common. The skin becomes dry, thin and wrinkled and senile bruises (senile ecchymoses) appear spontaneously, mainly on the forearms and on the legs. While the hair becomes white and sparse, degrees of deafness ensue, teeth fall out, the jaw gradually shrinks and dentures become loose. All organs tend to shrink in size and the functional reserve, which allows adaptation to stress, declines. While cardiac output decreases there is a rise in blood pressure, which, with the effects of atheroma, may lead to myocardial infarction, heart failure or a stroke. The lungs are more rigid and are predisposed to chronic bronchitis and pneumonia. The gastrointestinal tract diminishes in function resulting in constipation, which is common and troublesome. The enlarged prostate gland in men and the atrophic vagina in women may lead to urinary tract infections (UTIs), contributing to incontinence and impaired health. Other physical ailments to which the elderly are especially prone include diabetes, dehydration, anaemia, cancer and hypothermia (Pitt, 1974; Wicht, 1990). The key constituent being cartilage; the ears and nose will enlarge, while a larger shoe size is necessitated by the laxity of pedal ligaments and the resultant splaying of the pedal bones both lengthwise and sideways

## 30.2.5 Central nervous system

Mental function in the elderly is spared more than the dramatic microscopic changes in the brain would suggest. Cell loss approaches 50% in some cortical areas while fewer dendritic interconnections remain between neurons. All senses decline – deafness and failing vision lead to social isolation, while loss of sense of smell and taste lead to a decrease in appetite.

## 30.2.6 Intellectual function

A small percentage of elderly persons maintain a stable IQ even at an advanced age, although the majority demonstrate a gradual decline. Memory, contrary to belief, is not static throughout one's lifetime, nor is it dramatically altered in healthy, emotionally stable elderly persons. Fast mapping (in young children) is followed by fluid intelligence (excellent rote memory and the ability to acquire new information) which is more susceptible to the effects of ageing than crystallised intelligence (which synthesises and integrates acquired information with the person's educational and past experience). The memory lapses that increasingly occur from the fourth decade onwards are therefore to be considered physiological rather than pathological, as these are offset by a deeper understanding of subject matter (Pitt, 1974; Wicht, 1990).

## 30.2.7 Sexual function

Although all phases of the sexual act tend to be slowed down and prolonged in the elderly, decreased sexual interest and activity in this age group – in part hormonal in aetiology and in part due to a lack of partner – are generally psychological rather than physiological. While some are sexually active others find intimacy sufficient.

## 30.2.8 Personality changes

There is a natural tendency from extroversion towards **introversion** with ageing; as the circle of friends diminishes, so does the interest in social and current affairs (Pitt, 1974). The elderly become more set in their ways and are often preoccupied with bodily functions (such as the bowels), which may lead to hypochondriasis.

## 30.2.9 Life changes

Specific life changes and losses are associated with this stage of life (Pitt, 1974):

- Contemporary Western society with a tendency towards materialism holds senior citizens in lower status than their working counterparts. Thus, retirement can age a person, and those with a high investment in a work role more easily lose self-esteem and become depressed.
- Income drops substantially after retirement and careful budgeting and adjustments for inflation are necessary.
- Health deteriorates, often accompanied by discomfort or pain, which, apart from restricting mobility and reducing social interaction, generally impairs the enjoyment of life. This increasingly leads to dependency.
- Colleagues, friends and spouse (company) are lost with advancing years, resulting in progressive isolation with the loss of meaningful communication with others and especially the support of confidants. Elderly men living alone are the most vulnerable to suicide.

- As the standard of accommodation declines because of dwindling financial resources, the elderly may find themselves placed considerable distances away from shopping areas, access to transport and health services.
- The above contributes to a loss of independence as family and other social support systems increasingly have to be called in to maintain a semblance of independent living. This results in a role reversal that is frequently uncomfortable or painful to the elderly as well as those near to them.
- With impending closure of life there is a re-evaluation of past experiences and achievements, their meaning and purpose. The unfulfilled frequently become very difficult and bitter in temperament (Pitt, 1974).

### 30.2.10 Styles of ageing

Some maintain that the elderly cope best if they accept the inevitability of ageing, a quieter life and reduced social contact. Others stress that the elderly, aware of certain failing skills, must make all the more effort to counteract this deterioration in order to maintain a sense of purpose and satisfaction. The answer probably lies between the two, dependent on factors such as personality type, cultural background and former interests. In practice, the mental health worker will frequently find the style of ageing dominated by anxiety and hypochondriasis, bewilderment and indecision, irritability and frustration, defiance, denial and dependency (Pitt, 1974). Research has shown that any fieldworker who acts as a close friend or confidant and sounding board to the elderly has a pivotal role to play in relieving the above. Fortunately, some 70% of elderly adapt constructively (Fries, 1990; Katona and Robertson, 1995).

### 30.2.11 Needs of the elderly

The basic needs of the elderly are those of people generally, but unfortunately, are usually not met. They consist of physical needs such as nutrition, shelter, warmth, comfort and cleanliness, while their psychological needs encompass respect, security and self-determination (Pitt, 1974).

## 30.3 Principles of assessment

### 30.3.1 History taking

Firstly, it must be established what illness is present. This may be difficult since the individual's reaction to the illness, the presence of medication, physical illness, emotional upheavals and depression may all complicate the picture. Collateral information from a spouse, family or friends is essential and patients should be reminded to bring along their glasses and/or hearing aids, medication, and medical reports to the first interview.

### 30.3.2 Functional and social assessment

This is mandatory in order to plan future care. The aim is to assess the degree of impairment as well as the retained abilities, in order to maintain the person in the community. It involves the assessment of mobility, ability to communicate needs, ability to relate to others, ability to wash, dress and feed oneself, bladder and bowels control and the presence of aggression and other socially unacceptable behaviour. The patient's present social functioning and ability for self-care must be evaluated with regards to supervision required, ability to prepare meals, ability to go shopping, ability to do housework and compliance with medication.

The social assessment takes into consideration accommodation, employment, economic resources and evaluates the degree of available social support. The social assessment also incorporates financial and medico-legal matters such as testamentary capacity, wills, **power of attorney** and need for **curatorship**. With knowledge of the above, each patient's future can be projected and planned with regard to care and placement.

### 30.3.3 General principles

The general principles of including collateral information and the involvement of family or friends are pivotal in most cases. The illness in question determines the scope and depth of examinations and investigations required. This often entails both a physical and a neuropsychological assessment concentrating on neurological deficits. The Mini-Mental Status Examination (MMSE) (see Section 30.14.6) should be administered routinely (Folstein *et al.*, 1975).

Generally, in typical or advanced cases of neurocognitive decline, investigations may have little to offer towards clinical diagnosis, treatment and health benefit. Cost restraints often dictate that investigations cannot routinely be performed. However, a positive result is more likely to be obtained when:

- the patient is younger than 65
- the neurocognitive decline has been of recent and rapid onset
- the course of the disease fluctuates markedly
- the physical examination reveals a neurological deficit.

Baseline investigations consist of a so-called organic work-up (see Table 30.1).

## 30.4 Depressive disorder

See also Chapter 12: Depressive disorders, for a further discussion.

### 30.4.1 Epidemiology

The World Health Organization predicts that depression will be the leading general burden of disease impacting on human well-being by the year 2020. Not only is the number of elderly set to double over the next 25 years, the current 1946 cohort (the so-called baby boomers) has exhibited higher rates of depression and increased rates of suicide throughout their life cycle (World Health Organization, 2002).

In the elderly, depression is the second-most common psychiatric disorder after sleep disturbances, and affects 18% of women and 12% of men. It is more common in urban than in rural areas and in the working classes. It is usually multifactorial in aetiology with a broad range of contributory factors being present at any given time (Djernes, 2006).

**Table 30.1** Baseline investigations[1]

- Full blood count (haemoglobin, white cell count, mean cell volume)
- Random blood sugar and urea and electrolytes [fingerprick sugar test, urea and creatinine, sodium, potassium]
- Thyroid function tests and liver function tests [thyroid stimulating hormone, albumin, alkaline phosphatase and gamma-GT]
- Calcium
- Vitamin $B_{12}$
- Lipogram [total cholesterol]
- Syphilis serology
- HIV if suspected (informed consent)
- Urine dipstix
- Computerised tomography (CT) scan of the brain (if underlying neurocognitive disorder, focal or space-occupying lesions are suspected)
- Mini-Mental State Examination (MMSE) to exclude an underlying neurocognitive illness (depressed patients should lose at most 1–2 points).

[1] Text in square brackets denote the more economical options.
More specialised investigations include psychometric testing when there are difficulties with clinical assessment or for medico-legal purposes. A CT or MRI (magnetic resonance imaging) scan measuring the width of the medial temporal lobes is a useful adjunct in the assessment of Alzheimer's disease. If still in doubt a SPECT (single-photon emission computed tomography) may be a useful diagnostic pointer.

## 30.4.2 Aetiology

Physical stresses that may precipitate depression include viral brain infections (occurring especially during the post-influenza period), any condition that affects the brain (Parkinson's disease, early Alzheimer's disease or vascular neurocognitive disorder), as well as other physical disorders such as anaemia, chronic obstructive pulmonary disease and coronary heart disease. Depression is also commonly found in people who abuse or are dependent on alcohol and is a leading risk factor for cerebrovascular disease and will further complicate the picture in early neurocognitive disorder. The DSM-5 categorises these associations with depression as 'depressive disorder due to another medical condition' and 'substance/medication-induced depressive disorder', respectively (American Psychiatric Association, 2013).

Depression is present in about 30% of elderly patients who suffer from an acute or a chronic illness, hence the need to rule out organic causes of depression.

Psychological stressors are usually more important in depression. Predisposing factors consist of traumatic childhood experiences, bereavement during childhood and personality. Obsessional, conscientious individuals who are unable to display their emotions are more at risk, as are individuals who lack a close friend or confidant. Social issues, such as living with a younger, disliked family member are frequently overlooked. Genetic factors are less important with depression in late life and even less so with increasing age.

## 30.4.3 Presentation

Depression in the elderly appears in numerous guises, ranging from those with accompanying psychotic symptoms to the more common vague, somatic or neurotic complaints with little or no overt sadness. In practice, one or more of the following features will dominate the picture: physical symptoms, anxiety, irritability or aggression and depression (see Figure 30.2). Sleep disturbance and a decline in function are vital clues. The physical symptoms are often vague or hypochondriacal (Djernes, 2006).

**Figure 30.2** Depression quadrangle

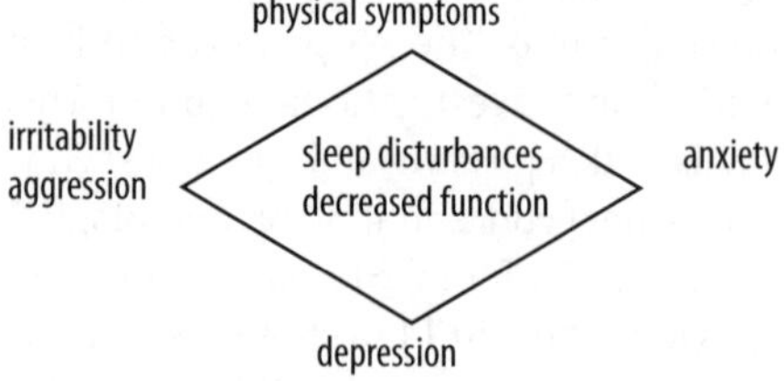


Commonly, we find the elderly patient's underlying physical ailments exacerbated by depression, and the unpopular patient who goes from doctor to doctor is often a patient suffering from depression. Alternatively, the patient may merely be extremely agitated, anxious or tense, and is then incorrectly treated with benzodiazepines and other tranquillisers. Others again present with irritability or in its extreme, aggression (Potocnik, 2014).

Note that there is interplay between affective symptoms, depression and cognitive disorders. A first-onset major depressive episode or anxiety disorder in a person in his or her 50s may herald a cognitive disorder up to two decades later on. This cognitive disorder is often (though not always) vascular in nature. The inter-leading years may be marked with intermittent bouts of depression of varying degrees of severity, becoming all the more frequent when the earliest signs of cognitive deficit become apparent (Alexopoulos, 1997). Most cognitive disorders are associated with a high rate of depression (20–40% in their early phases) and mask the underlying disorder, often giving way to apathy over a matter of months to years. An early sign of an impending cognitive disorder may also be an acute bout of anxiety or a hypomanic or manic episode. These patients may benefit from augmentation with low-dose cognitive enhancers and should be referred for specialist psychiatric care.

Lastly, some patients will only admit to feeling depressed or down after direct questioning. The reason for this may be the ability of the elderly to compartmentalise their mood state (thus making it possible for them to continue with their daily tasks) rather than a lack of insight into their depressed condition (Potocnik, 2014). Others see depression as a sign of moral weakness and will not readily admit to being depressed.

As in younger adults, depression may occur in the context of a range of mood disorders, including major depressive disorder, dysthymic disorder and bipolar disorder. (See Chapter 12: Depressive disorders, for the core criteria for the presentation of major depression.)

Regardless of the presentation, a common finding is a **decompensation** in function: the person no longer seems to care about the state of his or her dwelling, bodily hygiene, pastimes or friends. In addition, the elderly will frequently express excessive concern regarding their bodily health or financial state. The more usual case seen in general practice will be suffering from minor (or subsyndromal) depression (see Table 30.2) (American Psychiatric Association, 2013). The ratio of minor to major depression is roughly 10:1.

Depression is responsible for the majority of suicides in the elderly. Though this group only constitutes a small proportion of the population, they account for a third of all suicides. Most at risk is an elderly, single or recently bereaved male with a poor social support system. Agitated depressives and those with early cognitive decline are also at greater risk than apathetic or retarded depressives.

### 30.4.4 Management

The treatment of depression ranges from the manipulation of social circumstances and resources, psychotherapy, antidepressants and tranquillisers, to electroconvulsive therapy and psychosurgery.

Investigations are based on the organic work up.

Following an empathic hearing, active and firm intervention is usually indicated, preferably involving the patient's spouse, family members and friends. Guidance and pragmatic advice must be spelled out clearly. The choice of antidepressant is individual, based on experience with the medication, contraindications, cost, tolerability and medication availability. A suggested schedule is outlined in Table 30.3. Should the depression, agitation or insomnia not settle, specialist opinion should be sought.

On reaching the highest level of tolerance or maximum dose – and provided some benefits are seen – treatment should be continued for at least three months before deciding that the patient has not responded. Should the depressed elderly person not respond adequately to the above regimens, consultation with, or referral

**Table 30.2** Core criteria for minor depression of the elderly (unspecified depressive disorder)

The mood may be depressed, but more commonly there is a feeling of dissatisfaction or an inability to enjoy life (usually worse in the evenings). Sadness may alternate with periods of normal mood.

At least **three** of the following symptoms must be present:

- bouts of tearfulness or crying (often worse in the evenings)
- irritability or bouts of anger
- loss of interest or pleasure in activities
- mild appetite disturbances, often with weight gain
- sleep difficulties (usually an inability to fall asleep because of excessive worrying)
- decompensation in function with neglect of home and bodily hygiene
- fatigue or loss of energy
- social withdrawal, avoidance of contact with friends
- gloomy outlook on the future accompanied by brooding on the past and feelings of self-pity.

**Source:** Author's own Table

**Information box**

**General pointers in the management of depression in the elderly**

- Avoid tricyclic antidepressants on account of cardiotoxicity (QTc lengthening) and anticholinergic effects.
- Titrate slowly upwards in small increments.
- Use sedating agents such as citalopram 20 mg, mirtazapine 15–30 mg or agomelatine 25–50 mg at night.
- Patients with treatment-resistant depression should have a trial of venlafaxine XR 150–225 mg given in the morning or mianserin 30–60 mg at night.
- The benefit of antidepressants in Alzheimer's disease with a MMSE score of 22/30 is questionable as neuropsychiatric symptoms, such as apathy, will now predominate, confusing the presentation.
- The elderly are susceptible to the occurrence of sedation, confusion, impaired psychomotor performance (falls) and amnestic episodes when given benzodiazepines.
- In some cultures (e.g. Xhosa) there is no word that specifically denotes depression. Feelings of sadness or emotional distress may be referred to in somatic terms such as *ukudakumba* or 'heavy spirit'.

**Table 30.3** Treatment schedule for depression in the elderly

**1. Selective serotonin reuptake inhibitors (SSRIs)**

1.1 Citalopram (Cipramil®)

- 10 mg at night
- review after four weeks
- increase to 20 mg if necessary

Side effects include headache, nausea, agitation, anxiety, tremor, insomnia, akathisia, sexual dysfunction.

1.2 Sertraline (Zoloft®)

- 50 mg at night.
- review after four weeks
- increase in four-weekly increments of 50 mg (to 150 mg maximum) if necessary

Side effects include headache, nausea, agitation, anxiety, tremor, insomnia, akathisia, sexual dysfunction.

1.3 Escitalopram (Cipralex®)

- 2,5 mg at night
- review after four weeks
- increase in four-weekly increments from 2.5 mg up to 10 mg, if necessary.

Side effects include headache, nausea, agitation, anxiety, tremor, insomnia, akathisia, sexual dysfunction.

**2. Noradrenergic and specific serotonergic antidepressants (NaSSAs)**

2.1 Mirtazapine (Remeron®)

- 15 mg at night
- review after four weeks
- increase to 30 mg if necessary.

Side effects include increased appetite, weight gain, somnolence, headache.

**3. Melatonin receptor modulator**

3.1 Agomelatine (Valdoxane®)

- 25 mg at night
- review after 4 (four) weeks
- increase to 50 mg if necessary.

Side effects include somnolence and infrequently raised liver function tests.

**4. Other agents (for second-line use) are**

4.1 Serotonin and noradrenaline reuptake inhibitors (SNRIs): venlafaxine (Efexor®)

- 75 mg in the morning
- review after four weeks
- increase at four-weekly intervals to 225 mg if necessary.

Side effects include hypertension, agitation, tremor, insomnia.

**Source:** Baldwin, 2010

**Information box**

**Referring for specialist opinion**

- When the diagnosis is in doubt.
- In cases of severe depression evidenced by:
  - prominent psychotic symptoms
  - severe risk to health because of failure to eat or drink
  - suicide risk
  - history of, or first onset of, major depression or anxiety disorder in a patient approximately 50 years of age.

When complex therapy is indicated (e.g. medical co-morbidity).

Treatment resistance (two antidepressants from different classes have been tried and both have failed).

**Source:** Baldwin, 2010

to, a more specialised centre should be sought. Electroconvulsive therapy (ECT) is still one of the most potent treatment applications in the armamentarium. Depression in the elderly is eminently treatable, but owing to the high relapse rate (80% in the following two years) prolonged after-care and maintenance therapy for this period is mandatory (Anderson, 2010; Baldwin, 2010).

## 30.5 Bereavement late in life

Bereavement late in life may become a complicated process. While mourning for six months is the norm, it often takes up to two years (excluding anniversary phenomena) for the person's life to stabilise (Parkes, 1996).

Yearning or pining is a key feature with varying symptoms of depression. Should these symptoms interfere with social or occupational functioning, psychiatric intervention is indicated. The aim is for the person to find some degree of closure allowing him or her to move forward from this life event.

In its section on 'conditions for further study', the DSM-5 describes a proposed condition termed 'persistent complex bereavement disorder'. The proposed criteria (American Psychiatric Association, 2013) are listed in Table 30.4.

(See also Chapter 15: Acute reactions to adverse life events.)

**Table 30.4** DSM-5 Diagnostic Criteria for Persistent Complex Bereavement Disorder

| **Proposed Criteria** |
|---|
| A. The individual experienced the death of someone with whom he or she had a close relationship. |
| B. Since the death, at least one of the following symptoms is experienced on more days than not and to a clinically significant degree and has persisted for at least 12 months after the death in the case of bereaved adults and 6 months for bereaved children: |
| 1. Persistent yearning/longing for the deceased. In young children, yearning may be expressed in play and behavior, including behaviors that reflect being separated from, and also reuniting with, a caregiver or other attachment figure. |
| 2. Intense sorrow and emotional pain in response to the death. |
| 3. Preoccupation with the deceased. |
| 4. Preoccupation with the circumstances of the death. In children, this preoccupation with the deceased may be expressed through the themes of play and behavior and may extend to preoccupation with possible death of others close to them. |
| C. Since the death, at least six of the following symptoms are experienced on more days than not and to a clinically significant degree, and have persisted for at least 12 months after the death in the case of bereaved adults and 6 months for bereaved children: |
| **Reactive distress to the death** |
| 1. Marked difficulty accepting the death. In children, this is dependent on the child's capacity to comprehend the meaning and permanence of death. |
| 2. Experiencing disbelief or emotional numbness over the loss. |
| 3. Difficulty with positive reminiscing about the deceased. |
| 4. Bitterness or anger related to the loss. |
| 5. Maladaptive appraisals about oneself in relation to the deceased or the death (e.g., self-blame). |
| 6. Excessive avoidance of reminders of the loss (e.g., avoidance of individuals, places, or situations associated with the deceased; in children, this may include avoidance of thoughts and feelings regarding the deceased). |
| **Social/identity disruption** |
| 7. A desire to die in order to be with the deceased. |
| 8. Difficulty trusting other individuals since the death. |
| 9. Feeling alone or detached from other individuals since the death. |
| 10. Feeling that life is meaningless or empty without the deceased, or the belief that one cannot function without the deceased. |
| 11. Confusion about one's role in life, or a diminished sense of one's identity (e.g., feeling that a part of oneself died with the deceased). |
| 12. Difficulty or reluctance to pursue interests since the loss or to plan for the future (e.g., friendships, activities). |
| D. The disturbance causes clinically significant distress or impairment in social, occupational, or other important areas of functioning. |
| E. The bereavement reaction is out of proportion to or inconsistent with cultural, religious, or age-appropriate norms. |
| *Specify* if: |
| **With traumatic bereavement:** Bereavement due to homicide or suicide with persistent distressing preoccupations regarding the traumatic nature of the death (often in response to loss reminders), including the deceased's last moments, degree of suffering and mutilating injury, or the malicious or intentional nature of the death. |

**Source:** Reprinted with permission from the *Diagnostic and Statistical Manual of Mental Disorders*, Fifth Edition, (Copyright 2013). American Psychiatric Association.

The disorder is more common in females and innately susceptible individuals.

Attachment issues (childhood separation anxiety) are salient in creating vulnerability for prolonged grief.

A persistent complex bereavement disorder is more likely to occur when:

- the dependent personality loses his or her pillar of admiration and support, which results in anger or inability to come to terms with the loss

- an unexpected death arises in an otherwise fit and healthy individual (e.g. through an accident which is difficult to come to terms with)
- the bereaved was in a love-hate relationship with the deceased. (In such a case, the tussle between relief, guilt and regret for missed opportunities does not allow for resolution to occur.)

A more complex form of bereavement, which in part involves a re-evaluation of societal usefulness, occurs especially in men. Men have a raised incidence of death in the two years following retirement and the loss of their wives. The cause of death, though mainly cardiovascular by nature, also includes cancer.

The treatment of bereavement involves counselling or psychotherapy with antidepressant medication when indicated.

## 30.6 Bipolar disorder

Most elderly patients with bipolar disorder have a past history of manic or depressive illness and thus graduate into this age group. Their treatment stays much the same or is merely adjusted (most often, decreased) with advancing age.

First-onset hypomania or mania in the 60-plus age group is almost invariably a frontal release phenomenon and, being non-responsive to anticonvulsants or mood stabilisers, is best treated with neuroleptics. Confirm an underlying physical illness (e.g. stroke, early neurocognitive disorder or substance abuse such as alcohol) as the precipitating cause. In many patients with bipolar disorder the features of mania are replaced by lability of mood, irritability and often symptoms of paranoia. Not infrequently, both hypomania and depression co-exist (mixed bipolar). Both the therapeutic and toxic effects of lithium occur at lower blood levels in old age. This necessitates closer monitoring and lithium levels of no higher than 0,4–0,6 mmol/ℓ are recommended (Pitt, 1974; Katona, 1995) for maintenance therapy, while higher levels may be required in the acute phase. Anticonvulsants, such as sodium valproate (Epilim®) and lamotrigine (Lamictin®), may yield better results than lithium.

(See also Chapter 13: Bipolar disorders.)

## 30.7 Anxiety and agitation

Anxiety is prevalent in 15% of elderly and as a symptom often co-exists with another disorder, such as depression or neurocognitive disorder. Anxiety disorders, such as panic disorder, phobia, obsessive compulsive disorders, generalised anxiety disorders, acute stress reactions and post-traumatic stress disorder, do occur in the elderly. Anxiety disorders may make their first appearance after the age of 60 but must be closely monitored should they herald an impending neurocognitive disorder. Treatment of choice are antidepressants; failing this, the use of cognitive enhancers is indicated when a neurocognitive disorder is present. This may then also require augmentation with major tranquillisers. The elderly are susceptible to the occurrence of sedation, confusion, impaired psychomotor performance and amnestic episodes when given benzodiazepines (Pitt, 1974).

Marked agitation in the elderly occurs in more than 70% of patients who suffer from delirium and is treated with major tranquillisers and the appropriate medication for any associated medical condition. About a third of elderly depressed patients without an overt underlying neurocognitive disorder present with agitated depression and in this situation antidepressants remain the treatment of choice, but augmentation with cognitive enhancers may be indicated.

(See also Chapter 14: Anxiety, fear and panic.)

## 30.8 Sleep disturbances

A third of the elderly suffer from sleep disorders. Insomnia, drowsiness during the day, daytime naps and the use of hypnotics are common. The causes of sleep disturbances include primary sleep disorders, mood disorders (e.g. depression), medical conditions and environmental factors. Of the primary sleep disturbances the dysomnias are the most common – these include primary insomnia, nocturnal myoclonus, restless leg syndrome and sleep apnoea. Pain, nocturia, dyspnoea and heartburn are the medical symptoms that most affect sleep. Patients with vascular dementia frequently exhibit nocturnal urinary frequency/urgency necessitating two or more visits to the bathroom at night. This is remedied by treatment with chlorpromazine or quetiapine at night. In institutions elderly often go to bed very early (e.g. 18h00) and then find themselves insomniac in the early morning hours. More commonly, extended afternoon naps (in excess of 20 minutes) lead to disturbed sleep-cycle rhythms with somnolence during the day, mild confusion and incontinence at night. Re-establishing the normal circadian rhythm cannot be over-emphasised. Enquire about pre-morbid sleepwalking (in the patient's youth) as a cause of nocturnal confusion as this condition is prone to recur in old age. In sleepwalking nocturnal activities are usually less disorganised and more purposeful (e.g. pulling blankets off fellow residents' beds, but then folding them). Sleepwalking and restless leg syndrome may be treated with benzodiazepines which pre-empt their occurrence.

Alcohol, even in small quantities, may affect the quality of sleep through fragmentation and early-morning wakening. It may also precipitate or worsen sleep apnoea.

When prescribing hypnotics, give consideration to side effects such as cognitive impairment, drowsiness, psychomotor retardation, ataxia and falls, morning hangovers and blurring of biological day/night rhythms.

For short-term treatment of insomnia:

- clonazepam 0,5–2 mg at night
- zolpidem 5–10 mg at night
- zopiclone 3,75-7,5 mg at night.

For long-term treatment of insomnia:

- citalopram 10–20 mg at night
- mirtazapine 15 mg at night
- agomelatine 25 mg at night.

For insomnia in patients with psychosis:

- chlorpromazine 25–100 mg at night
- quetiapine 25–100 mg at night

(See also Chapter 22: Eating and sleep disorders.)

## 30.9 Paraphrenia

Paraphrenia is also known as late-onset schizophrenia or persistent persecutory states in the elderly. As a symptom, paranoia (ranging from vague suspiciousness to delusions of persecution) may be seen in the elderly and are not uncommonly associated with mood disorder (such as depression) and acute or chronic brain disorder (delirium and dementia), or are found to have been present as a personality trait (personality disorder) throughout life (Pitt, 1974; Post, 1979).

### 30.9.1 Clinical features

Paraphrenia is a distinct psychiatric disorder occurring for the first time in life in 1% of the population over the age of 60. It is characterised by systematised (highly circumscribed) paranoid (usually persecutory) delusions and hallucinations, which may occur in a variety of sensory modalities, in the absence of a primary affective illness or obvious organic aetiology.

The paraphrenic patient is typically female, solitary, partially deaf and eccentric (hostile and prickly), but without a history of serious psychiatric illness. There may, however, be an excess family history of psychiatric illness as a whole and particularly schizophrenia. The clinical picture is one in which an old person becomes convinced that her neighbours or family are interfering with her and are attempting to harm her. Delusions usually involve high-tech devices such as satellites that spy on her, but the exact mechanisms remain unclear. Misidentification syndromes are common, as are partition delusions, in which the walls or other boundaries of the home are inexplicably breached by observers and tormentors. Persecutory hallucinations may occur, the situation deteriorates, and ultimately the patient is referred for treatment by long-suffering neighbours and health staff.

While the DSM-5 has omitted paraphrenia as a separate disorder, the authors do acknowledge the following: 'Late-onset cases (i.e. onset after age 40 years) … can still meet the diagnostic criteria for schizophrenia, but it is not yet clear whether this is the same condition as schizophrenia diagnosed prior to mid-life (e.g. prior to age 55 years)' (American Psychiatric Assocation, 2013).

By virtue of its omission from DSM-5, paraphrenia is likely to straddle the diagnostic categories of delusional disorder, schizophreniform disorder and schizophrenia, depending on the severity and range of symptoms of the presenting illness, respectively (American Psychiatric Association, 2013):

- Delusional disorder, where the patient's delusions are strictly localised to one particular neighbour who is sometimes heard talking to her and is believed to enter the patient's dwelling and interfere with her belongings.
- A schizophreniform type where delusions are more widespread, often extending into the neighbourhood and the street. There are ideas of reference so that people seen talking together are thought to be talking about the patient, car lights are flashed ominously and special optical and bugging devices are used to spy on the patient. There may also be delusions of jealousy about the spouse; erotic delusions occur.
- A schizophrenic type, almost identical with schizophrenia in younger patients, in which the subject hears herself discussed in the third person and experiences passivity feelings, for example being influenced from a distance or having her thoughts read. Personality tends to be better preserved than in schizophrenia and thought disorder is confined to occasional neologisms (private words) and metonyms (ordinary words used with a private meaning). These differences and the more appropriate emotional and behavioural responses are explicable by the paraphrenic's more established and mature personality at the age when the disease first develops.

### 30.9.2 Treatment

Major tranquillisers or neuroleptics are indicated. Do not over-treat – delusions or delusional activity will diminish (but not disappear as it does in the younger age group). Lack of insight and judgement usually necessitate depot neuroleptics and even placement that gives greater supervision and care. Watch out for neuroleptic sensitivity and/or emerging depression after 6-12 weeks of treatment and treat accordingly (Potocnik, 2005).

## 30.10 Abuse of the elderly

In the USA it is estimated that 10% of the elderly are abused. Figures for South Africa are not readily available. Abuse of the elderly is notifiable by law. Abuse of the elderly includes physical abuse as well as acts of omission or negligence that lead to the detriment of the health and wellbeing of the person. This includes physical, psychological, financial and material aspects. Examples are the denial of food, visits, medication, clothing and other essentials. Note that sexual abuse and incest also occur. Signs of abuse must not be confused with naturally occurring senile ecchymoses seen mainly on the forearms and the legs.

Cases can be reported to Action on Elder Abuse at 0800 00 3081.

## 30.11 Hypersexuality

Hypersexuality is a form of sexual disinhibition characterised by excessive and socially inappropriate sexual behaviour. It may occur in both the very early and more advanced stages of dementia. Though it occurs in both genders it is more common in men. Control is rapidly obtained within a few days with the use of an anti-androgen cyproterone acetate available in oral tablets (50–100 mg three times daily) and depot injection (300 mg/2–4 weeks). Initiate and maintain treatment for a period of approximately six months. If, on cessation of therapy, symptoms recur, a further course of treatment for another three to six months is indicated.

(See also Chapter 23: Disorders of sexual function, preference and identity.)

## 30.12 Catatonia

A small percentage of all admissions present with catatonia, a non-specific syndrome with multiple aetiologies (Kaplan and Sadock, 2003). It may be secondary to substance abuse (alcohol, cocaine), iatrogenic (neuroleptic-induced extrapyramidal syndromes and neuroleptic malignant syndrome (NMS)) or psychiatric (mood disorders, schizophrenia, dementias).

The DSM-5 diagnostic criteria for catatonic disorder are listed in Chapter 11: Schizophrenia spectrum and other psychotic disorders. Patients are usually immobile, mute, withdrawn, refusing to eat or drink, and staring; on responding to treatment they may later describe having experienced intense anxiety and fear usually related to psychotic ideation (Hawkins, 1995).

Between 70-80% of catatonics will respond dramatically within 1–3 hours to low-dose benzodiazepines (ideally lorazepam 1–2 mg given intramuscularly or intravenously (least preferred orally)). Occasionally a second dose is required as well as maintenance medication of carbamazepine 400–600 mg or another anticonvulsant or mood stabiliser, yielding variable results.

## 30.13 Delirium in the elderly

### 30.13.1 Epidemiology

Cases of delirium increase in direct proportion to the increase in number of elderly in the population. Of all age groups the elderly, and especially the NCD compromised, are uniquely prone to delirium. Some 10–15% of elderly general surgical patients become delirious after an operation, and 30–50% of all elderly admissions are likely to be delirious at some point during their stay in hospital. The death rate for delirium varies from 10–30 % and is as high as 50% within the year that the patient has had delirium. Despite representing an acute organ failure syndrome, 50–60% of cases of delirium go undetected. It is also more common in the presence of hypo-activity rather than hyperactivity, patients older than 80 years, and in the presence of visual impairment and/or a pre-existing neurocognitive disorder (Butler, 2013; Pitt, 1974).

### 30.13.2 Predisposing factors

Predisposing factors for the development of delirium in the elderly consist of the stressors that accompany ageing, extremes of age (the elderly and children), previous brain insults (head injuries, stroke, Parkinson's disease), current neurocognitive disorder, a past history of delirium, alcohol dependence, diabetes, cancer, sensory impairment (poor vision or hearing) and malnutrition (Pitt, 1974).

These factors render the person vulnerable to an adverse interaction between their cognitive reserves, cognitive compensation mechanisms, the disease process, the effect of the therapeutic intervention and the environment of care (Butler, 2013).

### 30.13.3 Aetiology

The aetiology of delirium in the elderly is typically multifactorial in origin, involving organic factors, psychosocial stressors, unfamiliar environments and excessive or diminished sensory input (e.g. from reduced visual acuity and hearing) (Van Gool *et al.*, 2010).

Common causes of delirium in the elderly include:

- Medication (American Geriatrics Society, 2012): It is generally conceded that iatrogenics are responsible for up to 20% of cases of delirium in the elderly
  - sedatives and tranquillisers (benzodiazepines)
  - antidepressants and, less commonly, the anticholinergic effects of tricyclic antidepressants
  - oral hypoglycaemic agents (note that in asymptomatic diabetics random blood glucose levels of up to 15 mmol/l are acceptable)
  - corticosteriods
  - L-DOPA
  - antihypertensives and digoxin (note that in the elderly mildly higher blood pressure readings are acceptable)
  - alcohol – delirium tremens or alcohol withdrawal syndrome usually occurs on the second to third day after cessation or a marked reduction in drinking
  - heavy metals and other toxins.
- Infection (Van Gool *et al.*, 2010), commonly by a bacterial urinary tract infection or

bronchopneumonia. Acute psychotically ill elderly are frequently dehydrated, predisposing them to urinary tract infections; this is especially common during hot summer days.
  - Metabolic: uraemia, hypoglycaemia and hyperglycaemia, dehydration due to inadequate fluid intake, diuretics, laxatives or diarrhoea
- trauma: both psychological and organic (post-traumatic stress, concussion or subdural haematomal in origin), head injuries with diffuse axonal degeneration and post-operative complications
- oxygen deficit of any nature, such as what occurs in cardiovascular and respiratory disorders, especially strokes
- psychological, perceptual and post-ictal: anything that lessens the elderly person's contact with familiar surroundings or visual cues can increase confusion (reality testing), such as moving to a new room, an emotional shock, dim lights and the loss of glasses or a hearing aid. Postictal confusion presents as delirium and requires medical attention.

(See Chapter 10: Cognitive disorders, for a comprehensive discussion of the aetiology of delirium.)

## 30.13.4 Clinical features in the elderly

The core clinical features of delirium in the elderly are the same as in younger persons (see Chapter 10: Cognitive disorders, for details). In the elderly, good collateral information is especially important, including a history of nocturnal behaviour as well as that seen during the day. Nocturnal restlessness is more pronounced in delirium, while daytime restlessness is more pronounced in major neurocognitive disorder. The most reliable informants are roommates, night nurses and domestics doing night shift rather than senior staff on call during the day.

Note that delirium can be envisaged as a symptom of an underlying disorder. It is a very sensitive indicator of a disease in progress and is usually present before fever, pain or tachycardia: delirium can precede any sign of an acute illness by up to two days. The usual history is that of an elderly person suddenly becoming increasingly psychotic and unmanageable, especially during the night, while being quiet and drowsy during the day (reversal of the sleep-wake cycle). The patient may then become increasingly restless in the late afternoon, referred to as **sundowning**. In more subtle cases the relatives will claim that the patient is just not himself or herself, or the staff may report that the patient has become a 'little odd'.

A sudden and recent onset of incontinence may be the only sign. A sudden decompensation in function and change in psychomotor activity are indicators of delirium. In the latter the patient is either hypo-active, stuporous and apathetic or hyperactive and restless, though a mixed picture may often be present.

Once the cause is found and correctly treated the response is rapid and the patient will usually be well within a week (and at most four weeks), unlike the patient with major neurocognitive disorder whose intellectual and behavioural deficits will persist. Once a patient has recovered his or her recall of events during the delirious episode are usually patchy.

## 30.13.5 Management in the elderly

Since urinary tract infections are a common cause in the elderly, one must be especially vigilant for a urinary tract infection in an elderly person with delirium. Importantly, the initial one or two mid-stream urinary specimens for testing may be normal, only to be followed by a positive result within a further day or two. Patients in this age group tend not to report dysuria, frequency of micturition or pelvic pain; the only clue may be the sudden occurrence of incontinence or smelly urine. A urine dipstick test that includes testing for nitrates and leucocytes is helpful in these cases. Immediately start treatment with an appropriate antibiotic. The nocturnal upheaval to family, roommates or ward staff caused by an untreated patient is not justified. Cotrimoxazole is readily available and is administered in a dosage of two tablets twice daily for 10 days to combat the often accompanying pyelonephritis.

Alternatively, ciprofloxacin 500 mg *stat*, or 500 mg daily over five days will resolve most urinary tract infections. With repeated infections, laboratory results obtained from microscopy, culture and sensitivity may serve as a further guide to treatment. (See Chapter 10: Cognitive disorders, for a comprehensive discussion of the management of delirium.)

**Information box**

**Suitable dosages of drugs for treating delirium in the elderly**

- lorazepam: 1–2 mg imi or 0,5–1,5 mg ivi
- haloperidol: 2,5 mg p.o. or ivi
- quetiapine: 12,5–50 mg imi p.o. at night

### 30.13.6 Prognosis

The one-year mortality of a frail older person who has suffered an episode of delirium is 30–40%. Follow-up and discharge planning of this high-risk patient population is mandatory. Even in more robust persons delirium doubles mortality risk. Patients with vulnerable neurocognitive status (e.g. a major neurocognitive disorder) demonstrate a more rapid cognitive deterioration trajectory after an episode of delirium, regardless of age. This is thought to be due to an inability to reduce over-activation of microglial cells via cholinergic inhibition resulting in neuro-degeneration. Clinically this translates into a higher need for institutional care and long-term functional decline. Delirium results in longer hospital stays and increased health care cost (Butler, 2013).

## 30.14 Dementia and mild cognitive impairment in the elderly

### 30.14.1 Definitions

The term 'major neurocognitive disorder' has replaced the term 'dementia' in the DSM-5 and has various aetiologies that can occur across the adult lifespan. Whereas dementia was typically associated with impairment in the elderly, especially in memory, major neurocognitive disorder refers to an acquired decline in cognitive functioning in at least one cognitive domain with associated impairment in the activities of daily living. In this chapter, the terms 'major neurocognitive disorder' and 'dementia' will be used interchangeably to denote this condition in the elderly. (See Chapter 10: Cognitive disorders, for diagnostic criteria for major neurocognitive disorder as well as a description of the cognitive domains.)

Mild cognitive impairment (MCI) is now called mild neurocognitive disorder and describes a condition with a lesser degree of impairment in cognitive domains and without associated impairment in the activities of daily living. In the elderly, it is also referred to as age-associated memory impairment and describes those 'doddery' elderly whose decline in cognitive function falls short of major neurocognitive disorder. Approximately 20–30% of the elderly fall within this group. Two-year follow-up of this group usually reveals that a third have returned to a more normal level of functioning, a third remain static and the remaining third will have progressively declined and are now classified as major neurocognitive disorder. (See Chapter 10: Cognitive disorders, for the diagnostic criteria of mild neurocognitive disorder.)

### 30.14.2 Epidemiology

The prevalence of major neurocognitive disorder in the elderly population is 5–7%. Starting at 1% for 60 year olds, the incidence of dementia doubles every five years, rising to 30–40% for those over the age of 85 years (Jorm *et al.*, 1987).

Worldwide the prevalence of dementia currently exceeds 35 million people, a figure set to reach 115 million by 2050. Two-thirds of individuals with neurocognitive disorder live in developing countries, where the sharpest increase in numbers is said to occur. Of South Africa's 4 million elderly (60 years and older) an estimated 250 000 are suffering from a dementing illness. Of these, some 35 000 are thought to be suffering from Alzheimer's disease. Individuals may die within six months of diagnosis or live as long as 20 years. The mean duration of the illness being some 10–12 years, 20% of Alzheimer's patients are alive after a 15-year period. Bronchopneumonia or urinary tract infections (giving rise to septicaemia) are the common causes of death in Alzheimer's disease. The costs of the illness are enormous in both financial (exceeding US$ 420 billion in 2009) and human terms. While direct costs include the patient's use of health products and services, indirect costs involve, among many components, unpaid caregiving and lifestyle modifications.

## 30.14.3 Aetiology

The syndrome of major neurocognitive disorder becomes a diagnosis once the cause of the neurocognitive disorder has been established, often only definitively at a post-mortem examination. In developed countries, Alzheimer's disease accounts for some 50% of all cases of major neurocognitive disorder, vascular dementia for 20%, and mixed causes (i.e. both Alzheimer's and vascular dementia) for 15%. Note that HIV infection is steadily on the increase in sub-Saharan Africa, accounting for the highest number of major neurocognitive disorder in the overall population (i.e. across the lifespan). Among elderly South Africans, major vascular neurocognitive disorder is the most prevalent, followed by Alzheimer's disease which is on the increase. Lewy bodies, identical to those found in Parkinson's disease, are found in as many as 20% of people with dementia giving rise to neurocognitive disorder with Lewy bodies.

Major neurocognitive disorder is progressive and irreversible (cures are often misdiagnosed cases of delirium), but its profound psychosocial effects may be amenable to intervention, as may the co-morbid factors that hasten or complicate the disease process (e.g. depression). Such intervention will not only help the patient and alleviate the stress on the caregiver, but can also help in delaying institutionalisation. Early diagnosis is thus essential.

## 30.14.4 Clinical evaluation

### 30.14.4.1 Preamble

This entails taking a history, performing both a mental state and physical examination and doing investigations as indicated. A reliable informant (preferably family) is required to attend in order to assess the diagnostic, functional and social aspects of the patient.

The initial differential evaluation is usually between memory impairment, depression and delirium. Though these can co-exist with a neurocognitive disorder or even be a warning sign of its presence, they must be ruled out as they require treatment in their own right. Also, delirium constitutes a medical emergency.

In order to seal the co-operation of the patient, address their secret fear of abandonment by explaining to them that they will not be staying in, or be admitted to, hospital.

Explain to the informant that memory is not static throughout one's lifetime. As a child, fast-mapping (absorbing everything) gives way to fluid intelligence in young adulthood, which refers to the ability to memorise easily, integrate new information and switch from topic to topic and which gives way to crystallised intelligence around the fourth decade. This refers to the integration of information with the person's existing knowledge and experience, leading to a better understanding of matters, but possibly at the expense of a sharp memory. Unfortunately, it is people in this age group that often bring their parents for evaluation, the former secretly fearing that they have also inherited the illness on account of the changes they have noticed in their own memory.

Subjects with mild neurocognitive disorder must be followed up regularly as statistics show that over the next few years approximately a third of the patients in this group will deteriorate progressively.

### 30.14.4.2 Diagnostic assessment

A. The presence or absence of neurocognitive disorder is determined as well as the co-existence of depression and delirium, and indications of the cause and modifiable features of the neurocognitive disorder.

- Memory impairment: poor memory must interfere with daily functioning. The patient is forgetful, repetitive, articles are mislaid and there is some disorientation for time or place. Initially, short-term memory is affected with the later involvement of long-term memory.
- Personality and behavioural changes: emotions are shallow and easily influenced by environmental factors. There is an underlying irritability and emotional outbursts are common. Symptoms of anxiety, depression and paranoia occur. Usually pre-morbid traits become more accentuated. A suspicious person will become paranoid, a dependent person helpless and a previously difficult person 'impossible'. The person enters a 'second childhood', displaying self-centered, impulsive, argumentative behaviour, and is lacking in self-care. There is a loss of initiative and the person becomes increasingly apathetic and withdrawn: features that may be mistaken for depression.
- Intellectual impairment: thinking becomes more concrete and the person cannot cope with novel or difficult tasks. There are word-finding and other difficulties with language (dysphasia), the person may no longer recognise familiar faces or objects (agnosia) and may be unable to carry out simple manual tasks, such as fixing a plug or dressing themselves (apraxia). A key feature is the impairment in executive function (executive dysfunction). A person may no longer be able to plan and cook a meal without making numerous mistakes and forgetting ingredients or struggle to operate the TV set and DVD recorder.
- Physical changes: as the disease progresses, the patient appears unduly frail and weak, is stooped in posture with a slow, shuffling gait and mild tremor of the hands. There is weight loss regardless of appetite, increasing bouts of restlessness and confusion, and reduced sphincter control.

B. The course and nature of the neurocognitive disorder may give an indication of its aetiology. Patients with vascular (especially multi-infarct) neurocognitive disorder and, to some extent, an alcohol-induced neurocognitive disorder will present with:
   - a patchy memory loss and fluctuating disturbances in language and behaviour, with a relatively well-preserved personality in the earlier phases, characterised by appropriate social interaction
   - a sudden rather than a slow, insidious onset of the neurocognitive disorder
   - a step-wise deterioration rather than a steady even pattern
   - attacks of dizziness, frequent falls/fainting spells, nocturnal confusion and urinary frequency, particularly at night.

(Potocnik, 2014)

### 30.14.4.3 Neuropsychiatric symptoms and functional assessment

Neuropsychiatric symptoms and functional assessment determine the degree of severity of illness and the level of care required. The aim is to assess the degree of disability as well as the retained abilities in order to re-integrate the individual into the community.

Broadly speaking, NCD patients present clinically with overlapping cognitive (memory and intellect), behavioural and psychiatric symptoms. The behavioural symptoms usually consist of wandering, aggression, disinhibition, restlessness, apathy, abnormal eating and insomnia; while psychiatric symptoms consist of disturbances in mood (anxiety, depression, agitation and mania), and in perceptual abnormalities (hallucinations) or disorders of thought content (delusions).

The neuropsychiatric symptoms start early in the disease process and have an impact on the patient, caregiver, community and medical services. Neuropsychiatric symptoms are one of the most important determinants of entry into institutional care.

Cognition and behaviour also impact on the patient's level of function. Thus, determine whether patients can still perform more complicated tasks such as taking medication, shopping, cooking and managing finances (instrumental activities of daily living (IADL)) as opposed to merely washing, dressing, feeding and using the toilet themselves (basic activities of daily living (BADL)) (Cummings *et al.*, 1994; Galasko *et al.*, 1997).

## 30.14.5 Social assessment

Social assessment includes information regarding where the person lives, under what circumstances, who takes care of the individual and to what extent they are coping. The social assessment takes into consideration accommodation or placement, employment and economic resources, the degree of social support and medico-legal matters.

- Accommodation and level of supervision: the global move away from residential institutions is reflected in South Africa. Fewer beds are available at ever-rising cost. Patients and their families and caregivers increasingly have to rely on their own resources. To help them in this task are the primary care facilities, social clubs, seniors' centres, daycare centres and respite-care facilities. Welfare organisations and non-profit organisations that offer support, counselling and education are invaluable. Refer all families to Dementia South Africa (0860 636 679) for counselling and support.
- Financial resources and the administration of the patient's affairs: awareness of abuse in this area is of paramount importance. It should be determined who draws, administers and dispenses the pension.
- Medico-legal issues such as the need for a power of attorney, curatorship, the drawing up of a will and the need to stop driving must be explored (see Section 13.14.10).
- Teamwork is essential and should utilise as many members from the community (helpful family members, church groups) and medical resources (social worker, community nurse) as possible.

## 30.14.6 Mini-Mental Status Examination (MMSE) (Gauthier, 1999; Potochik, 2014)

The MMSE is done routinely at 6–12 month intervals in elderly individuals to quantify and evaluate cognitive aspects of mental function. Patients must be literate (a minimum of seven years' schooling) and alert, and impediments such as 'hard of hearing' or 'dominant hand weakness' must be clearly indicated next to the final score. The test is standardised and cannot reliably be repeated within less than three-monthly intervals because of practice-effect. The MMSE was originally designed to distinguish neurocognitive disorder from the 10% of patients with depressive pseudo-dementia that mimic neurocognitive disorder. While depressed patients will obtain a high MMSE score, patients with neurocognitive disorder will usually score 26 or less out of a maximum score of 30. While one or two mistakes are allowed, the nature of the mistakes is of importance (e.g. an accountant failing to do the serial sevens). A MMSE score of 27 generally indicates mild NCD or NCI, a MMSE score of 26–21 major NCD (mild severity), 20–11 major NCD (moderate severity) and 10–0 major NCD (severe severity).

The watershed between IADL and BADL usually occurs at 16 out of 30 while incontinence of urine will occur at a score of around 8. A person presenting with major NCD (MMSE 21–26), shuffling gait and urinary incontinence should therefore be suspected of having normal-pressure hydrocephalus and be referred immediately, as would be appropriate for any person showing atypical or uncharacteristic features. The clinician should also be alert to the possibility of an early neurocognitive disorder when a person achieves a score of 30/30 with enormous difficulty, while currently holding a high position in working life. There is no time limit for the completion of the test and the results are useful for monitoring progress. Patients with Alzheimer's disease lose an average of 2–3 points per year.

[Note to reader: For further information on the MMSE see Folstein reference in the reference section.]

## 30.14.7 Physical examination

A physical examination with the emphasis on the neurological examination must be undertaken in all elderly patients.

## 30.14.8 Special investigations

For a list of tests refer to 'baseline investigations' in the beginning of this chapter.

Cost restraints and other practicalities often dictate the number of investigations that can be performed. Generally, in typical or advanced cases of dementia, investigations have little to offer towards treatment. A 'positive' result is more likely to be obtained when:

- the patient is 65 years and younger
- the onset has been recent and the course rapid
- the course of disease fluctuates markedly
- physical examination reveals a neurological deficit.

## 30.14.9 Aetiological subtypes of neurocognitive disorder most commonly found in the elderly (American Psychiatric Association, 2013; Potocnik, 2013)

In the South African population, neurocognitive disorder due to the HIV/Aids complex (affecting mainly the younger age group) is the most common. Among the elderly the most prevalent is major neurocognitive disorder due to vascular disease (VaNCD, VaD), followed by Alzheimer's disease (Alzheimer's disease), which is on the increase (Gauthier, 1999).

### 30.14.9.1 Major or mild neurocognitive disorder due to Alzheimer's disease

The neuropathological hallmarks of Alzheimer's disease are amyloid plaques, neurofibrillary tangles, synaptic and neuronal loss with subsequent brain atrophy. Macroscopically, and with neuro-imaging (MRI and CT scan), this shows as flattening of gyri, widening of sulci, atrophied medial temporal lobes and enlarged ventricles. Pathology at micro-vascular level has increasingly been implicated in the aetiology of Alzheimer's disease, blurring the boundaries with VaNCD in many cases. Alzheimer's disease – and possibly most other dementias – tend to follow a sinusoidal course in that the initial slow, progressive deterioration accelerates rapidly before flattening out towards the end, in keeping with the three stages of mild, moderate and severe (Folstein *et al.*, 1975).

The illness may be as short as six months or as long as 20 years, with an average of 12 years. The cause of death is usually bronchopneumonia (also aspiration-induced pneumonia) or urinary tract infection (with septicaemia).

Neurochemically there are deficits in neurotransmitters including acetylcholine, noradrenaline, serotonin and somatostatin.

Specific mutations on chromosomes 21, 14 and 1 inherited as familial autosomal dominant traits with full penetrance are found in some 1% of all Alzheimer's disease patients. Here the illness usually presents itself in the 40s or early 50s and is essentially pre-senile in onset (i.e. before the age of 65 years). More than 90% of cases of Alzheimer's disease occur in individuals older than 60. Individuals carrying one or both alleles coding for apolipoprotein E-4 (APOE4) on chromosome 19 bear an elevated risk for late-onset Alzheimer's disease, although this gene is not itself a cause of the disorder and genetic testing is not recommended. Figure 30.3 represents the course of Alzheimer's disease (Potocnik, 2014).

### 30.14.9.2 Major or mild vascular neurocognitive disorder or vascular dementia – with or without stroke

Among the VaNCDs, multi-infarct neurocognitive disorder, associated with multiple areas of cortical infarction, patchy cognitive impairment, focal neurological signs and a stepwise rather than a steady, continuous deterioration as in Alzheimer's disease, is more easily diagnosed than a neurocognitive disorder due to vascular damage of the deep white matter (angiopathy or leukoairosis).

After each shower of mini-strokes producing a sudden deterioration in the individual's functioning, there is a partial recovery which stabilises within approximately 3–12 weeks until the next stroke or step occurs several weeks or months later. It is hypothesised that in both vascular and alcohol-induced neurocognitive disorders, presumably temporary vascular spasms may result in intermittent or fluctuating intellectual and personality changes with unpredictable bouts of irritability and mood swings. In all types of VaNCDs, assess the risk factors for stroke such as hypertension, arrhythmias, hypercholesterolaemia, diabetes, smoking and alcohol. Figure 30.4 represents the course of multi-infarct neurocognitive disorder compared to Alzheimer's disease (Potocnik, 2014).

The combination of Alzheimer's disease and vascular neurocognitive disorder are referred to as AD with cerebrovascular disease (CvD).

**Information box**

**Patterns of vascular events and cognitive decline**

There is a wide variation in cognitive deficits related to cerebrovascular disease. Cognitive decline is generally temporally related to a cerebrovascular event (Moorhouse and Rockwood, 2008).

- Large vessel disease is associated with clear, focal neurological signs.
- Multiple infarctions are associated with a stepwise decline in cognition.
- Stepwise cognitive decline may exhibit plateaus and even improvement in-between cerebrovascular events.
- Small vessel disease is generally associated with a gradual onset and slow progression of cognitive impairment.
- Small vessel disease typically affects fronto-subcortical circuitry and frontal lobe functioning (especially complex attention and executive functioning).

**Figure 30.3** Course of Alzheimer's disease

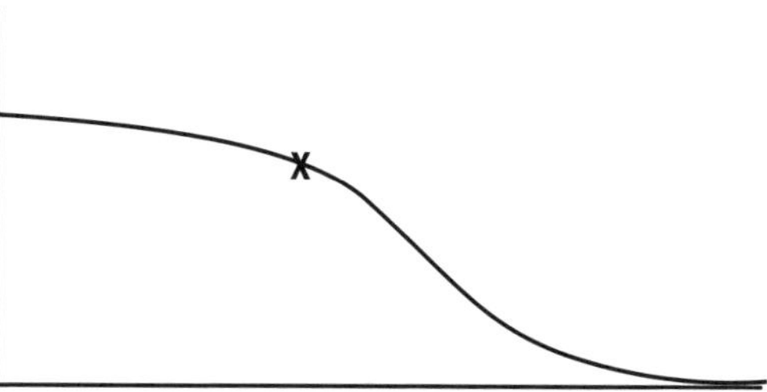


**Source:** Potocnik, 2014

**Figure 30.4** Course of vascular dementia

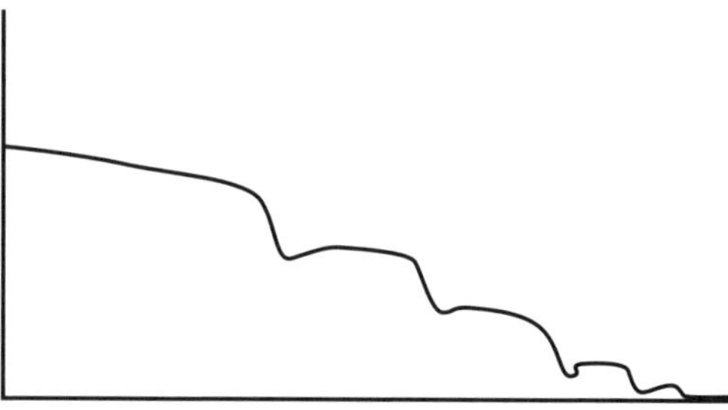

**Source:** Potocnik, 2014

### 30.14.9.3 Major or mild neurocognitive disorder with Lewy bodies

In Lewy body disease, there is a build-up of Lewy bodies (accumulations of alpha synuclein protein) in the brain (Perry *et al.*, 1990). This can manifest clinically as a major neurocognitive disorder (otherwise known as Lewy body dementia) or a mild neurocognitive disorder in the earlier stages of the disease.

Neurocognitive disorder with Lewy bodies usually exhibits as fluctuations in cognition (mimicking a sub-acute delirium or multi-infarct dementia) with pronounced variation in attention and alertness, recurrent well-formed visual hallucinations (especially sundowning), and then followed by motor features of parkinsonism (See Chapter 32: Neuropsychiatry, for a further discussion.)

Due to its effect on the motor and autonomic system, you may find that a patient with Lewy body disease does far worse functionally than a patient with Alzheimer's disease with the same cognitive deficit. The course of the illness tends to be rapidly progressive, interspersed with repeated falls, syncope, transient loss of consciousness, other hallucinations and congruent delusions. These patients tend to be sensitive to the side effects of neuroleptic agents (requiring treatment with drugs like clozapine or newer neuroleptic agents). They may be responsive to cholinesterase inhibitors.

### 30.14.9.4 Major or mild frontotemporal neurocognitive disorder

Pick's disease is a progressive neurocognitive disorder that chiefly affects the frontal cortex. Pick's disease most commonly manifests itself between the ages of 50–60 years, although age of onset does vary and you may find patients presenting with the disorder anywhere between their fourth and ninth decade of life. Survival is shorter than with Alzheimer's disease (about 5–10 years after diagnosis).

Pick's disease is distinguished from frontotemporal neurocognitive disorder by the presence of characteristic intraneuronal argentophilic Pick inclusion bodies found at autopsy. There are a number of syndromic variants of frontotemporal degeneration, and the classification system is constantly evolving as we better understand the underlying pathology. Symptoms are broadly divided into behavioural and language variants (Gorno-Tempini *et al.*, 2011).

Behavioural symptoms:

- apathy (presenting with decreased motivation, poor self-care, impact on work)
- disinhibition (e.g. new onset substance abuse, illicit affairs)
- change in religious or political beliefs
- lack of empathy
- hyperphagia or hyperorality
- stereotypies or compulsive behaviour
- poor insight.

Language symptoms:

- poor speech production
- difficulty naming
- poor comprehension.

It presents with prominent personality changes and impaired executive function. There is relative sparing of learning and memory and perceptual-motor function. Early primitive reflexes and incontinence, rigidity and tremor may be present. Affective symptoms may include depression, anxiety and somatic preoccupation. Clear cognitive decline, especially in the early stages, may be absent or difficult to assess. The early symptoms of behavioural variants often have tragic consequences. Individuals frequently lose their jobs, are ruined financially, face divorce and test close relationships because of the behavioural changes. The behavioural variant in particular may not get to a doctor till the condition is far progressed. Even when these individuals reach a doctor, the diagnosis may be mistaken for depression, bipolar mood disorder, schizophrenia, substance use disorder or antisocial personality disorder.

### 30.14.9.5 Major or mild neurocognitive disorder due to Prion disease (Creutzfeldt-Jakob's disease)

Prion disease encompasses a group of subacute spongiform encephalopathies, the most common being Creutzfeldt-Jakob disease (CJD) (Will, 2003). Creutzfeldt-Jakob disease is brought about by a virus-like infective agent called a **prion**. It causes a rapid progressive dementia also affecting the pyramidal and extrapyramidal systems. These include myoclonus or ataxia. A new variant of Creutzfeldt-Jakob's disease described in England in 1995 is transmitted to humans by eating contaminated beef products and is associated with bovine spongiform encephalopathy or 'mad cow disease'. It appears to express itself under certain conditions in individuals under the age of 40 years. Most cases of Creutzfeldt-Jakob disease are sporadic.

Initial symptoms are non-specific (fatigue, insomnia, poor concentration), which rapidly progress within weeks to incoordination, ataxia, abnormal movements (myoclonus, **choreoathetoid**, ballistic) and a dementia. The condition reaches a critical level of impairment typically within months, leading to death within a year.

## 30.14.10 Management

Management of neurocognitive disorder involves a quadrangle, viz. doctor-patient-caregiver-community support organisations. Take the time to fully discuss the illness with the caregiver and patient. Not only is this therapeutic but it also prevents'doctor-shopping'. Relatives may blame the dementia on a non-causal incident such as a severe flu, a mugging or motor vehicle accident (without head injury), a son or daughter leaving home or some other emotional or financial stressor. Attempt to establish that the onset of dementia occurred prior to the event and that the latter incident may at most have acted as a possible contributing factor in exposing the underlying illness. Be sympathetic but firm in handling a stubborn patient who is no longer coping and requires relocation to premises offering more supervision and care. Be prepared to act the role of'bad wolf'by firmly recommending admission to an old age home when it is necessary, since families are more often than not both guilt-ridden and intimidated by this decision. Discuss the genetics of the illness. Treatment of neurocognitive disorder is aimed at symptom alleviation and optimising maximum health.

### 30.14.10.1 Course

Explain to caregivers that neurocognitive disorder is a progressive disease that ultimately lead to death, commonly within eight to twelve years. Death is usually from a stroke or myocardial infarct in vascular and alcohol-induced neurocognitive disorder, while bronchopneumonia and urinary tract infections, giving rise to septicaemia, are the common causes of death in Alzheimer's disease and other dementias. Note that the patient in a'persistent vegetative state' does not appreciate the sensation of hunger or thirst. For this reason nasogastric tubes in these terminal patients are not recommended. Involve and discuss with family in all cases.

### 30.14.10.2 Non-pharmacological treatment

Non-pharmacological treatment should be implemented prior to attempting medication and involves:

- the psycho-education, support – and if necessary, treatment – of the caregiver, as well as arranging periods of respite.

**Information box**

**Cross-reference to other aetiologies of neurocognitive disorders covered in this book**

| Major or mild NCD due to: | Cross reference to chapter: |
|---|---|
| Huntington's disease | 32 – Neuropsychiatry |
| Parkinson's disease | 32 – Neuropsychiatry |
| traumatic brain injury | 32 – Neuropsychiatry |
| HIV infection | 33 – HIV and mental health |
| Substance-induced, medication-Induced | 20 – Addictions 1: Alcohol-related disorders |
| Another medical condition | 32 – Neuropsychiatry |
| Multiple aetiologies | 32 – Neuropsychiatry |
| Unspecified | 32 – Neuropsychiatry |

- the assessment of the patient's environment with particular emphasis on optimising orientation and handling by caregivers. Establish a safe and familiar routine, restricting the patient to a maximum of 20 minutes' afternoon nap. Remove precipitating factors and restrict the area of wanderers. Avoid restraints if possible.
- implementing validation/affirmative therapy, reminiscence therapy and 24-hour reality orientation with the patient. Diversion tactics are very important; keep the patient occupied (Ames *et al.*, 2010.

### 30.14.10.3 Pharmacological treatment

Pharmacological treatment is indicated as augmentation to the above or when non-pharmacological intervention has failed. The choice of medication is individual, based on experience, contraindications, tolerability, availability and especially costs. Under ideal conditions the regimens as set out in Tables 30.5, 30.6, 30.7 and 30.8 should be implemented.

Three acetylcholinesterase inhibitors are currently available for Alzheimer's disease: donepezil, rivastigmine and galantamine. These medications are acetylcholine esterase inhibitors resulting in increased acetylcholine levels in the brain. An alternative strategy is the inhibition of excitotoxic amino-acid neurotransmitters (e.g. glutamate, aspartate, homocysteine) by administering memantine which is an N-methyl-D aspartate (NMDA) receptor antagonist. These medications improve memory, behaviour and function; initially above baseline for approximately the first nine months, after which the deterioration of the disease appears to be slowed down by roughly half its usual rate for the remainder of its course. In general terms patients lose 2–3 points on MMSE per year. On treatment they can expect to have lost this amount after 2 years.

A combination of an AChEI with memantine is more effective than either agent on its own and is well tolerated, there being no pharmacokinetic or pharmacodynamic interaction between the two.

**Table 30.5** Pharmacological treatment schedule for Alzheimer's disease

1. One of the following acetylcholinesterase inhibitors:
   - donepezil 5–10 mg at night
   - rivastigmine 3–6 mg twice daily
   - galantamine 16–24 mg daily

   and/or
2. NMDA receptor antagonist:
   - memantine 10–20 mg daily
3. Psychotropic agents for residual neuropsychiatric symptoms, i.e. mood (depression, irritability) and behavioural disturbances (restlessness, agitation, psychotic symptoms, insomnia). (Also see Tables 30.7, 30.8 and 30.9.)
4. Control of cardiovascular risk factors such as hypertension, diabetes mellitus, dyslipidaemia and smoking (see Table 30.10)

**Source:** Potocnik, 2013

Patients must adapt to the medications, thus slow titration is recommended to the maximum dose tolerated. The higher the maximum dose, the better the results.

Use the maxim 'start low, go slow, end high'. Increase donepezil from 5 mg to 10 mg after eight weeks, and rivastigmine in increments of 1,5 mg twice daily, every four weeks, to a total of 6–12 mg per day. Galantamine is similarly titrated upwards in increments of 8 mg every four weeks to an effective dose of 16–24 mg per day. Metabolism is via the cytochrome P450 system. Memantine is given in the morning with a starting dose of 5 mg, then raised in increments of 5 mg on a weekly basis to an effective dose of 10–20 mg per day. Metabolism is primarily non-hepatic.

Most indications for the above agents are AD-specific but may also benefit AD patients with cerebrovascular disease. Other indications include mild neurocognitive disorder (MCI), neurocognitive disorder due to diffuse Lewy bodies (DLB), and neurocognitive disorder due to Parkinson's disease. These indications are, however, country-specific as is their range of applications for the mild, moderate and severe stages of Alzheimer's disease. The mode of administration (slow-release capsules, transdermal patches) further impacts more positively on tolerability, compliance and efficacy, as do ease of titration, price of product and familiarity with medication. Under ideal circumstances, treatment should start in the prodromal/symptomatic/MCI phase of Alzheimer's disease, bearing in mind that patients only tolerate the minimum effective dose in the early stages. With positive results, treatment may continue uninterrupted to a MMSE as low as 5/30, after which continuing benefit becomes increasingly questionable and difficult to evaluate in research or where the patient's neurocognitive disorder has progressed to a stage where there is no signficant benefit from continued therapy.

Side effects of AChEI's are usually transitory and include nausea, vomiting, bouts of diarrhoea, gastric discomfort, sedation, agitation, sweating, dizziness and headache. Note that the AChEIs may potentially have vagotonic effects on the heart (i.e. bradycardia); this is of importance in patients with sick sinus syndrome or other dysrhythmias, including the exaggeration of bradycardia medication such as beta-blockers, amiodarone and calcium channel antagonists (Lovestone and Gauthier, 2001).

Side effects of memantine are usually transitory and include confusion, dizziness, headache and fatigue. Uncommon are anxiety, hypertonia and vomiting. Being an amantadine derivative memantine may enhance the action of L-DOPA and dopaminergic agonists.

Generally, both groups of medications interact with anticholinergic medications and cholinomimetics to a variable extent. Failure to benefit from any one AChEI or memantine does not necessarily mean that the patient will not respond to another of these medications.

The inherent symptoms of apathy and social withdrawal mimic depression in the AD patient, making it difficult to distinguish between the two. In addition, depression frequently accompanies some 20% of AD patients in the early stages. Generally the diagnosis of depression is clinically relevant in the higher ranges of the MMSE, while the benefit of doubt should swing towards the patient being socially withdrawn and not depressed as one approaches a MMSE of 20–22/30.

Guidelines for the treatment of depression has been discussed earlier.

### 30.14.10.4 The caregiver

A most vital link in the pharmacotherapy and general care of neurocognitive disorder is the caregiver. Caregivers are estimated to spend an average of 70–100 hours per week on providing care. Caregivers utilise 45% more physician visits and 70% more prescription drugs than non-caregivers, and are more likely to be hospitalised. Caregivers are 50% more likely than those in the general population to become depressed. A recent study showed that caregivers of NCD spouses have a six times higher rate of developing major neurocognitive disorder themselves compared with other non-NCD couples. Judicious use of pharmacotherapy, therefore, not only alleviates the stress on the caregiver but also delays the institutionalisation of the NCD patient.

All caregivers should be referred to non-profit organisations such as Dementia South Africa (Toll-free line: 0860 636 679) or Alzheimer's Association South Africa (011 792 2511). Not only do these organisations assist in supporting caregivers and monitoring their well-being but they also explain how to care for the patient, provide support services (home help or respite care) wherever possible, provide counselling and medico-legal advice, and continually update the caregiver by means of newsletters, meetings or workshops, on the latest developments (Potocnik, 2013; Lovestone, 2001; Folstein *et al.*, 1975).

## 30.14.11 Medico-legal matters

See Chapter 35: Legal and ethical aspects of mental health, for information on competence/capacity, contractual or financial capacity, testamentary capacity, power of attorney and curatorship.

**Figure 30.5** Course of dementia with or without memory enhancer

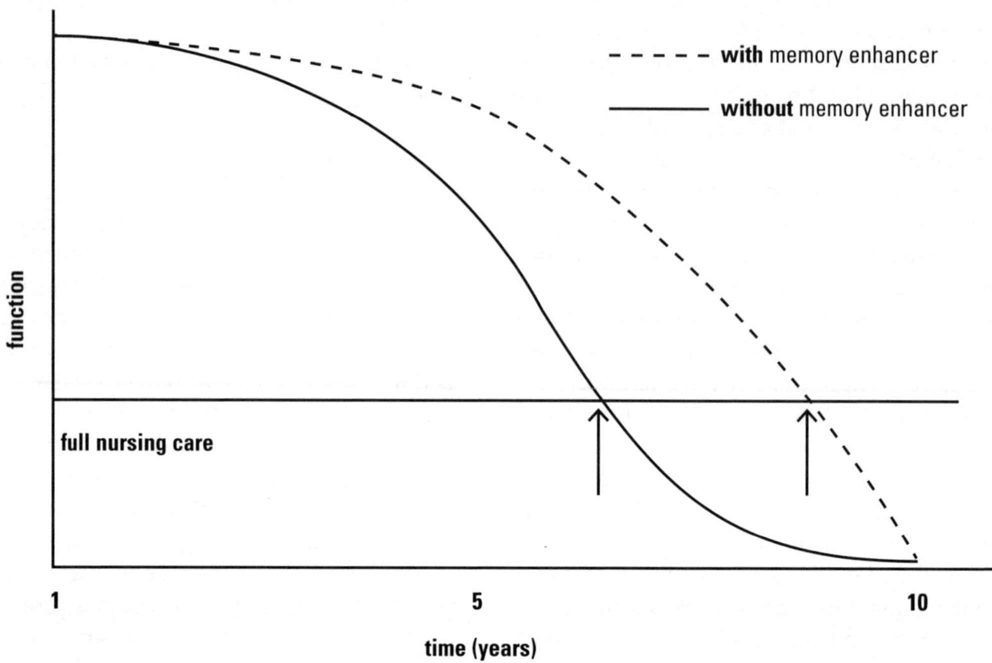


**Source:** Potocnik, 2014

**Table 30.6** Example of a neuroleptic regimen (treatment schedule for neuropsychiatric symptoms such as restlessness, psychotic symptoms, agitation and insomnia)

Haloperidol/risperidone 0,5 mg/0,25–0.5 mg respectively, at 8h00 and 17h00.

Increase the dose to 0,75 mg, 1,0 mg and 1,5 mg, if necessary, for daytime control. Wait a day or two between increases.

Together with:

- chlorpromazine or quetiapine 25 mg at night 20h00
- increase the dose to 50 mg, 75 mg and 100 mg at night, if necessary, for nocturnal control.
- wait a day or two between increases.

Or:

- alanzapine 2,5–5 mg at 17h00

Or:

- ziprasidone 20 mg at 08h00 and 17h00

**Source:** Potocnik, 2013

**Table 30.7** Psychotropics for acute sedation

One of the following agents:

- lorazapam
  1–2 mg po/IMI
  0,5–1,5 mg IVI

Do not exceed 8 mg over 24 hours.

- haloperidol
  2,5 mg IMI/IVI

Do not exceed 10 mg over 24 hours.

**Table 30.8** Depot neuroleptics

Depot agents are indicated in most paranoid and non-compliant patients and comprise:

- fluphenazine decanoate 12,5–25 mg administered every four weeks
- zuclopenthixol decanoate 200–400 mg administered every four weeks
- risperidone depot 25–50 mg administered every two to four weeks.

#### 30.14.11.1 Driving and firearms (Potocnik, 2006)

Driving a car relies on implicit memory, praxis and executive functioning. In the early phases of the illness patients can usually still drive a car because these abilities remain relatively intact. With time, however, they are unable to pay attention to all aspects of driving, become impulsive and exercise the wrong options. Should the dementia render the person incapable of driving safely, he or she is medico-legally disqualified from driving. Where the patient will not refrain from driving, doctors have a legal obligation under the National Road Traffic Act 1996 (No. 93 of 1996) to report such individuals to the local traffic authorities.

In general:

- assess all cases on individual merit
- patients must drive in conditions affording good visibility and then in day time only, on non-busy suburban roads and always accompanied by a caregiver.
- their MMSE should be at least 20–22/30 or above and they must still be able to do the pentagon test, which tests for visuospatial ability, or the Trail-making B test, which measures the ability to multitask.
- re-assess at three-monthly intervals.

Similarly, gun licences should be revoked for the same reason.

### 30.14.12 Prevention, delay and amelioration of neurocognitive disorder (Potocnik, 2013)

It is estimated that that the neurodegeneration in Alzheimer's disease starts some 20–30 years before the appearance of the first clinical symptoms, reflecting the need for earlier intervention while minimal brain damage has occured.

A delay in the onset of Alzheimer's disease by only five years will halve the prevalence of the disease, resulting in enormous savings of human misery and cost to society (Breitner, 2015). More than 70% of NCD in the elderly in developed countries are due to Alzheimer's disease, VaNCD or a combination of the two. The microvascular pathology common to all three has been addressed through better management of cardio-vascular risk factors and lifestyle. Though this was essentially aimed at reducing cardiovascular disease the spin-off has resulted in early signs of an overall leveling off of neurocognitive disorder in the elderly

Note that the preventative measures mentioned below offer no benefit to people whose preclinical Alzheimer's disease is very advanced or the neurocognitive disorder is clinically evident:

- Hormone replacement therapy (oestrogen with or without progesterone) is only effective if initiated at the time of menopause where a deficiency in female sex hormones has clearly been established. Treatment should not exceed 2–4 years.
- Vitamin E (<400IU) and vitamin C (400 mg) daily, preferably in combination. Note that high-dose vitamin E (+400 IU daily) supplementation is associated with an increased mortality risk (Breitner, 2011).
- Red wine (e.g. Bordeaux blend 250–500 ml daily). The benefits are ascribed to resveratrol and other aliphatic compounds.
- Non-steroidal anti-inflammatory drugs (NSAIDs). Conventional NSAIDs such as ibuprofen and voltaren as well as naproxen used for as little as 2-3 years may protect against Alzheimer's disease.
- Consuming 3-5 cups of coffee (not decaffeinated or instant) a day decreases the risk of neurocognitive disorder or Alzheimer's disease later in life.
- Cocoa. The equivalent of 40 grams of 80% dark chocolate per day
- A diet rich in vitamins B, C, D and E (fruit and vegetables) and omega-3 fatty acids (fish) and low in high trans-fat (processed foods) reflects in beneficial blood nutrient biomarker patterns influencing both cognitive function and brain volume.

- Intellectual stimulation and higher education improve brain reserve by improving synaptic connectivity.
- Reduction in stress is also linked to having close friends or confidants, a good social network and leisure activities and hobbies.
- The control of vascular risk factors as these are closely linked to the pathophysiology of Alzheimer's disease. These risks factors are linked to transient ischaemic attacks (TIAs), and vascular risk factors for neurocognitive disorder and Alzheimer's disease (see Table 30.9).

## 30.14.13 When to refer

Subjective complaints of memory impairment should always be taken seriously, especially when they impinge on daily social or occupational functioning. A full organic work-up (see Table 30.1) with careful monitoring of the complaint is indicated in most cases. Patients with an MMSE above 26/30 in whom dementia is suspected should be referred.

Patients not responding adequately to AChEIs, antidepressants or neuroleptics should be referred.

**Table 30.9** Management of vascular risk factors for vascular NCD, TIAs and Alzheimer's disease

Treatment of risk factors:

- Hypertension (age-acceptable blood pressure readings must be taken into account).
- Diabetes: in asymtomatic diabetes random blood-glucose levels of up to 15 mmol/ℓ are acceptable.
- Smoking should be stopped (also because it is a fire hazard).
- Reduce alcohol consumption to an equivalent maximum of three units per day.
- Prevent platelet aggregation (aspirin 80–150 mg per day).
- Control dyslipidaemia and peri-vascular inflammation through diet and medication (i.e. serum lipid-reducing agents such as the HMGCoA reductase inhibitors (statins); recommended dosage still under dispute).
- Control body mass index through dietary modification and regular exercise.
- Treat endothelial stress and inflammation with a thiamine supplementation.
- Treat hyperhomocysteinaemia with folic acid and vitamin $B_6$ and $B_{12}$ supplementation.

## Conclusion

The management of elderly patients and their ailments has increasingly been demistified over the past decades, attracting ever-younger health and allied professionals into this field of expertise. The combined efforts have resulted in not only an increase in life expectancy but dramatically improved the quality of life of the older person.

# References

Adamchak DJ (1996) Population ageing: Gender, family support and the economic condition of older Africans. *Southern African Journal of Gerontology* 5(2): 3–8

Alexopoulos GS, Meyers BS, Young RC (1997) Vascular depression hypothesis. *Archives of General Psychiatry* 1997: 54; 915–922

American Psychiatric Association (2013) *Diagnostic and Statistical Manual of Mental Disorders* (5th edition). Washington DC: American Psychiatric Association

Ames D, Chen E, Lindesay J, Shulman K (2010) *Guide to the Psychiatry of Old Age.* Cambridge, UK: Cambridge University Press

Anderson NH, Woodburn K (2010) Old-age psychiatry. In: Johnstone EC *et al.*, (Eds). *Companion to Psychiatry Studies* (8th edition). Edinburgh: Churchill Livingstone

Baldwin RC (2010) *Depression in Later Life.* Oxford: Oxford University Press

Breitner JCS (2015) *Changing the Trajectory of Alzheimer's Disease: How a Treatment by 2025 Saves Lives and Dollars.* Alzheimer's Association 800.272.3900alz.org 2015

Breitner JC, Baker LD, Montine T, , Meinert CL, Lyketsos CG, Ashe KH, Brandt J, Craft S, Evans DE, Green RC, Ismail MS, Martin BK, Mullan MJ, Sabbagh M, Tariot PN; ADAPT Research Group (2011) Extended results of the Alzheimer's disease anti-inflammatory prevention trial. *Alzheimer's and Dementia* 7: 402–411.

Butler I, Sinclair L, Tipping B (2013) Current concepts in the management of delirium. *Continuing Medical Education* u 31, n 10:363–366. Available at http://www.cmej.org.za/index.php/cmej/article/view/2793/3241

Campanelli CM (2012) American Geriatrics Society Updated Beers Criteria for Potentially Inappropriate Medication Use in Older Adults *Journal of American Geriatrics Society* April: 60(4): 616–631

Cummings JL, Mega MS, Gray K, Rosenberg-Thompson S, Carusi DA, Gornbein J (1994) The neuropsychiatric inventory: Comprehensive assessment of psychopathology in dementia. *Neurology* 44: 2380–2314

Djernes JK (2006) Prevalence and predictors of depression in population of elderly: A review. *Acta Psychiatrica Scandinavia* 113: 372–87

Folstein MF, Folstein SE, Mc Hugh PR (1975) 'Mini-Mental State:' A practical method for grading the cognitive state of patients for clinician. *Journal of Psychiatry Research* 12: 185–98

Fries JF (1990) The sunny side of ageing. *JAMA* 263(17): 2354–5

Galasko D, Bennett D, Sano M, Ernesto C, Thomas R, Grundman M, Ferris S (1997) An inventory to assess activities of daily living for clinical trials in Alzheimer's disease: The Alzheimer's co-operative study. *Alzheimer's Disease and Associated Disorders* 11 (Suppl 2): S33-S39

Gauthier S (1999) *Alzheimer's Disease in Primary Care* (2nd edition). London: Martin Dunitz.

Gorno-Tempini ML, Hillis AE, Weintraub S, Kertesz A, Mendez M, Cappa SF, , Ogar JM, Rohrer JD, Black S, Boeve BF, Manes F, Dronkers NF, Vandenberghe R, Rascovsky K, Patterson K, Miller BL, Knopman DS, Hodges JR, Mesulam MM, Grossman M (2011). Classification of primary progressive aphasia and its variants. *Neurology* 76(11): 1006–14

Hawkins JM, Archer KJ, Strakowski SM, Keck PE (1995) Somatic treatment of catatonia. *The International Journal of Psychiatry in Medicine* 25(4): 345–369.

Hayflick L (1985) Theories of biological ageing. *Experimental Gerontology* 20:145–59

Jorm AF, Korten AE, Henderson AS (1987) The prevalence of dementia: A quantitative integration of the literature. *Acta Psychiatrica Scandinavia* 76: 464–79

Kaplan HJ, Sadock BJ (Eds) (2003) *Synopsis of psychiatry* (9th edition). London: Williams and Williams

Katona C, Robertson M (1995) *Psychiatry at a glance.* Oxford: Blackwell Science

Lovestone, S, Gauthier S (2001) *Management of Dementia.* London: Martin Dunitz

Moorhouse P, Rockwood K (2008) Vascular cognitive impairment: Current concepts and clinical developments. *The Lancet Neurology* 7(3): 246–55

Parkes CM (1996) *Bereavement: Studies of Grief in Adult Life* (3rd edition). New York: Routledge

Perry RH, Irving D, Blessed G, Fairbairn A, Perry EK (1990) Senile dementia of Lewy body type: A clinically and neuropathologically distinct form of Lewy body dementia in the elderly. *Journal of the Neurological Sciences* 95(2): 119–39

Pitt B (1974) *Psychogeriatrics: An Introduction to the Psychiatry of Old Age*. Edinburgh: Livingstone

Post F (1979) The functional psychoses. In: Isaacs Alzheimer's disease, Post F (Eds.) *Studies in Geriatric Psychiatry*. Chichester: Wiley

Potocnik FCV (1992) Successful treatment of hypersexuality in AIDS dementia with cyproterone acetate. *South African Medical Journal* 81: 433–5

Potocnik FCV (2005) Psychogeriatrics. In: Emsley RA, Pienaar WP (Eds.) *Textbook of Psychiatry* (2nd edition). Tygerberg: Mental Health Information Centre of South Africa

Potocnik FCV (2013) Dementia. *South African Journal of Psychiatry* 19(3): 141–52

Potocnik FCV (2014) Psychogeriatrics. In: Emsley RA, Pienaar WP, Seedat S (Eds). *Textbook of Psychiatry.* Tygerberg: Mental Health Information Centre of South Africa

Potocnik FCV, Pienaar W (2006) The elderly. In: Kaliski S (Ed). *Psycholegal Assessment in South Africa.* Cape Town: Oxford University Press

Statistics South Africa (2013) *Mid-year population estimates.* Pretoria: Statistics South Africa

Tipping B Delirium. In: Cassim B (Ed) (2014) *South African Geriatric Society Guidelines*

Van Gool WA, van de Beek D, Eikelenboom P (2010) Systemic infection and delirium: When cytokines and acetylcholine collide. *The Lancet* 375: 773–5

Wicht CL (1990) The physiology of ageing. In: Meiring P de V (Ed.) *Textbook of geriatric medicine.* Cape Town: Juta

Will RG (2003) Acquired Prion disease: Iatrogenic CJD, variant CJD, kuru. *British Medical Bulletin* 66: 255–65

World Health Organization (2002) *The World Health Report 2002. Reducing Risks, Promoting Healthy Life*. Geneva: World Health Organization

CHAPTER

# 31 Psychiatry and medicine

Yasmien Jeenah, Yusuf Moosa

## 31.1 Introduction

This chapter deals with the interface between psychiatry and medicine. Medical symptoms may be either physical (e.g. back pain, headache, bowel disturbances, dizziness, palpitations, fatigue) or psychological (e.g. depressed mood, anxiety, guilt).'Physicians, who deal mainly with medical disorders, tend to label such symptoms as"physical". Mental health specialists tend to use the term'somatic'. Nonetheless, the two adjectives are synonymous and can be used interchangeably. It is inaccurate to always equate physical symptoms with medical disorders: many patients with physical symptoms do not have a medical disorder that can explain the presence and/or severity of their physical symptoms' (Kroenke, 2003). Psychiatric disorders may present primarily with somatic symptoms in a medical setting and may be misdiagnosed as a medical disorder. Some of the common symptoms will be elaborated upon later in this chapter. According to the fifth edition of the *Diagnostic and Statistical Manual of Mental Disorders* (DSM-5),'individuals with somatic symptoms may or may not have a diagnosed medical condition. They will usually meet DSM-5 criteria for somatic symptom disorder only if they have the maladaptive thoughts, feelings, and behaviors that define the disorder, in addition to their somatic symptoms' (American Psychiatric Association, 2013). Similarly, medical illnesses may also present with psychiatric symptoms. The psychiatric presentation of a medical disorder is defined in the DSM-5 as 'the presence of mental symptoms that are judged to be the direct physiological consequences of a general medical condition' (American Psychiatric Association, 2013). Failure to identify the medical cause of symptoms can be potentially dangerous because serious, and frequently reversible, diseases can be overlooked.

The chapter will also address psychiatric disorders that occur co-morbidly with medical disorders. Medically ill patients with co-existing psychiatric disorders pose several challenges to the health professional in the general hospital, including the appropriate treatment strategy (Eastwood, 1975). (Also see Section 31.5 and Section 31.6 for a discussion of the management of psychiatric disorders in the medically ill and the special role of **consultation-liaison psychiatry** respectively.)

The 1920s saw the establishment of general hospital psychiatric units in the USA and the founding of consultation liaison psychiatry (CLP), which is a result of the convergence of psychiatry and medicine (Lipowski and Wise, 2002). By the 1950s, consultation-liaison units were found in many US hospitals, while in the 1960s out-patient psychiatric clinics, which included social workers and psychologists as members of the treatment team and a bio-psycho-social model of patient management, were being set up (Kornfeld, 2002; Gitlin *et al.*, 2004).

## 31.2 Epidemiology

Various approaches have been used to calculate the incidence and prevalence of mental disorders. One approach is records of first and subsequent admissions, discharges, and movements of the patient in public institutions. The limitation of this approach includes the inability to calculate the number of mentally ill who

## 31.1 Advanced reading block

Some recent advances in the area of psychiatry and medicine include:

**Hypothalamic-pituitary-adrenal (HPA) axis**

'Abnormalities of the HPA axis are found in a number of neuropsychiatric disorders, including depression and post-traumatic stress disorder' (Yehuda *et al.*, 1995). 'The neuroendocrine response to chronic stress may lead to damage in intracranial structures, which in turn exacerbates congenital tendencies toward affective instability and the development of affective disorders' (Duman *et al.*, 2000). 'Patients with psychotic depression tend to show higher levels of serum cortisol levels inducing decreases in dopamine function which may underlie the cognitive deficits' (Schatzberg *et al.*, 2000).

**Psychoneuro-immunology**

There are three main regulatory systems in the body: the nervous, the endocrine and the immune system. These interact in complex bi-directional pathways, thus providing biological evidence that the mind and body cannot be separated into two discrete systems. Diseases, ranging from cardiovascular disease, osteoporosis to Alzheimer's disease, may be influenced by pro-inflammatory cytokines, such as interleukin-6 (Kiecolt-Glaser *et al.*, 2002; Ursin, 1994). Stress appears to enhance production of these injurious pro-inflammatory cytokines and is particularly important at the initial onset of recurrent psychiatric illnesses, such as depression. Further, sensitization of the limbic system to stress, mediated through the immunological and endocrine systems, results in changes in the genetic expression of the neurone, increasing the genetic vulnerability to depression (Kiecolt-Glaser *et al.*, 2002).

**Pathological emotional states and cardiac morbidity**

'Depression and other pathological emotions have been linked to altered cardiac function and the development of ischemic heart disease' (Glassman and Shapiro, 1998). 'In pre-existing cardiovascular disease, depression is associated with adverse cardiac outcome, including enhanced cardiac mortality and morbidity' (Tucker *et al.*, 1997). 'Ventricular arrhythmias and myocardial ischemia can be induced by stress and that major depression is associated with exaggerated platelet reactivity, which can increase the chance of ischemic events in patients prone to cardiac and cerebrovascular disease' (Krantz *et al.*, 1996). 'The presence of major depression negatively affects the outcome of some illnesses such as myocardial infarction' (Lesperance *et al.*, 1996). Patients with post-stroke depression have a poorer prognosis and lower rates of functional recovery than patients who are not depressed (Schulberg *et al.*, 1996) as well as increased expenditures (Katon *et al.*, 1995).

**Brain circuitry and emotion**

'Our brains respond to the world via three intricately connected neural systems: the limbic system, the prefrontal cortex and the paralimbic system' (Mesulam, 2000). 'Damage to these mediating structures interferes with the ability of emotion and visceral state to guide behaviour' (Mesulam, 2000).

remain in the community, the number institutionalised in private hospitals, those treated by private physicians and other factors that contribute to the under-reporting of mental illness. An additional limitation to the use of admission records involves the great variability in diagnoses within a hospital and between different hospitals. Given the above and the lack of consensus regarding the definition of terms and operationally defined criteria for diagnosis, reliable information regarding the epidemiology of this group of disorders is difficult to obtain.

Despite these methodological and sampling difficulties in epidemiological research, recent studies have been able to overcome these.

- In a general medical setting, up to 30% of patients have a psychiatric disorder (Al-sayyad *et al.*, 2010).
- Delirium is detected in 10% of all medical inpatients and in more than 30% of some high-risk groups (Levitan and Kornfield, 1981).

- Epidemiological studies that use standardised instruments for diagnosis report that the prevalence of mental disorders range from 41,3–46,5% in a general medical setting (Rothenhäusler, 2006).
- Two-thirds of frequent health care users have a psychiatric disturbance: 23% have depression, 22% have anxiety, and 20% have somatisation (Al-sayyad *et al.*, 2010).
- Depression and delirium are associated with longer stays in hospital.

(Also see Chapter 3: Psychiatric epidemiology and genetics.)

## 31.3 Presentation of psychiatric disorders in medical settings

More than 50% of patients with depression or anxiety present to primary care with complaints of somatic symptoms (e.g. pain, headache, fatigue, lethargy) rather than volunteering psychological symptoms (such as 'I'm depressed' or 'I've been feeling anxious'). Other psychiatric disorders that commonly present with somatic symptoms include panic disorders, somatoform disorders, personality disorders and factitious disorders. Irrespective of culture, presentation with somatic symptoms is common. Most patients with a psychiatric disorder will admit to psychological symptoms if specifically asked about them: while somatic symptoms may be the initial complaint, they also present an opportunity for the clinician to inquire about co-existing psychological distress (Kroenke, 2003).

With regards to somatic symptoms, pain has to be highlighted for the following reasons:

- Complaints about pain (including back pain, knee or hip pain, abdominal pain, headache, chest pain, and neck pain) account for more than half of all outpatient visits for somatic symptoms.
- There is a close association between pain and depression.
- More than half of depressed patients suffer from pain, and more than a quarter of patients with pain report significant depression.
- Pain is a risk factor for poor treatment response in depression.
- The prevalence of pain in depressed patients and its adverse impact on treatment response imply that attention to both pain

### Factors that increase the likelihood of a psychiatric disorder in patients with somatic symptoms

- Symptoms that remain medically unexplained after initial evaluation: up to two-thirds of patients with medically unexplained symptoms have a depressive disorder, and 40-50% have an anxiety disorder.
- Total number of somatic symptoms: the risk of psychiatric co-morbidity increases with both an increasing total somatic symptom count and an increasing medically unexplained symptom count.
- Somatic symptoms increase in prevalence with increasing severity of psychological distress: the prevalence of individual pain and non-pain somatic symptoms is highest in those with major depressive disorder, intermediate in those with other depressive disorders (dysthymia, minor depression) and lowest in those with no depressive disorder.
- History of recent stress.
- Self-rated overall health of poor or fair on a 5-point scale (excellent, very good, good, fair, poor); self-rated severity of presenting somatic symptom of 6 or greater on a 0 (none) to 10 (unbearable) scale.
- The clinician's perception that the patient encounter is difficult.

**Source:** Kroenke, 2003

and depressive symptoms from the outset of therapy are required to optimise patient outcomes (Kroenke, 2003).

Adverse consequences of psychiatric disorders presenting with somatic symptoms include:

- recurrence of symptoms
- excessive or unnecessary surgery or other expensive and increased health care utilisation
- overuse of non-opiate analgesics, which also is a risk for tolerance or addiction
- both patient and physician discontent, evidenced as 'difficult' encounters and/or therapeutic nihilism
- a decline in physical, mental, social, and work functioning that result in increased disability days and temporary and permanent work disability (Kroenke, 2003).

'Understanding common psychiatric symptoms and the medical diseases that may cause or mimic them is complex yet important. Failure to assess patients with psychiatric symptoms (which can be time-consuming and difficult) may lead to symptoms being prematurely dismissed as psychiatric in nature. This failure to identify the medical cause of symptoms can be potentially dangerous, since serious and reversible diseases can be overlooked. Proper diagnosis of a psychiatric illness necessitates investigation of all possible medical causes of the symptoms' (Kroenke, 2003).

## 31.4 The co-occurrence of psychiatric disorders and medical conditions

More than 68% of adults with a mental disorder in the general population have at least one medical condition (Valderas *et al.*, 2009). Co-morbidity is defined broadly as 'the co-occurrence of mental and physical disorders in the same person, regardless of the chronological order in which they occurred or the causal pathway linking them' (Valderas *et al.*, 2009). Mental disorders include a spectrum of conditions, such as depression, anxiety disorders, schizophrenia and bipolar disorder. Co-morbidity is associated with a heightened symptom burden, functional impairment, decreased length and quality of life and increased costs.

The pathways that result in co-morbidity are complex and bi-directional. Medical disorders may lead to mental disorders, mental conditions may place a person at risk of certain medical disorders and mental and medical disorders may share common risk factors. Exposure to early trauma and chronic stress may be a risk factor for both mental and medical disorders (Black and Garbutt., 2002). 'A possible mechanism responsible for the relationship between stress and illness is exposure to stressors resulting in a compromise of the immune system and

### Features suggestive of a medical origin for psychiatric symptoms

- Late onset of initial presentation.
- Known underlying medical condition.
- Absence of personal and family history of psychiatric illnesses.
- Illicit substance use.
- Medication use.
- Treatment resistance or unusual response to treatment.
- Sudden onset of psychiatric symptoms.
- Abnormal vital signs.
- Waxing and waning mental status.

**Source:** Kroenke, 2003

an increase in the inflammatory responses and activation of the hypothalamo-pituitary-adrenal axis leading to chronic hypersecretion of cortisol' (Black and Garbutt, 2002). 'Low socioeconomic status reduces available resources, such as social support, and increases the chances of exposure to adverse environmental conditions' (Phelan *et al.*, 2004). Individuals with little social support have higher levels of depressive symptoms, schizophrenia and bipolar disorder. Low levels of social support are also negatively linked to medical conditions. Modifiable health-risk behaviour, such as tobacco use, excessive alcohol and illicit drug consumption, lack of physical activity and poor nutrition, is responsible for the high rates of co-morbidity, burden of illness and early death related to chronic diseases (Centers for Disease Control and Prevention, 2010). Many of the most common treatments for diseases may actually worsen the co-morbid mental or medical problems. Most psychotropic medications, particularly antipsychotic medications, can cause weight gain, obesity and diabetes (Muench and Hamer, 2010). At the same time, many treatments for common medical conditions may have psychological side effects that may exacerbate or complicate underlying psychiatric conditions.

Some system-based examples of such co-occurrences include:

- cardiovascular: brief changes in blood pressure may occur in association with emotional states, but there is insufficient evidence that it can result in sustained hypertension. Common psychiatric disorders associated with cardiovascular disease are panic attacks, anxiety and depression. Antihypertensive treatment (such as reserpine and alpha-methyl dopa) may also result in depression. Anxiety and emotional disorders may precede ischaemic episodes. Recovery from a myocardial infarction (MI) may be complicated by denial or anxiety and depression. By the same token, untreated depression post-MI is associated with a higher risk of repeat infarction and poor outcome.
- respiratory: breathlessness is a common feature of anxiety and panic attacks. It is likely that emotional states may precipitate or exacerbate individual attacks in those with established asthma and complicate its management. Cystic fibrosis is associated with symptoms of anxiety, depression and adjustment disorders. Anxiety and uncertainty regarding the future in patients with cystic fibrosis may impact on both the sufferer and his or her family. In cases of pulmonary tuberculosis, associated depressive symptoms may be due to chronic ill health, adverse social circumstances (e.g. loss of employment), or other illnesses such as HIV/Aids (particularly in southern Africa). Antituberculosis treatment, in particular isoniazid, may cause or exacerbate depressive symptoms.
- gastroenterology: loss of appetite and weight often accompany depressive states; the sensation of a lump in the throat may be a feature of an anxiety disorder. Irritable bowel syndrome involves non-specific pain or discomfort, with or without an alteration of bowel habit, which persists for longer than three months in the absence of a demonstrable physical disease. It is unclear whether the symptoms are caused by a physiological disturbance (e.g. a motility disorder), dietary problems or any other physical factors. Similarly, there is no consistent evidence to prove an association with life events, social factors or a psychiatric disorder, although psychological and social factors are likely to lead patients to seek treatment.
- neurology: there is a clear association between headache and depression, but the relationship is complex and controversy persists as to whether the depression predates the headaches or is a response to a painful chronic disorder. Depression is the most common psychiatric disorder in multiple sclerosis. Parkinson's disease is associated with a wide range of neuropsychiatric conditions, including cognitive decline, affective disorders, psychoses and personality changes. Antiparkinsonian agents may precipitate or cause depression. Huntington's disease is also characterised by a wide range of psychiatric morbidity, including cognitive decline, dementia, mania, depression and

personality changes. Depression is a common complication following a cerebrovascular accident and may worsen the outcome if untreated. Risk factors for the development of depression include a left anterior lesion, dysphasia, persisting disability, previous psychiatric and physical disability and social isolation. Psychiatric disorders are common in epilepsy. Psychiatric symptoms may be an expression of an underlying pathology that gives rise to both a psychiatric disorder and the epilepsy or may be a result of the psychological and social impacts of a chronic and often stigmatised illness. Anti-epileptic treatment can also cause or precipitate a wide range of neuropsychiatric symptoms.

- endocrine: stressful experiences may alter blood glucose levels in individuals with diabetes mellitus and affect self-care and compliance with treatment. The medical complications of diabetes are also likely to have severe psychological and social consequences that further undermine optimal diabetic control. Sexual problems are common and are likely to be related to a complex interaction of psychological and physical factors, such as depression and autonomic neuropathy. Delirium is associated with both hypoglycaemia and hyperglycaemia. Thyrotoxicosis may present as a 'crisis' with an acute medical syndrome or as an anxiety state. Hypothyroidism, because of its associated slowness, apathy and memory impairments, may be misdiagnosed as a dementia or a depressive disorder; it may also precipitate depressive symptoms. Addison's disease presents with psychological symptoms such as slowness, withdrawal and fatigue, and may therefore be misdiagnosed as a dementia or a depressive illness. A wide range of psychological symptoms may be observed in Cushing's syndrome, but depression is the most common and is not related to plasma cortisol levels. Steroid therapy can also produce a wide range of manic, depressive, delirious and psychotic symptoms. Phaeochromocytomas are rare causes of episodic anxiety and possibly delirium. A variety of psychological symptoms may also be encountered in the porphyrias, including anxiety, depression, delirium and psychotic symptoms.
- dermatological: depression is common and its causation is multifactorial, including the alcohol misuse, social withdrawal and isolation, adverse effects of many of the treatments and sleep disturbances caused by pain or itching. The relationship between psychological disturbance and dermatological conditions is circular: it is widely acknowledged that stressful events may provoke eczematous lesions, which in turn lead to anxiety and depression.
- cancer: psychological factors, such as denial, may affect the course of the illness (e.g. by leading to delays in seeking treatment) and a range of emotions, including anger, disbelief, anxiety and depression, may accompany the diagnosis. Major depressive episodes are particularly common at the time of diagnosis. Relapse and the incidence of suicide are high. Pain, past psychiatric illness and lack of social support are risk factors. Mental disorders may arise from cerebral metastases and may present before the primary lesion has been identified (more commonly in cases of cancers of the breast, lung, and gastrointestinal tract). Several forms of cancer treatment can lead to psychiatric disorder. Mastectomy surgery, other mutilating procedures and the uncertainty of the final outcome are particularly associated with depression.
- Auto-immune disease: neuropsychiatric symptoms occur in approximately two-thirds of all lupus patients at some time during the course of their illness; it can vary from mild symptoms to life-threatening complications. Lupus patients are at risk of developing psychiatric symptoms due to a combination of physical, environmental, medication-related and psychosocial phenomena. Psychosis occurs in at least 10% of patients and may present in a variety of ways, ranging from a brief psychotic episode that lasts for a few hours to treatment-resistant psychosis that continues for several months. Clinical features

are equally variable and range from affective symptoms (with either psychotic depression or mania) to symptoms suggestive of schizophrenia. It is often difficult to determine whether the depression arises from the direct effect of the illness on the brain, or a medication effect or whether the stress of living with lupus precipitated the depressive episode. Recurrent severe episodes of cerebral lupus eventually lead to widespread cortical damage and result in dementia with marked impairment in short-term and long-term memory and disturbance in executive function and activities of daily living.

## 31.5 Management of psychiatric disorders in the medically ill

Medically ill patients with co-existing psychiatric disorders can be difficult to manage in the general hospital. A major challenge is to determine the appropriate treatment strategy: this requires a careful history, a mental status examination, and the use of bedside screening and diagnostic instruments. Treatment options include pharmacotherapy, psychotherapy, psycho-education and psychosocial support. All these interventions can improve the patient's mental health and have the potential to shorten the hospital stay and reduce the burden on health services.

### 31.5.1 Pharmacotherapy

Psychopharmacological interventions are an essential part of the management of the medically ill; it is reported that at least 35% of psychiatric consultations are treated with medication (Trijsburg *et al.*, 1992). The use of medication should follow immediately after a diagnosis. It is important to recognise when to use other somatic therapies, such as electroconvulsive therapy or trans-cranial magnetic stimulation in depressed, catatonic or critically ill patients.

- Appropriate use of psychopharmacology necessitates a careful evaluation of the underlying medical illness, drug interactions and contraindications.
- Some patients will require the reduction or discontinuation of psychotropic medications, as these may be contributing to the clinical presentation.
- Many medications used in the treatment of medical or surgical illness are associated with psychiatric syndromes (e.g. hallucinations with L-DOPA, anxiety with bronchodilators, psychosis with steroids). The psychiatric effects of medication as well as the specific indications for psychopharmacological interventions must be considered.
- Modifications may be necessary because of liver, kidney or cardiac disease or because of the potential for multiple drug–drug interactions.
- Pharmacotherapy of the medically ill often involves a modification in dosage (e.g. to account for older patients with an increased **volume of distribution**, a decreased rate of metabolism and an increased physiological reactivity).
- Pregnancy presents another challenge, with concerns regarding potential teratogenicity (Trijsburg, *et al.*, 1992).

### 31.5.2. Psychotherapy

A review of the literature supports the benefits of a wide range of psychotherapeutic modalities. 'They must be structured for the specific illness or condition (e.g. cancer or heart disease) and the specific medical or surgical setting (e.g. the cardiac care unit, cancer service, otolaryngology service)' (Bronheim *et al.*, 1998).

Medical psychotherapy includes different modalities techniques that may be applied singly, in combination, or alternately in different stages of an illness, such as:

- crisis interventions
- supportive therapy
- interpersonal therapy
- group therapy
- cognitive behavioural therapy (CBT).

An individual's innate defence, cognitive style and interpersonal style must be considered when recommending appropriate psychotherapeutic strategies. An individual with a personality disorder is at risk of stereotypical maladaptive behaviour and emotions when exposed to medical illness. These may generate negative or hostile reactions from the clinicians. For the patient with a terminal illness, complex medical conditions and chronic pain, goal-directed CBT has been proven to improve co-operation and compliance. Supportive psychotherapy can be beneficial to those undergoing repeated testing. 'The psychotherapeutic approach to the medically ill should be considered carefully and the modality used introduced should be appropriate to the patient's needs. No single psychotherapeutic modality will be effective with all patients, at all times, in the medical setting. The treating doctor would benefit by having knowledge and clinical experience with the psychological stresses inherent in medical illness (e.g., separation anxiety, fear of pain, fear of loss of control, impending death, guilt about dependency and grief)' (Bronheim *et al.*, 1998).

### 31.5.3 Constant observation and restraints

Using constant observation and restraints is a serious decision. Because of the delicate balance between medical necessity and individual liberty, the use of these measures requires documentation of the need, follow-up monitoring and reporting of consequences in accordance with the Mental Health Care Act (MHCA). These interventions must not be done solely for the convenience of medical staff. Constant observation and restraints should be implemented for the shortest possible time and with the least restrictive, though effective, means available. Constant observation is often necessary to ensure patient safety in a medical or surgical setting. It is typically provided by nursing staff and at times with the assistance of family members. Patients who require constant observation and restraints typically include those:

- with an altered mental state or restlessness (e.g. secondary to dementia or delirium) who may inadvertently harm themselves or others
- who have attempted suicide or with psychopathology (e.g. severe depression or psychosis) and are at risk for suicide or assaultive behaviour
- who are attempting to leave the hospital against medical advice and at risk of injury (University of Texas Health Science Center, 2015).

Restraints should be applied in accordance with the MHCA and should be monitored as a special treatment procedure that requires specific justification. The doctor should be knowledgeable about:

- the physical and emotional risks of restraints
- the need to implement the least-restrictive alternatives in managing agitation
- the most conservative level of assessment methodology
- the highest guidelines of documentation (i.e. doctor's orders and progress notes)
- the need to frequently re-evaluate the patient, allowing for the earliest and safest possible release from restraints.

One form of restraint is mechanical restraint. The various types of mechanical restraints include: anklet, wristlet, mittens, and chair or bed fixation (University of Texas Health Science Center, 2015). Commonly used in South African are the anklet and wristlet restraints, which are used in conjunction with a stationery object. It is acceptable to use the specifically manufactured products, which are the right size for the patient, soft and have either a velcro or buckle type fasteners. It is dangerous and unacceptable to simply use bandages or pieces of material as mechanical restraints. It is important to make sure that the restraints are securely applied yet not so tight that they may compromise circulation (ideally two fingers width should fit between the cuff and the skin of the patient) (University of Texas Health Science Center, 2015).

### 31.5.4 Referral

Other professionals (including from the fields of neurology, pain, substance abuse, geriatrics, and neuropsychology) should be brought in to consult when additional expertise is required.

Expertise may also be provided by practitioners from a variety of disciplines (e.g. psychology, social work, occupational therapy, physical therapy, pastoral care, behavioural medicine, electroconvulsive therapy).

## 31.6 Consultation-liaison psychiatry

Consultation-liaison psychiatry is the branch of psychiatry that specialises in the interface between medicine and psychiatry, usually taking place in a hospital or medical setting (Bronheim *et al.*, 1998). In South Africa, there are few such services outside the academic and metropolitan centres; the majority of psychiatric disorders associated with physical illness are managed by general practitioners.

Consultation-liaison psychiatry usually provides a service to patients in a general medical hospital, either as in-patients, out-patients or attendees at the emergency department. Referrals are made to a psychiatrist when the treating medical team has questions about a patient's mental health or how a patient's mental health is affecting his or her care and treatment. Alternatively, in specialist units, he or she may be a member of the clinical team advising on psychological aspects of general medical care.

An important function of the consultation-liaison psychiatrist is to train other members of the clinical team (medical doctors, nursing and paramedical staff). Given the limited resources in southern Africa, all medical staff must be trained to detect and manage psychopathology in their patients and to adopt a holistic view towards every patient. Consultation-liaison psychiatrists also play a role in breaking down barriers that exist between the discipline of psychiatry and the rest of the hospital community. Because the everyday work of the consultation-liaison psychiatrist is located within medical units and clinics resolving clinical problems, and involves the sensitisation of other staff to the psychiatric aspects of medical illnesses, this can have a positive effect on public relations with all of the hospital community. Furthermore, the consultation-liaison psychiatrist often works with the hospital staff, resolving and providing psychological support for the staff's personal problems, such as problems related to burn-out syndrome (Bronheim *et al.*, 1998).

### 31.6.1 Knowledge and skills of a consultation-liaison psychiatrist

A consultation-liaison psychiatrist should be have the following knowledge and skills:

- ability to liaise with medical colleagues and other members of the health care team (e.g. nursing, psychology)
- clinical skills to conduct a comprehensive psychiatric assessment of patients on non-psychiatric wards of a general hospital and to obtain collateral history
- ability to prescribe and carry out bio-psycho-social treatments in an effective manner in liaison with medical colleagues and other health professionals in a multi-disciplinary framework
- ability to expertly deal with psychiatric emergencies on medical or surgical wards
- familiarity with medical or surgical conditions frequently encountered in a CLP practice, principles of treatment of psychiatric patients with medical illness and disorders and the psychiatric sequelae of medical conditions and medical treatments
- knowledge of the interaction between psychotropic medication and commonly used medical drugs, including psychiatric symptoms that arise from medical drugs, metabolic factors and complications following surgery
- familiarity with psychological tests as well as neuro-imaging scans imaging
- knowledge of medico-legal issues such as assessment of competency, testamentary capacity, etc. (Bronheim *et al.*, 1998).

### Typical areas in which the consultation-liaison psychiatrist may be involved

- Evaluation of a patient with suspected psychiatric disorder, a psychiatric history or history of use of psychotropic medication to properly assess the underlying psychiatric syndrome and to determine its effect on the medical or surgical condition.
- Evaluation and management of a patient who is acutely agitated to review the medical and psychiatric reasons for agitation (e.g. psychosis, intoxication, withdrawal, dementia, delirium) and to delineate possible aetiologies (e.g. toxic metabolic disturbances, cardiopulmonary disorders, endocrine disorders, neurological disorders).
- Evaluation of a patient who expresses suicidal or homicidal ideation, including one who requests hastened death, physician-assisted suicide or euthanasia.
- Evaluation of a patient in an emergency situation to prevent harm to himself or herself or others.
- Evaluation of a patient with a medico-legal problem (e.g. where there is a question of a patient's capacity to consent to or refuse medical or surgical treatment).
- Supporting the management of patients with mental disorders who have been admitted for the treatment of medical problems and who are experiencing distress related to their medical problems.
- Assisting with the diagnosis, treatment and functional assessment of people with dementia, including advice on discharge planning or the need for long-term care.
- Assisting with assessment of the capacity of a patient to consent to treatment.
- Assessment of a patient prior to certain specified medical or surgical procedures, including pre-heart transplant assessment and assessment prior to treatment related to gender reassignment.

**Source:** Bronheim *et al.*, 1998

### Problems that commonly lead to requests for psychiatric consultation in the medical or surgical setting

- Psychiatric manifestations of medical and neurological illness, including delirium and dementia.
- Psychological factors that affect a medical illness.
- Acute stress reactions and post-traumatic stress disorder.
- Depression and anxiety.
- Psychosis.
- Aggression or impulsivity.
- Agitation.
- Sleep disorders.
- Suicide.
- Sexual abuse.
- Eating disorders.
- Factitious disorders and malingering.
- Personality disorders.
- Somatoform disorders.
- Determining capacity and other forensic issues as well as ethical issues.

**Source:** Bronheim *et al.*, 1998

## 31.7 Management of psychiatric disorders that present with medical symptoms in primary care settings

In a general practice, the tendency is to give priority to the detection of physical pathology when a patient presents with a physical symptom. While this is understandable, a possible consequence of this approach is that psychiatric diagnoses are made by exclusion. It could be argued that identifying psychiatric illness is equally important, or alternatively, that the clinician should focus on the interaction of physical and psychological factors in the presentation of physical symptoms (Edwards *et al.*, 2010).

### 31.7.1 Identifying and managing psychiatric disorders that present with physical symptoms (reattribution model)

- The first step is to acknowledge the symptom, or make the patient feel understood. This involves taking a full history, identifying emotional cues, considering social and family factors and the patient's health beliefs, and performing a focused physical examination.
- The second stage is described as 'broadening the agenda', which includes informing the patient of the results of the assessment, again acknowledging the reality of the symptoms, and then reframing the symptoms by drawing in psychological and social stresses and linking these to the physical complaints.
- The third stage involves establishing links between life events and the onset of the complaint, and explaining this carefully to the patient. Part of this process may include an explanation of how emotional states can lead to physical symptoms through physiological mechanisms. Illness behaviours are often supported and reinforced by family members or partners who are also most commonly the principal caregivers, and who bear the burden of the patient's suffering (Edwards *et al.*, 2010; Goldberg *et al.*, 1989).

### 31.7.2 Basic management skills required of a primary care doctor when treating medically unexplained physical symptoms

- Avoid reassuring the patient by stating that nothing is wrong. Similarly, a challenging or confrontational approach is not helpful. The patient requires understanding as much as symptom relief.
- The shift in emphasis should be away from the symptom and towards the level of functioning. Appropriate goals, rather than the simple expectation of a cure, should be established.
- Diagnostic tests should be limited, the patient's family and colleagues in the primary treatment team should be involved and regular appointments should be made and kept to effectively manage these difficult but common presentations (Edwards *et al.*, 2010; Goldberg *et al.*, 1989).

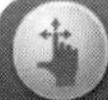

**Case study 31.1**

Mrs N is a 50-year-old woman with a long history of numerous physical complaints. Possibly as a result of her symptoms, she seems miserable and dissatisfied with her lot in life. She lives alone and has little support, and the nurses have formed the impression that a motivation for her attending the clinic is to obtain care and attention. She was abandoned by her mother at birth, and spent her childhood years in an orphanage. She has never seemed capable of meeting the challenges of life, and attributes this to her many ailments.

Consider the interplay between the patient's depression and the somatic symptoms that she presents with.

**Case study 31.2**

Mrs B, a 45-year-old recently divorced woman, presents with abdominal pain. After a brief history and examination, the practitioner declares that there is nothing wrong. This does not reassure Mrs B for long, and the pain recurs. She returns to the general practitioner a week later, increasingly anxious and somewhat depressed. He refers her to a gastroenterologist, who performs a number of investigations, all of which are negative. She is then referred to a gynaecologist who, noting her distress, asks whether there are significant stresses in her life. Mrs B responds angrily, 'Are you saying that the pain is all in my mind?' The exasperated gynaecologist refers Mrs B for a surgical opinion. An exploratory laparotomy is negative, but sepsis and adhesions develop, and these require further surgery. The abdominal pain is now worse, Mrs B is depressed and disabled, and in addition requires large amounts of opiate analgesics.

Consider the interplay between the patient's somatic symptoms and the possibility of underlying depression.

## Conclusion

It is evident that the interplay between psychiatry and medicine is significant. To adequately manage a patient who presents with somatic symptoms, the treating physician must consider the psychiatric component when planning the treatment of the patient. Similarly, a patient with a medical illness that has a high prevalence of co-morbid psychiatric illness may easily be overlooked, which will have an impact on the response of the medical illness to treatment.

# References


Al-Sayyad HH, Saddick EA, Al-Omer DK (2010) Prevalence rate of somatization and psychological disorder among patients consulting outpatient clinic in Nasiriyah general hospital. *Thi-Qar Medical Journal* 4(2): 1–13

American Psychiatric Association (2013) *Diagnostic and Statistical Manual of Mental Disorders* (5th edition). Washington, DC: American Psychiatric Association

Black PH, Garbutt LD (2002) Stress, inflammation and cardiovascular disease. *Journal of Psychosomatic Research* 52(1): 1–23

Bronheim HE, Fulop G, Kunkel E, Muskin PR, Schindler BA, Yates WR, Shaw R, Steiner H, Stern TA, Stoudemire A (1998). The Academy of Psychosomatic Medicine practice guidelines for psychiatric consultation in the general medical setting. *Psychosomatics* 39: S8-S30. Quotations on pages 584 and 585 reprinted with permission from Elsevier.

Centers for Disease Control and Prevention (2010) *Chronic diseases and health promotion*. Available at: www.cdc.gov/chronicdisease/overview/ (Accessed 9 August 2013.)

Duman RS, Malberg J, Nakagawa S, and D'Sa C (2000) Neuronal plasticity and survival in mood disorders. *Biological Psychiatry* 48(8): 732–9

Eastwood MR (1975) Epidemiological studies in psychosomatic medicine. *The International Journal of Psychiatry in Medicine* 6(1–2): 123–32

Edwards TM, Stern A, Clarke DD, Ivbijaro G, Kasney LM (2010) The treatment of patients with medically unexplained symptoms in primary care: A review of the literature. *Mental Health in Family Medicine* 7(4): 209–221

Gitlin DF, Levenson JL, Lyketsos CG (2004) Psychosomatic medicine: A new psychiatric subspecialty. *Academic Psychiatry* 28(1): 4–11

Glassman AH, Shapiro PA (1998) Depression and the course of coronary artery disease. *American Journal of Psychiatry* 155(1): 4–11

Goldberg D, Gask L, O'Dowd T (1989) The treatment of somatization: Teaching techniques of reattribution. *Journal of Psychosomatic Research* 33(6): 689–95

Katon W, Von Korff M, Lin E, Walker E, Simon GE, Bush T, Robinson P, Russo J (1995) Collaborative management to achieve treatment guidelines. Impact on depression in primary care. *Journal of the American Medical Association* 273: 1026–31

Kiecolt-Glaser JK, McGuire L, Robles TF, Glaser R (2002) Psychoneuroimmunology and psychosomatic medicine: Back to the future. *Psychosomatic Medicine* 64(1): 15–28

Kornfeld DS (2002) Consultation-liaison psychiatry: Contributions to medical practice. *American Journal of Psychiatry* 159(12): 1964–72

Krantz DS, Kop WJ, Santiago HT, Gottdiener JS (1996) Mental stress as a trigger of myocardial ischemia and infarction. *Cardiology Clinics* 14: 271–87

Kroenke K (2003) The interface between physical and psychological symptoms. Primary care companion. *Journal of Clinical Psychiatry* 5(7): 11–18

Lesperance F, Frasure-Smith N, Talajic M (1996) Major depression before and after myocardial infarction: Its nature and consequences. *Psychosomatic Medicine* 58: 99–110

Levitan SJ, Kornfeld D (1981) Clinical and cost benefits of liaison psychiatry. *American Journal of Psychiatry* 138: 790–3

Lipowski ZJ, Wise T N (2002) History of consultation-liaison psychiatry. In: Wise MG, Rundell JR (Eds). *Textbook of Consultation-Liaison Psychiatry: The Practice of Psychiatry in the Medically Ill*. Washington: American Psychiatric Publishing

Mesulam MM (2000) Neuropsychological assessment of mental state. In: Mesulam MM (Ed). *Principles of Behavioral and Cognitive Neurology* (2nd edition). New York: Oxford University Press

Muench J, Hamer AM (2010) Adverse effects of antipsychotic medications. *American Family Physician* 81(5): 109

Phelan JC, Link BG, Diez-Roux A, Kawachi I, Levin B (2004) 'Fundamental causes' of social inequalities in mortality: A test of the theory. *Journal of Health and Social Behavior* 45(3): 265–85

Rothenhäusler HB (2006) Mental disorders in general hospital patients. *Psychiatria Danubina 18*(3–4): 183–92

Schatzberg AF, Posener JA, DeBattista C, Kalehzan BM, Rothschild AJ, Shear PK (2000) Neuropsychological deficits in psychotic versus nonpsychotic major depression and no mental illness. The *American Journal of Psychiatry* 157(7): 1095–100

Schulberg HC, Magruder KM, deGruy F (1996) Major depression in primary medical care practice. Research trends and future priorities. *General Hospital Psychiatry* 18: 395–406

Trijsburg DW, Van Knippenberg FCE, Pijpma SE (1992) Effects of psychological treatment on cancer patients: A critical review. *Psychosomatic Medicine* 54: 489–517

Tucker P, Adamson P, Miranda R (Jr), Scarborough A, Williams D, Groff J, McLean H (1997) Paroxetine increases heart rate variability in panic disorder. *Journal of Clinical Psychopharmacology* 17(5): 370–6

University of Texas Health Science Center (2015) Patient Care Procedures, Seclusion / Restraint process: July 2015 version

Ursin H (1994) Stress, distress, and immunity. *Annals of the New York Academy of Sciences* 741: 204–211

Valderas JM, Starfield B, Sibbald B, Salisbury C, Roland M (2009) Defining comorbidity: Implications for understanding health and health services. *Annals of Family Medicine* 7(4)

Yehuda R, Boisoneau D, Lowy MT, Giller EL (Jr). (1995) Dose-response changes in plasma cortisol and lymphocyte glucocorticoid receptors following dexamethasone administration in combat veterans with and without posttraumatic stress disorder. *Archives of General Psychiatry* 52(7): 583–93

CHAPTER

# 32 Neuropsychiatry

Suvira Ramlall, Howard King

## 32.1 Introduction

While it may be argued that brain dysfunction forms the basis of all psychiatric disorders, the anatomic, genetic and chemical aetiology of psychiatric disorders is defined by the term 'biological psychiatry'. Neuropsychiatry concerns itself with understanding the neurological basis of psychiatric disorders, as well as with the diagnosis and management of the psychiatric (behavioural, emotional and cognitive) manifestations of neurological disorders. The association between several specific neurological disorders and particular constellations of psychiatric and behavioural disturbances justifies a separate category of neuropsychiatric disorders. The International Neuropsychiatric Association (2005) offers the following definition: 'Neuropsychiatry is a field of scientific medicine that concerns itself with the complex relationship between human behavior and brain function, and endeavours to understand abnormal behavior and behavioural disorders on the basis of an interaction of neurobiological and psychological–social factors. It is rooted in clinical neuroscience and provides a bridge between the disciplines of Psychiatry, Neurology and Neuropsychology' (Sachdev, 2005). The clinician who deals with neuropsychiatric disorders is therefore tasked with understanding and treating the patient with a neuropsychiatric disorder comprehensively, integrating the bio-psycho-social dimensions of aetiology, clinical manifestations and management in order to treat the patient optimally and holistically. This distinguishes the neurologist (who focuses on the motor-sensory manifestations of brain dysfunction) from the general psychiatrist (who focuses on the cognitive, behavioural and emotional manifestations of brain dysfunction).

## 32.2 Clinical assessment and diagnostic classification

### 32.2.1 Clinical assessment

The basis of accurate diagnosis and management of neuropsychiatric disorders lies in the comprehensive clinical assessment and appropriate investigation of the patient. Clinical assessment begins with a thorough, detailed and focused diagnostic interview with the patient followed by corroboration by a collateral source of information. It includes the examination of the patient, which has four components: the general physical examination, a detailed and systematic neurological examination, mental state examination (MSE) and the bedside evaluation of higher cognitive functions. (See Chapter 7: Clinical assessment in psychiatry, for a discussion of the MSE.) A neuropsychiatric mental state examination necessitates knowledge of, and skill in, the identification of the specific psychiatric manifestations of neurological diseases. While hallucinations are a common psychiatric symptom, for example, visual hallucinations in a patient who has spontaneous Parkinson's-like motor symptoms and fluctuations in attention and concentration would suggest Lewy body disease.

Neuropsychiatric assessment includes multiple domains as listed in Table 32.1.

Bedside cognitive testing requires a clear understanding of normal higher-brain functions and their neuro-anatomical basis. It may be conducted systematically based on functional domains (e.g. language, memory) or according to neuro-anatomical regions (e.g. frontal lobe, temporal lobe).

Appropriate investigations are necessary to confirm the clinical findings and include relevant haematological and biochemical tests, a lumbar puncture, electrophysiological and neuro-imaging tests.

**Table 32.1** Neuropsychiatric assessment – items of specific importance in the neuropsychiatric patient (including bedside neurocognitive evaluation)

| General component of assessment | Specific component of assessment | Specific symptoms, signs and tests |
|---|---|---|
| History | Past medical and surgical history | seizures or spells<br>significant head trauma |
| | Medication | drugs with neuropsychiatric adverse effects (e.g. extrapyramidal side effects)<br>drug-drug interactions |
| | Substances | short- and long-term neuropsychiatric effects of substance use |
| | Family history | family history of neurological disorders with familial basis (e.g. Huntington's disease) |
| | Systematic review of symptoms | behavioural problems (motivation, apathy, impulsivity, violence, aggression, etc.)<br>affective problems (emotional incontinence, **catastrophic reactions**, abulia)<br>cognitive problems (with attention, language, memory, praxis, recognition, complex cognition)<br>physical problems (headache, pain, visual disturbances, difficulty swallowing, tinnitus, ataxia, gait disturbance, weakness, paraesthesia, urogenital dysfunction, etc.) |
| Physical examination | General physical | dysmorphic features<br>soft neurological signs (e.g. Waldrop's Scale)<br>signs of self-harming behaviour<br>dermatological and ocular signs of specific neurological disorders |
| | Neurological | level of consciousness or **sensorium**<br>cranial nerves<br>motor (muscle bulk, power, tone)<br>sensory (light touch, vibration, proprioception, pain, temperature)<br>coordination (finger-to-nose, fine finger movements, rapid alternating movements, heel-to-shin)<br>gait (base/station, toe walking, heel walking, tandem gait, turning, assess for **Romberg's** sign)<br>reflexes (upper and lower limbs)<br>primitive reflexes (glabellar, snout, palmo-mental, grasp, rooting, suck, Hoffman's) |

| General component of assessment | Specific component of assessment | Specific symptoms, signs and tests |
|---|---|---|
| Mental state examination | General MSE | see Chapter 7: Clinical assessment in psychiatry |
| | Cognitive assessment | level of arousal<br>attention (serial sevens, months of year backwards, registration of three items, digit span forwards and reverse, trail-making A and B)<br>language (fluency, comprehension, naming, repetition, writing, reading)<br>memory (recent: spontaneous recall of three items; remote)<br>orientation (time, place, person, context)<br>praxis (limb-kinetic, ideomotor, ideational)<br>recognition (stereognosis, graphaesthesia)<br>visuo-spatial skills (figure copy, clock-drawing test, intersecting pentagons, folstein's mmse) |
| | Higher cognitive assessment (executive function) | word fluency (three letters: F, A, S)<br>trail-making B<br>reverse digit span<br>alternating sequences (Luria's 'fist-edge-palm' sequence)<br>conflicting instructions ('tap twice when I tap once')<br>go/no go ('tap once when I tap once; do not tap when I tap twice')<br>prehension behaviour ('do not take my hands')<br>abstraction (similarities, proverbs)<br>fund of information (general knowledge, semantic memory)<br>problem-solving (mathematical, real-life situations) |
| Investigations | Laboratory, imaging, neurophysiological, neuropsychological | see Chapter 9: Investigating psychiatric disorders |

**Sources:** Folstein *et al.*, 1975; Luria, 1976; Luria, 1980; Roth *et al.*, 1986; Huppert *et al.*, 1995

Note: A comprehensive assessment of the neuropsychiatric patient includes all aspects of the general psychiatric assessment (see Chapter 7: Clinical assessment in psychiatry).

Table 32.2 lists the common clinical features of lobar diseases.

## 32.2.2 Diagnostic classification

In recognition that psychiatric disorders themselves are medical conditions, the fifth edition of the *Diagnostic and Statistical Manual of Mental Disorders* (DSM-5), now requires that where there are other associated medical conditions, both the psychiatric and the medical condition be recognised diagnostically. In the case of neuropsychiatric disorders, this entails the listing of the primary condition (e.g. Parkinson's disease) with the psychiatric disorder (e.g. major depressive disorder); thus a diagnosis of major depressive disorder due to Parkinson's disease. In the ICD code the general medical disorder 'X' will be named first, followed by the psychiatry disorder-specific ICD code for 'X Disorder due to Another Medical Condition.'

# 32.3 General management principles

Neuropsychiatry is distinguished by its rejection of the 'mind-body' dualism and its adoption

**Table 32.2** Neuropsychiatric manifestations of cerebral lobar lesions

| Cortical lobe | Syndrome | Clinical features |
|---|---|---|
| Frontal lobe | Orbitofrontal syndrome | anosmia |
| | | primitive reflexes |
| | | disinhibited or pseudopsychopathic (impulsive and agitated behaviour, tactless, overfamiliar, inappropriate jocular affect, fatuous, euphoria, emotional lability or incontinence, poor judgement and insight, distractibility, inattention, perseveration, memory impairments) |
| | Dorsolateral (convexity) syndrome | contralateral hemiparesis |
| | | Broca's aphasia (dominant) |
| | | conjugate eye dysfunction |
| | | frontal lobe seizures |
| | | executive function deficits |
| | | motor perseveration and **impersistence**, **echopraxia**, stereotypy |
| | | stimulus-bound (utilisation) behaviour |
| | | apathy, indifference, abulia |
| | Medial frontal syndrome (apathetic-akinetic syndrome) | incontinence |
| | | movement (aspontaneous, akinetic, catatonic) |
| | | verbal (poverty, alogia, mutism) |
| | | cognitive (impersistence, avolition) |
| | | docile, apathetic, flat affect, abulia, pseudodementia |
| Temporal lobe | | temporal lobe epilepsy/ complex partial seizures |
| | | hallucinations (auditory, gustatory, olfactory) |
| | | Wernicke's aphasia (dominant) |
| | | **aprosody**, **dysprosody** |
| | | contralateral upper quadrantonopia |
| | | cortical deafness |
| | | emotional, personality, behavioural changes |
| | | memory impairment |
| | | Kluver-Bucy syndrome |
| Parietal lobe | | simple and complex partial seizures |
| | Dominant | **astereognosia** |
| | | **agraphaesthesia** |
| | | 2-point discrimination |
| | | lower quadrantonopia |
| | | Wernicke's aphasia |
| | | movement and colour agnosia |
| | | **prosopagnosia** |
| | | apraxia |
| | | **alexia** |
| | | Gerstmann's syndrome (**acalculia**, **agraphia**, finger agnosia, left-right disorientation) |

| Cortical lobe | Syndrome | Clinical features |
|---|---|---|
| | Non-dominant | astereognosia<br>agraphaesthesia<br>2-point discrimination<br>lower quadrantonopia<br>movement and geographic agnosia<br>prosopagnosia<br>hemineglect<br>apraxia (dress, construction)<br>**anosagnosia** |
| Occipital lobe | | simple and complex partial seizures<br>contralateral scotomata<br>cortical blindness<br>elementary visual hallucinations<br>Balint's syndrome (visual disorientation, ocular apraxia, optic ataxia) |

of an integrative approach. In order to address the complexity of neuropsychiatric disorders, proficiency in general medicine, neuroscience and psychiatry are essential and requires that the patient be treated by a multidisciplinary team that delivers competent, consistent, collaborative and individualised care (Sachdev and Mohan, 2013). Psychiatric symptoms impact on functional abilities, interpersonal relationships, quality of life and the ability to adhere to treatment. Because physical and psychiatric symptoms mutually impact upon recovery, simultaneous attention to both is necessary to ensure the effectiveness of either.

The following general principles apply:

- A holistic and individualised care plan is formulated that addresses the medical, psychological, social, physical and medico-legal needs of patient and caregiver for both the acute and rehabilitative phase of the illness; this plan is systematically addressed and reviewed over time.
- Comprehensive assessment and optimum treatment of the neurological disorder.
- Accurate diagnostic determination of the nature and cause of the associated psychiatric symptoms or syndromes.
- Careful evaluation of the pharmacological options available for both the neurological and psychiatric conditions to ensure that, in particular, neurological and psychiatric side effects are avoided and drug-drug interactions minimised.
- A team approach is adopted and case conferencing includes relevant health care professionals as needed, including a psychiatrist, neurologist, social worker, occupational therapist, speech therapist and physiotherapist. Where the required resources or service providers are not available within an institution, links with outside agencies (e.g. support groups for patients or caregivers) that specialise in, or cater for, the special needs of specific clinical groups must be identified as partners.
- The forensic implications of the neuropsychiatric disorder (e.g. dangerousness, safety to drive, testamentary capacity) are anticipated, assessed and appropriately managed.

The treatment of patients with neuropsychiatric complications requires the expertise of a physician, a neurologist and a psychiatrist as well as relevant paramedical practitioners depending on the specific physical and sensory deficits arising. Psychiatric symptoms are treated as for the underlying psychiatric disorder (e.g. an antidepressant for depression) with special regard for the side effect and drug-drug interaction profile in relation to the medical status and concomitant drug therapies that the patient is receiving. While certain neuropsychiatric symptoms (e.g. apathy) may appear relatively innocuous, the implications of such untreated symptoms on rehabilitation efforts and caregiver burden must be considered. Occupational and physical therapy are equally important for the management of the physical and mental components of stroke sequelae and are necessary for the optimal symptomatic and functional recovery and rehabilitation of the patient and to minimise dependence and assisted-living needs.

## 32.4 Neuropsychiatric aspects of cerebrovascular disorders

Cerebrovascular diseases are the commonest neurological disorder in adults and may arise from hypertensive atherosclerosis, intracranial or systemic inflammatory, infective or traumatic causes such as syphilitic arteritis, systemic lupus erythematosis (SLE), polycythaemia, aneurysms and trauma to the carotid artery. Associated risk factors are age, hypertension, ischaemic and valvular heart disease, atrial fibrillation, smoking and diabetes mellitus (Kaplan and Sadock, 1995).

From the perspective of neuropsychiatric manifestations, parenchymal changes in the brain occur as a result of ischaemia, with or without infarction, and include transient ischaemic attacks (TIAs), atherosclerotic thrombosis, cerebral embolism and haemorrhage. Haemorrhage may cause direct parenchymal damage by extravasation into surrounding tissue or indirect damage by bleeding occurring into the ventricles, subarachnoid space, extradural area or subdural space. The common clinical result of all these mechanisms of parenchymal change is a sudden, focal neurological deficit, called a stroke or cerebrovascular accident (CVA), the commonest manifestation of cerebrovascular disease (Yudofsky and Hales, 2008). The ratio of infarcts to haemorrhages is approximately 5:1, with atherosclerotic thrombosis and cerebral embolism accounting for almost a third of all incidents of stroke (Kaplan and Sadock, 1995).

The categories of cerebrovascular disease, based on Yudofsky and Hales (2008), are:

- atherosclerotic thrombosis: atheromatous plaques lead to stenosis or complete occlusion of cerebral arteries by a thrombus. The presence of a thrombotic process is almost always indicated by the occurrence of TIAs (or ministrokes). TIAs are transient focal ischaemic events that are associated with reversible neurological deficits. They commonly last for 2–15 minutes but can range from a few seconds to 24 hours. Neurological examination between episodes may be normal but thrombosis leads to infarction and permanent neurological deficits. TIAs may precede, accompany or follow a stroke or occur on their own.
- cerebral embolism: cerebral embolisms account for a third of all strokes; they are caused by a fragment of an atheromatous plaque breaking away from a thrombus (which may be located in the carotid artery or the heart). Strokes due to cerebral embolism develop most rapidly, generally without warning. Infarction occurs distal to the embolic site with the pattern of neurological deficit corresponding to the area of blood supply of the occluded vessel. A TIA may result if the embolus fragments and travels into smaller distant vessels.
- lacunae: lacunar infarcts, accounting for a fifth of strokes, result from the occlusion of small, penetrating cerebral arteries. They may result in no recognisable deficits or be associated with motor or sensory deficits related to the site of occlusion. Lacunae are strongly associated with atherosclerosis and hypertension.
- intracerebral haemorrhage (ICH): the fourth most frequent cause of stroke, ICH is the result of hypertension, rupture of saccular aneurysms or arteriovenous malformations, haemorrhagic disorders and trauma. ICH can vary from tiny petechial haemorrhages of less than a millimetre in diameter to massive bleeds several centimetres in diameter. It carries a poor prognosis with a high mortality.

- aneurysms and arteriovenous malformations (AVM): ruptured aneurysms and AVMs are the next most frequent type of cerebrovascular disease. Although most AVMs are silent, haemorrhage from aneurysms and AVMs may occur into the subarachnoid space or within brain parenchyma resulting in hemiplegia or death.
- subdural and epidural haematomas: haematomas behave as space-occupying lesions and may produce signs and symptoms of a stroke. Chronic subdural haematomas (SDH) most frequently result from trauma and lead to a gradual progression of signs and symptoms over days to weeks. Headache is the most frequent symptom, accompanied by neuropsychiatric manifestations that correspond to the gradually increasing intracranial pressure: confusion, inattention, apathy, memory loss, drowsiness and coma. The level of consciousness fluctuates and patients may present with hemiparesis, hemianopia, cranial nerve deficits, aphasia or seizures. Patients may present with the clinical picture of dementia; the dementia symptoms are potentially reversible. Ultimately, chronic SDHs may continue to expand, leading to death or may reabsorb spontaneously (Yudofsky and Hales, 2008).

Although stroke-related mortality is decreasing, it has led to an increasing prevalence of stroke survivors with mental and physical sequelae. The neuropsychiatric sequelae of cerebrovascular disease include a wide range of emotional and cognitive disturbances (Yudofsky and Hales, 2008). The clinical manifestations of a stroke vary according to the type of stroke, the type of vessel affected, the specific location of the insult in the brain, patient health and patient risk factors (Kaplan and Sadock, 1995; Schoenberg and Scott, 2011). The course of the psychiatric sequelae is determined by the severity of the stroke. Symptoms generally improve gradually as the acute effects of the stroke resolve (David *et al.*, 2009).

## 32.4.1 Clinical features

The clinical manifestations of a stroke are neurological as well as psychiatric. Psychiatric disturbances may arise directly from brain damage or may represent psychological reactions to the cerebral insult and the resultant physical handicaps. The premorbid personality and psychiatric risk profile require careful assessment in the determination of the precise aetiology of any emergent psychiatric symptomatology (David *et al.*, 2009). Regardless of the cause, psychiatric sequelae are important factors that influence the individual's clinical course, prognosis, response to treatment and rehabilitation.

The common neurological deficits that may arise following cerebrovascular disease are determined by the location of the lesion in the brain. The neuropsychiatric manifestations are also localisable to specific brain regions (though less accurately compared with the neurological deficits). Certain neuropsychiatric and neurobehavioural changes are more commonly associated with certain anatomical regions. Psychiatric assessment of post-stroke patients may be hindered by the neurological deficits (e.g. aphasic patient unable to verbalise feelings, facial paralysis affecting the expression of affect) (Kaplan and Sadock, 1995).

The common neuropsychiatric sequelae associated with cerebrovascular disease are major depression or post-stroke depression (PSD) (20%), minor depression (19%), mania, bipolar disorder and anxiety disorder (27%), psychotic disorder, apathy (with or without depression) (11%), pathological emotionalism (20%), catastrophic reaction (19%) and motor or sensory aprosodies (32%) (Yudofsky and Hales, 2008).

### 32.4.1.1 Epilepsy

In the first week after an ischaemic stroke, epileptic seizures occur in 3–6% of patients, with a fourfold greater risk in patients with intracerebral haemorrhage. Although 2–4% of patients will develop epilepsy in the long term, a stroke is the commonest cause of late-onset epilepsy. Post-stroke epilepsy carries a poorer prognosis and greater risk of psychosis, with early seizures posing a possible risk factor for cognitive impairment (David *et al.*, 2009).

### 32.4.1.2 Post-stroke depression

The commonest neuropsychiatric sequelae of cerebrovascular disease is depression, affecting up to 30% of stroke patients (Kaplan and Sadock, 1995). Prevalence is highest in the first weeks after the stroke and declines over the next 6–24 months (House, 1987). An increasing number of studies show that post-stroke depression (PSDs) is due to neurophysiological processes and not just to psychological reactions to brain injury (Robinson, 1987). Left hemisphere strokes are associated with significantly more depression than right hemisphere strokes.

Depression is recognised as a risk factor for cardiovascular disease (psychocardiology) (Koch, 2014) and for strokes. Depression is also associated with increased stroke mortality, poorer functional outcomes, worse patient and caregiver outcomes and increased health care use (Williams, 2005). The vascular depression hypothesis has been advanced to explain the co-morbidity of depression, vascular disease and vascular risk factors and the association of ischaemic lesions with distinctive behavioural symptoms (Alexopoulos *et al.*, 1997). The diagnostic criteria for major depression are frequently met, even when the neuro-vegetative symptoms may be attributable to the stroke and physical disabilities may limit proper assessment due to restricted language functions (Kaplan and Sadock, 1995). PSD delays recovery in activities of daily living and cognitive functions. Antidepressants have a beneficial effect on both depressive and cognitive symptoms; initiation within two months post the event is superior to later treatment in addressing recovery of activities of daily living (Yudofsky and Hales, 2008).

### 32.4.1.3 Post-stroke mania and bipolar disorder

Patients who develop mania after a stroke manifest similar symptoms to patients with primary mania. Risk factors include right hemispheric limbic area involvement and a family history of mood disorders. Some patients may develop depression in addition to the manic episode/s and meet criteria for a bipolar disorder. Bipolar disorder is associated with subcortical lesions, while manic episodes are associated with cortical lesions. Mania responds to mood stabilisers and neuroleptics (Yudofsky and Hales, 2008).

### 32.4.1.4 Post-stroke anxiety disorder

While anxiety is a frequent accompaniment of depression, anxiety symptoms may also commonly arise separately following a stroke. Generalised anxiety disorder is found in 25% of stroke patients. Anxiety is often associated with cortical lesions and, except when accompanied by depression, is more commonly found with right hemispheric lesions. The presence of generalised anxiety disorder (GAD) has also been associated with cortical and subcortical atrophy three years post-stroke. Post-stroke GAD is associated with greater social impairment in functioning than PSD (Kaplan and Sadock, 1995). The presence of anxiety delays resumption of activities of daily living and social functioning. Antidepressants with anxiolytic properties have been shown to be effective in the treatment of post-stroke anxiety (Yudofsky and Hales, 2008, David *et al.*, 2009, Moore, 2008).

### 32.4.1.5 Post-stroke psychosis

Psychotic symptoms may occur in the context of post-stroke delirium, but psychosis is rare in stroke patients. Secondary psychoses are associated with right hemisphere lesions in the temporoparietal region, subcortical atrophy or a seizure disorder (Yudofsky and Hales, 2008).

Depression with psychotic features may develop as a result of a stroke; manic psychoses may similarly result, more commonly from right hemispheric lesions. Delusional syndromes are frequently paranoid in nature and often arise from temporal lobe lesions. Specific time-limited delusional syndromes may arise less commonly (e.g. Capgras syndrome, where there is the belief that somebody familiar has been replaced by an impostor, or erotomanic delusions that one is secretly loved by a famous person) (Cummings and Trimble, 2002). Visual or auditory hallucinations in the presence of insight (hallucinosis) may complicate midbrain or pontine lesions (Yudofsky and Hales, 2008).

The use of antipsychotics in the elderly may be associated with an increased risk of stroke. Psychosis that occurs in the first few days after a stroke may resolve spontaneously. Should antipsychotics be required, they should be used after consultation with the family and, where possible, the patient (David *et al.*, 2009).

### 32.4.1.6 Apathy

Apathy is a decrease in motivation, which is expressed as reduced motor, cognitive and emotional activity as well as interest. Apathy is more prevalent in older patients and negatively impacts on the performance of activities of daily living. It may be associated with a diagnosis of depression or manifest in the absence of depression (Yudofsky and Hales, 2008).

### 32.4.1.7 Catastrophic reaction

Catastrophic reactions refer to the manifestation of anxiety, tears, aggressive behaviour, swearing, displacement and refusal in response to an inability to cope with physical or cognitive deficits. It has been found to be more frequent in stroke patients with a family or personal history of psychiatric disorder, usually depression, and is not significantly associated with aphasia (Yudofsky and Hales, 2008).

### 32.4.1.8 Pathological emotions

A not uncommon, but disabling and distressing complication of stroke is the development of pathological emotionalism or emotional lability or **emotional incontinence** (David *et al.*, 2009). This condition is also referred to as involuntary emotional expression disorder (Yudofsky and Hales, 2008). It may be attributed to pseudobulbar palsy as a result of bilateral lesions to the corticobulbar tracts. Pathological emotionalism is characterised by a heightened tendency to cry uncontrollably and unexpectedly, often with minimal or no triggers. The symptoms usually improve over months but more severe or persisting cases may require antidepressant treatment (David *et al.*, 2009). Serotonin specific reuptake inhibitors (SSRIs) have been shown to be effective in reducing the frequency of crying episodes (Yudofsky and Hales, 2008).

### 32.4.1.9 Aprosody

Aprosody refers to the abnormality in the affective components of language. In motor aprosody, difficulty in the spontaneous use of emotional inflection is evident in speech, whereas sensory aprosody is characterised by impairment in the comprehension of emotional inflection. It has been associated with right hemisphere lesions and subcortical atrophy (Yudofsky and Hales, 2008).

### 32.4.1.10 Cognitive impairment

Deficits in cognitive impairment are a serious complication of a stroke and compromise rehabilitation efforts. After a stroke, there is an initial clouding of consciousness, which varies in severity and duration depending on the extent of the cerebral damage and the presence of co-existing medical complications, such as respiratory insufficiency or cardiac failure. The longer the clouding lasts, the greater the likelihood of residual cognitive deficits persisting. Global cognitive impairment or major neurocognitive impairment (dementia) may follow a single extensive cerebral insult, while focal neuro-anatomical lesions may manifest with aphasias, apraxias, agnosias and amnestic syndromes. More commonly, multiple strokes over time result in a stepwise deterioration in cognition, referred to as multi-infarct dementia. The additional presence of significant functional impairment resulting from the cognitive deficits will determine the presence of 'major' versus 'minor' neurocognitive deficit according to the DSM-5. Assessment of intellectual functions is difficult in the presence of dysphasia, constructional difficulties, visual disturbances, agnosias, apathy, agitation and depression. These, in turn, also compromise rehabilitation efforts (David *et al.*, 2009; Yudofsky and Hales, 2008; Schoenberg and Scott, 2011). (See Chapter 30: Psychogeriatrics, for a discussion of vascular dementia and multi-infarct dementia.)

Post-stroke dementia refers to global cognitive impairment that follows a stroke; the risk of new-onset dementia doubles after a stroke, with left hemisphere lesions carrying a greater risk. Dementia usually follows in those who have had silent infarcts, global atrophy or diffuse white matter disease (leucoaraiosis). Although rare, dementia may follow a single, strategically located stroke (David *et al.*, 2009; Yudofsky and Hales, 2008).

#### 32.4.1.11 Transient global amnesia

Transient global amnesia refers to episodic disturbances in late middle age or old age. It is characterised by the sudden onset of anterograde memory loss in an alert and responsive individual. It is more common in males. Patchy retrograde amnesia may also extend to days, weeks or even years before the incident. The pathogenesis is not clear and symptoms last for several hours before gradually returning to normal (David *et al.*, 2009).

#### 32.4.1.12 Personality change

Changes in personality are often the most troublesome of sequelae and commonly precede the development of a progressive dementing illness. Changes range from inflexibility to apathetic dullness, paranoid traits and varying degrees of verbal and physical aggression. Irrational reactions to the dependency induced by the stroke include either excessive dependency or unrealistic assertions of independence. Sexual dysfunctions, usually due to physical limitations, may also be due to central factors that inhibit desire and arousal (David *et al.*, 2009).

## 32.5 Neuropsychiatric aspects of tumours, hydrocephalus and benign intracranial hypertension

### 32.5.1 Tumours

Intracranial masses include tumours that arise from the brain parenchyma, blood vessels, cranial nerves, pituitary, meninges and the skull. Also included are metastases from extracranial tumours, parasitic cysts, granulomas, haematomas and lymphomas (Kaplan and Sadock, 1995).

Patients with brain tumours present with headache, papilloedema, seizures, focal neurological deficits or non-specific cognitive or personality changes. The clinical presentation depends on the location, histology and rate of growth of the tumour. Neuropsychiatric symptoms are common in patients with brain tumours, with reported prevalence rates varying from 10-100% (David *et al.*, 2009). Psychiatric symptoms (as opposed to neurological symptoms) may be the presenting feature in 18-21% of patients (Oosthuizen, 2005). However, mental symptoms vary even when arising from common locations and therefore have little localising value; neurological signs and neuro-imaging are more reliable in locating the site of a tumour.

Patients with psychiatric disorders have a higher prevalence of malignancy and brain tumours than the general population, even though in up to half of psychiatric patients with brain tumours this is only discovered at post mortem (Oosthuizen, 2005). Conversely, brain tumours may exacerbate the clinical effect of pre-existing psychiatric disorders (Yudofsky and Hales, 2008).

Neuropsychiatric symptoms may arise from primary brain tumours, metastases, remote pressure effects, circulatory disturbances, the effects of increased intracranial pressure or from paraneoplastic syndromes. Most metastatic tumours arise from the lungs (50%). Primary brain tumours are twice as common in children, while metastases twice as common in adults. A paraneoplastic syndrome develops as a result of an auto-immune reaction to tumours and may precede the diagnosis of malignancy. Neuropsychiatric paraneoplastic presentations include those of a dementia and limbic encephalitis in which neuropathological changes in the limbic areas give rise to an encephalitic picture characterised by a chronic confusional state, profound amnesia, hallucinations, anxiety and depression (Kaplan and Sadock, 1995; David *et al.*, 2009; Moore, 2008).

However, certain symptoms and signs may alert the clinician to the possibility of a tumour underlying a psychiatric presentation (Yudofsky and Hales, 2008):

- the presence of concomitant focal neurological signs
- the new onset of seizures, especially in adults; in 50% of cases this may be the initial manifestation of a tumour
- the emergence of new-onset headaches, especially those that are generalised and dull, of increasing severity and/or frequency, positional, nocturnal or present immediately upon awakening
- the presence of nausea and vomiting, especially when accompanied by headaches, should alert one to the possibility of raised intracranial pressure
- sensory changes, either visual (diplopia, reduction in visual acuity) or auditory (tinnitus, hearing loss especially if unilateral and vertigo)
- other focal neurological signs such as focal weakness or sensory loss and ataxia
- personality changes or a first episode of psychosis after the age of 45 warrant appropriate investigation to exclude a primary medical basis for the psychiatric presentation (Yudofsky and Hales, 2008; Oosthuizen, 2005).

Presenting neuropsychiatric symptoms may be indistinguishable from those of a 'true' psychiatric illness, with any tumour type, at any location in the brain, presenting with any psychiatric symptom. A very general pattern is that slow-growing tumours produce changes of personality and allow premorbid traits to manifest, while fast-growing tumours cause cognitive deficits. Very rapid tumour growth can precipitate acute organic reactions and impaired consciousness (David *et al.*, 2009). However, the following factors may affect the clinical presentation (Oosthuizen, 2005):

- rate of growth: rapidly growing tumours are more likely to cause psychiatric symptoms, psychosis and agitation. Conversely, slow-growing tumours (such as meningiomas )may allow for more adaptive changes in the brain allowing the tumour to be 'neurologically silent' with the only signs being psychiatric in nature such as personality changes, apathy, depression and cognitive changes.
- location: in general, right hemisphere tumours are more likely to cause affective symptoms and left hemisphere tumours are more likely to be associated with psychotic symptoms. Supratentorial tumours and those located in the frontal and temporal lobes are more frequently associated with psychiatric symptomatology. Left-sided frontal tumours are associated with higher rates of depression and right-sided frontal tumours with manic-like presentations.
- pressure effects: the association of raised intracranial pressure with the tumour is likely to cause more psychiatric presentations through several possible mechanisms.
- premorbid factors: as with other insults to the brain, individuals with higher premorbid IQ levels and better psychological resilience are less vulnerable to the neuropsychiatric sequelae of tumours. The psychological adaptation to the diagnosis is also superior

in those with good premorbid psychosocial functioning.
- tumour type: the rate of growth, location and number of tumours in the brain will impact on the psychiatric sequelae (Oosthuizen, 2005).

### 32.5.1.1 Clinical features

The clinical features associated with intracranial tumours arise due to alterations in neural function after parenchymal invasion, mass effect on local and distant structures, oedema, raised intracranial pressure (RICP), hydrocephalus or stroke (Kaplan and Sadock, 1995; Schoenberg and Scott, 2011).

The neuropsychiatric symptomatology associated with brain tumours may be divided into the following domains (Kaplan and Sadock, 1995):
- headaches: headaches may be generalised or unilateral, in which case they may have some lateralising value. They are dull and may be severe in nature; classically they are worst in the morning and are worsened by recumbency. Headaches arising from raised intracranial pressure may be associated with projectile vomiting.
- seizures: seizures may be the presenting symptom in 20% of patients with brain tumours and may be present at some stage of the disease in 62% of patients (David *et al.*, 2009). One-third of all brain tumours manifest seizures that may be simple partial, complex partial or grand mal in type (Oosthuizen, 2005).
- non-focal symptoms: these arise from RICP and may include dizziness, fuzzy thinking and somnolence.
- focal signs: compression of brain tissue by the tumour mass or peri-tumour oedema may give rise to focal signs such as hemiplegia, aphasia, apraxia, cranial nerve palsies and hemianopia.
- specific syndromes: the most common syndromes associated with tumours are dementia and personality change followed, less commonly, by delirium, amnesia, mania, depression and psychosis (Moore, 2008). Post-irradiative encephalopathy may appear three months to three years after radiotherapy for cerebral or pituitary tumours and manifests as dementia, seizures and RICP (Kaplan and Sadock, 1995).

#### Cognitive change

Subtle cognitive changes such as impaired attention and concentration span, poor memory, reduced psychomotor speed, impaired visuospatial functioning and fatigability are the most common (and often the first) manifestations of a lesion. More severe cognitive impairment may present as dementia, which can be steadily progressive or fluctuating in severity. However, focal cognitive deficits are more common with amnesia, dysphasia, apraxia and visuospatial defects reported. The treatment of cerebral tumours also impacts on cognitive functioning. With improved treatment outcomes and longer survival times, these cognitive changes impact significantly on the quality of life. The impact of surgery depends on the impact on remaining brain tissue. Neurological complications of chemotherapy range from headache to cognitive slowing and encephalopathy (David *et al.*, 2009). (See Section 32.5.1.2 for the effects of radiation.)

#### Affective and anxiety symptoms

Depressive symptoms have an overall incidence of 20–25% with biological factors and psychosocial (disability and end-of-life) issues being contributory. Depressive changes are often accompanied by anxiety, intellectual changes, apathy, irritability, mood lability or euphoria. Suicidal tendencies occur in approximately 10% of cases (David *et al.*, 2009).

#### Psychotic symptoms

Hallucinations may occur in any modality, depending on the location of the tumour, and may also occur as part of a seizure. Generally, occipital tumours are associated with simple visual hallucinations and temporal lobe tumours with complex visual and auditory and sometimes olfactory and **gustatory hallucinations**. Parietal lobe tumours are associated with localised tactile and kinaesthetic hallucinations and frontal lobe tumours with visual, auditory or gustatory hallucinations. Delusions may occur early or late in the illness in the context of schizophrenic or affective psychoses and are characteristically poorly elaborated, shallow or fleeting (David *et al.*, 2009).

### Hypertensive encephalopathy

Hypertensive encephalopathy is an uncommon condition that occurs in those with malignant hypertension (diastolic blood pressure may be in excess of 140 mmHg). Its incidence has declined with improved hypertension management. It is

**Information box**

**Clinical features related to specific brain locations**

Specific brain locations are frequently associated with certain classic symptoms and signs (Yudofsky and Hales, 2008; Kaplan and Sadock, 1995; David *et al.*, 2009).

**Frontal lobes**

Frontal lobe tumours often present in the guise of primary dementing illnesses due to the absence of neurological signs and the early manifestation of mental signs. Impairment in consciousness and intellectual deterioration are frequently seen with left lobe lesions associated with greater cognitive disturbance than right lobe lesions. Generalised dementia is more common than isolated memory loss. Depression, irritability, euphoria and apathy can all be manifestations of frontal lobe pathology. Behavioural and personality changes may occur in the absence of any intellectual impairment.

- Orbitofrontal area: patients present with a pseudopsychopathic profile characterised by disinhibition, impulsiveness, inappropriate jocularity, euphoria, emotional lability, distractibility, impaired social and financial judgement and poor insight. Even in the presence of extensive tumour invasion intelligence may be preserved and it is only assessment of executive functions that may reveal the dysfunction that is present.
- Frontal convexity: patients present with a pseudo-depressed profile characterised by psychomotor retardation, apathy and indifference, with occasional unprovoked and sudden aggressive outbursts. Cognitive assessment may reveal several deficits, including perseveration, poor word list generation, motor programming deficits and impaired abstract thinking and visuospatial abilities.
- Medial frontal lobes: patients present with akinetic mutism characterised by a marked reduction in spontaneous speech and movement, incontinence and sensorimotor deficits in the lower extremities.

**Temporal lobes**

Dominant hemisphere tumours are associated with Wernicke's aphasia combined with schizophrenia-like symptoms: visual, tactile, and olfactory hallucinations, mood swings and intrusive suicidal thoughts with relative preservation of affect, unlike in true schizophrenia. These may be episodic in nature. Neuropsychological deficits include difficulties with verbal, nonverbal and visuospatial memory as well as a reduced ability for new learning. Temporal lobe tumours are often associated with seizures.

**Parietal lobes**

Complex psychiatric presentations, predominantly with cognitive symptoms, may lead to misdiagnoses of somatoform or conversion disorders. Dominant hemisphere lesions are associated with dysphasia, ideomotor and/or ideational apraxia or features of Gerstmann's syndrome (finger agnosia, dyscalculia, dysgraphia and right-left disorientation). Non-dominant parietal lobe tumour symptoms include visuospatial deficits, dressing apraxia, astereognosis, anosognosia, unilateral inattention, marked inappropriate indifference and social isolation.

**Occipital lobes**

Patients commonly present with visual hallucinations, which are simple and unlike those seen in psychotic illnesses. Psychiatric symptoms are less common but cognition and perceptual functions may be impaired. Visual agnosia, homonymous hemianopia and prosopagnosia may be present.

**Diencephalon**

Limbic system involvement will give rise to psychiatric symptoms as well as deficits in memory and new learning.

**Corpus callosum**

Patients present with a variety of behavioural, affective, psychotic and personality disturbances with greater association of the anterior part with psychiatric symptoms. Splenium involvement can give rise to memory and visual perception abnormalities.

**Pituitary gland**

Disruption in the wide variety of endocrine and physiological functions co-ordinated by the pituitary gland can give rise to corresponding changes in sleep, thermoregulation and sexual functioning, which may be associated with disturbances in mood and behaviour (Kaplan and Sadock, 1995, Yudofsky and Hales, 2008).

characterised by an acute onset of headache, drowsiness, apprehension and mental confusion. Seizures, focal neurological signs, vomiting and papilloedema may manifest. It evolves rapidly over 24 hours, progressing to coma and death if untreated; full recovery can follow successful treatment (David *et al.*, 2009).

The commonest presentations to neurologists or neurosurgeons of cerebral tumours are symptoms related to raised intracranial pressure, focal neurological signs or seizures. However, the frequency of neuropsychiatric symptoms range from 10-100% of cases (Kaplan and Sadock, 1995).

The evaluation of a suspected brain tumour requires careful neurological examination, neuro-imaging, electrophysiological and neuropsychological testing. Tumour-related psychiatric symptoms are to be treated like primary psychiatric disorders, using both pharmacotherapy and psychotherapy and the provision of psycho-educational support to both patient and family. Like other organic states, brain tumour patients with psychiatric symptomatology and disorders tolerate and respond to lower doses of psychotropic medication than are required for primary psychiatric disorders (Yudofsky and Hales, 2008).

### 32.5.1.2 Radiation neurotoxicity

Cognitive deficits have been reported in children and adults receiving radiotherapy to the brain for leukaemia or brain tumours. Vascular damage and demyelination are the main effects of radiation damage. An acute radiation encephalopathy can occur within two weeks, caused by vasogenic oedema and disruption of the blood–brain barrier. Presenting symptoms include headache, somnolence and a worsening of pre-existing neurological symptoms. This acute encephalopathy responds to corticosteroids. An 'early-delayed' radiation encephalopathy may develop one to six months after completion of radiotherapy and manifest with drowsiness, worsening of neurological symptoms and transient cognitive deficits involving short-term memory and attention. It may resolve completely after six months to a year but the 'late-delayed' encephalopathy is more serious and irreversible. Memory, attention and new learning, as well as processing speed, are affected by radiotherapy. Common neurological sequelae include urinary incontinence, ataxia, pyramidal and extrapyramidal signs. Improvements in technology, such as intensity-modulated radiation therapy (IMRT) and stereotactic surgery, deliver high doses of radiation to tumours while significantly sparing the surrounding healthy structures, offering a more circumscribed approach to the treatment of brain tumours and the promise of fewer adverse effects (David *et al.*, 2009).

### 32.5.1.3 Management of psychiatric sequelae of cerebral tumours

In view of the significant impact on cognition, comprehensive baseline and periodic assessments of cognition and activities of daily living and quality of life must be conducted on all patients. Patients will require treatment of depression and anxiety symptoms. Suicide risk must be assessed and managed, especially during the terminal stages of the illness. SSRIs are the drugs of choice, although the side-effect profile of drugs are a determining factor. There is some evidence that methylphenidate may benefit cognitive impairment in certain patients. Psychotherapeutic support, palliative care, pain relief, caregiver support and anticipatory grief counselling must be provided. End-of-life issues, spiritual needs and ethical aspects of care must be addressed (David *et al.*, 2009).

## 32.5.2 Hydrocephalus and normal-pressure hydrocephalus

Hydrocephalus refers to an enlargement of one or more ventricles due to an increase in cerebrospinal fluid (CSF) pressure. Depending on the ability of the CSF to flow between the ventricles and the subarachnoid space it may be communicating or non-communicating. Normal-pressure hydrocephalus (NPH) is a form of idiopathic chronic communicating hydrocephalus; it presents with the classic triad of gait disturbance, dementia and urinary incontinence. The cognitive deterioration often results in psychiatric referral, with the patient presenting with forgetfulness, psychomotor slowing, apathy and indifference. Personality change, depression, aggression and mania may be less common presenting symptoms. The gait disturbance is often the initial and striking feature. The distinctive 'magnetic' gait is described as short steps on a widened base with shuffling due to difficulty initiating steps – it looks as if the feet are held on the floor by magnets. Urinary incontinence or urgency may be intermittent. An examination may reveal generalised hyper-reflexia, positive Babinski signs and the presence of snout-and-grasp reflexes. The condition may progress to a state of akinetic mutism. Although the response varies, ventriculoperitoneal shunting is a treatment option (Moore, 2008).

## 32.5.3 Benign intracranial hypertension

Benign intracranial hypertension (BIH or idiopathic intracranial hypertension) is a syndrome of unknown aetiology. It is characterised by raised CSF pressure in the absence of an intracranial mass lesion or ventricular dilatation, normal spinal fluid composition, usually normal findings on neurological examination except for papilloedema and sixth nerve palsy, in the absence of impairment in consciousness (Soler *et al.*, 1998). The non-specific nature of symptoms, often in the absence of localising neurological signs, may suggest a psychiatric disorder.

The symptoms most commonly described are headaches (94%), visual disturbances (75%) and pulsatile intracranial noises (58%). Headaches are usually insidious with increasing intensity. They are daily, severe and pulsatile and often wake the patient during the early hours of the morning. Headaches are accompanied by nausea rather than vomiting (Shah, 1994). Headaches may be generalised or frontal in location. Visual symptoms include transient (less than 30 seconds) unilateral or bilateral visual obscurations, **photopsias**, diplopia and photophobia. Visual loss rarely occurs (Soler *et al.*, 1998; Shah, 1994). Intracranial noises are subjective, pulsatile, commonly unilateral and may be attenuated by compression of the ipsilateral jugular vein (Shah, 1994).

Other presenting symptoms may include lethargy, tiredness, dizziness and mood, sleep and behavioural changes. The neurological examination is usually normal except for papilloedema or a sixth nerve palsy. The management of BIH is focused on the changes in visual function and range from conservative symptomatic care to the use of acetazolamide and steroids and, ultimately, the insertion of a lumbar peritoneal shunt. The condition generally runs a self-limiting course although the threat of visual loss is significant (Shah, 1994).

## 32.6 Neuropsychiatric aspects of epilepsy

Prior to the invention of the electroencephalogram (EEG) all seizure disorders were classified with mental disorders (Yudofsky and Hales, 2008). The association of abnormal behaviour with epilepsy dates back to antiquity, while the behaviour of epileptics has been ascribed to spiritual or demonic possession (Kaplan and Sadock, 1995). Epilepsy adversely affects the quality of life of sufferers and it has biological, psychological, social and economic consequences. The aetiology, clinical manifestations and bio-psycho-social consequences of seizures predispose the sufferer to a variety of psychiatric sequelae. It is estimated that 20-30% of patients with epilepsy have psychiatric disturbances (Vuilleumier and Jallon, 1998).

Epilepsy is defined by the International League against Epilepsy as a disorder of the brain characterised by an enduring predisposition to generate epileptic seizures and by the neurobiological, cognitive, psychological and social consequences of this condition. An epileptic seizure is a transient occurrence of signs and/or symptoms due to abnormal excessive or synchronous neuronal activity in the brain. An understanding of the psychiatric manifestations of epilepsy begins with a clear description of the nature and frequency of seizures. A seizure is referred to as an ictus; it is preceded by the pre-ictal phase and followed by the post-ictal phase, together referred to as the peri-ictal phase. The **aura** refers to a distinct visual, motor, sensory or psychological perception occurring a few seconds to an hour before a seizure. The inter-ictal period refers to the interval between ictal events. Status epilepticus refers to a state of prolonged or repetitive seizures without an intervening period of recovery (Kaplan and Sadock, 1995).

A diagnosis of epilepsy is made on clinical grounds; the history obtained from the patient and family is therefore crucial. While characteristic EEG findings can confirm a diagnosis, 20% of epileptics will have a normal EEG and 2% of patients without epilepsy will evidence spike and wave formations (Engel and Rocha, 1992). Finding an elevated prolactin level is the only specific laboratory test that may be useful in epilepsy. An abrupt rise in prolactin levels (three to four times the normal level) occurs 15–20 minutes after a generalised tonic-clonic seizure and returns to normal within 60 minutes. Blood must be drawn within 15–20 minutes after a suspected seizure. However, a recent study found its diagnostic accuracy to be 60% (Vukmir, 2009) and it has not been found to be helpful in differentiating true seizures from non-epileptic seizures (Shukla *et al.*, 2004). Neuroleptic use is known to increase prolactin levels. The use of prolactin as a diagnostic test is therefore limited and can merely serve a confirmatory role supported by history and clinical observations.

### 32.6.1 Classification of epileptic seizures

Since the brain mediates a wide variety of functions, the clinical manifestations of a seizure include motor, sensory, autonomic, emotional, behavioural and psychic phenomena. These phenomena vary according to the locus of origin of the seizure as well as its spread to other brain areas. Seizures are classified as being, firstly, generalised or partial in origin: generalized seizures have initial widespread bihemispheric involvement, while partial seizures emanate from a focus in one hemisphere. Partial seizures may become secondarily generalised. Secondly, seizures may be complex or simple in nature: complex seizures are characterised by some degree of impairment in, or alteration of, consciousness or the presence of psychic symptoms (David *et al.*, 2009). See Table 32.3 for an international classification of epilepsies.

### 32.6.2 Psychiatric symptoms and syndromes in epilepsy

Although most patients with epilepsy are psychologically normal, there is an increased prevalence of psychosis, depression, borderline personality disorder and hyposexuality amongst epileptic patients (Kaplan and Sadock, 1995). In patients with severe complex partial seizures, 70% have one or more psychiatric diagnosis,

**Table 32.3** Classification of epileptic seizures

| | |
|---|---|
| *I* | *Partial seizures* |
| A | Simple partial seizures |
| B | Complex partial seizures |
| C | Partial seizures evolving to secondarily generalised seizures |
| *II* | *Generalised seizures* |
| A1 | Absence seizures |
| A2 | Atypical absence seizures |
| B | Myoclonic seizures |
| C | Clonic seizures |
| D | Tonic seizures |
| E | Tonic–clonic seizures |
| F | Atonic seizures |
| *III* | *Unclassified epileptic seizures* |

**Source:** Adapted from the Commission on Classification and Terminology of the International League against Epilepsy (1981)

58% have a history of depression, 32% agoraphobia and 13% have psychoses (Tucker, 1998). Epilepsy patients have a 6–12 times greater risk of psychosis than the general population, with a prevalence of 7–8%; the prevalence in those with treatment refractory temporal lobe epilepsy ranges from 0–16% (Torta and Keller, 1999).

The increased prevalence of psychiatric disturbances in epileptic patients can be explained by the psychosocial sequelae of having a chronic stigmatised illness and by several possible biological links between epilepsy and mental illness. The locus of pathology in the brain that gives rise to the seizure may also manifest psychiatric symptoms, for example temporal lobe lesions that give rise to seizures (which in themselves may have psychic symptoms such as auditory hallucinations as part of the pre-ictal, ictal or post-ictal symptomatology) as well as psychosis. Subclinical or subthreshold neuronal electrical firing may give rise to cognitive and behavioural symptoms through the mechanism of kindling. Seizures may also give rise to neurochemical and neuro-endocrine changes that may precipitate psychiatric presentations. Anti-epileptic drugs are known to cause cognitive impairment and psychiatric symptoms (e.g. vigabatrin causes psychosis). Psychiatric manifestations in epileptic patients therefore represent a heterogeneous group of disorders with a variety of causes (Kaplan and Sadock, 1995). The most common psychiatric conditions in epilepsy are depression, psychosis and anxiety and, together with suicide, these conditions are more prevalent in epileptics than in the general population (Algreeshah and Benbodis, 2013). Furthermore, the severity of depression among epilepsy sufferers is more severe (Blum, 1999). A clinically systematic approach to determine the cause, and hence the approach to treatment, of psychiatric symptoms in epileptic patients is to begin with a clear definition of the seizure event and its frequency.

A clear description of what constitutes the ictal phenomenon will enable ictal-related psychic phenomena to be correctly diagnosed and appropriately treated. While ictal psychic phenomena are generally brief, non-convulsive status epilepticus (simple partial seizures, complex partial seizures) may less commonly present as episodes of a psychiatric disorder. Peri-ictal psychic phenomena refer to the pre-ictal prodromal symptoms (e.g. anxiety, dysphoria) as well as post-ictal confusion, delirium and psychosis. The consistent relationship of these manifestations to the ictus distinguish them from primary psychiatric diagnoses (Kaplan and Sadock, 1995). Approximately 10–20% of persons with epilepsy have a prodrome consisting of a depressed-irritable mood that may be associated with anxiety, tension or headaches. However, post-ictal mood syndromes are not well researched (Algreeshah and Benbodis, 2013). Psychiatric conditions such as a schizophrenia-like psychosis and personality disorders may be unrelated to the ictal phenomenon. Using Fenton's classification system, the following categories of psychiatric symptoms and syndromes are found in relation to epilepsy (David *et al.*, 2009):

- disorders clearly attributable to the underlying brain disorder causing the epilepsy: a known underlying brain disorder gives rise to both the epilepsy and psychiatric, cognitive or behavioural symptoms (e.g. Lennox Gestaut syndrome)
- disorders temporally related to the seizures.

### 32.6.2.1 Pre-ictal disorders

The prodrome refers to subjective symptoms that occur hours to days prior to a seizure; they do not form part of a seizure. Of gradual onset and prolonged duration, symptoms of a prodrome include poorly defined malaise, headaches, fatigue, irritability, dysphoria or depression; they are reported by 7-20% of patients (David *et al.*, 2009).

### 32.6.2.2 Ictal disorders

Epileptic auras are brief, paroxysmal and highly stereotyped distinct perceptions – either visual, motor, sensory or psychological – that occur a few seconds to an hour before a seizure. They mostly occur in individuals who suffer from complex or generalised seizures. Auras vary from person to person, and can manifest as hallucinations, aberrations of thinking, depersonalisation or anxiety attacks. There may be brief periods of clouding of consciousness of which the patient has no memory (David *et al.*, 2009).

Epileptic automatisms refer to somewhat co-ordinated, repetitive motor activity (usually occurring while cognition is impaired) and for which patients have amnesia. Most automatisms are brief (seconds to minutes) and range from simple movements to complex semi-purposeful actions. Examples of automatisms include lip-smacking, tooth grinding, bursts of laughter or giggling (gelastic), vocal utterances, dysphasias and hypo- or hyper-kinetic movements (David *et al.*, 2009; Yudofsky and Hales, 2008).

Non-convulsive status epilepticus refers to a prolonged electrographic seizure activity that results in non-convulsive seizure symptoms. It accounts for 40% of all status epilepticus. Complex partial status is the most common type of non-convulsive status. The classic presentation is one of fluctuating delirium with motor automatisms. Non-convulsive status should be suspected in a known epileptic who has a protracted change in behaviour or mental state, especially if there is associated clouding of consciousness (David *et al.*, 2009).

### 32.6.2.3 Post-ictal disorders

**Delirium**

Normal function resumes very gradually after an epileptic seizure. The transition from a state of unresponsiveness and confusion to complete alertness occurs over minutes; it may, however, be longer in older adults and those with learning difficulties. The patient may complain of headache, drowsiness and mental slowing after the delirium resolves (David *et al.*, 2009; Kaplan and Sadock, 1995).

**Psychosis**

Post-ictal psychosis refers to brief, self-limiting episodes of psychosis that has a sudden onset after a seizure; it probably is the most common psychotic disorder seen in epilepsy. It has a prevalence of 6% and is typically seen in temporal lobe epilepsy. It is characterised by a sudden onset of mixed psychotic and affective features, following a brief lucid interval after seizures. Individual episodes resolve within days but tend to recur. Between 14–20% of post-ictal psychosis sufferers will develop chronic inter-ictal psychoses. It must be differentiated from non-convulsive status where there is an impairment of consciousness and intermittent motor signs. Episodes of post-ictal psychosis are self-limiting and antipsychotics are usually not required. Benzodiazepines may be used to control agitation and behavioural disturbances but the main focus should be to improve seizure control (Kaplan and Sadock, 1995; David *et al.*, 2009).

### 32.6.2.4 Inter-ictal disorders

Depression and anxiety are the most frequently encountered inter-ictal psychiatric disorders in epilepsy. Depression is the most prevalent neuropsychiatric disorder associated with epilepsy: patients with uncontrolled seizures have a prevalence of depression up to ten times greater than the general population and up to five times greater than in patients with controlled seizures. Depression is more common in temporal lobe epilepsy. Epileptics have higher rates of depression than other chronic illnesses such as asthma and diabetes mellitus and have much higher health care use (Yudofsky and Hales, 2008). The contribution of anti-epileptic drugs such as phenobarbitone and vigabatrin to the aetiology of depression in epileptics must be explored where appropriate. The clinical picture is one of chronic, low-grade depression interrupted by brief periods of normal mood. Irritability and somatic symptoms feature prominently; the atypical presentation results in the depression often going unnoticed. Optimum seizure control must be aimed for and the depression must be treated as a priority (David *et al.*, 2009; Kaplan and Sadock, 1995).

Anxiety is as frequent as depression; agarophobia, generalised anxiety disorder and social phobia are the most common. Anxiety disorders are more prevalent among epileptics than in the general population, ranging from 14–25%. Anxiety disorders and epilepsy share many similarities: both are episodic disorders with a sudden onset and without precipitating events, both may present with dissociative symptoms such as depersonalisation, derealisation and **déjà vu**, both present with perceptual and emotional abnormalities such as intense fear and terror and both have associated physical symptoms (Yudofsky and Hales, 2008). Seizure phobia refers to a situation where a patient's fear of having a seizure is more disabling than the seizure itself (David *et al.*, 2009).

The chronic inter-ictal psychosis of epilepsy occurs in individuals who have had 11–15 years of generally poorly controlled epilepsy, usually of the complex partial type with secondarily generalised tonic-clonic seizures, with auras and automatisms. The seizures arise from a left temporal focus, usually mediobasal. The psychosis is an atypical paranoid type, which lacks the affective blunting, negative signs and personality deterioration of schizophrenia. Patients are less socially isolated and do not have a family history of schizophrenia (Kaplan and Sadock, 1995). Epilepsy is associated with an increased risk of schizophrenia. Patients with chronic epilepsy, associated with significant disability requiring specialist attention, are two to three times more likely to develop schizophrenia than the general population (David *et al.*, 2009).

Although there is no specific epileptic personality type, patients with complex partial seizures, especially those that originate from temporal limbic foci, are predisposed to characteristic personality traits (Kaplan and Sadock, 1995). The term Geschwind syndrome has been suggested to describe a group of behavioural phenomena characterised by circumstantiality (increased verbal output, stickiness, hypergraphia), altered sexuality (usually hyposexuality), and intensified mental life (deepened cognitive and emotional responses) (Benson, 1991). Classically, individuals with this syndrome may be humourless, excessively religious or preoccupied with moral or philosophical issues (Kaplan and Sadock, 1995).

Epileptic patients, apart from the biological reasons for their personality traits, are vulnerable due to the stigma and fear associated with epilepsy. The condition also gives rise to financial, interpersonal, vocational and social limitations and stressors. Epileptic patients often suffer from unstable personalities, low self-esteem, impulsivity and dependency. Borderline personality is the most frequent personality type found among epileptics (Yudofsky and Hales, 2008).

Dissociative disorders, mood disorders, suicide, changes in sexuality, aggression and violence may be variably related to the ictus. Epileptic patients present with a wide variety of altered states of consciousness described as fugue, possession, dissociative or twilight states. Periods of amnesia, either psychogenic or biogenic, may give rise to identity disturbances or compulsive wandering (David *et al.*, 2009).

Cognitive impairment in epileptics may be due to the pathogenesis or aetiology of the seizure disorder, anatomical location of the seizure foci, severity and clinical course of the disorder (Yudofsky and Hales, 2008), associated co-morbid intellectual disability, the subtle cognitive effects of seizures, or the effects of anti-epileptic drugs. Cognitive deficits are associated with several types of epilepsy. Generalised tonic-clonic seizures are more likely to cause cognitive impairment than are focal seizures. Status epilepticus can cause severe and persistent amnesia (Yudofsky and Hales, 2008). Temporal lobe epilepsy is associated with deficits in memory and is related to hippocampal atrophy. Deficits in working memory and frontal executive tasks are associated with frontal lobe epilepsy (Blum, 1999). Although the long-term cognitive outcome is largely unknown, seizure remission can result in an arrest or a reversal of cognitive decline (Yudofsky and Hales, 2008).

Suicide is the cause of death in 10% of all patients with epilepsy compared to 1% in the general population (Jones, 2006); the risk is increased 25-fold if the epileptic focus lies in the temporal lobe (Kaplan and Sadock, 1995). The relationship between suicide and epilepsy is multifactorial and bidirectional (Kanner, 2009). A wide variety of factors contribute to the increased risk of suicide, including borderline personality traits, psychosocial stressors, command hallucinations during ictal states and psychotic states related to the seizures (Kaplan and Sadock, 1995). Ictal-related sexual events are rare: epileptics commonly manifest a lowered libido (David *et al.*, 2009).

Although epileptics are often perceived by the public to be violent, they rarely commit premeditated acts of violence. Violence as a direct consequence of seizures is rare and often represents a confused defensive reaction to attempts at restraining or assisting a patient. Patients may misconstrue this as threatening and act out violently. Such behaviour is brief, but prolonged non-directed aggression may occur in the context of post-ictal psychosis, or manifest in the context of automatisms, post-ictal confusion or delirious states (David *et al.*, 2009).

Crimes committed during peri-ictal or ictal states may exonerate patients from culpability. However, this conclusion must be supported by a sound history of epilepsy and objective clinical evidence (video-EEG telemetry) of seizure activity characterised habitually by similar aggressive behaviour (Yudofsky and Hales, 2008). In legal terms, if an act was committed but was neither intended as, nor the result of, recklessness it is regarded an an automatism (David *et al.*, 2009).

## 32.6.3 Treatment of epileptics with psychiatric disorders

Episodic psychotic conditions usually respond to optimal anticonvulsant drugs. The treatment of chronic psychosis requires the additional use of antipsychotics, at low doses. All antipsychotics can lower the seizure threshold, but atypical antipsychotics are less implicated. Clozapine is highly epileptogenic and should rarely be used and only in specialist settings. Combining carbamazepine with clozapine is contraindicated due to the high risk of agranulocytosis. Anti-epileptic drugs are most effective at the upper levels of the therapeutic range (Yudofsky and Hales, 2008).

Depression must be treated in conjunction with the elimination of anti-epileptic drugs that may be depressogenic, by replacing them with anti-epileptics with mood stabilising properties. All antidepressants are proconvulsive, with buproprion likely to cause seizures, although the incidence of seizures in healthy individuals is low. SSRIs are recommended as the first line of treatment. In most cases, treatment of depression often improves seizure control (Yudofsky and Hales, 2008).

Anxiety disorders respond to SSRIs but due regard must be given to interactions with hepatically metabolised anti-epileptic drugs that inhibit cytochrome P450 enzymes. Benzodiazepines may also be used while guarding against their potential to cause sedation, impaired cognition, psychomotor slowing, tolerance, addiction and withdrawal seizures (Yudofsky and Hales, 2008).

### 32.6.3.1 Basic principles of treatment

When treating patients with a seizure disorder and concomitant psychiatric symptoms, the following basic principles should apply (Yudofsky and Hales, 2008):

- perform a comprehensive assessment of aggravating bio-psycho-social factors
- review the type and dose of the anti-epileptic
- consider specific and appropriate psychotherapeutic interventions – individual, group or family

- aim for anti-epileptic monotherapy where possible
- introduce psychotropic medication by targeting specific symptoms
- 'start low, go slow' when using psychotropic agents
- be aware of and prevent adverse interactions between anti-epileptic and psychotropic medication
- employ a multidisciplinary approach and involve caregivers in the management.

### 32.6.3.2 Psychiatric effects of anti-epileptic drugs

Anti-epileptic drugs are psychotropic agents that act on the mind and can affect behaviour adversely or positively by virtue of their effects on brain electrochemical systems. Behavioural effects on cognition and mood associated with anti-epileptic drugs are complex and vary between patients, with epilepsy patients being more susceptible than the general population. It is not possible to predict whether an individual will tolerate a drug or experience adverse effects. Positive or negative behavioural effects may accompany suppression of seizures or inter-ictal epileptiform activity. Sedating anti-epileptic drugs, such as valproic acid and carbamazepine, generally have anxiolytic, antimanic and sleep-promoting effects but may lead to fatigue, impaired attention and depression of mood. Activating anti-epileptic drugs, such as lamotrigine, may have attention-enhancing efficacy but may cause anxiety, insomnia and agitation. Approximately 5–10% of adults and 12–25% of children on levetiracetam may display irritability, anxiety, depression and other behavioural disorders. Acute encephalopathy with seizures and a chronic cumulative encephalopathy after long-term exposure to high doses of phenytoin have been described. Patients on topiramate may manifest impaired attention, word-finding, verbal fluency and memory, as well as psychomotor slowing, depression, irritability and, although rare, psychosis. Depression, hyperactivity and aggressive behaviour may be associated with valproic acid, while vigabatrin may cause depression, psychosis and exacerbate hyperactivity. However, these generalisations are limited by a wide variability in clinical responses (Nadkarni and Devinsky, 2005). Conversely, the effects of antidepressants and antipsychotics on seizure threshold must be considered in patients with co-morbid epilepsy and psychiatric disorders.

### 32.6.3.3 Psychogenic non-epileptic seizures

Psychogenic non-epileptic seizures (also referred to as pseudoseizures or a conversion reaction) are paroxysmal events that mimic epileptic seizures (and are often misdiagnosed as such). They are psychogenic in origin. Paroxysmal non-epileptic events of organic origin may be due to syncope, migraine or transient ischaemic attacks. Psychogenic non-epileptic seizures are more prevalent in females (approximately 70%) and are common in epilepsy clinics, representing 20–30% of referrals. However, differentiating between true seizures and pseudoseizures is complicated by the fact that 15% of psychogenic non-epileptic seizures patients also have epilepsy (Benbadis, 2013).

Patients with pseudoseizures differ from seizure disorder patients in that they may have significantly more stress, more negative life events, a history of child abuse, more somatic symptoms and a high incidence of anxiety and psychotic disorders (Yudofsky and Hales, 2008).

Distinguishing psychogenic non-epileptic seizures from true seizures is challenging, especially in the absence of EEG or visual telemetry. However, the following criteria, adapted from Kaplan and Sadock suggest the presence of a psychogenic event:

- pre-ictal: the presence of an emotional stressor, an epileptic who can serve as a 'model', the ability to induce an event, the availability of an audience, anxiety symptoms featuring in the aura
- ictal: atypical clinical features or sequence, gradual onset, prolonged duration, abrupt cessation, asymmetric and out-of-phase limb movements, pelvic thrusting, avoidance of injury or eye opening, screaming and crying,

normal EEG, no increase in prolactin level, absence of whole-body rigidity, absence of autonomic signs, absence of incontinence and tongue biting, presence of corneal reflex, presence of a normal plantar response
- post-ictal: no confusion, normal EEG, ability to recall events occurring during ictus (Kaplan and Sadock, 1995).

The diagnosis of a psychogenic non-epileptic seizure must be made after a comprehensive evaluation of historical information (especially from witnesses of the event), a thorough clinical examination and investigation. The presence of atypical clinical presentations are insufficient to warrant a diagnosis of a psychogenic event as unusual or atypical seizures may not infrequently originate from frontal or other sites in the brain.

Note: See Chapter 18: Somatic symptom and related disorders, for a discussion of non-epileptic seizures.

## 32.7 Neuropsychiatric aspects of traumatic brain injury

Annually, 200–300 per 100 000 of the population in the UK attend hospital after a head injury. Approximately one-sixth are admitted: 80% with mild head injuries, 10% with moderate head injuries and 10% with severe head injuries. Head injury imparts both physical and psychological trauma (Lishman, 1988).

Traumatic brain injury results in a mixture of cognitive, emotional, behavioural and physical symptoms, which may lead to a psychiatric consultation. At this consultation, the interplay between the individual's pre-injury constitution, the brain and its injuries, as well as the psychodynamic processes that follow from the injury must be taken into account.

### 32.7.1 Classification of traumatic brain injury

The neuropathological changes associated with head injuries depend on the type and severity of the injury.

#### 32.7.1.1 Cause of the trauma

Non-missile injuries (or blunt head injuries) are usually due to rapid acceleration or deceleration of the head, with or without impact, or, less commonly, crushing of the head. Most often, non-missile injuries occur as a result of road traffic accidents or falls.

Missile injuries are due to penetration of the skull by a rapidly moving external object (e.g. gunshot wounds) and result in a different pattern of brain injury.

#### 32.7.1.2 Site and neuropathology of the trauma

Focal (or localised) lesions include contusions, haemorrhages and skull fractures.

Diffuse lesions include diffuse axonal injury, diffuse vascular injury, brain swelling (oedema) and ischaemia.

#### 32.7.1.3 Open versus closed brain injury

In an open head injury there is penetration of the skull, often with considerable destruction of brain tissue local to the trauma, but relatively less at a distance. Therefore, there is often little, if any, loss of consciousness. (See Section 32.7.2 for a discussion of closed head injuries.)

Note: A traumatic brain injury can result in primary (immediate) and secondary (delayed) injury to the brain. The primary injury results from the mechanical forces (acceleration-deceleration and rotational) transmitted to the brain tissue and the secondary injury from subsequent biochemical changes, including inflammation.

### 32.7.2 Closed head injury

In a closed head injury there is no penetration of the skull and injury commonly results from acceleration-deceleration, with or without impact (if impact occurs it is typically blunt). The neuropathological consequences will now be discussed.

#### 32.7.2.1 Contusions

In contusions the soft brain tissue moves within its bony box (skull) and is damaged locally. *Coup* injuries occur beneath the site of impact whereas *contrecoup* injuries at the site opposite. Bleeding into the contusion is usually seen; this appears as a high signal on computed tomography (CT) brain scans. However, the contusion later ends up as a localised atrophy more readily seen on magnetic resonance imaging (MRI) brain scans.

The frontal poles and the tips and under-surface of the temporal lobes are particularly vulnerable to contusions; damage to these areas may be responsible for much of the cognitive impairment and personality change commonly associated with traumatic brain injury.

#### 32.7.2.2 Diffuse axonal injury

The stretching of the brain parenchyma produces diffuse axonal injury of the white matter, particularly in the corpus callosum and in long tracts of the brainstem; axons break up over the course of the first 24–48 hours.

#### 32.7.2.3 Intracranial haemorrhages

Intracranial haemorrhages are classified depending on their site in relation to the brain and surrounding durae. In traumatic brain injury it may be difficult to predict outcome from the location and size of intracerebral haemorrhage.

Extradural haematomas, being arterial bleeding under high pressure, can rapidly cause coma and death. The patient may 'talk and die' (regain consciousness after the injury, only to lapse a few hours later into a severe coma that requires urgent surgery to evacuate the blood). It is important to realise that in traumatic brain injury it may be difficult to predict outcome from the location and size of intracerebral haemorrhage.

Subdural haematomas run a subacute course with a propensity to recur. They are characterised by a failure to improve, or fluctuating drowsiness or deterioration in mental state, and as such are of particular interest to the neuropsychiatrist. They may regress spontaneously. A chronic subdural haematoma is demonstrated by a low signal and an acute haematoma by a high signal on a CT scan.

Intracerebral haemorrhages occur in the brain parenchyma and overlap with contusions (bruising of the brain). In some cases, the size of the haemorrhage suggests that it itself is the cause of focal brain injury around the haemorrhage, as occurs in spontaneous intracranial haemorrhages associated with hypertension. Intracerebral haemorrhages are commonly found in the frontal and temporal lobes but also in deep cerebral structures such as the thalamus.

### 32.7.3 Late effects of traumatic brain injury

Hydrocephalus may be due to cerebral atrophy, which develops weeks or months after injury. Of greater importance is hydrocephalus that results from residual subarachnoid blood blocking the egress of cerebrospinal fluid (CSF); this may require the insertion of a ventriculo-peritoneal shunt.

Meningitis and cerebral abscesses may sometimes develop months and years after injury following basal skull fractures, particularly if they are associated with CSF leaks.

### 32.7.4 Clinical indicators of traumatic brain injury severity

There are several clinical indicators of head injury severity:

- the duration of retrograde amnesia (the period leading up to the injury of which memories have been lost)
- the depth of unconsciousness as assessed by the worst score on the Glasgow Coma Scale (GCS): score of 3 indicates absent responses (i.e. deep coma), 15 indicates normal consciousness, and a score of less than 9 generally indicates unconsciousness
- the duration of coma: this may be difficult to ascertain because of the routine sedation and ventilation that follow severe head injuries
- the duration of post-traumatic amnesia (the interval between injury and the return of normal continuous day-to-day memories).

Duration of post-traumatic amnesia can be measured retrospectively by asking the patient several months post-injury, about their memories of the post-injury period.

The duration of post-traumatic amnesia and the duration of loss of consciousness are probably the best markers of injury severity and therefore outcome. However, caution is always necessary when predicting outcome in individual patients. A majority of patients with a post-traumatic amnesia of less than one week will be left with little, if any, obvious disability.

A duration of more than one month indicates that there is likely to be enduring and significant disability. Age has a powerful effect on outcome: young patients generally recover much better for a given injury severity.

## 32.7.5 Cognitive sequelae of traumatic brain injury

There is a strong association between the duration of post-traumatic amnesia and the severity of cognitive impairment. Common cognitive impairments following moderate to severe traumatic brain injury include:

- impaired information processing
- difficulties with executive control
- impaired memory
- disorders of speech and language – in some
- disorders of executive control function can be of great importance to the neuropsychiatrist, as the dysexecutive syndrome can mimic some common psychiatric disorders.

### 32.7.5.1 Dysexecutive syndrome

A disturbance of the executive system can result in difficulty organising, planning, scheduling, prioritising and monitoring cognitive activities (Shallice and Burgess, 1991), and is particularly associated with damage to the frontal lobes and their connections.

In the real world, impairment of the executive system may be catastrophic. Dysexecutive syndrome can impair the organisation of everyday life, yet sometimes not be picked up by neuropsychological tests that draw on well-established or overlearned behaviours.

A few neuropsychological tests, such as the Behavioural Assessment of Dysexecutive Syndrome (BADS), have been developed to specifically assess executive control function (Wilson *et al.*, 1996). This is particularly useful in assessing changes in the emotional, motivational, behavioural and cognitive domain. The Multiple Errands Test (Shallice and Burgess, 1991) is used to demonstrate the severity of multitasking problems in a way that was not possible before and is important for assessment, treatment and rehabilitation.

**Information box**

**Clinical grading of severity of traumatic brain injury**

The severity of head injury is graded mild, moderate and severe based on the GCS score, duration of loss of consciousness and duration of post-traumatic amnesia:

- Mild head injury
  - GCS score 13 to 15
  - loss of consciousness of less than 30 minutes
  - post-traumatic amnesia of less than 24 hours.
- Moderate head injury
  - GCS score 9 to 12
  - loss of consciousness of between 30 minutes and 6 hours
  - post-traumatic amnesia of more than one day but less than one week.
- Severe head injury
  - GCS score 3 to 8
  - loss of consciousness of more than six hours
  - post-traumatic amnesia of more than 1 week.

**Sources:** Fleminger and Demjaha, *s.d.*; Folstein *et al.*, 1975; Roth *et al.*, 1986; Huppert *et al.*, 1995

### 32.7.5.2 Memory impairment

Amnesia, one of the commonest sequelae of traumatic brain injury, probably results from damage to several areas. Damage to the frontal lobes can, in some cases, result in failure of the executive processes required for normal memory (e.g. memory retrieval). Damage to the hippocampus is also seen. Amnesia following brain injury is for explicit memory; whereas implicit memory is generally well preserved. Confabulations are often seen.

#### 32.7.5.3 Communication

Dysphasia and dysprosody and word-finding difficulties are common in patients with a traumatic brain injury and contribute significantly to the disruption of social communication.

#### 32.7.5.4 Behavioural and personality change

The most troublesome sequelae of TBI are usually changes in behaviour or personality. Apathy and impairment of motivation and ambition are seen. Antisocial behaviour with irritability and sudden loss of temper is particularly difficult for carers, making integration back into the community very difficult.

In acquired antisocial personality disorder, the person is likely to be tactless, offensive, rude, self-centred, impulsive and aggressive. These traits are often accompanied by the dysexecutive syndrome. Patients may be fatuous and facetious. Traumatic brain injury is also a risk factor for borderline personality disorder (Streeter *et al.*, 1995).

### 32.7.6 Psychiatric sequelae of traumatic brain injury

#### 32.7.6.1 Depression

Depression is very common following a traumatic brain injury and may represent both biological and psychological factors. The diagnosis of depression relies heavily on identifying a depressive mood. Associated self-deprecation and guilt are very helpful in diagnosis. Apathy, anhedonia and slowness secondary to brain injury may resemble depression.

Be careful to distinguish between depression and demoralisation, grief reaction or emotional lability, which occurs commonly after brain injury. It is important to establish if there was an episode of depression prior to the accident, in which case the brain injury might have occurred as a result of depression or suicidal ideation.

#### 32.7.6.2 Suicide

Studies consistently report an increased risk of suicide in individuals with a traumatic brain injury (Achte *et al.*, 1970; Harris & Barraclough, 1997).

#### 32.7.6.3 Bipolar disorder

The occurrence of manic illness after a brain injury is less frequent than that of depression, but a brain injury can, nevertheless, result in mania. Careful evaluation is required to distinguish between disinhibition and fatuous behaviour following frontal injury. Mania is particularly associated with aggressive and assaultive behaviour after brain injury. Some patients develop rapid-cycling bipolar disorder.

#### 32.7.6.4 Anxiety disorders

Anxiety after traumatic brain injury is common. Anxiety symptoms related to post-traumatic stress disorder or travel anxiety may be specific to the trauma. On the other hand, many patients show elevated levels of anxiety and agoraphobia may develop in some cases. Although perhaps less common, obsessive-compulsive disorder has been reported following a traumatic brain injury.

#### 32.7.6.5 Psychosis

Psychosis can occur immediately or may develop long after a traumatic brain injury. Early psychosis is usually characterised by delusional misidentification of place, persons, objects and events.

Reduplicative paramnesia is perhaps the most pathognomic of brain injury; patients will often believe that the hospital is changed and is a duplicate of the original or may report that their home is no longer the same. Capgras and Fregoli syndromes may also be observed following a traumatic brain injury. Delusional misidentification syndromes can best be understood as the result of an interaction between organic brain disease and psychological disorder (Fleminger and Burns, 1993). Paranoid psychosis may occur relatively early, particularly in patients with cognitive impairment and personality change.

Later in the course, the patient may develop a typical schizophrenia indistinguishable from idiopathic schizophrenia, though there is uncertainty about the degree to which the risk of schizophrenia is raised after a traumatic brain injury.

## 32.7.7 Other factors that may be associated with traumatic brain injury

### 32.7.7.1 Drug and alcohol abuse

Drug and alcohol abuse are common in some patients and may be related to poor impulse control and anxiety symptoms.

### 32.7.7.2 Insight and capacity

Insight (self-awareness) and capacity to consent to treatment in the brain-injured patient, who often lacks awareness of deficits, should be assessed (Prigatano, 2005). Capacity to consent to treatment and capacity to manage finances and affairs should be evaluated independently of one another. Poor self-awareness can have a significant negative effect on the rehabilitation outcome.

### 32.7.7.3 Neurological sequelae

The neuropsychiatrist should be aware of neurological complications that may occur after a traumatic brain injury and that may exacerbate psychological problems. Patients are often troubled by ataxia, hemiplegia, slurred speech, visual and hearing impairments, frequent headaches, dizziness or persisting coldness. Many of these problems are due to damage of the brainstem white matter pathways.

### 32.7.7.4 Post-traumatic epilepsy

Depending on the severity, type and location of the brain injury, a variable proportion of patients will experience seizures. Seizures in the first week post-injury do not markedly increase the risk of chronic epilepsy. Only about 5% of patients with closed head injuries will develop late seizures, compared with 30% after an open head injury. After five years without seizures, any subsequent seizure may be unrelated to the head injury (Annegers *et al.*, 1980).

Risk factors for post-traumatic epilepsy include penetrating head injuries, chronic alcohol use, intracranial haematoma, early seizure and the severity of the injury.

Children are at increased risk of post-traumatic epilepsy. Post-traumatic epilepsy is associated with psychiatric morbidity and may increase the risk of late dementia.

## 32.7.8 Assessment of the neuropsychiatric consequences of traumatic brain injury

### 32.7.8.1 Neuro-imaging

Skull radiographs are rarely performed nowadays.

CT brain scanning is the preferred investigation in the trauma unit because of its faster acquisition time and safety and ability to pick up bleeding.

MRI is the better instrument in the post-acute setting. It is superior to CT in detecting cerebral contusions found near the bone-brain interface, changes in signal associated with a diffuse axonal injury (white matter appears normal on CT) and has a better image resolution.

Gradient echo sequences may be particularly valuable in demonstrating residual haemosiderin in areas that have suffered haemorrhagic contusions but that are not visible on T2 MRI images.

### 32.7.8.2 Electroencephalography (EEG)

Non-specific changes are seen on EEG after head injury. Suppression of the alpha rhythm is an early sign, while more severe injuries produce diffuse slowing.

EEG is largely confined to the investigation of deteriorating conscious level and unusual behavioural disturbances that may be attributed to epilepsy.

EEG is not a good predictor of post-traumatic epilepsy and is not a valuable prognostic marker (i.e. a normal EEG at follow-up may be seen in patients with a poor outcome).

## 32.7.8.3 Cognitive assessment

An assessment of potential cognitive impairments can either be performed by a bedside (clinical) assessment or by administering structured, neuropsychological tests with reference scores from the normal population.

Attention and concentration can affect higher-level functions, such as executive control function, and must be taken into account in the interpretation of test results.

Generally speaking, any cognitive assessment of a patient with a history of traumatic brain injury should cover at least the following areas: orientation, concentration and attention, language functions, memory, constructional ability, perceptual functions and executive control function including insight (see Table 32.4).

### Bedside cognitive assessment

There are structured approaches to the bedside cognitive assessment, for example the Mini-Mental State Examination (MMSE) and the Cambridge Cognitive Examination (CAMCOG).

### Neuropsychological testing

Performance on individual cognitive functions are, where possible, interpreted against the person's pre-morbid general intellectual ability.

### Rating scales and questionnaires

Rating scales or questionnaires often provide invaluable data about the patient's difficulties following a traumatic brain injury. Examples include the Health of the Nation Outcome Scale for Acquired Brain Injury (HoNOS-ABI) (Fleminger *et al.*, 2005) and the Neurobehavioral Rating Scale (Levin *et al.*, 1987). Some of these questionnaires provide an indication of potential problems of self-awareness. (A family member completes a parallel form of the questionnaire, which provides a potentially more objective view of difficulties experienced in the real world by the patient.) It is also good practice to interview a family member or carer to provide additional information on actual functioning in the community.

**Table 32.4** Neuropsychological tests

| Domain | Tests |
|---|---|
| **Pre-morbid intellectual ability** | National adult reading test (NART) or Wechsler test of adult reading (WTAR) gives an estimate of pre-injury IQ, which can be compared with present performance to ascertain the drop in performance as a result of the head injury |
| **General intellectual ability** | Wechsler adult intelligence scale (WAIS-III) |
| **Concentration and attention** | Trail making test, digit span (WAIS-III) |
| **Language functions** | COWAT, Boston naming test |
| **Memory** | Immediate and delayed recall, for both visually and verbally presented stimuli: Wechsler memory scale (WMS-III) |
| **Constructional ability** | Rey complex figure, block design (WAIS-III) |
| **Perceptual functions** | Block design (WAIS-III), Hooper visual organisation test |
| **Executive control function** | Delis-Kaplan executive function system |

## 32.7.9 Employment outcome following traumatic brain injury

Most patients who have sustained a mild or moderate head injury recover within weeks to months, without specific therapy (Van der Naalt, 2001). However, a proportion of patients are left with a residual disability that affect the psychosocial outcome, in particular their ability to return to work. Patients with post-traumatic amnesia of longer than one month are very likely to have difficulties returning to work. Those in employment at the time of injury are more likely to have returned to work by the post-injury follow-up visit. Return to work is determined more by the neuropsychiatric sequelae of the brain injury than the neurophysical sequelae.

## 32.7.10 Impairment, disability and handicap

The ideas encapsulated in the International Classification of Impairments, Disabilities and Handicaps (ICIDH) (WHO, 1980) are important in understanding recovery from brain injury.

Impairments are abnormalities of structure or physiological function (e.g. poor memory on a list-learning task). Disabilities refer to the behaviour of the person and their ability to perform activities. Handicap reflects the limitations in fulfilling the person's normal social role and participation in society.

Recovery of impairment is usually complete after one to two years, however, the level of disability may continue to fall long after the recovery of impairment has stopped.

Great caution is necessary when attempting to predict outcome following a traumatic brain injury, especially during the early days and when speaking to family members.

In general, neuropsychological rehabilitation aims to reduce disability by learning strategies to compensate for impairments; there may sometimes be little change in the underlying impairment.

For some patients, psychotherapy can assist with emotional adjustment. Once the person is back to living in the community, the multidisciplinary team can focus on minimising any handicaps.

## 32.7.11 Assessment of a patient who has sustained a traumatic brain injury

In assessing a person after a traumatic brain injury, it is important to consider a range of information related to the history of the injury, current symptoms, signs and risk, as well as level of functioning. Table 32.5 provides a checklist for a thorough post-traumatic brain injury assessment.

**Table 32.5** Checklist for the assessment post-traumatic brain injury

| Category of information | Checklist |
|---|---|
| History of injury | ▸ date, cause, nature, severity<br>▸ death or injuries of others from accident<br>▸ associated injuries |
| Investigation | ▸ intoxication<br>▸ lowest Glasgow Coma Scale neurosurgical intervention<br>▸ length of coma (ventilated or not?), treatment, rehabilitation and advice<br>▸ duration of hospitalisation<br>▸ retrograde and post-traumatic amnesia |

| Category of information | Checklist |
|---|---|
| Current risk identification | ▶ self-harm<br>▶ potential for exploitation by others<br>▶ assault, violence, threat to others<br>▶ wandering, falling, choking<br>▶ criminal behaviour, fire risk<br>▶ awareness of danger/road safety<br>▶ sexually inappropriate behaviour<br>▶ family cohesion<br>▶ alcohol or drug misuse<br>▶ able to self-medicate |
| Symptoms and signs: sequelae of injury:<br>▶ Physical | <br>▶ vision<br>▶ hearing<br>▶ speech, intelligibility<br>▶ swallowing (choking)<br>▶ pain<br>▶ neck and back symptoms<br>▶ headaches |
| ▶ Other | ▶ gait<br>▶ weakness, spasticity<br>▶ dizziness, balance<br>▶ epilepsy (type, frequency and time post-injury)<br>▶ other disturbances of consciousness<br>▶ adverse effects of medication, movement disorder<br>▶ skin/autonomic |
| ▶ Cognitive: general | ▶ conscious level (fluctuating); perceptual neglect<br>▶ dysexecutive - organisational ability; mental capacity (consent to treatment/ management of property and affairs) |
| ▶ Communication/thinking | ▶ verbal, non-verbal, social skills<br>▶ confabulation<br>▶ perseveration |
| ▶ Behavioural | ▶ drive, motivation, fatigue<br>▶ compliance<br>▶ disinhibition<br>▶ perseverative behaviour<br>▶ wandering, absconding<br>▶ irritability, aggression<br>▶ disruptive, noisy |

| Category of information | Checklist |
|---|---|
| ▶ Emotional | ▶ dysphoria<br>▶ lability, emotionalism<br>▶ catastrophic reaction<br>▶ PTSD |
| Activities of daily living:<br>▶ Personal | ▶ mobility<br>▶ eating and drinking<br>▶ continence<br>▶ washing and dressing |
| ▶ Community | ▶ ability to use transport<br>▶ fitness to drive<br>▶ leisure |
| ▶ Domestic | ▶ cooking<br>▶ laundry<br>▶ shopping<br>▶ money management |
| ▶ Available support | ▶ relatives, friends<br>▶ headway<br>▶ day centres<br>▶ social worker, benefits, legal representation |

**Source:** Fleminger and Demjaha, 2014

## 32.8 Neuropsychiatric aspects of movement disorders

Movement disorders are neurological conditions in which the primary problem is one of abnormal motor control. They are broadly categorised into those with excess movement (hyperkinetic disorders) or those with insufficient movement (hypokinetic disorders).

In hyperkinetic disorders there is an abnormally low inhibitory outflow from the basal ganglia, which results in a reduced inhibition of cortical motor areas and an abnormal increase in movement (e.g. chorea in Huntington's disease).

In hypokinetic disorders, there is an abnormally high inhibitory outflow from the basal ganglia, which results in an increased inhibition of cortical motor areas and hence suppression of movement (e.g. parkinsonism).

The basal ganglia consist of the:

- caudate nucleus and putamen (striatum or dorsal striatum or neostriatum)
- globus pallidum: internal and external segment
- substantia nigra: contains the dopaminergic neurons in the pars compacta and the GABA-ergic neurons of the pars reticulata
- subthalamic nucleus.

### 32.8.1 Parkinson's disease

#### 32.8.1.1 Clinical features

The classical manifestations of Parkinson's disease are resting tremor, rigidity (of the 'lead pipe' variety, or with 'cogwheeling' if tremor is present), bradykinesia, postural instability or loss of postural reflexes. Symptoms tend to present unilaterally

**Table 32.6** Symptoms and causes of movement disorders

| Symptom | Definition | Causes |
|---|---|---|
| Tremor | A rhythmic sinusoidal movement of a body part caused by regular muscle contractions. Defining the type of tremor assists in narrowing down the underlying aetiology | At rest: parkinsonism, drug-induced<br>Postural: essential tremor, hyperthyroidism, physiological<br>Related to specific actions: dystonic tremor<br>Action or intention: cerebellar disease (in patients with chorea and/or myoclonus it may look as though there is an action component to the tremor) |
| Bradykinesia | A slowness of movement characterised by reduced amplitude and early fatiguing | A key feature of parkinsonism |
| Parkinsonism | A triad consisting of bradykinesia, tremor and rigidity (and/or postural instability) | Parkinson's disease<br>Other neurodegenerative causes – PSP, MSA, CBD, DLB (see below)<br>Secondary to vascular disease, drugs (anti-emetics, lithium, sodium valproate, neuroleptics) and rarely tumours, infection and hydrocephalus |
| Chorea | A continuous flow of irregular, jerky and explosive movements, which flit randomly from one part of the body to another. Each muscle contraction is brief, often appearing as a fragment of what might have been a normal movement, and unpredictable in timing or site | Huntington's disease<br>Drug-induced (L-dopa, anti-epileptics)<br>Sydenham's chorea – post streptococcal, typically involving younger patients with frontal disinhibition<br>Pregnancy, systemic lupus erythematosis (SLE), anti-cardiolipin syndrome<br>Thyrotoxicosis and polycythaemia rubra vera |
| Dystonia | Sustained muscular contraction, which distorts the limbs and trunk into various characteristic postures. Causes depend on the anatomical pattern of involvement, age of onset and presence or absence of characteristic additional features | Primary generalised dystonia (see below)<br>Dystonic tremor (e.g. spasmodic torticollis, blepharospasm, dystonic tremor, writer's cramp): onset in adult life, aetiology unclear<br>Secondary: brain injury, stroke, neuroleptic drugs<br>Neurodegenerative conditions: Wilson's disease, neuroacanthocytosis, Parkinson's disease, advanced Huntington's disease, corticobasal degeneration |
| Tics | Sudden stereotyped movements, which often have a premonitory urge and are suppressible. Simple tics are confined to a few muscles, whereas complex tics may include quasi-purposeful movements (see Chapter 27: Child and adolescent psychiatry 1: Assessment and the young child, for discussion of tic disorders) | Transient tic disorders are common in young boys with a benign course<br>Tourette syndrome<br>Chronic multiple tics: motor or phonic tics, but not both<br>Secondary to drugs, cerebral palsy, Wilson's disease, Huntington's disease, neuroacanthocytosis, vascular disease |
| Myoclonus | Rapid shock-like muscle jerks, often repetitive and at times rhythmic | Secondary to hypoxic brain injury, metabolic or toxic encephalopathies, neurodegenerative conditions such as corticobasal degeneration, Alzheimer's disease, Creutzfeldt-Jakob disease |

**Source:** Barker *et al.*, 2014

or with an asymmetrical severity. Age at onset is usually between 50 and 65 years, although early- and late-onset cases are often described. In the majority of cases, Parkinson's disease is sporadic, but in the last few years a number of genetic factors have been identified. Environmental factors have also been proposed. Other clinical signs and symptoms of Parkinson's disease include masked face, hypophonia, **micrographia**, reduced arm swing, shuffling gait, festination (a tendency to accelerate in gait or speech), and positive glabellar tap (Myerson's sign).

### 32.8.1.2 Histopathology

Parkinson's disease presents with depigmentation, loss of dopaminergic neurons and presence of Lewy bodies in neurons of the substantia nigra and the ventral tegmental area (affecting dopaminergic pathways), locus coeruleus, nucleus basalis and the raphe.

### 32.8.1.3 Treatment

The main pharmacological treatments for Parkinson's disease are L-DOPA, dopamine agonists, catechol-O-methyl-transferase (COMT) inhibitors and anticholinergics. Subcutaneous (s.c.) apomorphine is also used in cases of severe motor impairment. Some patients may benefit from neurosurgical interventions such as pallidotomy and **deep-brain stimulation** of subcortical nuclei.

About half of the patients with Parkinson's disease treated with long-term L-DOPA will develop motor fluctuations (including on–off phenomena) and dyskinesias at some point during the illness.

### 32.8.1.4 Differential diagnosis

The main differential diagnoses of Parkinson's disease are drug-induced parkinsonism, vascular parkinsonism, progressive supranuclear palsy, multisystem atrophy, corticobasal degeneration, dementia with Lewy bodies, Alzheimer's disease with parkinsonism and parkinsonism associated with frontotemporal degeneration.

### 32.8.1.5 Neuropsychiatric disorders in Parkinson's disease (Serra-Mestres and Mukhopadhyay, *s.d.*)

The most common neuropsychiatric disorders and symptoms in Parkinson's disease are depression, anxiety, psychosis, apathy, mild cognitive impairment, dementia and psychiatric and cognitive consequences of neurosurgery for Parkinson's disease.

#### Depression

Depression is the most common psychiatric problem in Parkinson's disease, occurring in up to 50% of cases (Cummings, 1992). The majority of patients suffer from minor depression or dysthymia. Approximately 20% suffer from major depressive episodes (Nuti *et al.*, 2004). The identification of depressive phenomena is complicated by the overlap of certain symptoms with those of Parkinson's disease proper, such as fatigue, psychomotor retardation, flat facial expression, impaired concentration and sleep disturbances. Patients with Parkinson's disease and depression appear more cognitively impaired than those without depression, especially in executive functions. Patients with Parkinson's disease with depression and dementia have increased mortality rates (Hughes *et al.*, 2004). Depression in Parkinson's disease increases functional disability (Weintraub *et al.*, 2005).

Antidepressants and electroconvulsive therapy (ECT) (which can also improve motor function) are effective for depression in Parkinson's disease, while cognitive behavioural therapy (CBT) has also proven helpful (Dobkin *et al.*, 2011). SSRIs and serotonin and noradrenalin reuptake inhibitors (SNRIs) are preferred to tricyclics, especially in elderly patients with cognitive impairment.

#### Anxiety

Up to 40% of patients with Parkinson's disease suffer from anxiety problems that are often co-morbid with depression. Generalised anxiety disorder may occur in 11% of patients, and panic disorder in 30% (Ehrt and Aarsland, 2005). Psychosocial factors and noradrenergic and serotonergic deficits have been proposed for its aetiology. In some patients, paroxysmal anxiety in the form of panic attacks may occur in anticipation of, or during, 'freezing' or 'off' episodes. Anxiety, as low mood, can fluctuate with the motor state.

Antidepressants and psychological interventions such as CBT may be effective.

### Psychosis

Psychotic phenomena occur in 30–40% of cases of Parkinson's disease (Ring and Serra-Mestres, 2002) and are mainly related to treatment with dopaminergic and/or anticholinergic drugs. When unrelated to the treatment for Parkinson's disease, they are generally associated with the onset of dementia. Visual hallucinations are the commonest psychotic phenomena in Parkinson's disease, occurring in approximately 20% of cases. Hallucinations in other sensory modalities are rare. Hallucinations can develop soon after the start of dopaminergic treatment (especially with dopamine agonists) but they can also occur after several years of treatment. Delusions are infrequent (6–10%) in Parkinson's disease and tend to appear two years and more after the initiation of treatment and when dosages of dopaminergic drugs are high. They are typically paranoid, but delusions of jealousy have been reported. Formal thought disorder is very rare.

If psychotic symptoms are caused by a confusional state or delirium, the appropriate treatment for the relevant aetiology must be given. The first approach to treatment of psychosis in Parkinson's disease is to attempt to reduce or rationalise the dose of dopaminergic drugs if possible. This will require close collaboration with the treating neurologist or physician. Typical antipsychotics are not recommended because of their side-effect profile, especially in respect of worsening of motor symptoms. There is evidence from randomised clinical trials for the efficacy of clozapine, even at small doses (French Clozapine Parkinson Study Group, 1999; Parkinson Study Group, 1999). However treatment with this drug is complicated by the necessity to strictly monitor the white cell count. There is evidence from only one randomised clinical trial on the efficacy of quetiapine in Parkinson's disease psychosis without worsening motor function (Ondo *et al.*, 2005). Clozapine and quetiapine, in this order, would seem to be the antipsychotics of choice in patients with Parkinson's disease (Miyasaki *et al.*, 2006). There is also some evidence that discontinuation of clozapine or quetiapine in patients with Parkinson's disease who were previously psychotic is associated with a high rate of relapse (rebound psychosis) (Fernández *et al.*, 2004).

### Apathy

Apathy, a frequent symptom, can be associated with depression. It has been defined as lack of motivation relative to previous level of functioning, diminished goal-directed behaviour, diminished goal-directed cognition, diminished concomitants of goal-directed behaviour, unchanging affect and lack of emotional responsivity (Starkstein, 2002). Apathy tends to be associated with cognitive impairment, especially with executive dysfunction, and is probably caused by dysfunction of mesocortical dopaminergic pathways (Ring and Serra-Mestres, 2002).

The treatment of apathy is challenging, especially in Parkinson's disease. In those cases where it is associated with depression, apathy can improve with antidepressant treatment. Dopamine-enhancing drugs, such as L-DOPA, and other dopaminergic drugs, such as bromocriptine or amantadine, or stimulants such as methylphenidate have been used in the treatment of apathy in other neuropsychiatric conditions with variable success (Marin *et al.*, 1995; Van Reekum *et al*, 2005), but there are no available randomised clinical trial data. There is some indication that cholinesterase inhibitors may be helpful, as they have been shown to improve apathy in patients with Alzheimer's disease.

### Cognitive impairment

Cognitive deficits are present in a significant proportion of patients, even at the time of diagnosis. These deficits are heterogeneous and may range from a mild cognitive disorder to frank dementia.

Mild cognitive impairment may be present in up to 36% of patients without dementia living in the community (Foltynie *et al.*, 2004) even in the early stages of Parkinson's disease. It is probably caused by disruption of fronto-subcortical circuits and of the mesocortical dopaminergic pathway

(Ring and Serra-Mestres, 2002). It presents with reduced speed of information processing (bradyphrenia), executive dysfunction and attentional problems, visuospatial dysfunction and retrieval-related memory problems.

Significant widespread cognitive impairment amounting to dementia occurs in 15–40% of patients with Parkinson's disease according to earlier studies (e.g. Aarsland *et al.*, 1996). New clinical diagnostic criteria for Parkinson's disease dementia were proposed in 2007 (Emre *et al.*, 2007) and the cut-off score in the Mini-Mental State Examination (MMSE) in relation to Parkinson's disease dementia was set at 26/30.

The mean annual decline on the MMSE in patients with Parkinson's disease who suffer from dementia is 2,3 points, similar to that of patients with Alzheimer's disease (Aarsland *et al.*, 2004). The risk of developing dementia increases with disease progression (Braak *et al.*, 2005). Dementia in Parkinson's disease is characterised by impairment of attention, memory, executive and visuo-spatial functions, as well as apathy, hallucinations and affective changes (Emre *et al.*, 2007).

NICE guidelines for Parkinson's disease (NICE, 2006) state that there is evidence of the clinical effectiveness and safety of acetylcholinesterase inhibitors in the treatment of Parkinson's disease dementia, for both cognitive impairment and psychosis.

## 32.8.2 Huntington's disease (Wild and Tabrizi, 2014)

Huntington's disease is a slowly progressive autosomal dominant neurodegenerative disorder associated with an expansion of the trinucleotide CAG (often called a CAG repeat) in the Huntington gene on Chromosome 4, encoding the protein huntingtin (MacDonald *et al.*, 1993). The abnormal protein contains an excess of glutamine residues. There is a direct correlation between the CAG repeat size and the age of onset: the larger the size of the repeat the earlier the onset of disease.

Onset is usually in adult life with a mean age of about 40 years, although juvenile onset and onset in the elderly are well described. Huntington's disease progresses gradually, with death occurring 15–20 years after onset. Worldwide prevalence is about 2,5 per 100 000 people.

Huntington's disease prominently affects the basal ganglia but is increasingly recognised as a whole-brain disease. Early on, the brain looks normal but later there is marked cortical atrophy with ventricular dilatation. There is severe atrophy of the caudate, and also the putamen, globus pallidus and substantia nigra. Histology reveals striatal neuronal loss and gliosis. There is selective depletion of medium spiny neurons.

### 32.8.2.1 Clinical features

Huntington's disease produces a wide range of presentations; the manifestations often change as the disease progresses. Key symptoms are a triad of motor (especially chorea), cognitive and psychiatric symptoms. Typically motor symptoms manifest first, although psychiatric and cognitive symptoms can predate the motor symptoms by many years. A definitive diagnosis is usually made when unequivocal motor abnormalities are seen.

Early motor signs are restlessness, hyperreflexia and fidgety movements of extremities during stress or when walking. Extrapyramidal signs are invariable. Chorea is seen in 90% of adult-onset patients with varying degrees of dystonia, parkinsonism and bradykinesia. A key problem is impairment of voluntary motor function with clumsiness, disturbances in fine control, gait disturbance and falls. Postural instability and ataxia are common, as are dysarthria and dysphagia, so it is essential to ask about swallowing symptoms. Death is often due to aspiration pneumonia.

Oculomotor abnormalities are often the earliest sign. Delayed saccade initiation with unsuppressible blinks, slow **saccades** and inability to suppress reflexive glances at novel stimuli are seen. Later, head thrusting is used to initiate saccades, pursuit is impaired and there is gaze impersistence.

Cognitive abnormalities are an invariable feature of Huntington's disease. The term 'dementia' may not be appropriate, as many functions remain intact even in advanced disease. Early cognitive changes include deterioration in executive functioning, representing disruption to frontostriatal circuits. Patients initially display impaired concentration and attention, poor planning and judgement, impulsive behaviour and difficulty in multi-tasking. Psychomotor slowing with apathy and loss of initiative make caring for patients difficult.

In contrast to other disease features, psychiatric problems are often reversible if treated. Psychiatric symptoms include disinhibition, irritability, conduct symptoms, impulsivity, depression, apathy and even psychosis. Regarding psychopathology in Huntington's disease:

- depression and anxiety are common and can make patients withdrawn with poor self-care
- irritability is frequent and some individuals become aggressive
- obsessions together with compulsions can be challenging
- psychosis, though well recognised, is relatively rare, while mania and hypomania are seen
- attempted suicide rates of more than 25% have been reported
- aggressive management of drug and alcohol problems is recommended as these compound disease symptoms
- although hypersexuality is often assumed to be common, is actually less prevalent than hyposexuality.

## 32.8.2.2 Clinical management

Huntington's disease patients are best managed by specialist multidisciplinary teams comprising clinical geneticists, neurologists, neuropsychiatrists, psychologists, nurse specialists, dieticians, physiotherapists and speech and language therapists.

### Psychiatric symptoms

Psychiatric symptoms are amenable to treatment and should, therefore, be actively managed. The SSRIs citalopram and mirtazapine appear particularly effective in the management of depression, especially if anxiety is a co-factor. Risperidone, olanzapine and quetiapine are useful for psychotic symptoms, severe anxiety and aggressive or impulsive behaviour and should be commenced at the lowest possible dose and titrated up slowly. Mood-stabilising drugs, such as valproate and carbamazepine, are useful for symptoms of mania. Benzodiazepines are useful for short-term anxiety or long-term agitation. Many patients benefit from CBT, particularly in early stages of the disease.

### Cognitive symptoms

Integrated care with the involvement of social services, the general practitioner and caregivers is essential for cognitive symptoms. A fairly common problem in practice is patients with little insight who insist that they are able to care for themselves. Formal neuropsychological and clinical assessments are important to help advise on optimum care.

### Motor symptoms

Chorea is hardly the most functionally disabling motor symptom, despite being a common feature. Anti-choreic medication should be used sparingly as no drug is particularly efficacious. Motor side effects may actually worsen functional impairment. For disabling chorea, sulpiride, olanzapine and risperidone are useful. Voluntary motor impairment and gait disturbance are difficult to treat but patients benefit from physiotherapy input. Falls tend to become a problem and walking aids and adapted wheelchairs become necessary. In the later stages, the chorea abates and patients become more rigid and dystonic. Here, anti-spasticity drugs such as baclofen and clonazepam have some efficacy, although none is greatly beneficial and the importance of safe bedding and good nursing become paramount.

Juvenile Huntington's disease patients and adults with parkinsonian features may benefit from treatment with levodopa.

### Speech and language

Dysarthria contributes to communication difficulties and as the disease advances, patients become mute. Early referral to speech and language therapists can maximise communication ability. Dysphagia and choking episodes are common, even early in the disease, and should prompt speech and language therapy referral.

**Other management issues in Huntington's disease**

Weight loss is common in Huntington's disease, and the aetiology is usually multifactorial, including poor nutritional intake, swallowing problems and increased resting energy expenditure. It is important that patients maintain their weight, as a slower disease progression is associated with a higher pre-morbid body mass index. Dentition contributes to co-morbidity in Huntington's disease and may worsen dysarthria and dysphagia. Motor symptoms can make dental care difficult but many dentists are able to treat such patients.

## 32.8.3 Wilson's disease (Svetel, *et al.*, 2009)

Wilson's disease or hepatolenticular degeneration is a rare autosomal recessive disease caused by mutation in the ATP7B gene, coding for a protein important for copper transport and the elimination of excess copper from the body (Bull *et al.*, 1993; Tanzi *et al.*, 1993). Since the mutated gene prevents the transport protein from functioning properly, copper accumulates in the liver, brain, kidneys and skeletal system.

### 32.8.3.1 Medical conditions associated with copper accumulation in Wilson's disease

- Kayser–Fleischer rings (KF rings), a pathognomonic sign, may be visible in the cornea of the eyes (either directly or on slit-lamp examination) as deposits of copper in a ring around the cornea. They are due to copper deposition in Descemet's membrane.
- Renal tubular acidosis leads to nephrocalcinosis (calcium accumulation in the kidneys), a weakening of bones, and occasionally amino-aciduria (Bull *et al.*, 1993).
- Cardiomyopathy is a rare but recognised problem that may lead to heart failure and cardiac arrhythmias (Bull *et al.*, 1993).
- Hypoparathyroidism leads to low calcium levels, infertility and habitual abortion (Bull *et al.*, 1993).

### 32.8.3.2 Neuropsychiatric symptoms

In 40% of the patients the first symptoms are related to the liver, in 40% they are neurologic and in 20% of the cases the disease begins with behavioural or psychiatric disorders, for example depression, phobias, compulsive and antisocial behaviour, schizophrenia-like psychosis (Bearn 1972). Specific neurological symptoms are often in the form of parkinsonism, with cogwheel rigidity, bradykinesia and postural instability being the most common parkinsonian features (Medalia and Scheinberg, 1989) with or without a typical hand tremor, masked facial expressions, slurred speech, ataxia or dystonia. A characteristic tremor described as 'wing-beating tremor' is encountered in many people with Wilson's disease; this is absent at rest but can be provoked by extending the arms (Ala *et al.*, 2007). Patients with Wilson's disease who are neurologically impaired often have cognitive deficits and psychiatric disturbances, while neurologically asymptomatic patients generally do not (Medalia and Scheinberg, 1989). Subtle signs can appear before the characteristic neurological features, including changes in behaviour, deterioration of school work or an inability to carry out activities of daily living (Ala *et al*, 2007). Behavioural and personality changes and affective disorders, including depression, are the most common psychiatric manifestations (Lishman, 1987). Substance abuse, catatonia and sexual preoccupation in Wilson's disease have also been reported. Psychiatric manifestations of Wilson's disease can be categorised into five groups: personality changes, affective disorders, psychosis, cognitive impairment and others (Akil and Brewer, 1995). Cognitive disturbances give rise to two categories that are not mutually exclusive: frontal lobe disorder (may present as impulsivity, impaired judgement, promiscuity, apathy and executive dysfunction with poor planning and decision making) and subcortical dementia (may present as slow thinking, memory loss and executive dysfunction, without signs of aphasia, apraxia or agnosia). Dening and Berrios (1990) note that schizophrenia-like psychosis, often described in case reports, is infrequent and the common psychiatric manifestations included personality change, depression and cognitive impairment. These often co-occur with neurological symptoms, but not with hepatic manifestations. Psychosis has been described at various points in the course of Wilson's disease and includes frank delusions and/or thought disorder or disorganised thinking. Cases have been reported of patients carrying a diagnosis of schizophrenia for years, prior to being diagnosed with Wilson's disease.

A study of 195 cases of Wilson's disease (Dening and Berrios, 1989) found that an organic condition had not been suspected in 50% of patients who were first seen by a psychiatrist, which might lead to diagnostic misinterpretation and inadequate treatment.

Wilson's disease is treated with medication that reduces copper absorption or removes the excess copper from the body, but occasionally a liver transplant is required. Delay in the diagnosis and institution of chelating therapy adversely affects the outcome. Two treatment approaches to psychiatric symptoms of Wilson's disease have been described. First, the primary treatment of Wilson's disease, namely chelating therapy, alone leads to an improvement in the psychiatric symptoms (Bachmann *et al*, 1989). Second, psychotropic medications or psychotherapy may be used to address specific psychiatric presentations independent of medical therapy for Wilson's disease.

### 32.8.4 Other movement disorders

#### 32.8.4.1 Essential tremor

Essential tremor is one of the most common movement disorders. It can occur at any age, but with bimodal peaks between the ages of 15–20 and 50–70 years. It is not associated with increased mortality.

#### 32.8.4.2 Restless legs syndrome

Restless legs syndrome consists of abnormal sensory feelings in the legs that occur at rest (e.g. in bed at night) and are relieved by moving the legs (e.g. walking around). It can be associated with periodic limb movements of sleep. It is a very common condition, which responds well to a low-dose dopaminergic therapy. Restless legs syndrome is more common in women than men and can begin at any age. Symptoms may progress over time and in some cases become disabling.

#### 32.8.4.3 Dystonias

Primary dystonia is a rare condition with the majority being of the adult-onset focal dystonias.

Primary generalised dystonia is associated with a DYT1 mutation, has an early onset, and typically begins in the legs, spreading to involve the whole body.

The frequency of secondary dystonias is difficult to estimate.

#### 32.8.4.4 Other parkinsonian syndromes

Multiple system atrophy is the commonest parkinsonian syndrome, making up about 10% of cases with parkinsonism, whilst corticobasal degeneration and progressive supranuclear palsy account for around 5% each. Onset of multiple system atrophy, progressive supranuclear palsy and dementia with Lewy bodies is typically in the sixth decade. Dementia with Lewy bodies becomes more prevalent with increasing age. These syndromes typically present with parkinsonism, often bilateral and symmetrical, with poor response to L-DOPA, as well as additional characteristic neurological features.

## 32.9 Neuropsychiatric aspects of multiple sclerosis and other white-matter disorders (Muhlert and Ron, 2014)

Multiple sclerosis and other white-matter disorders are a group of conditions that predominantly or exclusively affect the white matter.

They are subdivided into:

- demyelinating diseases: normally developed myelin is damaged by inflammatory, infective, ischaemic or toxic processes

- dysmyelinating and hypomyelinating diseases (other white-matter disorders): the process of myelination is abnormal or arrested.

## 32.9.1 Demyelinating diseases

Clinical features of demyelinating diseases are determined by:

- the acuteness of the clinical presentation
- whether the disease is monophasic or not
- single episode (e.g. acute disseminated encephalopathy, posterior reversible encephalopathy syndrome)
- recurrent or progressive (e.g. multiple sclerosis, cerebral autosomal dominant arteriopathy with subcortical infarcts and leuko-encephalopathy (CADASIL))
- localisation of lesions.

Cognitive impairment is common and is usually preceded or accompanied by other neurological symptoms, such as motor and sensory symptoms, epilepsy, myoclonus, ocular problems, impaired consciousness and paralysis.

## 32.9.2 Dysmyelinating and hypomyelinating disorders

Dysmyelinating and hypomyelinating disorders are characterised by abnormal or arrested myelination. They are usually inherited conditions with onset in early childhood. Most display non-neurological manifestations.

Dysmyelinating disorders are a group of inherited conditions, such as mucopolysaccharidoses and leukodystrophies, that usually have an onset in childhood.

Hypomyelinating disorders include prematurity and a number of rare hereditary conditions with early childhood onset, such as Pelizaeus-Merzbacher disease, spastic paraplegia and 18q syndrome.

## 32.9.3 Multiple sclerosis

Multiple sclerosis is the most common disabling neurological condition that affects young adults. Multiple sclerosis presents with a clinically isolated syndrome and tends to follow a course with relapses and remissions. The level of disability then typically enters a stage of sustained worsening: the secondary progressive stage. For some patients the disease progresses from onset; in these cases it is termed primary progressive. Multiple sclerosis is characterised by demyelinated plaques with glial scar formation and inflammatory reaction with T cells and macrophages. The inflammatory reaction is reversible and accounts for clinical remissions. The primary target of the autoimmune reaction is myelin, but axons, neurones and astrocytes are also affected.

### 32.9.3.1 Cognitive impairment in multiple sclerosis

Cognitive impairment affects 50-60% of patients with multiple sclerosis. Cognitive impairment tends to be more severe in those with advanced disease, but it may be present at onset. For the majority of patients, deficits are mild to moderate, although a small minority will present with severe cognitive impairment. Cognitive impairment is often overlooked, despite being associated with unemployment, greater care needs and social isolation.

Disease modifying treatments (e.g. beta interferon) may slow down cognitive impairment but evidence to date is insufficient. Acetylcholinesterase inhibitors are linked to better outcomes. Cognitive rehabilitation may lead to modest improvements on test performance

### 32.9.3.2 Affective disorders in multiple sclerosis

Depression and anxiety are common in multiple sclerosis; they have a profound impact on quality of life and also impair cognitive performance. The lifetime prevalence of major depression in multiple sclerosis is 50%. People with multiple sclerosis are also twice as likely as the general population to abuse alcohol, to experience bipolar affective disorder and to commit suicide.

Depression in multiple sclerosis responds to antidepressants (e.g. SSRIs) and/or CBT aimed at improving coping strategies.

**Table 32.7** Infectious causes of neuropsychiatric disease – direct effect on central nervous system

| Bacteria | Viruses | Parasites | Spirochaetes | Rickettsiae | Fungi |
|---|---|---|---|---|---|
| ▶ meningococcus<br>▶ streptococcus<br>▶ haemophilus influenzae<br>▶ tuberculosis<br>▶ leprosy<br>▶ mycoplasma pneumonia<br>▶ typhoid fever | ▶ arboviruses<br>▶ herpes viruses<br>▶ enteroviruses<br>▶ rabies | **Protozoans**<br>▶ malaria<br>▶ African trypanosomiasis<br>▶ toxoplasmosis<br>▶ amoebiasis<br>**Trematodes (flukes)**<br>▶ paragonimiasis,<br>▶ schistosomiasis<br>**Cestodes (tapeworms)**<br>▶ cysticercosis,<br>▶ hydatidosis<br>**Nematodes (roundworms)**<br>▶ ascariasis<br>▶ parastrongyliasis<br>▶ gnathostomiasis<br>▶ trichinosis | ▶ neurosyphilis<br>▶ Lyme disease<br>▶ leptospirosis<br>▶ louse-borne/ epidemic relapsing fever<br>▶ tick-borne/ endemic relapsing fever | ▶ epidemic/ louse-borne typhus<br>▶ endemic/ murine/flea-borne typhus<br>▶ scrub typhus<br>▶ Rocky Mountain spotted fever | ▶ cryptococcosis<br>▶ histoplasmosis<br>▶ aspergillosis<br>▶ coccidiomycosis<br>▶ candidiasis<br>▶ paracoccidiomycosis<br>▶ blastomycosis<br>▶ nocardiasis[1] |

[1]Nocardia are *Actinomycete* bacteria that are grouped with fungi because of their morphology and behaviour

**Source:** Solomon and Jung, 2014 (adapted)

### 32.9.3.3 Anxiety disorders in multiple sclerosis

Anxiety disorders (most commonly generalised anxiety disorder) are present in about a third of multiple sclerosis patients. The development of anxiety disorders is significantly related to patient's perception of increased psychosocial stressors and decreased social support. Anxious patients are more likely to be depressed, to drink to excess and to become suicidal.

### 32.9.3.4 Psychosis in multiple sclerosis

The prevalence of schizophrenia-like psychosis and delusional disorders is twice that of the general population (2–3% to 1,3%).

## 32.10 Neuropsychiatric aspects of central nervous system infections

Infectious organisms can play an important role in pathophysiology of neurodegenerative and neurobehavioural diseases. They may enter the brain within infected migratory macrophages, or they may cross the blood-brain barrier by the process of transcytosis or by intraneuronal transfer from peripheral nerves.

Psychiatric symptoms can be part of the clinical presentation of several systemic and central nervous system (CNS) infections. On the other hand, psychological stress can affect the function of the immune system and predict susceptibility for infectious diseases. These symptoms may be the initial presenting symptoms without neurological signs or symptoms, as seen in some cases of viral encephalitis. These symptoms could also be part of the clinical picture, as in cases of psychotic or mood symptoms secondary to toxoplasmosis and brucellosis. Neuropsychiatric complications can also occur several years after the infection, as in subacute sclerosing panencephalitis secondary to measles. Accumulated evidence has implicated a possible role of infectious diseases in the pathogenesis of psychiatric disorders such as schizophrenia and psychosis following the influenza virus and herpes simplex virus-1 (HSV-1). Neuropsychiatric adverse effects can occur due to drugs used for the treatment of infectious diseases (e.g. mefloquine and interferon-alpha). Reactivation of psychiatric symptoms can follow on from chronic, complicated and severe infections such as HIV. This can give rise to adjustment, anxiety and depressive disorders, but a direct effect on the CNS by the agent itself may also be a possible aetiological factor. Even a small focus of chronic infection can result in a psychiatric disorder with symptoms of subtle cognitive dysfunction, irritability, depression, psychosis and delirium. Occult infections are concealed infections that may occur anywhere in the body, and can be associated with various psychiatric symptoms. Examples include urinary tract infections, abscesses, sinusitis, chronic otitis, bronchiectasis, cholecystitis, parasitosis, osteomyelitis, endocarditis, sinusitis and subclinical systemic infections (such as tuberculosis and HIV). A wide range of psychiatric symptoms can occur in febrile illnesses, including disorganised thinking and disorientation, depression, mutism, and catatonia.

Patients who suffer from primary psychiatric disorders, especially mania and schizophrenia, are at an increased risk of contracting infections related to their high-risk behaviour and co-morbid substance abuse. Keep in mind that the co-occurrence of psychiatric symptoms and infectious diseases could also be totally incidental. To avoid unnecessary long-term psychiatric treatment and complications of possible misdiagnosis or delayed diagnosis of the primary condition, early identification of the underlying aetiology of secondary psychiatric symptoms is essential for appropriate early treatment of the primary condition that could be the cause of the psychiatric symptoms.

Clinicians should carefully consider the relevant aspects of patients' histories, including immune status, regions of origin and residence, travel, high-risk behaviour, occupation and recreational activities. They should also consider which infectious diseases are endemic in the local area and in the areas where the patient has travelled or resided.

A past history of brain injury or degeneration of all types renders patients more vulnerable to the effects of infectious diseases.

The relation between infectious diseases and psychiatric features can be summarised as follows:

- infectious diseases that cause psychiatric symptoms
- infectious diseases with a possible aetiological role for major psychiatric disorders
- psychiatric symptoms due to adverse effects of drugs used in the treatment of the infectious disease
- the primary psychiatric disorders can increase the risk of contracting infection
- psychiatric symptoms reactive to chronic and serious infections

This section is broadly divided into bacterial, viral, fungal and parasitic infections, followed by a section on the psychiatric side effects of antimicrobial drugs and on drug interactions with psychotropic medications.

## 32.10.1 Overview of central nervous system infections

**Table 32.8** Infectious causes of neuropsychiatric disease – indirect effect on central nervous system

| Toxin-mediated infectious diseases | Immune-mediated post-infectious conditions |
|---|---|
| ▸ tetanus<br>▸ diphtheria<br>▸ shigellosis | ▸ Guillain-Barré syndrome<br>▸ acute disseminated encephalomyelitis |

**Source:** Mufaddel *et al.*, 2014; Ferrando and Freyberg, 2008

## 32.10.2 Bacterial infections

Bacteria are unicellular organisms classified, according to the Gram stain, into Gram-positive and Gram-negative organisms. With the use of light microscopy, they can be divided into cocci and bacilli (rods). Infections caused by bacteria may be confined to a particular body organ or system, while other infections can affect several systems or the entire body. Under unusual circumstances, these infections may become systemic. Bacteraemia and septicaemia may follow on the initial infection. Cell wall-deficient bacteria (e.g. mycoplasma, chlamydia, borrelia and brucella) may play important roles in neurodegenerative and neurobehavioural diseases.

## 32.10.3 Viral infections

Viruses gain entry to the CNS through several mechanisms:

- they may replicate outside the CNS and then invade by haematogenous spread (e.g. enteroviruses)
- viral particles pass directly across the blood-brain barrier or through infected leukocytes (e.g. mumps, measles, herpes viruses) and then infect vascular endothelial cells
- other viruses invade through peripheral nerves (e.g. polio) and cranial nerves (e.g. herpes simplex virus)
- viruses may spread through the subarachnoid space leading to meningitis
- they may also spread directly or via inflammatory leukocytes through neural tissue to neurons and glial cells.

Most viruses that cause encephalitis can also cause meningitis. Psychiatric symptoms are very common in the acute phase of viral encephalitis and they are also common after recovery.

Occasionally, psychiatric symptoms without neurological symptoms can be the initial presentation of viral encephalitis. Psychiatric symptoms may occur as psychosis, catatonia, psychotic depression, or mania.

## 32.10.4 Fungal infections

The frequency of fungal infections has steadily increased, and is coincident with the growing number of immunosuppressed patients who survive for longer periods of time. The following have also contributed to the increased frequency of fungal infection:

- an aging population
- an increased number of malignancies
- the spread of HIV/Aids
- the use of immunosuppressive and cytotoxic drugs
- IV-catheters
- hyperalimentation
- illicit drug use
- extensive surgery
- the development of burn units.

CNS symptom development depends on the size and shape of the fungi. The smallest fungi have access to the cerebral microcirculation and infect the subarachnoid space. Large hyphae obstruct large and intermediate arteries giving rise to infarcts (e.g. aspergillosis). Fungi with pseudohyphae occlude small blood vessels producing small infarctions and micro-abscesses (e.g. candida). Most fungi, such as aspergillosis, mucormycosis and candidiasis, are opportunistic. Others (e.g. coccidioidomycosis, cryptococcosis) are pathogenic, irrespective of the hosts' defences.

## 32.10.5 Parasitic infections

Protozoa are unicellular eukaryotic organisms and are more complex than bacteria. In order to be transmitted to a new host, some protozoa transform into cyst forms, while others are transmitted by an arthropod vector. Certain parasites are capable of selectively altering host behaviour to enhance their transmission.

## 32.10.6 Spirochaetal infections

With the advent of epidemic proportions of HIV infection, spirochaetal infections are often not thought of, or completely ignored, as a cause of

**Table 32.9** Bacterial infections that can be associated with neuropsychiatric symptoms

| Infection | Clinical features | Neuropsychiatric symptoms | Diagnosis |
|---|---|---|---|
| **Paediatric autoimmune neuropsychiatric disorders associated with streptococcal infections (PANDAS)**<br>Group A beta-haemolytic streptococci | ▶ abrupt onset<br>▶ episodic course<br>▶ sudden and dramatic exacerbations<br>▶ common neurological signs include motor abnormalities such as choreiform movements | ▶ distractibility<br>▶ impulsivity<br>▶ hyperactivity<br>▶ separation anxiety<br>▶ enuresis<br>▶ deterioration in handwriting<br>▶ increased risk of OCD, Tourette's syndrome and tic disorder | ▶ rapid increase in anti-streptococcal (ASO) titre<br>▶ throat culture |
| **Tuberculosis meningitis**<br>tubercular bacillus | ▶ fever<br>▶ generalised malaise<br>▶ headache<br>▶ neck stiffness<br>▶ encephalopathy<br>▶ focal neurological signs | ▶ fatigue<br>▶ personality change<br>▶ confusion | ▶ N.B. presence of HIV<br>▶ chest X-ray<br>▶ CSF – decreased glucose<br>▶ increased protein<br>▶ increased WBCs<br>▶ MRI scan |
| **Bacterial meningitis** | ▶ headache<br>▶ nausea<br>▶ vomiting<br>▶ confusion<br>▶ neck stiffness<br>▶ lethargy<br>▶ apathy | ▶ changes in personality, motivation and cognition | ▶ CSF low glucose<br>▶ high protein<br>▶ high WBCs with staining of responsible causative organism |
| **Bacterial abscess** | ▶ headache<br>▶ fever<br>▶ focal neurological deficits | ▶ personality change<br>▶ seizures<br>▶ encephalopathy<br>▶ affective disorder<br>▶ cognitive impairment<br>▶ psychosis<br>▶ aggression | ▶ CT and MRI brain scans |

**Source:** Mufaddel *et al.*, 2014; Ferrando and Freyberg, 2008

intracranial infections leading to unnecessary morbidity and mortality.

## 32.11 Neuropsychiatric aspects of headaches

Headache is a symptom and not a disease. It is one of the commonest clinical symptoms, presenting in more than 70% of the Western population. However, its diagnosis is complicated by the complex anatomy and physiology of the head and neck, the confusing nomenclature of headache syndromes and the host of psychosocial factors that influence the manifestation, severity and response to pain (Kaplan and Sadock, 1995).

The true prevalence of headaches in general is not known, as most sufferers do not present

**Table 32.10** Viral infections that can be associated with neuropsychiatric symptoms[1]

| Infection | Clinical features | Neuropsychiatric symptoms | Diagnosis |
|---|---|---|---|
| **Herpes simplex virus (HSV)**<br>HSV-1<br>HSV-2 | ▶ stomatitis<br>▶ genital herpes<br>▶ conjunctivitis<br>▶ encephalitis<br>▶ systemic infections in the immunocompromised | ▶ delirium<br>▶ personality change<br>▶ seizures<br>▶ psychosis<br>▶ hypomania<br>▶ Kluver-Bucy syndrome | ▶ HSV DNA by PCR |
| **Epstein-Barr virus (EBV)**<br>EBV – one of the herpes viruses | ▶ infectious mononucleosis: headache<br>▶ fatigue<br>▶ sore throat<br>▶ cervical LNs<br>▶ splenomegaly<br>▶ hepatitis | ▶ chronic fatigue syndrome<br>▶ dysthymia<br>▶ depressive disorder | ▶ atypical WBCs in peripheral smear<br>▶ positive Paul-Bunnell reaction |
| **Cytomegalovirus (CMV)**<br>CMV – one of the herpes viruses | ▶ generally asymptomatic, can mimic symptoms of infectious mononucleosis<br>▶ fever<br>▶ hepatitis | ▶ depressive disorder<br>▶ dementia | ▶ negative Paul-Bunnell reaction<br>▶ PCR<br>▶ direct immunofluorescence<br>▶ characteristic intracellular inclusions |
| **Measles**<br>paramyxovirus | ▶ two phases: catarrhal stage and the exanthematous stage | ▶ encephalomyelitis following infection, with SSPE = behaviour change<br>▶ cognitive impairment<br>▶ myoclonic jerks | ▶ clinical diagnosis |
| **Rabies**<br>RNA virus of *lyssavirus* genus | ▶ initial phase: fever, hyperaesthesia at site of inoculation excitatory phase: hydrophobia<br>▶ paralytic phase: generalised flaccid paralysis | ▶ generalised anxiety<br>▶ **melancholia** | ▶ serology for immunoglobulins |

[1] See Chapter 33: HIV and mental health, for a discussion of HIV diseases and Chapter 30: Psychogeriatrics, for Prion disease.

**Source:** Mufaddel *et al.*, 2014; Ferrando and Freyberg, 2008

for treatment. Although some headaches, such as cluster headaches, are more common in men, headaches are generally commoner in women. The two commonest types of headaches are tension and migraine headaches (Kaplan and Sadock, 1995). Although these are highly prevalent they are easily overlooked and underestimated because they are not 'dramatic' (World Health Organization, 2008).

The most important tool in making a diagnosis is eliciting a detailed and comprehensive history. It is necessary to obtain information about the location of the pain, its quality, the time course (duration, frequency and changes over time within and across headache episodes), age of onset, precipitating, relieving or exacerbating factors and associated physical and

**Table 32.11** Fungal infections that can be associated with neuropsychiatric symptoms

| Infection | Clinical features | Neuropsychiatric symptoms | Diagnosis |
|---|---|---|---|
| **Cryptococcosis**<br>cryptococcus | ▶ headache<br>▶ cerebellar signs<br>▶ cranial nerve deficits<br>▶ motor deficits.<br>This pathogen has a predilection for the subarachnoid space. Cryptococcus is the most common form of fungal meningitis. | ▶ irritability to psychosis<br>▶ lethargy to coma | ▶ serological testing reveals cryptococcal antigen in serum, CSF or both 90% of the time. |
| **Candidiasis**<br>*Candida albicans* | Symptoms are nonspecific:<br>▶ confusion,<br>▶ drowsiness,<br>▶ lethargy and headache.<br>May cause meningitis, microabscesses, microabscesses or vasculitis | Psychiatric symptoms occur from the 'toxic' effects of fungemia or from direct invasion of the CNS | |

**Source:** Mufaddel *et al.*, 2014; Ferrando and Freyberg, 2008

psychological symptoms. Also important are details of co-morbid medical and psychiatric illnesses, family history of headaches, concomitant medication use or cessation (withdrawal headaches) and acute or chronic stressors. A detailed and thorough physical examination, guided by the history elicited and followed by relevant medical investigations will facilitate the establishment of an appropriate diagnosis (Kaplan and Sadock, 1995).

Psychological factors such as psychological stressors, personality style, conditioning and psychodynamic issues play a role in the aetiology of migraine and tension headaches. Psychiatric disorders such as depression, anxiety, somatic symptom disorder and personality disorders may be co-morbid with headaches and impact on the course, treatment and prognosis of headaches (Shulman, 1991).

## 32.11.1 Classification of headaches

The International Headache Society classifies headaches into three broad categories:

- primary headaches, such as migraine, tension-type headache and trigeminal autonomic cephalgia
- secondary headaches, such as those attributable to a head or neck injury, infection, substance use or substance withdrawal, a psychiatric disorder
- painful cranial neuropathies, other facial pains and other headaches (International Headache Society, 2013).

The classification offers a hierarchical approach to headaches, with full sets of diagnostic criteria and minimum numbers and frequencies of headaches described for each headache subtype. Patients may experience more than one type of headache. Both headaches and psychiatric disorders are common, therefore frequent co-existence by chance may occur. However, the International Headache Society formally recognises headache attributed to somatisation disorder (a category previously found in the DSM IV-TR but not included in the DSM-5) or to a psychotic disorder (International Headache Society, 2013). Somatisation disorder is included under the diagnostic category of somatic symptom disorder in the DSM-5. Headaches may be classified under the latter category or the categories of psychological factors affecting other medical conditions.

**Table 32.12** Parasitic infections that can be associated with neuropsychiatric symptoms

| Infection | Clinical features | Neuropsychiatric symptoms | Diagnosis |
|---|---|---|---|
| **Cysticercosis** *taenia solium* | Neurocysticercosis (NCC) is the most frequent and widely disseminated human neuroparasitosis.<br>Clinical features are determined in part by the number of cysticerci, the location in the CNS, and the intensity of the host immune inflammatory response. Most frequent manifestation of NCC is seizures. | ▶ dementia<br>▶ other cognitive dysfunction<br>▶ a broad spectrum of other psychiatric manifestations | Rests on a high index of suspicion.<br>Neuro-imaging – MRI is superior to CT given its ability to demonstrate cysticerci and the inflammatory response.<br>Positive immunological CSF tests:<br>complement fixation<br>indirect immunofluorescence<br>passive hemagglutination<br>ELISA.<br>CSF may show an inflammatory response with elevated protein and pleocytosis. |
| **Toxoplasmosis** *toxoplasma gondii* | zPrimary toxoplasmosis infection during pregnancy may cause severe damage to the foetus, including microcephaly, hydrocephalus, encephalitis, mental retardation, seizures, blindness, and death. | ▶ disorientation<br>▶ anxiety<br>▶ depression<br>▶ schizophreniform psychoses<br>▶ cognitive impairment<br>▶ delirium<br>▶ dementia | Magnetic resonance scanning reveals toxoplasma abscesses as areas of increased signal intensity on T2 – weighted or FLAIR imaging, which typically show ring enhancement with gadolinium. The CSF may be normal or may display a mild lymphocytic pleocytosis and a mildly elevated total protein. Polymerase chain reaction assay for toxoplasma DNA is generally positive. Serologic testing may or may not be helpful |
| **Malaria** *plasmodium* species | Cerebral malaria, the most catastrophic complication of malaria.<br>Fever, headache, myalgia.<br>Focal signs, such as hemiparesis, may occur, but are uncommon. Rapidly progresses to seizures and coma with decerebrate posturing | ▶ disorientation<br>▶ stupor<br>▶ coma or even psychosis | Peripheral blood smear |

**Source:** Mufaddel *et al.*, 2014; Ferrando and Freyberg, 2008

**Table 32.13** Spirochaetal infections that can be associated with neuropsychiatric symptoms

| Infection | Clinical features | Neuropsychiatric symptoms | Diagnosis |
|---|---|---|---|
| **Syphilis** *treponema pallidum* | Primary stage: hard chancre, regional lymphadenopathy<br>Secondary stage: fever, malaise, arthralgia, sore throat, generalised lymphadenopathy, maculopapular rash, mucous patches, snail-track ulcers<br>Tertiary (late) stage: gummas, aortitis, neurosyphilis | neurosyphilis (general paralysis of the insane): symptoms similar to Alzheimer's disease or commonly frontal lobe syndrome, progressive cognitive decline, seizures, personality change, encephalopathy | Dark ground microscopy, serological, CSF examination for evidence of neurosyphilis, chest X-ray |

**Source:** Mufaddel *et al.*, 2014; Ferrando and Freyberg, 2008

### 32.11.2 Migraine

Migraines are common and carry high socio-economic and personal impact. The Global Burden of Disease Study 2010 ranked migraine as the third most prevalent disorder and the seventh-highest specific cause of disability (Murray *et al.*, 2012).

The International Headache Society defines migraines as a 'recurrent headache disorder manifesting in attacks lasting 4–72 hours. Typical characteristics of the headache are unilateral location, pulsating quality, moderate or severe intensity, aggravation by routine physical activity and association with nausea and or photophobia and phonophobia' (International Headache Society, 2013). Migraines may also be accompanied by auras (migraine with aura is also called classical migraine) characterised by 'unilateral, fully reversible visual, sensory or other central nervous system symptoms that usually develop gradually and are usually followed by headache and associated migraine symptoms' (International Headache Society, 2013) An aura refers to neurological symptoms that generally precede the headache but may begin after the pain commences or continue into the headache phase. Auras need not occur in every migraine episode, even in migraine with aura. Visual auras (e.g. zigzag figure spreading across visual fields, scotomas) are the commonest, and occur in more than 90% of patients with migraine with aura. Next in frequency are sensory disturbances, such as pins and needles affecting one side of the face or body and numbness. Less frequently, speech disturbances, such as aphasias, and motor weakness (hemiplegic migraine) occur. Auras of these different types usually follow each other in the order 'visual-sensory-aphasia' or in reverse order. They generally last an hour, except for motor symptoms, which may persist for longer.

Migraine arising from the basilar artery may be accompanied by brainstem symptoms such as dysarthria, vertigo, tinnitus, hyperacusis, diplopia, ataxia and a decreased level of consciousness (International Headache Society, 2013). Treatment requires the avoidance of trigger factors, learned control over the autonomic nervous system to prevent or abort attacks and pharmacotherapy. Most drugs act on the serotonergic receptor subtypes. Prophylactic treatment is indicated when more than two attacks occur per month or attacks are disabling (Kaplan and Sadock, 1995).

#### 32.11.2.1 Tension-type headache

Tension-type headaches (TTH) are very common, with a lifetime prevalence in the general population reported to be as high as 78% (International Headache Society, 2013). They are more common in women and the peak age of onset is between 20–40 years. Although headaches may occur daily and sometimes last for years, few patients seek medical attention (Kaplan and Sadock, 1995). Tension-type headaches are characterised by bilateral pressing or tightening of pericranial muscles without associated nausea, although photophobia and phonophobia may be present. The pain does not increase with routine physical activity. Although previously thought to be psychogenic in origin, recent studies suggest a neurobiological basis, at least for the moderate-severe subtypes. Tension-type headaches may be frequent or infrequent and acute or chronic in nature (International Headache Society, 2013). Most patients treat themselves with rest, hot or cold packs, and non-prescription analgesics. Frequent or disabling headaches may respond to low-dose tricyclic antidepressants, benzodiazepines (muscle relaxant) and physical therapies (Kaplan and Sadock, 1995).

#### 32.11.2.2 Trigeminal autonomic cephalalgia

Trigeminal autonomic cephalalgia (TAC or cluster headaches) occur in cluster periods lasting for weeks or months and, except for the chronic subtype, are separated by periods of remission lasting months or years (International Headache Society, 2013).

According to the International Headache Society, cluster headaches are characterised by 'attacks of severe, strictly unilateral pain which is orbital, supraorbital, temporal or in any combination of these sites, lasting 15–180 minutes and occurring from once every other day to eight times a day. The pain is associated with ipsilateral conjunctival injection, lacrimation, nasal congestion, rhinorrhea, forehead and facial sweating, miosis, ptosis and/or eyelid oedema and/or with restlessness or agitation' (International Headache Society, 2013). The pain may be excruciating: patients are usually unable to lie down and thus resort to pacing the floor. Pain usually recurs on the same side of the head during an individual cluster period. Age at onset is usually 20–40 years and men are three times more likely to suffer from cluster headaches than women (International Headache Society, 2013). Cluster headaches are treated almost exclusively pharmacologically; behavioural therapies are ineffective. Prophylaxis may also be utilised (Kaplan and Sadock, 1995).

#### 32.11.2.3 Secondary headache: medication-overuse headache

Medication-overuse headache is a common and debilitating disorder. It is characterised by the generation, perpetuation and persistence of headache caused by the frequent and excessive use of symptomatic drugs (International Headache Society, 2013). Medication-overuse headache was previously referred to as rebound or drug-induced headache. Overuse is defined in terms of treatment days per month and depends on the drug. Medication-overuse headache may complicate each type of headache and can be caused by all the drugs employed for headache treatment. Management of medication-overuse headache focuses on withdrawal of the overused drugs and detoxification, which help to stop the chronicity of the headache and improve the patient's responsiveness to acute or prophylactic drugs (Negro and Martelletti, 2011).

### 32.11.3 Headaches and psychiatric co-morbidity

Although the average headache patient does not have a psychiatric disorder, it is important to address psychological patterns such as headache-relevant stressors, coping strategies and beliefs that impact upon the headache. Assessing and monitoring levels of stress, cognitive and behavioural coping strategies, emotional reactivity and dysfunctional beliefs about headaches, personal control over headaches and headache-related disability are worthy of exploration and attention in clinical management (Shulman, 1991).

Although headache has been associated with psychiatric illness in the medical literature for more than a century, the relationship remains poorly understood and under-researched. Psychiatric co-morbidity is common among headache patients who present for treatment, especially in specialist settings. The presence of a psychiatric disorder complicates headache management and portends a poorer prognosis for the treatment of headache. Patients with migraine and tension-type headache have a higher prevalence of psychiatric illness than individuals with no history of recurrent headache. Affective disorders are three times more common among migraine sufferers than in the general population, with the prevalence increasing in clinical populations (Lake *et al.*, 2005).

Women are significantly more likely than men to receive lifetime diagnoses of both migraine and major depression by the age of 30. Longitudinal data indicate that women are four times more likely to develop migraine and two times more likely to develop major depression (Breslau *et al.*, 1994b; Breslau *et al.*, 1994a). Epidemiological and clinical research shows associations between depressive, bipolar and anxiety disorders and migraine as well as TTH. Although the exact relationship between migraine and mood disorders is unclear, it is unlikely that depression and anxiety are secondary to the burden of disease or that psychiatric distress causes the headache. Epidemiological genetic studies link anxiety, depression and migraine across generations. There is also evidence that headache can be a manifestation of somatoform (DSM IV-TR) disorder, with headache representing one of several medically unexplained somatic symptoms. Headache sufferers are at risk of substance abuse and dependence with nicotine dependence and illicit drug use significantly more common in migraineurs (Lake *et al.*, 2005). Conversely, medication-overuse headaches are increasing in prevalence. Prevalence ranges from a simple overuse of analgesics to a more complex pattern of overuse caused by behavioural factors such as the search for sedation, altered consciousness and wilful disregard of prescription guidelines (Saper *et al.*, 2005).

Increasing evidence implicates neuropathic mechanisms linked to the cortico-limbic system, which suggests an integrated relationship between migraine or pain and psychiatric disturbance in susceptible individuals (Lake *et al.*, 2005).

Personality disorder has been less extensively researched in relation to headache. However, significant headaches are reported by almost 60% of patients with personality disorder who present to emergency departments (Hogarty, 1993). Borderline personality disorder may be disproportionately common amongst migraine patients. In one study of migraine sufferers with borderline personality disorder, patients were more likely to be female, suffer more severe and disabling headaches, have a higher prevalence of self-reported depression and medication-overuse headache and a poorer response to pharmacological treatments (Rothrock *et al.*, 2007). Due to their impulsivity and propensity to abuse substances, patients with borderline personality disorder would benefit from specific management guidelines that address their special needs (Saper and Lake, 2002).

The presence of a co-morbid psychiatric illness adversely influences treatment outcomes and the prognosis for headache. There is emerging evidence that behavioural and psychological risk factors are more strongly associated with the progression of headache from episodic to chronic and daily than with analgesic overuse and abuse (Lake *et al.*, 2005). There is currently no evidence that treating depression or anxiety per se improves headache outcomes. However, there is evidence that optimal outcomes are achieved when multi-modal, multidisciplinary approaches are used. Differential headache outcomes have been shown to be related to treatment modalities that are appropriate to the co-morbid psychiatric disorder (Lake *et al.*, 2005). Significantly superior outcomes have been shown when behavioural treatment is combined with pharmacotherapy (Holroyd *et al.*, 2001). Patients with headaches, especially of a chronic nature, benefit from regular re-evaluation, education, reassurance as well as setting reasonable expectations for response. The aim should be to control pain to tolerable levels while optimising social, occupational and personal functioning.

Tricyclic antidepressants were first shown to be effective in preventing headaches in 1964 and have become a standard modality in headache prevention. A recent systematic review and meta-analysis (Jackson *et al.*, 2010) concluded that they are effective in preventing migraine and tension-type headache and are more effective than SSRIs, although their side-effect profile is worse than that of the SSRIs. Moreover, the effectiveness of the tricyclic antidepressants appeared to increase over time (Jackson *et al.*, 2010). The analgesic effect of tricyclic antidepressants is independent of its antidepressant effect and occurs at a lower dose. Doses of amitryptiline should be started at low doses of 10-25 mg/day and titrated slowly until optimum control is achieved or side effects preclude higher doses.

Note: should there be co-morbid depression, low doses of amitryptiline may not be the treatment of choice (Chetty *et al.*, 2012, Yudofsky and Hales, 2008).

## Conclusion

Rapid and major advances in the field of neurosciences will contribute to an improved understanding of the pathophysiology of brain disorders. This in turn will pave the way for improved therapeutic options.

However, good clinical practice requires a focus on treating *patients* as opposed to *diseases*. While advances in biological psychiatry enhance the understanding of the psychiatric sequelae of brain diseases, psychosocial factors are being increasingly recognised as playing a pivotal role in the initiation, maintenance, response to treatment, course and prognosis of a growing number of conditions that were traditionally regarded as being purely 'biomedical' in nature. The principles underlying neuropsychiatric practice are therefore relevant to the holistic and optimum assessment and management of both brain and non-brain-related disorders.

# References


Aarsland D, Andersen K, Larsen JP, Perry R, Wentzel-Larsen T, Lolk A, Kragh-Sørensen P (2004) The rate of cognitive decline in Parkinson's disease. *Archives of Neurology* 61: 1906–11

Aarsland D, Tandberg E, Larsen JP, Cummings JL (1996) Frequency of dementia in Parkinson's disease. *Archives of Neurology* 53: 538–42

Achte KA, Lonnqvist J, Hillbom E (1970) Suicides of war brain-injured veterans. *Psychiatrica Fennica* 1: 231–9

Akil M, Brewer GJ (1995) Psychiatric and behavioral abnormalities in Wilson's disease. *Advances in Neurology* 65: 171-78

Ala A, Walker AP, Ashkan K, Dooley JS, Schilsky ML (2007) Wilson's disease. *The Lancet* 369: 397–408

Alexopoulos GS, Meyers BS, Young RC, Campbell S, Silbersweig D, Charlson M (1997) 'Vascular depression' hypothesis. *Archives of General Psychiatry* 10: 915–22

Algreeshah FS, Benbadis SR (2013) Psychiatric disorders associated with epilepsy. *Medscape Medical News* http://emedicine.medscape.com/article/1186336-overview (Accessed 8 June 2014.)

Annegers JF, Grabow JD, Groover RV, Laws ER Jr, Elveback LR, Kurland LT (1980) Seizures after head trauma: A population study. *Neurology* 30: 683–9

Bachmann H, Lössner J, Kühn HJ, Biesold D, Siegemund R, Kunath B, Willgerodt H, Teichmann B, Wieczorek V, Mühlau G (1989) Long-term care and management of Wilson's disease in the GDR. *European Neurology* 29 (6): 301–30

Barker RA, Williams-Gray CH, Breen DP (2014) *Classification and Epidemiology of Movement Disorders.* http://www.ebrainjnc.com/learning/-- an e-learning resource by the British Neuropsychiatric Association, October

Bearn AG (1972) Wilson's disease. In: Stanbury JB, Wyngaarden JB, Fredrickson DS (Eds). *The metabolic basis of inherited diseases* (3rd edition). New York: McGraw-Hill

Benbadis SR (2013) Psychogenic nonepileptic seizures. *Medscape Reference - Drugs, Diseases and Procedures.* Available at: http://emedicine.medscape.com/article/1184694-overview (Accessed 19 January 2015.)

Benson DF (1991) The Geschwind syndrome. *Advances in Neurology* 55: 411–21

Blum D (1999) *Total impact of epilepsy: Biological, psychological, social, and economic aspects.* Available at: http://www.thebarrow.org/Education_And_Resources/Barrow_Quarterly/204913 (Accessed 19 January 2015.)

Braak H, Rüb U, Jansen Steur EN, Del Tredici K, de Vos R (2005) Cognitive status correlates with neuropathologic stage in Parkinson disease. *Neurology* 64: 1404–10

Breslau J, Lipton RB, Stewart WF, Schulz R, Welch KM (1994a). Joint 1994 Wolff Award Presentation. Migraine and major depression: a longitudinal study. *Headache,* 34: 387–93

Breslau N, Merikangas K, Bowden CL. (1994b) Co-morbidity of migraine and major affective disorders. *Neurology,* 44: S17–22

Bull PC, Thomas GR, Rommens JM, Forbes JR, Cox DW (1993) The Wilson disease gene is a putative copper transporting P-type ATPase similar to the Menkes gene. *Nature Genetics* 5: 327–37

Chetty S, Baalbergen E, Bhigjee AI, Kamerman P, Ouma J, Raath R, Raff M, Salduker S (2012) Clinical practice guidelines for management of neuropathic pain: Expert panel recommendations for South Africa. *South African Medical Journal* 102: 312–25

Cummings JL (1992) Depression in Parkinson's disease: A review. *American Journal of Psychiatry* 149: 443–54

Cummings JL, Trimble MR. (2002) *Neuropsychiatry and Behavioral Neurology,* Washington, DC: American Psychiatric Publishing

David AS, Fleminger S, Kopelman MD, Lovestone S, Mellers JDC (2009) *Lishman's Organic Psychiatry - A Textbook of Neuropsychiatry.* United Kingdom: Wiley-Blackwell

Dening TR, Berrios GF (1989) Wilson's disease. Psychiatric symptoms in 195 cases. *Archives of General Psychiatry* 46: 1126–34

Dening TR, Berrios GE (1990) Wilson's disease: A longitudinal study of psychiatric symptoms. *Biological Psychiatry* 28(3): 255–65

Dobkin RD, Menza M, Allen LA, Gara MA, Mark MH, Tiu J, Bienfait KL, Friedman J (2011) Cognitive-behavioral therapy for depression in Parkinson's disease: A randomized, controlled trial. *American Journal of Psychiatry* 168: 1066–74

Ehrt U, Aarsland D (2005) Psychiatric aspects of Parkinson's disease. *Current Opinion in Psychiatry* 18: 335–41

Emre M, Aarsland D, Brown R, Burn DJ, Duyckaerts C, Mizuno Y, Broe GA, Cummings J, Dickson DW, Gauthier S, Goldman J, Goetz C, Korczyn A, Lees A, Levy R, Litvan I, McKeith I, Olanow W, Poewe W, Quinn N, Sampaio C, Tolosa E, Dubois B. (2007) Clinical diagnostic criteria for dementia associated with Parkinson's disease. *Movement Disorders* 22: 1689–707

Engel JJ, Rocha LL (1992) Interictal behavioral disturbances: a search for molecular substrates. *Epilepsy Research* Suppl, 9: 341–9

Fernández HH, Trieschmann ME, Okun, MS (2004) Rebound psychosis: Effect of discontinuation of antipsychotics in Parkinson's disease. *Movement Disorders* 19: 831–3

Ferrando SJ, Freyberg Z (2008) Neuropsychiatric Aspects of Infectious Diseases. *Critical Care* 24: 889–919

Fleminger S, Burns A (1993) The delusional misidentification syndromes in patients with and without evidence of organic cerebral disorder: A structured review of case reports. *Biological Psychiatry* 33: 22–32

Fleminger S, Demjaha A (2014) *The assessment of traumatic brain injury*. http://www.psychiatrycpd.org/ - CPD Online from Royal College of Psychiatrists, November

Fleminger S, Leigh E, Eames P, Langrell L, Nagraj R, Logsdail S (2005) HoNOS-ABI: A reliable outcome measure of neuropsychiatric sequelae to brain injury? *Psychiatry Bulletin* 29: 53–5

Foltynie T, Brayne C, Robbins TW, Barker RA (2004) The cognitive ability of an incident cohort of Parkinson's patients in the UK: The CamPaIGN study. *Brain* 127: 550–60

Folstein M, Folstein S, McHugh P (1975) Mini-Mental State Examination: a practical method for grading the cognitive state of patients for the clinician. *Journal of Psychiatric Research* 12: 189–198

French Clozapine Parkinson Study Group (1999) Clozapine in drug-induced psychosis in Parkinson's disease. *The Lancet* 353: 2041–2

Harris ED, Barraclough B (1997) Suicide as an outcome for mental disorders: A meta-analysis. *British Journal of Psychiatry* 170: 205–28

Hogarty, A. (1993) The prevalence of migraine in borderline personality disorder. *Headache* 33: 271

Holroyd KA, O'Donnell, FJ, Stensland M, Lipchik GL, Cordingley GE, Carlson BW (2001) Management of chronic tension-type headache with tricyclic antidepressant medication, stress management therapy, and their combination: a randomised controlled trial. *Journal of the American Medical Association* 285: 2208–15

House A (1987) Depression after stroke. *British Medical Journal* 294: 76–8

Hughes TA, Ross HF, Mindham RH, Spokes EG (2004) Mortality in Parkinson's disease and its association with dementia and depression. *Acta Neurologica Scandinavica* 110: 118–23

Huppert FA, Brayne C, Gill C, Paykel ES, and Beardsall L (1995) CAMCOG-A concise neuropsychological test to assist dementia diagnosis: socio-demographic determinants in an elderly population sample. *Journal of Clinical Psychology* 34: 529–41

International Headache Society (2013) The International Classification of Headache Disorders, 3rd edition (beta version). *Cephalalgia* 33: 629–808. Quotations on pages 636 and 637 reproduced with permission from Sage Publications Ltd.

International League Against Epilepsy (1981) Proposal for revised clinical and electroencephalographic classification of epileptic seizures. From the Commission on Classification and Terminology of the International League Against Epilepsy. *Epilepsia* 22(4): 489-501

Jackson LJ, Shimeall W, Sessums L, Dezee KJ, Becher D, Diemer M, Berbano E, O'Malley PG (2010) Tricyclic antidepressants and headaches: Systematic review and meta-analysis. *British Medical Journal*. Available at: DOI: http://dx.doi.org/10.1136/bmj.c5222

Jones HB (2006) Intractable epilepsy and patterns of psychiatric comorbidity. *Advances in Neurology* 97

Kanner AM (2009) Suicidality and epilepsy: A complex relationship that remains misunderstood and underestimated. *Epilepsy Currents* 9: 63–6

Kaplan HI, Sadock BJ (1995) *Comprehensive Textbook of Psychiatry*. Maryland: Williams & Wilkins.

Koch HJ (2013) Psychocardiology: the spectrum of stress in the genesis of heart disease: A point of view. *Research Reports in Clinical Cardiology* 4: 153–157

Lake AE, Rains JC, Penzien DB, Lipchik GL (2005) Headache and psychiatric comorbidity: Historical context, clinical implications, and research relevance. *Headache* 45: 493–506

Levin HS, High WM, Goethe KE, M, Kalisky Z, Gary HE (1987) The neurobehavioral rating scale: Assessment of the behavioural sequelae of head injury by the clinician. *Journal of Neurology, Neurosurgery and Psychiatry* 50:183–193

Lishman WA (1987) *Organic psychiatry*. London, England: Blackwell Science Publication

Lishman WA (1988) Physiogenesis and psychogenesis in the 'post-concussional syndrome'. *British Journal of Psychiatry* 153: 460–9

Luria, AR (1976) *Cognitive development, its cultural and social foundations*. Cambridge: Harvard University Press

Luria, AR (1980) *Higher cortical functions in man*. New York: Basic Books

MacDonald ME, Ambrose CM, Duyao MP, Myers RH, Lin C, Srinidhi L *et al*., (1993) A novel gene containing a trinucleotide repeat that is expanded and unstable on Huntington's disease chromosomes. *Cell* 72(6): 971–83

Marin RS, Fogel BS, Hawkins J, Duffy J, & Krupp B. (1995) Apathy: A treatable syndrome. *Journal of Neuropsychiatry and Clinical Neuroscience* 7: 23–30

Medalia A, Scheinberg IH (1989) Psychopathology in patients with Wilson's disease. *American Journal of Psychiatry* 46: 662–4

Miyasaki JM, Shannon K, Voon V, Ravina B, Kleiner-Fisman G, Anderson K, Shulman LM, Gronseth G, Weiner WJ; Quality Standards Subcommittee of the American Academy of Neurology (2006) Practice parameter: Evaluation and treatment of depression, psychosis, and dementia in Parkinson disease (an evidence-based review). *Neurology* 66: 996–1002

Moore DP (2008) *Textbook of Clinical Neuropsychiatry*. London: Hodder Arnold

Mufaddel A, Omer AA, Salem MO (2014) Psychiatric aspects of infectious diseases. *Open Journal of Psychiatry* 4: 202–17 http://dx.doi.org/10.4236/ojpsych.2014.43027

Muhlert N, Ron M (2014) *Neuropsychiatric Aspects of Multiple Sclerosis and White Matter Disorders*. http://www.ebrainjnc.com/learning/ – an e-learning resource by the British Neuropsychiatric Association, August

Murray JL, Vos T, Lozano R *et al*., (2012). Disability-adjusted life years (DALYs) for 291 diseases and injuries in 21 regions, 1990–2010: A systematic analysis for the Global Burden of Disease Study 2010. *The Lancet* 380: 2197–223

Nadkarni S, Devinsky O (2005) Psychotropic effects of antiepileptic drugs. *Epilepsy Currents* 5: 176–81

National Institute for Health and Clinical Excellence (2006) *Parkinson's disease: diagnosis and management in primary and secondary care*. NICE Clinical Guideline 35. Available at: http://www.nice.org.uk/guidance/cg35/resources/guidance-parkinsons-disease-pdf (Accessed 18 March 2015.)

Negro A, Martelletti P (2011) Chronic migraine plus medication overuse headache: Two entities or not? *Journal of Headache and Pain* 12: 593–601

Nuti A, Ceravolo R, Piccinni A, Dell'Agnello G, Bellini G, Gambaccini G, Rossi C, Logi C, Dell'Osso L, Bonuccelli U (2004) Psychiatric comorbidity in a population of Parkinson's disease patients. *European Journal of Neurology* 11: 315–20

Ondo WG, Tintner R, Voung KD, Lai D, Ringholz G (2005) Double-blind, placebo-controlled, unforced titration parallel trial of quetiapine for dopaminergic-induced hallucinations in Parkinson's disease. *Movement Disorders* 20: 958–63

Oosthuizen P (2005) The neuropsychiatry of brain tumours. *South African Journal of Psychiatry* Vol 11, (1): 6–11

Parkinson Study Group (1999) Low-dose clozapine for the treatment of drug-induced psychosis in Parkinson's disease. *New England Journal of Medicine* 340: 757–63

Prigatano GP (2005) Disturbances of self-awareness and rehabilitation of patients with traumatic brain injury: A 20-year perspective. *Journal of Head Trauma Rehabilitation* 20: 19–29

Ring HA, Serra-Mestres J (2002) Neuropsychiatry of the basal ganglia. *Journal of Neurology Neurosurgery and Psychiatry* 72: 12–21

Robinson RG (1987) Depression and stroke. *Psychiatric Annals* 17: 731–40

Roth M, Tym E, Mountjoy Q (1986) CAMDEX: a standardized instrument for the diagnosis of mental disorder in the elderly with special reference to the early detection of dementia. *British Journal of Psychiatry* 149: 698–709

Rothrock J, Lopez I, Zweilfer R, Andress-Rothrock D, Walters N (2007) Borderline personality disorder and migraine. *Headache* 47: 22–6

Sachdev P (2005). International Neuropsychiatric Association. *Journal of Neuropsychiatric Disease and Treatment* 1: 191–2 Quotation on page 591 reprinted with permission from Dove Press

Sachdev P, Mohan A (2013) Neuropsychiatry: Where are we and where do we go from here? *Mens Sana Monographs* 11(1): 4–15

Saper J, Hamel R, Lake AE (2005) Medication overuse is a biobehavioral disorder. *Cephalalgia* 25: 545–6

Saper JR, Lake AE (2002) Borderline personality disorder and the chronic headache patient: Review and management recommendations. *Headache* 42: 663–74

Schoenberg MR, Scott JG (Eds) (2011) *The Little Black Book of Neuropsychology - A Syndrome-Based Approach.* New York: Springer

Serra-Mestres J, Mukhopadhyay S (2014) *Neuropsychiatric problems in Parkinson's disease.* http://www.psychiatrycpd.org/ – CPD Online from Royal College of Psychiatrists, September

Shah N (1994) Idiopathic intracranial pressure. *Specialist Medicine Neurology Forum* April 1994: 28–35

Shallice T, Burgess PW (1991) Deficits in strategy application following frontal lobe damage in man. *Brain* 114: 727–41

Shukla G, Bhatia M, Vivekanandhan S, Gupta N, Tripathi M, Srivastava A, Pandey RM, Jain S (2004) Serum prolactin levels for differentiation of nonepileptic versus true seizures: Limited utility. *Epilepsy Behaviour* 5(4):517–21

Shulman BH (1991) Psychiatric aspects of headache. *Medical Clinics of North America* 75: 707–15

Soler D, Cox T, Bullock P, Calver DM, Robinson RO (1998) Diagnosis and management of benign intracranial hypertension. *Archives of Disease in Childhood* 78: 89–94

Solomon T, Jung A (2014) *Introduction to Neurological Infectious Diseases.* http://www.ebrainjnc.com/learning/ – an e-learning resource by the British Neuropsychiatric Association, August

Starkstein SE (2002) Apathy and withdrawal. *International Psychogeriatrics* 12: 135–8

Streeter CC, Van Reekum R, Shorr RI, Bachman DL (1995) Prior head injury in male veterans with borderline personality disorder. *Journal of Nervous and Mental Disease* 183: 577–81

Svetel M, Potrebić A, Pekmezović T, Tomić A, Kresojević N, Ješić R, Dragašević N, Kostić VS (2009) *Parkinsonism & Related Disorders.* New York: Elsevier

Tanzi RE, Petrukhin K, Chernov I, Pellequer JL, Wasco W, Ross B, Romano DM, Parano E, Pavone L, Brzustowicz LM, *et al.* (1993) The Wilson disease gene is a copper transporting ATPase with homology to the Menkes disease gene. *Nature Genetics* 4: 344–50

Torta R, Keller R (1999) Behavioral, psychotic, and anxiety disorders in epilepsy: Aetiology, clinical features, and therapeutic implications. *Epilepsia* 40 (suppl 10): S2–20

Tucker GJ (1998) Seizure disorders presenting with psychiatric symptomatology. *Psychiatric Clinics of North America* 21: 625–35

Van der Naalt J (2001) Prediction of outcome in mild to moderate head injury: A review. *Journal of Clinical and Experimental Neuropsychology* 23: 837–51

Van Reekum R, Stuss DT, Ostrander L (2005) Apathy: why care? *Journal of Neuropsychiatry and Clinical Neuroscience* 17: 7–19

Vuilleumier P, Jallon P (1998) Epilepsy and psychiatric disorders: Epidemiological data. *Revue Neurologique (Paris)* 154: 305–17

Vukmir RB (2009) Does serum prolactin indicate the presence of seizure in the emergency department patient? *Journal of Neurology* 25: 736–9

Weintraub D, Newberg AB, Cary MS, Siderowf AD, Moberg PJ, Kleiner-Fisman G, Duda JE, Stern MB, Mozley D, Katz IR (2005) Striatal dopamine transporter imaging correlates with anxiety and depression symptoms in Parkinson's disease. *Journal of Nuclear Medicine* 46: 227–32

Wild E, Tabrizi S (2014) *Huntington's disease.* http://www.ebrainjnc.com/learning/ – an e-learning resource by the British Neuropsychiatric Association, August

Williams LS (2005) Depression and stroke: Cause or consequence? *Seminars in Neurology* 25: 396–409

Wilson BA, Alderman N, Burgess PW, Emslie H and Evans JJ (1996) *BADS: behavioural assessment of the dysexecutive syndrome.* Burt St Edmonds: Thames Valley Test Company

World Health Organization (2008) *Global Burden of Disease.* Geneva, Switzerland. WHO Press. Available at: http://www.who.int/healthinfo/global_burden_disease/GBD_report_2004update_full.pdf (Accessed 19 January 2015.)

World Health Organization (1980) *International Classification of Impairments, Disabilities, and Handicaps. A manual of classification relating to the consequences of disease.* Geneva: World Health Organisation

Yudofsky SC, Hales RE (2008) *The American Psychiatric Publishing Textbook of Neuropsychiatry and Behavioral Sciences.* Washington DC: American Psychiatric Publishing

CHAPTER

# 33 HIV and mental health

Greg Jonsson, Sibongile Mashaphu, Rethabile Mataboge

## 33.1 Introduction

As we enter the fourth decade of HIV/Aids, it is clear that the global impact of the virus has been vast. Although this condition occurs worldwide, sub-Saharan Africa is worst affected. South Africa has more than 6,3 million people living **with HIV/Aids (PLWHA)** (Joint United Nations programme on HIV/Aids: South Africa, *s.d.*). This has serious mental health implications, as mental illness and distress associated with the condition are very common. Moreover, severely mentally ill and intellectually disabled people are vulnerable and at high risk of contracting HIV as a result of sexual abuse and assault, poor information-processing capabilities, poor reality testing, social drift and poor impulse control. There is growing evidence that mental disorders impact significantly on people living with HIV/Aids and that ongoing intervention by mental health professionals is needed (Thom, 2012).

## 33.2 The burden of HIV

Although the advent of combination **anti-retroviral therapy (cART)** has had a major impact on the morbidity and mortality of the HIV-infected person, HIV still exerts an enormous burden and has an impact on social, political, personal and economic levels. The general health care system in South Africa is also under strain due to the financial burden of managing HIV/Aids and lack of sufficiently trained healthcare professionals. Even though close to one million people are currently accessing antiretroviral treatment (ART) in South Africa, there is still limited access to care and treatment as this represents fewer than 40% of patients in need of treatment (Rossouw, 2011).

Psychiatrists must understand and be aware of the clinical features of HIV/Aids and its management. Physicians also must understand the psychiatric, neuropsychiatric and psychological consequences of HIV/Aids.

## 33.3 Pathophysiology

The relationship between HIV infection and mental disorders is complex and intertwined. There is growing evidence for an increased prevalence of mental disorders in people living with HIV/Aids compared with the general population (Olley *et al.*, 2006). There are two groups of people who manifest with psychiatric illness and HIV infection:

- those with a pre-existing mental illness who become secondarily infected with HIV
- those who are HIV positive and present with or develop psychiatric disorders, either directly or indirectly.

In most cases of co-existing HIV infection and psychiatric conditions, the exact cause cannot be established and the symptom profile may be more complex than in uninfected individuals.

HIV infection can result in psychiatric disorders through a variety of mechanisms:

- The stress of the diagnosis may precipitate a psychiatric illness, such as a major depressive episode or an adjustment disorder.
- The virus affects the brain directly, possibly by entering the brain substance through endothelial gaps in brain capillaries or through infiltration of infected macrophages and leucocytes. The virus causes neuronal injury through a complex cascade of events, including irreversible binding to calcium channels,

alterations in brain glucose metabolism, neurotoxin production, altered immune modulation in the central nervous system (CNS), the release of glutamate and other free radicals and the acceleration of apoptosis (programmed cell death). Astrocytes and glial cells are predominantly affected.
- Complications of the immune-compromised state (infections, malignancies, hypoxia, septicaemia, etc.) may have psychiatric consequences.
- Medication (e.g. zidovudine (AZT), efavirenz (EFV)) has many psychiatric side effects, including mania and depression. Izoniazid (INH), which is often used in the treatment of associated tuberculosis (TB), can cause psychosis.
- A person with a pre-existing psychiatric illness (e.g. untreated depression, mania, intellectual disability), including an illness related to, or arising from, substance abuse, may become HIV+ due to their vulnerable mental status and risky behaviour (see Figure 33.1).

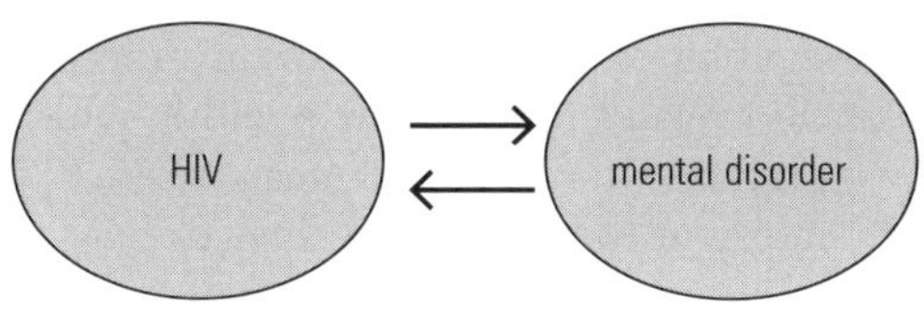


**Figure 33.1** The relationship between HIV and mental illness

**Source:** Adapted from Treisman, 2007

## 33.4 Screening and diagnosis in people living with HIV/Aids

Common mental disorders are often under-diagnosed and under-treated in a primary health care setting. This may be a result of busy clinics, overburdened health care workers and a feeling of helplessness as to where to refer an individual when a syndrome is identified. Many health care workers feel under-trained in dealing with mental disorders and would often ignore them (Mall *et al.*, 2012). The solution lies in simple screening tools that are easy and quick to administer and that do not require large amounts of training and expertise to implement and administer. The screening tools do, however, have to be adequately sensitive and specific to prevent false positives and to ensure detection of all those patients who need further screening. There are a number of self-report and clinician-initiated questionnaires available. The K-10 and PHQ-9 questionnaires are easy to implement and administer. The K-10 is a self-report questionnaire, which may also be administered by the interviewer and takes 2–3 minutes to complete (Spies *et al.*, 2009). A validation study conducted in Cape Town found the K-10 to be a useful measure of both depression and anxiety disorders, including post-traumatic stress disorder (PTSD) among patients who are HIV+. Another quick and relatively easy test to administer in a clinic that handles both common mental disorders and substance abuse, is the Substance Abuse and Mental Illness Symptoms Screener (SAMISS). It is a 13-item screening questionnaire developed for use in HIV+ populations and has been found to have a sensitivity of 86% and a specificity of 95% in diagnosing DSM-IV defined substance use, depressive and anxiety disorders (Thom, 2009). Screening tests for neurocognitive disorders have been validated both in Uganda and South Africa. The International HIV Dementia Scale (IHDS) is easy and relatively quick to administer but has some limitations (Joska *et al.*, 2011). (Also see Section 33.7.6.)

## 33.5 Testing for HIV in patients with mental illness

While informed consent prior to testing for HIV is important, issues of capacity always arise when testing for HIV in patients with mental illness. One should remember that capacity to consent to HIV testing is not defined by the presence of a mental illness, but by the patient's ability to comprehend the information presented to him or her and to draw reasonable conclusions from that information presented.

While in the pre-cART era, informed consent and confidentiality were vitally important to protect against stigma and discrimination, many feel that in the era of cART, these outdated policies of informed consent prohibit access to care and treatment and that a medical justification should be sufficient to test. This medical justification and discretion should lie with the treating clinician. Provider-initiated counselling and testing, sometimes synonymously used with opt-out testing, is generally accepted as the testing policy in use in South Africa. This policy is not routinely followed with mentally ill patients, however, as many clinicians feel that patients who lack capacity to consent also have no voice to opt out of the testing procedure. Many providers therefore wait for the individual's mental status to improve, ask family or next of kin for permission or receive permission from the head of the health establishment. None of these options are realistic for a patient with a serious mental illness:

- patients must receive HIV and psychopharmacological treatment concomitantly
- involving family or next of kin may exacerbate stigma and discrimination and in some cases lead to partner violence
- many heads of health establishments are not clinically trained, and may not realise the urgency of such a test
- testing may alter individual management strategies, as more in-depth investigations (e.g. lumbar puncture) and different psychotropic agents (e.g. second-generation antipsychotics) may be indicated because of contraindications for the use of other agents.

One needs to respect the informed consent process at all times but patients also have the right to receive appropriate, and often lifesaving, therapy. It is therefore recommended that in making the decision to test, the patient's condition be categorised as either a common mental disorder or a serious mental illness. In both cases it is important to assess the patient's capacity to provide consent. In the case of a common mental disorder where the patient gives consent for testing, provider-initiated counselling and testing may be offered and the informed consent process be followed as far as possible. In patients with a serious mental illness, one should distinguish between patients who have the capacity to consent and those who lack the capacity. In patients who lack capacity, one should also distinguish between patients who actively refuse and those who don't. It has been suggested that the onus, especially in patients who lack capacity to consent, falls on the senior treating clinician (Joska *et al.*, 2008). The senior clinician therefore weighs the benefits of testing against the benefits of not testing and thereby decides on what action should be taken. It is vital to document all stages of the process very clearly in patient records. Once capacity is regained, one should repeat the informed consent process. Confidentiality with regard to results of the test is vital and lies within the sanctity of the patient-clinician relationship (see Figure 33.2).

## 33.6 Investigations

Distinguishing between a primary and a secondary psychiatric illness in the context of HIV often proves difficult. This is not only as a result of the prohibitive costs of various investigative tests but relates to the context within which one practices. In many rural areas, access to a laboratory or to radiological services may be limited. Nevertheless, it is vital to distinguish between a primary and a secondary illness as it has serious implications, which may include prescription of antiretroviral drugs, prolonged morbidity and adherence issues. HIV-related psychopathologies may not be a clear and distinct group of symptoms: they often overlap as is seen with maniform psychosis and neurocognitive disorders.

In order to diagnose a secondary psychiatric illness, one often looks for a clear personal or family psychiatric history, age of onset and a close temporal proximity to the insult to the brain (i.e. HIV acquisition) (Nakimuli-Mpungu *et al.*, 2006). In a study looking at primary mania and first-episode secondary mania, it was found that those patients with secondary mania were more likely to be older and female, have an irritable

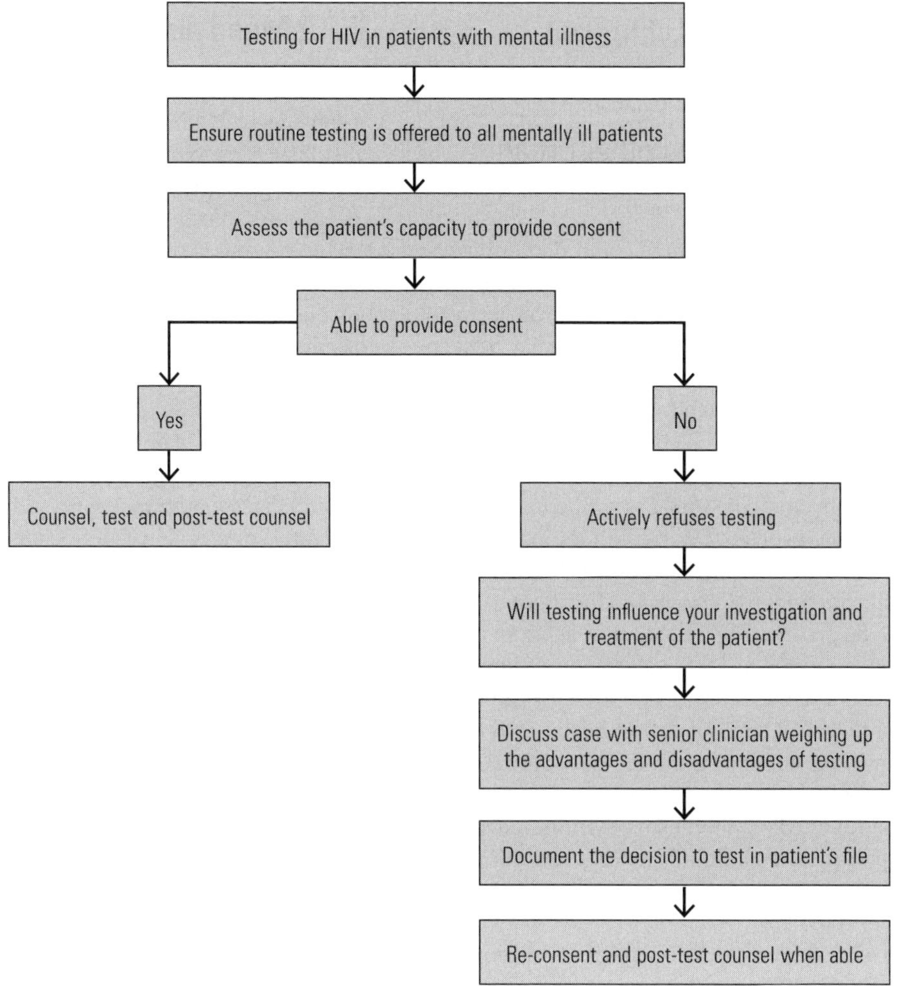


**Figure 33.2** Algorithm for testing for HIV in a patient with mental illness
**Source:** Jonsson *et al.*, 2013

mood (rather than an elevated mood), be aggressive, be over-talkative, have a decreased need for sleep, have more paranoid delusions and visual and auditory hallucinations and greater cognitive impairment. These clinical distinctions have important implications in terms of diagnosis, initiation of treatment and early intervention for adherence and reduction of risk behaviours.

It is vital to perform a full physical and neurological examination on all patients with a dual diagnosis (i.e. HIV and mental illness) after a full history is taken. Of particular importance is the elucidation of previous opportunistic infections (OIs) and treatment for these, diagnosis of HIV and to establish whether or not the patient is antiretroviral therapy (ART) naïve. Any patient who presents with an acute or sub-acute change in his or her mental status should be evaluated thoroughly. Investigations are often costly and may not always shed light on whether the psychiatric illness is due to HIV or not. It is therefore important that investigations and treatment are guided by findings on physical examination, rather than by blood results alone.

# 33.7 Clinical psychiatric syndromes

## 33.7.1 Delirium and other organic syndromes

Delirium is often the most common neuropsychiatric diagnosis in hospitalised or critically ill HIV+ patients, with a prevalence of up to 65% (Gallego *et al.*, 2011). Delirium may be seen in the acute infective stage, up to and including the late stages where it is often associated with opportunistic infections. It may even occur superimposed on dementia. Delirium is characterised by an acute onset of a fluctuating level of consciousness, disorientation, inattention, confusion and sleep-wake cycle abnormalities. Hallucinations, delusions and incoherence may also be present. The treatment of delirium is primarily directed towards identifying and treating the underlying cause. In the case of the HIV+ mentally ill patient, all opportunistic CNS infections must either be excluded or treated (i.e. TB, cryptococcal disease, toxoplasmosis, cytomegalovirus (CMV), neoplasms (lymphoma)). It is important to exclude substance intoxication and withdrawal, as these are easily treated (Vlassova *et al.*, 2009).

Delirium may present in the form of **immune reconstitution inflammatory syndrome (IRIS)**, which occurs when the immune system produces an inflammatory response as it reconstitutes on cART treatment. The result may be the paradoxical worsening of a known or underlying infection or the unmasking of a subclinical infection (Singer *et al.*, 2010). This may take place within the first two months of commencing cART. A number of risk factors predict the development of IRIS, including an active or subclinical opportunistic infection, low CD4 count, anaemia and a rapid decline in viral load (VL). The most common manifestations are HIV encephalopathy (HIVE), TB, tuberculous meningitis (TBM), cryptococcal meningitis (CCM) and progressive multifocal leuko-encephalopathy (PML).

## 33.7.2 Mood disorders in HIV

Major depression is one of the most commonly observed psychiatric conditions in people living with HIV/Aids. Not only do HIV+ individuals have a higher prevalence of depression than HIV negative individuals, but depression can lead to a greater risk of contracting HIV. This may be due to the negative effects depression has on behaviour, impulsivity, judgement and insight. Similarly, antiretroviral and opportunistic infection medication, as well as the psychosocial effects of HIV, may lead to depressive disorders. Depression is debilitating as it has severe effects on quality of life, adherence to medication and disease progression (Verdeli *et al.*, 2003). Untreated depression is associated with substance abuse and, alone or together, may increase risky sexual behaviour, which in turn results in increased transmission of HIV. Prevalence rates of depression in people living with HIV/Aids range from 12–71% in high-income countries, depending on the study, cohort and measures used (e.g. BDI, CES-D, HAM-D) (Sherr *et al.*, 2011). South African studies report prevalence rates of depression in PLWHA from 25–38% (Pappin *et al.*, 2012; Kagee and Martin, 2010). In South Africa, not enough is being done to integrate mental health and HIV care (Freeman *et al.*, 2005). As antiretroviral drugs are rolled out, health care providers are faced with many health priorities and tend to neglect mental health. It is vital to identify depression and treat it appropriately. Innovative approaches to the screening for and diagnosis and treatment of depression in the HIV+ population are required.

Diagnosing depression may present some difficulties, as symptoms of severe HIV disease progression (fatigue, loss of weight, poor concentration) overlap with the neuro-vegetative features of depression. A complete history and physical examination are thus critical, as screening tools are only useful to alert one to a possible disorder that requires further evaluation. Table 33.1 delineates an approach to the differential diagnosis of mood symptoms in the HIV+ patient. It is important to categorise the differential diagnosis as a primary mood disorder, a secondary mood disorder and other, including life stressors and psychosocial issues.

A full examination is not complete without the assessment of risk, including suicide risk. Asking about suicidal thoughts, plans or intent will not increase suicidal behaviour. There are specific times in a patient's life when these questions are vital, such as just after a diagnosis is given, recent losses, anniversary of a partner's death, uncontrolled pain, worsening of a patient's physical condition, loss of a job and where there is poor social support. One of the biggest predictors of suicide risk is a history of past suicide attempt(s).

Patients with HIV who are at a higher risk of developing depression are those with a personal or family history of mood disorder, substance abuse, suicide attempts or anxiety disorders. Other risk factors include exposure to chronic stress, inadequate social support, passive coping style, non-disclosure of HIV status, multiple losses, female gender, advanced illness and treatment failure (Ruiz, 2006).

## 33.7.3 Anxiety disorders

Anxiety disorders are more prevalent in people living with HIV/Aids than in the general population. As in the HIV negative patient, the key features that differentiate anxiety from normal physiological reactions in the HIV+ patient are anxiety symptoms that are difficult to control, marked impairment or distress and having a specified duration. Anxiety disorders may impair the social skills needed to ensure good attendance at follow-up health visits and adequate adherence to treatment regimens. They may also result in increased rates of high-risk behaviour and increased use of health care services. Anxiety disorders can occur at any stage of infection or phase of the illness. Mental health care providers must therefore be ready to address them as they arise. A Nigerian study found the prevalence of anxiety disorders in patients with HIV to be 22%: much higher than the 5,7% lifetime and 4,1% 12-month prevalence rates for anxiety disorders observed in the general community sample (Olagunju and Adeyemi, 2012). Interestingly, most high-income country studies suggest that HIV+ patients have rates of anxiety disorders similar to the general population, with the exception of slightly higher rates of generalised anxiety disorder. The Nigerian study found that those diagnosed with anxiety disorders were less likely to have family support, to be married or to be employed. A lack of previous mental illness and younger age seemed to be protective against developing an anxiety disorder. The HIV+ population is at particular risk for PTSD. Certain

**Table 33.1** Differential diagnosis

| Primary mood disorders | Secondary mood disorders | Psychosocial and other life stressors | Other |
|---|---|---|---|
| major depressive disorder | mood disorder due to another medical condition (HIV) | bereavement | medication effects:<br>efavirenz, antituberculosis drugs, hepatitis C drugs, other treatment for OI treatments |
| bipolar mood disorder (depressed episode) | HIV-associated neurocogntive disorder | relationship issues | |
| adjustment disorder with depressed mood | OI-TB, CCM, hepatitis C | adjustment issues due to stigma, disclosure, rejection, changes in body shape | |
| anxiety disorders | | | |
| PTSD | | | |

**Source:** Adapted from Stolar *et al.*, 2005. Reprinted with permission from Cambridge University Press.

sub-populations may be at even higher risk for complex PTSD as a result of multiple traumatic experiences. Having PTSD predicts worsened morbidity, more health-related complaints and more HIV-related illnesses (Matthews and Trujillo, 2006). It is important to recognise anxiety disorders in those with HIV, since pharmacological and non-pharmacological treatment can improve quality of life, decrease transmission and improve health outcomes.

## 33.7.4 Psychotic disorders and HIV

The pathophysiology of psychosis and other forms of severe mental illness in HIV infection is complex; a multifactorial causation is likely in most instances. It may be useful to categorise psychosis in the HIV+ person into one of five scenarios:

### 33.7.4.1 Psychotic disorders predating HIV

Major psychiatric disorders that present with psychosis and predate HIV infection include schizophrenia, bipolar mood disorder and major depressive disorder with psychotic features. Substance abuse may predispose and/or precipitate a substance-induced psychotic disorder.

### 33.7.4.2 New-onset psychotic disorders

New-onset psychosis in the HIV infected patient may occur with the development of psychotic symptoms, such as hallucinations, delusions, disorganised behaviour and acute or sub-acute altered forms of thought. This occurs in the absence of concurrent substance abuse, opportunistic infections, space-occupying lesions, cognitive impairment or various medications.

### 33.7.4.3 Psychotic disorders associated with medical conditions

Neurological conditions such as seizures, vascular lesions, space-occupying lesions, infections or neoplasms, endocrine conditions, metabolic abnormalities and systemic infections related to the pathophysiological changes caused by HIV infection, can trigger psychosis. Delirium can also present with psychotic symptoms.

### 33.7.4.4 Psychotic disorders associated with substance intoxication or withdrawal

Substance intoxication and withdrawal are reversible substance-specific syndromes and may present with a delirium-type picture.

### 33.7.4.5 Psychotic disorders associated with complications of treatment

Some medications used to treat HIV or the medical complications of HIV/Aids may cause psychiatric disorders to present with psychotic symptoms. Efavirenz is associated with a wide range of neuropsychiatric side effects, including psychosis. Other medications commonly used in HIV medicine that can be associated with psychosis include corticosteroids, ganciclovir, antifungal agents, and some antibacterials such as antituberculosis drugs.

### 33.7.4.6 Evaluation of a patient with HIV and psychosis

- Obtain a comprehensive history, including medication and substance use history.
- Perform a physical examination, including a full neurological examination.
- Perform a mental state examination.
- Evaluate for all possible causes using biochemical and radiological investigations. A lumbar puncture may be indicated in some cases, provided it is not contraindicated.
- An electroencephalograph (EEG) may have a diagnostic benefit in distinguishing a hyperactive delirium (Jonsson and Joska, 2009).

## 33.7.5 Adjustment disorders

HIV/Aids is a chronic and life-changing illness and adjusting to the illness may be a lifelong process. Adjustment disorders have been reported to occur in 5-20% of patients infected with HIV (Sadock BJ and Sadock VA, 2005).

Data on the prevalence of adjustment disorders in HIV+ patients is sparse, but common sense dictates that most individuals will suffer some form of adjustment symptoms during the course of HIV disease. After testing positive for HIV, individuals will have to address a number of issues common to those suffering any other chronic life-threatening illness. Shock, anger, denial, guilt and anxiety are just some of the emotions one could expect. Disclosure issues, possible exclusion from social circles, fear of loss of health and the possibility of death are some of the practical worries that confront the patient. It is often tricky to separate depressive symptoms associated with an adjustment disorder from those of a major depressive episode. Major depression can be conceptualised as a disease of the brain that affects those neural systems that control mood. Adjustment disorders arise from a patient's meaningful reaction to a particular life circumstance or event.

Patients with an adjustment disorder occurring within the context of HIV should be closely monitored since the symptoms may progress to depression and other anxiety disorders.

## 33.7.6 HIV-associated neurocognitive disorders (HAND)

**HIV-associated neurocognitive disorders (HAND)** is a term used to describe the spectrum of neurocognitive impairment seen in HIV/Aids. The diagnostic criteria of HAND was revised and amended in 2007 (Antinori *et al.*, 2007). The revisions emphasised that documented neurocognitive disturbance was an essential feature in the diagnosis of HAND, and specified more precise criteria for three categories. These three HAND categories, listed in a hierarchy of progressive severity, range from asymptomatic neurocognitive impairment (ANI), to minor neurocognitive disorder (MND), to the more severe HIV-associated dementia (HAD) (see Figure 33.3).

### 33.7.6.1 Epidemiology

HIV-associated neurocognitive disorders remain amongst the most common disorders in people infected with HIV, even in an era when cART is widely used. The incidence of HIV-associated neurocognitive disorders has declined by approximately 75% since the introduction of cART (McArthur *et al.*, 2010). Despite this remarkable reduction in incidence rates, the prevalence of HIV-associated neurocognitive disorders continues at high rates, presumably owing to incomplete reversal or prevention of cognitive impairment, longer survival on cART and an increasing HIV prevalence. HIV-associated dementia occurs in approximately 10-15% of all individuals with HIV/Aids and is more common in late stages of infection.

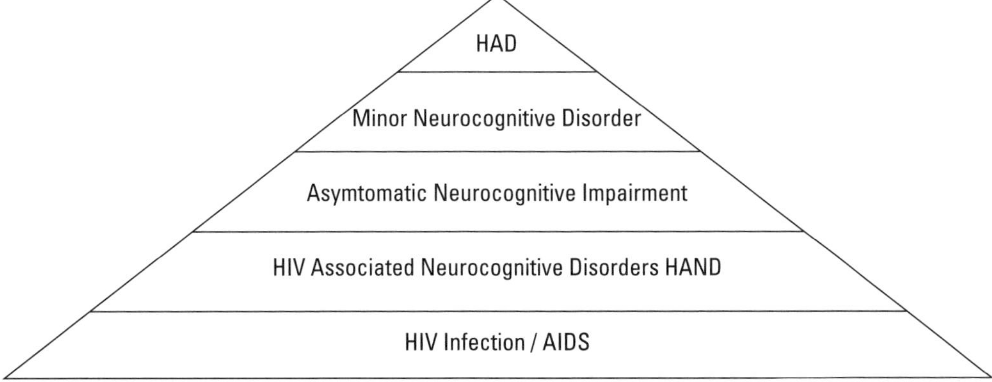


**Figure 33.3** Human immunodeficiency virus (HIV)-associated neurocognitive disorders (HAND): hierarchical relationship of different neurocognitive disorders associated with HIV/acquired immunodeficiency syndrome (AIDS). HAD = HIV-associated dementia

**Source:** McArthur *et al.*, 2010. This material is reproduced with permission from John Wiley and Sons Inc.

Depending on the stage of the disease, less severe forms of HIV-associated neurocognitive disorders occur in 30-60% of people infected with HIV (Singh, 2009).

### 33.7.6.2 Classification

The classification of HIV-associated neurocognitive disorder is shown in Table 33.2.

### 33.7.6.3 Clinical work-up

HIV-associated neurocognitive disorder is a diagnosis of exclusion. Other diseases that affect central nervous system functioning have to be systematically ruled out. The diagnosis of HIV-associated neurocognitive disorders requires testing the six cognitive domains using neuropsychological tests. Two-stage screening is commonly used in psychiatry. In the first stage

**Table 33.2** Revised research criteria for HIV-associated neurocognitive disorders (HANDS) (modified from HIV Neurobehavioral Research Center criteria)

| **HIV-associated asymptomatic neurocognitive impairment (ANI)*** |
|---|
| 1. Acquired impairment in cognitive functioning, involving at least two ability domains, documented by performance of at least 1.0 SD below the mean for age –education-appropriate norms on standardized neuropsychological tests. The neuropsychological assessment must survey at least the following abilities: verbal/language; attention/working memory; abstraction/executive; memory (learning; recall); speed of information processing; sensory-perceptual, motor skills. |
| 2. The cognitive impairment does not interfere with everyday functioning. |
| 3. The cognitive impairment does not meet criteria for delirium or dementia. |
| 4. There is no evidence of another preexisting cause for the ANI.† |
| * **If there is a prior diagnosis of ANI, but currently the individual does not meet criteria, the diagnosis of ANI in remission can be made.** |
| † **If the individual with suspected ANI also satisfies criteria for a major depressive episode or substance dependence, the diagnosis of ANI should be deferred to a subsequent examination conducted at a time when the major depression has remitted or at least 1 month after cessation of substance use.** |
| **HIV-1-associated mild neurocognitive disorder (MND)*** |
| 1. Acquired impairment in cognitive functioning, involving at least two ability domains, documented by performance of at least 1.0 SD below the mean age-education-appropriate norms on standardized neuropsychological tests. The neuropsychological assessment must survey at least the following abilities: verbal/language; attention/working memory; abstraction/executive; memory (learning; recall); speed of information processing; sensory-perceptual, motor skills.<br>Typically, this would correspond to an MSK scale stage of 0.5 to 1.0. |
| 2. The cognitive impairment produces at least mild interference in daily functioning (at least one of the following):<br>a) Self-report of reduced mental acuity, inefficiency in work, homemaking, or social functioning.<br>b) Observation by knowledgeable others that the individual has undergone at least mild decline in mental acuity with resultant inefficiency in work, homemaking, or social functioning. |
| 3. The cognitive impairment does not meet criteria for delirium or dementia. |
| 4. There is no evidence of another preexisting cause for the MND.† |
| * **If there is a prior diagnosis of MND, but currently the individual does not meet criteria, the diagnosis of MND in remission can be made.** |
| † **If the individual with suspected MND also satisfies criteria for a severe episode of major depression with significant functional limitations or psychotic features, or substance dependence, the diagnosis of MND should be deferred to a subsequent examination conducted at a time when the major depression has remitted or at least 1 month after cessation of substance use.** |

| HIV-1-associated dementia (HAD)* |
|---|
| 1. Marked acquired impairment in cognitive functioning, involving at least two ability domains; typically the impairment is in multiple domains, especially in learning of new information, slowed information processing, and defective attention/concentration. The cognitive impairment must be ascertained by neuropsychological testing with at least two domains 2SD or greater than demographically corrected means. (Note that where neuropsychological testing is not available, standard neurological evaluation and simple bedside testing may be used, but this should be done as indicated in algorithm; see below). Typically, this would correspond to an MSK scale stage of 2.0 or greater. |
| 2. The cognitive impairment produces marked interference with day-to-day functioning (work, home life, social activities). |
| 3. The pattern of cognitive impairment does not meet criteria for delirium (e.g., clouding of consciousness is not a prominent feature); or, if delirium is present, criteria for dementia need to have been met on a prior examination when delirium was not present. |
| 4. There is no evidence of another, preexisting cause for the dementia (e.g., other CNS infection, CNS neoplasm, cerebrovascular disease, preexisting neurologic disease, or severe substance abuse compatible with CNS disorder).[†] |
| *** If there is a prior diagnosis of HAD, but currently the individual does not meet criteria, the diagnosis of HAD in remission can be made.** |
| **† If the individual with suspected HAD also satisfies criteria for a severe episode of major depression with significant functional limitations or psychotic features, or substance dependence, the diagnosis of HAD should be deferred to a subsequent examination conducted at a time when the major depression has remitted or at least 1 month has elapsed following cessation of substance use. Note that the consensus was that even when major depression and HAD occurred together, there is little evidence that pseudo dementia exists and the cognitive deficits do not generally improve with treatment of depression.** |

**Source:** Antinori *et al.*, 2007. Reprinted with permission from Wolters Kluwer.

a brief cognitive screening test is administered; people who screen positive then undergo more detailed testing in the form of a neuropsychological battery.

### Cognitive screening tests

Cognitive screening tests for HIV-associated neurocognitive disorders include the following:

- Mini-Mental State Examination (MMSE): this test consists of items that specifically check for cortical functions. It is not ideal for the assessment of HIV-associated neurocognitive disorder as sub-cortical processes are primarily affected in HIV-associated neurocognitive disorder. Milder forms of HIV-associated neurocognitive disorder cannot be detected, and performance is influenced by age, education and cultural background (Tombaugh and McIntyre, 1992).
- HIV Dementia Scale (HDS): this test is more sensitive to subcortical functions and has been validated in South Africa (Ganasen *et al.*, 2008). However, it can be difficult for non-neurologists to administer without the necessary training.
- International HIV Dementia Scale (IHDS): The test has been validated in the United States, Uganda and South Africa (Saktor *et al.*, 2005; Joska *et al.*, 2011). It is easy and relatively quick to administer. However, its low sensitivity of 45% and specificity of 79% (at a cut-off of 10) means that this tool has limitations as a screen for HIV-associated neurocognitive disorders (Joska *et al.*, 2011). It has been recommended that extra executive function tests be included in the screening battery (Joska *et al.*, 2011).
- Montreal Cognitive Assessment (MOCA): the MOCA is particularly adept at assessing milder forms of cognitive impairment; more so than the MMSE (Vally, 2011). It screens for cortical and subcortical impairment and may be useful to screen for HIV-associated neurocognitive disorders.

### Neuropsychological test batteries

Various neuropsychological test batteries have been proposed; the absence of local population norms may limit their utility. They range from longer batteries, which may take as long as nine hours, to brief batteries that may take one to two hours. These tests require training and expertise and are likely to be beyond the reach of a busy primary care HIV clinical service. They may have an important role to play as part of a specialist referral service to diagnose HIV-associated neurocognitive disorders.

#### 33.7.6.4 Diagnosis, assessment and management of HIV-associated neurocognitive disorders

Screening tools are used to screen for HIV-associated neurocognitive disorders while further neuropsychological tests and other investigations are used to diagnose and further clarify the diagnosis of HIV-associated neurocognitive disorder. Diagnosis guides the appropriate management strategy (see Figure 33.4).

### 33.7.7 Substance-related disorders

Drug use, whether by injection or not, substantially increases the risk of HIV infection. Patients with co-morbid substance misuse are more likely to engage in HIV high-risk behaviour and more often lack adequate knowledge about HIV. Some drugs of abuse can exacerbate the central nervous system effects of HIV infection. The mechanisms responsible for neuronal injury caused by substance abuse and HIV overlap. Inflammatory cytokines, increased oxidative stress and increased permeability of the blood-brain barrier have been implicated in the mechanisms of neuronal injury (Kumar, 2012).

Not only is alcohol use common in people living with HIV/Aids, but it has a severe impact on adherence to cART (Chander, 2011). Screening for substance use disorders and other

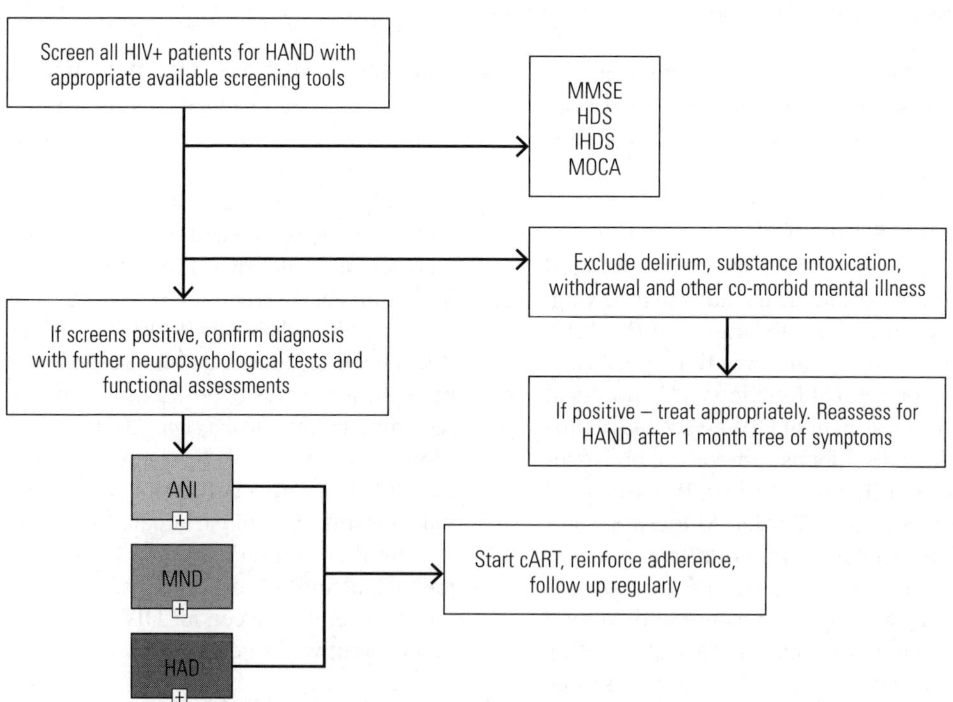


**Figure 33.4** Summary of the assessment and management of neurocognitive function in newly diagnosed people living with HIV/Aids
**Source:** Singh, 2009

common mental disorders is critical in ensuring appropriate intervention in cases where elevated risk is present. Identifying other mental health disorders is vital in people living with HIV/Aids, as these disorders have an impact on substance use disorder treatment, increase hospitalisation, and worsen co-morbid mental health disorders. Studies in the developing and developed world show that substance use is high in people living with HIV/Aids, with hazardous rates of up to twice that of the general population (Chander, 2011).

It is important to screen for alcohol-use disorders at baseline and at least annually thereafter if negative. If positive, this should be followed by a CAGE questionnaire or similar. Drinking becomes problematic when:

- it exceeds seven units per week for women and 14 units per week for men
- binge drinking occurs
- it has an impact on functioning
- it has an impact on interpersonal relationships
- it results in medical consequences.

Alcohol dependence is defined when the person displays three or more of the following signs: tolerance, withdrawal, unsuccessful efforts to cut down, great expenditure of time spent in acquiring alcohol, withdrawal from social or occupational functions or continued use that results in physical and psychological problems. Patients who screen positive for alcohol dependence should either receive a brief intervention (psycho-education, elucidating the effects of alcohol on health, recommendations for treatment, offering follow-up appointments) or be referred for pharmacological and psychological intervention in a facility adequately equipped to deal with such cases (see Chapter 20: Addictions 1: Alcohol-related disorders, for further information). A combination of psychopharmacological therapy and behavioural therapy may help to reduce relapse and maintain adherence to cART. Patients with mental health disorders, substance use disorders and HIV face a triple stigma and often have to navigate a very complex medical system. Many health care providers have little tolerance for such patients; care is often best in an integrated setting where the staff members are interested and specialise in such care. An integrated approach to prevention and treatment of these two co-morbid conditions is essential. HIV risk-reduction interventions must be offered to these individuals who are at high risk of contracting or transmitting HIV.

## 33.7.8 Pain syndromes

Pain is especially common in patients with HIV/Aids; various studies show ranges in prevalence of 28–97% (Cohen *et al.*, 2010; Tsao and Soto, 2009). It is recognised as a source of considerable distress and disability among persons living with HIV. Under-treated pain leads to an increase in psychological distress and a reduction in quality of life.

Pain in the context of HIV may derive from multiple and varied sources, including the HIV infection itself, complications from the infection such as malignancy, iatrogenic treatment effects such as the side effects of antiretroviral medication and factors unrelated to HIV (e.g. pre-existing conditions). Neuropathic pain related to HIV usually presents as a persisting, painful sensori-motor neuropathy with dysaesthesia, stocking-and-glove sensory loss, diminished distal reflexes and distal weakness. Similarly, post-herpetic neuralgia may involve pain of the face or trunk. Chronic headache may appear as a residual symptom of acute aseptic meningitis or as a result of chronic tension-type headaches.

All types of pain are associated with an increased risk of suicide, depression and self-medication with substances. Multidisciplinary pain treatment approaches, which employ coordinated efforts of experts in various disciplines, may be very useful in treating chronic HIV-related pain.

## 33.7.9 Personality and HIV

There is a significantly higher prevalence of personality disorders in HIV-infected individuals (30%) compared with the general population (10%) (Gallego *et al.*, 2011; Lenzenweger, 2008). Borderline, antisocial, dependent and histrionic personality disorders are some of the most frequently diagnosed in HIV-positive individuals (Gallego *et al.*, 2011).

Research suggests that the presence of personality traits or disorders may potentiate the risk of HIV infection and transmission, adversely affect adherence to HIV treatments due to serious interpersonal problems, contribute to disease progression and increase the risk of substance abuse (Gerhadstein *et al.*, 2011). Personality disorder (most notably antisocial personality disorder) is a risk factor for HIV infection specifically among substance users. The higher rate of HIV infection among drug users with antisocial personality disorder is related to the higher incidence of HIV-related risk behaviour, specifically more sexual contacts, needle use and injection-equipment sharing. Research offers support for the notion that personality pathology and substance abuse have an additive effect on the expression of HIV-related risk behaviour. Recognition of the impact of personality disorder on the individual's ability to cope with HIV infection is also important for comprehensive, sensitive and effective clinical care.

## 33.8 Prevention

A large proportion of patients with mental illness engage in behaviour that places them at high risk of contracting HIV. Although clinical factors such as poor reality perception, affective instability and impulsiveness play a major role in such behaviour, lack of knowledge and/or inaccurate information about HIV infection is also a significant variable.

As a result of the lower level of education and cognitive impairment often associated with mental illness, many mentally ill patients have largely been left out of HIV-prevention campaigns in the past. A call has been made to include this vulnerable group of patients and to target them specifically (Jonsson *et al.*, 2011). Studies have shown that levels of knowledge about HIV and AIDS are sub-optimal in patients with mental illness and that these levels differ between in-patients and out-patients and are influenced by psychiatric diagnosis (Grassi *et al.*, 2001; Melo *et al.*, 2010; Wainberg *et al.*, 2008). A study that assessed knowledge of HIV in a group of Indian patients with mental illness at baseline and again five days later after an HIV risk reduction programme, showed that brief HIV-focused educational interventions can improve knowledge (Chandra *et al.*, 2006). HIV-risk reduction interventions that target South Africans with psychiatric illnesses remain few and far between. Promotion of HIV testing and counselling of psychiatric patients and their families are needed and should further enable this group to receive the appropriate psychological support (Knox and Chenneville, 2006).

Risk assessment is an important tool to master; it should form part of each and every encounter with a patient. Within this assessment, maintaining a good rapport with a patient is very important, as is keeping the results and the discussion confidential.

Positive prevention aims to help infected individuals from spreading HIV. Small-group cognitive behavioural risk reduction interventions may be very effective among mentally ill HIV+ patients. Behavioural skills training methods are important to increase self-efficacy to change risky behaviours.

Other important prevention strategies include treatment as prevention, post-exposure prophylaxis (PEP), and pre-exposure prophylaxis (PrEP). Treatment of sexually transmitted diseases, medical male circumcision (MMC) and treatment of substance abuse are important in reducing acquisition and transmission of HIV amongst mentally ill patients.

## 33.9 Psychosocial treatment

Psychosocial interventions are important tools to help patients during their initial response to diagnosis and treatment, treatment adherence, adjustment to illness and stigmatisation and navigation through changes in identity and life.

### 33.9.1 Cognitive behavioural therapy

Cognitive behavioural therapy (CBT) promotes changes in thinking and behaviour in an attempt to change mood and anxiety symptoms (Zilber,

2006). CBT helps patients to examine their perceptions of HIV and to alter their response to it. CBT has been used to help patients with HIV cope with their diagnosis and to improve adherence to cART. A randomised controlled trial that evaluated CBT for adherence and depression (CBT-AD) in HIV-infected individuals found that those who received CBT-AD showed significantly greater improvements in medication adherence and depression relative to the comparison group. This type of therapy is potentially efficacious for individuals with HIV and who are struggling with depression and adherence (Safren *et al.*, 2009).

## 33.9.2 Interpersonal therapy

Interpersonal therapy (IPT) is a short-term therapy (12–20 weeks) aimed at developing problem-solving techniques. It also helps one acknowledge the exacerbating role that interpersonal problems have on coping. It specifically addresses grief, interpersonal role disputes, role transitions and interpersonal deficits (Markowitz and Weissman, 2004).

## 33.9.3 Psychodynamic psychotherapy

Psychodynamic psychotherapy helps explore and resolve conflicts interfering with optimal functioning. While it is aimed at 'restructuring patients' intrapsychic world', it also provides support and containment (Zilber, 2006). This type of therapy may not be an entirely cost-effective approach in low-income or developing countries and necessitates highly trained professionals to administer it.

## 33.9.4 Group therapy

Group therapy may be particularly valuable and seen as cost effective, especially where there are long waiting lists for psychotherapeutic interventions. Group therapy may be beneficial in recovery from substance abuse, stress management and coping, support and bereavement.

## 33.9.5 Family therapy

HIV affects families and it is important to address the feelings of helplessness, fear, stigma and grief within families of those with HIV. Family therapy is an intervention that can address these issues and ultimately help improve social support.

## 33.9.6 Community-based initiatives

### 33.9.6.1 The friendship bench

A innovative model to help deal with problems and stressors in people living with HIV/Aids is the friendship bench project (Chibanda *et al.*, 2011). Initiated in Zimbabwe, lay workers are trained in problem-solving therapy and to lead peer-support groups. This intervention consists of six structured sessions.

### 33.9.6.2 Support groups and food security

**Food insecurity** is a very real problem in resource-limited sub-Saharan Africa. The uncertainty it causes can lead to depression, while lack of food impacts on adherence to cART. A Ugandan study found that food insecurity was associated with severe symptoms of depression in women and that social support helped to alleviate the effects of food insecurity on depression (Tsai *et al.*, 2012).

Social and familial support are very important, however, since this requires disclosure of one's HIV status, a fear of stigma may preclude this. Nevertheless, peer-led support groups for people living with HIV/Aids are helpful in terms of adherence, disease outcomes and the alleviation of depression. Identification of substance-related issues and referral to groups like Alcoholics Anonymous (AA) and Narcotics Anonymous (NA) are useful.

### 33.9.6.3 HIV treatment-related adherence and prevention interventions

Groups run by peers and lay persons that deal with adherence and prevention issues may be useful as adjuncts to other interventions.

Psycho-education and other medically based education initiatives are important for patients to gain insight into their illness.

## 33.10 Psychopharmacological treatment of specific conditions

There are a number of basic principles that should guide the prescribing of psychotropic agents to patients with HIV. These can be delineated as follows:

- Conduct a thorough medication history, including other prescriptions, over-the-counter medication, herbal medication and recreational drugs.
- Classify substrates of the CYP 450 enzyme system, and classify the inducers and inhibitors of these substrates.
- Identify food drug interactions and other dietary restrictions.
- The motto to 'start low, go slow' should always be followed. Start at the lowest possible dose required and titrate up according to tolerability and response. HIV+ patients are often more sensitive to the side effects of psychotropic agents as they may have different rates of metabolism and have altered body mass due to the illness.
- Select the simplest dosing regimen possible.
- Select the agent with the fewest side effects and drug interactions possible.

Figure 33.5 delineates a basic approach to the treatment of delirium, mood disorders, psychotic disorders and HIV-associated neurocognitive disorders.

### 33.10.1 Major medication groups used in PLWHA with mental disorders

#### 33.10.1.1 Antidepressants

The use of fluoxetine and citalopram for the pharmacological treatment of mood and anxiety disorders is generally safe. Sertraline, citalopram and escitalopram generally have little effect on CYP enzyme systems. Doses of antidepressants used are generally similar to those used in non-infected patients. Be aware of interactions between fluoxetine and some non-nucleoside reverse transcriptase inhibitors (NNRTIs) and protease inhibitors (PIs). Tricyclic antidepressants may be useful in the patient with co-morbid pain or a sleep disorder. Consider the anticholinergic side effects of these drugs, lethality in overdose and some drug interactions with ritonavir. It is best to avoid the monoamine oxidase inhibitors due to the dietary restrictions and other side effects. Serotonin–norepinephrine reuptake inhibitors (SNRIs), such as venlafaxine and duloxetine, may be useful alternatives when response to first-line agents is not sufficient or in patients with co-morbid pain and anxiety disorders. Bupropion may have interactions with some of the PIs but has an advantage in that there are less sexual side effects and weight gain (Ferrando, 2009; Reid *et al.*, 2012). It is important to be aware of the potential to develop serotonin syndrome in patients with HIV, especially in the case of patients on two antidepressants and PIs.

#### 33.10.1.2 Mood stabilisers

The use of sodium valproate and lamotrigine are generally safe in patients infected with HIV. Caution is necessary in patients on AZT and sodium valproate as there have been a number of case reports describing neutropaenia. Also exercise caution with regard to possible drug interactions between lamotrigine and the PIs: doses may have to be adjusted accordingly. With lamotrigine, always be alert for the development of **Stevens-Johnson syndrome**. Although lithium is the gold standard drug to treat bipolar mood disorder and is not absolutely contraindicated for patients with HIV, one does need to be cautious with its use as it has a narrow therapeutic index. It should be avoided in patients with renal dysfunction and dehydration and possibly also in patients on tenofovir. It has been suggested that the use of lithium be restricted to physically stable patients with higher CD4 counts; careful and close monitoring of lithium levels is mandatory. It is best to avoid the use of carbamazepine in patients

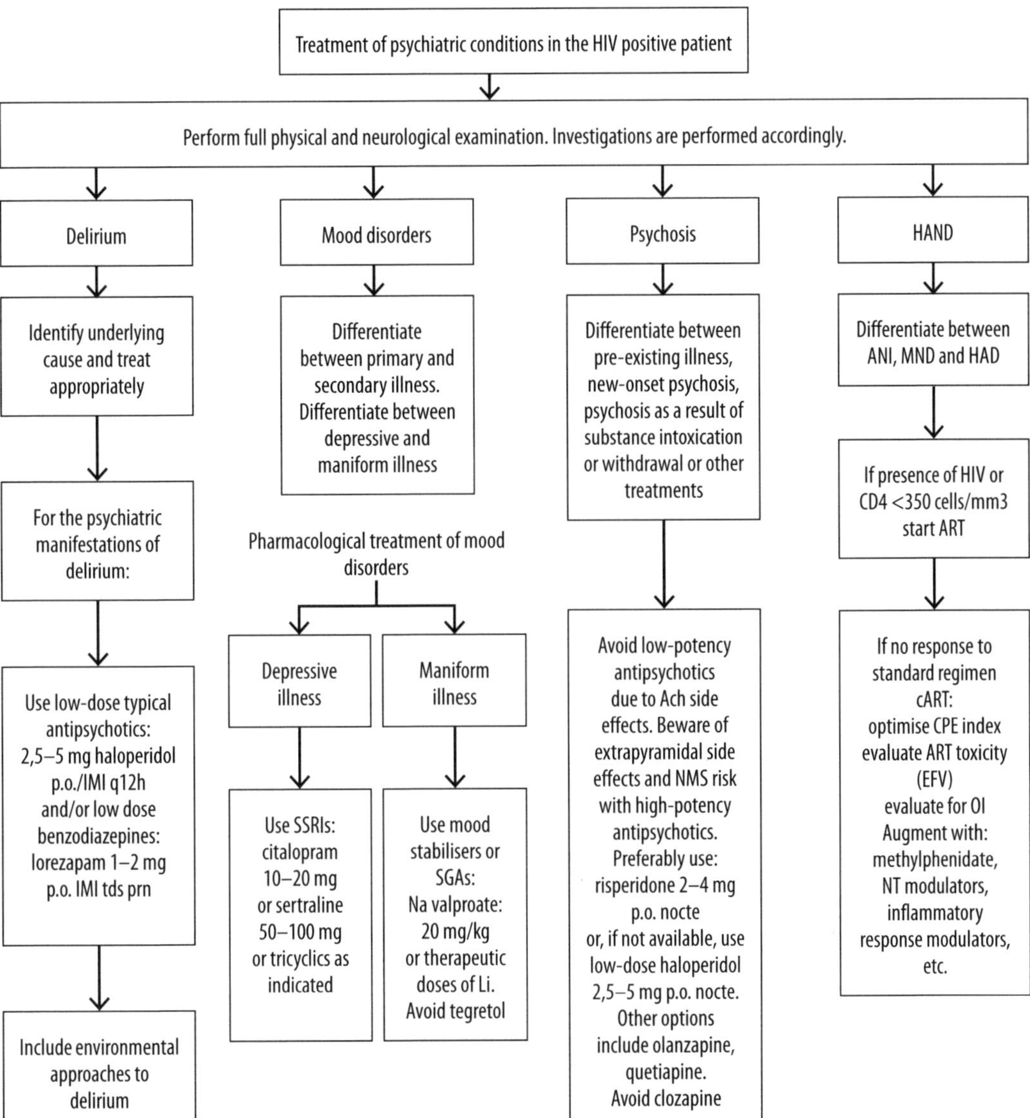


**Figure 33.5** Algorithmic approach to the treatment of delirium, mood disorders, psychotic disorders and HIV-associated neurocognitive disorders

on cART as there are numerous CYP 450 drug interactions as well as the added dilemma of neutropaenia. Consideration can also be given to using second-generation antipsychotics (SGAs), as their mood-stabilising properties have been well established. Here one should consider possible drug interactions, the development of dyslipidaemia, vascular risk factors, weight gain and glucose intolerance.

### 33.10.1.3 Antipsychotics

Generally, patients with HIV are more sensitive to the development of extrapyramidal side effects (EPSEs), neuroleptic malignant syndrome and tardive dyskinesia. Where available, SGAs should be used. However, where these are not available, typical antipsychotics (low doses of haloperidol 2,5–5 mg) should be used. It is important to monitor for EPSEs. One may also use low-potency antipsychotics (e.g. chlorpromazine); exercising caution regarding anticholinergic side effects and sedation. Risperidone is often the SGA of choice. It is used in low doses of between 2 mg and 4 mg. There have been reports of transaminitis and interactions with PIs, which may predispose patients to EPSEs. Quetiapine and aripiprazole have been used with good effect. Drug interactions with olanzapine and ritonovir result in a decreased concentration of olanzapine and may precipitate a psychotic episode or increase morbidity. Although the use of clozapine in the HIV+ patient is not absolutely contraindicated, it is not recommended. It is not known whether HIV+ patients have an increased risk of agranulocytosis, but clozapine is best restricted to patients who are physically stable, with higher CD4 counts and possibly for those with HIV psychosis and drug-induced parkinsonism. It is vital to closely monitor the white cell count of these patients.

#### 33.10.1.4 Anxiolytics

As there are drug interactions with alprazolam, midazolam and the PIs, it is best to avoid these agents and to rather prescribe agents with less active metabolites. The use of lorazepam and oxazepam is safe in the HIV+ patient, with the least likelihood of drug interactions. The dose of lorazepam for the agitated patient is usually prescribed as 1–2 mg p.o./IMI t.d.s. with a maximum dose of 12 mg/day. Oxazepam is a useful sleep aid but should only be prescribed for short periods of time.

## 33.11 Electroconvulsive therapy

The effectiveness of electroconvulsive therapy (ECT) for patients with major depression and major depressive disorder with psychotic features has been firmly established, especially in patients who respond poorly to medication or have contraindications for the use of oral medication. ECT is not contraindicated for patients with HIV. It is important, however, to exclude central nervous system pathology and perform a thorough physical and neurological examination. A lumbar puncture and neuro-imaging are indicated prior to commencement of ECT. The decision regarding the use of ECT in the patient with HIV is based on the clinical severity of the episode and the absence of contraindications. It is indicated as a therapeutic option in a patient who is cognitively intact, depressed, suicidal and deluded, who has not responded to other treatment, and in whom central nervous system pathology has been excluded (Schaerf *et al.*,1989).

## 33.12 Antiretroviral therapy and psychiatry

There are multiple barriers in accessing care for patients with mental illness. These include double or triple stigma (having to contend with the stigma related to two or three different illnesses) and navigating a complex health care system. Interestingly, a study in an integrated care setting in the United States showed that adherence in seriously mentally ill patients could equal that of the general population (Himeloch *et al.*, 2009). A further study showed that, compared with the general population, individuals with psychiatric disorders were significantly less likely to discontinue cART in the first and second years of treatment. In this case, mental health visits were associated with a decrease in the risk of discontinuing cART (Himeloch *et al.*, 2009). This, however, occurred in an integrated care setting where mental health services were on-site within the HIV clinic. Sadly there are not many such integrated care settings in South Africa.

Two distinct integrated care models exist: one in which HIV services are taken to the mental health clinic and the other where mental health services are taken to the HIV clinic. Sustainability, infrastructure and human resources limit the roll-out of integrated care settings in low- and middle-income countries.

Initiating cART within the mentally ill population is easily attainable, and they should not be discriminated against in terms of initiating cART. It is vital, however, that the importance of mental health visits is stressed and that adequate family support is present prior to initiation of cART. Adherence counselling must be stepped up and reinforced at every visit. The first goal is to initiate treatment of mentally ill patients on cART; once this is achieved one can optimise regimens depending on response and according to side effects. Generally, one should follow the Department of Health's cART initiation guidelines in the patient with mental illness, however, it is important to note when one should not use them. This may only be applicable in a handful of patients (e.g. efavirenz usage in a patient who develops psychosis soon after efavirenz initiation).

Initiation of antiretroviral therapy (ART) in the patient with mental illness is guided by three general principles:

- **pharmacokinetics** and **pharmacodynamic** drug-drug interactions between psychopharmacological agents and antiretroviral drugs
- neurotoxicity of certain antiretroviral therapy drugs (e.g. efavirenz toxicity in poor metabolisers of efavirenz)
- improved central nervous system penetration-effectiveness index of certain antiretroviral therapy drugs.

In some limited cases it may be necessary to change the drug to improve the central nervous system penetration-effectiveness score. One may do this in accordance with the central nervous system penetration effectiveness (CPE) index (see Table 33.3).

It is important to achieve the highest score possible with drug selection, as this not only provides more effective penetration of the blood-brain barrier (BBB), but also helps to eliminate sanctuary viral reservoirs that possibly are implicated in ongoing CNS disturbance. One should always weigh up the improved CPE score against the toxicity produced with better penetrating agents. Efavirenz has been implicated in this case. Most importantly, in cART therapy of patients with mental illness and HIV, one must consider the potential for synergistic effects resulting in dyslipidaemia, other vascular risk factors (including metabolic syndrome) and impaired glucose tolerance. This is most evident with some of the second-generation antipsychotics and the protease inhibitors (e.g. olanzapine and lopinavir boosted with ritonavir (LPV/r)).

Efavirenz deserves a mention, as many healthcare providers are reluctant to prescribe efavirenz in patients with a mental illness. While efavirenz does have neuropsychiatric side effects, they may not necessitate substitution of the drug. Neuropsychiatric side effects have been reported in up to 50% of patients, but only 2–6% required discontinuation of the drug (Vrouenraets *et al.*, 2007). Discontinuation rates are not higher in patients with a history of psychiatric disorder, or in patients currently on psycho-active medication. In most cases, once efavirenz is stopped, mental health disturbances prove to be transient with supportive care (Kennedi and Goforth,

**Table 33.3** The CPE Index

| **Penetration of ART through the blood-brain barrier: The CPE score** | | | | |
|---|---|---|---|---|
| **Agent** | **Penetration score** | | | |
| | 4 | 3 | 2 | 1 |
| **NRTI** | AZT | ABC, Emtircitabine | 3TC, D4T | DDI, TDF (NtRI) |
| **NNRTI** | NVP | EFV | Etravirine | |
| **PI** | Indinavir | DRV, FosAPV, LPV | AZV | SQV, unboosted AZV |
| **ENI** | Vicriviroc | Maraviroc | | Enfurvitide |
| **INI** | | Raltegravir | | |

**Key:**

NRTI: Nucleoside reverse transcriptase inhibitors
AZT: Zidovudine
ABC: Abacavir
3TC: Lamivudine
D4T: Stavudine
DDI: Didanosine
TDF: Tenofovir
NtRI: Nucleotide reverse transcriptase inhibitor
NNRTI: Non-nucleoside reverse transcriptase inhibitor
NVP: Nevirapine
EFV: Efavirenz
PI: Protease Inhibitor
DRV: Darunavir
FosAPV: Fosamprenavir
LPV: Lopinavir
AZV: Atazanavir
SQV: Saqinavir
ENI: Entry inhibitors
INI: Integrase Inhibitors

**Source:** Letendre, 2011

2011). It is important to remember that withholding efavirenz from patients with a mental illness results in these individuals having less effective, less convenient options and often drugs with more side effects. This may reduce adherence and add to the progression of the disease. One particular area that needs more investigation is the use of efavirenz in patients with neurocognitive disorders. In a trial of ART-naïve patients with no neuropsychological impairment, patients who were randomised to the efavirenz arm, showed a deterioration in neuropsychological functioning (Winston *et al.*, 2010). A second study showed that efavirenz use was associated with an increase in neurocognitive impairment (Ciccarelli *et al.*, 2011). These two studies highlight the neurotoxicity profile of efavirenz, which requires further study.

Drug-drug interactions between psychopharmacological agents and cART are important to discern. Although one has to be vigilant for these, it is important to appreciate that better adherence to cART through better mental health treatment far outweighs the negative impact psychotropic drugs might have on cART blood levels. Table 33.4 highlights the most common drug interactions between psychotropic agents and ART. A **clinically significant drug interaction (CSDI)** is one that produces at least a 30% change in pharmacokinetic parameters (Yiu *et al.*, 2011). Importantly, an actual CSDI requires intervention, whereas a theoretical interaction requires monitoring. Intervention could take the form of changing the dose interval, changing the dose frequency, or substituting a drug for one with fewer interactions.

Adherence to cART is of utmost importance in mentally ill patients with HIV. It is well known that patients need to be >95% adherent to their cART to remain virologically suppressed.

Non-adherence is associated with:

- decreased CD4 count
- increased viral load
- higher mortality and morbidity
- poorer quality of life.

Patients are often non-adherent because of various factors:

- treatment related: attitude towards treatment, side effects, dosing regimen
- patient related: age, sex, social status, level of motivation, forgetfulness, lack of insight, health status
- health-care related: patient/health-care provider relationship
- socioeconomic: education, literacy, access to clinic, support systems, stigma.

### 33.12.1 Strategies to improve adherence

While educating patients about their illness and medication is always necessary and plays a vital role in promoting adherence, there are a number of other strategies one can use to help support adherence in patients. These are often based on many of the factors mentioned above. Peer support and reminders, which may include pillboxes and setting reminders on cellphones, are some examples.

Treatment fatigue is a real problem in HIV care settings. HIV has all the components of an illness that predisposes a patient to non-adherence.

The doctor-patient relationship is something providers always should work on and improve. A patient must trust his or her health-care provider, especially in busy clinics where it is not always possible to communicate all the information in one sitting. It is always important to include as many family members or social support members in this process as possible.

Ultimately it is the integration of mental health and HIV care that will improve adherence and outcomes. Community-based projects aimed at improving and establishing community-based psychosocial support are helpful in improving adherence. These include community income-generating projects, food gardens for food security, support groups, peer-led defaulter tracing, and psycho-education programmes.

**Table 33.4** Common drug interactions between psychotropic medication and ART

| Agent | ARV | Effect | Recommend |
|---|---|---|---|
| bupropion | LPV/r | AUC⇓, LPV/r is unchanged | ⇑dose of bupropion if required |
| paroxetine | DRV/r | AUC⇓ | ⇑dose of paroxetine if required |
| sertraline | DRV/r | AUC⇓ | ⇑dose of sertraline if required |
| | EFV | AUC⇓ | ⇑dose of sertraline if required |
| trazodone | RTV | AUC⇑ | ⇓dose by 50% |
| fluoxetine | RTV | RTV AUC ⇑ | Effect likely not clinically significant |
| | NVP | fluoxetine AUC ⇓ | ⇑dose of fluoxetine if required |
| | EFV | no interaction | Use standard doses of both drugs |
| alprazolam | RTV | ⇓Alprazolam clearance | give lowest dose possible |
| lamotrigine | LPV/r | ⇓Lamotrigine AUC | ⇑lamotrigine |
| phenytoin | LPV/r | LPV/r and phenytoin AUC ⇓ | ⇑LPV/r and monitor anticonvulsant levels |
| carbamazepine | EFV | EFV and carbamazepine AUC ⇓ | monitor carbamazepine levels, may also require higher doses of efavirenz |
| olanzapine | LPV/r | olanzapine AUC ⇓ | ⇑olanzapine dose if required |
| valproate | LPV/r | AUC⇓ | Monitor anticonvulsant levels and increase dose of valproate if required |
| methadone | LPV/r | methadone AUC ⇓ | monitor for opiate withdrawal. May require increase in methadone dose |
| | NVP | | |
| | EFV | | |

**Key:** LPV/r: Lopinavir boosted with ritonavir; AUC: Area under the curve; DRV/r: Darunavir boosted with ritonavir; EFV: Efavirenz; RTV: Ritonavir; NVP: Nevirapine.

**Source:** Foisy and Tseng, 2015; Meemken *et al.*, 2015

## 33.13 Psychosocial issues common amongst people living with HIV/Aids

Common transition points in HIV syndromes may be delineated as follows:

- **sero-testing phenomena**: as with other life-threatening illnesses, there is shock, anger, anxiety, guilt, and denial
- emergence of physical symptoms: the idea of a shortened life expectancy and death may be confronted for the very first time when patients become symptomatic
- disclosure: fear of loss of control, of abandonment by family and friends, of the inability to work, of medical expenses and of pain may be evident
- commencing treatment: the HIV+ person often has questions and feels ambivalence about regular monitoring of lymphocytes and viral load, the need for regular review of medical symptoms, and the pros and cons of treatment with antiretroviral agents
- adverse events related to treatment: side effects to medication may have an impact on adherence, while some side effects (e.g. lipoatrophy) may be stigmatising.

### 33.13.1 Double stigma, double challenge

Stigma not only makes it more difficult for people to come to terms with HIV and to manage their illness, but also interferes with attempts to fight the Aids epidemic. Both HIV and mental illness are associated with stigma and high levels of discrimination. This may result in being shunned by family, peers and the wider community, poor treatment in health care, limited provision of health-related education, an erosion of rights, psychological damage and a negative effect on the success of HIV testing and treatment.

### 33.13.2 Children and adolescents living with HIV

Worldwide, about 2,7 million children younger than 15 and more than 10 million aged 15–24 are afflicted. Half of all new infections occur in young people. Despite improvements in antiretroviral therapies, child mortality due to Aids remains significant. Fortunately, recent developments in antiretroviral therapy have helped to decrease the incidence of vertical transmission and reduce the treatment burden on those infected. Depression is also very common in children and adolescents infected with HIV because they have to cope with the emotional distress of social stigmatisation, isolation and hopelessness, forced disclosure, loss and bereavement and anxiety about their medical prognosis.

### 33.13.3 Suicidal behaviour in patients living with HIV

People with HIV, like others with serious diseases, may have thoughts about suicide. They may also engage in self-harming behaviour that have a significant suicide risk. These thoughts or actions may not be just a measure of distress or desperation, but may strongly suggest the presence of a severe depressive disorder. People with HIV have a greater risk of suicide and deliberate self-harm than those without the infection. The risk of deliberate self-harm is greater in people who have a previous history of self-harm, substance abuse and personality disorders and a current or past psychiatric history. Mental health-care providers should be able to assess suicidal ideas, recognise the presence of a suicide risk and its degree, and formulate an intervention plan.

### 33.13.4 Couples and HIV

The majority of people living with HIV, no matter their sexual orientation, live at least some of the time with a partner. The introduction of HIV into a relationship usually results in a change of dynamics. Each partner may be confronted by multiple losses such as loss of health, independence, intimacy, privacy and the possibility of death.

Not all couples have a **sero-concordant relationship** (where both are either HIV positive or negative). There is growing evidence that **sero-discordant couples** are on the increase. These couples face unique challenges, such as:

- deciding on a comfortable level of sexual activity
- the possible risk of transmission
- care-giving responsibilities
- survivor guilt
- decision to have children.

Couples therapy can be very useful for these individuals. Difficulties that may require attention include dealing with conflict and disagreement, balancing the needs of both individuals and dealing with negative emotions such as anger, guilt and sexual problems. In addition to couples therapy, either partner may benefit from individual therapy, thereby creating a private space in which to address his or her own emotional needs (Robert *et al.*, 2010).

### 33.13.5 Criminal transmission of HIV

Can a person who is believed to have intended to infect someone, be charged with a crime? This is a controversial issue, giving rise to differences of opinion all over the world. Aids organisations are generally opposed to attempts to use criminal law in this way. This is because there are many social reasons why people with HIV may sometimes have unsafe sex, such as fear, denial, prejudice and even ignorance. Laws relating to various crimes, such as murder, attempted murder and assault, could be used to charge a person with harmful HIV-related behaviour.

In South Africa, there has not yet been a criminal case where a person has been convicted for deliberately infecting another person with HIV (Mokgoro, 2001).

### 33.13.6 Ethics, disclosure and workplace issues

HIV/Aids has raised many ethical issues relating to the basic rights and fair treatment of people infected with HIV. Health care workers must be knowledgeable about policy related to proper conduct, and work towards reducing denial and stigmatisation.

The South African Constitution affords every person the right of access to health care, the right to non-discrimination, the right to privacy and confidentiality, and the right to an environment that is not harmful to their health and well-being.

The ethical rules of the Health Professions Council of South Africa (HPCSA) make provision for protection of confidentiality: patient information may only be divulged with the patient's express (and preferably written) consent. A family does not have the right to know the patient's HIV status. However, the advantages of telling one's family should be pointed out during counselling, before the patient becomes too ill. Doctors are often harassed by third parties to provide information on a patient's HIV status. These parties should be informed that patient confidentiality is safeguarded by legislation and ethical rules binding medical practitioners, and that unless the patient provides consent, no medical information may be divulged.

A medical practitioner is not permitted to provide false information on a medical certificate. However, the practitioner may state that the employee is, in his or her opinion, not capable of working, owing to injury or illness, for a period of time, without disclosing the sensitive nature of the illness. Information may only be made available to the employer if the employee (patient) consents.

## Conclusion

There is a complex interrelationship between mental health and HIV. HIV affects mental health by means of its direct neurobiological action, the impact of having the illness, treatment for it and its impact on the family (Jayarajan and Chandra, 2010). The prevalence of mental health disorders is increased among people living with HIV/Aids. Psychiatrists must be aware of the varied psychiatric manifestations of HIV and how HIV may impact on existing psychiatric conditions. Mental health professionals must screen for common mental health disorders among patients with HIV and be aware of the dynamic relationship between treatment of mental disorders and HIV treatment, including drug interactions and complications of its treatment. We must be acutely aware of the role stigma plays in our patients' lives as well as the psychosocial consequences of this devastating disease. We should strive for integrated care, the provision of better access to multidisciplinary care, and the improvement of the quality of life of this vulnerable group of individuals.

# References

Antinori A, Arendt G, Becker JT, Brew BJ, Byrdt DA, Cherner M, Clifford DB, Cinque P, Epstein LG, Goodkin K, Gisslen M, Grant I, Heaton RK, Joseph J, Marder K, Marra CM, McArthur JC, Nunn M, Price RW, Pulliam L, Robertson KR, Sacktor N, Valcour V, Wojna VE (2007) Updated research nosology for HIV-associated neurocognitive disorders. *Neurology* 69(18): 1789–99

Chander G (2011) Addressing alcohol use in HIV infected persons. *Topics in Antiviral Medicine* 19(4): 143–7

Chandra PS, Krishna VAS, Carey MP (2006) Improving knowledge about HIV and AIDS among persons with a severe mental illness in India. *Indian Journal of Social Psychiatry* 22: 104–9

Chibanda, D, Mesu, P, Kajawu, L, Cowan, F, Araya, R, Abas, MA (2011) Problem solving therapy for depression and common mental disorders in Zimbabwe: Piloting a task shifting primary mental health care intervention in a population with a high prevalence of people living with HIV. *BMC Public Health* 11: 828–38

Ciccarelli N, Fabbiani M, Di Giumbenedetto S, Fanti I, Baldonero E, Bracciale L (2011) Efavirenz associated with cognitive disorders in otherwise asymptomatic HIV infected patients. *Neurology* 76(16): 1403–9

Cohen MA, Goforth HW, Lux JZ, Khalife S, Cozza KL, Soffer J (2010) *Handbook of Aids Psychiatry*. Oxford, England: Oxford University Press

Ferrando SJ (2009) Psychopharmacologic treatment of patients with HIV/AIDS. *Current Psychiatry Reports* 11(3): 235–42

Foisy M, Tseng A (*s.d.*). *Predicted interactions between psychotropics and antiretrovirals*. Available at: www.hivclinic.ca/main/drugs_interact_files/psych-int.pdf. (Accessed 1 February 2015.)

Freeman M, Patel V, Collins PY, Bertolote J (2005) Integrating mental health in global initiatives in HIV/AIDS. *British Journal of Psychiatry* 187: 1–3

Gallego L, Barreiro P, Lopez-Ibor JJ (2011) Diagnosis and clinical features of major neuropsychiatric disorders in HIV infection. *Aids Reviews* 13: 171–9

Ganasen KA, Fincham D, Smit J, Seedat S, Stein D (2008) Utility of the HIV Dementia Scale (HDS) in identifying HIV dementia in a South African sample. *Journal of Neurological Sciences* 269(1–2): 62–4

Gerhadstein KR, Griffin PT, Hormes JM (2011) Personality disorders lead to risky behaviour treatment obstacles. *HIV Clinician* 23(2): 6–9

Grant I (2002) The neurocognitive complications of HIV infection. In: Ramachandran VS, (Ed). *Encyclopedia of the Human Brain*. San Diego: Academic Press: 475–489

Grassi L, Biancosino B, Righi R, Finotti L, Peron L (2001) Knowledge about HIV transmission and prevention among Italian patients with psychiatric disorders. *Psychiatric Services* 52(5): 679–81

Himeloch S, Brown CH, Walkup J, Chander G, Korthuis PT, Afful J (2009) HIV patients with psychiatric disorders are less likely to discontinue HAART. *AIDS* 23(13): 1735–42

Jayarajan N, Chandra PS (2010) HIV and mental health: An overview of research from India. *Indian Journal of Psychiatry* 52(S1): S269-S273

Joint United Nations programme on HIV/Aids: South Africa (2013) *HIV and AIDS estimates*. Available at: http://www.unaids.org/en/regionscountries/countries/southafrica (Accessed 1 February 2015.)

Jonsson G, Davies N, Freeman C, Joska J, Pahad S, Thom R, Thompson K, Woollett N, Furin J, Meintjies G (2013) Management of mental health disorders in HIV-positive patients. *Southern African Journal of HIV Medicine* 14(4):155–65

Jonsson G, Joska J (2009) Assessment and treatment of psychosis in people living with HIV/AIDS. *Southern African Journal of HIV Medicine* 10(3): 20–27

Jonsson G, Moosa MYH, Jeenah Y (2011) Knowledge, attitudes and personal beliefs about HIV and AIDS among mentally ill patients in Soweto, Johannesburg. *Southern African Journal of HIV Medicine* 12(3): 14–20

Joska JA, Kaliski SZ, Benatar SR (2008) Patients with severe mental illness: A new approach to testing for HIV. *South African Medical Journal* 98(3): 213–7

Joska JA, Westgarth-Taylor J, Hoare J, Thomas KGF, Paul R, Myer L, Stein, DJ (2011) Validity of international HIV dementia scale in South Africa. *AIDS Patient Care and STDs* 25(2): 95–101

Kagee A, Martin L (2010) Symptoms of depression and anxiety among a sample of South African patients living with HIV. *AIDS Care* 22(2): 159–65

Kennedi CA, Goforth HW (2011) A systematic review of the psychiatric side effects of Efavirenz. *AIDS and Behavior* 15(8): 1803–18

Knox MD, Chenneville T (2006) Prevention and education strategies. In: Fernandez F, Ruiz P (Eds). *Psychiatric aspects of HIVAIDS*. Philadelphia: Lipincott Williams and Wilkins

Kumar A (2012) HIV and substance abuse. *Current HIV research* 10: 365

Lenzenweger M (2008) Epidemiology of personality disorders. *The Psychiatric Clinics of North America* 31(3): 395

Letendre S (2011) *The CPE Score*. Available at: http://www.neurohiv.com/PUB/FILE/letendre.pdf (Accessed 30 October 2012)

Mall S, Sorsdahl K, Swartz L, Joska J (2012) 'I understand just a little…' Perspectives of HIV/AIDS service providers in South Africa of providing mental health care for people living with HIV/AIDS. *AIDS Care* 24(3): 319–23

Markowitz JC, Weissman MM (2004) Interpersonal psychotherapy: principles and applications. *World Psychiatry* 3(3): 136–9

Matthews A, Trujillo M (2006) Anxiety disorders. In: Fernandez F, Ruiz P (Eds). *Psychiatric aspects of HIVAIDS*. Philadelphia: Lipincott Williams and Wilkins

McArthur JC, Steiner J, Sacktor N, Nath A (2010) Human immunodeficiency virus associated neurocognitive disorders: Mind the gap. *Annals of Neurology* 67(6): 699–714

Meemken, L Hanhoff N, Tseng A, Christensen S, Gillessen A (2015) Drug-drug interactions with antiviral agents in people who inject drugs requiring substitution therapy. *Annuls of Pharmacology* 49(7): 796–807

Melo APS, Cesar CC, De Assis Acurcio F, Campos LN, Ceccato M, Wainberg ML, McKinnon K, Guimaraes MDC (2010) Individual and treatment setting predictors of HIV/AIDS knowledge among psychiatric patients and their implications in a national multisite study in Brazil. *Community Mental Health Journal* 46: 505–16

Mokgoro JY (2001) Criminal law and harmful HIV-related behavior. The South African Law Commission. Project 85: *Fifth Interim Report on Aspects of the Law relating to AIDS*. Available at: http://www.justice.gov.za/salrc/reports/r_prj85_harmb_2001apr.pdf (Accessed 30 October 2012.)

Nakimuli-Mpungu E, Musisi S, Mpungu SK, Katabira E (2006) Primary versus secondary mania in Uganda. *American Journal of Psychiatry* 163: 1349–54

Olagunju AT, Adeyemi JD (2012) A study on epidemiological profile of anxiety disorders among people living with HIV/AIDS in a sub-Saharan Africa HIV clinic. *AIDS Behavior* 16: 2192–7

Olley B, Seedat S, Stein, D (2006) Persistence of psychiatric disorders in a cohort of HIV/AIDS patients in South Africa: A 6-month follow-up study. *Journal of Psychosomatic Research* 60: 479–84

Pappin M, Wouters E, Booysen LR (2012) Anxiety and depression amongst patients enrolled in a public sector antiretroviral treatment programme in South Africa. A cross-sectional study. *BMC Public health* 12: 244.

Reid E, Stolloff K, Joska J (2012) Psychotropic prescribing in HIV. *Southern African Journal of HIV Medicine* 13(4): 188–94

Robert M, Kairana R, Gray RH, Kiwanuka N, Makumbi F, Sewakambo NK, Serwadda D, Naugoda F, Kigozi G, Semanda J, Wawer MJ (2010) Disclosure of HIV results among discordant couples in Rakai, Uganda. *AIDS Care* 22(9): 1041–51

Rossouw TM (2011) HIV management in practice. *Continuing Medical Education* 29(5): 200–2

Ruiz P (2006) Mood disorders. In: Fernandez F, Ruiz P (Eds). *Psychiatric aspects of HIVAIDS*. Philadelphia: Lipincott Williams and Wilkins

Sadock BJ, Sadock VA (2005). In: Cancro R, Mitchell CW, (Eds). *Kaplan and Sadock's pocket handbook of clinical psychiatry*. Philadelphia: Lippincott Williams & Wilkins: 67–77

Safren S, O'Cleirigh C, Tan J, Raminani S, Reilly LC, Otto MW, Mayer KH (2009) A randomized controlled trial of cognitive behavioural therapy for adherence and depression (CBT-AD) in HIV infected individuals. *Health Psychology* 28(1): 1–14

Saktor NC, Wong M, Nakasujja N, Skolasky RL, Selnes OA, Musisi S, Robertson K, McArthur JC, Ronald A, Katabira E (2005) The International HIV Dementia Scale: a new rapid screening test for HIV dementia. *AIDS* 19(13): 1367–74

Schaerf FW, Miller RR, Lipsey JR, McPherson RW (1989) ECT for major depression in four patients infected with Human Immunodeficiency Virus. *American Journal of Psychiatry* 146(6): 782–4

Sherr L, Clucas C, Harding R, Sibley E, Catalan J (2011) HIV and depression – a systematic review of interventions. *Psychology, Health and Medicine* 16(5): 493–527

Singer EJ, Sueires MV, Commins, D (2010) Neurologic presentation of AIDS. *Neurologic Clinics* 28(1): 253–75

Singh D (2009) Neurocognitive impairment in PLWHA: Clinical features and assessment. *Southern African Journal of HIV Medicine* 10(3): 30–4

Spies G, Kader K, Kidd M, Smit J, Myer L, Stein D, Seedat, S (2009) Validity of the K-10 in detecting DSM-IV defined depression and anxiety disorders among HIV infected individuals. *AIDS Care* 21(9): 1163–68

Stolar A, Catalano G, Hakala SM (2005). Mood disorders and psychosis in HIV. In: Citron K, Brouillette MJ, Beckett A (Eds). *HIV and psychiatry: Training and resource manual*. Cambridge: Cambridge University Press: 88-109

Thom R (2009) Common mental disorders in people living with HIV/AIDS. *Southern African Journal of HIV Medicine* 35: 8–13

Thom RGM (2012) *HAART and MIND: Common mental disorders in people living with HIV/AIDS*. (The access series.) Johannesburg: Wits University Press

Tombaugh TN, McIntyre, NJ (1992) The mini-mental state examination. A comprehensive review. *Journal of the American Geriatric Society* 40: 922–35

Treisman GJ (2007) *Adherence, psychiatric disorders and HIV*. Available at: www.medscape.org/viewarticle/552857 (Accessed 1 February 2015)

Tsai AC, Bangsberg DR, Frongillo EA, Hunt PW, Muzoora C, Martin JN, Weiser SD (2012) Food insecurity, depression and the modifying role of social support among people living with HIV/ AIDS in rural Uganda. *Social Science and Medicine* 74: 2012–19

Tsao JCI, Soto T (2009) Pain in persons living with HIV and comorbid psychological and substance use disorders. *The Clinical Journal of Pain* 25(4): 307–12

United Nations Programme on HIV/AIDS (UNAIDS) and World Health Organisation (2009) *AIDS Epidemic Update*. Geneva: World Health Organisation: 7

Vally Z (2011) HIV-associated neurocognitive disorders. *South African Journal of Psychiatry* 17(4): 98–102

Verdeli H, Clougherty K, Bolton P, Speel- Man L, Lincoln N, Bass, J (2003) Adapting group interpersonal psychotherapy for a developing country. Experience in rural Uganda. *World Psychiatry* 2(2): 114–20

Vlassova N, Angelino AF, Treisman GJ (2009) Update on mental health issues in patients with HIV infection. *Current Infectious Disease Reports* 11: 163–9

Vrouenraets SM, Wit FW, Van Tongeren J, Lange JM (2007) Efavirenz: A review. *Expert Opinion on Pharmacotherapy* 8(6): 851–71

Wainberg ML, Mckinnon K, Elkington K, Mattos PE, Mann CG, De Souza Pinto D, Otto-Salaj L, Cournos F (2008) HIV risk behaviours among outpatients with severe mental illness in Rio de Janeiro, Brazil. *World Psychiatry* 7: 166–72

Winston A, Duncombe C, Li PC, Gill JM, Kerr SJ, Puls R (2010) Does choice of cART alter changes in cerebral function testing after 48 weeks in treatment naïve, HIV 1 infected individuals commencing cART? A randomized controlled study. *Clinical Infectious Diseases* 50(6): 910–9

Yiu P, Nguyen NN, Holodniy M (2011) Clinically significant drug interactions in younger and older human immunodeficiency virus positive patients receiving antiretroviral therapy. *Pharmacotherapy* 31(5): 480–9

Zilber C (2006) Psychotherapeutic strategies. In: Fernandez F, Ruiz P (Eds). *Psychiatric aspects of HIVAIDS*. Philadelphia: Lipincott Williams and Wilkins

CHAPTER

# 34 Suicide and the aggressive patient

*Shamima Saloojee, Naseema Vawda*

## 34.1 Introduction

An emergency is a serious, unexpected and often dangerous situation that requires immediate action. Psychiatric emergencies arise when individuals pose an immediate threat to themselves or others. This chapter will deal with the evaluation and management of psychiatric emergencies

The emergency situation requires a brief but thorough evaluation of the physical as well as the mental status of the individual, followed by an appropriate short-term management plan based on the clinical assessment.

## 34.2 The aggressive patient

### 34.2.1 Introduction and definition of terms

The evaluation and management of the patient with severe behavioural disturbance (the aggressive patient) by a skilled health care professional is important to ensure the safety of the community and the protection of the mentally disturbed individual. The reasons for violent and aggressive behaviour in society are manifold; in many instances, they do not involve the mental health professional. Violent acts that arise from deliberate criminal activity, for example, are more appropriately dealt with by the criminal justice system.

Individuals can present to the emergency department of a hospital, clinic or a family practitioner with a broad range of disturbances in behaviour that range from agitation and irritability to severe behavioural disturbance. Agitation can be defined as increased motor or verbal activity combined with subjective feelings of tension. Aggression, on the other hand, is defined as any verbal, non-verbal or physical behaviour that threatens or harms others or property (Morrisson, 1990). Violence is behaviour that involves the use of physical force with the intention of causing harm to people or damage to property. All individuals with severe behavioural disturbance present a complex clinical challenge in the emergency department.

### 34.2.2 Evaluation of the aggressive patient

The family practitioner may be the first point of care for patients with disturbed behaviour in the community. With appropriate knowledge and skill, many emergencies can be handled by competent doctors at all levels of the health care system.

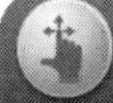

**Case study 34.1**

JD is a 22 year old university student. He is brought to hospital by the police because he suddenly jumped up during a lecture, smashed the data projector and tried to strangle the lecturer, whom he accused of transmitting personal information about him at the lecture. In the hospital he is abusive and angry; he further believes that hospital staff members are colluding with the university to have him killed. He is HIV positive but is not on antiretroviral treatment. He threatens to hit back at anyone who messes around with him.

The primary objectives in the management of patients with severe behavioural disturbance are to contain the behaviour, exclude any acute medical illnesses and institute definitive treatment and care. In order to achieve these objectives the situation requires a thorough physical as well as a mental state assessment.

Evaluation of these patients is essential because a behavioural disturbance is not a psychiatric diagnosis: it can be a manifestation of a psychiatric illness or a medical illness (Talbort *et al.*, 2000; O'Brien *et al.*, 2006). The behavioural disturbance can be caused or exacerbated by a medical illness (Henneman *et al.*, 1994; Hall *et al.*, 1978) or can occur coincidentally with a medical illness (Koran *et al.*, 2002). Previous studies have reported variable rates of medical illness in patients presenting to the emergency department with psychiatric symptoms: prevalence rates ranging from 7–63% have been reported (Gregory *et al.*, 2004).

The co-morbidity of psychiatric and medical illness is under-recognised in the emergency setting. Missed medical illnesses can result in significant morbidity and even mortality (Reeves *et al.*, 2000). Delirium presents with psychiatric and behavioural manifestations; it is important to exclude delirium in all patients who present with aggressive or violent behaviour. A high degree of suspicion for a medical cause for aggressive behaviour must be maintained for elderly patients in particular (Inouye *et al.*, 2014). Factors that should alert one to an underlying medical cause for the disturbed behaviour are:

- older than 40 years
- no past psychiatric history
- visual, tactile or olfactory hallucinations
- illusions
- disorientation.

Clinical features that may be used to differentiate between delirium and acute psychosis are listed in Table 34.1.

Throughout this chapter, a thorough physical assessment is emphasised as an essential component of the emergency psychiatric evaluation. If the violent behaviour is not due to a medical condition and is not substance-related, it can be assumed that the cause is psychiatric. A comprehensive psychiatric history and mental status examination must be conducted, and biological and psychosocial predisposing and precipitating factors identified.

## 34.2.3 Management of the aggressive patient

In the acute situation, it is seldom possible to obtain a reliable history and perform an adequate physical examination, as the patient may be threatening violence, or already be engaged in an assaultive or destructive act. The first objective in such a situation is to ensure the safety of the patient and others in the immediate vicinity. The physician should attempt to prevent the patient from harming himself or herself or others. The small, cluttered consulting rooms of the emergency department of many general hospitals in South Africa are overcrowded and structurally unsuitable to manage aggressive patients. A management plan must therefore be designed to accommodate the deficiencies in infrastructure and all members of the health care team must be educated and informed about the plan. It is important to make representations to the hospital management to employ security personnel to assist in the management of behavioural emergencies. Certain basic steps to prevent a crisis situation from developing within the emergency department are discussed below.

### 34.2.3.1 Step 1: Ensure that the environment is secure

- Devise a policy for the management of the aggressive patient.
- Security staff should be present in the department or must be readily available.
- Objects that have the potential to be used as weapons (e.g. portable blood pressure monitors) must be kept out of reach of the patient.
- The clinician should have immediate access to an exit from the consultation room.
- An alarm system (or even a simple bell) should be available in the consultation room.

**Table 34.1** Clinical features of delirium and acute psychosis

| Factor | Delirium | Psychotic illness |
|---|---|---|
| Onset | sudden: hours to days | gradual: days to weeks |
| Course | fluctuating, worse at night | continuous |
| Consciousness | impaired | patient alert and awake |
| Orientation | impaired in all spheres | usually preserved for person and place |
| Hallucinations | usually visual | mainly auditory |
| Illusions | may be present | very rare |
| Involuntary movements | may have coarse tremor | usually none |

**Table 34.2** Some medical causes associated with aggressive behavioural disturbance

| |
|---|
| **Infective:** meningitis, encephalitis, HIV, syphilis, pneumonia, urinary tract infections, tuberculosis, typhoid |
| **Central nervous system conditions:** epilepsy, tumours, cerebrovascular accidents |
| **Metabolic:** hypoglycaemia, hyponatraemia, hypocalcaemia, hypercalcaemia, hypomagnesemia, hypoxia, acidosis, uraemia, hepatic encephalopathy |
| **Substances of abuse:** alcohol, cannabis, mandrax, amphetamines, cocaine, phencyclidine, other hallucinogens |
| **Drugs:** steroids, anticholinergics, antiretrovirals, antiparkinsonian drugs, some antibiotics, antifungals, cimetidine |
| **Endocrine:** hyperthyroidism, hypothyroidism, hypoparathyroidism, hyperparathyroidism, hypopituitarism |
| **Nutritional:** vitamin B12 deficiency, folate deficiency |
| **Systemic disorders:** SLE (systemic lupus erythematosus), porphyria |
| **Traumatic:** head injury |

### 34.2.3.2 Step 2: De-escalation

**De-escalation** is the use of verbal and non-verbal techniques to calm down the disturbed patient and thereby attempt to defuse the situation. Respect for the patient and his or her dignity are integral to this process. The interaction between the patient and the practitioner is crucial for a successful resolution of the disturbed behaviour. The purpose of this step is to negotiate and collaborate, rather than maintain authority and control. De-escalation strategies that should be used are to:

- approach patients with caution
- avoid abrupt movements or vulnerable positions (e.g. turning your back to the patient)
- speak clearly and slowly but firmly
- introduce yourself and others involved in the process
- reassure the patient of your intention to help
- use open-ended sentences
- not threaten or humiliate the patient
- not make promises you cannot keep
- not challenge or collude with the patient: maintain neutrality
- give the patient choices.

### 34.2.3.3 Step 3: Physical restraint

The restraint of an aggressive patient should be undertaken by an experienced team. Firstly, a group of five trained staff should approach the patient cautiously and calmly, as a 'show of force'. This alone is sometimes enough to bring the behaviour under control. The team leader may attempt to contain behaviour by speaking firmly but respectfully to the patient, asking him or her to co-operate with staff. If verbal intervention and the show of force fail to halt the violent or destructive behaviour, physical restraint of the patient becomes essential. This procedure must be undertaken by an experienced restraining team of at least five staff members (one for each limb, and a designated leader). The leader should inform the patient of the team's intention to restrain him or her and continue to speak to the patient respectfully and calmly, telling him or her that he or she is being restrained for his or her own safety, and that no harm will come to him or her. The patient should be continually informed of each step of the procedure. Following restraint, a decision must be made about emergency sedation. Mechanical restraint must be used for as short a time as possible. If the patient is to be placed in a mechanical restraint, the patient must be monitored continuously. Care must be exercised to prevent aspiration problems, decreased limb perfusion and nerve compression injuries. (See Chapter 31: Psychiatry and medicine, for a full discussion of physical restraints.)

### 34.2.3.4 Step 4: Sedation

In an emergency situation, it is often necessary to sedate a patient under circumstances that are not ideal, that is, with insufficient historical information and no opportunity to carry out an adequate physical examination. The choice of effective and safe medication will therefore depend on the attending physician's clinical judgement.

The two classes of drugs that are used to sedate violent patients are antipsychotics and benzodiazepines (Battaglia *et al.*, 1997; Dubin and Feld, 1989; Yildiz *et al.*, 2003). It is always safer to administer sedative drugs orally or intramuscularly and to avoid the intravenous route.

The following sedative drugs are recommended as safe and effective in an emergency situation. It is common practice to use lorazepam (2–4 mg) alone or in combination with haloperidol (5 mg) to sedate aggressive patients in a hospital setting (see Table 34.3). These drugs may be administered intramuscularly for rapid and effective sedation. When using benzodiazepines, lorazepam is preferred, as it has a rapid onset of action when given intramuscularly. Diazepam is ineffective when administered intramuscularly, due to unreliable absorption. It is effective when administered intravenously or rectally, but it is recommended that intravenous use be avoided, due to the risk of respiratory depression.

It is important to note that the benzodiazepines, although useful sedative agents in a crisis, may have the paradoxical effect of increasing aggression, especially in medically ill or elderly patients. The patient's pulse, blood pressure and respiratory rate must be monitored every 15 minutes for the first hour and then hourly until the patient is ambulatory.

If an underlying medical condition is suspected as the cause of the aggressive behaviour, or if the patient is over the age of forty and lorazepam monotherapy is not effective, it is advisable to use haloperidol, which is generally safe, and is not accompanied by profound sedation or adverse cardiovascular and respiratory effects (Clinton *et al.*,1987). Haloperidol can cause *torsade de pointes* and sudden death; this is more common with intravenous use (Wilt *et al.*, 1993; Ozeki *et al.*, 2010). Clothiapine and chlorpromazine, although effective sedating agents, may cause undesirable cardiovascular effects such as tachycardia, arrhythmia, hypotension, and a lowering of the seizure threshold.

After sedating a patient, it is essential that regular monitoring of vital signs – pulse rate, blood pressure, respiration, temperature, pupillary reactions, and level of consciousness – is carried out by trained personnel. A sedated patient will also need correct positioning to ensure an open airway. Haloperidol can cause extrapyramidal side effects and patients must be monitored for these, especially acute dystonia. Once the patient is adequately sedated, it is necessary to carry out a thorough medical examination (if this could not be done previously) and appropriate investigations to exclude a medical cause for the aggressive behaviour.

### 34.2.3.5 Legal and ethical considerations

The patient must be admitted as an involuntary patient in accordance with the procedure for the admission of involuntary patients of the Mental Health Care Act (No. 17 of 2002).

**Table 34.3** Drugs used in the sedation of the aggressive patient

| |
|---|
| 1. In antipsychotic naïve patients and those patients where a general medical condition or a substance related disorder is likely, administer lorazepam (Ativan) 2–4 mg. A combination of Lorazepam 4 mg intramuscularly and haloperidol 5 mg intramuscularly may be administered if there is a documented history of a past psychiatric illness and the patient does not have a co-morbid general medical condition. |
| 2. If the patient still not sedated after 15–20 mins, administer haloperidol 5 mg intramuscularly. |
| 3. Haloperidol 5 mg intramuscularly may be administered at 60 minute intervals if required. |
| 4. Monitor the blood pressure (hypotension is a side effect) and look out for extra-pyramidal symptoms. |
| 5. The maximum dose of haloperidol is 10 mg in 24 hours. |
| 6. Use lower doses in elderly patients (haloperidol 2 mg and lorazepam 1–2 mg). |

#### 34.2.3.6 Post-violence counselling

Post-violence counselling prior to discharge is important for patients with a previous history of violence. The aim is to help the patient and his or her family identify the precipitating factors of violence before it occurs, to strengthen their understanding of the negative consequences of further violent episodes and motivate them to prevent these, and to equip them with non-violent alternatives to deal with conflict situations.

**Injury to health workers**

In the clinic and ward setting, staff members are often the victims of violence. It is important that a traumatised staff member is physically assessed and provided with emotional support immediately after the event. The incident should be investigated and thoroughly documented, as legal advice and possibly compensation may be sought in the case of injury. Follow-up treatment, including the debriefing of the traumatised person, is essential to prevent post-traumatic stress disorder or other negative psychological consequences. Encourage the staff member to speak about the experience and his or her feelings in the days following the event. The team should also spend time together to review the episode, share feelings of vulnerability and provide one another with support.

All staff members who work in an environment where they are at risk of physical injury should, ideally, be required to complete a course in violence management training. Such a course could enable them to take routine precautions to protect themselves in their daily interactions with patients, to detect the potentially violent patient at an early stage, to interact with such patients in a way that minimises the risk of violent behaviour and to manage situations of acute violence. Staff training in violence management must be updated on a regular basis. At present, such courses are relatively uncommon in South Africa. Institutions should consider providing such training on a regular basis.

## 34.3 Suicide and suicidal behaviour

### 34.3.1 Introduction and definition of terms

History, literature and the arts are filled with examples of suicide such as that in William Shakespeare's Othello and in Romeo and Juliet. The painter Vincent van Gogh, the writers Virginia Woolf and Ernest Hemingway and the actor Robin Williams are examples of famous people who have committed suicide. Suicidal behaviour (encompassing suicidal ideation, suicidal plans and suicide attempts) has been popularised in movies, books and songs. The term 'suicide' was originally coined by the physician and philosopher Thomas Browne in 1642 (Bertolote and Wasserman, 2009). Terms such as **parasuicide**, self-harming behaviour and attempted suicide are often used interchangeably.

#### 34.3.1.1 Suicide

The World Health Organization (1998) proposed the following operational definition of suicide: 'For the act of killing oneself to be classed as suicide, it must be deliberately initiated and performed by the person concerned in the full knowledge, or expectation, of its fatal outcome.'

Most contemporary definitions of suicide rely on two elements: a precise outcome (death) and a prerequisite (the intention or wish to die) (Bertolote and Wasserman, 2009).

#### 34.3.1.2 Suicidal ideation

Suicidal ideation is frequently described as a person's thoughts about killing himself or herself. Suicidal ideation is not restricted to merely thinking about committing suicide but can also include an individual writing or talking about and or planning his or her suicidal behaviour (Schlebusch, 2005).

#### 34.3.1.3 Suicidal plans

Suicidal plans involve an individual making preparations to kill himself or herself, such as planning how to commit the act (the method), place, purchase of items to commit the act, plans for discovery etc.

#### 34.3.1.4 Suicide attempt

Platt *et al.*, 1992 defined suicide attempt as: 'An act with a nonfatal outcome, in which an individual deliberately initiates a non-habitual behaviour that without intervention from others will cause self-harm, or deliberately ingests a substance in excess of the prescribed or generally recognized therapeutic dosage and which is aimed at realizing changes which the subject desired via the actual or expected physical consequences.'

This definition is descriptive and does not take into consideration the individual's intention. It also does not make a distinction between serious and non-serious suicide attempts. The term 'attempted suicide' thus encompasses all intentional self-inflicted injuries and poisonings (Bertolote and Wasserman, 2009).

The literature indicates that more people entertain ideas about killing themselves (suicidal ideation) than plan to kill themselves or make suicide attempts (Bertolote and Wasserman, 2009).

### 34.3.2 Epidemiology

Suicide and suicidal behaviour are significant public health problems both internationally and in South Africa. Suicide is one of the leading causes of death worldwide, with estimates indicating that approximately one million people commit suicide every year (Bruwer *et al.*, 2014). It is estimated that by 2020, this figure will increase to approximately 1,53 million per year (Bertolote, 2001). At least ten times as many people engage in suicide attempts, frequently ending up disabled by the psychological, physical and social consequences of their action (Sartorius, 2009).

In South Africa, an understanding of the phenomenon of suicidal behaviour (including completed suicide) has been hampered by a lack of systematic data collection, lack of research or under-research in certain ethnic groups, lack of collection of cases seen in general practice, the unwillingness of health practitioners to certify a death as suicide for fear of stigmatising the survivors, etc. (Schlebusch, 2005; Schlebusch and Burrows, 2009). The statistics collected by national organisations are often years out of date. There are wide differences in the ranges of the statistics reported for both adults and child and adolescents, possibly due to factors such as community versus clinical sampling, differences between rural and urban areas and cultural factors.

#### 34.3.2.1 Suicide

The National Injury Mortality Surveillance System (NIMSS) was established in 1999 to provide more comprehensive information about deaths due to violence and injury, including data on suicides. Data are obtained from most mortuaries throughout South Africa. The most recent national statistics available (for the year 2008) indicate that of the 31 177 deaths reported, 10,02% (n = 3 125) were suicides. Hanging accounted for the 46,2% (n = 1 444) of the 3 125 suicides, followed by poisoning (17,0%, n = 530) and firearms (13,5%, n = 422). Nearly 70% (69,2%, n = 2 164) of all suicide victims were aged between 15–44 years. Deaths due to suicide were highest among youth aged 15–29 years (35,9%, n = 1 122), followed by adults aged 30–44 (33,3%, n = 1 042). There were more than four male suicides for every female suicide. The major external causes of suicide among males were hanging (50,2%) and firearms (14,7%), while poisoning (38,2%) and hanging (29,5%) were methods of choice among females. While ethnic differences are not available in the 2008 NIMMS report, other research indicates that the highest percentage of suicides were amongst whites (26,7%), followed by Indians (18%), blacks (7,6%) and coloureds (6,8%) (Prinsloo, 2002).

More recent statistics are available for certain provinces (NIMSS, 2011). Estimates given for suicide in South Africa indicate that the rate is 15,4 per 100 000 (Burrows and La Flamme, 2006)

### 34.3.2.2 Suicidal plans and attempts in adults

There is no single primary data source for nationally representative information on non-fatal suicidal behaviour (suicidal ideation, plans and attempts), with reliance placed on small-scale local studies to obtain data. One big study, the South Africa Stress and Health Study (SASH) attempted to address this by using a national probability sample to look at the prevalence and trends of non-fatal suicidal behaviour in a national sample in South Africa. The study found an estimated prevalence rate of 9,1% for lifetime suicidal ideation and 2,9% for suicide attempts among South Africans (Joe *et al.*, 2008a). Significant differences were established for the different ethnic groups in terms of suicide attempts: Coloured South Africans had the highest rates at 7,1%, Indians 2,5%, with whites and blacks at 2,4% each (Joe *et al.*, 2008a).

One of the biggest studies worldwide, The World Health Organization's Multisite Intervention Study on Suicidal Behaviours (SUPRE-MISS), explored suicidal behaviour among approximately 20 000 subjects in nine cities (including Durban). The findings indicated that 25,4% of the Durban sample reported suicidal ideation, while suicidal plans were at 15,5% and suicide attempts were less than 5% (Bertolote *et al.*, 2009).

Gender differences have consistently been reported in the literature, with females reporting more attempts than males (Atwoli *et al.*, 2014; Schlebusch 2005). Being in the 18–34 age group and having low to medium education levels have also been identified with suicide attempts (Joe *et al.*, 2008b). Ingestion (overdose) of a wide variety of substances including over-the-counter medication, analgesics and household poisons such as paraffin, insecticides and corrosives, is the most common method used in most attempts (Schlebusch 2005; Schlebusch *et al.*, 2003).

### 34.3.2.3 Suicidal ideation, plans and attempts among children and adolescents

Suicidal behaviour (ideation, plans and attempts) amongst children and adolescents are largely under-researched in South Africa. However, various researchers have identified the downward trend in the age of patients who present with suicidal attempts at government-funded hospitals in South Africa. Up to one third of non-fatal suicidal behaviour involves children and adolescents (Schlebusch and Bosch, 2000; Vawda, 2005). Non-hospital-based studies on children and adolescents in South Africa have reported figures ranging from 4–47% for suicidal ideation (Pillay, 1995; Madu and Matla, 2003; Mashego and Madu, 2009; Mayekiso and Mkhize, 1995; Flisher *et al.*, 1992; Peltzer *et al.*, 2008; Vawda, 2014).

Suicide plans were reported by 5,9–18% of scholars (Madu and Matla, 2003; Mayekiso and Mkhize, 1995; Vawda, 2014), while the literature indicates that 5,4–21% of scholars reported having made suicidal attempts (Madu and Matla, 2003; Mayekiso and Mkhize, 1995; Flisher *et al.*, 1992; Shilubane *et al.*, 2013a; Mashego and Madu, 2009; Vawda, 2014). Among this group, ingestion of over-the-counter medication such as paracetamol and household poisons such as insecticides, cleaners and battery acid is common (Vawda, 2005).

Studies have generally found that more females attempt suicide (Joe *et al.*, 2008b; Schlebusch, 2005). Among those who have attempted suicide, only a small proportion is hospitalised (Shilubane *et al.*, 2013a).

## 34.3.3 Risk factors and risk assessment

Suicidal behaviour is a complex phenomenon with an interplay of multiple factors. Risk factors and the causes of suicidal behaviour are multifactorial and multidimensional (Schlebusch, 2005) and range from psychological, social and biological to cultural and environmental. Identification of risk factors can assist in risk assessment. While some authors argue that pre-existing psychopathology for both adults and children is an important risk factor, others argue that suicide attempts are not necessarily associated with prior psychopathology (Bruwer *et al.*, 2014; Vawda, 2005).

### 34.3.3.1 Adults

Within psychopathology, a diagnosis of a mood disorder (and depression in particular) (Schlebusch *et al.*, 2003) and any mood disorder, anxiety disorder or substance use disorder increases the risk of suicide attempts. One study found that respondents who confirmed at least one mental disorder were four times more likely to attempt suicide than those who did not (Joe *et al.*, 2008a). Schizophrenia and substance induced psychoses have also been identified as risk factors for suicide attempts (Schlebusch *et al.*, 2003).

For adults, factors such as physical abuse, sexual abuse (including incest) and parental divorce have emerged as significant risk markers for lifetime suicide attempts, while physical abuse and parental divorce were identified as significant correlates of suicidal ideation: an indication that intrusive and aggressive experiences in childhood may have long-term effects (Bruwer *et al.*, 2014; Schlebusch and Burrows, 2009).

Different associations have been detected between parental psychopathology and suicidal behaviour in their adult offspring. In one study, parental panic disorder and parental antisocial personality disorder were associated with adult offspring suicidal ideation, while parental panic disorder and generalised anxiety disorder were associated with suicide attempts (Atwoli *et al.*, 2014).

Physical illnesses such as cancer (Schlebusch, 2005) and HIV/Aids (Schlebusch and Vawda, 2010; Govender and Schlebusch, 2012) have been identified as risk factors for suicide ideation and attempts. The risk of suicidal behaviour for HIV/Aids may be higher at particular stages of the disease (eg. after testing but before the diagnosis is known, within 3-6 months after diagnosis and in later stages of the disease) (Schlebusch and Burrows, 2009). While the diagnosis of HIV/Aids in itself may be a risk factor, relational problems that stem from the diagnosis can also trigger suicidal behaviour (Schlebusch and Burrows, 2009).

Social and contextual factors such as unemployment, financial problems, problems at work, relationship problems and chronic and acute perceived stress have all been identified as risk factors (Mpiana *et al.*, 2004; Schlebusch, 2005; Schlebusch and Burrows 2009).

### 34.3.3.2 Children and adolescents

Various risk factors for suicidal behaviour have been identified in children and adolescents. Precipitants of suicidal behaviour in adolescents include:

- family conflict as a stressor (Pillay, 1995; Pillay & Wassenaar, 1997)
- interpersonal conflict (Schlebusch and Bosch, 2000)
- child abuse and school-related problems such as failing and bullying (Noor Mahomed *et al.*, 2000; Schlebusch, 2005)
- rigid problem-solving behaviour, over-controlling parental styles and lack of tolerance by parents or caregivers for developmental or role changes (Pillay & Wassenaar, 1997).

Parental loss through divorce or parental death can also be risk factors for suicidal behavior (Schlebusch, 2005).

A family history of psychopathology (including substance abuse) (Schlebusch, 2005) a family history of suicide (Vawda, 2012), as well as poor perceived parental support and negative feelings about the family, forced sexual intercourse and physical violence by partners (Shilubane *et al.*, 2013b) all increase suicidal behaviour. Substance use (alcohol use in particular), a mood disorder (depression), perceived stress and a friend or peer's suicidal ideation have also been identified as risk factors of suicidal behaviour (Vawda, 2014). Smoking cigarettes has also emerged as a significant risk factor in suicide attempts (Shilubane *et al.*, 2013a).

Anger (Vawda, 2014) and anger control problems (Peltzer *et al.*, 2008), low self-esteem and perceived stress (Vawda, 2014; Peltzer *et al.*, 2008) and unmet school goals (Peltzer *et al.*, 2008) have also been identified as predictors of suicide risk in adolescents. Feelings of hopelessness (Vawda, 2014; Shilubane *et al.*, 2013a), feeling unsafe and being a participant in or victim of violent behaviour all emerged as significant factors in suicidal ideation (Shilubane *et al.*, 2013a). Being involved in bullying, either as perpetrator or victim, can also lead to suicidal ideation (Liang *et al.*, 2007).

Suicidal behaviour has also been viewed as an inappropriate method of communicating and problem solving, with poor coping and problem solving skills and rigid thinking also being identified as risk factors. Suicidal behaviour is possibly seen as a viable option by someone who is unable to see alternative solutions to engage help for his or her problems (Schlebusch, 2005; Peltzer *et al.*, 2008). The risk factors are:

- male gender (for completed suicide)
- female gender (for suicide attempts)
- younger age for suicide attempts (18-34)
- past history of suicide behaviour (including suicide attempt(s))
- presence of a mood disorder, in particular depression
- presence of other psychiatric disorders, including substance abuse
- diagnosis of terminal illness such as cancer, HIV/Aids history of physical or sexual abuse
- parental divorce
- parental psychopathology, including substance abuse
- a family history of suicidal behaviour, including completed suicide
- presence of chronic and acute stressors such as unemployment, financial problems, relationship problems, perceived stress and lack of perceived social support
- presence of hopelessness, helplessness, anger, impulse-control problems/impulsivity, aggressiveness, poor problem-solving ability or cognitive rigidity, impaired coping.

## 34.3.4 Management

As the majority of the population have limited access to mental health services in South Africa, individuals in a suicidal crisis (often with somatic symptoms and masked suicidal ideation) are more likely to visit a general practitioner than a mental health specialist in the days, weeks or months that precede a suicide attempt (Burrows and Schlebusch, 2009). Primary health care practitioners, who are often the first port of call, can play an important role in the early detection and prevention of suicidal behaviour. Family practitioners are often influential members of their community and have an important role to play in facilitating referrals to other health professionals (Vawda, 2013) such as psychiatrists, psychologists and social workers.

Some individuals who make a suicide attempt are brought to accident and emergency departments in general hospitals or clinics for treatment. As these individuals make significant demands on clinical services they often receive little sympathy or support from health care providers when compared to other patients who do not have self-inflicted injuries. However, it is imperative that these individuals receive appropriate care and treatment, as failure to do so may result in a completed suicide and leave the treating medical staff open to litigation on grounds of negligence. Professionals who treat the patient may not wish to engage in frank and open discussion of suicidality for fear of enhancing the patient's suicidal behaviour. However, in most cases, patients with suicidal behaviour welcome opportunities to express their distress.

Questions to ask when assessing for continued **suicidal intent** include:

- detailed information on the events leading up to the attempt
- the method used
- whether there were opportunities for discovery following the attempt (for example, sending a text message or using social media such as Facebook)
- whether the patient put his or her affairs in order in preparation for death (for example, made a will or gave away their possessions).

A thorough history and mental status examination keeping the above identified risk factors in mind will help identify individuals at high risk of suicide attempts. Inappropriate or inadequate treatment in emergency settings often leads to failure to adhere to after-care prescriptions and an increase in subsequent suicidality (Dunne, 2009). While there are scales that assess suicidal risk, some questions to ask individuals who present with suicidal ideation or attempts are given in the Information box.

It is essential to have a protocol to manage suicidal patients. One such protocol developed in hospitals in the Durban municipal area is to have all patients with suicidal behaviour seen at the accident and emergency department of a hospital (Schlebusch, 2005). It is recommended that all patients who present with suicide attempts be hospitalised, where they are stabilised and seen by clinical psychologists or psychiatrists. This should occur usually within 24-48 hours of admission and again prior to discharge (Schlebusch *et al.*, 2003). During this period, when they are in a general medical ward, it is recommended that these individuals be placed on strict 24-hour suicide observation or watch, with a view to transferring them to a closed psychiatric unit for their own safety and protection, especially if they continue to verbalise or display suicidal ideation, plans or behaviour. If necessary, in the face of a suicidal patient's refusal to be admitted, involuntary admission procedures for a 72-hour period under the Mental Health Care Act of 2002 can be utilised by the health care professional. The relevant forms for such a procedure are usually available in all accident and emergency departments of hospitals to expedite admission of patients deemed a danger to themselves or others.

Admission in a psychiatric unit provides health care professionals with opportunities to interview and obtain collateral from family, friends or colleagues of the patient regarding the precipitant(s) of the attempt, information about the lethality and intent (as some patients may deny the attempt or may feel too embarrassed to provide such information) and to verify the patient's account of the attempt as well as his or her mental status. Patients with a continuing suicidal intent or ideation may minimise the current episode and may even deny it completely.

Admission may also provide a respite or time-out from stressful situations for the patient and offer opportunities to the patient to problem solve and identify sources of support with the help of health care professionals. More importantly, patients can be screened for mental disorders such as depression or schizophrenia and be referred to a psychiatrist and the mental health team for appropriate management (which may include pharmacological and other biological treatments) (Moller, 2009) and psychotherapy (individual or group). Other members of the multidisciplinary team, such as social workers, can also be mobilised to assist the patient to access, for example, social services, the various social care grants, a referral to legal aid, if necessary. Opportunities to engage the family in psycho-education (e.g. the signs and symptoms of mental disorder) must be maximised to prevent further suicidal behaviour.

While many patients who present with suicidal attempts are given follow-up appointments, the literature indicates that very few keep these: one study found that only 43,5% of all patients kept their follow-up appointments (Pillay *et al.*, 2004). Thus it is important to maximise the initial consultation (Schlebusch, 2005) to engage in considerable preventative work. To this end structured psychotherapy, such as brief cognitive behavioural therapy, problem-solving therapy and interpersonal psychotherapy, can be considered (Schlebusch, 2005; Beskow *et al.*, 2009). Effective treatment also emphasises the importance of crisis management and access to

**Information box**

1. Distinguish between active suicidal ideation versus passive suicidal ideation (e.g. 'Have you ever wished that you were dead or wished you could go to sleep and not wake up?')
2. Assess dimensions of current suicidal thoughts including:
   i) Frequency, intensity, duration of and reasons for suicidal ideation:

   'Do you ever have thoughts of killing yourself…thoughts of suicide?'

   'How often do you think of suicide (daily, weekly, monthly)?'

   'How many times a day?' 'How long do the thoughts usually last?' 'How severe, intense or overwhelming are these thoughts?' 'Can you stop thinking about killing yourself or wanting to die if you want to?' 'Were you drinking or using any substance?' 'Can you rate how much in control you feel on a scale of 1 to 10?'

   'Are there things – anything or anyone – such as your family, religious beliefs or pain of death, that stopped you from wanting to die or acting on thoughts of killing yourself?' 'What keeps you going?' 'What keeps you alive right now?'

   'What reasons do you have for thinking about wanting to kill yourself? Was it to end the pain you are in or to get attention, revenge or reaction from others, or both?' 'Can you rate the intensity or severity on a scale of 1 to 10?'

   ii) Specificity of the plans (how, where, when):

   'What exactly do you think about?'

   'When people think about suicide, it's not unusual to think about how, when or where…… have you had these kinds of thoughts?'

   'Do you have any intention to act on these thoughts of suicide?'

   'Have you thought about the method?'

   'Have you thought about other methods of suicide?'

   iii) Availability of methods, availability of opportunity:

   'Do you have a method?'

   'Do you have access to the method?'

   iv) Preparatory behaviour of any type:

   'Have you acted on these thoughts in any way?'

   'Have you taken any steps in preparation for killing yourself such as giving your things away, writing a suicide note, texting, making a will?'
3. Suicide attempt:

   'Have you made a suicide attempt?'

   'What did you do? Did you___________ as a way to end your life?'

   'What made you feel that you wanted to kill yourself?'

   'What did you hope to achieve by doing this?'

   'Do you still feel like killing yourself?'

   'What has happened or changed that does not make you want to kill yourself anymore?'

**Source:** Adapted from Rudd and Joiner, 1998

available emergency services during and after treatment with a clear plan of action being identified (Rudd *et al.*, 2009) particularly in the face of continuing suicidal ideation, plans or attempts. After-care plans with suicide attempters must focus on immediate short-term safety and the avoidance of subsequent attempts – something in which the family can play a major part (Dunne, 2009).

Post-discharge referrals for patients and their families to organisations such as the South African Depression and Anxiety Support Group (SADAG) and Survivors of Loved Ones (SOLOS) are also useful in preventive efforts. Schlebusch (2005) provides a useful organisational system for the management and prevention of suicidal behaviour.

Access to health care services for individuals at risk of suicidal behaviour, early diagnosis and treatment of conditions such as mood disorders, psychoses and substance use, identification of psychosocial risk factors, and follow up and rehabilitation for suicide attempters and those with a mental disorder, all assist in management and prevention.

### 34.3.5 Ethical and legal considerations

Suicidal behaviour is an emotional issue and because it can lead to completed suicide, it presents a number of clinical and ethical dilemmas in clinical practice.

Schlebusch (2005) states that a conceptual struggle between promoting individual freedom and autonomy versus protecting people from self-harm or self-injury underlies the ethical and legal aspects of suicide and the clinical management of suicidal persons. While the assessment and treatment of suicidal patients involves a clinical judgement, conflicting ethical principles and ambiguities as well as the threat of litigation often compromise clinical judgement.

Two questions dominate this issue:

- Does the patient have the moral right to commit suicide?
- What is the moral obligation of the clinician and others to intervene to prevent the suicide?

The prevailing traditional approach to suicide, often called the scientific or determinist view, proposes that factors beyond the patient's control cause suicidal behaviour. Thus the patient's decision to commit suicide is not seen as rational or autonomous. The patient is thus not responsible and therefore does not face a moral decision. Society has a moral obligation to intervene and save the patient and is permitted or mandated to prevent the suicide (Bosch, 2000).

Bosch (2000) states that legally the standard is that the suicidal person should receive prudent and reasonable care (whatever is the prevailing standard in the community). One issue of responsibility of care is that patients should be informed of the limitations of confidentiality through standard informed consent: patients have the ethical and legal right to be informed about measures and to participate in measures to prevent their suicide. The responsibility to obtain information is not obviated by the patient's self-destructive state. The second issue is assessing imminent danger of suicide: the prediction of suicide is fraught with uncertainty. Risk creates an obligation to intervene. Is the individual (an adult) capable of making decisions for himself or herself? What are the limits on the clinician's obligation to prevent suicide?

The clinician's moral obligations are not unlimited. Truly suicidal patients often complete their suicide; involuntary commitment is often only a temporary, partial and unsatisfactory answer. Some patients (e.g. those with a personality disorder) are resistant to treatment. Repeated attempts at treatment may not succeed and involuntary hospitalisation and forced treatment may reinforce the patients 'regressive dependency' (Bosch, 2000) or may create feelings in the patients that they are a burden (which may in turn lead to further feelings of depression and hopelessness).

Issues such as failure to diagnose properly may arise; with the first question being whether or not the evaluation was sufficiently thorough to assess suicidality. Few – if any – tests have been useful in the assessment of suicidal behaviour. The clinician's own skills are the most useful assessment tool. Hence the clinician must have a very good knowledge of the risk factors for the various patient populations (for example, children or the aged) in terms of evaluating and formulating suicidal potential and instituting suicide prevention. It is therefore recommended that case consultation with other health care professionals be used to assist in diagnosis and responsible and proper assessment.

Failure in care can lead the treating clinician open to liability in terms of negligence and malpractice. Failure in care involves the following:

- failure to predict or diagnose suicidality
- failure to control, restrain or supervise
- failure to administer tests and evaluations of the patient to establish suicidal intent
- failure to medicate properly
- failure to observe or supervise the patient continuously or on a sufficiently frequent basis
- failure to take an adequate history
- failure to remove dangerous objects (e.g. belt, rope, medication)
- failure to place in a secure room (Bosch, 2000).

Clinicians must properly document the process of suicide assessment and intervention through case note or reports (Brems, 2000). In South Africa, negligent failure of a professional to prevent a patient from committing suicide is usually regarded as professional negligence. The professional could be held liable for loss of support by the deceased's dependents and criminally liable for culpable homicide. Dereliction of duty has application to hospital suicide, outpatient suicide, suicide after release, misuse or non-adherence to medication (Bosch, 2000).

Liability prevention involves prudent and responsible assessment and intervention, durable documentation and consultation. In the case of a malpractice suit, the injured party must prove the following four elements: duty, dereliction of duty, damages and direct causation.

In terms of duty, once a professional relationship has been established between a clinician and a patient, the clinician assumes the legal duty to provide care. Appropriately discharging the patient or arranging alternative care (e.g. admission to a closed unit) ends the duty to provide care.

Dereliction of duty involves the failure to meet the applicable standard of care either by commission or omission (such as failure to take a proper history or failure to evaluate a patient's depression or past suicidal behaviour), failure to treat a patient's psychiatric condition, negligent release or discharge, and failure to communicate the patient's condition to other hospital staff. Clinicians can be held responsible for direct causation; with some of the following defences being offered in response to allegations of malpractice: patient's concealment of suicidal intent, compliance with standard of care, proper assessment despite adverse outcome, impossibility of suicide prediction.

Ethically, most principles focus on autonomy (respect for the individual's self-determination including beliefs, principles and actions), beneficence (doing the greatest good possible), non-maleficence (doing no harm), justice (fairness and equality between individuals) and fidelity (trustworthiness and faithfulness to commitments). It is strongly recommended that post-vention or debriefing be made available to all staff including treating clinicians (including those in individual general practice) who lose a patient to suicide. Institutions must ensure that mechanisms are in place in case such an event occurs.

## Conclusion

Clinicians cannot be expected to prevent the suicide of every at-risk or high risk patient. However, clinicians do have to ensure that they act professionally, ethically and consistently, keeping all the above factors and issues in mind when suicidality is present.

# References


Atwoli L, Nock M, Williams DR and Stein DJ ( 2014) Association between parental psychopathology and suicidal behaviour among adult offspring: results from the cross sectional South African Stress and Health Survey. *BMC Psychiatry* 14: 65. Available at: http://www.biomedcentral.com/1471-244X/14/65

Battaglia J, Moss S, Rush J, Kang J, Mendoza R, Leedom L, Dubin W, Mc Glynn C, Goodman L (1997) Haloperidol, lorazepam, or both for psychotic agitation? A multi-center, prospective, double-blind, emergency department study. *The American Journal of Emergency Medicine* 15: 335–40

Bertolote JM (2001) Suicide in the world: An epidemiological overview, 1959–2000. In: Wasserman D (Ed.) *Suicide: An Unnecessary Death.* London: Martin Dunitz.

Bertolote, JM, Fleischmann A, De Leo D, Wasserman D (2009) Suicidal thoughts, suicide plans and attempts in the general population on different continents. In: Wasserman D, Wasserman C (Eds). *The Oxford Textbook of Suicidology and Suicide Prevention.* Oxford: Oxford University Press

Bertelote JM, Wasserman D (2009) Development of definitions of suicidal behaviours. In: Wasserman D, Wasserman C (Eds). *The Oxford Textbook of Suicidology and Suicide Prevention.* Oxford: Oxford University Press

Beskow J, Salkovskis P, Beskow AP (2009) Cognitive treatment of suicidal adults In: Wasserman D, Wasserman C (Eds). *The Oxford Textbook of Suicidology and Suicide Prevention.* Oxford: Oxford University Press

Bosch BA (2000) Workshop on ethics and suicide. In: Schlebusch L, Bosch BA (2000) Suicidal behaviour 4: Proceedings of the Fourth South African Conference on Suicidology. Department of Medically Applied Psychology, Faculty of Medicine, University of Natal.

Brems C (2000) *Dealing with challenges in psychotherapy and counselling.* Belmont, CA: Wadsworth

Bruwer B, Govender R, Bishop M, Williams DR, Stein DJ, Seedat S (2014) Association between childhood adversities and long term suicidality among South Africans from the results of the South African Stress and Health study: A cross-sectional study. *British Medical Journal* Open 2014, 4e004644.doi:10.1136/bmjopen-2013-004644.

Burrows S, La Flamme L (2006) Suicide mortality in South Africa. *Social Psychiatry and Psychiatric Epidemiology* 41:108–14

Burrows S, Schlebusch L (2009) Suicide prevention in South Africa. In: Wasserman D, Wasserman C (Eds). *The Oxford Textbook of Suicidology and Suicide Prevention.* Oxford: Oxford University Press

Clinton JE, Sterner S, Stelmachera Z, Ruiz E (1987) Haloperidol for sedation of disruptive emergency patients. *Annals of Emergency Medicine* 16: 319–22

Dubin WR, Feld JA (1989) Rapid tranquilization of the violent patient. *The American Journal of Emergency Medicine* 7:313–20

Dunne EJ (2009) Family psycho-education with suicide attempters. In: Wasserman D, Wasserman C (Eds). *The Oxford Textbook of Suicidology and Suicide Prevention.* Oxford: Oxford University Press

Flisher AJ, Ziervogel CF, Chalton DO, Roberston BA (1992) In: Schlebusch L (Ed.) Suicidal behaviour 2. Proceedings of the second South African Conference on Suicidology. Department of Medically Applied Psychology, Faculty of Medicine, University of Natal

Govender RD, Schlebusch L (2012) Suicidal ideation in seropositive patients seen at a South African HIV voluntary counselling and testing clinics. *African Journal of Psychiatry* 15: 94–98

Gregory RJ, Nihalani ND, Rodriguez E (2004) Medical screening in the emergency department for psychiatric admissions: a procedural analysis. *General Hospital Psychiatry* 26: 405–10

Hall RC, Popkin MK, Devaul RA, Faillace LA, Stickney SK (1978) Physical illness presenting as psychiatric disease. *Archives of General Psychiatry* 35: 1315–20

Henneman PL, Mendoza R, Lewis, RJ (1994) Prospective evaluation of emergency department medical clearance. *Annals of Emergency Medicine* 24: 672–677

Inouye SK, Westendorp RG, Saczynski JS (2014) Delirium in elderly people. *The Lancet* 383: 911–22

Joe S, Stein DJ, Seedat S, Herman A, Williams DR (2008a) Prevalence and correlates of non-fatal suicidal behaviour among South Africans. *British Journal of Psychiatry* 192: 310–1

Joe S, Stein DJ, Seedat S, Herman A, Williams DR (2008b) Non- fatal suicidal behaviour among South Africans: Results from the South African Stress and Health Study. *Social Psychiatry and Psychiatric Epidemiology* 43: 454–461

Koran LM, Sheline Y, Imai K, Kelsey TG, Freedland KE, Mathews J, Moore M (2002) Medical disorders among patients admitted to a public-sector psychiatric inpatient unit. *Psychiatric Services* 53: 1623–5

Liang H, Flisher AJ, Lombard CJ. (2007) Bullying, violence and risk behavior in South African school students. *Child Abuse and Neglect* 31(2): 161–71

Madu SN, Matla MP (2003) The prevalence of suicidal behaviours among secondary school adolescents in the Limpopo Province, South Africa. *South African Journal of Psychology* 33: 126–32

Mashego TAB, Madu SN (2009) Suicide-related behaviours among secondary school adolescents in the Welkom and Bethlehem areas of the Free State province (South Africa). *South African Journal of Psychology* 39(4): 489–97

Mayekiso TV, Mkize DL (1995) The relationship between self-punitive wishes and family background. In: Schlebusch L (Ed). Suicidal behaviour 3: Proceedings of the Third Southern African Conference on Suicidology. Department of Medically Applied Psychology, Faculty of Medicine, University of Natal

Moller HJ (2009) Pharmacological and other biological treatments of suicidal individuals In: Wasserman D, Wasserman C (Eds). *The Oxford Textbook of Suicidology and Suicide Prevention.* Oxford: Oxford University Press

Morrison E (1990) Violent psychiatric patients in a public hospital. *Scholarly Inquiry for Nursing Practice* 4: 65–82

Mpiana MP, Marincowitz GJO, Ragavan S, Malete N (2004), Why I tried to kill myself – An exploration of the factors contributing to suicide in the Waterberg District. *South African Family Practice 46*(7): 21–5

National Injury Mortality Surveillance System (2008) *National Injury Mortality Surveillance Systems Report.* Available from: http://www.mrc.ac.za/crime/nimss. (Accessed 20 January 2010.)

National Injury Mortality Surveillance Systems (2011) *A profile of fatal injuries in Gauteng.* NIMMS Gauteng.pdf (Accessed 1 August 2014.)

Noor Mohamed, S B, Selmer CA and Bosch B A (2000) Psychological profiles of children presenting with suicidal behaviour, with a specific focus on psychopathology. In Schlebusch L and Bosch B A (Eds) Suicidal Behaviour 4: Proceedings of the Fourth South African Conference on Suicidology, 56–70. Department of Medically Applied Psychology, Faculty of Medicine, University of Natal

O'Brien RF, Kifuji K, Summergrad P (2006) Medical conditions with psychiatric manifestations. *Adolescent Medicine Clinics* 17(1): 49–77

Ozeki Y, Fujii K, Kurimoto N, Yamada N, Okawa M, Aoki T, Takahashi J, Ishida N, Horie M, Kunugi H (2010) QTc prolongation and antipsychotic medications in a sample of 1 017 patients with schizophrenia. *Progress in Neuro-psychopharmacology and Biological Psychiatry* 34: 401–5

Peltzer K, Kleintjies S, van Wyk B, Thompson EA, Mashego TAB ( 2008) Correlates of suicide risk among secondary school students in Cape Town. *Social Behaviour and Personality* 36(4): 493–502

Pillay AL, Wassenaar DR, Kramers AL (2004) Attendance at psychological consultants following non-fatal suicidal behaviour: An ethical dilemma. *South African Journal of Psychology* 34: 350–63

Pillay BJ (1995) A study of suicidal behaviour at a secondary school. In: Schlebusch L (Ed.) Suicidal behaviour 3. Proceedings of the Third Southern African Conference on Suicidology. Department of Medically Applied Psychology, Faculty of Medicine, University of Natal

Platt S, Bille-Brahe U, Kerkhof A, Schmidtke A, Bjerke T, Crepet P, De Leo D, Haring C, Lonnqvist J, Michel K, Philippe A, Pommereau X, Querejeta I, Salander-Renberg E, Temesvary B, Wasserman D, Sampaio Faria J (1992) Parasuicide in Europe: the WHO/EURO multicentre study on parasuicide. I. Introduction and preliminary analysis for 1989. *Acta Psychiatrica Scandinavica* 85(2): 97–104

Prinsloo, M (2002) Manner of non-natural death. In: Matzopouloos R (Ed.) *A profile of fatal injuries in South Africa: The third annual report of the National Injury Mortality Surveillance System.* Tygerberg: Medical Research Council

Reeves RR, Pendarvis EJ, Kimble R (2000) Unrecognized medical emergencies admitted to psychiatric units. *The American Journal of Emergency Medicine* 18: 390–3

Rudd MD, Joiner T (1998) The assessment, management, and treatments of suicidality: towards clinically informed and balanced standards of care. *Clinical Psychology: Science and Practice* 5(2): 135–149

Rudd MD, Williams B, Trotter DRM (2009) The psychological and behavioural treatment of suicidal behaviour. In: Wasserman D, Wasserman C (Eds). *The Oxford Textbook of Suicidology and Suicide Prevention.* Oxford: Oxford University Press

Sartorius N (2009) Foreword. In: Wasserman D, Wasserman C (Eds). *The Oxford Textbook of Suicidology and Suicide Prevention.* Oxford: Oxford University Press

Schlebusch L (2005) *Suicidal behaviour in South Africa.* Scottsville, South Africa: University of KwaZulu-Natal Press

Schlebusch L, Bosch BA. (2000) Suicidal behaviour 4: Proceedings of the Fourth South African Conference on Suicidology. Department of Medically Applied Psychology, Faculty of Medicine, University of Natal.

Schlebusch L, Burrows, S (2009) Suicide attempts in Africa. In: Wasserman D, Wasserman C (Eds). *The Oxford Textbook of Suicidology and Suicide Prevention.* Oxford: Oxford University Press

Schlebusch L, Vawda NBM (2010) HIV-infection as a self-reported risk factor for attempted suicide in South Africa. *African Journal of Psychiatry* 13(4): 280–3

Schlebusch L., Vawda NBM, Bosch BA ( 2003) Suicidal behaviour in black South Africans. *Crisis* 24: 24–28

Shilubane HN, Ruiter RAC, Bos AER, Van den Borne B, James S, Reddy PS (2013a) Psychosocial correlates of suicidal ideation in rural South African adolescents. *Child Psychiatry and Human Development* 45(2) 153–62

Shilubane HN, Ruiter RAC, Van den Borne B, Sewpaul R, James S, Reddy PS (2013b) Suicide and related health risk behaviours among school learners in South Africa: Results from the 2002 and 2008 National youth Risk Behaviour Surveys. *BMC Public Health* 13: 926. Available at: http:/www.biomedcentral.com/1471-2458/13/926

Talbort-Stern JK, Green T, Royle TJ (2000) Psychiatric manifestations of systemic illness. *Emergency Medicine Clinics of North America* 18: 199–209

Vawda NBM (2005) Suicidal behaviour among black South African children and adolescents. In: Malhotra S (Ed). *Mental disorders in children and adolescents: Needs and strategies for intervention.* New Delhi: CBS Publishers

Vawda NBM (2012) Associations between family suicide and personal suicidal behaviour in youth. *South African Family Practice Journal* 54(3): 244–9

Vawda NBM (2014) The prevalence of suicidal behaviour and associated risk factors in Grade 8 learners in Durban. *South African Family Practice Journal* 56(1): 37–42

Wilt J, Minnema A, Johnson R, Rosenblum AM (1993) *Torsades de pointes* associated with the use of intravenous haloperidol. *Annals of Internal Medicine* 119: 391–4

World Health Organization. (1998). *Primary prevention of mental, neurological and psychosocial disorders. Ch 4: Suicide.* Geneva: WHO. http://whqlibdoc.who.int/publications/924154516X.pdf (Accessed 15th May 2015)

Yildiz A, Sachs G, Turgay A (2003) Pharmacologic management of agitation in emergency settings. *Emergency Medicine Journal* 20: 339–346

CHAPTER

# 35 Legal and ethical aspects of mental health

*Paul de Wet, Carla Kotzé, Funeka Sokudela*

## 35.1 Introduction

Forensic mental health is the interface between mental health care practice and the law. It is a field in health care that encompasses several factors including the health professional's ethical and legal duty to care for patients competently, the patient's right to choose to receive treatment, court, legislative and governmental matters affecting the provision of care to patients, and ethical principles and codes that affect the way health practitioners conduct themselves as professionals and towards the population they serve.

The legal protection and management of people considered to be mentally ill or mentally disordered has been around since the 17th century. Regarding most international mental health legislation before the year 2000, the overriding concern and focus were the welfare and safety of the community. Mental health services revolved around large mental institutions that were centralised in peri-urban tertiary psychiatric institutions, far from the homes and communities of most patients. People with mental health problems were institutionalised.

The emphasis of care was mostly psychopharmacological and mental health services were separated from general health care. Responsibility for mental health care was left to psychiatrists and a few medical practitioners.

In addition, the human rights of people with mental health problems were often violated and the individuals were discriminated against and subjected to stigmatisation. People with medical problems and emergencies, such as delirium, meningitis or metabolic disturbances who presented with behavioural disturbances, were often referred and admitted inappropriately to mental health facilities.

In South Africa, as in many other countries, the needs of people with mental health problems have been largely unmet. A high estimated global burden of disease attributed to neuropsychiatric disorders (14%) and considerable co-morbidity with physical illnesses and substance abuse, have necessitated a call for the well-integrated and purposeful participation of all stakeholders and practitioners in serving the needs of persons with mental health problems. In addition, the mental health context in South Africa is complex due to HIV rates, high levels of substance abuse and a high prevalence of violence and injury (Bateman, 2006).

Health professionals in general should have adequate knowledge and skills in the management of persons with mental health needs including psychiatric emergencies. Some of these emergency conditions are addressed in Section 35.4 and in Chapter 33: HIV and mental health, of this textbook. To this end, there is a need to integrate mental health care into general health care systems and to promote the implementation of coordinated community-based mental health care services and the destigmatisation thereof. Moreover, health care practitioners should have the know-how and the wherewithal to apply basic procedures, regulations, legal and ethical principles that govern forensic mental health care in the country. They should be able to complete the relevant Mental Health Care Act (MHCA) forms and to liaise appropriately with relevant stakeholders within and outside their field.

Mental health care features in various South African policies, pieces of legislation and their amendments, including the following:

- Constitution of the Republic of South Africa
- Mental Health Care Act (No. 17 of 2002)
- National Health Act (No. 61 of 2003)
- Children's Act (No. 38 of 2005)
- Child Justice Act (No. 75 of 2008)
- Older Persons Act (No. 13 of 2006)
- Medicine and Related Substances Amendment Act (No. 72 of 2008)
- Promotion of Access to Information (Act No. 54 of 2002)
- Protection of Personal Information Act (No. 4 of 2013)
- Road Accident Fund (Transitional Provisions) Act (No. 15 of 2012)
- Compensation for Occupational Injuries and Diseases Act (No. 130 of 1993)
- Consumer Protection Act (No. 68 of 2008)
- Prevention and Treatment of Substance Abuse Act (No. 70 of 2008)
- Traditional Health Practitioners Act (No. 22 of 2007)
- Choice of Termination of Pregnancy Amendment Act (No. 1 of 2008)
- Sterilization Amendment Act (No. 3 of 2005)
- Domestic Violence Act (No. 116 of 1998)
- Criminal Procedures Act (No. 51 of 1977)
- Criminal Law (Sexual Offences and Related Matters) Amendment Act (No. 32 of 2007).

## 35.2 Basic medico-legal considerations in mental health

The forensic or medico-legal aspects of mental health refer to the interaction between mental health and the law. Forensic mental health is the arm of practice related to the evaluation of an individual for legal purposes. In such evaluations, it is thus inferred that the individual is not necessarily a patient but a subject of the law. The role of the doctor is not that of one who is providing therapy, but that of one who is performing a duty for another party (in this instance, the court or another agency) and not necessarily the patient. For the general practitioner, it is important to be familiar with medico-legal matters that can form part of basic medical practice and matters that can guide the referral to specialist services.

The interaction between mental health and the law can be split roughly into criminal matters and civil matters.

- Criminal matters include instances when an individual is referred in terms of mental health issues related to an alleged crime.
- Civil matters include instances when a person is referred in terms of mental health issues related to noncriminal matters.

Often the issue in question relates to the mental capacity of the individual to be assessed at the time of, or prior to the time of, the inquiry. The medical assessor is strictly confined to the question of the person's mental capacity at a given time and not in solving a legal enigma. One way of viewing this is that the doctor is called upon to consider the ethics of being involved in a case where neither objectivity nor lack of bias can be maintained. This scenario illustrates the very sensitive and intertwined relationship between ethics, medical practice and the law.

## 35.3 Basic ethical considerations in mental health

Ethics deals with the relationship between people in different groups and may entail a balancing of rights. It is the philosophical study of morality that determines what one ought to do to achieve a certain prescribed good (Deigh, 2010). Medical ethics are the moral codes of practice in medicine.

As an introduction to medical ethics and in relation to their relationships with patients, there are four generally recognised basic ethical principles that health practitioners must bear in mind. These are: respect of autonomy, beneficence, non-maleficence and justice. These principles must be weighed against each other constantly in the doctor-patient interaction.

- Respect for autonomy refers to the instances when a doctor has to respect the patient's right to make choices when the patient has a clear understanding of the options involved in his or her health care. In this context, choices made by a patient who has full capacity to make decisions about his or her life have to be respected, even if those choices go against the opinion of the doctor.

- Beneficence refers to the protection of the interest of the patient as far as possible. It is based on the principle of paternalism where the doctor supposedly knows best and acts in the interest of the patient. It may at times be in conflict with other ethical principles (e.g. respect for autonomy) when the doctor acts against the wishes of the patient in a life-death or a high-risk situation.
- Non-maleficence refers to the principle of doing no harm to the patient as far as possible. The doctor is expected to ensure that no harm befalls the patient due to inappropriate clinical decisions.
- Justice in the context of mental health practice refers to the fair distribution of health resources and fairness of treatment. The principle includes the weighing up of the most equitable ways of taking care of the needs of the patient vs. those of the community or society at large. It comes into play in the example of **involuntary care treatment and rehabilitation** where the mentally ill individual's right to autonomy and treatment in the least restrictive environment is weighed against the rights of those who may come to harm should the individual not be compelled to receive treatment against his or her will in a highly restrictive environment. (See Section 35.4.)

The four basic principles discussed above are not exhaustive of ethical considerations in medicine in general and in mental health in particular. Some of the other considerations are referred to below. All these must be applied with the awareness of cross-cultural values in the context within which a doctor practices. Ethics cannot be entirely separated from values within the system they guide (Fulford *et al.*, 2006). (See also Chapter 6: Culture and psychiatry.)

## 35.3.1 Confidentiality

Confidentiality refers to the medical premise that binds medical practitioners to keep secret all information divulged by patients during a doctor-patient interaction. In the context of mental health care it can apply to a multidisciplinary group of professionals caring for the same patient without the need to receive the patient's permission for individual professionals. The individual professionals caring for the patient are each bound by the principle.

In the South African mental health context, the divulging of medical information by medical practitioners to other parties regarding a patient is regulated by the Promotion of Access to Information Act (No. 2 of 2000), the Protection of Personal Information Act (No. 4 of 2013) (POPI) and the MHCA and other relevant pieces of legislation.

Confidentiality can be breached under specific conditions, including a court order. A health care practitioner is then obliged, even under protest, to divulge confidential information. The patient may or may not be required to give informed consent for this breach to take place. Another condition under which a doctor may have to breach confidentiality is when the patient gives away the right to keep the information confidential to another party (e.g. a medical health care fund). There are other obligations that bind a practitioner to divulge information. The Children's Act applies in case of abuse of a minor and the Older Person's Act applies in case of abuse of an elderly person. The Domestic Violence Act (No. 116 of 1998) also puts the health practitioner in a position to identify and assist at-risk individuals by reporting abuse to the appropriate officials with the patient's informed consent. Confidentiality can also be breached when the doctor is in a legal battle with the patient and needs to raise self-defence issues that may have emerged previously during clinical consultations with the patient. (Also see Section 35.4 and Chapter 27: Child and Adolescent psychiatry 1: Assessment and the young child.)

## 35.3.2 Privilege

Privilege is the right of a health practitioner not to comply with a court order and to maintain confidentiality in certain special circumstances. In South Africa no specific law protects the practitioner but certain case laws have emerged whereby the health practitioner is granted privilege rights not to divulge information that is potentially harmful to the patient or is not relevant to the legal question at hand (Gauteng High Court Judgments – *State vs. Van Ameron* cc83/2006 and *State vs. Thobejane* cc352/2006). Patient-doctor, marital spouse, and priest-penitent relationships are examples of situations that may be protected against forced disclosure.

## 35.3.3 Informed consent

Informed consent is a term that refers to a process that ascertains that an individual is fully and mentally competent to give consent to enter into a procedure at a specific time. The individual is aware of his or her rights and the options available to him or her prior to making a choice. The process of giving informed consent has to be voluntary, irrespective of the medico-legal status of the patient (see Section 35.4) and is situation and time-specific. Once given, by a fully competent person, informed consent can be withdrawn.

A person who is not fully competent can assent to a procedure nonetheless, even if a legal guardian's informed consent will still be required. In this case the individual agrees to the procedure but is clinically and/or legally not fit to give informed consent.

## 35.3.4 Expert witness

Forensic mental health experts are from various disciplines within mental health care who have trained specifically in the field or have worked in the field for a long enough time to gain worthwhile experience. Placement in an academic environment offers an added advantage. The MHCA defines a mental health practitioner and includes psychiatrists, registered medical practitioners, nurses, clinical psychologists, social workers and occupational therapists that are trained accordingly (see Section 35.4.)

An expert witness is a health practitioner who is called upon to present an objective report or finding of an investigation in court. While a factual witness is required by the court to give evidence on the factual contents of the case, an expert witness only has to answer questions directed to his or her specific field of expertise and in some instances his or her professional and truthful opinion about the disposition of the matter at hand. General practitioners can only give professional opinions regarding areas in which they are experts. For anything more specialised they ought to refer to relevant specialists.

## 35.3.5 Human rights

Human rights are a universal set of rights supposedly granted automatically to any individual, irrespective of the person's status in society. Some might claim that there are conditions attached to the granting of these rights and that they come with responsibilities. In mental health, human rights issues illustrate a spectrum that stretches between morality, values and ethics. Without the consideration of any of these factors, a practicing health practitioner may fall into a trap where he or she might be accused of disregard of the human rights of the patient. South Africa has a long history of violations of human rights generally but shares a wider platform with most of the world when it comes to the violation of the rights of those who are mentally ill. Historically, medical practice in the African continent and elsewhere has been fraught with the violation of the rights of mentally ill patients.

The Nazi atrocities of population cleansing that led to the killing of those who were deemed weaker led to a wide-ranging set of guidelines and codes of conduct that were an attempt to prevent any further gross mistreatment by medical doctors against vulnerable individuals or communities (see Section 35.5.4.9). In South Africa, although not reported on widely, the role of certain medical personnel during the time of apartheid has come under scrutiny in the not-so-distant past. The case of Steve Biko served to illustrate what could go wrong when medical personnel become involved in roles other than their professions, where an individual, because of his or her political affiliation, may be treated differently from a mere patient (Dowdall, 1991; Jenkins and Mclean, 2004). The Health Professions Council of South Africa (HPCSA) is the main referee between patients and medical professionals in maintaining fair and ethical clinical practice.

When compared to other disabilities due to medical disorders, mental health disorders pose a bigger challenge as they are shadowed by considerable stigma (also see Chapter 39: Public mental health). There is bias against mentally ill individuals and differential treatment that comes not only from some of their family or community members but even from health practitioners from within and outside the mental health sphere. Discrimination according to the mental health status of a group is systematic and includes public and private health policy omissions or budgetary restrictions. Budget allocations for mental health care funding are still comparatively low in most low- and middle-income countries (Patel, 2007).

The improvement of legislation focusing on the rights of mentally ill individuals and their caregivers in South Africa through the MHCA has been an attempt at redressing violations of the past. It is hoped that the attempt will improve the lot of mentally ill individuals in the South African context in terms of their rights. Preservation of the human dignity of the mentally ill person by various means is one of the core emphases of the Act. Improvement of access to mental health services at community level is another. A move away from unnecessary and prolonged institutionalisation, through involuntary care, treatment and rehabilitation (CTR), is also strongly emphasised. The Act, in itself, has good intentions but has yet to be followed fully by strong implementation plans in all spheres of government. Medical professionals operating in the health care system in South Africa cannot proceed to deliver their services without being aware of the glaring deficits as far as equal rights and opportunities for mentally ill individuals are concerned.

The establishment of global networks working on the improvement of human rights has culminated in the creation of global policies like the United Nations Convention on the Rights of Persons with Disabilities (CRPD) to which South Africa became a ratified signatory in November 2007 (United Nations, 2006).

## 35.4 Mental health legislation and the health practitioner

The Mental Health Care Act (No. 17 of 2002) and its regulations replaced the previous Mental Health Act (No. 18 of 1973). It was promulgated in December 2004 and was enacted from January 2005. The Act is consistent with international human rights standards. The Act is essential for monitoring mental health services, improving the quality of care and protecting the human rights of people with mental disorders.

The overall aim of the Act is to:

- provide for the appropriate care, treatment and rehabilitation of persons who are mentally ill
- set out different procedures to be followed in the admission of such persons to treatment facilities
- establish mental health review boards in respect of every mental health establishment
- provide the care and administration of the property of mentally ill persons.

The Act attempts to collaborate and coordinate different stakeholders' duties towards people with mental health problems or mental disabilities.

The preamble to the Act recognises:

- that health is a state of physical, mental and social well-being and that mental health services should be provided as part of primary, secondary and tertiary health services
- that the Constitution of the Republic of South Africa prohibits the unfair discrimination of people with mental or other disabilities

- that the person and property of the person with mental disorders or mental disabilities may at times require protection and similarly to protect members of the public and their property
- further to provide and coordinate mental health services within general health services and the community in which the mentally ill person resides. (Mental Health Care Act).

The MHCA has 10 chapters and 76 sections with subsections that set out the obligations of the different role-players and the rights of persons with mental health problems or mental disabilities. The regulation section of the MCHA has 12 chapters with 48 annexures. The MHCA, the regulations and amendments thereof can be found with government notices or on the national gazette's website (www.sagazette.co.za and www.gov.za).

It is important to note that a good knowledge of the first three chapters of the Act is essential to be able to apply the necessary procedures for the CTR of persons with mental health problems or a mental disability.

## 35.4.1 Definitions in terms of the MHCA and regulations

The first chapter of the MHCA defines various concepts including places, role-players and procedures to be considered. Most of the terminology originates from the National Health Act. Additional matters related to the MHCA are defined in the regulations. For practical purposes, some of the important definitions and other noteworthy issues have been grouped together for further discussion.

### 35.4.1.1 Basic terminology

- Mental health status refers to the holistic mental well-being of an individual as affected by physical, social and psychological factors.
- Mental illness means a positive diagnosis of a mental health related illness in terms of accepted diagnostic criteria made by a mental health care practitioner authorised to make such diagnosis
- Intellectual capacity: only persons with a severe or profound intellectual disability are defined in terms of the Act. These categories of disability refer to a specific range of intellectual functioning.
- Severe intellectual disability refers to a person with partial self-maintenance under close supervision, limited self-protection skills in a controlled environment, limited self-care and requiring constant aid and supervision.
- Profound intellectual disability refers to a person with severely restricted sensory and motor functioning requiring nursing care.

**Points to ponder**

Although not specified in the MHCA, the needs and abilities of persons with a mild to moderate degree of intellectual disability have to be carefully considered as well when applying care, treatment and rehabilitation in terms of the Act.

### 35.4.1.2 Role-players

- Mental health care practitioner (MHCP): per definition, a mental health care practitioner is a psychiatrist or a registered medical practitioner. Additionally, a nurse, occupational therapist, psychologist and social worker who have been trained to provide prescribed mental health care, treatment and rehabilitation are included in the list. This acts to expand the human resources available and is an attempt to improve access to mental health care services for those in need. It also ensures that mental health care is provided by people who are able and qualified to do so. The minimum requirements for training have not been defined by the Act. Networks of mental health care practitioners in an area are encouraged. These role-players are included in the group defined as:
  - mental health care provider: refers to any person who provides mental health care services (including the mental health care practitioners listed above)

  - mental health care user (MHCU): a person with mental health needs or a mental disability, his or her next of kin and any other supportive role-player as listed below. In the context of the MHCA, the term mental health care user does not just refer to the patient or person with mental health problems or mental disability who receive care, treatment and rehabilitation but to a more holistic inclusion of caregivers. It is also important to remember the order of the hierarchy in the next-of kin-list. The spouse is always the closest followed by a parent, brothers and/or sisters, uncles, aunts, and so forth
  - custodian: a person who actually lives with and physically cares for a mental health care user
- administrator: a person who looks after a mental health care user's affairs and finances. Per definition, an administrator means a person appointed in terms of the Act to care for and administer the property of a mentally ill person and, where applicable, includes an interim administrator. An administrator may not necessarily live with the mental health care user. Any person over the age of 18 may apply to the Master of the High Court for the appointment of an administrator for a mentally ill person
- head health establishment (HHE): a person who manages a health establishment offering any health services including mental health care. The tasks of the heads of health establishments in terms of the MHCA are more managerial and administrative than clinical. The HHEs are also to ensure the appropriateness of the legal and ethical processes in terms of the Act. Heads of health establishments who do not have any clinical expertise must act in consultation with a relevant mental health care practitioner if a decision falls outside their scope of professional practice. In the absence of a head of a health establishment, the duties and functions can only be performed by an officially designated manager at that health establishment
- the Mental Health Review Board (MHRB): an entity made up of at least one mental health care practitioner, a representative of the legal field and a member of the community. They review all assessments, applications, transfers and periodical reports. They also have to consider any appeals against decisions made by mental health care practitioners or heads of health establishments. At any stage during the care, treatment and rehabilitation of a mental health care user, a mental health care practitioner may be subpoenaed to appear before the MHRB. The mental health care practitioner's role is to assist in promoting and protecting international, regional and nationally determined human rights of people with mental disorders and intellectual disability.

### 35.4.1.3 Some procedures and tasks from the MHCA

- Admission, discharge and transfer: In terms of the Act, these concepts do not have the same meaning as found elsewhere in the field of health. In this context they mean the admission, discharge and transfer of a person in terms of the legal procedures related to the MHCA. For instance a person is admitted as a mental health care user legally in terms of the Act and not necessarily physically into a hospital. The same applies for discharges; a person is discharged from a section of the MHCA and not necessarily from a hospital. Admission may apply to a legislated process in terms of the MHCA. For example, a person is admitted as an assisted mental health care user in terms of the MHCA to be treated as an outpatient at a clinic on a monthly basis. Admission does not necessarily imply that a mental health care user has to be admitted to a hospital ward as such. In case of a transfer, a person can be transferred from a section of the Act into another (see Section 35.4.3). A mental health care practitioner therefore must be constantly aware of the differences in meanings of these terms in relation to the MHCA versus their meaning in terms of general health admissions, discharges and transfers.

- Seclusion and physical and/or mechanical restraint: Seclusion means the isolation of a user in a space where his or her freedom of movement is constricted and restricted. Physical and/or mechanical restraint means the use of any instrument or appliance whereby the movements of the body or any of the limbs of a user are restrained or impeded. It means temporary physically restraining the movements of the body by one or more persons in order to prevent the person so restrained from harming self, others or destroying property.

Procedures related to seclusion and physical/mechanical restraint are described in the Regulations to the MHCA.

**Points to ponder**

For guiding principles, indications, contraindications, special considerations and procedures also see the National Department of Health's policy guidelines on seclusion and restraint.

**Periodical reports**

Periodical reports are measures to regulate long-term admissions and to prevent unnecessary limitations to a person's ability to decide on care, treatment and rehabilitation. The mental health status of a person who cannot give informed consent or who is a state patient or a mentally ill prisoner has to be reviewed and reported on within six months of being admitted under the MHCA and then yearly thereafter. A summary report of the review must be submitted to the MHRB and other relevant authorities as regulated by the MHCA. All mental health care practitioners are responsible for the writing of periodical reports.

### 35.4.1.4 Health establishments

Hospitals, clinics and any other place where persons receive care, treatment, rehabilitative assistance and diagnostic or therapeutic interventions as part of a mental health care service are referred to as health establishments in terms of the Act. It is important to note that different health establishments perform different roles in terms of the various procedures described in the MHCA. This allows for much greater accessibility to varying mental health services. Also, a distinction ought to be made between general psychiatric hospitals and rehabilitation units that provide care, treatment and rehabilitation to persons with severe or profound intellectual disabilities. Some health establishments have been designated as 72-hour assessment centres.

## 35.4.2 Ethical considerations

The MHCA has included a chapter on the rights and duties related to mental health care users. The ten sections in the chapter are very important to acknowledge and bear in mind whenever dealing with a person with a mental health related problem.

The Act aims to protect the rights of mentally ill people and to protect the community whilst providing appropriate treatment. The rights and duties of persons, bodies or institutions set out in Chapter III of the MHCA are in addition to any rights and duties that mental health care users may have in terms of any other law. The best interest of the mental health care user must be considered at all times.

The mental health care user's person, human dignity and privacy must be respected and any care, treatment and rehabilitation have to intrude as little as possible to give effect to the appropriate care, treatment and rehabilitation and be proportionate and improve the mental capacity. A person has to be allowed to develop to his or her full potential and be integrated back into community life.

Informed consent to care, treatment and rehabilitation and admission to and in terms of the Act (or for that matter any medical treatment) is arguably the most important right of a mental health care user to be acknowledged by all health care providers.

A health establishment may provide care, treatment and rehabilitation services to a mental health care user only if he or she has consented to such. The only exceptions to this requirement are when care, treatment and rehabilitation are authorised by a court order, a MHRB or if it is considered to be an emergency.

The emergency clause of the MHCA states that a heath care provider or a health establishment may provide care, treatment and rehabilitation without consent if, due to mental illness, any delay in providing care, treatment and rehabilitation may result in death or irreversible harm or when inflicting serious harm to self or others, cause serious damage to or loss of property belonging to self or others.

The typical clinical set-up where the emergency clause applies involves a scenario where the mental health status of the individual and therefore his or her suitability to be declared a mental health care user is not certain. This individual is then admitted to elucidate whether the presenting signs and symptoms are part of a recognisable psychiatric disorder or should be clinically managed otherwise.

Due to the nature of mental illness, mental health care users may at times display aggressive behaviour to themselves or to others and to property. This may warrant emergency intervention in the form of restraint or seclusion. Seclusion and restraint, mechanical or otherwise, are emergency interventions that involve the curtailment of freedom of the mental health care user. These procedures should only be used in extreme circumstances and as a last resort. Physical restraint should be limited to brief periods during which medication to control the behaviour is administered and while awaiting the medication to take effect. Always exclude serious treatable medical conditions as the underlying cause.

Other rights and duties toward mental health care users that must be followed are:

- Section 10 – No unfair discrimination on the grounds of mental health status.
- Section 11 – Exploitation, abuse, degrading treatment, forced labour or punishment, for the convenience of other people, have to be reported.
- Section 12 – The health status may not be based on socio-political or economic status, cultural or religious background or affinity.
- Section 14 – This deals with the limitation on intimate adult relationships. Such limitation may only be considered if, due to mental illness, the ability of the user to consent is diminished.
- Section 15 – A mental health care user is entitled to a representative, including a legal representative, when submitting an application, lodging an appeal, appearing before a magistrate, judge or a review board, subject to the laws governing rights of appearances in a court of law. An indigent mental health care user is entitled to legal aid provided by the State in respect of any proceeding, instituted or conducted in terms of this Act, subject to any condition fixed in terms of Section 3(d) of the Legal Aid Act (No. 22 of 1969).
- Section 16 – This refers to a discharge report. The application of such notice informs the mental health care user, the applicant and all regulated role-players, of the mental health care user's discharge from the Act.
- Section 17 – This acknowledges a mental health care user's right to knowledge of his or her rights and must, before administering any services, be informed of them in an appropriate manner, unless admitted under circumstances referred to in Section 9(1)(*c*).

Confidentiality under the MHCA falls under the auspices of the national health department, the head of the provincial department or the head of the health establishment. Disclosure of information, with or without a person's consent, should always be with special care and according to the Promotion of Access to Information Act (No. 2 of 2000) and the MHCA as described earlier in this chapter.

A mental health care practitioner may temporarily deny a mental health care user access to information contained in his or her health records if disclosure is likely to seriously prejudice the user and/or cause the user to conduct himself or herself in a way that may seriously prejudice the mental health care user or the health of others.

An information officer should regulate such procedures at a health establishment.

It is important to note that the ability to give informed consent to treatment and operations for illnesses other than psychiatric disorders must be considered separately. A loss of capacity to give informed consent in terms of the MHCA does not automatically imply a loss of capacity to consent to other procedures. Where a mental health care practitioner assesses a user as not capable of consenting to treatment or an operation due to mental illness or intellectual disability, then a curator (if a court has appointed one), spouse, next of kin, parent or guardian can give consent.

## 35.4.3 Application of the MHCA

The general scenario in practice in all health establishments and with all health care practitioners is to examine a person who presents with a problem, be it a physical, social or mental health related problem, and then to decide on the appropriate treatment and management. Mental health care practitioners have to deal with emergencies within the scope of their expertise and facilities in which they work. If they cannot attend to the appropriate level of care the person needs, the person has to be referred to a hospital, clinic or HE where such services can be provided.

The procedures and terms that heads of health establishments and mental health care practitioners have to apply when a person is considered to be a mental health care user and has to be managed in terms of the MHCA are set out in Chapter V of the MHCA. Additionally, the regulations have to be adhered to and the Fundamental Provisions of the Act (Chapter II), The Rights and Duties of the mental health care user (Chapter III), and the duties toward the Mental Health Review Board have to be considered.

It is important to realise that this is not a procedural act – meaning that a mental health care practitioner can assess a patient, fill in a form and have the person processed. In practice, the admission procedures in terms of the Act, set out in Chapter V (Voluntary, Assisted and Involuntary mental health care), have to be applied when a person presents with mental problems or mental disabilities and is considered in need of management in terms of the Act. However, these procedures can only be applied together with a clear understanding and consideration of the extremely important issues in the first three chapters – the defining issues, fundamental principles and human rights obligations.

Contact and proper liaison with the mental health care practitioner at the referral health establishments should always be followed. This should include booking notices, transport arrangements, copies of clinical notes and copies of special investigations.

Mental health care practitioners have to make enquiries regarding, and be familiar with, the resources of the health establishments in which they work – including the internal guidelines on movement of forms, transport management and referral routes. They have to know who is responsible for keeping copies of the forms at the health establishment and where these copies are kept.

The above provisions are all-important to be able to apply the MHCA procedures.

## 35.4.4 The fundamental provisions

The fundamental provisions of the MHCA set out objectives and implementation policies and measures. Together with the regulations, they must be integrated within the level of service of the different health establishments. The expectations, requirements and responsibilities that emerge from the different sections in this chapter are very important.

All role-players have the obligation to provide the best possible mental health care, treatment and rehabilitation services to the population equitably, efficiently and in the best interest of the mental health care user within the limits of the available resources.

By recognising primary, secondary and tertiary care, treatment and rehabilitation, much greater accessibility to various mental health services are available and the responsibility is divided between more health care providers and integrated in a general health care setting. The provision for the control and protection of the person and the public is recognised.

The regulations to the MHCA states clearly that if a person requires care, treatment and rehabilitation services, such a person has to be assessed and treated at a community-based or primary care facility (considered the point of entry for health services). If the primary care or community facility cannot manage the assessment and management, only then may the mental health care user be referred to a secondary care level and, if necessary, from there to tertiary level care (being considered as the more restricted environment furthest from his or her community). Therefore, it is important at all times to consider and implement primary, secondary or tertiary level of care and promote community-based care.

Some hospitals have been designated to provide certain services. Some health establishments are designated as 72-hour assessment service centres. A few secondary health establishments provide a tertiary level of psychiatric care in a unit as part of a health establishment, not specifically a psychiatric hospital. Some health establishments have the facilities to provide a wider scope of mental health care, treatment and rehabilitation and are obliged by the fundamental provisions, set out in the Act, to deliver such services. The heads of health establishments and provincial and national executives will be required to draw up protocols, guidelines and structures to provide expected services to the mental health care users. Mental health care practitioners have to be aware of the nature and scope of services provided by the health establishment where they are working.

The needs of a person with a mental health problem, as well as the nature of the disorder or mental disability, determine the procedures for admission in terms of the Act and the level of management provided at a health establishment. The procedure followed for management depends on the severity of the illness and the behaviour of the patient.

## 35.4.5 Care, treatment and rehabilitation procedures

Emergency and other categories of care, treatment and rehabilitation are regulated in the MHCA and its regulations. There are three categories to be applied for for the care, treatment and rehabilitation of a mental health care user: voluntary submission, non-opposing submission, and compulsory treatment and management.

Consider at least four main issues:

- the capacity of the mental health care user for informed consent for mental health care, treatment and rehabilitation
- at which health establishment can the appropriate level of care, treatment and rehabilitation be provided?
- should the mental health care user receive care, treatment and rehabilitation as an in-patient or out-patient (least restrictive environment)?
- can the health establishment provide the necessary treatment or should the mental health care user be referred to another facility?

### 35.4.5.1 Emergency care, treatment and rehabilitation

Mental health care users who urgently require care, treatment and rehabilitation and are a danger to self or others are treated under this section. In this case, examination and treatment are necessary but are against the person's will (without consent) for a period of up to 24 hours. The management, treatment and differentiation (if further mental health care, treatment or rehabilitation is required) must be reported in terms of the MHCA and on a regulated annexure (MHCA 1) after the set 24-hour period. If further care, treatment and rehabilitation in terms of the person's mental health status is required then an application in terms of the treatment procedures set out in the rest of this section must be followed.

### 35.4.5.2 Voluntary care, treatment and rehabilitation

The least restrictive and preferred situation is one in which the person has the ability to agree to admission and treatment. A voluntary mental health care user is required to understand the circumstances and the implications of the care, treatment, rehabilitation and admission to and in terms of the MHCA. The mental health care user has to agree to be admitted in terms of the MHCA and to be treated. Voluntary mental health care users are viewed and treated in the same manner as persons with other health problems.

### 35.4.5.3 Assisted (non-opposing) care, treatment and rehabilitation

**Assisted care, treatment and rehabilitation**, in terms of the Act, is the management of a person requiring mental health care that agrees to be treated, or does not object, but is unable to give informed consent due to mental illness, intellectual disability or is under the age of 18. It is important to keep in mind that even in the presence of a severe mental illness a person may have the ability to agree to treatment and that this must be evaluated.

For an assisted admission to the Act, an application is made on a prescribed and regulated form setting out the necessary detail and, in addition, setting out the relationship to the proposed assisted mental health care user. Only a spouse, next of kin, partner, associate, parent or guardian may apply. Where a mental health care user is younger than 18 years, the parent or guardian has to make the application. If the applicant is not a next of kin or if the next of kin is unwilling, incapable or not available, then a mental health care provider may apply. In such cases the steps taken to locate the relatives to determine their capability or availability to make the application has to be stated.

The reasons why the application is made must be stated, including the grounds on which the applicant believes that care, treatment and rehabilitation are required; and the date, time and place where the proposed assisted mental health care user was last seen by the applicant within the seven days before making the application. Although a mental health care practitioner can per definition apply, such practitioner may then not be a role-player in the following admission procedures. Considering the shortage of mental health care practitioners, preference given to

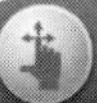

#### Case study 35.1

The SAPS presents at a large secondary care hospital a young man who was found roaming around half dressed, shouting at people passing by, kicking at cars and shop doors. The man refuses to say who he is, resists being properly examined and becomes threatening. The casualty officer is unable to evaluate him and uncertain if he is mentally ill. He wonders if the person is physically ill or maybe intoxicated. Is he a bad character?

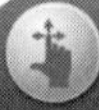

#### Case study 35.2

Mrs X is a 36-year-old woman who goes to a community service clinic. She presents with a major depressive disorder. You suggest admission and further treatment, which she voluntarily accepts.

#### Case study 35.3

Parents bring their 18-year-old severely intellectually impaired son to you. They want him to be admitted because they cannot control his behaviour.

another mental health care provider may be more appropriate. Often the next of kin may need some direction and/or assistance to complete the application form. An application has to be certified by a Commissioner of Oaths. An application may be withdrawn at any time.

Two mental health care practitioners, one of whom must be qualified to do a physical examination, are appointed by the head of the health establishment to examine the mental health care user. These mental health care practitioners then submit their examination findings independently and separately on the regulated annexure. The examination or assessment findings refer to the physical health, collateral information, mental health status and a provisional diagnosis. Consideration of homicidal tendencies, suicidality or dangerousness is also required. The mental health care practitioners will then recommend to the head of the health establishment, treatment of the person as an assisted mental health care user. If applicable, they may recommend that the person be considered for involuntary care, treatment and rehabilitation instead (see Section 35.4.5.4). It is important to note that the mental health care practitioner declares the information to be truthful.

The head of the health establishment checks whether the findings on the application and the examination reports are congruent and that the necessary ethical issues have been considered. If the findings of the two mental health care practitioners differ, the head of the health establishment must ensure that the mental health care user is examined by another mental health care practitioner who, on completion of such examination, submits a written report. The head of the health establishment will then approve, give written notice and direct the mental health care user for assisted care, treatment and rehabilitation at the closest available and appropriate facility. The prescribed forms forwarded to the MHRB note the mental health care user's admission to the MHCA. Any specific treatment, special investigations, laboratory results or other observations must be noted, added to the copies of the procedural forms and accompany the MHCU to the health establishment where the care, treatment and rehabilitation will take place.

#### 35.4.5.4 Involuntary (compulsory) care, treatment and rehabilitation

Some mental health care users will require involuntary care, treatment and rehabilitation to be provided without consent in terms of the MHCA. In this instance, the mental illness is of such a nature that the proposed mental health care user is likely to inflict harm to self or others and care, treatment and rehabilitation is necessary for protection of his or her financial interest or reputation; but the mental health care user refuses treatment. Such a decision should be made in the context of the longitudinal history, present mental state, and the need to intervene in the early stages of a relapse.

The procedure in this instance is initiated as with the assisted mental health care user above, but has extra requirements as described below. After the required application and examination have been completed as for the assisted mental health care user, and the two mental health care practitioners recommend involuntary care, treatment and rehabilitation, then a 72-hour assessment period must be completed at a designated health establishment. Introduction of a 72-hour assessment period prior to involuntary admission at a psychiatric hospital was added to the MHCA to allow increased accessibility and availability of mental health care services at the community level and to reduce the need for premature or unnecessary transfers to tertiary psychiatric hospitals. In addition, it allows screening of medical conditions disguised and presenting as psychiatric disorders. Note the involuntary and compulsory admission 72-hour assessment policy guidelines by the Director General: Health. Information on hospitals listed as designated 72-hour health establishments in terms of the Act can be sourced from the Mental Health and Substance Abuse Directorate of the National Department of Health.

At the commencement of the 72-hour process, two mental health care practitioners appointed by the head of the health establishment conduct the assessment, determine the treatment program and the place within the designated health establishment where the mental health care user is to be kept during the 72-hour assessment period. They have to ensure the safety of the user and others.

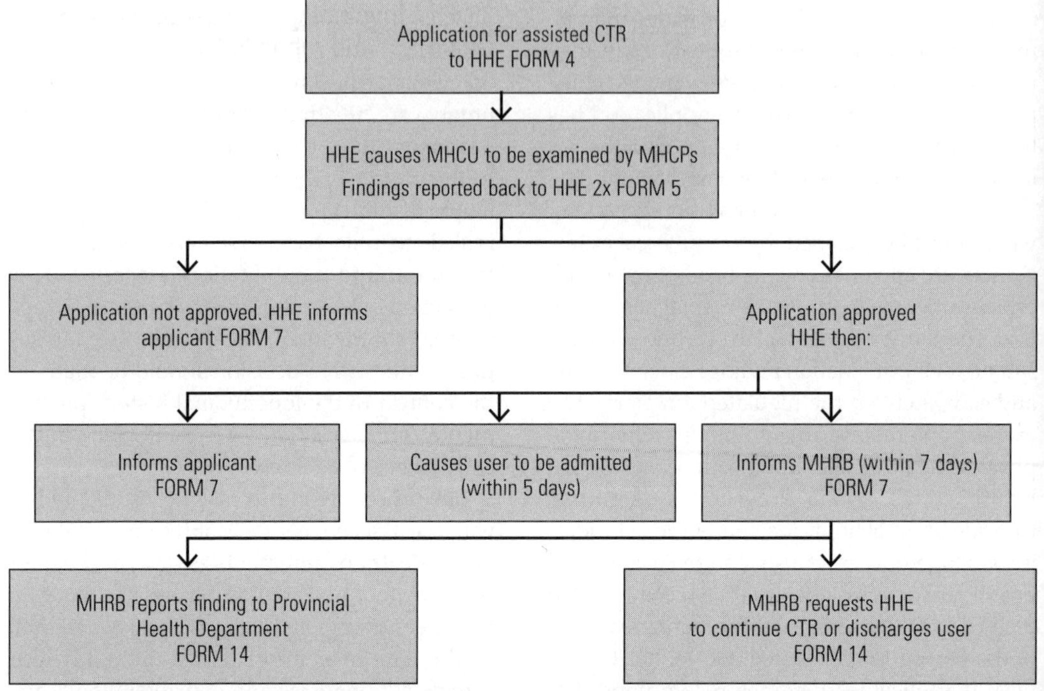


**Figure 35.1** Assisted care, treatment and rehabilitation

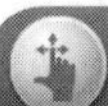

## Case study 35.4

After midnight on a Saturday evening the husband brings Mrs K, a well-known patient with schizophrenia, to the hospital. According to Mr K, his wife stopped her medication several months ago. She started to act aggressively and in a strange manner and threatened to kill her children. She says they are devils. She also accuses him of poisoning her food. She is untidy, threatening and appears to be listening to someone not in the room. She has been physically well otherwise. Mr K confirms that she has presented like this before.

They have to exclude other medical co-morbidity or problems that may require attention. They have to take care that the mental health care user is properly managed, not unnecessarily heavily sedated, not inadequately secured, not receiving the wrong treatment, or is medically neglected. The evaluation may redirect the clinical needs of the mental health care user after the 72-hour period to another field.

After the assessment period the mental health care practitioners submit their examination findings independently and separately on the regulated annexure.

If the head of the health establishment, following the assessment, is of the opinion that the mental health care user does not warrant involuntary admission, the user must be discharged immediately, unless the user consents to remain under voluntary or assisted care, treatment and rehabilitation. If the head of the health establishment accepts the need for further involuntary care, treatment and rehabilitation on an out-patient basis, the mental health care user can be transferred. In such a case, the mental health care user will be subjected to the prescribed conditions or procedures relating to his or her outpatient care, treatment and rehabilitation in writing. If the findings warrant further involuntary care on an in-patient basis, the head of the health establishment must, within 48 hours, cause the transfer to the nearest psychiatric hospital or psychiatric unit.

All the original applications, examination reports, opinions and notices have to be forwarded to the MHRB to approve further involuntary care, treatment and rehabilitation.

### 35.4.5.5 Appeals

An assisted and an involuntary mental health care user or their next of kin may appeal against the decision of the head of the health establishment for care, treatment and rehabilitation. The mental health care provider or the head of the health establishment has to provide the appellant with the necessary form to cause such an appeal (regulated annexure MHCA 14). The MHRB will consider the matter and may uphold the appeal and the mental health care user has to be discharged according to accepted clinical practice. If the MHRB does not uphold the appeal, the matter must be forwarded to the High Court for further orders. Reasons for an appeal may be the belief of the next of kin that the mental health care user does not have a mental disorder or the mental health care user believes he or she does not suffer from a mental disorder and demands to be discharged.

### 35.4.5.6 The role of the South African Police Services

If a member of the South African Police Service has reason to believe, from personal observation or from information obtained from a mental health care practitioner, that a person, due to his or her mental illness or mental disability, is likely to inflict serious harm to himself or herself or to others, the member must apprehend the person. The SAPS's obligation and assistance may be requested to apprehend a person considered to need mental health care intervention and cause such person to be examined at the closest health establishment with the appropriate infrastructure and facilities.

The member of the SAPS must cause that person to be taken to an appropriate health establishment administered under the auspices of the State for assessment of the mental health status of that person. The person has to be handed over into custody of the head of the health establishment or any other person designated to receive such persons. The necessary regulations and forms in terms of the MHCA apply (regulated annexure MHCA 22).

If an assisted mental health care user or an involuntary mental health care user has absconded, is deemed to have absconded, or if the user has to be transferred, the head of the health establishment may request assistance from the South African Police Service to locate, apprehend and return the user to the health establishment or transfer the user in a prescribed manner.

**Points to ponder**

To apply the above-mentioned procedures and level of care the following questions may be considered:

- What is the health establishment's designation of the mental health care practitioner attending to the mental health care user?
- What is the nature of, and/or level of care, treatment and rehabilitation the health establishment can offer the mental health care user?
- Are there mental health care practitioners with the necessary expertise to manage the mental health care user?
- Does the health establishment have the required medication and infrastructure?
- What is the appropriate referral route if your health establishment can only provide a part of the appropriate management or higher or more specialised level input is needed or, the appropriate management can be provided at lower level (down refer) or, the health establishment is full to capacity and a referral to another health establishment with the same facilities needs to be applied (lateral referral) – Regulation 2
- Are the contact person(s) and contact number(s) of the HHEs and health establishments and community health care clinics in the community and referral area available?

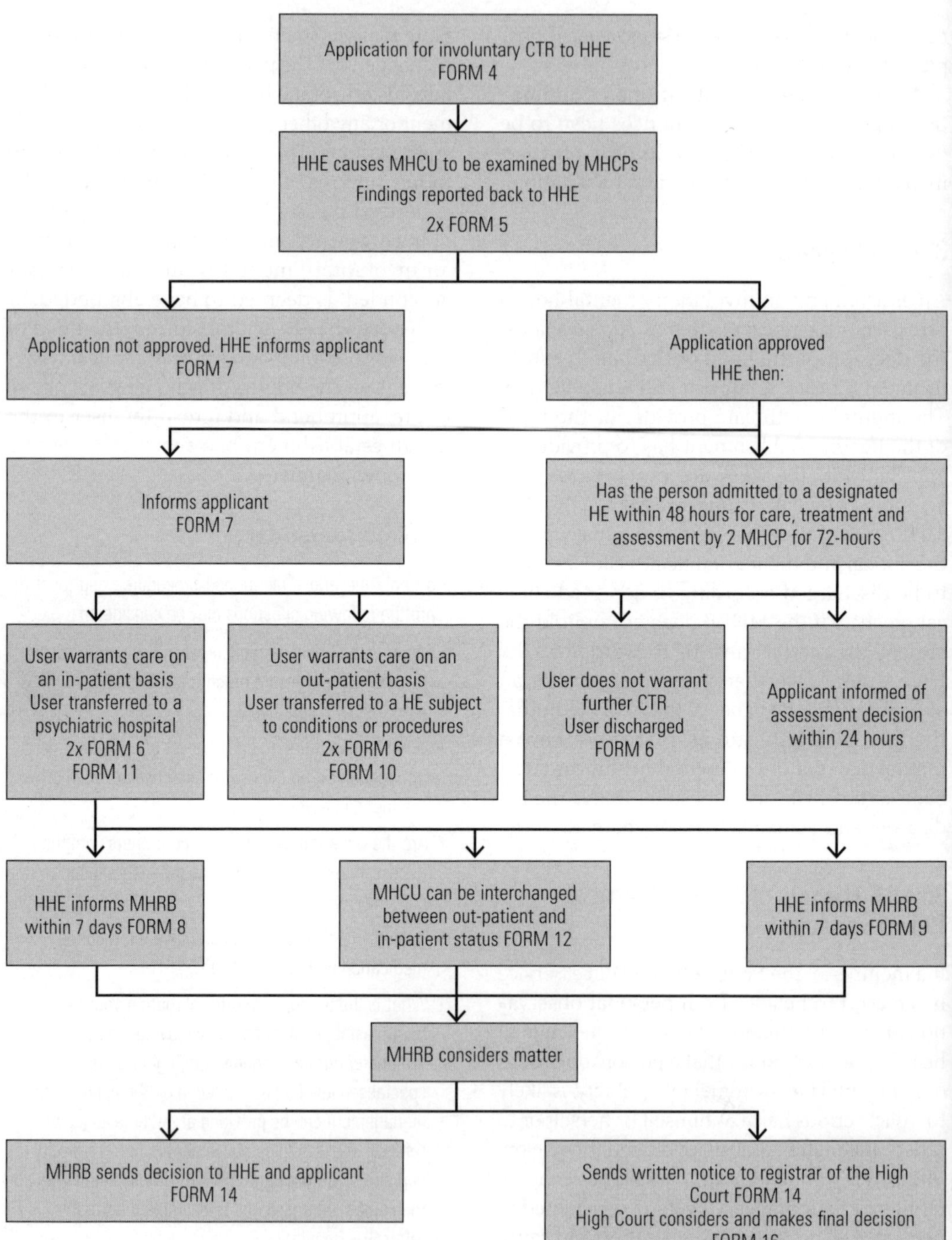


**Figure 35.2** Involuntary care, treatment and rehabilitation

## 35.5 Health care practitioners and other related legislative matters

### 35.5.1 The health practitioner and criminal matters

If the mental state and/or the history of mental illness of an accused are brought before the court the matter is referred for examination by a mental health expert according to relevant legislation. Most referrals are in terms of Sections 77, 78 and 79 of the the Criminal Procedure Act as amended. The assessment of young offenders whose mental capacity to offend is in question is regulated by the Child Justice Act. The management of matters related to the victims or perpetrators of sexual offences is regulated by the Criminal Law (Sexual Offences and Related Matters) Amendment Act.

#### 35.5.1.1 Referrals under the Criminal Procedure Act

The accused may be referred for a forensic mental health observation at a designated psychiatric hospital for up to 30 days (Section 79). During this period of observation, a psychiatric diagnosis, if any, has to be made. The mental capacity of the accused to follow court proceedings so as to defend himself or herself (Section 77) and his or her mental capacity to offend (Section 78 (*a*) and (*b*)) are assessed (Kaliski, 2006).

In South Africa, referrals are strictly legislated to be performed by registered psychiatrists and clinical psychologists, as well as other mental health experts within the field.

However, the general health practitioner may become involved in the clinical management of persons referred by the criminal justice system, including the following:

- Awaiting-trial prisoners who are in need of medical and/or mental health care at any stage, including during the bail period, of the criminal justice process. These individuals may be cared for in different establishments, such as prison hospitals, general hospitals or police holding cells, and the intervention will not be related to the Criminal Procedure Act processes referred to above.
- Mentally ill prisoners (MHCA, Chapter VII): individuals who are convicted prisoners and are in need of mental health care are generally treated in the correctional facility by mental health care practitioners, including medical practitioners and psychiatrists. In exceptional cases, where directed by a court order, they may be evaluated and managed by mental health care practitioner at a designated psychiatric hospital.
- State patients (MHCA, Chapter VI): individuals who are declared state patients by the court at the end of their trial are referred to designated psychiatric hospitals for care, treatment, rehabilitation and discharge pending the decision of the judge in chambers. State patients may be attended to by a general mental health care practitioner for follow-up during periods of leave of absence in the community, or when they have absconded and have to be referred back to the original designated psychiatric hospital. Chapter VI of the MHCA and its regulations give a stepwise approach to the admission procedures related to state patients.
- Involuntary mental health care users (MHCA, Chapter V): individuals who have committed minor offences, as defined in the Criminal Matters Amendment Act (No. 68 of 1998), may be referred back via a court order for further CTR as general psychiatric patients.

The mental health care practitioner's duty towards such a patient is that of good and objective clinical care, including the management of medical records.

In the case of state patients, mentally ill prisoners and involuntary mental health care users, periodical reports must be completed. (See Section 35.4.)

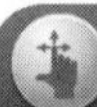

**Case study 35.5**

A medical officer at a primary care hospital attends to out-patients. One of the patients is an involuntary mental health care user booked for a follow-up. What are the duties of the mental health care practitioner towards the patient? What regulations must the mental health care practitioner consider?

## 35.5.2 The health practitioner and the Sterilization Act

In the context of mental health care, the Sterilization Act (No. 3 of 2005) seeks to provide regulations on how to proceed when a person is incapable of consenting or is incompetent to consent due to severe mental disability.

A panel made up of a multidisciplinary team comprising mental health professionals (a psychiatrist, a psychologist or a social worker and a nurse) must be appointed after an application has been presented to a person in charge of a health establishment or a delegate to review the conditions of an application to perform sterilisation. The panel must show that the individual is affected by a mental disability to a severe degree, will not be able to develop sufficiently to ever give informed consent, or will not be able to fulfil parenting responsibilities associated with giving birth. The affected individual has to be 18 years of age and it should be proven that there is no safer or more effective method of contraception available. An individual younger than 18 years of age may be considered in case of a threat to his/her physical well-being.

Sterilisation is performed at designated facilities only and with the consent of a parent, spouse, guardian or curator of the affected individual.

Individuals who can give a full informed consent are dealt with on a voluntary basis as in any other health care request.

This Act is read in conjunction with its amendments (Sterilization Amendment Act (No. 3 of 2005)).

## 35.5.3 The health practitioner and the Prevention and Treatment for Substance Abuse Act

The Drug Dependency Act (No. 20 of 1992) was replaced by the Prevention of and Treatment for Substance Abuse Act (No. 70 of 2008). The aim of the newer legislation was to simplify the systems that sought to eliminate substance abuse in South Africa. The Act aims to ensure a coordinated strategy to reduce abuse of substances and to regulate the establishment of treatment centres including in- and out-patient facilities and halfway houses. Prevention, early intervention, treatment and re-integration programmes would be enhanced. The Act also provides for the committal of individuals to treatment centres, research and the establishment of a Central Drug Authority.

## 35.5.4 The health practitioner and civil matters

In certain situations it has to be established whether a mental illness is affecting the ability of a person to manage his or her affairs or if a mental illness is impairing the occupational functioning of the individual. Mental health professionals can play an important role in assessments for these civil cases.

### 35.5.4.1 Psychiatric impairment for disability claims

Impairment is the clinical assessment of alteration in normal functioning due to an illness. Psychiatric illnesses are increasingly being recognised as an important cause of impairment. A clinician can only express an opinion regarding functional impairment and not about disability.

It is advised by the HPCSA that the treating clinician should not participate in these assessments. A thorough evaluation should be done taking into account, among other things, collateral information, activities of daily living, motivation and the response to optimal treatment. The claimant should be informed that the information obtained during these evaluations is not necessarily confidential. The evaluation report will be submitted to the relevant third party for the disability assessment.

Disability is defined as the alteration of capability to meet personal, social, or occupational demands because of impairment. This is determined by a non-clinical assessor, such as an insurer or employer, after considering the nature of the impairment. It is important to keep in mind that there are many ethical, social and clinical reasons to assist people with mental illness to work, and work rehabilitation should always be attempted. In South Africa, the Employment Equity Act (No. 55 of 1998) specifies that people with disabilities have a right to be protected against unfair discrimination and to expect all employers to make reasonable accommodation for people with disabilities who are suitably qualified for a job. It is also important to distinguish between individuals who are unable to work and those who are unwilling to work because of secondary gains.

#### 35.5.4.2 The Compensation for Occupational Injuries and Diseases Act

The Compensation for Occupational Injuries and Diseases Act (No. 103 of 1993) provides for the compensation for disability caused by occupational injuries or diseases sustained by workers in the course of their employment, or for death resulting from such injuries or diseases.

Generally specialists in the areas of the disabilities affecting the individual, including psychiatrists, become involved in the assessment. Experience in this area of medical assessment is mandatory before an individual health care practitioner becomes involved in the determination of the level of impairment resulting from the diseases or injuries.

#### 35.5.4.3 Impaired practitioner

The HPCSA, through the Health Professions Act (No. 56 of 1974), has established a Health Committee that oversees the evaluation and determination of competency of medical practitioners referred to it with a query of impairment of capacity to perform their duties. The Health Committee oversees the evaluation of fully qualified professionals and trainees (e.g. intern doctors and medical students). Specific prescripts are followed should there be a query about the mental or physical capacity of an individual who is duly registered and is practicing in South Africa under the auspices of the HPCSA.

The measures set out by the HPCSA through the committee are to ensure that the public is managed by competent health practitioners, the health care practitioner's welfare is maintained and the reputation of the profession is preserved.

The ethical duty to protect patients is of outmost importance when confronted with the possibility of an impaired health professional. Advice from senior members of staff within an establishment or practice may be necessary prior to approaching the HPCSA. Self-report is also encouraged. After impairment is confirmed, the individual health practitioner has several options, including working under supervision until fitness to practice is restored, receiving treatment and/or retirement from the field. These outcomes depend on individual case-assessments (Health Profession Council of South Africa, *s.d.*).

#### 35.5.4.4 Competence

Competence is the ability to make autonomous, informed decisions and to take the necessary action to put these decisions into effect. The terms 'competence' and 'capacity' are used interchangeably. The capacity requires several sub-capacities that include the ability to acquire, retain and understand information, to integrate this with personal preferences or values, to deliberate and make a reasoned choice and to communicate that choice together with, where necessary, the reasoning behind it.

Competency issues normally arise when those functions are impaired by mental illness, especially if chronic or irreversible. The question of whether a person is competent or not is complex. Competence is task-specific and not global. The criteria for someone's competence to, for example, stand trial, care for animals, write out cheques or teach a class are radically different. Competence is, therefore, relative to the particular decision to be made. Thus, a person who is incompetent to decide about financial affairs may be competent to decide to participate in medical research or be able to handle simple tasks easily.

Competence may vary over time, be eroded suddenly (as in stroke), gradually (as in dementia) or intermittently (as in delirium). The law regards all persons as competent until proven otherwise. While informal assessments of competency are made in everyday life, only a court can make formal legally binding determinations of incompetency.

### 35.5.4.5 Contractual or financial competence and testamentary capacity

Contractual capacity refers to the ability of a patient to make a valid contract. If an individual is not able to understand the nature of an agreement, then no contractual capacity is present. Presence of a mental illness does not automatically imply a lack of contractual capacity.

Note that if the patient has not yet drawn up a will or testament and now wishes to do so, referral to a psychiatrist is necessary to establish testamentary capacity. As far as civil law is concerned, competence is most commonly questioned with respect to money, and specificially the ability of the testator to make a will.

In all these cases the MMSE and good notes are vital. As an interim measure the general practitioner may wish to assess the following:

- a knowledge of income
- a knowledge of expenses (i.e. can he or she balance a household budget)
- an ability to handle everyday financial expenses and make change (MMSE's serial-sevens is useful)
- the ability to delegate financial wishes, but retain knowledge and details of finances

Testamentary capacity specifically covers the following points relevant to the patient:

- Understanding the nature and effect of a will. A simple statement such as 'When I die, my children get all my things' will do.
- A reasonable knowledge of the extent of his/her assets.
- Assessing the influence of the illness on the making of the will. The will is legally valid if made during a lucid interval.
- The will is reasonable, usually following the rules of intestate. In the latter, the assets devolve to the spouse, children, parents, siblings, nieces and nephews, respectively.
- If the will is unreasonable the testator gives explanations to this effect. Re-assess patient's wishes on more than one occasion (consistency) and then supply an affadavit regarding the assessment.

In summary: Testamentary capacity refers to the testator's mental state and corresponding capacity at the time of drawing up the will. To make a will the testator or testatrix must have sufficient mental capacity to understand the nature of the will, the extent of his or her property, the relation of those whose interests are affected by the will and must not be influenced by abnormal mental states, delusions or undue external influence. Evaluations to establish testamentary capacity can be tricky and the family practitioner is often called upon to take part in the process. Detailed notes of the evaluation should be kept in anticipation of possible disputes to the validity of the will at a later stage.

### 35.5.4.6 Power of attorney and curatorship

Should the patient be incapable of handling her or his financial affairs, urge a reliable and trustworthy member of the family to take control of the situation. Transfer of authority by means of power of attorney forms work well in early neurocognitive disorder where competency is still preserved. Power of attorney lapses when capacity is lost.

In these situations or where disputes are likely, or no family members are available, curatorship should be sought. This is a time-consuming and expensive process. The forms are obtainable from the court which, with a supporting affidavit from both a psychiatrist and a medical officer, will appoint a *curator bonis* and *ad persona* to attend to the patient's affairs, through a *curator ad litem*. A *curator personae* is usually a family member appointed by the court to control a person's personal care and welfare. A *curator ad litem* is someone who acts as a legal guardian and represents a patient's legal interests. Where the annual income is less than R24 000 or the estate is less than R200 000, the appointment of an administrator should be sought. These amounts are stipulated in the regulations of the MHCA. Social workers who are well-versed in these matters may have to be called in for advice and help with these cases (Kaliski, 2006).

### 35.5.4.7 Custody

Children's rights are enshrined in the Bill of Rights in the Constitution of the Republic of South Africa, which advances the principle of best interest. During divorce proceedings problems can arise when the parties cannot agree on what is in the best interest of their children, or when the court is not satisfied with the terms of the agreement. In these situations experts can be used to assist the court or to help resolve the issues. Clinicians should not make findings on legal issues (e.g. child abuse by a parent). These are highly specialised assessments and it should be conducted with as little intrusion to the family as possible by appropriately qualified experts.

### 35.5.4.8 Living wills and advanced directives

An advance medical directive is a statement or instruction given by a competent adult that enables people to refuse medical treatment in particular circumstances in the future when they are no longer capable of making decisions. A living will refers to such directives that can take the form of advance refusal of specified treatments or it can also contain information about the patient's values and beliefs. It can also consist of a lasting power of attorney in which the author appoints another person to refuse medical treatment in future on his or her behalf. In South Africa the legal validity of such advance medical directives is uncertain and although they are ethically acceptable, they are not legally enforceable.

For an **advanced directive** to be valid, the patient must be 18 years or older and must have the mental capacity to make their own decisions at the time when the directive is issued. The patient should also be fully informed about his or her condition and the proposed treatment before he or she can refuse treatment. The care provider must be satisfied that the patient did not change his or her mind after issuing the directive. If these conditions are met, from an ethical perspective, the directive should be followed, even when the patient later loses decisional capacity. Always ensure that you obtain a copy of the original living will before proceeding with or withdrawing treatment.

The South African Medical Association (SAMA) and the HPCSA have both issued guidance stating that all patients have a right to refuse treatment and that patients who have advance directives in place have constitutional rights to expect their living wills to be honoured. In cases where emergency treatment is necessary, you should provide the necessary treatment until you are notified of a directive and provided with a copy (Medical Protection Society, 2012).

### 35.5.4.9 Ethics and relationship with Pharma

Most ethical guidelines are based on the norms of respect for autonomy, non-maleficence, beneficence and justice. Respect for the dignity, safety and well-being of participants should be the primary concern in health research involving human participants.

In modern research ethics, the Helsinki Declaration has been adopted internationally. It reflects the fundamental commitment to protect the welfare of the human subject and to promote autonomy. The basic principles include that research must have scientific merit, that the objectives of the research must be proportional to the risks and that the participants' welfare and interests should be protected over those of society and science.

Decisionally impaired people may be competent to make some decisions, while simultaneously being incompetent to make others. Consequently an individual's capacity to make decisions should be evaluated for a specific decision rather than a judgement of global function.

All health research conducted in South Africa must be reviewed by a research ethics committee and should not commence until the ethics committee has granted approval. Before a clinical trial involving medicines may be conducted in South Africa, approval must be obtained from the Medicines Control Council and an accredited ethics committee. The Medicines Control Council must review all clinical trials of both registered and non-registered medicinal substances.

Through the National Health Act, 2003 (No. 61 of 2003), the National Health Research Ethics Council was established. It did not replace existing committees, but serves as a central body to regulate matters of research ethics and advises the Department of Health on the management of health research ethics.

A protocol for a clinical trial must conform to the following guidelines and international documents:

- World Medical Association Declaration of Helsinki
- The International Conference for Harmonisation Guideline for Good Clinical Practice
- The Association of the British Pharmaceutical Industry (ABPI) Guidelines for Medical Experiments in healthy volunteers if the study intends involving such volunteers
- Guidelines for Good Practice in the Conduct of Clinical Trials in Human Participants in South Africa.

The aims of every trial should be precisely stated and every trial should be conducted by competent researchers with suitable experience and qualifications (World Medical Association, 1964).

## Conclusion

Legislation and ethical practice surrounding those in need of mental health services has evolved. Mental health care is now back in the fold of general health care systems. It is imperative that all health care providers equip themselves with the knowledge of how to apply current legislation and policies governing the management of people in need of mental health care (World Medical Association, 1964).

# References


Bateman C (2006) Lack of capacity devitalizing SA's hospitals. *South African Medical Journal* 96(3): 168–170

Deigh J (2010) *An Introduction to Ethics* (e-book). New York: Cambridge University Press

Department of Health (Directorate: Mental Health and Substance Abuse), Republic of South Africa (2001). Update on the Mental Health Legislation. *Quarterly Newsletter* (second quarter 2001). Pretoria: Department of Health

Department of Health, Republic of South Africa (2012) *Policy Guidelines on: 72-hour Assessment of Involuntary Mental Health Care Users*. Pretoria: Department of Health

Department of Health, Republic of South Africa (2012) *Policy guidelines on: Seclusion and Restraint of Mental Health Care Users*. Pretoria: Department of Health

Dowdall TL (1991). Repression, health care and ethics under apartheid. *Journal of Medical Ethics*. Available at: http://www.ncbi.nlm.nih.gov/pmc/articles/PMC1378176/pdf/jmedeth00280-0053.pdf (Accessed 11 February 2013)

Fulford KWM, Thornton T, Graham G (2006). *Oxford Textbook of Philosophy and Psychiatry*. Oxford: Oxford University Press

Health Profession Council of South Africa (*s.d.*) *Professional Conduct and Ethics*. Available at: http://www.hpcsa.co.za/Conduct/Ethics (Accessed 15 July 2014.)

Jenkins T, Mclean GR (2004) The Steve Biko affair. *The Lancet* Available at: http://hmb.utoronto.ca/HMB303H/Case_Studies/USA-Torture/The_Biko_Affair.pdf (Accessed 11 February 2013)

Kaliski S (2006) *Psycholegal assessment in South Africa.* Cape Town: Oxford University Press

Medical Protection Society (2012) *Living wills/advanced directives.* Available at: http://www.medicalprotection.org/southafrica/factsheets/living-wills-advance-directives (Accessed 15 July 2014)

Patel V (2007) Mental health in low- and middle-income countries. *British Medical Bulletin* 1–16

United Nations (2006) Convention on the Rights of Persons with Disabilities, 13 December 2006. Available at: https://treaties.un.org/Pages/ViewDetails.aspx?src=IND&mtdsg_no=IV-15&chapter=4&lang=en (Accessed 15 July 2014.)

World Medical Association (1964) Declaration of Helsinki. Available at: http://www.wma.net/en/30publications/10policies/b3/index.html (Accessed on 12 March 2015)

# PART 6

## Management of psychiatric disorders

# CHAPTER 36 Pharmacological and other treatments in psychiatry

Gian Lippi, Liezl Koen, Ilse du Plessis

## 36.1 Introduction

Psychopharmacology remains an area of active research and development. Psychotropic medications are effective but should not be used in isolation, but always in conjunction with psychosocial interventions. Treatment failure can be related to many causes including incorrect diagnoses, inadequate prescriber knowledge and non-adherence. To optimise outcomes, prescribers should avail themselves of best current evidence, while also keeping patients informed and actively engaging them in their treatment plan.

The modern treatment era in psychiatry began with the introduction of effective psychotropic medication in the early 1950s, revolutionising the practice of the discipline. This chapter aims to provide an overview of biological treatments currently available for the management of psychiatric disorders.

### 36.1.1 Basic principles for use

Psychotropic medications are often classified according to their clinical use as detailed in this chapter. However, it is important to remember that a medication in one group often has uses in others as well. For example, fluoxetine (an antidepressant) is often used to treat anxiety disorders. The general principles for prescribing and discontinuing psychotropic medications are outlined in Tables 36.1 and 36.2. It is also important to note that **off-label prescription** of psychotropic medications commonly occur worldwide. When partaking in this practice clinicians should familiarise themselves with the evidence base, where possible include clients in decision-making and carefully consider potential risks and benefits (Sadock BJ and Sadock VA, 2007; Taylor *et al.*, 2012).

### 36.1.2 Special considerations

Best practice for clinicians includes prescribing treatments within their scope of expertise. Patients who have dual diagnoses or are treatment-resistant often need to be referred to higher levels of care. Other populations of special consideration include children and the elderly, pregnant and breastfeeding women (see Table 36.3 for general principles) as well as individuals with co-morbid medical conditions (e.g. porphyria). Some of these situations will be discussed here but others are only mentioned as a detailed discussion thereof falls outside the scope of this chapter.

## 36.2 Antipsychotics

### 36.2.1 Classification

There are different classes of antipsychotic medications, each differing in molecular structure, but having equal efficacy (Taylor *et al.*, 2012). However, their potencies and side-effect profiles differ. Antipsychotics are generally subdivided into two types: classical/typical/first-generation and atypical/second-generation (see Table 36.4).

### 36.2.2 Indications for use

Antipsychotics are primarily used to treat psychotic disturbances (such as schizophrenia), bipolar disorder and other serious, disruptive

**Table 36.1** General principles for prescribing psychotropic drugs

- Establish the psychiatric diagnosis.
- Establish medical co-morbidities, including pregnancy and prescribed medications.
- Consider the patient's age.
- Formulate a specific treatment plan identifying target symptoms to be monitored.
- Avoid polypharmacy if at all possible.
- Educate the patient about the medication, particularly its side effects.
- Use therapeutic dosages for a sufficient time period.
- Consider a gradual dosage increase to minimise side effects.
- Keep the dosage schedule simple as this increases the likelihood of adherence.
- Monitor drug interactions and unwanted effects.
- Arrange for the administration of the medication to be supervised if necessary.
- Monitor suicide risk and prescribe the minimum amount of medication to reduce the risk of serious complications in the event of an overdose.
- Limit use of potentially habit-forming drugs and use for limited periods (two to four weeks).
- Document all observations and reported effects carefully.

**Source:** Author's own Table

**Table 36.2** Basic principles for discontinuing psychotropic drugs[1]

- Identify a good reason for discontinuation:
  - appropriate period of remission; ongoing prophylaxis unnecessary
  - used for a sufficient time period at adequate dosage, but ineffective
  - relapse despite compliance and a further dose increase is not feasible
  - side effects unmanageable
  - drug interactions or a medical condition makes further use unacceptable
  - abuse of the medication
  - inappropriate polypharmacy is present
  - patient requests discontinuation.
- Optimise level of functioning prior to discontinuation.
- Choose an appropriate moment i.e., not during a period of new/increased stress
- Lower the dosage gradually. This could be over days/weeks/months depending on:
  - type of medication
  - duration of treatment
  - psychiatric diagnosis
  - patient factors (e.g. follow up intervals, motivation for co-operation)
  - inform the patient of possible withdrawal effects when discontinuing medications.
- Do regular follow-ups to monitor for signs/symptoms of early relapse.
- In case of relapse, restart the medication and increase to therapeutic dosages.
- Document all observations and reported effects carefully.

[1] These principles do not pertain to emergencies.

**Source:** Author's own Table

**Table 36.3** General principles for prescribing during pregnancy and breastfeeding

- Always discuss the possibility of pregnancy with all women of childbearing age
- In all pregnancies:
  - involve parents in all decision-making as far as possible
  - avoid medications if possible, but especially polypharmacy
  - use established medications at lowest effective dosage
  - adjust dosages as pregnancy progresses and medication handling is altered
  - ensure adequate foetal management including possible withdrawal effects after birth
  - work in conjunction with an obstetric team
  - document all decisions.
- First trimester:
  - optimise non-drug treatments; try to avoid all medications
  - where benefits outweigh risks use established medications at lowest effective dosage.
- Planning a pregnancy:
  - consider discontinuation if well and at low risk of relapse
  - if there is a high risk of relapse consider switching to medication with established safety in pregnancy at lowest effective dosage.
- Discovering pregnancy:
  - abrupt discontinuation in high-risk patients is not recommended
  - consider evidence for remaining with current medication versus switching.
- Breast feeding:
  - weigh benefits of breast feeding need against risk of drug exposure for infant
  - withholding treatment to continue breast feeding in high risk patients is not recommended
  - monitor infant for possible adverse effects.

**Source:** Adapted from Taylor *et al.*, 2012. This material is reproduced with permission from John Wiley and Sons Inc.

conditions. However, these medications are also commonly prescribed for a number of other indications with the evidence base differing greatly between individual agents. These indications include, but are not limited to, major neurocognitive disorder (MND) (especially behavioural symptoms), augmentation in major depressive disorder (MDD) and obsessive-compulsive disorder (OCD), generalised anxiety disorder (GAD) and tic disorders. All of these medications have significant side-effect profiles; the use of single agents at the lowest possible dose is always recommended (Taylor *et al.*, 2012; Stahl, 2008).

When choosing which agent to use many factors should be considered (e.g. patient profile, side-effect profile of agent, previous agents used, cost, patient preference). If adherence is likely to be an ongoing problem a depot preparation should be given serious consideration. When switching between two antipsychotics the following general principles apply:

- don't rush discontinuation
- no gaps between the two
- do not start the second agent at a full dose (Taylor *et al.*, 2012; Hasan *et al.*, 2012).

To date, only clozapine has been shown to have superior efficacy in treatment-resistant schizophrenia (Hasan *et al.*, 2013). However, clinicians who use clozapine must first familiarise themselves with this agent due to its dosing regime and side-effect profile (see Table 36.5).

**Table 36.4** Classification of antipsychotics and their suggested target dose ranges

| Medications | Daily dose range |
|---|---|
| **First-generation** | |
| haloperidol | 0,5–15 mg |
| chlorpromazine | 200–800 mg |
| trifluoperazine | 2–15 mg |
| zuclopenthixol decanoate | 2–40 mg |
| flupentixol dihydrochloride | 2–20 mg |
| pimozide | 1–12 mg |
| **Second-generation** | |
| risperidone | 1–8 mg |
| paliperidone | 3–12 mg |
| olanzapine | 5–20 mg |
| quetiapine | 300–800 mg |
| amisulpride | 100–800 mg |
| sulpiride | 200–800 mg |
| ziprasidone | 40–160 mg |
| aripiprazole | 10–30 mg |
| clozapine | 100–800 mg |
| **Depot preparations/long-acting injections** | |
| fluphenazine | 12,5–50 mg/month |
| flupentixol decanoate | 10–60 mg/month |
| zuclopenthixol decanoate | 100–400 mg/month |
| risperidone microspheres (2nd generation) | 25–50 mg/2 weeks |
| **Acute onset intramuscular preparations** | |
| haloperidol | 5–10 mg/2–4h (max 40 mg/24h) |
| olanzapine (not with benzodiazepines) | 10 mg/2–4h (max 30 mg/24h) |
| ziprasidone | 10mg-20 mg/4h (max 40mg/24h) |
| zuclopenthixol acetate | 50–150 mg/72h (max 400 mg over 2 weeks) |

**Source:** Author's own Table

**Table 36.5** Guidelines to follow when using clozapine

- Indicated in treatment-resistant schizophrenia, intolerable extrapyramidal side effects or tardive dyskinesia.
- Starting dose is 12,5/25 mg, titrating up by 25 mg every 2–3 days only.
- Life-threatening side effects include myocarditis, toxic megacolon, seizures at high doses, metabolic syndrome and agranulocytosis.
- Agranulocytosis is rare (<1%) but due to risk, do three white blood cell counts before starting treatment, then weekly for 18 weeks, then monthly (monitor for, and warn patient about, early signs of infection).
- Other common side effects include hypersalivation, weight gain and sedation.
- If agranulocytosis does occur, clozapine must be stopped and never again be reintroduced.

**Source:** Author's own Table

## 36.2.3 Mode of action

First-generation antipsychotics primarily work by blocking dopamine 2 receptors in the meso-limbic and meso-cortical pathways in the brain, with extrapyramidal symptoms resulting from a concurrent blockade of the nigro-striatal pathway. According to their affinity to the D2 receptors, the agents are further divided into high-potency and low-potency groups. Second-generation antipsychotics work by blocking both dopamine (DA) and serotonin (5-HT) receptors, but broadly exhibit a lower affinity for D2 and therefore have less extrapyramidal side effects (Stahl, 2008).

## 36.2.4 Side effects

In all cases, the management of undesirable side effects is to review, and if possible, reduce, the dose of the antipsychotic. Where this is not possible, the patient must be switched to another agent or a specific treatment for the side effect must be introduced.

Whilst the first-generation agents are particularly likely to cause movement disorders, the second-generation agents are prone to cause metabolic disturbances such as weight gain, diabetes mellitus and dyslipidaemia. Other important (although sometimes rare) side effects include hyperprolactinaemia, anticholinergic effects, QT prolongation, seizures, agranulocytosis and an immediately life-threatening condition, neuroleptic malignant syndrome (Taylor *et al.*, 2012; Stahl, 2008).

The following neuroleptic-induced movement disorders can occur:

### 36.2.4.1 Neuroleptic-induced acute dystonia

Neuroleptic-induced acute dystonia usually develops within a few days of starting or raising the dosage of a first-generation antipsychotic. Dystonia is a prolonged contraction of the muscles of the neck, mouth, tongue or, occasionally, other muscle groups that is subjectively distressing and often painful. Acute dystonia usually responds dramatically to a parenteral anticholinergic drug, e.g. biperidine 2–4 mg IV or IM. After dystonia resolves, a course of oral anticholinergics (e.g. biperidine 2 mg three times per day) will usually prevent recurrences. Patients with a history of dystonic reactions should be given prophylactic anticholinergics when starting on antipsychotics (Hasan *et al.*, 2013).

### 36.2.4.2 Neuroleptic-induced parkinsonism

Neuroleptic-induced parkinsonism comprises the parkinsonian triad of tremor, rigidity and akinesia/bradykinesia. It usually starts a few weeks after the patient begins treatment with high-potency antipsychotics, or after an increase in dosage (Hasan *et al.*, 2013). Treatment includes:

- an anticholinergic drug, e.g. orphenadrine 50 mg two or three times per day
- decreasing the neuroleptic drug dosage (especially in the case of high dosages)
- the neuroleptic drug may be replaced with one that is less likely to cause a movement disorder (e.g. a second-generation antipsychotic).

### 36.2.4.3 Akathisia

Akathisia does not appear immediately, but typically has an onset in the first few weeks of treatment with dopamine-blocking neuroleptics. This condition consists of subjective complaints of anxiety and tension and objective fidgetiness and agitation. Patients report that they feel compelled to pace, move around in their chairs, or tap their feet.

Treatment is similar to neuroleptic-induced parkinsonism. Benzodiazepines or beta blockers may also be of use (e.g. propranolol 30 mg three times per day) (Hasan *et al.*, 2013).

### 36.2.4.4 Neuroleptic-induced tardive dyskinesia

Tardive dyskinesia consists of abnormal involuntary movements, usually of the mouth and tongue (oro-bucco-lingual), although other parts of the body may become involved, including the trunk and extremities. In most patients, the movements are mild and tolerable; some patients develop a more malignant form of the disorder that may be disabling. It is often irreversible. As it is less likely to occur with the second-generation antipsychotics, the most effective treatment strategy is prevention. If intervention is necessary, decrease the dose of the neuroleptic, replace it with clozapine or stop it altogether (Taylor *et al.*, 2012; Hasan *et al.*, 2013).

### 36.2.4.5 Neuroleptic malignant syndrome

Neuroleptic malignant syndrome (NMS) is a potentially life-threatening syndrome characterised by rigidity, high fever, delirium, and marked autonomic instability. There are no pathognomonic laboratory abnormalities, although elevations of creatinine phosphokinase and liver enzymes are common. It usually starts one week after the patient begins neuroleptic treatment, or after increasing the dosage (in which case it may take longer to develop) (Tural and Önder, 2010) . (See Table 36.6 for treatment principles).

**Table 36.6** Management of neuroleptic malignant syndrome

- Upon clinical suspicion of neuroleptic malignant syndrome immediately stop all antipsychotic treatment
- Ideally the patient should be managed in a medical ward
- The diagnosis should be verified – exclude other serious neurological or medical conditions
- Supportive management, including cooling and monitoring of hydration, is essential
- Muscle rigidity may be relieved by a short course of a benzodiazepine such as diazepam – avoid anticholinergic agents which may exacerbate delirium
- Other treatment options such as dantrolene sodium and bromocriptine methylsate should only be used in consultation with a physician and when all other treatment measures have failed

**Source:** Author's own Table

Side effects of the antipsychotics other than movement disorders include the following:

### 36.2.4.6 Anticholinergic side effects

Anticholinergic side effects are particularly associated with compounds such as chlorpromazine, and include dry mouth, urinary retention, blurred vision, constipation and exacerbation of narrow-angle glaucoma. They can be treated by reducing the dose of medication or switching to a different agent. Anticholinergic drugs can exacerbate these side effects (Hasan *et al.*, 2013).

### 36.2.4.7 Metabolic side effects

Metabolic side effects include weight gain, dyslipidemia, and hyperglycaemia and are mostly associated with second-generation antipsychotics. These adverse effects are all risk factors for cardiovascular disease; in combination with hypertension, they form part of the conditions that are grouped together to make the diagnosis of metabolic syndrome.

It is recommended that, in addition to lifestyle interventions, patients are screened for the above parameters prior to initiating treatment and at regular intervals whilst on treatment in order to pro-actively manage the morbidity and mortality risk associated with these conditions (Taylor *et al.*, 2012; Hasan *et al.*, 2013).

### 36.2.4.8 Seizures

Seizures may be induced by low-potency drugs, especially at higher doses, or where dose titrations are too fast (e.g. increases of more than 400 mg chlorpromazine per day). Antipsychotics are not contraindicated in epileptic patients, as long as they are adequately treated with anticonvulsants (Taylor *et al.*, 2012).

### 36.2.4.9 Haematological effects

Agranulocytosis is a rare side effect associated with the use of low-potency antipsychotics. The incidence peaks during the first two months of treatment. Be alert to the possible appearance of malaise, fever or sore throat early in the course of therapy. Routine full blood counts are usually not necessary (Taylor *et al.*, 2012). An exception is clozapine (see Table 36.5).

### 36.2.4.10 Miscellaneous side effects

Sedation, non-specific skin rashes, retinitis pigmentosa, fever, pigmentary changes in the skin, postural hypotension, cholestatic jaundice, reduced libido, and inhibition of ejaculation can occur secondary to antipsychotic treatment (Taylor *et al.*, 2012).

Antipsychotics appear to be safe during pregnancy, but as a general rule, avoid them if the risks outweigh the benefits of treatment. Use high-potency antipsychotics at the lowest possible dose during pregnancy.

In order to pro-actively manage the side effects of antipsychotics, the clinician must continuously monitor for them and also know which side effects are more likely with which agent (see Table 36.7).

## 36.3 Antidepressants

Antidepressants are the most commonly prescribed class of medications in psychiatry. Although, as the name suggests, they are frequently prescribed for their antidepressant effects, these medications are used in the treatment of a wide range of psychiatric disorders. No class of antidepressant medication has consistently been shown to have superior antidepressant effect compared to another for the treatment of MDD. The choice of antidepressant prescribed should be according to individual patient needs.

**Table 36.7** Comparison of relative adverse effects of antipsychotic agents

| Medication | Sedation | Weight gain | Diabetes | Extra-pyramidal symptoms | Anticholinergic | Hypotension | Prolactin elevation |
|---|---|---|---|---|---|---|---|
| amisulpride | - | + | + | = | - | - | +++ |
| aripiprazole | - | +/- | - | +/- | - | - | - |
| chlorpromazine | +++ | ++ | ++ | ++ | ++ | +++ | +++ |
| clozapine | +++ | +++ | +++ | - | +++ | +++ | - |
| flupentixol | + | ++ | + | ++ | ++ | + | +++ |
| fluphenazine | + | + | + | +++ | ++ | + | +++ |
| haloperidol | + | + | +/- | +++ | + | + | +++ |
| olanzapine | ++ | +++ | +++ | +/- | + | + | + |
| paliperidone | + | ++ | + | + | + | ++ | +++ |
| perphenazine | + | + | +/- | +++ | + | + | +++ |
| pimozide | + | + | - | + | + | + | +++ |
| quetiapine | ++ | ++ | ++ | - | + | ++ | - |
| risperidone | + | ++ | + | + | + | ++ | +++ |
| sulpiride | - | + | + | + | - | - | +++ |
| trifluoperazine | + | + | +/- | +++ | +/- | + | +++ |
| ziprasidone | + | +/- | - | +/- | - | + | +/- |
| zuclopenthixol | ++ | ++ | + | ++ | ++ | + | +++ |

+++ high incidence/severity; ++ moderate; + low; -very low

Note: the table is made up of approximate estimates of relative incidence and/or severity, based on clinical experience, manufacturers' literature and published research. This is a rough guide.

**Source:** Adapted from Taylor *et al.*, 2012. This material is reproduced with permission from John Wiley and Sons Inc.

To discontinue or switch antidepressants, the dose of the antidepressant should be decreased slowly before it is stopped or switched to another antidepressant to prevent discontinuation syndromes which occur more frequently with certain classes of antidepressants.

## 36.3.1 Classification

Generally, antidepressants are classified according to their individual mode of action, although some of the first antidepressants are still classified according to their molecular structure.

## 36.3.2 Pharmacokinetics

Antidepressants are metabolised in the liver by the cytochrome P450 (CYP 450) system. Many antidepressants, especially selective serotonin reuptake inhibitors (SSRIs), are potent inhibitors of multiple CYP 450 enzymes and can therefore cause clinically significant drug interactions resulting in increased levels of anything from theophylline to clozapine. Similarly, serum levels of SSRIs can be increased by the co-administration of protease inhibitors in HIV positive patients. Clinicians should familiarise themselves with these potential drug interactions before prescribing antidepressants (Taylor *et al.*, 2012).

## 36.3.3 Mode of action

All antidepressants commonly cause an antidepressant effect by reversing both the down-regulation of synaptic receptors due to hypercortisolaemia caused by an over-activity of the hypothalamic-pituitary-adrenal axis (HPA axis) found in depressive states and by increasing the sensitivity of these receptors to specific neurotransmitters in monoaminergic neurons found in neural circuits involving the medial prefrontal cortex, medial and caudolateral orbital cortex, the amygdala, hippocampus and ventromedial parts of the basal ganglia. Antidepressants also promote dendritic regrowth in neurons that have undergone atrophy in the synaptic areas secondary to depressive states. Neuronal regrowth is increased in these areas secondary to increased protein synthesis stimulated by higher levels of neurotrophic factors such as neuregulin and brain derived neurotrophic factor (BDNF) that occur when the hypercortisolaemia is reversed.

Finally, synaptic availability of individual monoaminergic neurotransmitters is increased by different classes of antidepressants through differing, unique modes of action, which are discussed below.

## 36.3.4 Selective serotonin reuptake inhibitors (SSRIs)

SSRIs have become the first-line treatment option for MDD. They have a more tolerable side-effect profile compared with older antidepressants like the tricyclic antidepressants (TCAs) and monoamine oxidase inhibitors (MAOIs) and are safer than these medications when taken as an overdose in a suicide attempt (Sadock BJ and Sadock VA, 2007).

As the name of their class suggests, these medications selectively increase the synaptic availability of 5-HT through blocking of the 5-HT transporter enzyme, thus inhibiting its presynaptic reuptake (Stahl, 2008).

SSRIs are prescribed for the treatment of a wide range of psychiatric disorders or for symptoms of certain disorders, either as monotherapy or as adjunctive treatment (see Table 36.8).

Prescribed dosages of SSRIs differ according to the disorder for which they are prescribed – initial dosages for the treatment of anxiety disorders are low, while high dosages may be required for effective treatment of OCD or bulimia nervosa. Dose ranges and most common side effects of SSRIs are summarised in Table 36.9 and Table 36.10 respectively.

**Table 36.8** Indications for use of SSRIs

| Licensed indications | Other indications |
|---|---|
| ▶ MDD<br>▶ panic disorder<br>▶ social anxiety disorder (social phobia)<br>▶ GAD<br>▶ OCD<br>▶ post-traumatic stress disorder<br>▶ bulimia nervosa | ▶ amphetamine-induced depressive disorder<br>▶ depressive disorder due to another medical condition<br>▶ persistent depressive disorder (dysthymia)<br>▶ other specified depressive disorder<br>– recurrent brief depression<br>– premenstrual dysphoric disorder<br>– bipolar disorders (depressive phase)<br>– schizoaffective disorder (bipolar and depressed types)<br>– anxiety disorder due to another medical condition<br>– separation anxiety disorder<br>– body dysmorphic disorder (BDD)<br>– somatic symptom disorder with predominant pain<br>– depersonalisation/derealisation disorder<br>– premature (early) ejaculation<br>– paraphilic disorders<br>– other specified sexual dysfunctions<br>– hypersomnolence disorder<br>– intermittent explosive disorder<br>– kleptomania<br>– gambling disorder<br>– trichotillomania (hair-pulling disorder)<br>– others specified disruptive, impulse control, and conduct disorders<br>– schizoid personality disorder<br>– schizotypal personality disorder<br>– borderline personality disorder<br>– narcissistic personality disorder<br>– avoidant personality disorder<br>– dependent personality disorder<br>– obsessive-compulsive personality disorder<br>– other specified personality disorders<br>– personality change due to another medical condition<br>– tic disorders<br>– autism spectrum disorder |

**Source:** Authors' own Table

## 36.3.5 Tricyclic and tetracyclic antidepressants

As the original antidepressants, TCAs have been replaced by SSRIs as first-line antidepressants. This is due to the less tolerable side effects of the TCAs (most notably the anticholinergic and antimuscarinic side effects) and their potential to cause lethal arrhythmias when taken in overdose (although tetracyclic antidepressants are slightly safer in overdose compared to their tricyclic cousins).

**Table 36.9** Dose range of SSRIs

| | |
|---|---|
| ▸ fluoxetine | 10–80 mg |
| ▸ paroxetine | 10–60 mg |
| ▸ citalopram | 10–40 mg |
| ▸ escitalopram | 5–20 mg |
| ▸ sertraline | 25–200 mg |
| ▸ fluvoxamine | 50–300 mg |

**Source:** Author's own Table

**Table 36.10** Side effects of SSRIs

- nausea and vomiting
- dyspepsia
- diarrhoea
- abdominal pain
- headache
- agitation and anxiety
- sexual dysfunction
- insomnia
- rash
- sweating
- tremor
- hyponatraemia
- cutaneous bleeding

**Source:** Author's own Table

As a class, the TCAs do have effective antidepressant action. They are not receptor specific – all the TCAs increase the synaptic availability of noradrenalin (NA) through blocking of the noradrenalin transporter enzyme, thus inhibiting its presynaptic reuptake, whilst some of them also inhibit 5-HT reuptake by the same method. Their lack of specificity in receptor occupation results in many of their side effects as they are also antagonists at receptors such as the muscarinic and histaminergic types (Stahl, 2008; Sadock BJ and Sadock VA, 2007).

Mianserin is listed under the tetracyclic antidepressants due to its structure. It can also be classified according to its mode of action which most resembles that of mirtazapine (see NaSSAs in Section 36.3.10).

For more detailed information about the TCAs, refer to Table 36.12

## 36.3.6 Monoamine oxidase inhibitors (MAOIs) and reversible inhibitors of monoamine oxidase A (RIMAs)

Both MAOIs and reversible inhibitors of monoamine oxidase A (RIMAs) inhibit the function of monoamine oxidase A by binding **covalently** to this enzyme. Monoamine oxidase enzymes (A and B) metabolise synaptic DA, NA and 5-HT. Inhibition of the enzymes therefore increases the synaptic availability of the three monoaminergic neurotransmitters by decreasing their breakdown.

MAOIs bind irreversibly to monoamine oxidase enzymes, effectively deactivating the enzymes for the duration of their lifespan. Enzyme activity returns with the synthesis of new enzymes. RIMAs not only selectively inhibit monoamine oxidase A, but bind reversibly to the enzyme, making them safer medications to use (see the discussion on tyramine-induced hypertensive crisis below (Stahl, 2008; Sadock BJ and Sadock VA, 2007)).

Tyramine is an amino acid ingested as part of our diets. It is metabolised in the gastrointestinal tract by both monoamine oxidase enzymes. In unmetabolized form it is a potent releaser of NA, which causes elevation of blood pressure through vasoconstriction due to stimulation of $\alpha_1$ and other adrenergic receptors. Normally the NA levels don't rise sufficiently to cause this effect because it is broken down monoamine oxidase A. However, if the function of monoamine oxidase is inhibited by a monoamine oxidase inhibitor, NA accumulates, blood pressure rises and this can result in a tyramine-induced hypertensive crisis (Stahl, 2008).

Patients on MAOIs should therefore receive psycho-education about the importance of sticking to a low-tyramine diet (Stahl, 2008; Sadock BJ and Sadock VA, 2007). For a list of foods containing moderate to high levels of tyramine refer to Table 36.11.

For more information about the MAOIs and RIMAs, refer to Table 36.12.

**Table 36.11** Foods to be avoided when on a MAOI due to their tyramine contents

| Foods with a high tyramine content | Foods with a moderate tyramine content |
|---|---|
| **Cheese:**<br>▶ English stilton<br>▶ Danish blue<br>▶ mozzarella<br>▶ cheese spreads<br>▶ old cheddar and 3 year old white<br>**Meat and fish:**<br>▶ salami<br>▶ mortadella<br>▶ air-dried sausage ('droëwors')<br>▶ aged meats (biltong)<br>**Alcoholic drinks:**<br>▶ liqueurs<br>▶ fortified wines<br>**Other:**<br>▶ Marmite<br>▶ sauerkraut | **Cheese:**<br>▶ Swiss gruyère<br>▶ muenster<br>▶ feta<br>▶ parmesan<br>▶ gorgonzola<br>▶ blue cheese dressing<br>▶ black diamond<br>**Meat and fish:**<br>▶ chicken livers<br>▶ bologna<br>▶ aged sausages<br>▶ smoked meat<br>▶ salmon mousse<br>**Alcoholic drinks:**<br>▶ beer<br>▶ Rioja-type red wine |

**Source:** Adapted from Sadock BJ and Sadock VA, 2007; Himmelhoch JM, *s.d.*

## 36.3.7 Serotonin and noradrenalin reuptake inhibitors (SNRIs)

Serotonin and noradrenalin reuptake inhibitors (SNRIs) selectively increase the synaptic availability of both 5-HT and NA through blocking of both the 5-HT transporter enzyme and the NA transporter enzyme, thus inhibiting the presynaptic reuptake of both these neurotransmitters (Stahl, 2008; Sadock BJ and Sadock VA, 2007).

For more information about the SNRIs, refer to Table 36.13.

## 36.3.8 Selective noradrenalin reuptake inhibitors (NRIs)

Selective noradrenalin reuptake inhibitors (NRIs), also referred to in the literature as NaRIs, selectively increase the synaptic availability of NA through blocking of the NA transporter enzyme, thus inhibiting its presynaptic reuptake. They essentially work just like the SSRIs but selectively on NA and not 5-HT (Stahl, 2008; Sadock BJ and Sadock VA, 2007).

For more information about the NRIs, refer to Table 36.13.

## 36.3.9 Noradrenalin dopamine reuptake inhibitors (NDRIs)

Bupropion, the only medication in this class, selectively increases the synaptic availability of both NA and DA through blocking of both the NA transporter enzyme and the DA transporter enzyme, thus inhibiting the presynaptic reuptake of both these neurotransmitters. This medication has only weak blocking properties of the NA and DA enzyme but is metabolised to a number of active metabolites, some of which are more potent NA transporter blockers (Stahl, 2008).

For more information about the NDRIs, refer to Table 36.13.

**Table 36.12** Indications, side effects and dose ranges of TCAs, MAOIs and RIMAs

| Class/Medication | Daily dose range | Indications (licensed indications in bold print) | Most common side effects |
|---|---|---|---|
| **TCAs (tricyclics)** | | | |
| ▶ amitriptyline | 50–200 mg | **MDD** | dry mouth |
| ▶ clomipramine | 30–250 mg | **OCD** | constipation |
| ▶ imipramine | 50–200 mg | **narcolepsy with cataplexy (clomipramine)** | urinary retention |
| ▶ trimipramine | 50–300 mg | **enuresis** | blurred vision |
| ▶ lofepramine | 140–210 mg | somatic symptom disorder with predominant pain | tachycardia |
| ▶ dothiepin | 75–225 mg | PTSD | conduction abnormalities |
| **TCAs (tetracyclics)** | | panic disorder (clomipramine) | orthostatic hypotension |
| ▶ maprotiline | 25–150 mg | nightmare disorder | sedation |
| ▶ mianserin | 10–90 mg | intermittent explosive disorder | tremor |
| | | kleptomania | myoclonic jerks |
| | | gambling disorder (clomipramine) | rash |
| | | trichotillomania (hair pulling disorder) (clomipramine) | weight gain |
| **MAOIs** | | | |
| ▶ tranylcypromine | 10–30 mg | **MDD** | postural hypotension |
| | | **social anxiety disorder (social phobia)** | drowsiness |
| | | persistent depressive disorder (dysthymia) | insomnia |
| | | panic disorder | headaches |
| | | PTSD | oedema |
| | | bulimia nervosa | weight gain |
| | | | sexual dysfunction |
| | | | anxiety |
| | | | anticholinergic side effects |
| | | | hypertensive crisis |
| **RIMAs** | | | |
| ▶ moclobemide | 300–600 mg | | dizziness |
| | | | insomnia |
| | | | nausea |

**Source:** Author's own Table

## 36.3.10 Noradrenergic and specific serotonergic antidepressants (NaSSAs)

Because of its complex mode of action, mirtazapine, the antidepressant in this class, is also classified in the literature as an $\alpha_2$ antagonist or a serotonin and noradrenalin disinhibitor (SNDI). Due to its $\alpha_2$ antagonist properties it is in fact indirectly also a noradrenalin and dopamine disinhibitor (NDDI) (Stahl, 2008).

For more information about the NaSSAs, refer to Table 36.13.

## 36.1 Advanced reading block

### NaSSAs mode of action

The $\alpha_2$ receptor can be found presynaptically on 5-HT and NA neurons. When this receptor is occupied by these respective monoamine neurotransmitters, there is an activation of what is equivalent to a negative feedback mechanism. Occupation of $\alpha_2$ receptors causes inhibition of the presynaptic release of 5-HT and NA. When synaptic availability of these neurotransmitters is high or increased, more $\alpha_2$ receptors are occupied, resulting in less neurotransmitter being released through inhibition. When an $\alpha_2$ antagonist (such as mirtazapine) occupies the receptor, the negative feedback is blocked – there is no resultant inhibition of presynaptic neurotransmitter release despite adequate synaptic neurotransmitter availability, resulting in continued neurotransmitter release and subsequent increased synaptic neurotransmitter availability. This blocking of the inhibitory pathway causes what is essentially a disinhibitory effect – hence the term disinhibitor and the classification as a SNDI. Other psychotropic medications with this $\alpha_2$ antagonist action include the antidepressant mianserin and the second-generation antipsychotics clozapine, risperidone, paliperidone and quetiapine.

A second mechanism of action of mirtazapine is its increased postsynaptic release of 5-HT via $\alpha_1$ receptors. NA neurons from the locus coeruleus innervate 5-HT neurons in the midbrain raphe. The increased NA availability caused by the $\alpha_2$ antagonism causes enhanced 5-HT release via the $\alpha_1$ receptors further increasing synaptic 5-HT availability.

Finally, mirtazapine is also an antagonist at specific 5-HT receptors, namely 5-$HT_{2A}$, 5-$HT_{2C}$ and 5-$HT_3$, hence the term specific serotonin antidepressant and the classification as a NaSSA. The 5-$HT_{2A}$ and 5-$HT_{2C}$ antagonism of mirtazapine causes an indirect increase in NA and DA release and therefore also availability in the prefrontal cortex through a complex disinhibitory action similar to that of the $\alpha_2$ antagonist action – thus the term NDDI.

**Table 36.13** Indications, side effects and dose ranges of SNRIs, NRIs, NDRIs and NaSSAs

| Class/Medication | Daily dose range | Indications (licensed indications in bold print) | Most common side effects |
|---|---|---|---|
| **SNRIs**<br>▶ venlafaxine<br>▶ duloxetine | <br>37.5–375 mg<br>30–120 mg | **MDD**<br>**social anxiety disorder (social phobia) (venlafaxine)**<br>**panic disorder (venlafaxine)**<br>persistant depressive disorder (dysthymia)<br>GAD<br>attention-deficit hyperactivity disorder (venlafaxine)<br>OCD (venlafaxine)<br>intermittent explosive disorder (venlafaxine)<br>trichotillomania (hair pulling disorder) (venlafaxine) | nausea<br>anorexia<br>constipation<br>blurred vision<br>dry mouth<br>sedation<br>dizziness<br>hypertension<br>anxiety<br>sweating<br>erectile dysfunction |

| Class/Medication | Daily dose range | Indications (licensed indications in bold print) | Most common side effects |
|---|---|---|---|
| **NRIs**<br>▶ reboxetine | 4–12 mg | **MDD** | nausea<br>dry mouth<br>constipation<br>insomnia<br>sedation<br>dizziness<br>tachycardia<br>sweating<br>headache<br>urinary hesitancy |
| **NDRIs**<br>▶ bupropion | 150–300 mg | **MDD**<br>persistant depressive disorder (dysthymia)<br>tobacco-use disorder<br>attention-deficit hyperactivity disorder (ADHD)<br>male hypoactive sexual desire disorder | headache<br>insomnia<br>dry mouth<br>tremor<br>nausea |
| **NaSSAs**<br>▶ mirtazapine | 7.5–45 mg | **MDD**<br>GAD<br>panic disorder<br>social anxiety disorder (social phobia) | sedation<br>increased appetite<br>weight gain<br>dry mouth<br>constipation<br>dizziness<br>headache<br>oedema<br>blood dyscrasia |

**Source:** Author's own Table

## 36.3.11 Serotonin antagonist/reuptake inhibitors (SARIs)

SARIs are 5-$HT_{2A}$ and 5-$HT_{2C}$ antagonists that cause an indirect increase in NA and DA release and therefore also availability in the prefrontal cortex, just like mirtazapine. They also selectively increase the synaptic availability of 5-HT through blocking of the 5-HT transporter enzyme, thus inhibiting its presynaptic reuptake just like the SSRIs (Stahl, 2008).

For more information about the SARIs, refer to Table 36.14.

## 36.3.12 Melatonin agonists

Agomelatine is an agonist at the $MT_1$ and $MT_2$ melatonin receptors (which accounts for its sedating and sleep promoting properties) and an antagonist at the 5-$HT_{2C}$ receptors (thus causing an indirect increase in NA and DA release and therefore also availability in the prefrontal

**Table 36.14** Indications, side effects and dose ranges SARIs and melatonin agonists

| Class/Medication | Daily dose range | Indications (licensed indications in bold print) | Most common side effects |
|---|---|---|---|
| **SARIs** | | | |
| ▸ trazodone | 75–600 mg | **MDD**<br>GAD<br>panic disorder<br>social anxiety disorder (social phobia)<br>insomnia disorder<br>erectile disorder<br>bulimia nervosa<br>intermittent explosive disorder<br>kleptomania<br>trichotillomania (hair-pulling disorder) | sedation<br>dizziness<br>postural hypotension<br>tachycardia<br>headache<br>nausea and vomiting<br>priapism |
| **Melatonin agonists** | | | |
| ▸ agomelatine | 25–50 mg | **MDD** | sedation<br>dizziness<br>headache<br>migraine<br>nausea<br>elevated liver enzymes |

**Source:** Author's own Table

cortex). Its antidepressant effect is hypothesised to be attributable to both these mechanisms of action (Sadock BJ and Sadock VA, 2007).

For more information about the melatonin agonists, refer to Table 36.14.

# 36.4 Mood stabilisers

The term 'mood stabiliser' is used by psychiatrists to refer to a medication that stabilises the different phases of bipolar disorders. Included in this class of medications are lithium, anticonvulsants and antipsychotics. To be a foundational mood stabiliser a medication must be proven to stabilise acute manic symptoms, help in the management of depressive symptoms and to help prevent future relapses into mania or depression (Bauer *et al.*, 2012).

## 36.4.1 Lithium

Lithium (see Table 36.15) has been used in the treatment of bipolar disorders for more than 50 years. It is still the closest we get to an ideal mood stabiliser due to its effect in all the phases of bipolar disorder. It is also unique in its ability to prevent suicidality. Unfortunately its side-effect profile limits its use to a narrow spectrum of patients. The mechanism of action of lithium remains elusive, but being an element that the body handles in a similar way to sodium, it seems to alter sodium-dependent intracellular second messenger systems, modulates DA and 5-HT pathways, reduces activity of protein kinase C, reduces turnover of arachidonic acid and via NMDA-pathways and is neuroprotective (Sadock BJ and Sadock VA, 2007).

**Table 36.15** Lithium

| **Indications** |
|---|
| ▶ mood stabiliser: antimanic and antidepressive effects<br>▶ bipolar disorders: acute treatment of mania, prophylaxis for affective episodes<br>▶ MDD: augmentation of an antidepressant<br>▶ anti-aggressive effect<br>▶ antisuicidal effect<br>▶ protective effect in self-mutilation |
| **Dosage** |
| ▶ 20 mg/kg/day. Monitor 5–7 days after dose adjustments until therapeutic levels are achieved |
| **Plasma levels** |
| ▶ maintenance: 0,4–0,8 mmol/L<br>▶ acute episodes: 0,8–1,2 mmol/L |
| **Adverse effects** |
| ▶ dose-related gastrointestinal upset<br>▶ central nervous system (CNS): fine tremor<br>▶ kidneys: polyuria, polydipsia, renal toxicity, interstitial nephritis<br>▶ thyroid abnormalities<br>▶ other: teratogenic, metallic taste in mouth, ankle oedema, weight gain,<br>▶ dermatological problems, hyperparathyroidism, leucocytosis, cardiac conduction changes |
| **Toxicity** |
| ▶ Levels > 1,5 mmol/ℓ<br>– Gastrointestinal symptoms: nausea, diarrhoea, anorexia<br>– CNS: muscle weakness, drowsiness, ataxia, course tremor, muscle twitching, hyperreflexia<br>▶ Levels > 2 mmol/ℓ<br>– CNS: disorientation, seizures, coma, death |
| **Baseline tests** |
| ▶ β-hcg in females (pregnancy) – prescribe contraception if indicated<br>▶ thyroid stimulating hormone (TSH) (thyroid function)<br>▶ glomerular filtration rate (GFR) (kidney function)<br>▶ weight<br>▶ electrocardiogram (ECG) (cardiac function) – if indicated, or in patients above 50 years |
| **On-treatment monitoring** |
| ▶ lithium level three-monthly once on stable dosage<br>▶ thyroid and kidney functions six-monthly<br>▶ regular weight monitoring: do lipogram and serum glucose if there is an increase in weight |
| **Discontinuation** |
| ▶ high risk of relapse<br>▶ less effective with after multiple discontinuations |

| **Drug interactions** |
|---|
| ▶ ACE-inhibitors<br>▶ diuretics<br>▶ non-steroidal anti-inflammatory drugs (NSAIDs)<br>▶ monitor sodium levels if combined with SSRIs/carbamazepine |
| **Contraindications** |
| ▶ cardiac disease, renal impairment, CNS disorders such as epilepsy, pregnancy |
| **Other information** |
| ▶ teratogenic: **Ebstein's anomaly** or neonatal goitre<br>▶ lithium levels must be drawn 12 hours after last dose<br>▶ warn patients about risk of diarrhoea and severe sweating that can cause increased lithium levels due to haemoconcentration |

**Source:** Sadock BJ and Sadock VA, 2007; Taylor *et al.*, 2012

Lithium is unique in being water soluble and thus excreted exclusively through the kidneys. It has a narrow therapeutic index and routine blood sampling for lithium levels is essential. Drug interactions are common through the renal system and patients should be warned regarding symptoms of lithium-toxicity as it can be fatal.

## 36.4.2 Anticonvulsants

### 36.4.2.1 Classification

The anticonvulsants with registration for use in bipolar disorders include valproate, carbamazepine and lamotrigine.

### 36.4.2.2 Mechanism of action

Anticonvulsants are thought to diminish neuronal excitation and enhance inhibition by, among others, blocking low-voltage sodium ion channels, reducing glutamate activity (an excitatory neurotransmitter) and stimulating the effect of γ-aminobutyric acid, or GABA (an inhibitory neurotransmitter). They seem to alter synaptic plasticity by altering extracellular signal-regulated kinase (ERK) and changing intracellular signalling and by promoting BDNF. Apart from their registration for use in the treatment of different types of epilepsy, they are extensively used in psychiatry (Stahl, 2008; Schachter *et al.*, 2012).

### 36.4.2.3 Pharmacokinetics

Some anticonvulsants can cause gastric irritation during absorption and enteric-coated versions or co-administration with food might limit side effects. Most are lipophylic and highly protein-bound. Blood and tissue-levels do not correlate with clinical efficacy. Most anticonvulsants are metabolised in the liver and complex drug interactions are therefore possible (Schachter *et al.*, 2012).

### 36.4.2.4 Valproate

Valproate (see Table 36.16) has been used in the treatment of bipolar disorders, specifically mania, since the mid-1980s. Clinically it is often prescribed for maintenance treatment and to treat target symptoms associated with mood disorders, such as aggression, mood lability and impulsivity. It has been studied specifically in cases where lithium seems to lack efficacy (e.g. in the treatment of rapid cycling) but valproate has not been found to be superior to lithium in this aspect. It does, however, seem to be significantly more helpful in patients with multiple episodes where lithium lacks efficacy and in mixed states. Valproate is often better tolerated than lithium due to its more benign side-effect profile. Valproate is available as a salt, sodium valproate, and valproic acid, which is assumed to be the active component. As valproic acid is

**Table 36.16** Valproate

| **Preparations** |
|---|
| ▶ sodium valproate<br>▶ valproic acid |
| **Indications** |
| ▶ Bipolar disorders:<br>– acute treatment of mania<br>– mixed episodes<br>– rapid cycling<br>– multiple mood episodes, poor response to lithium<br>– prophylaxis of affective episodes.<br>▶ other psychiatric symptoms:<br>– aggression<br>– agitation<br>– impulsivity |
| **Plasma levels** |
| ▶ No evidence for usefulness of routine blood levels in bipolar disorders.<br>▶ To monitor compliance or confirm toxicity. |
| **Dosages** |
| ▶ Initial loading of 20–30 mg/kg/day or 600 mg/day in divided dosages<br>▶ Maximum 60 mg/kg/day |
| **Adverse effects** |
| ▶ Common: sedation, tremor, nausea, hair loss, weight gain<br>▶ Less common: ataxia, vomiting, diarrhoea, dysarthria, persistent elevation of hepatic enzymes, polycystic ovarian syndrome in females, pancreatitis, hepatotoxicity, haematological abnormalities |
| **Toxicity** |
| ▶ hepatotoxicity: lethargy, malaise, anorexia, oedema, abdominal pain, nausea and vomiting |
| **Baseline tests** |
| ▶ liver function test (LFT)<br>▶ full blood count (FBC)<br>▶ weight measurement. |
| **On-treatment monitoring** |
| ▶ LFT after two weeks, then six-monthly with FBC<br>▶ weight monitoring |
| **Discontinuation** |
| ▶ slowly titrate over one month. |
| **Drug interactions** |
| ▶ interacts with other anticonvulsants<br>▶ increases levels of lamotrigine, antidepressants, warfarin and aspirin<br>▶ lowers levels of olanzapine. |

| **Contraindications** |
|---|
| ▸ liver disease<br>▸ pregnancy<br>▸ breast feeding |
| **Other information** |
| ▸ teratogenic: neural tube defects<br>▸ woman of childbearing potential must be put on contraception and folate 5 mg/daily |

**Source:** Sadock BJ and Sadock VA, 2007; Taylor *et al.*, 2012; McIntyre and Yoon, 2012

already in the reduced form and does not need dissociation in the stomach, it is said to have less gastric side effects. There is no difference in efficacy (McIntyre and Yoon, 2012; Sadock BJ and Sadock VA, 2007; Mahli *et al.*, 2012).

### 36.4.2.5 Carbamazepine

Carbamazepine (see Table 36.17) is a tricyclic compound, related to imipramine and other antidepressants, which possibly explains its efficacy in bipolar depression. Its spatial configuration is again closely related to phenytoin. After valproate, carbamazepine is the second most commonly used anticonvulsant in bipolar disorder. The extended release formula is approved for use in acute manic and mixed episodes. Its pharmacokinetics complicates its prescription. Recent data suggest that it is falling out of favour with prescribers when compared to valproate and lithium.

Because carbamazepine is a potent liver enzyme inducer, the following is found:

- an increased clearance of oral contraceptives, corticosteroids, warfarin and theophylline
- clearance is inhibited by INH, erythromycin, cimetidine and valproate
- clearance is enhanced by barbiturates and phenytoin.

The pharmacokinetics of carbamazepine are thus affected in a complex way by use with other anticonvulsants, and care should be taken during prescription (Sadock BJ and Sadock VA, 2007; Taylor *et al.*, 2012; Schachter *et al.*, 2012).

### 36.4.2.6 Lamotrigine

Lamotrigine (see Table 36.18) shows good efficacy for treatment of acute bipolar I depression, prevention of recurrence in bipolar II rapid cycling and long-term (up to 18 months) prevention of recurrent mood episodes after an acute illness phase in bipolar I disorder. Lamotrigine has been shown to prevent relapses when used as monotherapy, with a greater efficacy against depressive episodes than manic episodes. It has been approved for bipolar I maintenance treatment, but not for treating bipolar depression, for which it is most commonly used.

Lamotrigine is metabolised in the liver and its metabolite is excreted in the urine as a glucoronide conjugate. Its **elimination half-life** ($t\frac{1}{2}\beta$) is drastically affected by drug interactions:

- $t\frac{1}{2}$ = 24 hours normally
- $t\frac{1}{2}$ = 15 hours with a CYP 450 inducer, such as carbamazepine
- $t\frac{1}{2}$ = 60 hours with a CYP 450 inhibitor, such as valproate.

Its relative benign side-effect profile makes it a popular choice in modern psychiatry. Dose titration is performed slowly in order to reduce the risk of Stevens-Johnson syndrome. This slow titration limits its use in the acute setting (Schachter *et al.*, 2012).

### 36.4.2.7 Newer anticonvulsant medications

None of the newer medications have shown benefits in treating acute mania or depression, or as long-term prophylactic agents in bipolar

**Table 36.17** Carbamazepine

| |
|---|
| **Indications**<br>▶ second-line treatment in bipolar disorders<br>▶ neuropathic pain<br>▶ intractable hiccups<br>▶ chronic dystonic disorders<br>▶ alcohol withdrawal<br>▶ aggression in non-psychotic patients. |
| **Plasma levels**<br>▶ No evidence for usefulness of routine blood levels in bipolar disorders<br>▶ To monitor compliance or confirm toxicity. |
| **Dosages**<br>▶ initial loading of 20 mg/kg/day or 400 mg/day in divided dosages twice a day<br>▶ slowly increase to 600–1200 mg/day. |
| **Adverse effects**<br>▶ Common: sedation, dizziness, ataxia, diplopia, nausea, erythematous rash, dry mouth<br>▶ Less common: hepatitis, oedema, hyponatreamia (inappropriate anti-diuretic hormone secretion), haematological abnormalities (agranulocytosis, aplastic anaemia), Stevens-Johnson syndrome. |
| **Toxicity** (correlates with blood levels)<br>▶ confusion, abnormal movements, nystagmus, diplopia, ataxia, drowsiness, speech disturbance, blurred vision and sometimes hallucinations. |
| **Baseline tests**<br>▶ urea and electrolytes (U&E), LFT, FBC. |
| **On-treatment monitoring**<br>▶ six-monthly U&E, LFT, FBC |
| **Discontinuation**<br>▶ slowly taper over a month. |
| **Drug interactions**<br>▶ complex drug interactions can increase or decrease plasma levels.<br>▶ induces CYP 450 system (CYP3A4), reducing levels of other anticonvulsants, oral contraceptives, antidepressants, antipsychotics and its own levels (auto-inducer). |
| **Contraindications**<br>▶ liver disease, pregnancy and breastfeeding |
| **Other information**<br>▶ teratogenic: neural tube defects. |

**Source:** Sadock BJ and Sadock VA, 2007; Taylor *et al.*, 2012; Schachter *et al.*, 2012

disorders. Psychotropic efficacy has been recognised for other symptoms often associated with bipolar disorders. Although there are studies that support their use, they do not have registration for these indications. Careful risk-benefit assessments must be conducted and patients must be informed before prescribing them for off-label use.

Topiramate is seen as an adjunct treatment in bipolar disorders. It has shown efficacy in

**Table 36.18** Lamotrigine

| **Indications** |
|---|
| ▶ bipolar disorders, especially prophylaxis for depressed phases. More commonly used in bipolar II disorder |
| **Plasma levels** |
| ▶ Not applicable |
| **Dosages** |
| ▶ 25 mg daily for 2 weeks, then 50 mg daily for 2 weeks; titrate according to clinical response up to maximum of 300 mg<br>▶ When on valproate: 25 mg for 4 weeks, then 50 mg for 4 weeks; titrate slowly upwards |
| **Adverse effects** |
| ▶ Common: sedation or insomnia, nausea, dizziness<br>▶ Less common: rash, headache, ataxia, diplopia |
| **Toxicity** |
| ▶ Stevens-Johnson syndrome (rare) |
| **Baseline tests** |
| ▶ LFT |
| **On-treatment monitoring** |
| ▶ monitor for skin rash |
| **Discontinuation** |
| ▶ abrupt withdrawal may provoke rebound seizures: taper slowly over 2-4 weeks |
| **Drug interactions** |
| ▶ Lamotrigine levels reduced by:<br>– anticonvulsant agents that induce hepatic enzymes (phenytoin, carbamazepine)<br>– oral contraception<br>– ritonavir.<br>▶ Lamotrigine levels increased by: valproate (lower dosages of lamotrigine needed). |
| **Contraindications** |
| ▶ liver disease<br>▶ pregnancy<br>▶ lactation |
| **Other information** |
| ▶ teratogenic: cleft palate and other central fusion disorders |

**Source:** Sadock BJ and Sadock VA, 2007; Taylor *et al.*, 2012; Mahli *et al.*, 2012

the treatment of bulimia nervosa, binge-eating disorder, alcohol dependence and migraine prophylaxis. An extended-release formulation has been approved in combination with phentermine for weight loss. According to the sparse research available on the subject, there are possible indications for its use in tobacco use disorder, certain disruptive, impulse-control and conduct disorders, PTSD and borderline personality disorder associated with aggression and/or self-harm. The side-effect profile often limits its use – these include teratogenicity, glaucoma, metabolic acidosis as well as cognitive and psychiatric side effects. The recommended daily oral dose for adults is between 25 mg and 500 mg (Joubert, 2008; Gitlin and Frye, 2012; MIMS, 2012–2013).

**Table 36.19** Second generation antipsychotics: evidence for use in bipolar disorder

| Medications | Mania | Depression | Mixed episodes | Rapid cycling | Maintenance |
|---|---|---|---|---|---|
| **olanzapine** | + | + (best evidence with fluoxetine) | | + | + |
| **quetiapine** | + | + | | + | + |
| **risperidone** | + | | | + | + |
| **aripiprazole** | + | + add-on by specialist | | + | + |
| **ziprasidone** | + | | + | | |

**Source:** Mahli *et al.*, 2012; Gitlin and Frye 2012; Taylor *et al.*, 2012; Stein *et al.*, 2012

Gabapentin has value in comorbid anxiety and alcohol-related features associated with bipolar disorders, but no effect on bipolar disorders themselves. Efficacy has been proven in the treatment of neuropathic pain. The recommended oral dose for adults is 300–600 mg p.o. t.d.s (Taylor *et al.*, 2012).

Pregabalin is registered for the treatment of neuropathic pain. It also has evidence of efficacy in the treatment of certain anxiety disorders. The recommended oral dose for adults is 50–200 mg p.o. t.d.s (Taylor *et al.*, 2012).

Oxcarbamazepine is the keto analogue of carbamazepine that does not induce the CYP 450 system the way carbamazepine does, which limits its hepatotoxicity, lessens its drug-interactions and increases its therapeutic index. Oxcarbamazepine has shown possible pharmacodynamic efficacy in bipolar disorders in open, but not controlled, trials. However, hyponatraemia is more common with oxcarbazepine than with carbamazepine, and serum sodium levels must be monitored. It has a similar mode of action to carbamazepine but is less potent and 50% higher dosages are needed. The recommended oral dose for adults is 300–1200 mg p.o. b.d (Sadock BJ and Sadock VA, 2007).

Levetiracetam has only anecdotal evidence for the treatment of bipolar disorders. Further research is needed before it can be used as a mood stabiliser. The recommended oral dose for adults is 300–1200 mg p.o. b.d. (Sadock BJ and Sadock VA, 2007).

### 36.4.3 Antipsychotics

All antipsychotics (see Table 36.19) have mood-stabilising effects to some degree. They are the safer choice during pregnancy. First-generation antipsychotics have long been used in the acute treatment of mania, especially in combination with another mood stabiliser. The second-generation antipsychotics have undergone more extensive testing for use as monotherapy and in combination with other mood stabilisers. Clozapine is indicated for resistant cases. Research on the specific mood-stabilising effects of antipyschotics is still evolving.

## 36.5 Sedatives, hypnotics and anxiolytics

### 36.5.1 Benzodiazepines

#### 36.5.1.1 Classification

Benzodiazepines are divided into two groups based on their elimination half-lives (t½). Those with short half-lives are used as hypnotics, and those with longer half-lives as anxiolytics. Due to their shared pharmacodynamics, the so-called Z-drugs (zolpidem and zopiclone) will also be discussed here. These non-benzodiazepines are used as hypnotics with relatively short half-lives (Sadock BJ and Sadock VA, 2007).

## 36.2 Advanced reading block

**Other medications with mood stabilising effects**

**Riluzole**

Riluzole is being investigated for the treatment of amyotrophic lateral sclerosis (ALS). It seems to act like lamotrigine. There is possible scope for future use as a mood stabiliser.

**Benzodiazepines**

Benzodiazepines can be added during the acute management of manic or mixed episodes. Lorazepam and clonazepam both have evidence of mood-stabilising properties in the acute setting.

Benzodiazepines are not indicated specifically for their use in bipolar disorders. By understanding their mechanism of action (see Section 36.5 for a discussion of sedatives, hypnotics and anxiolytics), it is understandable that they are useful in the early treatment of mania. One has to keep all the effects of benzodiazepines in mind, including the addictive, anxiolytic, anti-convulsant and additive effects with alcohol and antispasmodics.

It is thus very helpful that benzodiazepines are available in an injectable form for the emergency management and short-term treatment of intermittent agitation, insomnia, anxiety and mania, especially in the interim, until therapeutic efficacy of the prescribed mood stabilisers have been reached.

**Memantine, amantadine and ketamine**

These medications are not yet indicated in the treatment of bipolar disorders, but theoretically could be beneficial due to their effects on N-methyl-D-aspartate (NMDA) receptors, where they act as antagonists and thus reduce the glutamatergic activity, similar to other mood stabilisers. (See Sections 36.7.4.3 and 36.9.8 for a discussion of memantine and amantadine respectively.)

**Calcium channel blockers**

In view of the effect of anticonvulsants on voltage-dependent calcium channels, it is possible that dihydropyridine-type calcium channel blockers could aid in the treatment of bipolar disorders. They are used for treatment-resistant bipolar disorders and are not first-line medications. There is some evidence supporting the use of nimodipine, amlodipine, isradipine and verapamil for maintenance treatment of bipolar disorder, and verapamil for antidepressant-induced mania. However, studies are not yet conclusive regarding the benefits of this treatment option and should be seen as being for specialist use only for these indications.

**Tamoxifen**

In an interesting prospective study, tamoxifen was given to manic patients for three weeks, resulting in a reduction of manic symptoms. This may be because this anti-oestrogen medication used in the treatment of breast cancer, works on intracellular protein kinase C.

**Source:** Taylor *et al.*, 2012

### 36.5.1.2 Indications for use

Apart from their primary uses as hypnotics and anxiolytics, benzodiazepines are also used for rapid tranquillisation, epilepsy, severe muscle spasms, pre-medication in certain surgical procedures and as conscious sedation for certain procedures.

As anxiolytics, benzodiazepines reduce agitation, tension and pathological anxiety. Due to their addictive properties, they are not indicated for the long-term treatment of anxiety disorders. They are used to augment the effects of SSRIs, especially at the onset of treatment. For the management of an acute panic attack,

## 36.3 Advanced reading block

**Hormonal and nutritional products with mood-stabilising effects**

**Omega-3 fatty acids**

Omega-3 fatty acids, eicosapentaenoic acid (EPA) and docosahexaenoic acid (DHA), which is converted from EPA, are natural oils found in fish and seeds. They have few side effects and both are found in high concentrations in neural tissue. They are also recognised as anti-inflammatory precursors in the double phospholipid cell membrane in humans.

The possible mechanism of action could be the inhibition of phosphokinase C, in a way which differs from that of valproate. Studies are still ongoing with no conclusive evidence as yet.

**Inositol**

This carbohydrate is linked to second messenger systems which may play a role in bipolar disorders. It is also related to 5-$HT_{2A}$. Evidence is non-conclusive and more research is needed.

**Folic acid**

Folic acid is the synthetic form of folate. The centrally active form of folate is L-methylfolate (MTHF), which may have a dual role in bipolar disorders. Firstly, it boosts trimonoamine neurotransmitter function (5-HT, NA and DA) and may augment the function of antidepressants. Secondly, because anticonvulsive agents have an effect on folate metabolism, it may be beneficial in partial responders to treatment.

**Thyroid hormone**

The $T_3$ form of the hormone is thought to stabilise mood in bipolar disorders. This is not well researched and the long-term use of an exogenous hormone may have detrimental effects on the organ function.

Liothyronine, the levorotatory form of endogenous $T_3$, has been shown to be useful in cases of treatment-resistant MDD when added to an antidepressant as an augmenting agent at doses of 25-50µg p.o./day.

**Source:** Taylor *et al.*, 2012

benzodiazepines provide immediate symptom relief. The injectable forms have a quicker onset of action, limiting patient distress.

Benzodiazepines are effective hypnotics as they hasten sleep onset, decrease nocturnal awakenings, increase total sleeping time and often impart a sense of deep and refreshing sleep. However, slow-wave sleep and rapid eye movement (REM) sleep are reduced and the extra sleeping time is largely made up of relatively light sleep. It is recommended that, because of their addictive properties, benzodiazepines only be prescribed as hypnotics for up to a month. However, there are studies that have proven the effectiveness of Z-hypnotics over a period of six months. It remains to be seen whether this data can be extrapolated to other benzodiazepines (Sadock BJ and Sadock VA, 2007; Taylor *et al.*, 2012).

### 36.5.1.3 Basic pharmacodynamics and pharmacokinetics

Benzodiazepines work as positive **allosteric modulators** of GABA-A receptors. This means that they bind to a specific binding site on the receptor, enhancing the binding of GABA to its receptor, resulting in an increased influx of chloride into the neuron with subsequent hyperpolarisation. Z-drugs have selectivity for certain subunits of the GABA-receptor and this can possibly explain their relative selectivity for sedation and relative lack of muscle relaxation or anticonvulsant effects.

It is the pharmacokinetic characteristics that basically determine the indication and use of each benzodiazepine. When administered orally, the rate of absorption is crucial in the onset of pharmacological action, specifically when used as hypnotics. All benzodiazepines are absorbed unchanged from the gastrointestinal tract. Sublingual preparations are used for the rapid relief of panic attacks. Intravenous preparations are used during treatment of status epilepticus, for sedation to ventilate patients, for conscious sedation in anaesthetics or sometimes in the management of catatonia. Intravenous administration can be painful and carries a risk for thrombophlebitis. Midazolam and lorazepam are the only two with predictable intramuscular absorption and are thus often used for rapid tranquillisation.

Those benzodiazepines with short half-lives are mostly used as hypnotics and those with longer half-lives for anxiety. The risk of those with longer half-lives is accumulation with sedation, while those with a short half-life may have more severe withdrawal symptoms due to greater fluctuations in plasma levels. Benzodiazepines are metabolised in the liver with limited pharmacokinetic interactions. Interactions are mostly pharmacodynamic, when other sedating medications are co-prescribed, or with alcohol that augments their effects (Stahl, 2008) .

### 36.5.1.4. Side effects and contraindications

Sedation and drowsiness are the most common side effects, and patients must be informed about the risk. Even residual daytime sedation due to benzodiazepines poses a risk for driving the next day. Dizziness and ataxia can pose a risk of falling, especially in the elderly, with an increased risk of

**Table 36.20** Benzodiazepines

| Medications | t½ (hours) | Usual therapeutic daily dose | Time until onset (minutes) | Duration of action |
|---|---|---|---|---|
| triazolam# | 2–6 | 0,125–0,25 mg | 45 | Short (t½<6hours) |
| midazolam | | 7,5–15 mg | 20 | |
| zopiclone | | 7,5 mg | 15–30 | |
| zolpidem | | 10 mg | 7–27 | |
| alprazolam# | | 0,5–2 mg | 60+ | |
| brotizolam | | 0,25–2 mg | 30–60 | |
| oxazepam | 10–20 | 15–30 mg | 20–50 | Intermediate (t½ 6–24 hours) |
| flunitrazepam | 10–20 | 0,5–1 mg | | |
| loprazalam | 4,6–11 | 0,5–2 mg | 140 | |
| lormetazepam# | 8–12 | 0,5–1,5 mg | 30–60 | |
| temazepam* | 8–20 | 10–20 mg | 30–60 | |
| lorazepam# | 10–20 | 1–4 mg | 60+ | |
| clonazepam | | 0,25–4 mg | | |
| nitrazepam | 25–35 | 5–10 mg | 20–50 | Long (t½>24 hours) |
| flurazepam* | 48–120 | 15–30 mg | 60–120 | |
| quazepam* | 48–120 | 7,5–15 mg | 120 | |
| diazepam* | 20–80 | 5–10 mg | 60–120 | |
| clobazam | | 10–30 mg | 60+ | |
| prazepam | | 10–20 mg | 60–180 | |
| Elderly: Quarter to half the adult dose<br>*Active metabolite<br># High-potency benzodiazepines | | | | |

**Source:** Sadock BJ and Sadock VA, 2007; Taylor *et al.*, 2012

hip fractures. Paradoxical reactions of disinhibition are a risk, especially in the immature, young, aged or damaged brain. Anterograde amnesia is associated with high-potency benzodiazepines, which are used therapeutically in anaesthetics for certain procedures. Cognitive problems can persist long after the medication has been removed from the body compartments, and long-term use in middle age can predispose an individual to an earlier onset of MND. Respiratory depression is a risk, especially when blood levels increase rapidly as happens with intravenous administration. The benzodiazepine antagonist flumazenil can be of value diagnostically in cases of suspected benzodiazepine overdose, but has limited therapeutic value because of its short half-life.

Withdrawal, tolerance and dependence are risks of benzodiazepine use and are more common in drugs with a short half-life; however, a delayed withdrawal effect is described in those with longer half-lives. This can happen as early as two weeks into treatment; the use of benzodiazepines should be kept to short periods to prevent iatrogenic dependence. Tolerance can even develop to their anxiolytic effects, and higher dosages are then needed for treatment or maintenance. The appearance of withdrawal symptoms depends on the dosage, length of treatment, half-life of medication and rate of tapering. Severe withdrawal symptoms (e.g. paranoia, delirium, seizures) can be seen after abrupt discontinuation of benzodiazepines, especially in those with short half-lives and when persons on high dosages for long periods suddenly discontinue use. Some symptoms of withdrawal can develop in as many as 90% of persons who take the medication. When medication is discontinued, it must be tapered at a rate of 25% per week to prevent the development of withdrawal symptoms. Withdrawal symptoms can even develop after the use of Z-drugs, but the tolerance for the sedative effect is said to be low. This should not be confused with the natural rebound insomnia experienced for one to two days after discontinuation of hypnotics.

Withdrawal symptoms include anxiety, nervousness, irritability, depersonalisation, delirium and seizures, diaphoresis, hyperacusis, nausea, difficulty concentrating, myoclonus, tremor, weakness and fatigue (Sadock BJ and Sadock VA, 2007).

For more information on the benzodiazepines, refer to Table 36.20.

### 36.5.2 Buspirone

Buspirone is a 5-$HT_{1a}$ partial agonist. It has a delayed onset of its anxiolytic effect and is not addictive. It has a very short half-life of 2–6 hours, necessitating frequent dosing of three times a day. Therapeutic effect is implied after two to three weeks, comparable to the SSRIs. Its mild anxiolytic effect compared to that of benzodiazepines can be attributed to it not having any effect on GABA-receptors, thus having no subsequent hypnotic, muscle relaxant or acute anxiolytic effects. It is sometimes used for augmentation of antidepressants (Stahl, 2008; Sadock BJ and Sadock VA, 2007).

### 36.5.3 Etifoxine

Etifoxine is a non-benzodiazepine with little sedation, often used in the short-term treatment of anxiety.

### 36.5.4 Meprobamate

Meprobamate is highly addictive and is often present in combination analgesics, with a high potential for abuse. It is not indicated for the primary treatment of insomnia.

### 36.5.5 Chloral aldehyde

Chloral aldehyde is often used as a sedative in children undergoing painful procedures or investigations. It is not recommended for the management of sleep difficulties in children.

## 36.5.6 Melatonergic medications as hypnotics

### 36.5.6.1 Melatonin

Melatonin has been found to be effective in decreasing sleep latency in primary insomnia, but studies in secondary insomnia are not as convincing. Melatonin is not addictive. Short-term problems include worsening of nocturnal asthma and seizures. The effective dose seems to be 2 mg (Erman, 2006).

### 36.5.6.2 Agomelatine

Agomelatine improves sleep architecture in depressed patients, but daytime sedation can be problematic during the onset of treatment.

## 36.5.7 Antihistamines as hypnotics and anxiolytics

The sedative properties of antihistamines result from antagonism of central histamine-1 receptors ($H_1$), $\alpha$-adrenergic antagonism and anticholinergic effects. Some antihistamines with hypnotic properties include alimemazine, diphenhydramine, doxylamine and hydroxyzine. Antihistamines may cause troublesome antimuscarinic effects and those with longer half-lives may cause residual sedation the following day. Their efficacy seldom lasts longer than one week. They are commonly available as over-the-counter hypnotics (Sadock BJ and Sadock VA, 2007; Stahl, 2008).

## 36.5.8 Antidepressants and antipsychotics as hypnotics

Antidepressants with sedating effects include amitriptyline, mianserin, mirtazapine and trazodone. Sedation due to, amongst others, their $H_1$-antagonism, $\alpha_1$ adrenergic antagonism and antimuscarinic effects, can be used to treat insomnia. Antipsychotics also have their sedating effects via histamine receptors (Sadock BJ and Sadock VA, 2007; Stahl, 2008).

**Information box**

**Other substances commonly seen to be used as sedaties, hypnotics or anxiolytics**

**Valeriana officinalis**

Extracts of the roots of valerian are widely used to induce sleep and improve sleep quality. The evidence, however, is lacking, but there are suggestions that valerian might improve sleep quality without producing side effects. It is often sold in combination with diphenhydramine.

**Tryptophan**

Tryptophan, sometimes in the form of dietary supplements, has enjoyed some popularity in the treatment of insomnia. Its efficacy is difficult to substantiate and, since the publication of reports that linked tryptophan with the eosinophilic-myalgia syndrome, preparations indicated for insomnia have been withdrawn from the market in many countries.

**Alcohol**

Alcohol is not recommended for sleep because it has a short, weak hypnotic action, and rebound excitation can result in early-morning insomnia. Its diuretic effects can interrupt sleep and chronic use can lead to rapid development of tolerance and addiction. 'Natural products' available for infants usually have a high alcohol content.

**Kava, camomile and passionflower**

These products are often tried as self-medication, but apart from the placebo effect, no scientific evidence can support their use.

**Source:** Taylor *et al.*, 2012; Bent, 2006

## 36.6 Medications used primarily in the treatment of children

Children and adolescents can develop the same psychiatric illnesses as adults, but the symptoms may present atypically, respond less predictably, and be associated with more subtle cumulative impairment. Childhood-onset illness is at least as severe and functionally disabling as adult-onset disease. With few medications registered for use in children, the prescriber must be familiar with the available evidence and risks in order to obtain informed consent from parents and patients prior to initiating treatment.

## 36.6.1 Psychostimulants: methylphenidate

### 36.6.1.1 Indications

Methylphenidate is the first-line of treatment for ADHD. The initial dosage is 5 mg/day of the immediate release formulation. If there is a clinical response, it can be increased by 5 mg daily until it is given three times a day. If there is no clinical response, a higher dosage must be tried and increased in a similar manner until the total daily requirements have been established. It is advised to change to an extended-release formulation with once-daily administration to optimise compliance and limit disruption during the school day. The maximum dosage is 1 mg/kg/day (Sadock BJ and Sadock VA, 2007; Taylor *et al.*, 2012).

### 36.6.1.2. Basic pharmacodynamics and pharmacokinetics

Stimulants mimic the effect of naturally occurring sympathomimetic amines. They increase motivation, mood, energy and wakefulness. They act as indirect sympathomimetics by causing the release of presynaptic catecholamines. Their clinical efficacy relates to the presynaptic release of DA and NA. Methylphenidate is available in immediate-release preparations with a short half-life of 2–3 hours, while the extended-release preparation reaches peak concentration after 6–8 hours with efficacy for up to 12 hours. It is a Schedule 6 registered medication subject to specific prescription regulations (amount written in words and figures, maximum prescription for one month).

**Table 36.21** Principles of prescribing practice in childhood and adolescence

- **Target symptoms, not diagnoses.** Diagnoses can be difficult in children and co-morbidity is very common. Treatment should target key symptoms. While a working diagnosis is beneficial to frame expectations and help communication with patients and parents, it should be kept in mind that it may take some time for the illness to evolve.
- **Be aware of the technical aspects of paediatric prescribing.** The Medicines Act 1968 and European legislation make provision for doctors to use medicines in an off-label or out-of-licence capacity or to use unlicensed medicines. However, individual prescribers are always responsible for ensuring that there is adequate information to support the quality, efficacy, safety and intended use of a drug before prescribing it. It is recognised that the informed use of unlicensed medicines, or of licensed medicines for unlicensed applications ('off-label' use), is often necessary in paediatric practice.
- **Begin with less, go slow and be prepared to end with more.** In outpatient care, dosage will usually commence lower in mg/kg per day terms than adults and finish higher in mg/kg per day terms, if titrated to a point of maximal response.
- **Multiple medications are often required in the severely ill.** Monotherapy is ideal. However, childhood-onset illness can be severe and may require treatment with psychosocial approaches in combination with more than one medication.
- **Allow time for an adequate trial of treatment.** Children are generally more ill than their adult counterparts and will often require longer periods of treatment before responding. An adequate trial of treatment for those who have required in-patient care may well take 8 weeks for depression or schizophrenia.
- **Where possible, change one drug at a time.**
- **Monitor outcome in more than one setting.** For symptomatic treatments (such as stimulants for attention deficit hyperactivity disorder [ADHD]), bear in mind that the expression of problems may be different across settings (e.g. home and school); a dose titrated against parent reports may be too high for the daytime at school.
- **Patient and family medication education is essential.** For some child and adolescent psychiatric patients, the need for medication will be lifelong. The first experiences with medications are therefore crucial to long-term outcomes and adherence.

**Source:** Taylor *et al.*, 2012. This material is reproduced with permission from John Wiley and Sons Inc.

#### 36.6.1.3 Side effects and contraindications

Side effects include insomnia, growth deceleration, anorexia, headache, hypertension, nausea and gastric discomfort. Most side effects are transient. If growth is stunted, drug holidays are advised during weekends and school holidays. Monitoring should include weight and height measurements and recording of blood pressure and pulse rate. It is not recommended that all patients receive a baseline ECG but in the presence of cardiac symptoms or a family history of cardiac conduction problems or sudden cardiac events, specialist evaluation prior to initiation of treatment is recommended.

Methylphenidate is contraindicated in patients with a tic disorder or a family history of tic disorders, glaucoma, hyperthyroidism, tachyarrhythmias, anxiety, agitation, cardiomyopathy and structural cardiac abnormalities (Taylor *et al.*, 2012).

### 36.6.2 Atomoxetine

Atomoxetine is a good non-stimulating alternative for the treatment of ADHD if patients cannot tolerate methylphenidate or if it is contraindicated.

#### 36.6.2.1 Basic pharmacodynamics and pharmacokinetics

The clinical effect of atomoxetine is via the selective inhibition of the presynaptic NA transporter. Atomoxetine is metabolised primarily via $CYP_{2D6}$. Its half-life varies according to pharmacogenetics. In fast metabolisers, the half-life is 3–6 hours, but can be 21 hours in poor metabolisers. It has an active metabolite that is excreted through the kidneys. The initial dosage is 0,5 mg/kg/day and can be increased to 1,2 mg/kg/day after at least three days. It can be administered as a single dosage or divided into two dosages. The maximum dosage in adults or adolescents weighing 70 kg or more is 100 mg daily.

#### 36.6.2.2 Side effects and contraindications

Side effects include abdominal discomfort, decreased appetite with weight loss, dizziness, vertigo and irritability. Minor increases in pulse rate and blood pressure have been noted. A few cases of severe hepatic injury have been described and atomoxetine must be discontinued permanently in patients who develop jaundice.

It is contraindicated in hepatic impairment, uncontrolled hypertension and narrow angle glaucoma.

### 36.6.3 Third-line treatment for ADHD

It is recommended that a third line of treatment only be followed by specialists in the field. Available medications include TCAs, the $\alpha_{2A}$-adrenergic agonist clonidine, carbamazepine, bupropion and modafinil. They should never be used for ADHD alone. If behavioural problems are present, especially in an intellectually disabled person, risperidone can help to reduce the aggression. Second-generation antipsychotics have no supportive evidence in the treatment of ADHD.

## 36.7 Medications used primarily in the treatment of the elderly

### 36.7.1 General principles

Prescribing for the elderly has its own challenges due to the altered pharmacodynamics and pharmacokinetics of most medications in this population. It is further complicated by the use of concomitant medication to treat other medical problems, resulting in a higher risk of drug interactions. The risk of side effects is thus higher in the elderly.

### 36.7.2 Altered pharmacodynamics

Control over autonomic reflexes (e.g. blood pressure) changes with an increased sensitivity of receptors with aging. This leads to an increased incidence and severity of side effects. Medications that can affect blood pressure (e.g. TCAs) are more likely to cause falls. Constipation is a common side effect of medication that reduces gut motility (e.g. anticholinergics). The elderly are specifically more sensitive to benzodiazepines, with a higher risk of falling. Serious side effects like agranulocytosis with clozapine, bleeding with SSRIs and stroke with antipsychotics are also more common.

Therapeutic response can also be delayed in the elderly, and care should be taken not to increase dosages prematurely (Taylor *et al.*, 2012).

## 36.7.3 Altered pharmacokinetics

The rate of absorption is slower in the elderly due to decreased gastric secretions, resulting in a slower onset of action.

Due to the relative loss of lean body mass, the elderly have a higher volume of distribution, resulting in a smaller portion of medications being bound to plasma proteins (e.g. increased unbound fractions of warfarin), a higher concentration of some medications at the site of action (e.g. digoxin), and a longer duration of action of some fat soluble medications (e.g. diazepam).

Hepatic metabolism is unchanged in the absence of liver disease.

Excretion is affected as renal function declines with age – 35% of function is lost by the age of 65 and 50% by the age of 80. In the presence of other concurrent medical diseases, such as diabetes, hypertension and ischaemic heart disease, renal function is further impaired. Most metabolites are excreted renally and lithium and sulpiride are excreted unchanged. Accumulation can lead to toxicity and side effects, so dosages must be reduced. It should be kept in mind that serum creatinine and urea levels can be misleading in the elderly due to the loss of muscle mass leading to a decreased production of creatinine. GFR is more reliable (Taylor *et al.*, 2012).

## 36.7.4 Cognitive enhancers

### 36.7.4.1 Classification

Cognitive enhancers are used in the treatment of MND. Acetylcholinesterase (AChE) inhibitors are indicated for all levels of major neurocognitive disorder, while memantine is registered for moderate to severe major neurocognitive disorder.

### 36.7.4.2 Acetylcholinesterase inhibitors (AChE-Is)

There are three different types of AChE-Is on the market – donepezil, rivastigmine and galantamine. All three decrease the degradation of acetylcholine, implicated in the pathophysiology of MND, thereby increasing the levels of acethylcholine in the brain. Clinical efficacy is similar between all three medications. Main differences involve dosage frequency.

Side effects are related to the increased levels of acetylcholine peripherally. Common side effects include nausea, vomiting, diarrhoea, anorexia and headache. Less common side effects are agitation, syncope, dizziness, abdominal pain, dyspepsia, hyperhydrosis and urinary incontinence.

Donepezil binds AChE reversibly and selectively. The starting dose is 5 mg daily and can be increased to 10 mg after four weeks.

Rivastigmine binds AChE pseudo-irreversibly and also binds butyrylcholinesterase (BuChR). The dosage is twice a day, initially 1,5 mg bd, which can be increased to 6 mg b.d. A transdermal patch is available internationally.

**Table 36.22** Reducing risk of drug-related morbidity and mortality in the elderly

- Use drugs only when absolutely necessary.
- Avoid, if possible, medications that block $\alpha_1$-adrenoreceptors, have anticholinergic side effects, have a long half-life, or are potent inhibitors of hepatic enzymes.
- Start with a low dose and increase slowly, but do not undertreat. The full adult dose might be necessary.
- Try not to treat side effects with another medication: rather switch to an alternative that is better tolerated.
- Keep therapy simple, with preferably once daily dosages in order to ease administration and adherence.
- Be vigilant regarding drug-induced problems with any medical or cognitive decline.

**Source:** Adapted from Taylor *et al.*, 2012. This material is reproduced with permission from John Wiley and Sons Inc.

Galantamine binds AChE selectively and reversibly. It is also a nicotine receptor modulator. It has a twice daily dosage, initially 4 mg b.d, which can be increased to 12 mg b.d. A once-daily extended-release formulation is available internationally.

#### 36.7.4.3 Memantine

Memantine acts as an antagonist at the NMDA receptor. This action is said to be neuroprotective and possibly disease modifying. It also has antagonistic effects on the 5-$HT_3$ receptor. Side effects include drug hypersensitivity, somnolence, dizziness, hypertension, dyspnoea, constipation and headache. The starting dose is 5 mg daily, and can be increased weekly up to 20 mg daily.

#### 36.7.4.4 Other treatments

Although research in the treatment of Alzheimer's disease is ongoing, results are often disappointing. No treatment has yet been proven to be disease-modifying by targeting amyloid processing. Immunisation against amyloid had been unsuccessful as it resulted in meningoencephalitis. ß-amyloid antagonists, such as tramisrosate, were expected to prevent assembly of amyloid plaques, but have not yet been proven effective. Targeting of the γ-secretase enzyme to modulate or inhibit amyloid formation by selective amyloid lowering agents (SALAs) shows promising early results.

There is, however, research into the symptomatic treatment of MND and Alzheimer's disease, but the results are disappointing (Taylor *et al.*, 2012).

## 36.8 Medications used primarily in the treatment of substance-related and addictive disorders

Pharmacological interventions in the treatment of substance-related disorders and addictive disorders should generally always be used in conjunction with psychosocial interventions. General medications (e.g. benzodiazepines, antipsychotics) used to treat withdrawal or intoxication symptoms of different substances of abuse will not be discussed here; rather the focus will be on medications used specifically in the management of certain substance use disorders.

### 36.8.1 Tobacco-use disorder

Smoking carries significant health risks and complete cessation is therefore the treatment goal. It is however very important to keep in mind that stopping smoking could alter the pharmacokinetics and pharmacodynamics of other medications (e.g. clozapine, alprazolam, warfarin, insulin). Additional care should also be taken in patients suffering from mental illness who are attempting smoking cessation, due to a higher risk of emerging depression and some of the available treatments having possible neuropsychiatric side effects (Galanter and Kleber, 2008; Taylor *et al.*, 2012).

#### 36.8.1.1 Nicotine replacement therapies

These are designed to relieve nicotine craving and withdrawal symptoms and should preferably be used in conjunction with psychosocial interventions aimed at smoking cessation. Many different formulations are available including those sold over the counter (gum, patches, and lozenges) and those on prescription (inhaler and nasal spray).

#### 36.8.1.2 Varenicline

This medication is a partial agonist with high affinity to the $\alpha_4\beta_2$ nicotinic acetylcholine receptor. It significantly reduces nicotine withdrawal symptoms but also likely makes smoking less rewarding, potentially preventing one slip from becoming a full relapse. It is usually prescribed as a 12 week treatment – day 1–3: 0.5 mg/d; day 4–7: 0.5 mg b.d. and from day 8: 1 mg b.d. The main side effect is nausea but neuropsychiatric symptoms (including suicidality) have been reported and patients should therefore be carefully monitored (Galanter and Kleber, 2008; Taylor *et al.*, 2012).

#### 36.8.1.3 Bupropion

Bupropion significantly reduces the severity of withdrawal symptoms and also makes smoking less pleasurable. The increased seizure risk has to be considered before initiation of treatment. It is usually prescribed as a 12 week treatment – 150 mg/day for the first two weeks, then 150 mg twice per day for 8–10 weeks (Galanter and Kleber, 2008; Taylor *et al.*, 2012). (See Section 36.3 for a discussion of antidepressants.)

### 36.8.2 Alcohol-use disorder

Benzodiazepines are the mainstay of alcohol withdrawal regimes with monitoring of hydration status and prophylactic use of thiamine also generally advocated even for uncomplicated withdrawal syndromes. Importantly, benzodiazepines should not be prescribed beyond the acute withdrawal period, where necessary treatments such as acamprosate or disulfiram should be used in conjunction with psychosocial interventions (Galanter and Kleber, 2008; Taylor *et al.*, 2012; Sadock BJ and Sadock VA, 2007).

#### 36.8.2.1 Thiamine

Thiamine or vitamin $B_1$ is a water-soluble B-complex vitamin. It serves as an important co-factor in carbohydrate metabolism and as such is essential for numerous critical biochemical reactions in the body, including the synthesis of certain neurotransmitters. The human body cannot produce thiamine and chronic alcohol consumption can result in a deficiency by causing inadequate intake, decreased absorption and impaired utilisation. Although people show a differential sensitivity to thiamine deficiency, it is generally advocated that healthy uncomplicated alcohol-use disorder or heavy drinking should be treated with 100–200 mg orally per day for a month whilst treatment of detoxification requires higher dosages (Galanter and Kleber, 2008; Taylor *et al.*, 2012; Sadock BJ and Sadock VA, 2007).

#### 36.8.2.2 Disulfiram

Disulfiram inhibits aldehyde dehydrogenase with resultant acetaldehyde accumulation after drinking leading to very unpleasant physical side effects (e.g. vomiting, headaches, tachycardia, vertigo, dyspnoea). Patients should be made clearly aware of the mode of action and should only use it willingly. Reactions could continue to occur up until two weeks after discontinuation and could have serious or lethal consequences. It has no effect on the craving for alcohol; rather it is used as aversive conditioning. Start with 400 mg per day orally for the first two weeks, thereafter 200 mg per day orally. Special care should be taken where there is a history of convulsions, an abnormal EEG, known medical complications or additional substance abuse (Galanter and Kleber, 2008; Taylor *et al.*, 2012; Sadock BJ and Sadock VA, 2007).

#### 36.8.2.3 Acamprosate

The mechanism of action of acamprosate appears to be central on glutamate and GABA receptor systems, up-regulating NMDA receptors and down-regulating GABA receptors, thereby reducing craving. Treatment should be initiated as soon as possible after abstinence has been achieved and continued for up to six months at a dosage of 666 mg twice daily. Side effects include diarrhoea, abdominal pain, nausea and vomiting as well as pruritis (Galanter and Kleber, 2008; Taylor *et al.*, 2012; Sadock BJ and Sadock VA, 2007).

#### 36.8.2.4 Naltrexone

Naltrexone is an oral, relatively pure opioid antagonist. As such it could be useful in someone who is still using alcohol as it blocks the DA/endogenous opiate reinforcement of alcohol, making drinking less pleasurable. Recommended dosage is 50 mg per day (Galanter and Kleber, 2008; Taylor *et al.*, 2012; Sadock BJ and Sadock VA, 2007).

## 36.8.3 Opioid-use disorder

Whilst it is important to be aware of the available options, the treatment of opioid use disorder is a specialist intervention and further training is a prerequisite before use of these medications should be attempted by a generalist (Galanter and Kleber, 2008; Taylor *et al.*, 2012).

### 36.8.3.1 Methadone

Methadone is an oral long-acting opioid agonist that has been shown to be a cost-effective maintenance therapy intervention. The initial total daily dose, depending on the level of tolerance, will be in the range of 10–30 mg for most patients. Detailed information in terms of the patient's current use, use of other depressant drugs (e.g. alcohol, benzodiazepines) as well as hepatic and renal function is needed to make a dose determination. Regular review for signs of toxicity forms part of the initial dose titration against withdrawal symptoms (Galanter and Kleber, 2008; Taylor *et al.*, 2012).

### 36.8.3.2 Buprenorphine

Buprenorphine is a sublingual synthetic partial opioid agonist with low intrinsic activity and high affinity at the $\mu$ opioid receptors. Due to the phenomenon of precipitated withdrawal it is important that the first dose be administered when the patient is experiencing symptoms of opioid withdrawal. Recommended starting dose is based on whether the patient is in withdrawal, as well as the presence of any risk factors (e.g. medical condition, polysubstance misuse, uncertain severity of disordered use). Duration of action is related to dose, with higher doses (16–32 mg) exerting effects for as long as 48–72 hours (Galanter and Kleber, 2008; Taylor *et al.*, 2012; MIMS, 2012–2013).

### 36.8.3.3 Naltrexone

Naltrexone works best when used as part of a structured abstinence program, especially in those individuals highly motivated to remain on treatment. Users often experience adverse effects such as dysphoria, depression and insomnia with resultant increased risk of inadvertent overdose due to illicit opioid use. The minimum recommended interval between stopping the opioid and starting naltrexone depends on the opioid used and, in the case of methadone, could require a wash-out period of up to 10 days.

### 36.8.3.4 Naloxone

Naloxone is a non-selective short-acting opioid antagonist used to counter the effects of opiate overdose. A stat dose of 0,4 mg is given intramuscularly, and repeated 2–3 minutes later if needed. It can also be given intravenously at a slow initial rate of 0,8 mg per 70 kg of body weight. A total dose of as high as 15 mg may be necessary (Galanter and Kleber, 2008; Taylor *et al.*, 2012; MIMS, 2012–2013).

### 36.8.3.5 Buprenorphine/naloxone combinations

Buprenorphine/naloxone combinations are sometimes recommended in patients who are at high risk of diversion (i.e. buprenorphine abuse by injection or snorting). The rationale is that in the presence of naloxone, opioid withdrawal symptoms will be precipitated when buprenorphine is not used sublingually. Dosing schedules are as for buprenorphine (Galanter and Kleber, 2008; Taylor *et al.*, 2012).

## 36.8.4 Other

### 36.8.4.1 Clonidine

Clonidine is a centrally acting $\alpha_2$ adrenergic agonist that can ameliorate noradreneric overdrive in alcohol withdrawal and opioid detoxification. Only experienced clinicians should prescribe it for these and other indications such as ADHD and tic disorders. The adult dosage is 0,025–0,075 mg twice daily (Galanter and Kleber, 2008; Taylor *et al.*, 2012; MIMS, 2012–2013).

#### 36.8.4.2 Flumazenil

Flumazenil is a GABA antagonist injection that can be used as an antidote in the treatment of benzodiazepine overdose at a dosage of 200 μg slowly IV over 15 seconds. Another 100 μg can be given slowly IV over 10 seconds if a required level of consciousness was not achieved after the first dose. The maximum daily dose is 1 mg (Galanter and Kleber, 2008; Taylor *et al.*, 2012; MIMS, 2012–2013).

## 36.9 Other medications used in psychiatry

### 36.9.1 Anticholinergics

Anticholinergic medications are used in psychiatry for the treatment of neuroleptic-induced parkinsonism. Orphenadrine and biperidine tablets can be prescribed in daily dosages for the long-term treatment of dyskinetic and mild dystonic effects. Biperidine injection intravenously or intramuscularly is indicated for the treatment of medication –induced acute dystonia where the dose can be repeated half hourly to a maximum of three doses if clinically indicated.

Common side effects of these medications are a dry mouth and blurred vision. Due to other common side effects, such as constipation, urinary retention and their propensity to cause delirium in the elderly, these medications should be avoided in this patient population where possible – especially in patients with MND, where the cognitive dysfunction which these medications can cause, can have a detrimental effect on the overall cognitive functioning of these patients (Stahl, 2008).

- Biperidine 5 mg IM or slowly IV stat OR 2,5–5 mg p.o. 1–4 times/day
- Orphenadrine 50–100 mg p.o. 2–3 times/day (MIMS, 2012–2013).

### 36.9.2 Propranolol

Propranolol is a β-adrenergic receptor blocker (β-blocker). In psychiatry it is a commonly used β-blocker because of its lipid solubility, allowing it to cross the blood-brain barrier in sufficient concentrations to have an effect in the brain (Sadock BJ and Sadock VA, 2007).

Propranolol can be useful in the treatment of social anxiety disorder (social phobia), especially the performance type, where it must be taken 30 minutes before an anxiety-provoking situation. There are data available advocating its use in GAD, panic disorder and PTSD; it should, however, not be considered as a first-line treatment option in these disorders (Sadock BJ and Sadock VA, 2007).

Aggression secondary to an underlying psychiatric disorder has been shown to respond favourably to propranolol prescribed as an adjunct to the appropriate medications prescribed for the primary psychiatric disorder (Sadock BJ and Sadock VA, 2007).

The use of propranolol for medication-induced akathisia has also been shown to be beneficial (Sadock BJ and Sadock VA, 2007; Taylor *et al.*, 2012).

A further indication for use is in the treatment of medication-induced postural tremor, which can be caused by medications such as lithium, valproate and TADs (Sadock BJ and Sadock VA, 2007).

- Propranolol 10–40 mg p.o. 2–3 times/day (MIMS, 2012–2013).

### 36.9.3 Prazosin

Prazosin is an α-adrenergic receptor antagonist that can be effective in reducing nightmares and improving sleep in patients with treatment-refractory PTSD (Lanouette and Stein, 2010; Sadock BJ and Sadock VA, 2007; Taylor *et al.*, 2012).

- Prazosin 0.5 mg p.o. nocte (MIMS, 2012–2013).

### 36.9.4 Steroidal antiandrogens

Cyproterone acetate and medroxyprogesterone acetate have anti-androgenic effects and can be used therapeutically in the treatment or management of paraphilias, hypersexual or sexually deviant or inappropriate behaviour in paraphilias, MND, intellectual disability and sexual offenders (Assumpção *et al.*, 2014; Garcia and Thibaut, 2012; Joller *et al.*, 2013; Tucker, 2010; Sajith *et al.*, 2008).

- Cyproterone acetate 25–150 mg p.o. daily – b.d. OR 150–600 mg IM weekly or monthly
- Medroxyprogesterone acetate 150–900 mg IM weekly or monthly (MIMS, 2012–2013).

### 36.9.5 Phosphodiesterase-5 inhibitors

This class of medication is indicated for the treatment of erectile disorder, for which there is evidence of efficacy almost no matter what the underlying cause. Sildenafil has been described as being useful in the treatment of SSRI-induced sexual dysfunction in men and women and as having a positive effect on sexual inhibition in women. Vardenafil and tadalafil are newer medications in this class (Taylor *et al.*, 2012; Sadock BJ and Sadock VA, 2007; Balon, 2009).

- Sildenafil 25–100 mg p.o. 1/day, 30 minutes to an hour prior to sexual intercourse
- Vardenafil 5–20 mg p.o. 1/day, 1 hour prior to sexual intercourse
- Tadalafil 5–20 mg p.o. 1/day prior to sexual intercourse (MIMS, 2012–2013).

### 36.9.6 Alprostadil

Alprostadil is also used in the treatment of erectile disorder. Mode of administration is by direct injection into the corpora cavernosa of the penis about 2–3 minutes before sexual intercourse. An erection is achieved without sexual stimulation, unlike with the use of the phosphodiesterase-5 inhibitors (Balon, 2009).

- Alprostadil 10–20 µg, max 60 µg/day (MIMS, 2012–2013).

### 36.9.7 Modafinil

This psychostimulant is effective for the treatment of narcolepsy and can be used in an attempt to manage somnolence related to circadian rhythm sleep-wake disorder, shift-work type, obstructive sleep apnoea, hypopnoea and side effects of psychotropic medications. Modafinil can be used with positive results to treat patients with both bipolar and treatment-resistant unipolar depression with prominent hypersomnia and fatigue, when prescribed as an adjunctive agent to mood stabilisers and antidepressants respectively (Sadock BJ and Sadock VA, 2007; Taylor *et al.*, 2012; Ãkerstedt and Wright, 2009).

- Modafinil 100–400 mg p.o. 1/day(mane or divided into mane and noon dose) (MIMS, 2012–2013).

### 36.9.8 Amantadine

Amantadine is best known for its use in the treatment of Parkinson's disease. It is therefore not surprising that it is effective in the treatment of neuroleptic-induced parkinsonism where it is as effective as the anticholinergic medications. However, due to its effect of increasing synaptic DA, the risk of patients experiencing a relapse in psychotic symptoms is increased, limiting its use. It can be considered in elderly patients who cannot tolerate side effects like constipation and urinary retention on anticholinergic medications. Amantadine also causes less cognitive dysfunction (Sadock BJ and Sadock VA, 2007).

Other indications for which amantadine is less commonly used include SSRI-induced sexual dysfunction, neuroleptic malignant syndrome, tardive dyskinesia and behavioural disturbances in autism spectrum disorder (Sadock BJ and Sadock VA, 2007; Taylor *et al.*, 2012).

- Amantadine 100–200 mg p.o. b.d. (MIMS, 2012–2013).

### 36.9.9 Selegiline

Although not classified as an antidepressant, selegiline is also a MAOI, but inhibits monoamine oxidase-B and not monoamine oxidase-A like the other MAOIs and RIMAs.

Monoamine oxidase-B metabolises DA and tyramine. The inhibition of DA breakdown is used therapeutically in the treatment of Parkinson's disease, for which it is primarily indicated. The inhibition of tyramine makes patients susceptible to a tyramine-induced hypertensive crisis. Patients who take oral selegiline should therefore also stick rigidly to a low tyramine diet, especially at the higher doses used to treat MDD off-label, because it loses its selectivity for monoamine oxidase-B at these doses and also starts blocking monoamine oxidase-A (Stahl, 2008; Sadock BJ and Sadock VA, 2007).

Selegiline has some demonstrated benefit as an augmenting agent in the treatment of negative symptoms of schizophrenia. However, its DA-elevating effects can potentiate a relapse or worsening of psychotic symptoms. It should, therefore, be used with care for this indication and probably be reserved for specialist use (Taylor *et al.*, 2012).

- Selegiline 5–10 mg p.o. mane (MIMS, 2012–2013).

## 36.9.10 Dopamine receptor agonists

Medications in this class – bromocriptine, pergolide, pramipexole and ropinirole – have been used in the treatment of antipsychotic-induced extrapyramidal side effects, but, like amantadine, are rarely used for this purpose due to the risk of inducing a relapse in psychotic symptoms. This is due to their synaptic DA-increasing properties for which they are primarily used in the treatment of Parkinson's disease (Sadock BJ and Sadock VA, 2007).

Another indication is in the treatment of sexual dysfunction, but phosphodiesterase-5 inhibitors are better tolerated and more effective for this purpose (Taylor *et al.*, 2012).

Bromocriptine remains an effective treatment option for neuroleptic malignant syndrome, while pramipexole has shown some promise as an adjunct treatment option in bipolar disorders, but should be reserved for use by a specialist (Sadock BJ and Sadock VA, 2007; Taylor *et al.*, 2012).

Pramipexole and ropinirole are effective in the treatment of restless legs syndrome while bromocriptine may be effective in some patients (Varga *et al.*, 2009).

- Bromocriptine 1,25–40 mg p.o./day
- Pergolide 0,05–3 mg p.o./day
- Pramipexole 0,375–4,5 mg p.o./day
- Ropinirole 0,25mg–24 mg p.o./day (MIMS, 2012–2013).

## 36.9.11 Cyproheptadine

Cyproheptadine is a unique antihistamine because of its concomitant 5-$HT_2$ antagonist actions. It is prescribed for its anti-serotonergic properties for delayed orgasm, anorgasmia and impotence secondary to SSRI treatment, often, unfortunately, with a negative effect on the antidepressant effect of the SSRI. These properties are also utilised in the emergency setting in the treatment of serotonin syndrome (Sadock BJ and Sadock VA, 2007; Taylor *et al.*, 2012).

Other indications include the treatment of both nightmares associated with PTSD and antipsychotic-induced acute akathisia for which it is not a first-line option (Sadock BJ and Sadock VA, 2007; Taylor *et al.*, 2012).

There is support for its use in anorexia nervosa, restricting type, to aid weight gain (Aigner *et al.*, 2011; Sadock BJ and Sadock VA, 2007).

- Cyproheptadine 4–20 mg p.o./b.d (MIMS, 2012–2013).

## 36.9.12 Dantrolene

Dantrolene is a muscle relaxant used in the emergency setting in the treatment of neuroleptic malignant syndrome (along with appropriate supportive measures) where intravenous administration can reduce muscle spasms in about 80% of patients (Tural and Onder, 2010; Sadock BJ and Sadock VA, 2007) .

Other conditions where muscle rigidity can be prominent, like catatonia and serotonin syndrome, may well respond to dantrolene administration (Sadock BJ and Sadock VA, 2007).

- Dantrolene 1 mg/kg p.o. qds
- Dantrolene, mannitol combination 1 mg/kg via rapid IV infusion (MIMS, 2012–2013).

## 36.9.13 Orlistat

For the treatment of antipsychotic-induced weight gain orlistat can be useful when combined with a calorie-restricted diet. It is a selective gastric and pancreatic lipase inhibitor that reduces the absorption of fat from the diet (Ruelaz, 2009; Sadock BJ and Sadock VA, 2007; Taylor *et al.*, 2012.

- Orlistat 120 mg p.o. t.d.s (MIMS, 2012–2013).

## 36.9.14 Metformin

Valproate and antipsychotic-induced weight gain has consistently been shown to respond favourably to metformin, which has the added benefit of being effective in the treatment of type II diabetes mellitus (for which it is widely used). It thus combats the hyperglycaemia associated with metabolic syndrome which is associated with certain, mostly second-generation antipsychotics (Wu *et al.*, 2012; Sadock BJ and Sadock VA, 2007; Taylor *et al.*, 2012).

- Metformin 500 mg p.o. t.d.s. (MIMS, 2012–2013).

## 36.9.15 Ondansetron

This 5-$HT_3$ receptor antagonist can be used with positive benefit as an augmenting agent in the management of treatment-resistant schizophrenia, especially for negative symptoms. It may also be helpful in the treatment of OCD, mostly as an adjunct medication in treatment-resistant cases (Pallanti *et al.*, 2009; Soltani *et al.*, 2010; Taylor *et al.*, 2012).

- Ondansetron 0,25–4 mg p.o. b.d. (MIMS, 2012–2013).

# 36.10 Other treatments in psychiatry

## 36.10.1 Neuromodulation treatments

### 36.10.1.1 Electroconvulsive therapy (ECT)

ECT is still the most effective treatment for MDD and has longstanding proven efficacy in the treatment of the disorder. Several guidelines support the role of ECT as a first-line treatment of MDD, especially in psychotic and/or suicidal patients, or those with catatonia or treatment-resistant depression (Sadock BJ and Sadock VA, 2007; Stahl, 2008; Taylor *et al.*, 2012).

It is also a useful, rapidly effective treatment for certain other psychiatric disorders and life-threatening conditions. Refer to Table 36.23 where indications for ECT are listed (Sadock BJ and Sadock VA, 2007; Stahl, 2008).

The beneficial effects of ECT are attributable to a therapeutic generalised seizure which is induced by a potent electrical stimulus that

**Table 36.23** Indications and relative contraindications for ECT

| Indications | Relative contraindications |
|---|---|
| ▸ MDD (especially for cases accompanied by psychosis, catatonia, suicidal ideation and severe melancholic features including refusal to eat)<br>▸ manic episodes<br>▸ schizophrenia (more effective in the acute phase than for treatment of chronic schizophrenia)<br>▸ catatonia<br>▸ OCD<br>▸ neuroleptic malignant syndrome<br>▸ pregnant women (those in whom psychotropic medications are contraindicated)<br>▸ geriatric or medically ill patients (those who cannot tolerate or safely take psychotropic medications) | ▸ space occupying lesions in the central nervous system<br>▸ increased intracranial pressure<br>▸ recent myocardial infarction |

**Source:** Author's own Table

increases overall cortical activity. Increased cerebral blood flow and use of glucose and oxygen are accompanied by increased permeability of the blood-brain barrier during the seizure. After the seizure cerebral blood flow and glucose metabolism are decreased (Sadock BJ and Sadock VA, 2007.

The exact mechanism of action of ECT is only partially known. Antidepressant effects are related to several mechanisms including restoration of hemispheric balance, increased BDNF levels, enhanced neurogenesis and long-term up-regulation of 5-HT activity accompanied with down-regulation of muscarinic activity.

Delivery of the electrical pulse is through electrodes placed on the scalp in either a bilateral or unilateral pattern. Bilateral frontotemporal placement of electrodes yields a quicker therapeutic response but is associated with more cognitive side effects. In unilateral ECT, one electrode is placed over the frontotemporal region of the non-dominant hemisphere while the other electrode is placed adjacent to the vertex position on the same side (Sadock BJ and Sadock VA, 2007).

ECT is administered under general anaesthesia along with the administration of a muscle relaxant (Sadock BJ and Sadock VA, 2007).

The most noteworthy side effect of ECT is memory loss. Memory impairment occurs in most patients and occurs most frequently during the course of ECT. The memory impairment is almost always reversible but there are a minority of patients who complain of persistent difficulties with memory and other cognitive functions (Sadock BJ and Sadock VA, 2007).

Another frequent side effect is headache (Sadock BJ and Sadock VA, 2007).

There are no absolute contraindications for ECT. Relative contraindications are listed in Table 36.23.

ECT is usually administered two to three times a week and the number of treatments in a course varies according to the disorder being treated (usually one to four for catatonia, six to twelve for in MDD and eight to twenty for mania) (Sadock BJ and Sadock VA, 2007).

#### 36.10.1.2 Transcranial magnetic stimulation (TMS)

TMS is registered for the treatment of treatment-resistant MDD in a number of countries. It should be considered as a specialist treatment modality. Its efficacy when repeatedly administered (rTMS) is comparable to that of antidepressant medications. Although not registered for this purpose, TMS can be useful in the treatment of OCD, PTSD and panic disorder but should possibly be reserved for treatment-resistant cases (Pallanti *et al.*, 2009; Sadock BJ and Sadock VA, 2007).

Considered as being a non-invasive treatment technique, TMS is administered over the dorsolateral prefrontal cortex for the treatment of MDD. Local anaesthesia is applied to the scalp overlying the target area but the patient is awake during the treatment (Pallanti *et al.*, 2009).

TMS creates a magnetic field that induces focussed current in the area of the brain to which it is being applied. Low-frequency TMS administered over the right dorsolateral prefrontal cortex induces a decrease in cortical excitability which might modify interhemispheric imbalance (MDD possibly being associated with an imbalance of prefrontal cortex activity); while high-frequency TMS administered over the left dorsolateral prefrontal cortex increases cortical excitability, thus ameliorating depressive symptoms.

The most common side effects are headache and facial pain.

#### 36.10.1.3 Vagus nerve stimulation

Research into vagus nerve stimulation (VNS) as a treatment modality for psychiatric disorders is in its early days. It is approved in the United States for treating chronic or refractory depression in patients with no adequate response to four antidepressant treatments. Such patients suffering from MDD or bipolar depression may well benefit from this treatment modality (Sadock BJ and Sadock VA, 2007).

In VNS therapy, a bipolar helical electrode is placed around the left cervical vagal nerve

## 36.4 Advanced reading block

**Transcranial direct current stimulation (tDCS)**

MDD treatment with tDCS is still considered to be experimental at this stage and is not routinely used for this purpose.

Weak direct currents are applied to the brain via scalp electrodes in a simple, painless manner. The treatment is administered while the patient is awake. Anodal stimulation induces enhanced cortical excitability with resulting hyperpolarisation while cathodal stimulation decreases cortical excitability resulting in **depolarisation**.

at the level of about the fifth to sixth cervical vertebra and is stimulated in a regular cycle by pulses generated by a connected pulse generator placed in the chest wall. Both the electrodes and the pulse generator can be inserted via a minimally invasive surgical procedure (Beekwilder and Beems, 2010).

Although the exact mechanism of action of VNS is not known, it seems that impulses from the vagus nerve are transmitted to the locus ceruleus, raphe nuclei and nucleus tractus soliarious, which then project to other regions of the brain, including the limbic system and certain subcortical areas. Increased regional cerebral blood flow is found in the right parietal area and the orbitofrontal and anterior cingulate cortices. These regions are associated with depression and the afferent pathways of the vagus nerve. Therefore, this may be a less focal method of electrical stimulation than ECT or TMS.

Most common side effects are limited to the periods in which the stimulator is delivering pulses. These include hoarseness, throat pain and coughing. Other side effects that seem to be related to VNS are abdominal pain, nausea, shortness of breath and chest pain.

Although the present evidence supporting the use of VNS is still limited, it may be seen as a new promising form of treatment (Beekwilder and Beems, 2010; Sadock BJ and Sadock VA, 2007).

### 36.10.1.4 Deep brain stimulation

Deep brain stimulation (DBS) is a known treatment modality for a number of neurological disorders. It is most commonly used in the treatment of Parkinson's disease. It is also being studied as a treatment option for a number of psychiatric disorders from MND due to Alzheimer's disease to restless legs syndrome. However, it is primarily being studied as a treatment option in MDD, OCD and tic disorders (Lyons, 2011).

DBS is the most invasive neurostimulatory treatment. Electrodes connected to a pulse generator are implanted in target brain areas through a locally anaesthetised burr hole. This is done with the patient awake so that verbal feedback can be obtained in an attempt to prevent unwanted side effects. The pulse generator, implanted subdermally in the chest wall, generates regular high frequency pulses which excite the electrode causing a temporary halt in functioning in the target area and inducing long-term synaptic changes (Lyons, 2011; Tye *et al.*, 2009).

The major surgery-specific risks for DBS are haemorrhage, infection, fracture and misplacement or migration of the lead (Lyons, 2011).

Possible general side effects include nausea, paraesthesias, lethargy, sedation, sexual dysfunction, vertigo, syncope, mutism, mild dysarthria, whole-body dystonic jerks, hypertonia and hypotonia with increasing stimulation intensity. Other side effects are target-specific (Piedad *et al.*, 2012).

DBS treatment in psychiatry is currently still in the experimental phase but there are promising results for the treatment of selected disorders.

### 36.10.1.5 Psychosurgery

There has been a significant advance in psychosurgical techniques since the first frontal lobotomy was performed in 1935 (Sachdev and Chen, 2008).

## 36.5 Advanced reading block

**VNS for MND due to Alzheimer's disease and bulimia nervosa**

VNS is being investigated for treating MND due to Alzheimer's disease and has been shown to have a positive effect on cognitive functioning. Improvements in motor speed, psychomotor function, language and executive functions have been reported. VNS also affects the levels of neurotransmitters known to be depleted in MND due to Alzheimer's disease and activates brain regions that are usually degenerated in these patients. These effects seem to be sustained - behaviour and mood disturbances, usually associated with disease progress, are not being seen in patients receiving VNS (Beekwilder and Beems, 2010).

Patients with bulimia nervosa show a dampened satiety response to food intake. This satiety response is under vagus nerve control. In early research into severe unremitting bulimia nervosa attempts are made to dampen neural oscillations in the vagus nerve through VNS. Early findings are encouraging (Beekwilder and Beems, 2010).

VNS for MND due to Alzheimer's disease and bulimia nervosa is considered to be an experimental treatment.

Modern stereotactic neurosurgical equipment allows the discrete placement of lesions in the brain using radioactive implants, cryoprobes, electrical coagulation, proton beams or ultrasonic waves to make the lesions (Sadock BJ and Sadock VA, 2007).

The major indications for psychosurgery are chronic, debilitating MDD, OCD or tic disorders non-responsive to a wide range of treatment approaches over at least a five year period. Recently DBS, being less invasive, having mostly the same indications and often having the same or similar anatomical targets, is often attempted before psychosurgery (Sachdev and Chen, 2008; Sadock BJ and Sadock VA, 2007).

The most common psychosurgical procedures for these psychiatric indications are the anterior cingulotomy, anterior capsulotomy, subcaudate tractotomy, limbic leucotomy and bilateral amygdalotomy. These procedures result in an improvement in the majority of carefully selected patients. Furthermore, continued improvement is often seen one to two years after the surgery and patients often respond better to pharmacotherapy and behavioural therapy than they did before the surgery (Sachdev and Chen, 2008; Anderson and Lenz, 2009; Sadock BJ and Sadock VA, 2007).

The hypothalamotomy is being studied for its possible use in the treatment of sexual disorders and addictive and aggressive behaviours (Anderson and Lenz, 2009).

A uniquely psychosurgical side effect is post-operative seizures, which occur in less than 1% of patients. These are usually controlled by phenytoin (Sadock BJ and Sadock VA, 2007.

Regulations for psychosurgery are set out in the Mental Health Care Act (No. 17 of 2002).

### 36.10.2 Light therapy

The major indication for this therapy is MDD with a seasonal pattern (seasonal affective disorder), a disorder characterised by symptoms that appear on a seasonal basis, usually in the autumn and winter (Roos *et al.*, 2001; Sadock BJ and Sadock VA, 2007).

Light therapy involves exposing the patient to bright artificial light (2 500 lux), about 200 times brighter than the usual indoor lighting, on a daily basis during hours of darkness, usually the hours preceding sunrise (Roos *et al.*, 2001; Sadock BJ and Sadock VA, 2007).

Patients usually respond after two to four days of treatment, but may relapse within two to four days if the treatment is stopped during seasons when the days are short (Roos *et al.*, 2001).

### 36.10.3 Hormonal and nutritional products

Many hormonal and nutritional products have been and are being studied for their use in the treatment of psychiatric disorders. Not many of

## 36.6 Advanced reading block

**DBS for MDD, OCD and tic disorder**

Initial findings for DBS use for treatment-resistant MDD are promising. Targets for DBS in MDD with positive effects include the nucleus accumbens, internal capsule, subthalamic nucleus, internal globus pallidus, ventral striatum and subcallosal cingulate gyrus (Lyons, 2011; Tye *et al.*, 2009).

Preliminary studies indicate that DBS is a possible treatment option in severe, refractory OCD with the anterior limb of the internal capsule, subthalamic nucleus, right nucleus accumbens and the inferior thalamic peduncle being the reported targets (Lyons, 2011; Tye *et al.*, 2009; Sadock BJ and Sadock VA, 2007).

Stimulation of the thalamus, globus pallidus and nucleus accumbens have all shown positive effects in treating refractory tic disorders (Lyons, 2011; Piedad *et al.*, 2012; Tye *et al.*, 2009).

these have consistently been shown in research to be effective for the indications for which they are claimed to be effective or for which they were researched. However, there are a few exceptions.

As discussed earlier in the chapter (see Advanced reading block 36.3), $T_3$ can be used in the specialist setting as an augmenting agent for the management of treatment-resistant MDD; while melatonin can be useful in the treatment of insomnia. Patients should be warned that all over-the-counter forms of melatonin (and other hormonal supplementations) being sold as 'natural products' have not been reliably and vigorously tested for their efficacy and safety (Sadock BJ and Sadock VA, 2007).

## 36.10.4 Allied health care and alternative medicine

Certain allied health care sciences provide scientifically recognised interventions that are often incorporated with psychiatry in the treatment plans of patients. An example is occupational therapy, which is often used to improve the levels of functioning of patients with disorders such as schizophrenia and MDD.

Dieticians can be helpful in setting up dietary programmes for patients who gain weight on certain first-generation antipsychotics, while exercise can be effective for mild to moderate depression (Roos *et al.*, 2001).

There are a vast variety of practices available that are not widely recognised as being psychiatric treatments per se or having convincing evidence of efficacy in treating psychiatric disorders. For this reason it is not within the scope of this chapter to present detailed descriptions of these practices. However, clinicians are advised to be aware of these practices because some of them can be helpful in adjunctive management of some psychiatric symptoms.

Some practices, such as yoga and meditation, are in essence relaxation techniques and can be useful in the management of anxiety; while art and music therapy can, for example, help patients with disorders such as MND with relaxation (Roos *et al.*, 2001).

Alternative health care as a field is not as carefully regulated as the more conventional forms of medical care and cannot be advocated by the clinician as a treatment option for psychiatric disorders. However, large proportions of this country's population do consult religious, spiritual and traditional healers and firmly believe in their curative abilities. Knowledge of these practices is therefore advised because clinicians are likely to find that their patients may well be using alternative medicines instead of, or along with, their prescribed psychotropic medications. Finding a way to safely incorporate specific alternative medical practices (which the patient believes in) into his or her overall treatment plan may well be a way of best benefitting his or her mental health in the long run. Such a strategy may improve adherence to prescribed psychotropic medications (Roos *et al.*, 2001).

For a list of some of the most common and most well-known alternative medicine practices refer to the Information box.

**Information box**

**Alternative medicine practices**

- Traditional healing
- Spiritual healing
- Religious healing
- Homeopathy
- Herbal medicines
- Traditional Chinese medicine
- Acupuncture
- Chiropractic medicine
- Massage therapy
- Aromatherapy
- Reflexology
- Osteopathic medicine

**Source:** Adapted from Sadock BJ and Sadock VA, 2007

Herbal and homeopathic medicines do not have any evidence of efficacy in the treatment of psychiatric disorders. These products are often referred to as being 'natural' but not all of them are. Furthermore, they have not been tested as thoroughly and vigorously for their efficacy and safety as have conventional pharmaceutical medications. They are, therefore, potentially unsafe even though they are often referred to as being safe and having no side effects. These products cannot be endorsed for the treatment of psychiatric disorders. Even the minority of these products that have been adequately researched, such as St John's wort for depression and ginseng and gingko biloba for MND, have not been found to have efficacy above that of placebo in most trials.

## Conclusion

Pharmacotherapeutic and other treatment options (not related to psychotherapy) in psychiatry have increased vastly over the last few decades. A wide-ranging knowledge of established and newer psychotropic medications with regard to indications for use, efficacy, dose ranges, side effects, contraindications, drug interactions, pharmacodynamics and pharmacokinetics is essential for the proper treatment of patients. It is also important to know about other treatment options and their availability and appropriateness for the management of specific patients.

# References

Aigner M, Treasure J, Kaye W, Kasper S, The World Federation of Societies of Biological Psychiatry Task Force on Eating Disorders (2011) The World Federation of Societies of Biological Psychiatry Guidelines for the Pharmacological Treatment of Eating Disorders. *The World journal of Biological Psychiatry* 12: 400–43

Ãkerstedt T, Wright KP (Jr) (2009) Sleep loss and fatigue in shift work and shift work disorder. *Sleep Medicine Clinics* 4(2): 257–71

Anderson WS, Lenz FA (2009) Lesioning and stimulation as surgical treatments for psychiatric disorders. *Neurosurgery Quarterly* 19: 132–43

Assumpção AA, Garcia FD, Garcia HD, Bradford JMW, Thibaut F (2014) Pharmacologic treatment of paraphilias. *Psychiatric Clinics of North America* 37: 173–81

Balon R (2009) Medications and sexual function and dysfunction. *Journal of Lifelong Learning in Psychiatry* 7(4): 481–90

Bauer M, Ritter P, Grunze H, Pfennig A (2012) Treatment options for acute depression in bipolar disorder. *Bipolar Disorders* 14: (Suppl. 2) 37–50

Beekwilder JP, Beems T (2010) Overview of the clinical applications of vagus nerve stimulation. *Journal of Clinical Neurophysiology* 27: 130–8

Bent S (2006) Valerian for sleep: A systematic review and meta-analysis *The American Journal of Medicine* 119(12): 1005–12

Erman M (2006) An efficacy, safety and dose-response study of Ramelteon in patients with chronic primary insomnia. *Sleep Medicine* 7: 17–24

Galanter M, Kleber HD (2008) *American Psychiatric Publishing Textbook of Substance Abuse Treatment* (4th edition). Washington, DC: American Psychiatric Press

Garcia FD, Thibaut F (2011) Current concepts in the pharmacotherapy of paraphilias. *Drugs* 71(6): 771–90

Gitlin M, Frye MA (2012) Maintenance therapies in bipolar disorders. *Bipolar Disorders* 14 (Suppl. 2): 51–65

Hasan A, Falkai P, Wobrock T, Lieberman J, Glenthoj B, Gattaz WF, Thibaut F, Möller H-J, WFSBP Task Force on treatment guidelines for schizophrenia (2012) Guidelines for Biological Treatment of Schizophrenia, Part 1: Update 2012 on the acute treatment of schizophrenia and the management of treatment resistance. *The World Journal of Biological Psychiatry* 13(5): 318–78

Hasan A, Falkai P, Wobrock T, Lieberman J, Glenthoj B, Gattaz WF, Thibaut F, Möller H-J, WFSBP Task Force on treatment guidelines for schizophrenia (2013) Guidelines for Biological Treatment of Schizophrenia, Part 2: Update 2012 on the long-term treatment of schizophrenia and management of antipsychotic-induced side effects. *The World Journal of Biological Psychiatry* 14(1) 2–44

Joller P, Gupta N, Seitz DP, Frank C, Gibson M, Gill SS (2013) Approach to inappropriate sexual behaviour in people with dementia. *Canadian family physician/ Médecin de famille canadien* 59: 255–60

Joubert PM (2008) Psychiatric uses of topiramate: What is the current evidence? *South African Journal of Psychiatry* 14(2): 44–50

Lanouette, NM, Stein MB (2010) Advances in management of treatment-resistant anxiety disorders. *Journal of Lifelong Learning in Psychiatry* 8(4): 509–15

Lyons MK (2011) Deep brain stimulation: Current and future clinical applications *Mayo Clinic Proceedings* 86(7): 662–72

Malhi GS, Bargh DM, McIntyre R, Gitlin M, Frye MA, Bauer M, Berk M (2012) Balanced efficacy, safety and tolerability recommendations for the clinical management of bipolar disorders. *Bipolar Disorders* 14 (Suppl 2): 1–21

McIntyre R, Yoon J (2012) Efficacy of antimanic treatments in mixed states. *Bipolar Disorders* 14 (Suppl 2): 22–36

Monthly Index of Medical Specialities (MIMS) 2012–2013 Nov/Dec-Jan, 52(11)

Pallanti S, Bernardi S (2009) Neurobiology of repeated transcranial magnetic stimulation in the treatment of anxiety: A critical review. *International Clinical Psychopharmacology* 24: 163–73

Pallanti S, Bernardi S, Antonini S, Singh N, Hollander E (2009) Ondansetron augmentation in treatment-resistant obsessive-compulsive disorder: A prelimanary, single-blind, prospective study. *CNS Drugs* 23(12): 1047–55

Piedad JCP, Rickards HE, Cavanna A E (2012) What patients with Gilles de la Tourette syndrome should be treated with deep brain stimulation and what is the best target? *Neurosurgery* 71: 173–92

Roos JL, Joubert PM, Stein D (2001) Physical treatments. In: Robertson B, Allwood C, Gagiano C (Eds). *Textbook of Psychiatry for Southern Africa*. Cape Town: Oxford University Press

Ruelaz AR (2009) Psychiatric involvement in obesity treatment. *Journal of Lifelong Learning in Psychiatry* 7(3): 311–6

Sachdev PS, Chen X (2008) Neurosurgical treatment of mood disorders: Traditional psychosurgery and the advent of deep brain stimulation. *Current Opinion in Psychiatry* 22: 25–31

Sadock BJ, Sadock VA (2007) *Kaplan & Sadock's synopsis of psychiatry behavioral sciences/clinical psychiatry* (10th edition). Philadelphia: Lippincott Williams & Wilkins

Sajith SG, Morgan C, Clarke D (2008) Pharmacological management of inappropriate sexual behaviours: A review of its evidence, rationale and scope in relation to men with intellectual disabilities. *Journal of Intellectual Disability Research* 52(12): 1078–90

Schachter SC, Pedley TA, Wilterdink JL (*s.d.*) *Pharmacology of antiepileptic drugs*. Available at: http://0-www.uptodate.com.innopac.up.ac.za/contents/pharmacology-of-antiepileptic-drugs (Accessed 17 September 2012.)

Soltani F, Sayyah M, Feizy F, Malayeri A, Siahpoosh A, Motlagh I (2010) A double-blind, placebo-controlled pilot study of ondansetron for patients with obsessive-compulsive disorder. *Human psychopharmacology* 25(6): 509–13

Stahl SM (2008) *Stahl's Essential Psychopharmacology: Neuroscientific Basis and Practical Applications* (3rd edition). New York: Cambridge University Press

Stein DJ, Lerer B, Stahl SM (2012) *Essential Evidence-Based Psychopharmacology* (2nd edition). New York: Cambridge University Press

Taylor D (Ed.), Paton C (CoEd.), Kapur S (CoEd.) (2012) *The Maudsley Prescribing Guidelines in Psychiatry* (11th edition). Chichester: John Wiley & Sons. Inc.

Tucker I (2010) Management of inappropriate sexual behaviors in dementia: A literature review. *International Psychogeriatrics* 22(5): 683–92

Tural Ü, Önder E (2010) Clinical and pharmacological risk factors for neuroleptic malignant syndrome and their association with death. *Psychiatry and Clinical Neurosciences* 64(1): 79–87

Tye SJ, Frye MA, Lee KH (2009) Disrupting disordered neurocircuitry: treating refractory psychiatric illness with neuromodulation. *Mayo Clinic Proceedings* 84(6): 522–32

Varga LI, Ako-Agugua N, Colasante J, Hertweck L, Houser T, Smith J, Watty AA, Nagar S, Raffa RB (2009) Critical review of ropinirole and pramipexole – putative dopamine D3-receptor selective agonists – for treatment of RLS. *Journal of clinical pharmacy and therapeutics* 34(5): 493–505

Wu R, Jin H, Gao K, Twamley EW, Ou J, Shao P, Wang J, Guo X, Davis JM, Chan PK, Zhao J (2012) Metformin for treatment of antipsychotic-induced amenorrhea and weight gain in women with first-episode schizophrenia: A double-blind, randomized, placebo-controlled study. *American Journal of Psychiatry* 169(8): 813–21

CHAPTER

# 37 Psychological interventions

Ugasvaree Subramaney, Giada del Fabro

## 37.1 Introduction

Psychiatry, one of the first medical specialities to be recognised, literally means 'healers of the spirit' (Naidu and Ramlall, 2008). As such, it incorporates the use of both medication and psychotherapy in the treatment of clients. Psychotherapy is an important modality of treatment for people who suffer from emotional and mental disorders; even people with serious mental illnesses can benefit from psychotherapy. It is not merely 'talking therapy', although talking is the basis of how the treatment works. It is fair to say that some psychiatric disorders, such as schizophrenia, cannot be treated by psychotherapy alone. However, psychotherapy can be the sole form of treatment for some less serious psychiatric conditions, such as adjustment disorders. Usually though, psychotherapy is an important adjunct to many psychotropic agents. There are many types of psychotherapy modality, and this chapter will introduce some of the more important ones. Before presenting an in-depth review of the various psychological therapies, we begin with basic counselling skills, which form the basis of an effective psychotherapeutic relationship. The different psychological treatments will be discussed thus:

- definitions of the type of therapy
- indications
- basic principles (how to do it)
- some challenges.

In general, clients (or patients) have to be psychologically minded, have a fair amount of insight and motivation and be verbal enough so as to be able to engage with the therapist. They should not be acutely psychotic or severely cognitively impaired. There are some other provisos linked specifically with certain types of therapy, but these will be discussed in detail later.

## 37.2 Counselling skills

It is important for all doctors to develop sound counselling skills – even if they do not intend to specialise in psychiatry. Counselling skills essentially mean those verbal and non-verbal communication skills that are aimed at helping clients with important issues, life stressors and decision-making as well as an understanding of their ailments and treatments. Skills include the ability to convey empathy, establish rapport and communicate effectively with clients. Clients must feel comfortable enough to trust you as an individual to whom they can talk about their problems, difficulties and vulnerabilities, including topics about which they may feel embarrassed or guilty. In order to facilitate this, practitioners must be warm and non-judgemental towards their clients and allow them time and space to open up and talk about their problems.

## 37.3 Psychodynamic psychotherapy

Psychodynamic psychotherapy derives its methods and framework for understanding client problems from the school of psychodynamic and psychoanalytic psychology. This school emphasises the importance of intrapsychic factors and the unconscious in explaining the repetitive patterns and relationships in which individuals get involved. Intrapsychic factors are located within the person (i.e. their psychological make-up), as opposed to interpsychic (or interpersonal) factors that exist between people.

Early theorists, such as Sigmund Freud, emphasised the central role of sexual and aggression in shaping one's psychological make-up and relationships with others. Freud also postulated the **topography** of the psyche as consisting of an id, ego and super-ego (see Table 37.1) and spoke of stages of development which an individual has to negotiate across their early lifespan. Any interference with the successful negotiation of these phases result in fixations, which are the basis of psychological difficulties and problems in later life as an adult. These phases are the oral phase (0–2 years old), anal phase (3–5 years old), Oedipal phase (5–7 years old) and latency phase (7 years old until adolescence).

**Table 37.1** Freud's topographical model

| |
|---|
| **ID** |
| ▸ contains the basic, instinctual drives such as libido |
| ▸ acts according to the pleasure principle (seek to avoid pain) |
| ▸ unresponsive to the demands of reality |
| **EGO** |
| ▸ acts according to the reality principle (in ways that will bring benefit as opposed to negative consequences in the long terms) |
| ▸ organizing function |
| ▸ reality testing |
| **SUPEREGO** |
| ▸ made up of ego ideals (strivings and aspirations) as well as one's 'conscience' |
| ▸ strives to act in socially acceptable manner, according to what is right and wrong |

**Source:** Gabbard, 2010

Each phase consists of particular aspects that must be mastered by the young child, as well as conflicts that must be resolved in order to enable healthy or normal development. After the early work of Sigmund Freud, psychoanalytic work was expanded and differentiated by individuals such as Melanie Klein, Donald Winnicott, Wilfred Bion and Carl Jung.

## 37.3.1 Indications

Psychodynamic psychotherapy is useful for clients with a high degree of motivation, capacity for self-reflection and basic insight and relatively robust or intact psychological mechanisms and resources. Freud and other early analysts believed that certain conditions, such as psychosis, were not suitable for psychoanalysis. Later developments, however, have seen an adaptation of a more supportive model, especially by the interpersonal school and individuals such as Harry Stack Sullivan.

## 37.3.2 Basic approach

Therapeutic approaches include:

- working with the transference or counter-transference
- examining a client's psychological defences
- techniques such as interpretation, confrontation, and reflection.

Transference refers to the process whereby the client responds and relates to the therapist in a way that mirrors his or her early relationships with caregivers. Counter-transference is the therapist's response to the client, which may include the therapist's personal feelings and emotions regarding the client, as well as the feelings and emotions that the client is trying to evoke in the therapist. Many theorists and analysts operate on the fundamental principle that in order to help a client, one should increase his or her awareness of unconscious material, including fixations and conflicts that may be repeated in conscious life without realising why and with negative consequences. Clients are often reluctant to confront unconscious material and this manifests itself through an expression of their defences. One such defence is resistance to the therapeutic process (e.g. by missing sessions).

## 37.3.3 Challenges

Psychodynamic approaches require an accurate and detailed formulation of the client before developing a strategy with which to proceed to therapy. One has to understand the client's primary defences (see Table 37.2), their early relationships and dynamics and unconscious conflicts. This may take some time, practise and experience to be able to formulate in an accurate manner. As a result, beginner therapists may feel anxious in commencing with this type of therapy.

Psychodynamic psychotherapies tend to be longer than other types of therapy, even though shorter-term and brief models have been developed over the past years. Given that the client has to attend therapy for at least six months in these approaches, issues of compliance and cost become salient.

Certain types of client (such as those with severe personality disorders, severely traumatised or psychotic individuals) working with the transference may result in decompensation of the client due to a lack of psychological robustness and strength to manage this type of work and differentiate between reality and fantasy.

**Table 37.2** A hierarchy of defense mechanisms

| **Primitive defenses** | |
|---|---|
| Splitting | Compartmentalizing experiences of self and other such that integration is not possible. When the individual is confronted with the contradictions in behavior, thought, or affect, he/she regards the differences with bland denial or indifference. This defense prevents conflict stemming from the incompatibility of the two polarized aspects of self or other. |
| Projection | Perceiving and reacting to unacceptable inner impulses and their derivatives as though they were outside the self. |
| Projective identification | Both an intrapsychic defense mechanism and an interpersonal communication, this phenomenon involves behaving in such a way that subtle interpersonal pressure is placed on another person to take on characteristics of an aspect of the self or an internal object that is projected into that person. The person who is the target of the projection then begins to behave, think and feel in keeping with what has been projected. |
| Denial | Avoiding awareness of aspects of external reality that are difficult to face by disregarding sensory data. |
| Distortion | Significantly altering external reality to meet one's inner wish-fulfilling needs. |
| Dissociation | Disrupting one's sense of continuity in the areas of identity, memory, consciousness, or perception as a way of retaining an illusion of psychological control in the face of helplessness and loss of control. While similar to splitting, in extreme cases of disassociation, there is alteration of memory of events because of the disconnection of the self from the event. |
| Idealization | Attributing perfect or near-perfect qualities to others as a way of avoiding anxiety or negative feelings such as contempt, envy or anger. |
| Acting out | Enacting an unconscious wish or fantasy impulsively as a way of avoiding painful affect. |
| Somatization | Converting emotional pain or other affect states into physical symptoms and focusing one's attention on somatic (rather than intrapsychic) concerns. |
| Regression | Returning to an earlier phase of development of functioning to avoid the conflicts and tensions associated with one's present level of development. |
| Higher-level (neurotic) defences introjection | Internalizing aspects of a significant person as a way of dealing with the loss of that person. One may also introject a hostile or bad object as a way of giving one an illusion of control over the object. Introjection occurs in nondefensive forms as a normal part of development. |
| Identification | Internalizing the qualities of another person by becoming like the person. While introjection leads to an internalized representation experiences as an 'other', identification is experienced as part of the self. This, too, can serve nondefensive functions in normal development. |
| Displacement | Shifting feelings associated with one idea or object to another that resembles the original in some way. |

| | |
|---|---|
| Externalization | Disavowing personal responsibility for a behavior by attributing that responsibility to someone else. |
| Intellectualization | Using excessive and abstract ideation to avoid difficult feelings. |
| Isolation of affect | Separating an idea from its associated affect state to avoid emotional turmoil. |
| Rationalization | Justification of unacceptable attitudes, beliefs or behaviors, to make them tolerable to one's self. |
| Sexualization | Endowing an object or behavior with sexual significance to turn a negative experience into an exciting and stimulating one or to ward off anxieties associated with the object. |
| Reaction formation | Transforming an unacceptable wish or impulse into its opposite. |
| Repression | Blocking or expelling unacceptable ideas or impulses from entering consciousness. This defense differs from denial in that the latter is associated with external sensory data, while repression is associated with inner states. |
| Undoing | Attempting to negate sexual, aggressive, or shameful implications from a previous comment or behavior by elaborating, clarifying, or doing the opposite. |
| **Mature defences** | |
| Humor | Finding comic and/or ironic elements in difficult situations to reduce unpleasant affect and personal discomfort. This mechanism also allows some distance and objectivity from events so that an individual can reflect on what is happening. |
| Suppression | Consciously deciding not to attend to a particular feeling, state or impulse. This defense differs from repression and denial in that it is conscious rather than unconscious. |
| Ascetism | Attempting to eliminate pleasurable aspects of experience because of internal conflicts produced by that pleasure. This mechanism can be in the service of transcendent or spiritual goals, as in celibacy. |
| Altruism | Committing oneself to the needs of others over and above one's own needs. Altruistic behavior can be used in the service of narcissistic problems, but can also be the source of great achievements and constructive contributions to society. |
| Anticipation | Delaying of immediate gratification by planning and thinking about future achievements and accomplishments. |
| Sublimation | Channeling socially objectionable or internally unacceptable aims into socially acceptable ones. |

**Source:** Gabbard, 2010. Reprinted with permission from *Long-Term Psychodynamic Psychotherapy: A Basic Text*, Second Edition, (Copyright ©2010). American Psychiatric Association. All Rights Reserved.

## 37.4 Supportive psychotherapy

Supportive psychotherapy is, by definition, supportive in nature. In order to be a competent supportive psychotherapist, the therapist must have the ability to:

- assess regressive and adaptive shifts in ego functioning. This means the therapist must be able to determine when and why the client is behaving in a certain way. The behaviour is likely to be related to the client's developmental stage.
- make interventions specifically in support of a client's ego functions, including defensive operations. This means interpreting and guiding as well as advising appropriately to support the current functioning of the ego. Defenses are for the most part unchallenged and are maintained or even strengthened to promote a comfortable or solid adaptation to otherwise unexpressed or unacceptable conflict. The reason for this frequently is not that the client's defences are necessarily maladaptive but that they are useful measures to manage the crises or emotional difficulties in their lives. Defences can therefore be healthy and adaptive, serving to protect one psychologically.
- recognise internal conflict and help a client manage it without an emphasis on

interpretation. Here the therapist shows an awareness of the current difficulty the client is experiencing and gently and supportively guides the client to an acceptance and resolution without emphasising the deeper reasons for it. The focus is on issues that are already conscious for the client, rather than on the interpretation of the client's defences against previously unconscious conflict.
- be directive: give advice, set limits and educate a client when appropriate. This is something that doctors do in general. However, during emotional and psychiatric distress, this is particularly important.
- make appropriate manipulations of the environment or take action on behalf of the client. This would include practical things like phoning a spouse to inform them that they are recommending that the client be admitted to a hospital.

Therapists must be able to use a wide range of interventions, such as:
- minimal encouragement
- silence
- approval and reassurance
- provision of information
- direct guidance
- confrontation
- nonverbal reference
- self-disclosure.

It is important to be able to clarify, ask closed and open-ended questions, paraphrase and restate, summarise and reflect.

### 37.4.1 Indications

Supportive psychotherapy is especially suited to clients who have specific problems and where psychodynamic psychotherapy and cognitive behavioural therapy (CBT) are not indicated or appropriate. It may be used in the context of mood and anxiety disorders as well as psychotic disorders such as schizophrenia. In psychotic disorders, supportive psychotherapy may be particularly useful in the early stages of the first episode, during an acute relapse and during the maintenance phase. Many psychiatric patients on psychotropic agents have benefitted from supportive psychotherapy, regardless of their diagnosis, as have their families.

### 37.4.2 Challenges

It may be difficult for the therapist to adapt to the client's character organisation. It is important to be able to intervene in ways that are familiar to, and compatible with, the client's overall character structure (for example, if the client has an obsessional type of character structure, the therapist's interventions might include a cognitive and intellectualised style). Managing regression may also be challenging; in supportive therapy it is important to minimise regression or to reverse it where possible, or avoid promoting further regression through the therapist's behaviour, interventions or interactions.

## 37.5 Cognitive behavioural therapy

CBT is a relatively short-term, goal-directed, problem-focused treatment that is fundamentally based on the assumption that changing cognitions (thoughts) is possible and leads to behavioural change (Dobson, 1999). It involves active participation by the client, as well as homework assignments such as diarising thoughts, feelings and behaviour.

### 37.5.1 Indications

CBT can help clients with a variety of emotional conditions. Of the psychiatric disorders, it is mostly suited to clients with anxiety disorders, such as obsessive compulsive disorder (OCD), panic disorder, social anxiety disorder (SAD) and mood disorders such as depression. CBT is also a useful modality in the treatment of eating disorders. In order to benefit from CBT, clients must be able to engage adequately, and be relatively psychologically minded. They must be prepared to be an active partner in the therapeutic process, to complete homework assignments and to be subject to monitoring by the therapist.

### 37.5.2 Basic principles

Therapists should be able to:

- state the cognitive model (the mind or thinking and perceptions affect the way we behave and feel; therefore, changing our thoughts will change the way we feel and behave)
- socialise the client into the cognitive model
- use structured cognitive model activities (mood check, bridging to prior session, agenda setting, homework review, capsule summaries and client feedback)
- identify and elicit automatic thoughts (automatic thoughts are thoughts that 'jump' into the person's mind without them actively thinking about them)
- state and employ knowledge of the cognitive triad of depression. The triad of depression is Aaron Beck's concept of depression as consisting of a person's negative view of self, negative interpretation of experience and negative expectation of the future (Kaplan and Sadock, 1991)
- use the client's dysfunctional thought record as a tool in therapy. Dysfunctional thoughts are those thoughts that do not serve any useful function to the client. Since dysfunctional thoughts reinforce the client's patterns of thinking and behaviour, and hence the pathology, they are, in fact, counterproductive. A thought record is a record (e.g. diary) of dysfunctional thoughts that the person may experience, which is then brought to the therapy session and the client is assisted to manage these
- identify common cognitive errors in thinking. These are misinterpretations or evaluations of situations and thoughts that lead to patterns of thinking that are maladaptive (e.g. **catastrophising**)
- use activity scheduling as a tool in therapy. The therapist encourages the client to schedule activities that the client has to do but that normally makes them anxious, ranging from least anxiety provoking to most anxiety provoking
- use behavioural techniques as a tool in therapy
- plan booster sessions, follow-up and self-help sessions appropriately with clients when terminating active therapy.

### 37.5.3 Challenges

As clients have to be active participants, there may be difficulties if they are unable to verbalise their thoughts, feelings and emotions adequately, refuse to engage sufficiently and if homework tasks are not completed.

Clients who are not of a certain level of psychological mindedness and/or intellectual/cognitive capacity will also not be able to benefit fully and appropriately.

Clients with deep-seated emotional issues who are not willing to work in the 'here and now' may not derive optimal benefit from CBT and may be better suited to another form of therapy (e.g. psychodynamic psychotherapy).

Clients with severe medical conditions may not benefit from CBT either. For example, clients who suffer from cognitive disorders such as dementia or neurocognitive impairment due to HIV/Aids may not be able to engage and apply their minds appropriately.

The therapist should ensure that CBT is undertaken at an appropriate time: patients with psychiatric conditions who are currently too ill may not be able to engage adequately.

## 37.6 Dialectical behaviour therapy

Dialectical behaviour therapy (DBT) is a highly structured form of psychotherapy that was initially developed by Marsha Linehan (1993) to address the chronic parasuicidal behaviour of women with a diagnosis of borderline personality disorder (BPD). Linehan (1993) describes borderline personality disorder as a disorder of the emotional regulation system. Emotional dysregulation stems from high emotional vulnerability and an inability to regulate emotions. The key characteristics of emotional vulnerability include high sensitivity to emotional intensity and a slow return to emotional baseline levels. In short, a seemingly minor trigger event may provoke an extreme and enduring emotional reaction in the sufferer.

## 37.6.1 Indications

DBT has been subjected to thorough empirical exploration. At least two randomised control trials have demonstrated that DBT is more effective than other therapies in reducing self-harm, length of hospital admissions, inappropriate anger and in improving social adjustment and employment performance (Linehan, 1993).

Initially developed specifically to treat clients with borderline personality disorder, DBT is increasingly being adapted to treat a range of other seemingly intractable mental health problems that may involve emotional instability. These include substance dependence, binge eating, anger problems and depression.

## 37.6.2 Basic principles

DBT is usually implemented in a group setting over a period of 4–6 weeks. It is a highly standardised form of treatment with a manual for facilitators to use in implementing the programme. Group members are encouraged to share and discuss their progress and challenges with each other and to reflect on homework tasks that they are given after each session. Sessions normally take place twice a week.

DBT uses four key modules to equip clients with skills to address the problem areas of emotional regulation and interpersonal relationships. The four key modules include:

- mindfulness
- distress tolerance
- emotional regulation and
- interpersonal effectiveness.

### 37.6.2.1 Mindfulness

The core skills module of mindfulness addresses self-dysregulation and cognitive dysregulation. Mindfulness skills are psychological and behavioural versions of meditation skills usually taught in Eastern spiritual practices (Linehan, 1993). Often, clients with borderline personality disorder find themselves making emotional choices. An important treatment goal is to help them move away from exclusive reliance on their 'emotional mind' to using both emotional and rational input to make balanced decisions, called wise-mind decisions. Patients are taught to use six mindfulness skills to facilitate observing their experiences in non-judgemental ways and putting their observations into words to help make a transition from 'emotional mind' to 'wise mind'. Focused use of these skills ultimately increases their effectiveness in coping with difficult situations, for example:

- 'what' skills: observing, describing, participating
- 'how' skills: nonjudgementally, one thing at a time, effectively.

### 37.6.2.2 Distress tolerance

The distress tolerance skills module targets behavioural dysregulation and impulsivity and includes both crisis survival skills (distracting oneself, self-soothing using the five senses, making a list of pros and cons) and radical acceptance skills. These skills help the client to tolerate seemingly intolerable, painful circumstances without engaging in impulsive behaviour like parasuicide and/or high-risk sexual, substance-related or other dangerous behaviour.

### 37.6.2.3 Emotional regulation

The emotional regulation skills module addresses emotional dysregulation. The client is taught how to reduce emotional vulnerability, increase positive experiences (resulting in positive emotions) and change current emotions by acting oppositely. The goals are to understand and identify emotions so as to better manage these using the coping skills taught.

#### 37.6.2.4 Interpersonal effectiveness

The interpersonal effectiveness skills module addresses interpersonal problems and teaches clients how to negotiate to get what they want while maintaining good relationships and self-respect.

### 37.6.3 Challenges

Work with the client often has to be accompanied by similar interventions with family, friends and loved ones in order to enable a reinforcement of the skills learnt as part of DBT in the client's social and family context. It may be difficult at times to ensure compliance and involvement of family members who may have become frustrated or given up hope for the client.

In order for the intervention to be successful, the group has to remain consistent with regards to its members. Thus, once a group has started it is not possible for new members to join and existing members have to comply and be present for each session for the treatment to move along the standardised method. As a result, member drop-out can have consequences for group morale and the motivation of other group members.

## 37.7 Family therapy

Family therapy is a branch of psychotherapy that works with families and couples to enable change. Change is viewed in terms of the systems of interaction between family members as well as relationships between family members.

The origins of family therapy, as a branch of psychotherapy, can be traced to the early 20th century with the emergence of the child guidance movement and marriage counselling. The formal development of family therapy has taken place through the work of various independent clinicians and groups in the United Kingdom (John Bowlby at the Tavistock Clinic), the United States (John Elderkin Bell, Nathan Ackerman, Christian Midelfort, Theodore Lidz, Lyman Wynne, Murray Bowen, Carl Whitaker, Virginia Satir) and Hungary (DLP Liebermann), who began seeing family members together for observation or therapy sessions. There was initially a strong influence from psychoanalysis (most of the early founders of the field had psychoanalytic backgrounds) and social psychiatry, and later from learning theory and behaviour therapy.

The movement received an important boost in the mid-1950s through the work of anthropologist Gregory Bateson and colleagues – Jay Haley, Donald D. Jackson, John Weakland, William Fry, and later, Virginia Satir, Paul Watzlawick and others – at Palo Alto in the United States, who introduced ideas from **cybernetics** and general systems theory into social psychology and psychotherapy, focusing in particular on the role of communication.

By the mid-1960s, a number of distinct schools of family therapy had emerged. From those groups that were most strongly influenced by cybernetics and systems theory, there came Brief Therapy and, slightly later, Strategic Family Therapy, Salvador Minuchin's Structural Family Therapy and the Milan Systems model. Structural family therapy emphasises the readjustment of the structural aspects of the family to ensure effective functioning of the family unit. Interventions within this model may include making sure that parental sub-systems and child sub-systems are clearly defined and delineated in a family where children may find themselves called on to take a parental role which they experience as overwhelming.

Partly in reaction to some aspects of these systemic models, came the experiential approaches of Virginia Satir and Carl Whitaker, which downplayed theoretical constructs and emphasised subjective experience and unexpressed feelings (including the subconscious), authentic communication, spontaneity, creativity and total therapist engagement. Members of the extended family were often included.

### 37.7.1 Indications

Family therapy is useful in situations in which a client's problematic behaviour or psychological difficulty is influenced heavily by the family system of which that client is a member. For example, a child may present with severe anxiety symptoms that are largely related to the marital conflict between his or her parents. In addition to this, the child in question or 'identified patient' may also have an older sibling who presents with negative acting-out behaviour such as playing truant from school and getting into fights with peers and teachers. It may also be useful in cases where a child presents with symptoms as a result of feeling torn between his or her parents who may repeatedly try to draw the child into an alliance against the other parent.

## 37.7.2 Basic principles

The number of sessions depends on the situation, but the average is 5–20 sessions. A family therapist usually meets several members of the family at the same time. This has the advantage of making differences between the ways family members perceive mutual relations, as well as interaction patterns in the session, apparent to both the therapist and the family. These patterns frequently mirror habitual interaction patterns at home, even though the therapist is now incorporated into the family system. Therapy interventions usually focus on relationship patterns rather than on analysing impulses of the unconscious mind or early childhood trauma of an individual as a Freudian therapist would do. This approach involves a moving away from the traditional focus on individual psychology and historical factors (that involve so-called linear causation and content) and rather emphasises feedback and homeostatic mechanisms and 'rules' in here-and-now interactions (so-called circular causation and process) that are thought to maintain or exacerbate problems, whatever the original cause(s). Circular causation in a family refers to the process where each family member's behaviour influences and has an impact on the behaviour of the other members in a circular fashion. For example, a father's aggressive behaviour will influence the behaviour of the other members in the family whose actions in turn will have an impact on each other and the father's aggressive behaviour.

Some family therapists may also make use of the genogram (see Figure 37.1) to help to elucidate the patterns of relationship across generations.

Family therapists are relational therapists: they are generally more interested in what goes on between individuals rather than within one or more individuals. Depending on the conflicts at issue and the progress of therapy to date, a therapist may either focus on analysing specific previous instances of conflict (e.g. in reviewing a past incident and suggesting alternative ways family members might have responded to one another during it) or proceed directly to addressing the sources of conflict at a more abstract level (e.g. by pointing out patterns of interaction that the family might have not noticed).

Family therapists tend to be more interested in the maintenance and/or solving of problems rather than in trying to identify a single cause. Some families may perceive cause-effect analyses as attempts to allocate blame to one or more individuals, with the consequence that for many families a focus on causation is of little or no clinical utility. It is important to note that a circular way of problem evaluation is used as opposed to a linear route. Using this method, families can be helped by finding patterns of behaviour, what the causes are and what can be done to improve the situation.

## 37.7.3 Challenges

Family therapy requires the participation and commitment of the entire family. This can sometimes be difficult to carry out in practice. Some therapists adapt their technique to make constructive use of the absence of various members: for example, they may use an empty chair and ask other members to anticipate how the absent member may have reacted to things said.

The 'circular causality' approach can be difficult to implement in contexts where there is an emphasis on linear thinking and approaches in teaching and practice. It may take some time, training and supervision to adjust the manner in which one hypothesises and formulates problems.

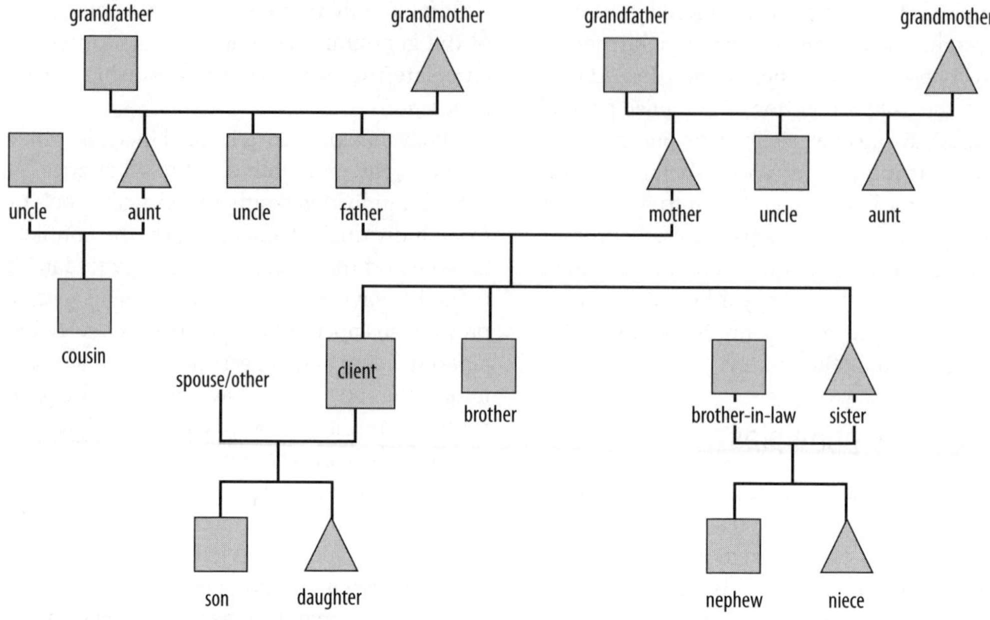


**Figure 37.1** Example of a genogram

In family therapy approaches that require two therapists (who act as co-therapists) or where a reflecting team (which observe the process behind a one-way mirror) is required, it may be difficult to find enough therapists to comply with these requirements in contexts where resources are minimal or limited.

# 37.8 Group therapy

Group therapy is a type of psychotherapeutic intervention that involves one or more therapists working with several people at the same time. Group therapy can stand alone as an intervention, but it is also commonly integrated into a multifaceted treatment plan that may include individual therapy, medication as well as other interventions. Group therapy also does not fall into one particular modality or another but can be implemented using various theoretical perspectives and orientations, for example, psychodynamic group therapy. Group therapy has often successfully incorporated techniques from art and music therapy (in the form of drawing, movement and drama) to facilitate the group members' negotiation and exploration of certain areas of difficulty.

## 37.8.1 Basic principles

*The Theory and Practice of Group Psychotherapy* (Yalom and Lesczc, 2005), outlines the key therapeutic principles that have been derived from self-reports from individuals involved in the group therapy process (see Table 37.3).

## 37.8.2 How does group therapy work?

Groups can be as small as three or four people, but group therapy sessions generally involve seven to twelve individuals (although it is possible to have more participants). The group typically meets once or twice each week for an hour or two.

The minimum number of group therapy sessions is usually six, but a full year of sessions is more common. These sessions may either be

**Table 37.3** Principles of group therapy

- The instillation of hope: the group contains members at different stages of the treatment process; seeing people who are coping or recovering gives hope to those at the beginning of the process.
- Universality: being in a group of people experiencing the same things helps people see that what they are going through is universal and that they are not alone.
- Imparting information: group members are able to help each other by sharing information.
- Altruism: group members are able to share their strengths and help others in the group, which can boost self-esteem and confidence.
- The corrective recapitulation of the primary family group: the therapy group is much like a family in some ways. Within the group, each member can explore how childhood experiences contributed to personality and behaviour. They can also learn to avoid behaviour that is destructive or unhelpful in their real life.
- Development of socialisation techniques: the group setting is a great place to practice new behaviour. The setting is safe and supportive and allows group members to experiment without the fear of failure.
- Imitative behaviour: individuals can model the behaviour of other members of the group or observe and imitate the behaviour of the therapist.
- Interpersonal learning: by interacting with other people and receiving feedback from the group and the therapist, each individual can gain a greater understanding of himself or herself.
- Group cohesiveness: because the group is united in a common goal, members gain a sense of belonging and acceptance.
- **Catharsis**: sharing feelings and experiences with a group of people can help relieve pain, guilt or stress.
- Existential factors: while working within a group offers support and guidance, group therapy helps member realize that they are responsible for their own lives, action and choices.

**Source:** Yalom and Lesczc, 2005

open or closed. In open sessions, new participants are welcome to join at any time. In a closed group, only a core group of members are invited to participate (Manor, 1994).

So what does a typical group therapy session look like? In many cases, the group will meet in a room where the chairs are arranged in a large circle so that each member can see every other person in the group (Dies, 1993). A session might begin with each member of the group introducing themselves and sharing why they are in group therapy, or members might share their experiences and progress since the last meeting.

The specific manner in which the session is conducted depends largely on the goals of the group and the style of the therapist. Some therapists might encourage a more free-form style of dialogue, where each member participates as he or she sees fit. Other therapists might have a specific plan for each session that might include having clients practise new skills with other members of the group.

## 37.8.3 Indications

Group therapy can be very effective, especially in certain situations. Studies have shown that group therapy can be an effective treatment choice for depression and traumatic stress (Etchegoyen, 2000). Group therapy allows people to receive the support and encouragement of the other members of the group. People participating in the group are able to see that others are experiencing the same thing, which can help them feel less alone. Group members can serve as role models to other members of the group. By seeing someone who is successfully coping with a problem, other members of the group can see that there is hope and recovery is possible. As each person progresses, they can in turn serve as a role model and support figure for others. This can help foster feelings of success and accomplishment. Group therapy is very cost effective: instead of focusing on just one client at a time, the therapist can devote his or her time to a much larger group of people. Group therapy offers a safe haven. The setting allows people to practice behaviours and actions within the safety and security of the group. By working in a group, the therapist can see first-hand how each person responds to other people and behaves in social situations. Using this information, the therapist can provide valuable feedback to each client.

## 37.9 Trauma counselling

Not everybody who experiences a traumatic event will develop post-traumatic stress disorder (PTSD), which is an anxiety disorder (see Chapter 15: Acute reactions to adverse life events). PTSD is a psychiatric condition with specific criteria and that develops after a traumatic event during which time the individual felt horror and out of control. Even people who do not experience all of the symptoms of PTSD may benefit from trauma counselling. Remember that most people will recover with minimal effects. Trauma counselling combines principles of supportive therapy and CBT and focuses on the actual trauma experience and how it has affected the person. Clients are encouraged to remember and focus on the experienced trauma (trauma-focused therapy). There is an emphasis on helping the client to increase his or her coping skills for current here-and-now stressors to improve daily functioning and decrease symptoms. There are three main stages:

- establishing trust and safety
- dealing with symptoms of trauma in a supportive manner
- integration.

### 37.9.1 Indications

Victims of trauma may experience symptoms of a sufficient magnitude such that intervention is required. In general, 'debriefing' (a singular cathartic experience, usually in a group format setting during which time victims of trauma tell their story) is contraindicated, as studies have shown that this may have an increased risk of re-traumatising the client, with the future development of PTSD. Trauma counselling is indicated when victims experience ongoing difficulties or symptoms such as sleep disturbances, thinking about the event a lot, re-experiencing the traumatic event as if it is happening again, nightmares, depression, irritability and aggression, numbing and avoidance symptoms. They do not necessarily need medication.

### 37.9.2 Challenges

Building trust can be difficult in the face of trauma, particularly when trauma was of an interpersonal nature (e.g. rape). It is of the utmost importance for the therapist to be patient and sensitive. If not conducted appropriately, there is the risk of symptoms worsening, particularly if the trauma was complex, or chronic and ongoing. It may be difficult to distinguish whether the symptoms are not better accounted for by serious mental illnesses (e.g. frank PTSD or major depression). It is important to know when to refer these particular clients for more appropriate therapies and/or medication. (Also see Chapter 15: Acute reactions to adverse life events.)

### 37.9.3 Basic principles of trauma counselling

Basic principles should include the following:

- telling and retelling the story
- normalising emotions
- psycho-education
- processing the trauma.

NB: Telling and retelling the story should not be confused with debriefing (see Advanced reading block 37.1). While the former is viewed as a necessary step in the trauma counselling process, aimed at getting the person to process the trauma and preparing them for the next step (normalising emotions) the latter is a once-off process, without sufficient emphasis on the processing of the trauma.

## 37.1 Advanced reading block

**Debriefing: Is it useful or harmful? Can it cause PTSD?**

Psychological debriefing is an intervention (often in the form of sessions that last two hours with 10–20 participants) that is conducted by trained professionals shortly after a traumatic event. It allows victims to talk about their experience and receive information of normal types of reactions to such an event. The best-known form of debriefing is critical incident stress debriefing (CISD). However, its many modifications and variations have led to the use of the more general term 'psychological debriefing'. Proponents of psychological debriefing believe it can abort the onset of a serious mental disorder, reduce the severity and duration of **serious mental disorders** once it has occurred or prevent acute stress reactions from progressing to a chronic and incapacitating PTSD or some other debilitating psychiatric disorder. During the intervention, the group shares facts about the traumatic event and collectively review their thoughts, impressions and emotional reactions. The facilitator normalises many of their emotions and provides resources such as materials related to the normal stress response and contact details of a mental health practitioner and treatment centres should their symptoms not subside.

Despite its popularity, research (several rigorous, randomised clinical trials) suggests that debriefing recipients either receive no benefit or actually experience a worsening of symptoms. Reasons for the consistent failure and possibly counterproductive effect of debriefing on recovery may be related to the following:

- forcing premature exposure to traumatic memories may actually interfere with a natural recovery process that allows the traumatic material to be consolidated and then to fade from conscious awareness
- debriefing may actually interfere with habituation and cognitive changes that are essential for normal recovery.

An early focus on acute post-traumatic symptoms may foster negative cognitions about oneself. Negative cognitions predict the later development of PTSD. (Friedman, 2012) (Also see Chapter 15: Acute reactions to adverse life events.)

## Conclusion

There are a wide range of psychological therapies available, some of which have a huge evidence base for the treatment of many psychiatric disorders. Many psychiatric clients and their families/caregivers can benefit from a form of psychotherapy that is tailored to their needs in terms of: diagnosis, timing with the course of their illness, character organisation, insight and desire for therapy.

# References

Dies RR (1993) Research on group psychotherapy: Overview and clinical applications. In: Alonso A, Swiller HI (Eds). *Group Therapy in Clinical Practice*. Washington, DC: American Psychiatric Press

Dobson KS (1999) *Handbook of Cognitive Behavioural Therapies* (2nd edition). New York: Guilford Press

Etchegoyen H (2000) *The Fundamentals of Psychoanalytic Technique*. London: Karnac Books

Friedman MJ (2012) *Posttraumatic and Acute Stress Disorders*. Ontario: Jones and Bartlett Learning

Gabbard G (2010) *Long-term Psychodynamic Psychotherapy: A Basic Text* (2nd edition). (Core Competencies in Psychotherapy. California: American Psychiatric Publishing

Kaplan H, Sadock B (1991) *Synopsis of Psychiatry: Behavioural Sciences in Clinical Psychiatry* (6th edition). Baltimore: Williams and Wilkins

Linehan MM (1993) *Skills Training Manual for Treating Borderline Personality Disorder.* New York: Guildford Press

Manor O (1994) Group psychotherapy. In: Clarkson P, Pokorny M (Eds). *The Handbook of Psychotherapy.* New York, NY: Routledge

McDermut W, Miller IW, Brown RA (2001) The efficacy of group psychotherapy for depression: A meta-analysis and review of the empirical research. *Clinical Psychology: Science and Practice* 8: 98–116

Naidu T, Ramlall S (2008) Establishing psychiatric registrars' competence in psychotherapy: A portfolio based model. *African Journal of Psychiatry* 11: 264–71

Yalom ID, Lesczc M (2005) *The Theory and Practice of Group Psychotherapy*. New York, NY: Basic Books

CHAPTER

# 38 Social interventions in psychiatry

John Parker, Orlando Alonso Betancourt

## 38.1 Introduction

As medical historians (Porter, 1987) and others (Foucault, 1971), have noted, the origins of psychiatry as a discipline are closely associated with the care (or at least detention) of people who suffer from mental illness in various forms of institutions and more recently, in hospitals. It thus follows that for most of its history, psychiatry has had an orientation that is primarily towards the medical and biological care of an isolated patient. The origin of the wide range of social interventions that are commonly described under the concept of **psychosocial rehabilitation** is therefore closely linked to the closure of the large institutions and the relocation of care to the community.

It should be noted however, as Foucault (1971) points out, that the creation of the institutions themselves was also an act of social intervention, if not one that was necessarily beneficial for those who were detained there. Any understanding of social interventions should, therefore, begin with the history of the large asylums, the rather extensive and rapid expansion of these institutions and their even more abrupt closure in the process of **deinstitutionalisation** (which led to a variety of new problems) but ultimately has driven community-based care.

These shifts are of course, reflective of a more general transformation in the field of health care provision from an emphasis on tertiary care to one that is focused at the primary level on treatment and prevention in the community. In the case of mental health care provision, the imperative for this change in focus has been given added impetus, both by epidemiological work that has shown that mental health disorders make a major and growing contribution to global disease burdens (Mayosi *et al.*, 2009), and also through an increasing recognition of the contribution of social factors towards the development of mental illness (Leff, 2010).

From a global perspective, it is clear that these processes are by no means uniform throughout the world, with a variety of experiences and circumstances described. Valuable lessons can be learnt from a range of systems in various stages of development and from innovations in approach that have emerged with increased focus on care in the community.

## 38.2 Deinstitutionalisation

### 38.2.1 Definition

Deinstitutionalisation essentially refers to the depopulation of large psychiatric institutions, which was an important component of policy in Europe and the USA in particular, beginning in the middle to late 20th century. As a component of the provision of comprehensive psychiatric care, however, it should be defined as the replacement of long-stay psychiatric hospitals with smaller, less isolated community-based alternatives for the care of mentally ill people (Bachrach, 1996). In this context it can be understood as consisting of three components:

- the release of persons residing in psychiatric hospitals to alternative placements in the community
- the diversion of potential new admissions to alternative facilities

- the development of special services for the care of a non-institutionalised mentally ill population (Lamb and Bachrach, 2001).

## 38.2.2 History of the institution

Perhaps the earliest purpose-built psychiatric hospitals were established in the Islamic empire between the eighth and tenth centuries. These were known as Bimaristans; records show that Ahmad ibn Tulun built one such hospital in 872 in Cairo to care for the 'insane' (Koenig, 2005) with early historical records suggesting that the humane care offered in these institutions made an impression on early European travellers.

This does not, however, seem to have been maintained in medieval Europe, when some of the most severely mentally ill were housed in institutional settings such as monasteries or, in some parts, in purpose-built settings known as *Narrentüme* (fools' towers) and occasionally in extensions to hospitals (Porter, 2006). The first purpose-built psychiatric institution in the United Kingdom, the Priory of Saint Mary of Bethlehem (which later became known as Bethlem or more notoriously as Bedlam) was founded in 1247, but records show it only housed six male inmates at the start of the 15th century. This pattern of relatively little hospital care for those with a mental illness was to be maintained until at least the start of the 18th century when Bethlem was still the only public asylum in Britain, with only 100 inmates.

The next two centuries saw a radical change, with the development of institutional confinement as the principal way of dealing with most individuals who were deemed to be mentally ill. By the end of the 18th century there were at least five public institutions and a far larger number of privately run ones. By 1900 there were more than 100 000 inmates in psychiatric institutions in the UK (Porter, 2006). Although a feature of this era was the development of more humane treatments as pioneered by Phillipe Pinel after the French Revolution, it has also been asserted that these large institutions were not only the birthplace of the discipline of psychiatry, but that psychiatrists (or alienists as they were then known) in these institutions were co-opted as agents of social control (Porter, 1987). This was a time of major cultural change that became known as the Age of Enlightenment. The philosopher Michel Foucault argues that the growth of the asylums occurred as an act of social exclusion that took place as a result of society's newly found obsession with rationality and its need to purge society of its unreasonable elements. He argues that the so-called moral treatments were, in effect, efforts at enforcing conformity (Foucault, 1971).

## 38.2.3 The era of deinstitutionalisation

With a rapid population growth and little in the way of effective treatment so that few patients were ever discharged, this situation could not go on forever. By the early to mid-1900s the demand for institutional places led to costs that were in excess of what governments were prepared to spend. Conditions deteriorated and the institutions became notorious as places of overcrowding, poor treatment, neglect and abuse. However, by the end of the 20th century, particularly in the United States and Europe, the number of in-patients in psychiatric hospitals had been radically reduced. To use the example of the US, the population of state and county psychiatric hospitals fell from 553 979 in 1954 to 61 722 in 1996; during the same period 120 hospitals were closed (Geller, 2000).

A number of factors seem to have led to this sudden change in the way psychiatry was practiced. These include the following:

- the pioneering work of former military psychiatrists in Britain after World War II, who, as a result of witnessing the rapid improvement of serious symptoms in soldiers removed from the battlefield, had developed a new optimism with regard to recovery from mental disorder. As a result they developed out–patient clinics and began to discharge patients (Leff, 2010)
- the advent of effective antipsychotic medication, following the first successful use of chlorpromazine for psychosis in 1952 (Kaplan *et al.*, 1994)

- the growing wave of public antipathy towards psychiatric institutions as the abuses and poor conditions became more widely known
- the growth of mental health care user/survivor groups and the development of disability activism
- an assumption that community-based care would both be more humane and more therapeutic than hospital-based care (Lamb and Bachrach, 2001)
- a variety of political arguments based to some degree on human rights concerns but also on the need to reduce spending (Stroman, 2003).

## 38.2.4 Sudden deinstitutionalisation and its consequences

The latter part of the 20th century saw the large-scale closure of psychiatric facilities in the United States and Europe, which led to fundamental changes in the way psychiatry was practiced. These changes have had a number of consequences, both good and bad, from which a number of critical lessons can be learnt. These are lessons that developing nations, such as South Africa, that were either not part of the deinstitutionalisation wave, or have adopted these policies more recently, would do well to consider.

Undoubtedly, the most positive outcome of deinstitutionalisation was the disappearance of the huge asylums and with them, the potential for human rights abuses, as well as the loss of individuality that came as a consequence of what is known as the 'total institution' (Goffman, 1961). This coincided with the development of a wider range of more effective medications, an expanded scope of practice outside of the asylums, and the diversification of care with both sub-specialisation and the advent of multiple venues where care of different forms can take place (Novella, 2010). The latter has given impetus to psychosocial rehabilitation and the recovery movement. De-linked from the profoundly negative association with the institutions, psychiatry has steadily gained recognition as a mainstream medical discipline and psychiatric treatment has become socially more acceptable. Where all three elements of deinstitutionalisation have been properly implemented, the result has been greatly improved quality of care and a significant degree of normalisation in the lives of those who were once condemned to a lifetime of confinement (Lamb and Bachrach, 2001).

The consequences of suffering from a severe mental illness were not entirely positive in countries where the enthusiasm for cost-cutting hospital closures was not matched in the development of alternatives (Bloom, 2010). The most obvious negative consequence has been the emergence of large numbers of people with severe mental illnesses becoming homeless after being discharged from psychiatric hospitals (Scott, 1993). There have also been increases in the numbers of mentally ill persons incarcerated in prisons (Bloom, 2010), whilst others have been housed in smaller, even less well-regulated facilities (Novella, 2010). It has even been argued that those who were meant to benefit most from the closure of the old institutions, the indigent severely mentally ill, have fared worst as a result of the new reforms (Grove, 1994).

The reasons why this has happened have become clearer in retrospect:

- The successful placement of a person living with a chronic mental illness in a community setting requires substantial effort and resources which, when properly assessed, are unlikely to translate into any substantial financial saving over a long-term hospital admission (Okin, 1978).
- Substance dependence disorders have emerged on a large scale amongst people with chronic and severe mental illness. Known as a dual diagnosis, this results in exacerbation of the primary disorder, which in turn complicates treatment of dependence. It also tends to reduce the likelihood of adherence to psychosocial rehabilitation programmes and leads to problems in areas such as accommodation and work.
- Throughout the world, deinstitutionalisation has happened at a time when social spending has generally been reduced, with fewer

funds available for housing schemes and other support systems.

- The ability of families and other community resources to provide support has also been reduced with social changes, such as urbanisation, the shift to smaller family size, higher divorce rates and declines in the number of 'stay at home parents' (Novella, 2010).
- The emergence of widespread unemployment has made vocational rehabilitation a far greater challenge than in the past.
- In some areas community resistance has emerged as a significant factor.
- Some authors have suggested that 'the new generation of severely mentally ill persons' (individuals who were not previously institutionalised) has proved far less willing to engage in community-based programmes than their predecessors who had, to various degrees, been conditioned into a state of relative compliance (Lamb and Bachrach, 2001).
- The scope of mental health care has broadened considerably and less severe forms of mental illness are increasingly recognised. The result is that many of the services that have been made available at community level have been taken up by a less disabled population, leaving many of those who most need it, without help (Grove, 1994).

### 38.2.5 Lessons learnt

Perhaps, more than anything else, we have learnt the true meaning of the bio-psycho-social approach to mental illness from the experience of deinstitutionalisation. It has become clear that creating conditions that allow for recovery to take place involves more than just attending to the biological needs of an individual such as medication, food and shelter. It requires that attention is paid to individual circumstances, needs and hopes and it also demands that we see care from a social context, one that attends to the wide range of factors in society that impact on a person with mental illness such as prejudice and discrimination.

Moving from a hospital-centred orientation to one focused in the community is thus a process of ongoing social change. It demands a far more individualised form of care that takes into account the fact that people with a mental illness are a highly diverse group and that they come from a variety of cultural backgrounds. This requires that services become more flexible and responsive to the needs of those who are living with a mental illness, which can only happen if their voices are taken into account in the planning of services.

Finally, it has become clear that whilst services need to diversify and broaden extensively, it is the most vulnerable that fall through the gaps if this happens in a fragmented way. Continuity of care thus becomes paramount in the planning and development of services. This continuity begins with the individual needs of each person living with a mental illness and extends into all spheres of their lives. This kind of care has been formulated under the concept of psychosocial rehabilitation and its more recent development, the recovery movement.

## 38.3 Psychosocial rehabilitation

### 38.3.1 Concept and history

Psychosocial rehabilitation is the process of restoring the social functioning and well-being of an individual who has a psychiatric disability. Psychosocial rehabilitation work undertaken by psychiatrists, social workers and other mental health professionals (usually psychologists and occupational therapists) aims to bring about changes in a person's ability to deal with his or her environment and the person's environment itself, and in doing so, to facilitate the improvement in symptoms or personal distress. These services often 'combine pharmacological treatment, independent living and social skills training, psychological support to clients and their families, housing, vocational rehabilitation, social support and network enhancement, and access to leisure activities' (National Institute for Mental Health, 1999).

The importance and validity of community-based rehabilitation programmes for patients with schizophrenia and other chronic psychotic disorders has been well documented in the literature under different names and approaches. The following broad types of social intervention have been studied:

- specialised modalities for the delivery of mental health care in the community, including the community mental health team (CMHT) approach and its refinements (such as crisis intervention (CI)), intensive case management (ICM) (including assertive community treatment (ACT) and early intervention)
- vocational support
- residential care and alternatives to hospital admission
- family interventions
- skills training and illness self-management
- cognitive interventions (cognitive therapy and cognitive rehabilitation)
- integrated treatment of substance use disorders and severe mental illness (International Journal of Psychosocial Rehabilitation, 2010).

## 38.3.2 Modalities for delivery of mental health care in the community

### 38.3.2.1 The community mental health team

The community mental health team (CMHT) approach involves the use of a specialised multidisciplinary team for the care of people with, primarily, severe mental illness in the community. These teams originated in France and Britain in the 1950s in conjunction with the closure of psychiatric hospitals and the advent of home-based care; they have since become a standard feature of community-based care in most high-income countries as well as many others.

Most commonly CMHTs consist of a psychiatrist, nurses and social workers and may also have occupational therapists, psychologists, vocational counsellors and substance dependence counsellors in the team. The role and degree of involvement of the psychiatrist may vary between that of team leader, occasional supervisor and team resource or team member. This multidisciplinary make-up allows for a rounded holistic approach, with the availability of specialised care, but the team approach also allows for personalised care with some overlap of roles in the care of individual patients. Case management is a characteristic feature of this personalised care, which involves the practice of individual team members carrying a discrete caseload. Caseload size is, however, a critical factor that must be controlled if the CMHT is to operate effectively. Additional important aspects of the CMHTs function is initial assessment by the team and regular team reviews with a system of determining the extent of care required by each client at any particular time (Burns, 2010). Most CMHTs operate as community-based secondary care, in that they require referral from another health professional rather than being directly accessible by members of the community.

Despite the widespread establishment of such teams, the evidence-base in support of their use is very thin, with most of the research being done in high-resource settings. A review (Malone *et al.*, 2007) found that CMHT management is not inferior to non-team standard care in any important respects and is superior in promoting greater acceptance of treatment. It may also be superior in reducing hospital admissions and preventing death by suicide; however, the lack of research into comparing CMHT management to standard care was highlighted as a serious concern. It should be noted, however, that most research has been done in resource-rich settings where primary care centres are not overburdened. It is likely that such teams offer an advantage in settings where patients with mental illness struggle to be seen in primary care (such as in much of southern Africa).

### 38.3.2.2 Intensive case management and assertive community treatment

Intensive Case Management (ICM) consists of the management of the mental health problem and of the rehabilitation and social support needs of the person concerned, over an indefinite period of time, by a team of people who have a fairly small group of clients (less than 20). It also offers 24-hour help and sees clients in a non-clinical setting.

A review (Dietrich *et al.*, 2010) showed that ICM was superior to standard care in terms of patient retention, general functioning, likelihood of getting a job, retaining accommodation and of length of stay in hospital (especially where there were previously very long stays in hospital).

Assertive community treatment (ACT) is understood as a specific form of ICM that was developed in the USA in the 1970s with the specific aim to help patients who struggle to remain out of hospital to live more successfully in the community. Following the extremely positive findings of the first randomised controlled trials on this form of care in the USA (Stein and Test, 1980) the model was adapted widely in the USA, the UK and elsewhere in the world.

Essential features of the ACT model include the following:

- a core team that is responsible for assisting patients in meeting all their needs and providing clinical care
- staff to patient ratios are small (no more than 1:15)
- engagement and follow-up are assertive
- the primary goal is improved patient functioning in the widest possible range of bio-psycho-social domains
- direct assistance with symptom management
- each patient is assigned a key worker but there is team involvement in all cases
- treatment plans are individualised and flexible
- treatment is provided in community settings
- care is continuous both over time and across functional areas
- the most likely criteria for referral include severe mental illness, heavy service use or multiple recent admissions (Kent and Burns, 2005).

Despite the extremely positive initial findings on the effectiveness of ACT as a mode of mental health care delivery, including a Cochrane review (Marshall and Lockwood, 2000) that led to its initial rapid uptake, the outcome of further research brought this into question (Killaspy *et al.*, 2009; Byford *et al.*, 2000). These findings, however, bear further interrogation, particularly in the context of southern Africa and other lower- and middle-income settings. A key finding in explaining such results has been that the 'standard care/treatment as usual' control groups have often been poorly defined and in many cases are reflective of what has been learnt from the early ACT and ICM programmes: that more comprehensive follow-up and the reduced caseloads that allow for this, lead to improved services. The differences between ACT programmes and this form of highly developed 'standard care' thus lose significance. In settings where standard care is markedly different from the ACT model, the findings have, predictably, been far more positive.

### Experience with ACT in South Africa – a modified assertive community-based treatment programme

In response to problems associated with pressures on psychiatric in-patient beds and the observation that one particular contributor to this was a cohort of patients who were admitted to these beds at a high frequency, the modified assertive community-based treatment (M-ACT) programme was introduced, with one team operating from each of three psychiatric hospitals in the Western Cape province of South Africa. Due to budgetary constraints the original ACT model was modified to allow for larger caseloads, a lower frequency of contacts, and teams that were based at the psychiatric hospitals but did most of their work in the community, rather than being primarily community-based. With an overall caseload of approximately 100 patients per team and a maximum of 35 cases per key worker, less frequent contacts and office-hours services with back-up from the psychiatric hospital, it is nevertheless still a vast improvement over local CMHT loads which typically consist of as many as 600 patients per (rather attenuated) CMHT and more than 250 caseloads per community psychiatric nurse. Not surprisingly, the intervention has proved highly effective with significantly improved outcome scores and reduced hospital admissions (Botha *et al.*, 2010).

### 38.3.2.3 Crisis intervention

Crisis intervention (CI) involves the provision of care outside of hospital by specialised teams during a crisis. These teams typically are made up of psychiatric nurses and social workers; the teams either have a psychiatrist on the team or the team has direct access to one. These teams evolved from the realisation that many individuals with a severe mental illness have poor networks of support in the community.

This model was developed in the United Kingdom as a way of reducing hospital admissions and length of stay in hospital. CI teams usually offer a 24-hour service that provides regular support, ongoing risk assessments and treatment in the home environment. In some cases admission to home-like environments outside of hospitals are offered.

Thus far, research (Murphy *et al.*, 2012) suggests that CI appears to reduce repeat admissions after the initial index crises. CI has also been shown to improve patient retention in programmes, to reduce the burden on the family and to result in an improved mental state over standard care, three months after the crisis. Not surprisingly, it is experienced as more satisfactory than hospitalisation by both patients and families. It seems to be a viable and desirable approach, although thus far there is insufficient evidence to determine its cost effectiveness.

### 38.3.2.4 Early intervention in psychosis

This model has a significant community-based component. This focused intervention is aimed primarily at preventing a potentially chronic course of illness and hospitalisation by ensuring early treatment and rehabilitation of individuals with early psychosis in a community setting.

### 38.3.2.5 Lessons for the southern African context

There can be little reason to suspect that any of the above-mentioned interventions would be anything but highly effective in local settings, particularly where large-scale deinstitutionalisation is either a relatively recent event or an ongoing one. However, in countries with such large treatment gaps, as is the case in southern African region (Seedat *et al.*, 2009; Jacobs *et al.*, 2007), the arguments for the cost effectiveness of such interventions often carry little weight with administrative and political authorities since they tend to have little immediate tangible effect on service use, unless provided on a massive scale. Additionally, as in the Western Cape, interventions tend to be based on existing services that remain highly centralised and focused on large hospitals. The major challenge is to develop models that are highly applicable to community-based settings and which can then be rolled out on a large scale. In this respect, the lessons are abundantly clear:

- community-based services for people with severe and enduring mental illnesses do require a certain degree of specialisation and cannot be provided generically
- meaningful recovery, with a markedly reduced need for hospitalisation, is achievable if the appropriate service is provided
- for recovery to take place, services must provide for a wide range of needs beyond simple treatment administration: this demands relatively small caseloads and multidisciplinary teams.

The challenge is to take the lessons learnt from high-income settings and to both motivate for adequate funding and find creative ways of applying these lessons in the realities that prevail.

### 38.3.2.6 Vocational programmes

Much of the early evidence on vocational programmes, and particularly on the model of sheltered workshops, did not demonstrate much success in improving prospects for competitive employment or, indeed, in stimulating recovery. More recently, however, extensive reviews have demonstrated that two particular models, the Clubhouse programme and individual placement and support, have been successful. Emerging research points to a number of important factors that differentiate successful programmes from weaker ones (Anthony and Furlong-Norman, 2011).

### The Clubhouse model

The Clubhouse model is one of the oldest existing models of social and vocational rehabilitation, having evolved from the original Fountain House, which was established in New York City in 1948, with at least 283 active Clubhouses in 28 countries by 2011. Clubhouses are intentional communities within which individuals with a mental illness can achieve or regain the confidence and support needed to lead vocationally productive and socially satisfying lives (Beard *et al.*, 1982). The model seeks to overcome barriers of stigma, dependency and isolation that hamper full community participation. Essential features of the model include low staff to member ratios, a partnership approach with staff and members working side by side, full member participation in decision-making, organisation around a work-ordered day that emulates a typical business day and the articulation of employment as a right of Clubhouse membership, with members involved in career development, job searches and job choice.

Transitional employment has been a defining feature of Clubhouses for more than 50 years. More recently, most clubhouses have incorporated a three-tier approach with a continuum of services, including transitional employment, supported employment and independent employment.

Transitional employment usually lasts 6–9 months in a part-time position. Transitional employment positions are negotiated between the clubhouse and employers: the clubhouse determines who will fill the position out of its members. Additionally, the clubhouse provides on-site training, support and absence coverage, thus allowing it to maximise opportunities for its members to gain work experience. Members are able to get as many opportunities to participate as is necessary.

Supported employment and independent employment are not designed to be time-limited, contracts are between the employer and the member and the employer determines the selection criteria. In supported employment, the clubhouse does not provide absence coverage but does provide on- and off-site support at the member's request. There is usually an existing relationship between the clubhouse and the employer. In independent employment there is no relationship between the clubhouse and the employer, no support is rendered on-site and employment takes place via a fully competitive process. Most members seem to remain in part-time employment. Research has shown this model to be very successful in vocational rehabilitation; the key features of successful outcomes seem to be ongoing contact and support from the clubhouse (McKay *et al.*, 2005).

### Individual placement and support

The individual placement and support model of supported employment for clients with a severe mental illness has been described as a standardisation of evidence-based supported employment (Bond *et al.*, 2001). The core principles of this model are:

- a focus on competitive employment
- eligibility based on consumer choice
- integration of mental health and employment services
- attention to consumer preference in job search
- individualised job support
- personalised benefits counselling (Bond 2004).

Individual placement and support services are typically delivered by supported employment teams that operate as part of community mental health services. When a client (user) expresses interest in working, that client is referred to an employment specialist on the individual placement and support team for an initial meeting. The employment specialist works with the client to learn about his or her goals and preferences and provides information about how individual placement and support work. They then begin to look for jobs together. Employment specialists are trained to provide people with support, coaching, résumé development, interview training and on-the-job support. They also develop relationships with businesses that have suitable jobs for their client base.

The choices of the client are central in individual placement and support. The client decides whether or not employers and potential employers should be informed of his or her mental illness and whether or not the employment specialist talks to employers on his or her behalf. The client also decides which jobs to apply for and how much he or she wants to work. People who try individual placement and support often get a number of jobs before finding one that is a good fit. In individual placement and support there is an orientation towards moving between jobs as part of a normal process. This process aims at convergence towards stable employment in a job that is fulfilling for the client (Bond, 2004).

This approach has been assessed in a number of randomised controlled trials; a number of reviews of the various trials have shown this approach to be effective. A review (Bond *et al.*, 2008) established this approach as one of the most robust psychosocial interventions available for persons with severe mental illness.

**What makes for successful vocational rehabilitation?**

The question of successful vocational rehabilitation was specifically considered in a 2004 study (Gowdy *et al.*, 2004), which found that the following factors were consistent in differentiating the highest from the lowest performing supported employment programmes:

- programme leaders emphasise the value of work in people's lives and the belief that they can return to work
- programme leaders emphasise strengths-based practices as an explicit part of supported employment work with consumers
- programme leaders use outcome data to guide their programming and practice
- staff do not view stigma against people with psychiatric disabilities as a barrier to consumers' ability to gain employment
- staff perceive that consumers have a desire and motivation to work
- there is a close working relationship between supported employment workers and members of the clinical team
- case managers participate in helping clients to find work
- therapists are involved in supporting consumer employment goals.

### 38.3.2.7 Residential support

**The problem of homelessness in chronic mental illness**

The term 'homeless' can refer to a wide variety of contexts, from someone sleeping in the open with minimal shelter, to someone sleeping in the yard or on the floor of an acquaintance's house. Additionally, the degree to which this is a particular problem associated with individual circumstances versus the degree to which it is a function of more general social circumstances, varies enormously between countries. Evidence from many Western nations is that urban homelessness has been on the increase for the past two decades with growing shortages of affordable accommodation, particularly in urban areas. This is associated with poverty and social disadvantages and significantly higher rates of psychiatric disorders in homeless populations. Indeed, the initial wave of deinstitutionalisation that in most cases was implemented with little investment in living support of any form has been strongly implicated in the subsequent development of large populations of homeless mentally ill individuals in many developed nations (Craig and Timms, 1992; Lamb, 1984). The situation in developing countries, including those in southern Africa, is more complex, with far larger populations of people defined as being homeless and factors such as urbanisation and housing shortages playing a much greater role (Tipple and Speak, 2009).

The problem of homelessness in developing countries is far less specific to those living with severe mental illness. Conversely, however, it is likely to be a far more common problem with even greater difficulties for people with mental illness who have to compete with many others from the general population for a smaller pool of resources. There are, nevertheless, a number of important lessons that can be learnt from the work that has been done primarily in developed nations.

#### The transition to independent living

Being able to live independently is considered to be a key step in recovery from severe mental illness, since it involves reintegration into communities (Anthony and Furlong-Newman, 2011). More specifically, qualitative work has revealed that it allows for a greater sense of stability, the re-establishment of supportive relationships and the restoration of a sense of personal identity (Nelson *et al.*, 2005). It has been proposed that transition to independent living involves three important processes: establishing a sense of control, establishing (and successfully managing) the relationship between illness and place and attaining a sense of belonging (Hill *et al.*, 2010).

#### Changing approaches to residential rehabilitation

The traditional approach to residential rehabilitation involved a notion of residential continuum, whereby people would gradually transition from more to less restrictive types of supervised housing, based on their condition (Anthony and Furlong-Newman, 2011). The continuum of settings included halfway houses and foster care settings. As our understanding of psychiatric rehabilitation grew, a new paradigm known as supportive housing has evolved. This model assists individuals to make use of mainstream housing resources by providing specific assistance with particular problems (Ridgway and Zipple, 1990).

#### Supported housing

Supported housing is broadly defined as independent housing in the community that is coupled with the provision of community mental health and support services (Carling, 1992). Key features include:

- the individual, rather than an agency, being the owner or leaseholder
- housing that is integrated into communities but is affordable
- a choice of housing options
- voluntary services from a community-based service that is independent of the housing
- 24-hour crisis services (Rog, 2004).

Available evidence suggests that this approach is most suitable for younger individuals and those without co-occurring substance-abuse problems and that those who have previously been homeless for extended periods are less likely to do well in such programmes. In these particular subgroups supported housing has been shown to be a powerful intervention that improves the stability of individuals with mental illness that is suitable even for those with a severe illness (Rog, 2004).

The lesson for the resource-scarce settings that are often the norm in southern Africa is that an approach that aims to empower the individual to participate in the general housing market through individual support has better recovery outcomes than the provision of sheltered housing. The challenge, however, is to provide suitable financial, emotional, social, legal and medical support to make this possible.

### 38.3.2.8 Hospitalisation in acute settings – is there an alternative?

With the closure of psychiatric institutions, the locus of care for those who need some form of care for an acute crisis has increasingly shifted to admission wards in general hospitals. Whilst this may have many positive implications, such as less segregation, there have also been some disadvantages, including less staff and client satisfaction, less continuity of care with rehabilitation services that were previously housed in the same institution and reductions in bed numbers (Leff and Warner, 2006). This result has led to growing pressure to find more suitable alternatives to admission to hospital in a crisis situation.

The range of alternatives that have been documented include some of the following:

- acute day hospitals that provide care during working hours as well as support and advice for family members

- crisis houses in the community that are staffed to the same level as a hospital ward, but which provide an open-door domestic environment which is less restrictive, but also seems to be associated with less aggressive behaviour than hospital settings
- crisis homes that are specially selected and prepared private homes that accept individual patients as 'guests' under the care of a team of professionals
- home treatment teams, which are specialised teams that administer care on a 24-hour basis to clients in crisis, in their home environment (Leff and Warner, 2006).

In southern African settings, with its vast treatment gaps (Seedat *et al.*, 2009; Jacobs *et al.*, 2007), it is highly likely that a large proportion of people with acute psychiatric crises are already finding some sort of support or care in community settings outside of the health care system. Of course, the reality is that many may also be at the receiving end of exploitative practices, abuse and exclusion. The challenge is to provide services that deal with the latter possibility whilst at the same time strengthening the former. This requires that existing cultural and social practices in caring for people with a mental illness are carefully examined before decisions are made to introduce models that may potentially undermine local practices or only be partially relevant.

### 38.3.2.9 Family interventions

Family intervention programmes are a relatively long-term approach (from six months to two years). These programmes focus on improving adherence to prescribed medication, improving relationships among family members and helping the family to better understand the patient's disorder. These take the form of cognitive behavioural therapy (CBT) with the individual or the family, psycho-education tailored towards the illness in question and exploration of family reactions with a view to reducing high levels of expressed emotion, where this may be present. This has been shown to reduce relapse rates, decrease readmission and improve medication adherence (Pharaoh *et al.*, 2006). Evidence from intervention studies in China (Li and Arthur, 2005; Xiong *et al.*, 1994) suggest that similar interventions are effective in developing nations.

### 38.3.2.10. Cognitive interventions

Cognitive intervention involves both the use of CBT, particularly for the management of residual symptoms in a severe mental illness, as well as cognitive remediation therapy. There is a substantial body of evidence in support of the use of CBT in severe mental disorders (Lynch *et al.*, 2009), where the focus is on treating residual symptoms, such persistent delusions or hallucinations, so that these are better managed to allow for better social function.

Cognitive remediation therapy is an umbrella term for a number of rehabilitation technologies that use computer programs and the intervention of a therapist to directly target cognitive deficits associated with schizophrenia (Brekke and Long, 2010). Early evidence would suggest that improvements in cognitive function, especially memory, can be achieved at little additional cost, with the improvements associated with changes in other aspects of social functioning, work skills and capacity for independent living (Wykes *et al.*, 2007).

### 38.3.2.11 Social interventions for people with severe personality disorders

Evidence from developed nations is that people with personality disorder suffer high levels of distress, suicide, self-harm, addiction, family breakdown and social exclusion, placing a high burden of cost on primary care (Rendu *et al.*, 2002). This has led to an increased emphasis on the provision of effective community-based services for such individuals (National Institute for Mental Health in England, 2003). Two interventions that have been shown to be effective are dialectical behaviour therapy (Verheul *et al.*, 2003) and problem solving therapy (Paris, 2007).

Dialectical behaviour therapy is the most widely evaluated treatment for individuals with borderline personality disorder. It is based on the premise that borderline personality disorder is typified by a failure to regulate emotions as a result of key early-life experiences. A combination of group and individual therapies, over a period of around a year, focuses on enhancing motivation to engage, building self-acceptance, developing distress tolerance, teaching skills for emotion regulation and improving interpersonal effectiveness (Linehan, 1993). Positive effects in randomised controlled trials include reduction of self-harming behaviour, reduction of substance use and improvement in global adjustment and treatment retention (Verheul *et al.*, 2003).

Problem-solving therapy is a cognitive-affective behavioural intervention that promotes the application of effective problem-solving skills to solve problems in everyday living (Nezu, 2004). This involves the use of psycho-education and group or individual approaches to teach social problem solving skills:

- problem recognition: learning to recognise negative emotions as signals that a problem exists and if used as information, can trigger a rational response
- problem definition: learning to define the problem clearly and accurately
- goal setting: learning to specify the desired outcomes
- generating alternatives: learning to be creative and generate a range of possible ways to achieve the set goals
- decision-making: learning to evaluate potential outcomes of a choice of decisions (for self and others) and to choose those most likely to lead to a favourable solution
- evaluation: learning to review the degree of success of the action plan so that it can be learnt from (McMurran *et al.*, 2008).

#### 38.3.2.12 Treatment of substance use disorders

Substance use disorders with co-occurring severe mental illness (i.e. dual diagnoses) are associated with a wide range of negative outcomes, including relapse and re-hospitalisation, housing instability, financial problems, violence, suicidality, increased service utilisation, family conflict and legal problems. This co-morbidity is highly prevalent in southern Africa and therefore it is inevitable that it should be included in the psychosocial rehabilitation approach.

## 38.4 From psychosocial rehabilitation to the philosophy of recovery

As the problems associated with deinstitutionalisation became more evident in countries where this took place on a large scale, such as in the US, a new way of thinking about how services should be organised and delivered began to emerge. It became clear that if people with chronic and severe mental illness were to live successfully in community settings, a wide range of needs had to be addressed, including:

- the need for treatment to relieve symptoms
- the need for crisis intervention from time to time when critical problems arose
- the need for personalised case management to address the different needs of each individual
- the need for rehabilitation to enable better role functioning as a member of society
- the need for opportunities for enrichment and self-development.
- the need to ensure rights protection through advocacy.
- the need for support in ensuring access to basic necessities such as food, shelter and health care
- the need for empowerment such that individuals can exercise choice and make their views heard.

For this to occur a wide array of services that responded to the variety of needs were required. This gave rise to the concept of psychosocial rehabilitation that was delivered within a comprehensive community support system; new concepts of recovery began to arise in this context (Anthony, 1993).

Although the concept of recovery was well established in the field of physical disability, it had previously received little attention in the field of mental health (Spaniol, 1991). It involved the basic understanding that recovery can occur even though an illness or disability has not been entirely cured (e.g. an amputee can recover even though he or she will not regain the lost limb). This understanding began to emerge primarily in the writings of self-identified mental health care users, such as Patricia Deegan, who described it as a process of recovering a new and valued sense of self and purpose that occur in people with psychiatric disabilities as they become active and responsible participants in their own rehabilitation project (Deegan, 1988).

At the same time, those working to reintegrate people with a serious mental illness into society began to shift their focus from pure symptom reduction to an emphasis on functional ability. Inevitably, this led to an increased understanding of rehabilitation to include social and psychological aspects rather than only purely medical ones. This, in turn, involved the realisation that not only was a broader attention to the resources of the individual required, but also to those of the society in which that individual is expected to live. As psychosocial rehabilitation gained more currency as a concept, with it came a better understanding of the importance of both consumer choice and of social mobilisation (Anthony *et al.*, 1990).

Recovery, according to Anthony (1993) 'is a deep personal, unique process of changing one's attitudes, values, feelings, goals, skills and roles. It is a way of living a satisfying, hopeful and contributing life, even with the limitations caused by illness. Recovery involves the development of new meaning and purpose in one's life as one grows beyond the catastrophic effects of mental illness.'

Recovery is therefore seen as a multidimensional process that involves much more than symptom improvement and that includes the recovery from stigma, from loss of self-belief and opportunity and from loss of a voice in society. Recovery can thus be seen as a critical goal that can serve to integrate all efforts to promote healing, from the individual level through to the levels of services and of society in general. On a personal level, Jacobson and Greenley (2001) emphasises four internal conditions:

- hope, both as a belief that recovery is possible and as a frame of mind that allows this to occur
- healing, as something distinct from cure, as something that emphasises self, as apart from illness and control
- empowerment as a corrective for the sense of helplessness and dependency that comes with both a severe mental illness and with prolonged contact with some of the less-transformed mental health services
- connection with broader society and with one's role as part of that society.

To promote these key conditions, Farkas (2007) suggests four key values that promote recovery within services:

- person orientation
- person involvement
- self-determination or self-choice
- hope.

This vision is thus critical for the further development of mental health services in southern Africa as it involves a huge range of role-players including consumers, their friends and family members, the multiplicity of non-governmental organisations and the private and public sectors. Indeed, as awareness improves and stigma is challenged, it will become apparent that improved mental health is everyone's business and that achieving this involves the empowerment of individuals and the transformation of society that has been the dream of many young democracies. Adopting the vision of recovery as a shared goal is the first step in developing a united and powerful force that will drive the development of the kind of health service and society that so many desire.

## 38.5 Global perspectives on social intervention

### 38.5.1 Evolution of mental health reforms: examples from around the world

#### 38.5.1.1 South America: Cuba and Chile

The first attempts at reforming mental health services in Latin America and the Caribbean took place in the 1960s, when the early effects of the community mental health movement in the United States and the psychiatric reform experiences in Italy and other European countries began to reach this region.

One important aspect of the newly implemented mental health policies in several countries was the integration of mental health into primary care.

Cuba was among the first countries to include mental health in primary care as the basis of the new mental health system, and to implement this strategy at the national level (Basauri, 2008). The strategy followed in Chile was different, to the extent that development of specific programmes was favoured in primary care to target problems identified as priorities, such as depression (Farmer, 2008). The main objective of national and regional projects in a number of countries was the development of a comprehensive, community-based mental health service. Important lessons that were learnt include the following:

- Collaboration between mental health services and other city institutions can provide a safety net for persons with serious mental disorders, reducing acute episodes of illness.
- Care for persons with mental illness in the community must include attention to all aspects of the person's life.
- Mental health services can function with primary care doctors who provide pharmacological interventions.
- Cohesive, committed mental health teams can form meaningful relationships with users that help sustain them in the community.
- Teams must remain up to date with advances in mental health care. The programme must develop methods for accessing and staying current with information on best practices.
- A programme of research and service evaluation could help the team to objectively identify areas of success and weakness.

Facilitating greater involvement of users in service delivery decisions would operationalise human rights ideas that underlie the programme.

- The need for supportive housing solutions must be addressed realistically, taking into account the objective needs of each community.
- Community mental health centres could be established at a very reasonable cost; these centres should be linked to the patients' families.
- There is a need to educate the people on the rationality of psychiatric community services otherwise the stigma usually associated with mental illness will push people to retain hospital-based services.
- A back-up legislation that brings together health, labour and social security authorities is important for the success of these programmes (Farmer, 2008).

#### 38.5.1.2 Psychosocial rehabilitation in Europe

In the majority of European countries the process of deinstitutionalisation and reform of psychiatry from a hospital-based model to a community-based model took place in the 1960s and 1970s. The type and quality of community psychiatry services varied widely between countries. Stigma and the population's attitude were identified as the major obstacles to community psychiatric service development (Monsalve, 2004).

#### 38.5.1.3 The special case of Italy

Italy was one of the most radical countries in the process of deinstitutionalization of psychiatric services. In 1978, the reform law established fundamental changes in the mental health care system (prohibiting admissions to state mental hospitals, stipulating community-based services and allowing hospitalisation only in small general-hospital units). At the beginning this process was unbalanced, but after a few years the new community approach was available for 80% of the population. Burti (2001) comments: '1998 marked the very end of the state mental hospital system in Italy.'

### 38.5.1.4 The South African situation

In the current South African situation, community psychiatry services are non-existent or poorly developed. Mental health services are slowly evolving from a hospital-based to a community-based approach (Hering *et al.*, 2008), but it seems that it will take some years to achieve the minimum number of desired psychiatrists and other mental health professionals.

Several authors (Moosa and Jeenah 2008; Szabo, 2010) have proposed the reshaping of the present psychiatric hospitals' functions and the organisation of hospital-based community psychiatry services, as the standard for psychiatry care in the country. Many psychiatric hospitals have existing outreach programmes: this could be the point of departure for a real community psychiatry approach that takes on board physicians in primary health care, psychiatric nurses, clinical associated staff and the community component: families, community leaders, NGOs, religious institutions and community business people.

There will be many challenges to overcome in this task, from the manner in which services are designed so that the system becomes integrated into primary care rather than a parallel one, to internal resistance among colleagues to changing old patterns of care. Even so, there will be rewards as well. For example, a model where the same team who takes care of the patient in the hospital also takes care of the psychosocial rehabilitation needs of the patient, will allow mental health care providers and their clients to co-manage the illness from in primary health care right through to the tertiary institution. The work satisfaction generated by this type of approach would provide a great incentive for mental health professionals to choose to practice within the often-challenging southern African public service context.

## Conclusion

The origins of most modern forms of psychosocial rehabilitation can be located in the changes that occurred in the aftermath of deinstitutionalisation. The resultant changes have been in keeping with a general shift in emphasis from tertiary care to primary-level treatment and prevention.

Whilst this shift has on the whole been a positive one, it has by no means been a simple or easy process. It is something that continues to evolve throughout the world and from which many valuable lessons can be learned. It is in the process of deinstitutionalisation that the true meaning of bio-psycho-social approaches to mental health begins to emerge and this demands an approach that is at once individualised, flexible and comprehensive.

The range of social interventions that have been developed include specialised modalities of delivery of mental health care in the community, vocational and residential support, skills training and illness self-management, focused therapeutic interventions for specific disorders and interventions that focus on the family as well as on the community as a whole.

In areas with large treatment gaps, such as those that exist in many southern African countries, it is likely that large numbers of people with mental illnesses do currently receive some form of support and care in the community, although many may also be experiencing exclusion and even abuse. It is thus critical that any existing social and cultural practices are carefully understood before additional services are developed in order to avoid undermining existing systems of care.

The philosophy of recovery has emerged as a key organising element in mental health care that expands the emphasis from a simple focus on symptomatic improvement to a range of outcomes that include the recovery of hope, individual empowerment and the restoration of one's rightful place in society. As such, in southern African settings, this philosophy has the potential to bring about far more than a simple improvement of mental health services. It is also a social transformation towards better mental health care that will be of benefit to all of society.

Although attempts to reform institution-based systems in different parts of the world have met with varying levels of success, a number of important lessons can be learned. Perhaps most vital is an understanding of the complexity of mental health care and of its multidimensional nature. Thus, any social intervention must arise out of a careful understanding of the cultural, political and socioeconomic circumstances of the country involved. Key to success is the realisation that, in order to be successful, social interventions must specifically be social in nature, rather than something carried out by certain identified practitioners in society. In developing nations such as those in the southern African region where treatment gaps are large, there is an inherent advantage to truly social approaches. When mental health-care users themselves, their family members, those in their communities and those involved in the provision of a wide range of services all understand that not only do they play a role in improving mental health outcomes but that they all stand to benefit from improved mental health outcomes, then society itself becomes an unstoppable force in the drive towards better mental health care for all.

# References


Anthony W, Cohen M, Farkas M (1990) *Psychiatric Rehabilitation*. Boston, Mass: Center for Psychiatric Rehabilitation

Anthony WA (1993) Recovery from mental illness: The guiding vision of the mental health service system in the 1990's. *Psychosocial Rehabilitation Journal* 16(4): 11–23. Quotation on page 775 reprinted with permission from the American Psychological Association.

Anthony WA, Furlong-Norman K (2011) Introduction to Chapter 4: Psychiatric rehabilitation and vocational outcomes. In: Anthony WA, Furlong-Norman (Eds). *Psychiatric Rehabilitation and Recovery*. Boston, MA: University Center for Psychiatric Rehabilitation.

Anthony WA, Furlong-Norman K (2011) Introduction to Chapter 5: Psychiatric rehabilitation and residential outcomes. In: Anthony WA, Furlong-Norman (Eds). *Psychiatric Rehabilitation and Recovery*. Boston, MA: University Center for Psychiatric Rehabilitation.

Bachrach LL (1996) Deinstitutionalization: promises, problems and prospects. In: Knudsen HC, Thornicroft G (Eds). *Mental Health Service Evaluation*. Cambridge, England: Cambridge University Press

Basauri VA (2008) Cuba: Mental health care and community participation. In: Caldas de Almeida JM, Cohen A (Eds). *Innovative mental health programs in Latin America and the Caribbean*. Washington, DC: Pan American Health Organisation

Beard JH, Propst RN, Malamud TJ (1982) Fountain House Model of Psychiatric Rehabilitation. *Psychosocial Rehabilitation* Journal 5: 47–53

Bloom JD (2010) 'The Incarceration Revolution': The abandonment of the seriously mentally ill. References to our jails and prisons. *Journal of Law, Medicine and Ethics: Conundrums and Controversies in Mental Health and Illness*, winter 2010: 727–34

Bond GR (2004) Supported employment: Evidence for an evidence-based practice. *Psychiatric Rehabilitation Journal* (27) 345–359.

Bond GR, Becker DR, Drake RE, Rapp CA, Meisler N, Lehman AF, Bell MD, Blyler CR (2001) Implementing supported employment as an evidence-based practice. *Psychiatric Services* (52) 313–322.

Bond GR, Drake RE, Becker DR (2008) An update on randomized control trial of evidence-based supportive employment. *Psychiatric Rehabilitation Journal* 31(4) 280–290.

Botha U, Koen L, Oosthuizen P, Joska J, Hering L (2008). Assertive community treatment in the South African context. *African Journal of Psychiatry* 11: 272–5

Botha UA, Koen K, Joska JA, Hering LA, Oosthuizen PP (2010) Assessing the efficacy of a modified assertive community-based treatment programme in a developing country. *BMC Psychiatry* 10: 73. Available at: http://www.biomedcentral.com/1471-244X/10/73 (Accessed 28 February 2013.)

Brekke JS, Long JD (2010). *Community-based psychosocial rehabilitation and perspective changes in functional, clinical and subjective experienced variables in schizophrenia*. Available at: http//schizophreniabulletin.oxfordjournals.org (Accessed 20 July 2010.)

Burns T (2010) Team structures in community mental health. In: Morgan C, Bhugra D (Eds). *Principles of Social Psychiatry* (2nd edition). Chichester, UK: Wiley and Sons

Burti L (2001) Italian psychiatric reform 20 plus years after. *Acta Psychiatrica Scadinavica* 104 (Suppl. 410): 41–6

Byford S, Fiander M, Torgerson DJ, Barber JA, Thompson SG, Burns T, Van Horn E, Gilvarry C, Creed F (2000) Cost-effectiveness of intensive v. standard case management for severe psychotic illness. UK700 case management trial. *British Journal of Psychiatry* 176: 537–43

Carling PJ (1992) Housing, community support, and homelessness: Emerging policy in mental health systems. *New England Journal of Public Policy* 8: 281–95

Craig T, Timms PW (1992) Out of the wards and onto the streets? Deinstitutionalization and homelessness in Britain. *Journal of Mental Health* 1(3): 265–75

Deegan PE (1988) Recovery: The lived experience of rehabilitation. *Psychosocial Rehabilitation Journal* 11(4): 11–9

Dieterich M, Irving CB, Park B, Marshall M (2010) Intensive case management for severe mental illness. *Cochrane Database of Systematic Reviews 2010*, Issue 10. Art. No.: CD007906. DOI: 10.1002/14651858.CD007906.pub2

Farkas M (2007) The vision of recovery today: What it is and what it means for services. *World Psychiatry* 6: 1–7

Farmer CM (2008) Chile: Reforms in national mental health policy. In: Caldas de Almeida JM, Cohen A (Eds). *Innovative mental health programs in Latin America and the Caribbean.* Washington, DC: Pan American Health Organisation

Foucault M (1971) *Madness and Civilisation: A History of Insanity in the Age of Reason*. London: Tavistock

Geller JL (2000) The last half century of psychiatric services as reflected in 'Psychiatric Services'. *Psychiatric Services* 51: 41–67

Goffman E (1961) *Asylums: Essays on the Social Situation of Mental Patients and Other Inmates*. New York: Doubleday

Gowdy EA, Carlson LS, Rapp CA (2004) Organisational factors differentiating high performing from low performing supported employment programs. *Psychiatric Rehabilitation Journal* 28(2): 150–156

Grove B (1994). Reform of mental health care in Europe. *British Journal of Psychiatry* 165: 431–433

Hering L, Dean C, Stein D (2008) Providing psychiatric services in general medical settings in South Africa: Mental health-friendly services in mental health-friendly hospitals. *South African Journal of Psychiatry* 14(1): 4–6

Hill A, Mayes R, McConnell D (2010) Transition to independent living accommodation for adults with schizophrenia. *Psychiatric Rehabilitation Journal* 33(3): 228–31

International Journal of Psychosocial Rehabilitation (2010). *Psychosocial rehabilitation – assertive community treatment* (Editorial). Available at: http://www.psychosocial.com/index.htm (Accessed 21 July 2010.)

Jacobs KS, Sharan P, Mirza I, Garrido-Cumbrera M, Seedat S, Mari JJ, Sreenivas V, Saxena S (2007). Mental health systems in countries: where are we now? (Global Mental Health Series No. 4). *The Lancet* 370:1062–77. DOI:10.1016/S0140-6736(07)61241-0

Jacobson N, Greenley D (2001). What is recovery? A conceptual model and explication. *Psychiatric Services* 52: 482–5

Kaplan HI, Sadock BJ, Grebb JA (1994) *Kaplan and Sadock's synopsis of psychiatry: behavioural/sciences, clinical psychiatry*, 7th ed. Baltimore: Williams and Witkins: 866

Kent A, Burns T (2005) Assertive community Treatment in UK practice. (Revisiting setting up an assertive community treatment team (series)). *Advances in Psychiatric Treatment* 11: 388–97

Killaspy H, Kingett S, Bebbington P, Blizard R, Johnson S, Nolan F, Pilling S, King M (2009) Randomised evaluation of assertive community treatment: 3-year outcomes. *British Journal of Psychiatry* 195: 81–2

Koenig HG (2005). *Faith and Mental Health: Religious Resources for Healing*. Philadelphia: Templeton Foundation Press

Lamb HR (1984) Deinstitutionalization and the homeless mentally ill. *Hospital and Community Psychiatry* 35(9): 899–907

Lamb HR, Bachrach LL (2001) Some perspectives on deinstitutionalisation. *Psychiatric Services* 52: 1039–45

Leff J (2010) The historical development of social psychiatry. In: Morgan C, Bhugra D (Eds). *Principles of Social Psychiatry* (2nd edition). Chichester, UK: Wiley and Sons

Leff J Warner R (2006) *Social Inclusion of People with Mental Illness.* Cambridge, UK: Cambridge University Press

Li Z, Arthur D (2005) Family education for people with schizophrenia in Bejing, China. *British Journal of Psychiatry* 187: 339–45

Linehan MM (1993) *Cognitive-Behavioral Treatment of Borderline Personality Disorder.* New York: Guilford Press

Lynch D, Laws KR, McKenna PJ (2009) Cognitive behavioural therapy for major psychiatric disorder: Does it really work? A meta-analytical review of well-controlled trials. *Psychological Medicine* 29: 1–16

Malone D, Marriott S, Newton-Howes G, Simmonds S, Tyrer P. (2007) Community mental health teams (CMHTs) for people with severe mental illnesses and disordered personality. *Cochrane Database of Systematic Reviews*, Issue 3. Art. No.: CD000270. DOI: 10.1002/14651858.CD000270.pub2

Marshall M, Lockwood A (2000) Assertive community treatment for people with severe mental disorders. *Cochrane Database of Systematic Reviews,* CD001089. Available at: http://www.ncbi.nlm.nih.gov/pubmed/10796415 (Accessed 26 February 2013.)

Mayosi BM, Flisher AJ, Lalloo UG, Sitas F, Tollman SM, Bradshaw D (2009) The burden of non-communicable diseases in South Africa. (Health in South Africa Series No. 4.) *The Lancet* 374: 934–47

McKay C, Johnsen M, Stein R (2005) Employment outcomes in Massachusetts clubhouses. *Psychiatric Rehabilitation Journal* 29(1): 25–33

McMurran M, Huband N, Duggan C. (2008) The role of social problem solving in improving social functioning in therapy for adults with personality disorder. *Personality and Mental Health* 2: 1–6

Monsalve MH (2004) La Psiquiatría Comunitaria. In: Ibor JJL, Cercós CL, Masiá CC (Eds). *Imágenes de la Psiquiatría Española. Asociación Mundial de Psiquiatría.* Barcelona: Ed. Glosa

Moosa MYH, Jeenah FY (2008) Community psychiatry: An audit of services in southern Gauteng. *South African Journal of Psychiatry* 14(2): 36–43

Murphy S, Irving CB, Adams CE, Driver R (2012) Crisis intervention for people with severe mental illnesses. *Cochrane Database of Systematic Reviews* Issue 5. Art. No.: CD001087. DOI: 10.1002/14651858.CD001087.pub4

National Institute for Mental Health (1999) *Psychosocial Rehabilitation Services. Mental Health: A Report of the Surgeon General*. Available at: www.surgeongeneral.gov/library/mentalhealth/chapter4/sec5.html#psychosocial. (Accessed 19 May 2011.)

National Institute for Mental Health in England (2003) *Personality Disorder: No Longer a Diagnosis of Exclusion.* London: Department of Health

Nelson G, Clarke J, Febbraro A, Hatzipantelis M (2005) A narrative approach to the evaluation of supportive housing: Stories of homeless people who have experienced serious mental illness. *Psychiatric Rehabilitation Journal* 29(2): 98–104

Nezu AM (2004) Problem solving and behavior therapy revisited. *Behavior Therapy* 35:1–33

Novella EJ (2010) Mental health care in the aftermath of deinstitutionalization: A retrospective and prospective view. *Health Care Annals* 18: 222–38

Okin RL (1978) The future of state mental health programs for chronic psychiatric patients in the community. *American Journal of Psychiatry* 135: 1355–8

Paris J (2007) Problem-solving therapy improves social functioning in people with personality disorder (Commentary). *Evidence-Based Mental Health* 10: 121

Pharoah F, Mari J, Rathbone J, Wong W (2006) Family intervention for schizophrenia. *Cochrane Database of Systematic Reviews*, (4), Art. No.: CD000088. http://www.ncbi.nlm.nih.gov/pubmed/21154340 (Accessed 30 March 2013.)

Porter R (1987) *A Social History of Madness: Stories of the insane.* London: Weidenfield and Nicholson

Porter R (2006). *Madmen: A Social History of Madhouses, Mad-Doctors and Lunatics* (Ill. ed.) Stroud: Tempus

Rendu A, Moran P, Patel A, Knapp M, Mann A (2002) Economic impact of personality disorders in UK primary care attenders. *British Journal of Psychiatry* 181: 62–6

Ridgway P, Zipple AM (1990) The paradigm shift in residential services: From the linear continuum to supported housing approaches. *Psychosocial Rehabilitation Journal* 13(4): 11–31

Rog DJ (2004) The evidence on supported housing. *Psychiatric Rehabilitation Journal* 27(4): 334–44

Scott J (1993) Homelessness and mental illness. *British Journal of Psychiatry* 162: 314–24

Seedat S, Williams DR, Herman AA, Moomal H, Williams SL, Jackson PB, Myer L, Stein DJ (2009) Mental health service use among South Africans for mood, anxiety and substance use disorders. *South African Medical Journal* 99(4):346–352

Spaniol L (1991) Editorial. *Psychosocial Rehabilitation Journal* 14(4): 1

Stein LI, Test MA (1980) Alternative to mental hospital treatment I. Conceptual model, treatment programme, and clinical evaluation. *Archives of General Psychiatry* 37: 392–7

Stroman D (2003). *The Disability Rights Movement: From Deinstitutionalization to Self-determination.* Lanham, MD: Press of America

Szabo CP (2010). Should state sector community psychiatry be hospital based? A local, and personal, perspective (Editorial). *African Journal of Psychiatry* 13(1): 1

Tipple G, Speak S (2009) *The Hidden Millions: Homelessness in Developing Countries.* London, New York: Routledge

Verheul R, Van den Bosch LM, Koeter MW, De Ridder MA, Stijnen T, Van Den Brink W (2003) Dialectical behaviour therapy for women with borderline personality disorder: 12-month, randomized clinical trial in the Netherlands. *British Journal of Psychiatry* 182: 135–140

Wykes T, Reeder C, Landau S, Everitt B, Knapp M, Patel A, Romeo R (2007) Cognitive remediation in schizophrenia: Randomized control trial. *British Journal of Psychiatry* 190: 421–7. DOI: 10.1192/ bjp.bp.106.026575

Xiong W, Phillips MR, Hu X, Wang R, Dai Q, Kleinman J, Kleinman A (1994) Family-based intervention for schizophrenic patients in China: A randomised controlled trial. *British Journal of Psychiatry* 165: 239–47

CHAPTER

# 39 Public mental health

*Yusuf Moosa, Surita van Heerden*

## 39.1 Introduction

Worldwide, mental health problems have a significant impact on individuals and their families, resulting in diminished quality of life, morbidity and mortality (World Health Organization, 2010a). 'The epidemiology of most mental disorders in South Africa is similar to that found in developed countries' (Stein *et al.*, 2008). 'However, continuous urbanisation has led to an over-utilisation of all resources, unemployment, malnutrition, re-emergence of infectious diseases, violence, substance abuse, child abuse and the break-up of traditional social support networks' (World Health Organization, 2010b). Public mental health services are one way in which services can be delivered for mental illness. These services must be organized in such that they are effective and meet the aims and objectives of the country's mental health policy. The plan of the service delivery depends on the country's social, cultural, political and economic situation (World Health Organization, 2013). The World Health Organization (WHO) broadly recommends the following forms of public mental health services (World Health Organization, 2013) (see Figure 39.1).

- Mental health services in primary care, which include treatment services (to detect and treat most common and acute mental disorders) and preventive and promotional activities delivered by primary care professionals such as doctors, nurses and community health workers.
- Mental health services in general hospitals, which include services offered in district, regional and tertiary academic hospitals that form part of the general health system. Such services include psychiatric in-patient wards, psychiatric beds in general wards and emergency departments and out-patient clinics. There may also be some specialist services (e.g. for children, adolescents and the elderly). These services are provided by

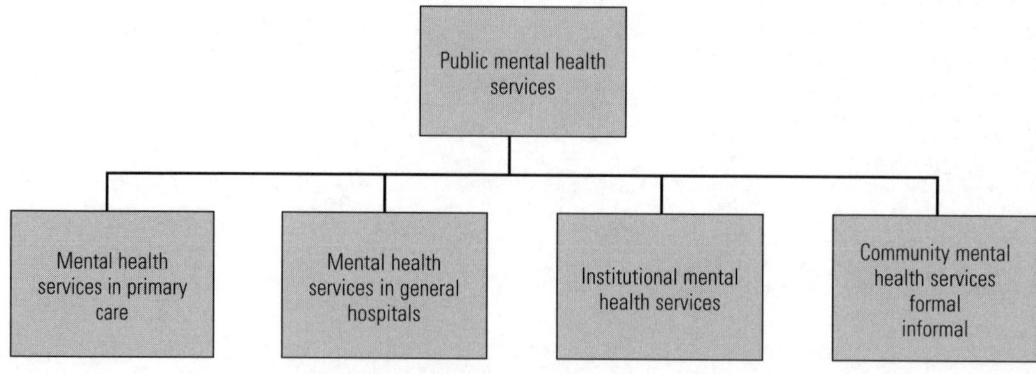


**Figure 39.1** Organisation of mental health services (WHO, 2003)

specialist mental health professionals such as psychiatrists, psychiatric nurses, psychiatric social workers and psychologists.

- Institutional mental health services, which include dedicated psychiatric hospitals and specialist institutional services. These institutions are usually independent stand-alone service style, although they may have some links with the rest of the health care system. These services include those provided by acute and high security units, units for children and elderly people and forensic psychiatry units.
- Community mental health services are intended for persons with mental disorders to continue living in the community and promote community integration. Formal community mental health services include community-based rehabilitation services, therapeutic and residential supervised services and support services. Primary health care workers can deliver these services with some training in mental health. Informal community mental health services are provided by local community members and are a useful complement to formal mental health services (World Health Organization, 2003). Health care is a partnership between all role players, including service users and their families. Citizens need to take more responsibility for developing and managing their own health care. Instead of being treated as recipients of care, patients and their families are viewed as partners in care and play an advocacy role in psychiatry and mental health. The formation of alliances for the mentally ill, support groups for those suffering from particular psychiatric disorders (e.g., groups for those experiencing post-natal depression and twelve-step programmes for addiction), and family advocacy associations, have resulted in greater attention to human rights issues and more rapid improvements in the mental health delivery system. Service users and their families are involved at all levels of service planning and implementation, including the governing and monitoring of services (e.g., through representation on district committees and hospital boards). Programmes offering training to service users and families in leadership and organizational skills are required for these tasks. Finally, in order to play an effective advocacy role, service user and family advocacy organizations should receive funding from the health budget (World Health Organization, 2003).

The World Health Report (2006) recommends that the current predominant utilisation of in-patient and specialised mental health care must evolve to a care that promotes self-management and community-based pre-hospital care. This would necessitate a review in how generalist health workforce is trained and deployed. There would also have to be training of other community stakeholders such as police officers, religious healers and social workers on mental health issues. This shift to community-based care must take cognisance of the specialist and sub-specialist care that, besides providing services, is required for the training and supervision of generalists.

## 39.2 Mental health policy and services development in South Africa

### 39.2.1 Mental health policy

Decentralisation of all health care became a cornerstone of the WHO's policy during the 1970s (World Health Organization, 1978). This policy was expressed in the recommendations of the International Conference on Primary Health Care at Alma-Ata in 1978, known as the Declaration of Alma-Ata (World Health Organization, 1978). The conference also affirmed that 'health is a state of complete physical, mental and social well-being, and not merely the absence of disease or infirmity. Primary health care was declared to be the key to attaining the target of health for all by the year 2000' (World Health Organization, 1978).

Efforts have been made since the 1970s to apply these principles to psychiatry and to integrate psychiatric care into general health care and the primary health care system, with varying degrees of success. Psychiatry and mental health services in South Africa were marginalised and stigmatised, a situation compounded by inadequate training and a lack of skills transfer to health, welfare, education, and other professionals. Collaboration between the health, welfare, education, justice, prisons, labour, housing, and non-governmental sectors was not taking place adequately.

## 39.2.2 The South African Mental Health Policy Framework and Strategic Plan, 2013–2020

Due to the morbidity, suffering and disability caused by mental illness, the WHO adopted the Comprehensive Mental Health Action Plan 2013–2020 (CMHAP) in May 2013. South Africa, being a member state of the WHO, agreed to take specific actions to reach the agreed targets set out by the CMHAP.

Following on the CMHAP, the National Health Council adopted the Mental Health Policy Framework (MHPF) for South Africa and the Strategic Plan 2013–2020 in July 2013.

The vision of the MHPF is: 'From infancy to old age, the mental health and well-being of all South Africans will be enabled, through the provision of evidence-based, affordable and effective promotion, prevention, treatment and rehabilitation interventions. In partnerships between providers, users, carers and communities, the human rights of people with mental illness will be upheld; they will be provided with care and support; and they will be integrated into normal community life.' (Department of Health, Republic of South Africa, 2013).

The MHPF is a comprehensive strategy that deals with epidemiology, costs of care for mental illness, recommended norms and standards and policy and legislation mandates. The MHPF also clearly delineates the responsibilities of the minister of health, provincial governments and non-governmental organisations.

The eight key objectives of the MHPF are:

- district based mental health services and primary health care re-engineering
- building institutional capacity
- surveillance
- research and innovation
- building infrastructure and capacity of facilities
- mental health technology, equipment and medicines
- intersectoral collaborations
- human resources for mental health

**Information box**

**Public mental health services in South Africa**

The delivery of public mental health services in South Africa has been developed based on the following South African legislative frameworks:

- The Constitution of the Republic of South Africa
- The White Paper for the Transformation of the Health System in South Africa, 1997
- The National Health Policy Guidelines for Improved Mental Health in South Africa, 1997
- National Mental Health Policy Framework and Strategic Plan 2013–2020
- National Health Act (No. 63 of 2003)
- Mental Health Care Act (No. 17 of 2002)
- Correctional Services Act (No. 111 of 1998)
- Medicine and Related Substances Control Act (No. 101 of 1965) as amended
- Pharmacy Act (No. 53 of 1974) as amended
- Nursing Act (No. 50 of 1978)
- Public Finance Management Act (No. 29 of 1999)
- The Children's Act (No. 38 of 2005)
- Prevention of and Treatment for Substance Abuse Act (No. 70 of 2008)
- National Drug Master Plan, 2012–2016
- Adolescent and Youth Health Policy Guidelines, 2001
- School Health Policy and Implementation Guidelines, 2003
- Child and Adolescent Mental Health Policy Guidelines, 2003
- Child Justice Act (No. 75 of 2008)
- Criminal Law (Sexual Offences and Related Matters) Amendment Act (No. 32 of 2007)
- Older Persons Act (No. 13 of 2006)

- advocacy
- mental health promotion and prevention of mental illness.

The MHPF clearly sets out a set of values and principles for the delivery of mental health services in South Africa (see Table 39.1).

See also Chapter 35: Legal and ethical aspects of mental health, for a discussion of the MHCA.

**Table 39.1** Values and principles in the delivery of mental health services

| Values | Principles |
|---|---|
| Mental health is part of general health | ▶ Mental health care should be integrated into general health care.<br>▶ People with mental disorders should be treated in primary health care clinics and in general hospitals in most cases.<br>▶ Mental health services should be planned at all levels of the health service. |
| Human rights | ▶ The human rights of people with mental illness should be promoted and protected.<br>▶ The rights to equality, non-discrimination, dignity, respect, privacy, autonomy, information and participation should be upheld in the provision of mental health care.<br>▶ The rights to education, access to land, adequate housing, health care services, sufficient food, water and social security, including social assistance for the poor, and environmental rights for adult mental health care users should be pursued on a basis of progressive realization. The non-conditional rights of mental health care users under the age of 18 years, including basic nutrition, shelter, basic health care services and social services, should be promoted and protected. |
| Community care | ▶ Mental health care users should have access to care near to the places where they live and work.<br>▶ Mental health care users should be provided with the least restrictive forms of care.<br>▶ Local community-based resources should be mobilized where ever possible.<br>▶ All avenues for outpatient and community-based residential care should be explored before in-patient care is undertaken.<br>▶ A recovery model, with an emphasis on psychosocial rehabilitation, should underpin all community-based services. |
| Accessibility and equity | ▶ Equitable services should be accessible to all people, regardless of geographical location, economic status, race, gender or social condition.<br>▶ Mental health services should have parity with general health services. |
| Intersectoral collaboration | ▶ Addressing the social determinants of mental health requires collaboration between the Health sector and several other sectors, including Education, Social Development, Labour, Criminal Justice, Human Settlements and NGOs. |
| Mainstreaming | ▶ Mental health should be considered in all legislative, policy, planning, programming, budgeting, and monitoring and evaluation activities of the public sector. |
| Recovery | ▶ Service development and delivery should aim to build user capacity to return to, sustain and participate in satisfying roles of their choice in their community. |
| Respect for culture | ▶ There are varying cultural expressions and interpretations of mental illness, which should be respected, insofar as they protect the human rights of the mentally ill. |
| Gender | ▶ Services should be sensitive to gender-related issues experienced by men and women, and boys and girls. |
| Social support and integration | ▶ Maximum support should be provided to families and carers of those with mental illness, in order to broaden the network of support and care. |

| | |
|---|---|
| Participation | ▸ Mental health care users should be involved in the planning, delivery and evaluation of mental health services.<br>▸ Self-help and advocacy groups should be encouraged. |
| Self-representation | ▸ Mental health care users and their associates should have support to enable them to represent themselves.<br>▸ The development of self-help, peer support and advocacy groups should be supported. |
| Citizenship and non-discrimination | ▸ Mental health care users should be given equal opportunities and reasonable accommodation to ensure full participation in society.<br>▸ Attitudinal and structural barriers to full participation should be overcome. Access to education, employment, housing, and social supports should receive particular attention. |
| Efficiency and effectiveness | ▸ The limited resources available for mental health should be used efficiently, for maximum effect.<br>▸ Interventions should be informed by evidence of effectiveness. |
| Comprehensiveness | ▸ Mental health interventions should be directed at mental health promotion, the prevention of mental illness, treatment and rehabilitation. |
| Protection against vulnerability | Developmental vulnerabilities to mental health problems associated with life stages of infancy, middle childhood, adolescence, adulthood and old age, as well as vulnerabilities associated with gender (including pregnancy), socioeconomic position, ill-health and disability should be protected against through the provision of targeted prevention interventions. |

**Source:** Department of Health, Republic of South Africa, 2013

## 39.2.3 Key components of mental health care services

Public mental health services in South Africa are based on the following components, as shown in Figure 39.2.

### 39.2.3.1 Promotion and prevention

The WHO defines mental health promotion as 'actions to create living conditions and environments that support mental health and allow people to adopt and maintain healthy lifestyles' (WHO, 2014). It is intended to enhance an individual's ability to cope with stressors, improve their self-esteem and ultimately a sense of mental well-being. This is usually achieved by coping strategies that are directed against various psychological and/or social stressors combined with some preventive activities (WHO, 2014; Mrazek and Haggerty, 1994). Most existing promotional and preventative activities are provided by the Department of Health, with support from non-governmental organisations (NGOs) such as the South African Federation for Mental Health (SAFMH) and the South African Depression and Anxiety Group (SADAG).

Mental health promotion includes educational activities directed at individuals, groups or whole populations. It is offered in schools, health service organisations, businesses and industries. The programmes include components such as awareness and appreciation of mental health, promoting healthy lifestyles, teaching life skills, addressing ignorance, prejudice and stigma, creating awareness of the impact of mental illness and promoting the use of mental health services. Health promotion activities target both physical health and mental health. Physical health promotion is crucial, considering that the leading causes of death and morbidity among individuals with serious mental illness are chronic diseases (e.g. cardiovascular disease, cancer, pulmonary disease, diabetes).

In primary prevention the goal is to prevent the development of mental illness. This is attained by a combination of reducing the risk factors that may contribute to the illness whilst at the same time increasing those factors that serve to protect one against developing the illness (Institute for

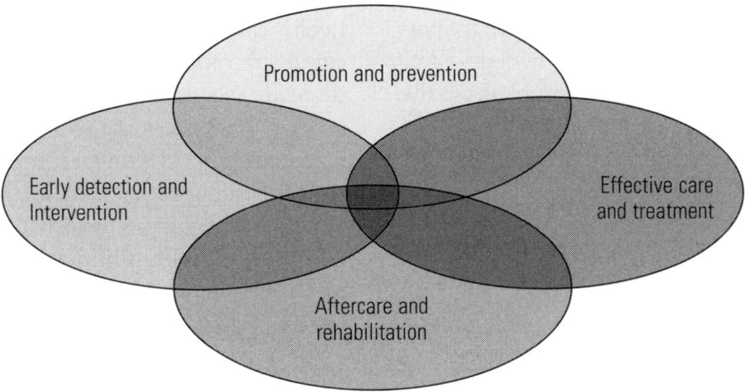


**Figure 39.2** Components of mental health services

Work and Health, 2015; Mrazek and Haggerty, 1994).

Risk factors can be modifiable (able to be changed through preventive interventions) or non-modifiable (e.g. age, race, sex, family history); and may or may not be causal of the illness (Mrazek and Haggerty, 1994). Protective factors on the other hand precede a disorder and are associated with a reduced risk of that disorder. Identifying and addressing these risk and protective factors through interventions is one of the ways of preventing the development of an illness (Mrazek and Haggerty, 1994).

Interventions may be 'universal', i.e. directed against the entire population (such as restrictions on the sale of alcohol, drugs, and firearms) or 'selective', i.e. it targets the at-risk groups (such as crisis and trauma intervention for victims of floods or airplane hijacking) (Desjarlais *et al.*, 1995). 'Indicated interventions', on the other hand focuses on high-risk individuals (such as substance abusers). In the field of psychiatry, predicting the risk for the development of a disorder is still not an exact science and further studies are required before 'selective and indicated preventive interventions' can be utilised in daily practice (Compton and Shim, 2014).

In general, secondary prevention is targeted at reducing the impact and progression of a disease once exposure has already occurred (Institute for Work and Health, 2015; Mrazek and Haggerty, 1994). With regards to mental illness, it is aimed at detecting it in the early stages and the prevention of the development of chronicity and complications (Mrazek and Haggerty, 1994). An example of secondary prevention is psycho-education, which involves providing both the patient and their families an understanding of the epidemiology, treatment options, and the course and prognosis of the disorder. This knowledge helps with adherence to treatment, rehabilitation and recovery.

Tertiary prevention aims to reduce the effect and impact of an ongoing illness that has long-term and complex effects and to improve their ability to function, their quality of life and their life expectancy (Institute for Work and Health, 2015; Mrazek and Haggerty, 1994). In mental illness it includes the reintegration into the community through rehabilitation (Mrazek and Haggerty, 1994).

Prevention efforts take place across the life span of the individual. However, because many mental disorders occur early in life, special emphasis must be placed on prevention in childhood and adolescence. Effective, high-quality prenatal care and screening of new mothers (e.g. using the Edinburgh depression rating scale) can have a robust impact on the risk and detection of postpartum depression. The STEP programme (systematic training on effective parenting) assists in preventing attachment disorders and behavioural and emotional problems in the child. In early and later adulthood, screening, brief intervention, and referral to treatment (SBIRT) is an effective, well-studied secondary prevention approach to alcohol and substance use. Similarly, screening for depression in primary care settings has a secondary prevention, or early detection and intervention, goal. Among older adults, screening for early depressive symptoms and other secondary prevention measures, such as psychosocial support, is useful in isolated persons.

See also Chapter 37: Psychological interventions, for a discussion of tertiary prevention, Chapter 20: Alcohol-related disorders, for a discussion of alcohol-related disorders and Chapter 21: Other substance-related and addiction disorders, for a discussion of other substance-related disorders.

### 39.2.3.2 Early detection and intervention

Although overlapping with secondary prevention, early intervention is about individual and group counselling and support groups for high risk and vulnerable groups with unique needs, such as children in conflict with the law, children living and working on the streets, youth with academic, family or peer problems, women and the elderly.

### 39.2.3.3 Effective and comprehensive treatment

The focus is on effective and comprehensive treatment of persons with an established mental illness. Services are provided at all health facilities and accommodate people of all ages. These services vary depending on the level of skill and competency at the facility. At a primary health level it is integrated with general health services (both out-patient and in-patient) and provided by non-specialised mental health workers. In-patient care includes short-term hospitalisation of patients with uncomplicated mental illness, admission of assisted mental health care users, 72-hour assessment of involuntary mental health care users, and treatment of uncomplicated substance withdrawal. In some districts, there are secondary level specialised psychiatric services that provide care for complicated mental illness and supervision and support for the generalists treating both out-patient and in-patients. Effective and comprehensive treatment of more complicated mental illness (out-patient and in-patient) is provided at tertiary academic and specialised psychiatric institutions.

### 39.2.3.4 Aftercare and reintegration

Psychosocial rehabilitation (PSR) aims to facilitate the optimal functioning of mentally ill and disabled people (World Health Organization, 1996). It implies improving individuals' competencies and introducing environmental changes with a view to improving the quality of life of persons with a mental disorder or impaired mental capacity and a certain level of disability. Aftercare and rehabilitative services are provided at primary, secondary and tertiary levels of care, and involve collaboration with the community and other stakeholders. The goal is to give people with disabilities the ability for social and economic participation, independence and self-reliance.'The five basic elements of psychosocial rehabilitation are psycho-education, case management, skills teaching, vocational rehabilitation and appropriate housing' (Robertson *et al.*, 1997).

Psychosocial rehabilitation can be achieved by:

- reducing symptomatology through appropriate treatment
- reducing the adverse effects of treatment, including institutionalisation
- improving social functioning
- reducing discrimination and stigma
- providing family support
- providing social support, including basic needs related to housing, employment, social network, and leisure
- providing consumer empowerment.

See also Chapter 37: Psychological interventions, for a discussion of psychosocial rehabilitation.

## 39.2.4 Roles and responsibilities of key stakeholders

The roles and responsibilities of key stakeholders in mental health are set out in the Constitution and the National Health Act (No. 63 of 2003) and are listed below.

### 39.2.4.1 Minister of Health

The Minister of Health is responsible for:

- developing national mental health policy and legislation, in consultation with a range of stakeholders
- developing national strategic plans for mental health, in collaboration with provincial health services, and in consultation with a range of stakeholders
- monitoring and evaluating the implementation of policy and legislation, in relation to specified targets and indicators
- evaluating the prevalence and incidence of mental illness
- identifying and driving the implementation of key priority areas
- mental health promotion and prevention
- promoting research in priority areas, and utilising research evidence to inform policy, legislation and planning
- coordinating an intersectoral approach to mental health, through engagement of other sectors, and providing technical support to other sectors
- ensuring equity between provinces in mental health service provision.

### 39.2.4.2 Director General

The Director General is responsible for:

- developing guidelines for human resources for mental health
- issuing guidelines to promote a multi-disciplinary team approach to the planning and delivery of services
- developing and implementing norms and standards for mental health care
- developing and monitoring the implementation of clinical protocols for mental health at all service levels.

### 39.2.4.3 Provincial departments of health

The provincial departments of health are responsible for:

- translation of national policy into provincial operational plans, which include clear targets, indicators, budgets and timelines
- monitoring and evaluation of the implementation of national mental health policy and legislation
- provision of a sustainable budget for mental health services, keeping parity with other health conditions, in proportion to the burden of disease, and based on evidence for cost-effectiveness
- working closely with district health managers to promote the equitable provision of resources and services for mental health at district level
- consulting with a range of stakeholders in the planning and delivery of services
- integrating mental health indicators into the general health information system, for the routine monitoring and evaluation of mental health care
- facilitating intersectoral collaboration, to bring together all sectors involved in mental health, including education, social development, labour, criminal justice, housing, agriculture and NGOs
- ensuring the integration of mental health care into all health services, particularly within the district health system
- expanding the mental health workforce in all provinces
- building capacity for provincial health management in mental health planning, service monitoring and the translation of research findings into policy and practice.

#### 39.2.4.4 District health services

The district health services are responsible for:

- providing mental health promotion and prevention interventions, in keeping with national and provincial priorities
- inclusion of mental health in the core package of district health treatment and rehabilitation services
- routine screening for mental illness during pregnancy, and provision of counselling and referral where appropriate
- medication monitoring and psychosocial rehabilitation within a recovery framework for severe mental illness
- detection and management of depression and anxiety disorders in primary health care clinics and referral where appropriate
- detection and management of child and adolescent mental disorders in primary health care clinics, and referral where appropriate
- conducting mental health training programmes for all general health staff for basic screening, detection and treatment, as well as referral of complex cases
- establishing and maintaining mental health supervision systems for health staff at primary health care level
- establishing and maintaining specialist mental health teams to support primary health care staff
- establishing and maintaining referral and back-referral pathways for mental health
- implementing clinical protocols for assessment and interventions at primary health care level
- establishing and maintaining community-based rehabilitation programmes, through trained community health workers
- developing intersectoral collaboration between a range of sectors involved in mental health, through the establishment of district multisectoral forums for mental health
- undertaking mental health education programmes in communities
- provision of psychotropic medication to all appropriate levels of the district health system, as determined by the essential drugs list.

#### 39.2.4.5 Other sectors

- NGOs play an active role in the provision of health education and information on mental health and substance abuse, and the targeting of vulnerable groups such as women, children, the elderly and those with disabilities.
- The national Department of Health actively pursues partnerships between other government departments and traditional, faith-based, non-governmental and other private sector organisations.
- The provincial departments of health license and regulate the provision of community-based mental health services by NGOs, such as community residential care, day services, halfway houses, etc.
- District health services support all public sector workers and civil society partners who contribute to mental health care in the district.

## 39.3 Levels of care in psychiatry and mental health

Based on policies already discussed, the mental health services are delivered at three levels namely primary, secondary and tertiary, as shown in Table 39.2.

### 39.3.1 Primary mental health care

The components of primary health care are illustrated in Figure 39.3.

Primary health care is defined as essential, universally accessible, affordable health care provided at the first level of contact, and which should ideally provide promotive, preventive, curative and rehabilitative services, including public health measures and essential drugs. The principles of the primary health care system include intersectoral collaboration, maximum community participation and self-determination, the involvement of traditional practitioners and a mutually supportive referral system. (This is also known as the district health system). Most curative primary level care is provided on an out-patient basis. Rehabilitative primary level care includes attendance at clinics

**Table 39.2** Levels of mental health care

| Level of care | Components | Staff complement | Examples |
|---|---|---|---|
| **Primary mental health care** | ▶ community-based services | ▶ community-based workers | ▶ community workers |
| | ▶ primary health care clinics | ▶ primary nurse practitioners | ▶ clinics |
| | ▶ community health care centres | ▶ health care centre occupational therapists, social workers and nurses<br>▶ mental health nurses<br>▶ medical officers<br>▶ family physicians | ▶ larger primary health care centres |
| | ▶ district hospitals | ▶ district hospital nurses, occupational therapists and social workers<br>▶ mental health nurses<br>▶ medical officers | ▶ general acute hospitals |
| **Secondary psychiatric care** | ▶ community specialised mental health services<br>▶ specialised outreach services | ▶ psychiatrists<br>▶ psychologists<br>▶ occupational therapists<br>▶ social work outreach to primary care | ▶ outreach clinics at primary care sites |
| | ▶ psychiatric units in regional hospitals (secondary level hospitals) | ▶ full dedicated multidisciplinary team<br>▶ dedicated psychiatric units | ▶ hospitals with specialists |
| | ▶ general psychiatry units in specialised psychiatric hospitals | ▶ full dedicated multidisciplinary team | ▶ psychiatric hospitals |
| **Tertiary psychiatric care** | ▶ specialised units in tertiary academic hospitals | ▶ full dedicated subspecialist multidisciplinary team | ▶ child and adolescent units<br>▶ geriatric units |
| | ▶ subspecialist units in psychiatric hospitals | ▶ full dedicated subspecialist multidisciplinary team | ▶ forensic units<br>▶ neuropsychiatry units |

for maintenance and relapse prevention activities, vocational training and activities for daily living programmes in sheltered workshops, group homes and institutions. Given the complex, multifactorial, context-bound and long-term nature of many psychiatric disorders, treating them effectively at the primary care level requires the allocation of adequate resources and the selection of appropriate service models. In industrialised countries, psychiatrists, psychologists, social workers, or psychiatric nurses work in the community in supportive, supervisory or consultative relationships with general practitioners, or as case managers. In developing countries, case management is often undertaken by nurses, who are usually more available and accessible than other professionals. In regions where psychiatry is poorly understood and services are difficult to access, community workers (supervised by a professional) may make the best case managers.

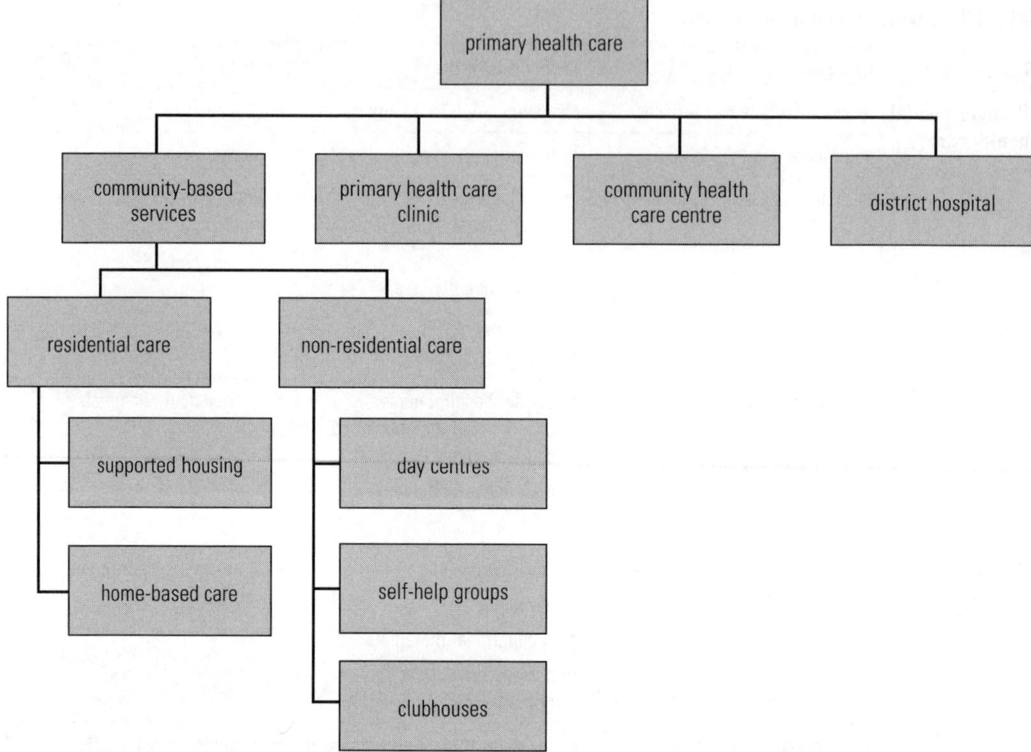


**Figure 39.3** Components of primary health care

## Information box

**Training**

Training and preparation of primary health care workers for these tasks includes training in knowledge and skills necessary to:

- elicit and detect mental health problems in all age and cultural groups
- arrange appropriate further investigations, including obtaining essential collateral information
- make a multi-axial diagnosis, and devising a multimodal, intersectoral treatment plan
- therapeutic skills appropriate for all ages, including basic counselling skills, basic cognitive behaviour strategies, and pharmacotherapy
- maintenance and rehabilitative skills, including case management
- basic promotive and preventive principles and strategies
- knowledge of when, where and how to refer
- a working knowledge of traditional healing practices and maintaining a dialogue with local traditional healers in which problem areas can be discussed, mutual education can occur and possible collaboration is facilitated.

### 39.3.1.1 Community-based services

Community-based services can either be provided at home, in the community or at primary health care centres. These services are usually provided by trained community workers and, in South Africa, mostly by NGOs. Areas of focus may include treatment adherence, relapse prevention, social skills, social interaction, rehabilitation and the early identification of imminent relapse. These services include home-based care and day centres.

### 39.3.1.2 Primary health care clinics

Primary health care clinics (PHCs) are easily accessible and are the entry level for all mental health users. Services are delivered at these facilities by primary care professionals, including community health workers, registered nurse practitioners, clinical nurse practitioners, medical officers, family physicians and other health staff (Department of Health, Republic of South Africa, 2000).

Here medical staff diagnose, investigate and initiate out-patient management options (at a biological, psychological and social level) of less complex and common mental health problems. If medical staff members are not available or the primary health care clinic does not have the necessary expertise, clinic staff will initiate emergency treatment and refer patients to a higher level of care (community health care centres). Primary health care staff members also provide long-term out-patient maintenance care of stable patients referred down from higher levels of care. This includes continued treatment, ongoing assessment (mental state, functional ability, social circumstances) and detection and monitoring of distress and relapse.

**Information box**

**Services at primary health care clinics**

- Information on mental health and mental illness to address ignorance, fear and prejudice.
- Community awareness programs for mental health according to the national and international calendar.
- Diagnosis, investigation and initiation of out-patient management options (biological, psychological, social level) of less complex and common mental health problems.
- Initiation of emergency treatment and referral of patients to a higher level of care (e.g. community health care centres).
- Recognition of the key features of more complex mental health problems (other than those listed above) and the expediting of referral to other levels or types of care (e.g. Community specialised mental health services (CMHS) or in-patient care).
- Provision of long term out-patient maintenance care of stable patients referred down from higher levels of care. This includes continued treatment and ongoing assessment (mental state, functional ability and social circumstances).

### 39.3.1.3 Community health care centres

Larger community health care centres often include general medical officers, dedicated mental health nurses and access to multidisciplinary team members, such as social workers and occupational therapists. The complement of staff are able to manage most mild to moderate psychiatric illnesses and can refer patients to higher levels of care (e.g. district hospitals, secondary hospitals, psychiatric hospitals, mental health outreach teams, community specialised mental health services) should they not be able to diagnose and stabilise patients. Staff at this level initiate emergency and out-patient treatment and make the necessary follow-up arrangements (i.e. booking with outreach specialist services). Here, long-term out-patient management of stable moderate to severely ill patients is offered, as well as acute and maintenance care of unstable mildly to moderately ill patients.

**Information box**

**Services at community health care centres**

- Information on mental health and mental illness to address ignorance, fear, and prejudice.
- Community awareness programs for mental health according to the national and international calendar.
- Emergency psychiatric care, including a good medical and psychiatric history, physical examinations, side-room tests and basic special investigations.
- Exclusion and treatment of medical illnesses causing psychiatric symptoms.
- Recognition of the key features of more complex mental health problems.
- Capacity to organise and refer patients for admission under the Mental Health Care Act at higher levels of care.
- Diagnosis, investigation and treatment of out-patients (biological, psychological and social level) with less complex and common mental health problems.
- Provision of long-term out-patient maintenance care of stable patients referred down from higher levels of care. This includes continued treatment and ongoing assessment (mental state, functional ability and social circumstances).

#### 39.3.1.4 District hospitals

The mental health services that are offered at a district hospital include in-patient psychiatric care in the general wards and emergency departments. Patients are up-referred to these hospitals by medical staff from primary health care clinics, community health care centres and community specialised mental health services, and are down-referred for continued in-patient care from regional and tertiary academic hospitals with designated psychiatric units. The services are provided by family physicians (who have received special training in psychiatry) as well as nurses (preferably at least one dedicated, mental health trained nurse) with support from specialised psychiatric outreach services and community specialised mental health services working in the district.

**Information box**

**Services at district hospitals**

- Information on mental health and mental illness to address ignorance, fear, and prejudice.
- Emergency psychiatric care, including a good medical and psychiatric history, physical examinations, side-room tests and special investigations.
- Exclusion and treatment of medical illnesses causing psychiatric symptoms and co-morbid medical conditions.
- Care and management of voluntary and assisted mental health users, including the admission of acutely ill patients under the MHCA for 72-hour hospital assessment periods.
- Diagnosis, investigation, initiation of emergency and non- emergency treatment and referral of patients with complex and serious mental illness for care at a higher level (e.g. hospitals with designated psychiatric units or psychiatric hospitals).
- Diagnosis, investigation and treatment of out-patients (biological, psychological and social level) with mild to moderate mental illness or problems.
- Provision of consultation/liaison services for general medical patients with psychiatric symptoms and planned out-patient programs for follow-up of some in-patients.
- Discharge of stable patients for out-patient maintenance care to primary health care clinics, community health care centres or community specialised mental health services and the ensuring of a seamless service delivery.
- Support groups for patients and families - training, education and assistance to family and carers of patients, encouraging them to play an active role in rehabilitation.
- Provision of outreach and support to primary health care and community health care levels.

### 39.3.2 Secondary mental health care

Secondary mental health care is general specialised psychiatric care provided at regional level and may be on an out-patient or in-patient basis. Secondary level public-sector psychiatric services are usually situated in general and psychiatric hospitals. In addition, in South Africa, the community mental health team provides specialised secondary services and support to the primary health care service.

### 39.3.2.1 Community specialised mental health services and specialised outreach services

These specialised secondary level services provide non-urgent assessments, treatment, case management, support and continuing care services to people with serious mental illnesses in the community. This specialised service can be based at district hospitals, community health care centres and some large primary health care clinics (where there are no community health care centres) and has close working links with district, regional, academic and psychiatric hospitals. Mental health users are referred to these services from the primary services at primary health care clinics, community health care centres and district hospitals, or are down-referred from in-patient facilities for continued out-patient care as per the referral pathways. The services are provided by dedicated psychiatric nurses, psychologists, social workers, occupational therapists, and psychiatrists or registrars (i.e. a multidisciplinary team).

**Information box**

**Services by community specialised mental health services**

- Provision of specialised out-patient services by referral from primary health care services.
- Diagnosis, investigation and initiation of out-patient management options (at biological, psychological and social level) of complex and moderate to severe mental illness.
- Initiation of emergency out-patient treatment and referral of patients for in-patient care if it is required.
- Down-referral of stable patients for long-term out-patient maintenance care to primary health care clinics and community health care centres.
- Rehabilitation of mentally ill patients.
- Support groups for patients and families in the form of training, education and assistance to family and carers of patients, encouraging them to play an active role in rehabilitation.

### 39.3.2.2 Regional hospitals with designated psychiatric units

Some regional hospitals have designated psychiatric units, which provide assessments, in-patient treatment, case management, support and continuing care to people with a moderate to severe mental illness. They have close working links with academic and psychiatric hospitals. Patients are up-referred to these hospitals by medical staff from primary health care clinics, community health care centres, community specialised mental health services and district and regional hospitals, or are down-referred for continued in patient care from tertiary academic hospitals. The services are provided by a dedicated multidisciplinary team which consist of psychiatric nurses, psychologists, social workers, occupational therapists, and psychiatrists or registrars.

**Information box**

**Services at regional hospitals**

- Information on mental health and mental illness to address ignorance and prejudice.
- Diagnosis, investigation and initiation of in-patient care (biological, psychological and social level) of complex and mild to moderate mental illness.
- Care of voluntary, assisted and involuntary mental health users.
- Conducting of 72-hour hospital assessment periods.
- Admission of involuntary mental health users beyond the 72-hour hospital assessment periods.
- Diagnosis, investigation, initiation of emergency treatment and referral of patients for in-patient care at a higher level (academic and psychiatric hospitals).
- Provision of consultation or liaison services.
- Provision of planned out-patient programs for follow-up of some in-patients.
- Discharge of stable patients for out-patient maintenance care.
- Support groups for patients and families – training, education and assistance to family and carers of patients, encouraging them to play an active role in rehabilitation.

### 39.3.2.3 Care and rehabilitation centres

The information box below illustrates the levels of services available at care and rehabilitation centres.

**Information box**

**Services at care and rehabilitation centres**

- Long-term in-patient services to individuals who are profoundly and severely mentally disabled where constant supervision and medical care is warranted. Care, treatment and rehabilitation needs are such that these individuals cannot be managed at home or at a NGO residential care facility.
- Medium-term in-patient services to individuals who are moderately mentally disabled who may benefit from a finite period of care, treatment and rehabilitation to the extent where they can be discharged to their families or to other community-based services.
- Day care or out-patient services for individuals whose degree of disability allows for them to be managed at home and whose families are capable of and willing to do this. Families bring the users in to the day care centres, which have programs designed for each user based on his or her disabilities.
- Respite care: week-end and/or weekly respite care for families who are capable of and willing to take care of users.

### 39.3.2.4 Tertiary care

Tertiary care is the highest level of referral, and becomes necessary when patients require highly specialised diagnostic and therapeutic techniques. It includes subspecialty areas and the most sophisticated medical technology. It can be provided in the private or public sector (usually academic or psychiatric hospitals), to both in- and out-patients. These services can be provided at both specialist psychiatric hospitals or at tertiary academic hospitals.

Psychiatric disorders requiring referral to the highest level of care are likely to be:

- any treatment-resistant disorder requiring tertiary intervention
- any complex disorder posing a diagnostic problem
- any disorder for which the required therapeutic intervention is not available outside the tertiary level. These would include disorders falling within the following sub-specialist fields in psychiatry:
  - forensic psychiatry
  - child and adolescent psychiatry
  - geriatric psychiatry
  - neuropsychiatry
  - substance-related disorders.

As at the other levels of care, psycho-education and psychosocial rehabilitation (where indicated) must be planned and provided from the beginning of the tertiary care process, together with the curative treatments. After the completion of tertiary level assessment or treatment, patients should be referred back to the lowest level of care able to provide appropriate follow-up.

### 39.3.2.5 Tertiary academic hospitals

These services provide short-term in-patient treatment and rehabilitation for users who have unremitting and severe symptoms of mental illness, together with associated significant disturbance, that inhibit their capacity to live in the community. They represent one of the highest levels of care on the continuum of mental health services and are mostly focused on sub-specialist disciplines within psychiatry. These specialised tertiary level services provide assessments, in-patient treatment, case management, support and continuing care to people with a serious mental illness.

This specialised service has close working links with psychiatric hospitals. Patients can be up referred to these hospitals by medical staff from primary health care clinics, community health care centres, community specialised mental health services, district and regional hospitals, or referred from psychiatric hospitals for both in-patient and out-patient care. The services are provided by a dedicated multidisciplinary team of psychiatric nurses, psychologists, social workers, occupational therapists, and psychiatrists or registrars. These multidisciplinary teams are often

**Information box**

**Services at tertiary academic hospitals**

- Information on mental health and mental illness to address ignorance, fear and prejudice.
- Diagnosis, investigation and initiation of in-patient care (biological, psychological and social level) of complex and moderate to severe mental illness.
- Care of voluntary, assisted and involuntary mental health users.
- Conduct of 72-hour hospital assessment periods
- Medium- to long-term admission of involuntary mental health users beyond the 72-hour hospital assessment periods.
- Provision of specialised in- and out-patient services to general adult and special population patients, including specialised therapeutic services, substance use services and eating disorder services.
- Discharge of stable patients for out-patient maintenance care to primary health care clinics, community health care centres, community specialised mental health services or regional services.
- Provision of planned out-patient programs for follow-up of some in-patients.
- Support groups for patients and families – training, education and assistance to family and carers of patients, encouraging them to play an active role in rehabilitation.

dedicated subspecialist teams, such as a child and adolescent subspecialist team.

#### 39.3.2.6 Specialised psychiatric hospitals

Specialised psychiatric hospitals are independent, stand-alone services that provide medium- to long-term in-patient treatment and rehabilitation for users who have unremitting and severe symptoms of mental illness, together with associated significant disturbance, that makes it difficult to manage them at other facilities. While they often represent the highest level of care on the continuum of mental health services and have medium-security and high-security units, they are not necessarily acknowledged as tertiary services in South Africa. General adult services (including therapeutic services) are managed as secondary services.

Tertiary services at specialised psychiatric hospitals include forensic services, child and adolescent services, neuropsychiatric services and geriatric psychiatry services. Patients will be referred to these hospitals by medical staff from district and regional hospitals and tertiary hospitals for continued in-patient care. The services are provided by a multi-disciplinary team of psychiatric nurses, psychologists, social workers, occupational therapists, psychiatrists or registrars. In a tertiary service unit the services will be provided by members of a multidisciplinary team and a registered subspecialist psychiatrist or subspecialist registrar.

## 39.4 Referral pathways

Figure 39.4 illustrates the appropriate referral pathways between different levels of care and different mental health services.

## 39.5 Resources for different contexts

Table 39.3 summarises what mental health services might be expected in contexts with differing levels of resources.

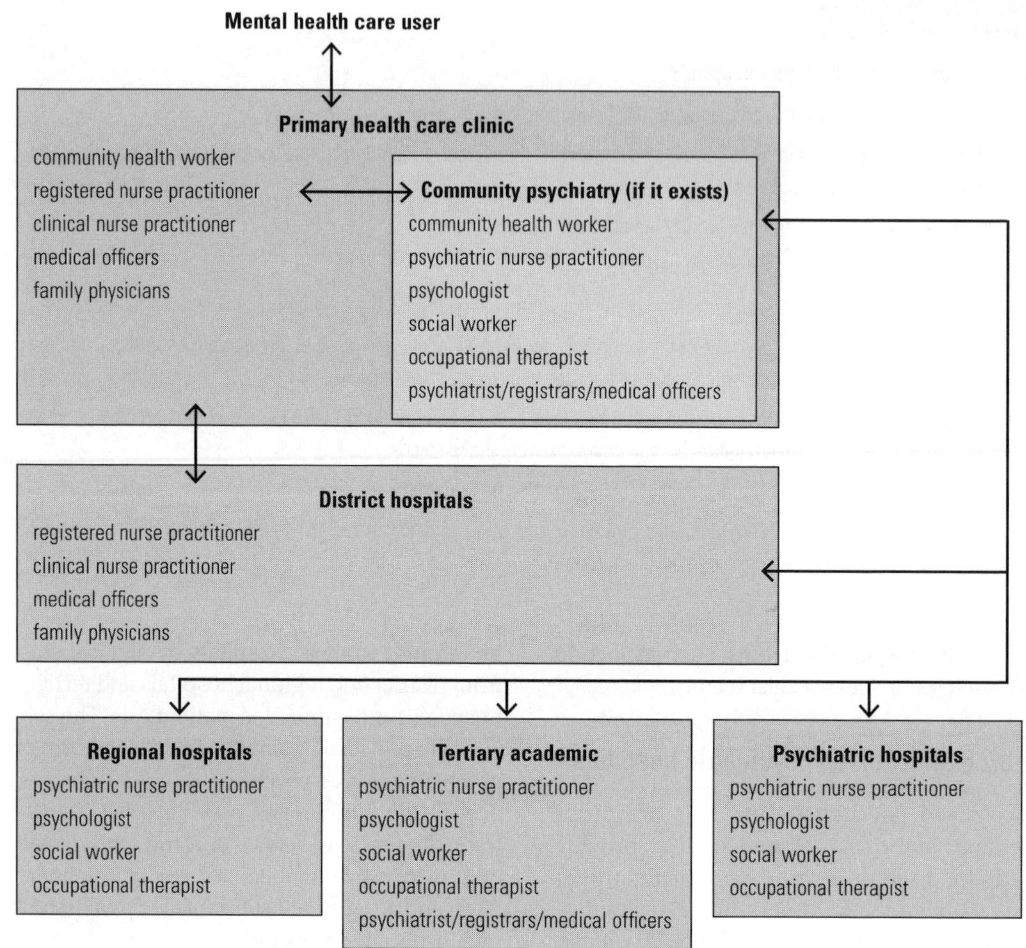


**Figure 39.4** Referral pathways

**Table 39.3** Mental health service components for low-, medium- and high-resource contexts

| Low-resource contexts | Medium-resource contexts | High-resource contexts |
|---|---|---|
| Primary care mental health with specialist backup | Primary care mental health with specialist backup and mainstream mental health care | Primary care mental health with specialist backup and mainstream mental health care and specialised or differentiated mental health services |
| Screening and assessment by primary care staff<br>Talking treatments, including counselling and advice<br>Pharmacological treatment | Out-patient/ambulatory clinics | Specialised clinics addressing specific disorders or patient groups, including:<br>▶ eating disorders<br>▶ dual diagnoses<br>▶ treatment-resistant affective disorders<br>▶ adolescent services |
| | Community mental health teams (CMHTs) | Specialised CMHTs, including:<br>▶ early intervention teams<br>▶ assertive community treatment (ACT) teams |

## Conclusion

South Africa has an excellent mental health policy that is aligned with most international mental health systems. It is evidenced based and ensures that all aspects of mental health care are included and provided for at all facility levels. It encompasses a fundamental prerequisite for effective care, which is the involvement of the community and community-based services, to help integrate mentally ill persons back within their communities. Full implementation of the policy, however, will take a few years and achievement of all the objectives is dependent on the availability of the necessary resources (infrastructure, human and financial).

# References


Compton MT, Shim R (2014). Considering Edison's predictions: Prevention as the next frontier for psychiatry. *Psychiatric Times*. Available at: http://www.psychiatrictimes.com (Accessed 1 August 2014.)

Department of Health, Republic of South Africa (2000) *The Primary Health Care Package for South Africa – a set of norms and standards*. Available at: http://bettercare.co.za/wp-content/uploads/2013/01/The-Primary-Health-Care-Package-for-South-Africa-a-set-of-norms-and-standards.htm (Accessed 9 August 2014.)

Department of Health, Republic of South Africa (2013) *The National Mental Health Policy Framework and Strategic Plan 2013–2020*. Available at: www.health-e.org.za (Accessed 14 January 2015.)

Desjarlais R, Eisenberg L, Good B, Kleinman A (Eds) (1995) *World Mental Health. Problems and Priorities in Low-Income Countries*. New York. Oxford: University Press.

Institute for Work and Health (2015) What researchers mean by … primary, secondary and tertiary prevention. *At Work* 80 Available at: http://www.iwh.on.ca/wrmb/primary-secondary-and-tertiary-prevention (Accessed 31 August 2015)

Mrazek PJ, Haggerty RJ (Eds) (1994) *Reducing risks for mental disorders: Frontiers for preventive intervention research*. Washington: The National Academics Press

Robertson IH, Manly T, Andrade J, Baddeley BT, Yiend J (1997) 'Oops!': Performance correlates of everyday attentional failures in traumatic brain injured and normal subjects. *Neuropsychologia* 35: 747–58

Stein DJ (2014) A new mental health policy for South Africa. *South African Medical Journal* 104(2):115–6

Stein DJ, Seedat S, Herman A, Moomal H, Heeringa SG, Kessler RC, Williams DR (2008) Lifetime prevalence of psychiatric disorders in South Africa. *The British Journal of Psychiatry* 192: 112–7

World Health Organisation (1978) *Declaration of Alma-Ata* International Conference on Primary Health Care, Alma-Ata, USSR. Available at: www.who.int/publications/almaata_declaration_en.pdf

World Health Organisation (1996) *Psychosocial rehabilitation: a consensus statement*. Geneva: World Health Organisation. Available at: http://apps.who.int/iris/handle/10665/60630

World Health Organization (2003) *Mental Health Policy and Service Guidance Package. Organization of Services for Mental Health*. Geneva: World Health Organization. Available at: http://www.who.int/mental_health/policy/services/4_organisation%20services_WEB_07.pdf?ua=1 (Accessed 16 May 2015.)

World Health Organization (2006) *The World Health Report: Working together for health*. www.who.int/whr/2006/en/. (Accessed 4 August 2014.)

World Health Organization (2010a) *Mental health and work: Impact, issues and good practices*. Available at: www.who.int/mental_health/media/en/712.pdf (Accessed 2 February 2014.)

World Health Organization (2010b) *Violence and Health in the WHO African Region - Regional Office for Africa*. Available at: www.afro.who.int/index.php (Accessed 2 December 2013.)

World Health Organization (2013) *The World Health Report*. Available at: www.who.int/whr/2013/en/ (Accessed 7 August 2014.)

World Health Organisation (2014) *Mental health: strengthening our response*. Fact sheet N°220. Updated August 2014. Available at: http://www.who.int/mediacentre/factsheets/fs220/en/ (Accessed 31 August 2015)

CHAPTER

# 40 Combating stigma in psychiatry

*Mashadi Motlana*

## 40.1 Introduction

The history of mental illness and society's treatment of those with mental illness is a regrettable story of stigmatisation, discrimination and social rejection.

In Ancient Greek medicine, the Hippocratic Corpus held a theory that the cause of mental illness was a blocked vein to the brain. The previous belief that epilepsy was a 'sacred disease' was denounced as a misnomer invented by charlatans who were not able to cure the disease. Rather, epilepsy was to be regarded as an illness like any other. Sadly, this enlightened explanation was not widely embraced and the mentally ill continued to be the subject of fear, shame and guilt.

Mental illness was attributed to the four humours: blood, yellow bile, black bile and phlegm; each of which was thought to be more prominent according to the respective season – spring, summer, autumn and winter. Black bile, in particular, was associated with mental illness and autumn in Graeco-Roman times.

The earliest writings that attributed the psychological manifestations of mental illness to physiological causes were those of Socrates.

The Greek and Hebrew explanation of mental illness was that of demon possession. Several millennia later, this theory of causality is still firmly held by certain segments of society.

Plato, in *The Republic,* describes madness or disease as injustice and health as justice. Mental illness is equated with cowardice and self-indulgence and sufferers are considered weak and socially deviant.

During the Middle Ages and well into the 17th century, the demonological explanation for mental illness was prominent.

One of the earliest known asylums in Europe, the Priory of St Mary of Bethlehem, was founded in the 13th century. Its name was later corrupted to Bedlam in colloquial language. The conditions, as the modern understanding of the word 'bedlam' infers, were ghastly. The 'insane' were manacled to walls and deprived of basic freedoms. In the absence of asylums, families treated their family members in a similar fashion, holding them in barns, chained to stakes and out of view of a society that was intolerant of any variation in rigid societal norms of the time.

It was not until the end of the 18th century and the Age of Enlightenment that the idea of a therapeutic asylum was proposed. Up until then the institutions had performed a custodial function only. William Battie, a British psychiatrist who published his *Treatise on Madness*, in 1758, was one of the first psychiatrists to argue for the therapeutic benefits of an asylum. He went on to propose the idea that mental illnesses were not uniformly incurable.

Phillippe Pinel, a 19th century Parisian psychiatrist, is credited with removing the shackles from the asylum (although Vincenzio Chiarugi, an Italian psychiatrist, may have been the first to unchain his patients) and supported the use of psychological treatment.

Biological psychiatry arose out of 'the desire of psychiatrists to lay bare the relationship between the brain and the mind through systematic research' (Shorter, 1998). In addition, for psychiatry to become a discipline to be taught and researched, it was necessary for mental illness to become medicalised. This required for mental illness to be 'de-demonised' by emphasing medical attributions to the illness. Historically this occurred at the same time that tuberculosis and nephritis were drawn into medicine in other medical disciplines.

## 40.2 Understanding stigma

The origin of the word stigma dates back to Ancient Greece when slaves were branded with a mark on their bodies to denote their status as belonging to an inferior class of citizens.

The stigma attached to cancer has diminished with the advent of effective treatment and similarly attitudes towards HIV/Aids have improved. Although mental illness is rarely fatal or contagious, and despite advances in treatment and knowledge, it remains highly stigmatised. The sociologist Gerhard Falk notes that 'the ability to think and act rationally and in a meaningful fashion has been declared mandatory by public opinion since the Age of Reason began in the 18$^{th}$ Century' (Falk, 2001). This requirement on the part of individuals makes the stigma attached to mental illness more severe.

Corrigan and Wassel (2008) use a cognitive behavioural construct to describe stigma and identify four social-cognitive processes – cues, stereotypes, prejudice, and discrimination – that can manifest as public stigma and self-stigma. In this model the first step in the evolution of stigma involves the identification of cues such as psychiatric symptoms, a deficiency in social skills, or a disheveled physical appearance and/or the use of labels (e.g. clinical diagnoses) that may suggest that an individual has a mental illness. Cues may trigger cognitive associations with negative stereotypes. An individual may either endorse the stereotypes by accepting them or rejecting them. Prejudice results when those who endorse the stereotypes hold negative attitudes about the mentally ill. Discrimination is the behavioural manifestation of prejudice.

### 40.2.1 Self-stigmatisation

Self-stigma describes the phenomenon that occurs when an individual identifies himself or herself with the stigmatising stereotypes associated with a mental illness. The idea that one is somehow responsible for one's mental illness, for example, may resonate with that individual. As a result he or she may experience low self-esteem and, feeling discouraged by daily experiences of discrimination, withdraw from trying to find a job or from entering into a meaningful relationship. The 'why try?' effect leads to a lack of self-efficacy and low self-confidence. The individual may also be affected emotionally and experience a depressed mood and low self-esteem (Corrigan and Wassel, 2008).

### 40.2.2 Perceived or felt stigma

Perceived stigma is the phenomenon where individuals with a (potentially) stigmatised health condition fear the negative perceptions and the possible enactment of discriminatory behaviour by society. This is not associated with shame as is the case with self-stigma. Felt stigma describes perceived stigma that is associated with shame and represents a combination of perceived and self stigma (Brohan *et al.*, 2010).

### 40.2.3 Experienced stigma

Experienced stigma is described by Van Brakel *et al.* (2006) as the 'experience of actual discrimination and/or participation restrictions on the part of the person affected'. Participation restriction refers to the social exclusion of individuals with mental illness and manifests itself most commonly in the socioeconomic marginalisation of this population group. An example of this is discriminatory labour practices that hinder the attempts of mentally ill individuals to find gainful employment.

### 40.2.4 Label avoidance

Label avoidance occurs when individuals who experience mental illness avoid seeking help. This is an attempt to escape the negative effects of stigma associated with receiving a diagnosis and thereby becoming a member of the group of 'the mentally ill'. Help-seeking behaviour is compromised as these individuals fear being stigmatised. This results in delays in presenting for treatment and has a negative impact on their prognosis.

### 40.2.5 Courtesy stigma

Families, caregivers and mental health professionals may experience stigma by virtue of their association with mentally ill people.

Perceived genetic liability for certain forms of mental illness may increase social distance (e.g. the marriage prospects of family members may be diminished by a family history of mental illness). Social distance describes the extent to which there is a reluctance to associate with an individual with a mental illness at various levels of interaction. Employing a mentally ill individual as a secretary for example, may be more acceptable that entrusting that individual with the job of a baby sitter.

### 40.2.6 Institutional stigma

Disparities in the allocation of resources (e.g. health care budgets allocate more resources towards communicable diseases, with mental health care services attracting a smaller slice of the pie) and the organisation of mental health care services (i.e. the resistance towards the integration of psychiatry with general medical services at primary levels of care) reflect how stigma influences the manner in which the needs of mental health users are addressed or neglected.

Health care professionals also contribute to the stigmatisation of the mentally ill. Patients feel stigmatised by the attitudes of their health providers and describe feeling punished, patronised, humiliated and spoken to as though they were children. They also describe feeling an unspoken threat of coercive treatment that could result in involuntary care and treatment. Of equal concern is that patients report feeling excluded from decision-making processes and not being adequately informed about treatment and medication side effects such as weight gain.

Key findings of a mortality analysis released by the UK Health and Social Care Information Centre in 2011 revealed that the mortality rate for mental health services users was 4 008 per 100 000 (83 390 deaths in total), compared to the general population rate of 1 122 per 100 000 (Health and Social Care Information Centre, 2013).

People with a mental illness are less likely to receive appropriate treatment for their general medical problems for a variety of reasons, including bias toward the individual. Lifestyle diseases feature prominently among the causes of higher than expected morbidity and mortality in this group. The metabolic side effects of some psychiatric medication and the increased rates of smoking put this vulnerable population group at risk.

Psychiatry is not seen as an important subject in some countries and this bias is reflected in the education of medical students. As a result, medical students often become dismissive of psychiatry and mentally ill patients.

The stigmatising attitudes of the general public is reflected in the widely held belief that the mentally ill are dangerous. The response is to react with fear. Reports in the media, for example, often sensationalise crimes committed by a mentally ill person. This further reinforces the fear that the mentally ill are dangerous. There is no evidence to support the belief that individuals with a mental illness pose more of a threat than members of the general public.

Movies often portray mental illness in ways that perpetuate the stigma that surrounds mental illness. The mentally ill are portrayed at times as childlike and requiring protection and benevolence and in other instances as being dangerous and unpredictable.

## 40.3 Strategies to address stigma in mental health

### 40.3.1 Education: improving the mental health literacy of the public

Raising awareness about mental illness leads to an improved recognition of signs and symptoms and increased health-seeking behaviour. In a review of the impact of education campaigns, it was found that mental health literacy had indeed improved. There was also an increased likelihood that the services of a mental health practitioner would be sought. However, the stigmatising attitudes towards those with a mental illness also increased. The attribution of illness to a biological cause appeared to have the unintended consequences of increasing the stigmatising attitudes of the general public towards the mentally ill (Spriggs *et al.*, 2008; Pattyn *et al.*, 2013).

### 40.3.2 Protest

Protest may take the form of a written objection to incorrect representations of mental illness in the media and other public forums. The opportunity to engage with both media and politicians on the issue of mental illness raises sensitivities to how these important public voices may be contributing to the negative perceptions of mental illness.

### 40.3.3 Contact-based education

Exposure to, and interaction with, an individual who has successfully managed mental illness is a powerful way to reduce stigma and to challenge the message of hopelessness that is often communicated to individuals with a mental illness by health professionals and the general public.

### 40.3.4 Legislative reform

Important actions include lobbying government to address the discrepancies in health care expenditure, pushing for legislation that makes discriminatory practice illegal, that protects the human rights of individuals with a mental illness, and calling for the enactment of laws that decrease social exclusion.

### 40.3.5 Advocacy

Advocacy makes use of various platforms to engage decision-makers on the needs of mental health care users. It involves education, training, mutual help, counselling, mediating and defending (Newbigging and McKeown, 2007; Arboleda-Floréz and Stuart, 2012). This is aimed at improving access to services such as housing, education, health care and increasing opportunities for employment.

The various types of advocacy include:

- self-advocacy, peer advocacy and citizen advocacy that aim to empower the individual to speak for him- or herself (Pandya and Jän Myrick, 2012). Consumer advocacy groups run by people with a mental illness have been quite powerful in challenging institutional and public stigma in many countries. Peer advocacy enables individuals to take control of their illness by engaging with their mental health care provider.
- professional advocacy, non-instructed advocacy and legal advocacy that maximise choices and enhance decision-making within a legal framework
- collective advocacy occurs when a group is formed to challenge inequalities
- community advocacy promotes better health services within the community

### 40.3.6 Self-management

Addressing self-stigma is an important part of the journey to recovery. One of the strategies employed to tackle this challenge is to encourage membership of the individual in a group where he or she affiliates for support and personal empowerment. Coming out with the disclosure of having a mental illness may be useful for the individual; this can be done privately or publicly. Public disclosures help to fight the roots of stigma by illustrating that a large number of people are, in fact, affected by the illness. The president of Norway, Kjell Magne Bondevik, became the highest ranking world leader to make public an episode of major depressive disorder and took leave of absence for three weeks during his first term in 1998. This declaration was well received by the Norwegian electorate and made a substantial contribution towards making depression less stigmatised in that country.

## 40.4 Tools to measure stigma in individuals with a mental illness

The most commonly used instrument to measuring stigma is the self-reporting perceived devaluation and discrimination scale (PDD), which measures perceived stigma, discrimination and devaluation (Brohan *et al.*, 2010).

Other tools that measure experienced stigma include the internalised stigma of mental illness scale (ISMI) (Boyd *et al.*, 2014), the consumer experiences of stigma questionnaire (CESQ) (Switaj *et al.*, 2013)) and the rejection experiences scale (RES) (Hansson and Bjorkman, 2005).

The ISMI and the depression self-stigma scale (DSSS) (Barney *et al.*, 2010) are examples of instruments that measure aspects of self-stigma.

## 40.5 Measuring mental health literacy

In a review of instruments used to measure mental health literacy, O'Connor and colleagues (2014) found that there was a paucity of information on the psychometric attributes measured by the mental health literacy scale. There also is very little information on how the scales were developed and the sample populations used to test the scales.

Recent studies reviewing anti-stigma interventions have reported some interesting findings. The results from the Stigma in Global Context Mental Health Study (SGC-MHS) conducted across 16 countries, including South Africa, showed that levels of recognition, acceptance of the neurobiological attribution and treatment endorsement were high, but that this did not correlate with lower levels of prejudice (Pescosolido *et al.*, 2013). The gains observed in mental health literacy rates translated into increased awareness of mental illness and also raised the likelihood that a mental health practitioner would be consulted. In another study, data from the 1996 US mental health modules of the General Social Survey were compared to data from the 2006 General Social Survey; it concluded that the biological conception of mental illness appeared to be associated with increased social distance and perceived danger (Pescoscolido *et al.*, 2010). Pescoscolido and colleagues hypothesised that the root causes of stigma were the moralistic, religious and unscientific attributions to the mental illness and that improvements in mental health literacy would counter the prejudicial attitudes towards the mentally ill. The hypothesis was not supported by the findings in this study. It would appear that stigma-reduction strategies will have to be reconfigured to target recovery; and inherent in that are the concepts of social inclusion and competence.

## Conclusion

In South Africa several pieces of legislation attempt to protect the rights of people with mental illness. The most pertinent of these is the Mental Health Care Act (No. 17 of 2002) that seeks to treat the mentally ill primarily in the community and limit the exercise of involuntary care. Safeguards that are in place include Mental Health Review Boards to which an individual or family member can appeal admission or report any abuses.

South Africa is a signatory to the UN Convention on the Rights of Persons with Disabilities (see http://www.un.org/disabilities/convention/conventionfull.shtml). The Employment Equity Act (No. 55 of 1998) protects people with disabilities from unfair discrimination in the workplace. The employer is expected to provide reasonable accommodations for disabled employees once he or she has become aware of the conditions. Reasonable accommodations in the case of a mentally ill individual may include, for example, redeploying an employee to a less stressful position or modifying his or her work hours.

In recognition of the fact that mental illness will be the leading cause of disability by 2020, the World Health Organization coined the slogan 'No health without mental health' to emphasise the importance of integrating mental health services with general medical services (World Health Organization, 2014). It is understood that mental health is not simply an absence of disease. Mental health is determined by socio-economic, biological and environmental factors. Efforts to advocate for the mentally ill necessitate cost-effective intersectoral strategies and interventions, global collaboration to share best practices, more research to support evidence-based treatment and improvements in the quality of mental health care services. In 2013 the World Health Assembly approved a 'Comprehensive mental health action plan for 2013–2020' to encourage member nations to take specific actions to improve mental health.

Recovery for individuals living with a mental illness is a central goal of treatment that mental health practitioners have only recently begun to embrace. Recent clinical outcome studies on schizophrenia have demonstrated that a reasonable quality of life can be achieved and have also challenged the messages of hopelessness that are driven by the traditional views on mental illness. Mental health care practitioners can play a pivotal role by inspiring, giving hope and empowering the individual. A helping or therapeutic relationship predicts better outcomes with less time spent hospitalised, improved medication adherence and improved functioning. The definition of recovery for an individual is personal but usually entails finding purpose and meaning in life through renewed hope and empowerment that is associated with improved self-confidence, self-efficacy and self-determination (Russinova *et al.*, 2011).

A person-centred integrative diagnosis has been embraced by several global organisations such as the World Psychiatric Association and the World Health Organization. This diagnostic model marries science and humanism and can be conceptualised as a 'diagnosis of the person (of the totality of the person's health, both ill and positive aspects), by the person (with clinicians extending themselves as full human beings), for the person (assisting the fulfillment of the person's health aspirations and life project), and with the person (in respectful and empowering relationship with the person who consults)' (Mezzich *et al.*, 2010). This model may provide mental health practitioners with some insight and competence in playing a role in the recovery of the mental ill and promoting mental health.

(Also see Chapter 38: Social interventions in psychiatry, for a further discussion of recovery and Chapter 8: Person-centred psychiatry, for a further discussion of the person-centered approach.)

# References


Arboleda-Floréz J, Stuart H (2012) From sin to science: Fighting the stigmatization of mental illnesses. *Canadian Journal of Psychiatry* 57(8): 457–63

Barney LJ, Griffiths KM, Christensen H, Jorm AF (2010) The Self-Stigma of Depression Scale (SSDS): Development and psychometric properties of a new instrument. *International Journal of Methods in Psychiatric Research* 19(4): 243–54

Boyd JE, Adler EP, Otilingam PG, Peters T (2014) Internalised Stigma of Mental Illness Scale: A multinational review. *Comprehensive Psychiatry* 55 (1) 221–31

Brohan E, Slade M, Clement S, Thornicroft G (2010) Experiences of mental illness, stigma, prejudice and discrimination: A review of measures. *BMC Health Services Research* 10: 80

Corrigan PW, Wassel A (2008) Understanding and influencing the stigma of mental illness. *Journal of Psychological Nursing* 46(1): 42–8

Falk G (2001) *Stigma: How We Treat Outsiders.* Amherst, NewYork: Prometheus Books

Hansson L, Bjorkman T( 2005) Empowerment in people with mental illness: Reliability and validity of the Swedish version of an empowerement scale. *Scandanavian Journal of Caring Science* 19: 32–8

Health and Social Care Information Centre (2013) *Mortality rate three times as high among mental health service users than in the general population*. Available at: www.hscic.gov.uk (Accessed 26 September 2014.)

Mezzich JE, Salloum IM, Cloninger CR, Salvador-Carulla L, Kirmayer LJ, Banzato CE, Wallcraft J, Botbol M (2010) Person-centred integrative diagnosis: Conceptual bases and structural model. *Canadian Journal of Psychiatry* 55(11): 701–8

Newbigging K, McKeown M (2007) Mental health advocacy with black and minority ethnic communities: Conceptual and ethical implications. *Current Opinion in Psychiatry* 20(6): 588–93

O'Connor M, Casey L, Clough B (2014) Measuring mental health literacy – a review of scale-based measures. *Journal of Mental Health* 23(4): 197–204

Pandya A, Jän Myrick K (2012) wellness and recovery programs: A model of self-advocacy for people living with mental illness. *Journal of Psychiatric Practice* 19(3): 242–6

Pattyn E, Verhaeghe M, Sercu C, Bracke P (2013) Medicalizing versus psychologizing mental illness: What are the implications for help seeking and stigma? A general population study. *Social Psychiatry and Psychiatric Epidemiology* 48(10): 1637–45

Pescosolido BA, Martin JK, Long JS, Medina TR, Phelan JC, Link BG (2010) A disease like any other? A decade of change in public reactions to schizophrenia, depression and alcohol dependence. *American Journal of Psychiatry* 167(11): 1321–30

Pescosolido BA, Medina TR, Martin JK, Long JS (2013) The backbone of stigma: Identifying the global core of public prejudice associated with mental illness. *American Journal of Public Health* 103(5): 853–60

Russinova Z, Rogers ES, Ellison ML, Lyass A (2011) Recovery promoting professional competencies: Perspectives of mental health consumers, consumer-providers and providers. *Psychiatric Rehabilitation Journal* 34(3): 177–85

Shorter E (1998) *A History of Psychiatry from the Era of the Asylum to the Age of Prozac*. New York: John Wiley and Sons

Spriggs M, Olsson CA, Hall W (2008) How will information about the genetic risk of mental disorders impact on stigma? *The Australia and New Zealand Journal of Psychiatry* 42(3): 214–20

Switaj P, Grygiel P, Wciorka J, Humenny G, Anczewska M (2013) The Stigma Subscale Questionnnaire ( CESQ): a psychometric evaluation in Polish psychiatric patients. *Comprehensive Psychiatry* 54(6): 713–719

Van Brakel WH, Anderson AM, Mutatkar RK, Bakirtzief Z, Nicholls PG, Raju MS, Das-Pattanayak RK (2006) The Participation Scale: Measuring a Key Concept in Public Health. *Disability and Rehabilitation* 28(4):193–203

World Health Organization (2014) *Mental health: strengthening our response*. http://www.who.int/mediacentre/factsheets/fs220/en/ (Accessed 25 September 2014)

# Glossary

**abulia:** a lack of will or initiative; can be seen as a disorder of diminished motivation or loss of volition.

**acalculia:** an acquired impairment in which patients have difficulty performing simple mathematical tasks, such as adding, subtracting, multiplying and even simply stating which of two numbers is larger. Acalculia is distinguished from **dyscalculia** in that acalculia is acquired late in life due to neurological injury such as stroke, while dyscalculia is a specific developmental disorder first observed during the acquisition of mathematical knowledge.

**acculturation:** a phenomenon which results when groups of individuals from different cultures come into continuous first-hand contact, with subsequent changes in the original cultural patterns of either one or both groups.

**acrophobia:** the pathological fear of heights.

**acting out:** performing an extreme behaviour in order to express thoughts or feelings the person feels incapable of otherwise expressing.

**activation site:** amino acid/s contained within the three-dimensional structure of a receptor protein that allows activation of the receptor following interaction with an agonist.

**adaptive functioning:** the ability to adapt to the needs of everyday living, requiring conceptual, social and practical skills, e.g. in intellectual **disability**.

**addiction:** an uncontrollable craving, seeking and using of a substance such as alcohol or an illicit drug or activity (e.g. **gambling**).

**adherence: compliance** with treatment as prescribed.

**administrator (medico-legal):** in South Africa a court may appoint an administrator to take care of and administer the property of a mentally ill person.

**advanced (health care) directive:** also known as a living will, personal directive, advance directive, or advance decision; a legal document in which a person specifies what actions should be taken for their health if they are no longer able to make decisions for themselves because of illness or incapacity.

**advocacy:** all forms of effort to ensure that the rights of vulnerable groups in particular are protected.

**affect:** observed expression of emotion.

**affective instability:** a psychophysiological symptom observed in some **psychopathologies**, characterised by dysfunctional modulation of emotions and rapid shifting from neutral **affect** to intense **affect**.

**affiliative behaviour:** behaviour that is enacted with the intent of supporting or improving individual union with others, or which are connected with a **drive** to build, maintain and improve close individual partnerships with others. Includes behaviour that promotes group cohesion (friendly/positive gestures), such as grooming, touching, and hugging.

**affinity:** describes how avidly an endogenous substance or xenobiotic binds to a receptor, being either a 'loose' or a 'tight' binding.

**agitation:** an increased frequency of non-goal-directed movements, as opposed to hyperactivity, which is goal-directed.

**agnosia:** the inability to process sensory information. Often there is a loss of ability to recognise objects, persons, sounds, shapes or smells while the specific sense is not defective nor is there any significant memory loss. It is usually associated with brain injury or neurological illness, particularly after damage to the occipitotemporal border, which is part of the ventral stream. Agnosia only affects a single modality, such as vision or hearing.

**agonist:** a pharmacologically active molecule that binds to a receptor and stimulates it to a similar degree as its neurotransmitter/physiological **ligand** would; it therefore can elicit a response at a receptor. It has full intrinsic activity at the receptor.

**agoraphobia:** an anxiety disorder often associated with panic disorder characterised by anxiety in situations where the sufferer perceives certain environments as dangerous or uncomfortable, often due to the environment's vast openness or crowdedness. There is fear of incurring a panic attack in such environments.

**agranulocytosis:** a marked decrease in granulocytes (white cells) that leads to an increased vulnerability to infection.

**agraphaesthesia:** a disorder of directional cutaneous kinesthesia or a disorientation of the skin's sensation across its space. It is a difficulty in recognising a written number or letter traced on the skin after parietal damage.

**agraphia:** a loss of the ability to communicate through writing, either due to some form of motor dysfunction or an inability to spell.

**akathisia:** a subjective feeling of inner and motor restlessness manifested by a compelling need to be in constant movement.

**akinetic:** inability to move.

**alexia:** a brain disorder in which a person is unable to understand written words. It refers specifically to the loss, usually in adulthood, of a previous ability to read.

**alexithymia:** difficulty experiencing, expressing and describing emotional responses. Instead, patients may describe emotions as **somatic** experiences or behavioural reactions.

**allele:** one of a number of alternative forms of the same gene or same genetic locus. Sometimes, different alleles can result in different observable **phenotypic traits**, such as different pigmentation. However, most genetic variations result in little or no observable variation. Most multicellular organisms have two sets of chromosomes; that is, they are diploid. These chromosomes are referred to as homologous chromosomes. Diploid organisms have one copy of each gene (and, therefore, one allele) on each chromosome. If both alleles are the same, they and the organism are homozygous with respect to that gene. If the alleles are different, they and the organism are heterozygous with respect to that gene.

**allosteric:** inhibition of an enzyme by binding of an inhibitor to a binding site thereby reducing the enzyme's binding **affinity** for the substrate.

**allosteric and steric interaction:** a binding site located in close proximity of a receptor that allows interference of that receptor's function, either positively or negatively.

**allosteric binding site:** a binding site that allows allosteric modulation of a receptor to take place.

**allosteric modulator:** any compound, endogenous or xenobiotic, that binds to an **allosteric binding site** in the close proximity of a known receptor, allowing it to either positively or negatively influence receptor activation.

**alogia**: also known as poverty of speech; a general lack of additional, unprompted content seen in normal speech. As a symptom, it is commonly seen in patients who suffer from schizophrenia, and is considered as a negative symptom. In conversation, alogic patients reply very sparsely and their answers to questions lack spontaneous content, sometimes failing to answer at all. Responses are brief, generally only appearing as a response to a question or prompt.

**alter/alter personality:** observable phenomena (sudden subjective experiences of self-alteration or objectively observable behaviour) that indicate the presence/activity of self-states (e.g. suddenly and oddly feeling like a different person, switching back and forth between feeling like a child and an adult, switching back and forth between feeling like a man and a woman, or seeing someone else in the mirror).

***amafufunyane*:** a broad construct used by black South Africans to describe a combination of symptoms that include **hallucinations**, **delusions**, outbursts of aggression, hysterical behaviour disorientation, and violent madness. It is conceptualised as a manifestation of spirit possession, mediated by witchcraft.

**ambivalence:** inability to choose between incompatible goals.

**amnesia:** inability to recall important autobiographical information, usually of a traumatic or stressful nature, that is inconsistent with ordinary forgetting.

**anhedonia:** inability to take pleasure in activities usually enjoyable.

**anorexia:** the lack or loss of appetite for food.

**anosagnosia: a** deficit of self-awareness, a condition in which a person who suffers a certain **disability** seems unaware of the existence of his or her disability. The condition does not seem to be directly related to sensory loss and is thought to be caused by damage to higher-level neurocognitive processes that are involved in integrating sensory information with processes that support spatial or bodily representations (including the somatosensory system).

**antagonist:** a pharmacological molecule that binds to a receptor without stimulating it and thus prevents the actions of its neurotransmitter/physiological **ligand**, effectively blocking and reversing the effect of an agonist at a receptor. It can bind to a receptor, but has no intrinsic activity.

**anterograde amnesia:** loss of the ability to create new memories after the event that caused the **amnesia**, leading to a partial or complete inability to recall the recent past, while long-term memories from before the event remain intact.

**anxiogenic:** anything that causes anxiety to increase (e.g. an axiogenic substance may cause anxiety).

**anxiolytic:** anything (e.g. substance or drug) that inhibits or reduces anxiety.

**apathy:** a lack of feeling, emotion, interest and concern. Apathy is a state of indifference, or the suppression of emotions such as concern, excitement, motivation, and/or passion. An apathetic individual has an absence of interest in or concern about emotional, social, spiritual, philosophical and/or physical life and the world.

**apoptosis:** programmed cell death by fragmentation into membrane-bound particles that are then eliminated by phagocytosis.

**apraxia:** the inability to execute learned purposeful movements, despite having the desire and the physical capacity to perform the movements. Apraxia is an acquired disorder of motor planning.

**aprosody (dysprosody):** an abnormality in the affective components of language. In motor aprosody, difficulty in spontaneous use of emotional inflection is evident in speech, whereas sensory aprosody is characterised by impairment in comprehension of emotional inflection.

**assimilation:** where one or more individual/s come into contact over a period of time with another culture and take on the cultural beliefs and habits of the host culture. The culture of origin is largely rejected, and the new culture is adopted as a replacement.

**assisted care, treatment and rehabilitation:** the provision of health interventions to people incapable of making informed decisions due to their mental health status and who do not refuse the health interventions.

**astasia-abasia:** a form of psychogenic gait disturbance in which gait becomes impaired in the absence of any neurological or physical pathology. The person usually walks in a bizarre manner, staggers and appears as if going to fall but always manages to catch hold of something in time. Sometimes a person cannot stand but is well able to move the legs while lying down or sitting. It is often associated with conversion disorder or somatisation disorder.

**astereognosia:** the inability to identify an object by active touch of the hands without other sensory input. An individual with astereognosis is unable to identify objects by handling them, despite intact sensation.

**ataxia:** a neurological sign that consists of a lack of voluntary coordination of muscle movements. Ataxia is a non-specific clinical manifestation implying dysfunction of the parts of the nervous system that coordinate movement, such as the cerebellum.

**athetosis:** slow, involuntary, convoluted, writhing movements of the fingers, hands, toes, and feet and in some cases, arms, legs, neck and tongue. Movements typical of athetosis are sometimes called athetoid movements.

**at-risk mental state (ARMS):** used predominantly in relation to psychosis, ARMS represents a state where an individual (often an adolescent or a young adult) manifests some attenuated features of psychosis that are insufficient to indicate a disorder, but are significant in that their presence increases a risk of future psychotic disorder.

**attachment:** the dynamics of long-term interpersonal relationships between humans. In infants, attachment as a motivational and behavioural system directs the child to seek proximity with a familiar caregiver when they are alarmed, with the expectation that they will receive protection and emotional support.

**attention:** the behavioural and cognitive process of selectively concentrating on a discrete aspect of information, whether deemed subjective or objective, while ignoring other perceivable information.

**atypical antipsychotic:** a class of drugs whose mechanism involves serotonin-dopamine antagonism, specifically $D_2$ and $5HT_{2A}$ receptors.

**augmentation:** when a medication from a certain class is added to a medication from another class to enhance the **efficacy** of that medication.

**aura:** a distinct visual, motor, sensory or psychological perception that occur a few seconds to an hour before a seizure.

**automatic thoughts:** negative thoughts that individuals have about themselves, the world and/or the future, which arise spontaneously and of which they are not aware (initially).

**automatism:** somewhat coordinated, repetitive motor activity that usually occurs while **cognition** is impaired and for which the patient has **amnesia**. Most automatisms are brief (seconds to minutes) and range from simple movements to complex semi-purposeful actions.

**autoreceptor:** receptor involved in the auto-inhibition of a neuron, usually located presynaptically. Activation will reduce transmitter release while inhibition will increase transmitter release.

**avoidance: maladaptive** coping mechanism characterised by the effort to avoid dealing with a stressor.

**avolition:** general lack of **drive** or motivation to pursue meaningful goals.

**behavioural phenotypes:** patterns of behaviour (e.g. self-injurious behaviour, **attachment** to specific objects) that present in syndromes caused by chromosomal or genetic abnormalities.

***belle indifférence*:** also known as *la belle indifférence*; characterised by a lack of concern and/or feeling of indifference about a **disability** or a symptom. It can be seen in conversion disorder.

**bereavement:** a culturally influenced, emotional and behavioural reaction to the death of a significant other, commonly referred to as grief.

**bias (statistical):** the introduction of unaccounted for, extraneous factors that may impact on the **validity** of results in a statistical analysis.

**bingeing:** a pattern of disordered eating that consists of episodes of uncontrollable eating. During a binge, a person rapidly consumes an excessive amount of food. Most people who have eating binges try to hide this behaviour from others, and often feel ashamed about being overweight or depressed about their overeating.

**biomarker:** a measurable indicator of some biological state or condition.

**bizarre delusions: delusions** that are clearly implausible, e.g. the belief that aliens have removed one's brain.

**black-out (alcohol):** phenomenon caused by the intake of any substance or medication in which long-term memory creation is impaired, therefore causing a complete inability to recall events. Black-outs can be caused by any substance, but are most frequently associated with GABA-ergic drugs. Black-outs are frequently described as having effects similar to that of **anterograde amnesia**, in which the subject cannot recall any events after the event that caused the **amnesia**.

**blunted (affect):** a lack of emotional reactivity (affect display) in an individual. It manifests as a failure to express feelings either verbally or non-verbally, especially when talking about issues that would normally be expected to engage the emotions. Expressive gestures are rare and there is little animation in facial expression or vocal inflection.

***bouffée délirante*:** a French term used in the past for acute and transient psychotic disorders (F23 in ICD-10). In the DSM-IV it is described as brief psychotic disorder (298.8). The symptoms usually have an acute onset and reach their peak within two weeks. The symptoms start resolving in a few weeks and complete **recovery** usually occurs within 2–3 months.

**bradykinesia:** slowness of movement characterised by reduced amplitude and early fatiguing.

**bradyphrenia:** reduced speed of processing information.

**brain fag:** a **culture-bound syndrome**. Once a common term for mental exhaustion, it is now encountered almost exclusively in West Africa. Seen predominantly in male students, it generally manifests as vague **somatic** symptoms, depression, and difficulty concentrating.

**capability:** the ability to perform or achieve certain actions or outcomes through a set of controllable and measurable faculties, features, functions, processes or services.

**capacity/competence:** clinical capacity to make health care decisions is the ability to understand the benefits and risks of the proposed health care, to understand possible alternatives and to make and communicate a health care decision.

**Capgras delusion (syndrome):** a disorder in which a person holds a **delusion** that a friend, spouse, parent, or other close family member (or pet) has been replaced by an identical-looking impostor. The Capgras delusion is classified as a delusional **misidentification syndrome**, a class of delusional beliefs that involves the misidentification of people, places or objects.

**cART (combination antiretroviral therapy):** combinations of antiretroviral agents used to keep the HIV infection under control. The drug combination usually consists of three drugs, with a minimum of two active drugs from two different classes.

**case management:** the coordination of community services for mental health care patients by allocating a professional to be responsible for the assessment of need and implementation of care plans. It is usually required for individuals who have a serious mental illness and need ongoing support in areas such as housing, employment, social relationships and community participation.

**catalepsy:** a nervous condition characterised by muscular rigidity and fixity of posture regardless of external stimuli, as well as decreased sensitivity to pain. Symptoms include rigid body and limbs, limbs staying in same position when moved (waxy flexibility), no response, loss of muscle control and slowing down of bodily functions, such as breathing.

**cataplexy:** a sudden loss of muscle tone, which is generally precipitated by a sudden emotional response.

**catastrophic reaction:** emotional outburst, sometimes accompanied by physical acting-out behaviour, that seems inappropriate or out of proportion to the situation. The reaction may be triggered by a present event or by one from the distant past.

**catastrophising:** automatically assuming a 'worst-case scenario' and inappropriately characterising minor or moderate problems or issues as catastrophic events.

**catatonia:** a state of apparent unresponsiveness to external stimuli in a person who is apparently awake. Catatonia is a syndrome and not just a single symptom. There are different degrees or variations of the syndrome, including episodes of **agitation** (catatonic excitement) to cases that show extreme rigidity and immobility in the same position for some time (catatonic **stupor**).

**categorical approach:** an approach to classifying mental disorders that involves assessing whether an individual has a disorder on the basis of symptoms and characteristics that are described as typical of the disorder.

**catharsis:** the purification and purgation of emotions, especially pity and fear. In therapy, the act of expressing, or more accurately, experiencing the deep emotions often associated with events in the individual's past that had originally been **repressed** or ignored and had never been adequately addressed or experienced.

**causal attribution:** explanation given for actions, behaviours or experiences (e.g. auditory **hallucinations** are attributed to being bewitched).

***cerea flexibilitas*:** meaning'waxy flexibility', this refers to people allowing themselves to be placed in postures by others, and then maintaining those postures for long periods even while being obviously uncomfortable. It is characterised by a patient's movements having the feeling of a plastic resistance, as if the person were made of wax. It is usually a feature of **catatonia**.

**chorea:** an abnormal involuntary movement disorder, one of a group of neurological disorders called **dyskinesias.** Chorea is characterised by brief, semi-directed, irregular movements that are not repetitive or rhythmic, but appear to flow from one muscle to the next. These'dance-like' movements of chorea often occur with **athetosis**, which adds twisting and writhing movements.

**choreoathetosis:** involuntary movements in a combination of **chorea** (irregular migrating contractions) and **athetosis** (twisting and writhing).

**chronobiology:** a field of biology that examines periodic (cyclic) phenomena in living organisms and their adaptation to solar- and lunar-related rhythms. These cycles are known as biological rhythms.

**circumscribed (delusion): delusion** that is limited to a narrow range and does not taint the mass of one's beliefs. It is a compartmentalised false belief.

**circumstantiality:** speech that is very indirect and delayed in reaching its goal due to the inclusion of tedious detail; sometimes referred to as over-inclusiveness.

**CMD (common mental disorders):** psychiatric disorders with a higher **prevalence** (e.g. major depressive disorder, anxiety disorders, substance use disorders).

**co-dependency:** a type of dysfunctional helping relationship where one person supports or enables another person's **addiction**, poor mental health, immaturity, irresponsibility or under-achievement. People with a predisposition to be a co-dependent enabler often find themselves in relationships where their primary role is that of rescuer, supporter and confidant. These helper types are often dependent on the other person's poor functioning to satisfy their own emotional needs.

**cognition:** operation of the mind by which we become aware of objects of thought and **perception**.

**cognitive distortions/errors:** excessive or irrational thought patterns that are believed to perpetuate the effects of psychopathological states such as depression or anxiety.

**cognitive behavioural therapy (CBT):** form of **psychotherapy** that is based on the theory that the way individuals perceive situations determines how they feel emotionally. CBT aims to assist individuals (or groups) to identify **automatic thoughts** and **cognitive distortions** and to change these in order to bring about behavioural change.

**co-morbidity:** the presence of one or more additional disorders (or diseases) co-occurring with a primary disease or disorder; or the effect of such additional disorders or diseases. The additional disorder may also be a behavioural or mental disorder.

**compartmentalisation:** a neural network concept operating as a mechanism of **dissociation** that involves the suspension of mental integration and the inability to bring into conscious awareness information typically accessible to consciousness and susceptible to conscious influence. Despite their disconnection from consciousness, compartmentalised processes continue to function.

**completed suicide:** successful suicide resulting in death.

**compliance:** the degree to which a patient correctly follows medical advice. Most commonly, it refers to medication or drug compliance, but it can also apply to other situations such as medical device use, self-care, self-directed exercises or therapy sessions.

**compulsions:** repetitive behaviours (e.g. hand washing, ordering, checking) or mental acts (e.g. praying, counting, repeating words silently) that the person feels driven to perform in response to an **obsession** or according to rules that must be applied rigidly.

**concentration:** the action or power of focusing all one's **attention**; the fixing of close, undivided attention.

**conditioning:** a process in which a previously neutral stimulus comes to evoke a specific response by being repeatedly paired with another stimulus that evokes the response.

**confabulation:** a plausible but imagined memory that fills in gaps in what is remembered; to fill in gaps in one's memory with fabrications that one believes to be facts.

**confidentiality**: ethical principle or legal right that a physician or other health professional will hold secret all information relating to a patient, unless the patient gives **consent** permitting disclosure.

**confounding:** in statistics, a variable that is not the risk factor under study but is independently associated with both the outcome and the risk factor under study.

**consent:** permission for something to happen or agreement to do something; the ethical requirement for an individual to agree to something.

**consultation-liaison psychiatry:** branch of psychiatry that specialises in the interface between medicine and psychiatry; it usually takes place in a hospital or medical setting.

**conversion:** a psychological **defence mechanism** where **repressed** ideas, conflicts or undesirable impulses – often sexual or aggressive – are manifested by various bodily or **somatic** symptoms of a neurological kind such as paralysis, sensory deficits and seizures that have no physical cause.

**coprolalia:** the involuntary utterance of socially inappropriate phrases. It is a phonic tic associated with Tourette's syndrome, although less than 15% of persons with Tourette's have coprolalia.

**counter-transference:** the therapist's response to the patient that may include the therapist's own personal feelings and emotions regarding the patient, as well as the feelings and emotions that the patient is trying to evoke in the therapist.

**covalent bond:** a bond that forms between two atoms when electrons from each atom combine to form an electron pair.

**crisis intervention:** the provision of care outside of hospital by specialised teams during a mental health crisis.

**CSDI (clinically significant drug interaction):** a drug interaction that produces at least a 30% change in **pharmacokinetic** parameters requiring intervention.

**culture-bound syndrome (culture-specific syndrome/reaction):** also known as a folk illness; a combination of psychiatric and **somatic** symptoms that are considered to be a recognisable disease only within a specific society or culture.

**curatorship:** the power given by authority of the law, to one or more persons to administer the property of an individual who is unable to take care of his or her own estate and affairs, either on account of his or her absence without an authorised agent, or in consequence of his or her mental health.

**cybernetics:** the discovery or design and application of principles of regulation and communication. Cybernetics treats ways of behaving and not things. In family therapy, it is based on the idea that all elements in a system are interdependent and that changes in one element result in changes in all the others.

**cytochrome P450:** microsomal liver enzyme complex responsible for the metabolism of a number of endogenous substances, as well as various xenobiotics.

**debriefing:** part of an emergency counselling intervention to help people who have recently experienced a major loss or suffering. It is intended to reduce the risk of post-traumatic stress disorder (PTSD) but its **efficacy** is doubtful; it is discouraged as it may, in fact, result in retraumatising the individual.

**decompensation:** the inability to maintain **defence mechanisms** in response to stress, which results in **personality** disturbance or psychological imbalance.

**deep-brain stimulation:** a neurosurgical treatment that involves the implantation of a medical device that sends electrical impulses to specific parts of the brain for the treatment of some neurological and psychiatric disorders such as Parkinson's disease, obsessive-compulsive disorder (OCD) and epilepsy.

**de-escalation:** the use of verbal and non-verbal techniques to calm down an agitated and/or aggressive patient.

**defence mechanisms: unconscious** mental processes used by the ego to resolve internal conflicts.

**deinstitutionalisation:** the replacement of long-stay psychiatric hospitals with smaller, less isolated community-based alternatives for the care of mentally ill people.

***déjà vu*:** phenomenon of having the strong sensation that an event or experience currently being experienced has been experienced in the past, regardless of whether it has actually happened.

**deliberate self-harm:** the intentional, direct injuring of body tissue; most often done without **suicidal intentions**.

**delusion:** a fixed, false belief, based on incorrect inferences about external reality that is not consistent with a patient's intelligence and cultural background and that cannot be corrected by reasoning.

**delusional jealousy:** false belief that a spouse or lover is having an affair, with no proof to back up this claim.

**dementia:** broad category of acquired brain diseases that cause a long-term and often gradual decrease in the ability to think and remember to such an extent that a person's daily functioning is affected. Other common symptoms include emotional problems, problems with language and a decrease in motivation. Level of consciousness is not affected. For the **diagnosis** to be present it must be a change from a person's usual mental functioning and a greater decline than one would expect due to ageing.

**denial:** a psychological **defence mechanism** postulated by Sigmund Freud, in which a person is faced with a fact that is too uncomfortable to accept and rejects it instead, insisting that it is not true despite what may be overwhelming evidence.

**dependence:** in relation to substance use, a state in which there is a compulsion to take a drug, either continuously or periodically, in order to experience its psychic effects or to avoid the discomfort of its absence.

**depersonalisation:** feeling detached from one's mental processes, body or actions (as if one's self is robotic or unreal).

**depolarisation:** the tendency of the cell membrane potential to become positive with respect to the potential outside the cell when stimulated, effectively reversing the resting potential of excitable cell membranes.

**derealisation:** feeling detached from one's surroundings (as if an observer of unreal objects).

**descriptive psychiatry:** the study of observable symptoms and behavioural phenomena rather than underlying psychodynamic processes, in which the clinical psychiatrist focuses on empirically observable behaviours and conditions, such as words spoken or actions taken.

**desensitisation:** diminished emotional responsiveness to a negative or aversive stimulus after repeated exposure to it.

**detachment:** neural network concept that operates as a mechanism of dissociation that may also confer survival advantage on an animal under threat through attenuation of the adverse emotional consequences of stress. Detachment rations the brain's finite capacity for **attention**, thereby freeing it to remain focused on the task at hand – to mitigate threat.

**detoxification:** physiological or medicinal removal of toxic substances from a living organism. It can also refer to the period of **withdrawal** during which a person returns to homeostasis after the long-term use of an addictive substance. In medicine, detoxification can be achieved by decontamination of poison ingestion and the use of antidotes as well as techniques such as dialysis and (in a limited number of cases) chelation therapy.

**devaluation:** in psychoanalytic theory, when an individual is unable to integrate difficult feelings, specific defences are mobilised to overcome what the individual perceives as an unbearable situation. When viewing people as all bad, the individual employs devaluation: attributing exaggeratedly negative qualities to the self or others.

**diagnosis:** the identification and classification of an illness; linking it to an existing understanding of the illness.

**dimensional classification:** the approach to classifying mental disorders that quantifies a person's symptoms or other characteristics of interest and represents them with numerical values on one or more scales or continuums, rather than assigning them to a mental disorder category. It assumes that symptoms exist on a continuum.

**disability:** the lack of ability to function normally, physically or mentally and to perform activities.

**discontinuation:** to stop or cease medication.

**discrimination:** prejudicial treatment of an individual based solely on their membership of a certain socially undesirable group or social category. Discrimination manifests in the inequitable distribution of resources.

**disinhibition:** state characterised by impulsiveness, inappropriate jocularity, euphoria, emotional lability, distractibility, impaired social and financial judgement and poor insight.

**displacement:** redirecting thoughts, feelings and impulses directed at one person or object to take it out upon another person or object.

**disorganisation:** thoughts, speech and/or behaviour that lack coherence and structure and that may be contradictory, inconsistent and seemingly purposeless.

**dissociation:** protective psychological process to manage overwhelming or conflictual affects and experiences, usually of a traumatic or stressful nature. Clusters of mental contents may be split off from conscious awareness or ideas may be separated from their emotional significance and affect. This may allow an individual to maintain allegiance to two contradictory truths while remaining unconscious of the contradiction. (Also see Advanced reading box 19.1, for additional definitions of dissociation.)

**dissociative disorders:** characterised by a disruption of and/or discontinuity in the normal integration of consciousness, memory, identity, emotion, **perception**, body representation, motor control and behaviour, dissociative disorder may reflect an incredible ability to subdivide or compartmentalise one's mind, to the point where it becomes dysfunctional rather than useful. They can also be thought of as a cluster of clinical syndromes where dissociative processes, symptoms and **defence**

**mechanisms** have become severe enough to be clinically significant, thereby affecting a person's level of functioning to the extent that he or she is diagnosable as mentally ill.

**dizygotic twins:** fraternal twins that develop from two eggs, each fertilised by separate sperm cells.

**double stigma:** having to contend with the synergistic effects of the **stigma** of two illnesses (e.g. mental illness and HIV).

**down-regulation:** a slowing of neurotransmitter receptor synthesis that results in fewer receptors at the synapse.

**drives (psychological):** an 'excitatory state produced by a homeostatic disturbance', an instinctual need that has the power to drive the behaviour of an individual. Drive theory is based on the principle that organisms are born with certain psychological needs and that a negative state of tension is created when these needs are not satisfied. When a need is satisfied, drive is reduced and the organism returns to a state of homeostasis and relaxation. Freud identified a number of **unconscious** drives including the life (*eros*) and death (*thanatos*) drives as well as the sexual and ego drives.

**dual diagnosis:** the condition of suffering from a mental illness and a **co-morbid substance abuse problem**.

**dualism:** drug that exhibits receptor activating or inhibiting properties that is dependent on the concentration of an endogenous **ligand**.

**dynamic psychiatry: person-centred psychiatry** that is concerned with what is unique about each patient and how a particular patient differs from others as a result of a specific life history. Symptoms and behaviour are seen as an expression of underlying psychological and biological forces with a hidden logic and meaning. It encompasses **descriptive psychiatry**, but is furthermore interested in the subjective and personal experiences of the individual.

**dynamics:** the forces or properties that stimulate growth, development or change within a system or process.

**dyscalculia:** difficulty in learning or comprehending arithmetic, such as difficulty in understanding numbers, learning how to manipulate numbers, and learning facts in mathematics. It is generally seen as a specific developmental disorder.

**dyskinesia:** a category of movement disorders that are characterised by involuntary muscle movements, including movements similar to **tics** or **chorea** and diminished voluntary movements.

**dysmorphic feature:** a difference of body structure that can be an isolated finding in an otherwise normal individual or can be related to a congenital disorder, genetic syndrome or birth defect.

**dysphasia:** a partial or complete impairment of the ability to communicate as the result of a brain injury.

**dysphoria:** a profound state of unease or dissatisfaction. In a psychiatric context, dysphoria may accompany depression, anxiety or **agitation**. Common reactions to dysphoria include emotional distress or indifference.

**dysprosody:** markedly abnormal tonal patterns in speech.

**dyssomnia:** a broad classification of primary sleep disorders that make it difficult to fall asleep or to remain sleeping.

**dystonia:** extrapyramidal motor disturbance that consist of slow, sustained contractions of the axial or appendicular musculature and that lead to relatively sustained postural deviations and acute dystonic reactions such as facial grimacing and torticollis.

**Ebstein's anomaly:** a congenital heart defect with a downward displacement of the tricuspid valve into the apex of the right ventricle.

**echolalia:** automatic repetition of vocalisations made by another person.

**echopraxia:** involuntary repetition, imitation or mirroring of an observed action. Imitated actions can range from simple motor tasks such as picking up a phone to violent actions such as hitting another person.

**ecological fallacy:** erroneous assumption of statistical association at the individual level based on an observed association at the group level.

**efficacy:** how well treatment works when measured in a controlled environment, such as in a clinical study.

**elimination half-life:** the time it takes for a plasma concentration of a drug to reduce by 50%.

**emic approach:** the view that society and culture play such an important role in the presentation of psychiatric disorders that traditional Western systems of classification and measurement cannot be assumed to be universally appropriate.

**empathy:** intellectual identification with the thoughts, feelings or state of another person; also the capacity to understand another person's point of view or the result of such understanding.

**epigenetics:** the study of changes in **gene expression** caused by certain base pairs in DNA or RNA being 'turned off' or 'turned on' through chemical reactions. Epigenetics is mostly the study of heritable changes that are not caused by changes in the DNA sequence. Examples of mechanisms that produce such changes are DNA methylation and histone modification, each of which alters how genes are expressed without altering the underlying DNA sequence.

**erotomania: delusion** in which a person falsely believes another person is in love with him or her.

**etic approach:** the assumption that psychiatric disorders are broadly similar throughout the world and that measurements are universally applicable.

**euphoria:** exaggerated or abnormal sense of physical and emotional well-being not based on reality or truth, disproportionate to its cause and inappropriate to the situation; it is commonly seen in the manic stage of bipolar disorder, some forms of schizophrenia, organic mental disorders and toxin- and drug-induced states.

**euthymia:** stable mood; a normal non-depressed, reasonably positive mood.

**excitation:** stimulation of a molecule through the addition of energy and absorption of photons.

**executive function:** an umbrella term for the management (regulation, control) of cognitive processes, including working memory, reasoning, task flexibility and problem solving, as well as planning and execution.

**exposure with/and response prevention: CBT** for conditions such as OCD; where 'exposure with' refers to confronting the thoughts, images, objects and situations typical of an individual's OCD, and 'response prevention' refers to not doing the compulsive behaviour after being exposed to the anxiety-provoking stimulus.

**extrapyramidal side effects:** movement disorders, such as **tardive dyskinesia** or **akathisia**, caused by taking dopamine **antagonists**, usually antipsychotic (neuroleptic) drugs. They are due to blockage of the dopamine receptors in the nigrostriatal dopamine pathway, which forms part of the extrapyramidal nervous system.

**extraversion**: a **personality** type described by Carl Jung, it is 'the act, state, or habit of being predominantly concerned with obtaining gratification from what is outside the self'. Extraverts enjoy human interactions and are enthusiastic, talkative, assertive and gregarious. They are energised and thrive on being around other people. They are prone to boredom when they are by themselves and enjoy activities that involve large social gatherings.

**fatuous (affect):** silly, superficial mood that resembles the moods of a child. This condition may be seen in schizophrenia.

**fixation:** the arresting of part of the **libido** at an immature stage that causes an obsessive **attachment**.

**flashback:** aspects of a traumatic event are **re-experienced** involuntarily as though they were reoccurring at that moment.

**flat affect:** dull, unresponsive expression of mood with little or no variation; there is a loss of range in expression of mood.

**flight of ideas:** thoughts following each other rapidly, but the connections between successive thoughts are understandable.

***folie á deux*:** French for 'a madness shared by two', or shared psychosis; a psychiatric syndrome in which symptoms of a delusional belief are transmitted from one individual to another. This is usually shared by two or more people who are closely related emotionally: one has a real psychosis while the symptoms of psychosis are induced in the other or others through a close **attachment** to the psychotic person. Separation usually results in symptomatic improvement in the non-psychotic person.

**food insecurity:** psychosocial problems (e.g. **adherence** to medication) that are the results of a lack of food and the uncertainty over food provision.

**formulation:** a theoretically-based explanation or conceptualisation of the information obtained from a clinical assessment, which offers a hypothesis about the cause and nature of the presenting problems. It is considered an alternative approach to the more **categorical classification** approach of psychiatric **diagnosis**.

**Frégoli syndrome:** a rare disorder in which a person holds a delusional belief that different people are, in fact, a single person who changes appearance or is in disguise.

**fugue:** apparently purposeful travel or bewildered wandering that is associated with **amnesia** for identity or for other important autobiographical information.

**gambling:** placing something of value at risk in the hopes of gaining something of greater value. Gambling requires three elements to be present: consideration, chance and prize.

**gambling problem:** friction or difficulty in any area of functioning as a result of some element of **gambling** behaviour. This friction may arise as a result of differences of opinion regarding amounts of money potentially risked, time away from the home or family in the absence of any excessive financial losses relative to disposable income, a **preoccupation** with gambling, absent or impaired control or other adverse consequences.

**gender:** the public lived role as boy or girl, man or woman.

**gender dysphoria:** the distress that may accompany the incongruence between one's experienced or expressed gender and the gender one has been assigned.

**gene-environment interaction** (or **genotype-environment interaction** or **g×e):** the **phenotypic** effect of interactions between genes and the environment. In psychiatry it is commonly observed that disorders cluster in families, but family members may not inherit these disorders as such; rather, they often inherit sensitivity or vulnerability to the effects of various environmental risk factors. Individuals may be differently affected by exposure to the same environment in clinically significant ways.

**gene expression:** the process by which information from a gene is used in the synthesis of a functional gene product. These products are often proteins, but in non-protein coding genes such as ribosomal RNA (RRNA), transfer RNA (TRNA) or small nuclear RNA (SNRNA) genes, the product is a functional RNA.

**genetic load:** the extent to which a population deviates from the theoretically fittest genetic constitution.

**genogram:** a pictorial display of a person's family relationships and medical history. It goes beyond a traditional family tree by allowing the user to visualise hereditary patterns and psychological factors that punctuate relationships.

**genotype:** the inherited instructions carried within an individual's genetic code.

**grandiose delusions:** fantastical beliefs that one is famous, omnipotent, wealthy or otherwise very powerful. The **delusions** are generally fantastic and often have a supernatural, science fictional or religious theme.

**grandiosity:** an unrealistic sense of superiority – a sustained view of oneself as better than others that causes one to view others with disdain or as inferior – as well as a sense of uniqueness: the belief that few others have anything in common with oneself and that one can only be understood by a few or very special people.

**guanosine (G) binding protein:** the regulatory protein common to all trans-membrane spanning receptors that binds guanosine, resulting in either inhibition (GI) or activation (GS) of the receptor.

**gustatory hallucinations: hallucinations** of taste.

**habit reversal therapy:** a type of therapy that forms the core of most behavioural treatments for hair-pulling disorder (HPD) and skin-picking disorder (SPD) and involves three primary components: awareness training, competing response training, and social support.

**half-life (t½):** the amount of time required for the concentration of drug in the blood to fall to half its value as measured at the beginning of the time period.

**hallucination:** a **perception** in the absence of an external stimulus that has qualities of real perception. Hallucinations are vivid, substantial and located in external objective space.

**handicap:** the limitations on fulfilling one's normal social role and participation in society due to a **disability**.

**harm reduction:** a range of public health policies designed to reduce the harmful consequences associated with both legal and illegal behaviour. Harm reduction policies are used in numerous settings (ranging from services through to geographical regions) to manage behaviour such as recreational drug use and sexual activity.

**health promotion:** defined by the World Health Organization as 'the process of enabling people to increase control over their health and its determinants, and thereby improve their health'.

**heritability:** the proportion of a **phenotypic** variance that can be attributed to genetic variance.

**heteroreceptor:** receptor involved in the inhibition of one neurotransmitter system upon another, usually located presynaptically.

**HIV-associated neurocognitive disorder (HAND):** the spectrum of neurocognitive impairments seen in HIV/Aids. It occurs in a hierarchy of progressive severity, which ranges from asymptomatic neurocognitive impairment (ANI), to minor neurocognitive disorder (MND), to the more severe HIV-associated **dementia** (HAD).

**hookah:** also known as a water pipe; a single or multiple stemmed instrument used to vaporise or smoke flavoured tobacco.

**Hoover's sign:** a physical test of compensatory movement in the legs in which a supine individual, when asked to raise one leg, involuntarily exerts counter-pressure with the heel of the opposite leg, even if that leg is paralysed.

**hyper-arousal:** also known as the 'fight-or-flight' response; a physiological reaction that occurs in response to a perceived harmful event, attack or threat to survival.

**hyperpolarisation:** an increase in the amount of electrical charge separated by the cell membrane and hence the strength of the transmembrane potential.

**hypersomnia:** excessive sleep or sleepiness that interferes with everyday life.

**hypervigilance:** an enhanced state of sensory sensitivity accompanied by an exaggerated intensity of behaviour with the purpose of detecting threats.

**hypnotics:** a class of medications/drugs that induce sleep.

**hypochondriasis:** also hypochondria; a belief that **physical symptoms** are signs of a serious illness, despite medical testing and reassurance to the contrary. It represents an erroneous appraisal of bodily experiences or states with excessive worry and **preoccupation** about health and having a feared illness.

**hypomania:** mood abnormality with the qualitative characteristics of **mania** but somewhat less intense.

**hysteria**: obsolete term, once used to describe a mental condition where excessive emotions or psychological conflict are experienced physically or in the body with no underlying bodily abnormality. It is expressed through a wide array of symptoms including paralysis, sensory losses and seizures.

**idealisation:** in psychoanalytic theory, when an individual is unable to integrate difficult feelings, specific defences are mobilised to overcome what the individual perceives as an unbearable situation. When viewing people as all good, the individual is said to be using the **defence mechanism** of idealisation: a mental mechanism in which the person attributes exaggeratedly positive qualities to the self or others.

**ideas of reference:** a **delusional** belief that general events are directed at oneself. Innocuous events are interpreting as personally highly significant. A person may believe that he or she is receiving messages from the TV that are directed especially at him or her, or that a red car passing by has a specific meaning.

**identity alteration:** discovering the fully-dissociated activities of another self-state (e.g. time loss, 'coming to', switches, being told of actions, finding evidence of one's recent behaviour).

**identity confusion:** a conscious feeling of uncertainty, puzzlement or conflict about one's identity as a result of **intrusions** from a dissociated self-state.

**illusion:** a false **perception** of a detectable stimulus, which may take the form of a misinterpretation of a stimulus (e.g. a moving curtain is misinterpreted as a face in the window).

**immune reconstitution inflammatory syndrome (IRIS):** a syndrome that occurs when the immune system produces an inflammatory response as it reconstitutes on **cART** treatment.

**impairment:** abnormalities of structure or physiological function.

**impersistence (motor):** the inability to maintain postures or positions (such as keeping the eyes closed, protruding the tongue, maintaining conjugate gaze steadily in a fixed direction, or making a prolonged 'ah' sound) without repeated prompts.

**impulsivity:** a multifactorial construct that involves a tendency to act on a whim, displaying behaviour characterised by little or no forethought, reflection or consideration of the consequences. Impulsive actions are typically 'poorly conceived, prematurely expressed, unduly risky, or inappropriate to the situation, often resulting in undesirable consequences', which imperil long-term goals and strategies for success.

**inappropriate affect:** an emotional response that does not correspond with the experience that triggers it (e.g. laughing during a serious conversation).

**incidence:** the number of people who develop a certain disorder during a given period of time, divided by the defined population at risk at the beginning of the period.

**incontinence (emotional):** also known as pathological emotions; involuntary crying or uncontrollable episodes of crying and/or laughing or other emotional displays, usually associated with organic brain syndromes such as **dementia** or pseudobulbar palsy.

**insight:** the extent to which an individual with a particular disorder, symptom or behaviour acknowledges and understands the excessive or irrational nature of the symptom or behaviour.

**insomnia:** sleeplessness or an inability to fall asleep or stay asleep as long as desired.

**intellectualisation:** an overemphasis on thinking when confronted with an unacceptable impulse, situation or behaviour without employing any emotions to help mediate and place the thoughts into an emotional human context.

**intelligence and intellect:** one's capacity for logic, abstract thought, understanding, self-awareness, communication, learning, emotional knowledge, memory, planning, creativity and problem solving. It can also be more generally described as the ability to perceive and/or retain knowledge or information and apply it to itself or other instances of knowledge or information, creating referable, understandable models of any size, density, or complexity, due to a conscious or subconscious imposed will or instruction to do so.

**intoxication:** an organic mental syndrome characterised by the presence in the body of an exogenous psycho-active substance that produces a substance-specific syndrome of effects on the central nervous system that leads to **maladaptive behaviour** such as belligerence or impaired social or occupational functioning.

**introspection:** looking inwards and directly consulting one's attitudes, feelings and thoughts for meaning.

**introversion:** a **personality** type described by Carl Jung; it is'the state of or tendency toward being wholly or predominantly concerned with and interested in one's own mental life'. The introvert prefers solitary activities, enjoys time spent alone, and finds less reward in time spent with large groups of people.

**intrusion (dissociative):** unwanted thoughts or impulses that enter the mind or unwanted emotions that arise.

**involuntary care, treatment and rehabilitation:** the provision of health interventions to people who are incapable of making informed decisions due to their mental health status and who refuse health intervention but require such services for their own protection or for the protection of others.

**ionophore:** a hydrophilic pore that transcends a cell membrane, allowing ions to pass through while avoiding contact with the membrane's hydrophobic interior.

**ionotropic receptor:** a receptor that is structurally associated with an ion channel and the influx of anions or cations.

**jargon aphasia:** incoherent, meaningless speech with **neologisms**.

**judgement:** the cognitive faculty that allows one to evaluate evidence to make a decision, to adjudicate, to decide or discern between various options.

**karyotype:** the general appearance (size, number and shape) of chromosomes.

**khat:** a drug that is derived from the young leaves of the *Catha edulis* shrub. A stimulant, its effects are similar to an amphetamine. It is believed to alleviate fatigue and reduce appetite if chewed in moderation. The leaves, twigs or shrub can be smoked, chewed, brewed as tea or sprinkled over food.

**kindling:** the effects of repeated seizures on the brain, whereby a first seizure may increase the likelihood of more seizures occurring. Although controversial as a model in epilepsy, it has also been used to describe the development over time of certain psychiatric illnesses, especially depression, whereby repeated episodes increase the chances of subsequent episodes.

**labelling:** a prejudgement or assumption about someone or something without having sufficient knowledge to do so with guaranteed accuracy.

***la belle indifférence*:** a naïve, inappropriate lack of emotion or concern in the face of perceptions by others of a patient's apparently grave symptoms, seen in conversion disorder.

**labile affect and emotions:** affect and emotions that are constantly undergoing change (e.g. from crying to laughter and from happiness to depression). There are rapid and dramatic shifts in emotional tone.

**libido:** a person's overall sexual **drive** or desire for sexual activity.

**ligand:** any compound (endogenous or xenobiotic) that binds to a given neuroreceptor. It may be either stimulate or block the receptor.

**lobotomy:** also known as a leucotomy; a neurosurgical procedure and a form of psychosurgery, which consists of cutting or scraping away most of the connections to and from the prefrontal cortex (the anterior part of the frontal lobes of the brain).

**loosening of associations:** also known as **derailment**; a thought disorder characterised by discourse consisting of a sequence of unrelated or only remotely related ideas. The frame of reference often changes from one sentence to the next.

**macropsia:** a neurological condition that affects human visual **perception**, in which objects within an affected section of the visual field appear larger than normal and which causes the person to feel smaller than he or she actually is.

**magical thinking:** the attribution of a causal relationships between actions and events that cannot be justified by reason and observation.

**maladaptive behaviour:** a type of behaviour that is often used to reduce one's anxiety, but with a dysfunctional and non-productive result.

**malingering:** fabrication or exaggeration of the symptoms of mental or physical disorders for a variety of 'secondary gain' motives, which may include financial compensation (often tied to fraud); **avoidance** of school, work or military service, the obtaining of drugs; the securing of a lighter criminal sentence or simply to attract attention or sympathy.

**mania:** a mood state characterised by elation, **agitation**, hyperactivity, hypersexuality and accelerated thinking and speaking.

**mannerism:** a habitual or characteristic manner, mode, or way of doing something; distinctive quality or style, as in behaviour or speech.

**melancholia:** a severe form of depression characterised by the presence of a specific combination of symptoms.

**mental health literacy:** the knowledge and beliefs about mental disorders, the ability to recognise specific disorders, to identify risk factors and to display help-seeking behaviour.

**metabotropic receptor:** a receptor that is structurally associated with a trans-membrane spanning guanosine (G)-protein coupled receptor, leading to the enzymatic conversion of membrane precursors to an active intracellular signalling molecule.

**micrographia:** an acquired disorder, usually associated with neurological conditions such as Parkinson's disease, where there is abnormally small, cramped handwriting or a progression to continually smaller handwriting.

**micropsia:** a condition that affects human visual **perception** in which objects are perceived to be smaller than they actually are.

**mindfulness:** the intentional, accepting and non-judgemental focus of one's **attention** on the emotions, thoughts and sensations occurring in the present moment, which can be trained by meditational processes.

**misidentification syndromes (delusional):** a group of delusional disorders that occur in the context of a mental or neurological illness. They all involve a belief that the identity of a person, object or place has somehow changed or has been altered. As these **delusions** typically only concern one particular topic they also fall under the category called monothematic delusions (e.g. **Capgras, Cotard, Fregoli syndromes**).

**misperception:** the incorrect or mistaken interpretation of a sensory stimulus (e.g. a moving curtain is mistakenly perceived as a face in the window).

**mode of action:** a change at the cellular level, brought about as a result of exposure to a pharmacologically active substance.

**monotherapy:** treatment of a condition by means of a single drug.

**monozygotic twins:** identical twins that develop from one zygote that splits and forms two embryos.

**mood-congruent delusion:** a **delusion** with mood-appropriate content (e.g. a depressed person believes that a TV news anchor disapproves of him or her, or a person in a manic state believes he or she is a powerful deity).

**mood-incongruent delusion:** a **delusion** with content that has no association to a mood or is mood neutral.

**mutation:** a change in the structure of a gene so that it alters the genetic message; this mutation may be transmitted to subsequent generations. These changes may include single-base alterations or larger deletions, insertions or rearrangements.

**mutism:** verbal unresponsiveness; an absence of the faculty of speech.

**myoclonus:** brief, involuntary twitching of a muscle or a group of muscles.

**negativism:** when, on examination, a patient resists attempts to move him or her and does the opposite of what is asked. Usually a sign of **catatonia**, it may progress to (catatonic) rigidity.

**neologism:** from the Greek words, *neos* (new) and *logos* (word); a new word or phrase of the patient's own making (e.g.'headshoe' to mean hat) or an existing word used in a new sense; often seen in schizophrenia. In psychiatry, such usages may have meaning only to the patient or be indicative of the patient's condition.

**neurodegeneration:** nervous tissue degeneration.

**neurodevelopment:** the processes that generate, shape and reshape the nervous system, from the earliest stages of embryogenesis to the final years of life.

**neurogenesis:** the development of nervous tissue.

**neuromodulation:** electrical stimulation of a nerve, the spinal cord or the brain for therapeutic effect.

**neuroticism:** a fundamental **personality trait** characterised by anxiety, fear, moodiness, worry, envy, frustration, jealousy and loneliness.

**neurovegetative:** pertaining to the autonomic nervous system.

**nihilism:** ideas of meaninglessness, transience or nonexistence.

**nociceptive/nociception:** the ability to induce or register pain.

**nucleoside:** a glycosylamine; essentially any nucleotide without a phosphate group; it includes cytidine, uridine, adenosine, guanosine, thymidine and inosine.

**nyaope:** also known as **whoonga**; a mixture of cannabis, heroin, ARVs, and rat poison or/and baking powder to give it bulk.

**obsessions:** recurrent and persistent thoughts, urges, or images that are experienced as intrusive and unwanted and that usually cause marked anxiety or distress.

**off-label prescription:** unapproved, but legal, prescribing of medications for uses other than their intended indications.

**olfactory hallucination:** false **perception** of smell.

**operant conditioning:** a method of learning that occurs through rewards (reinforcements) and punishments for behaviour. It encourages the subject to associate desirable or undesirable outcomes with certain behaviour.

**orientation:** a cognitive function that allows one to locate oneself temporally, geographically and in terms of personal identity; it involves awareness of three dimensions: time, place and person.

**overvalued ideas:** isolated, preoccupying beliefs, accompanied by a strong affective response, that are held strongly but are open to being corrected when evidence is provided to contradict them.

**paediatric auto-immune neuropsychiatric disorders associated with streptococcal infections (PANDAS):** a hypothetical disease in which a subset of children are thought to exhibit a rapid onset of OCD and/or **tics** subsequent to group A beta-haemolytic streptococcal (GABHS) infections.

**paranoia:** a mental condition characterised by **delusions** of, for example, persecution, which may be typical of a **personality** disorder, drug or **substance abuse** or of a psychotic disorder.

**paraphilia:** any intense and persistent sexual interest other than genital stimulation or preparatory fondling with phenotypically normal, physically mature, consenting human partners.

**paraphilic disorder:** a variation or disturbance of sexual preference that causes significant distress or dysfunction in the individual and/or entails a risk of harm or actual harm to others.

**parasomnias:** a category of sleep disorders that involve abnormal movements, behaviour, emotions, **perceptions** and dreams that occur while falling asleep, sleeping, between sleep stages, or during arousal from sleep.

**parasuicide:** derived from the Greek'near'; an act that resembles suicide, it is the deliberate infliction of injury on oneself or the taking of a drug overdose in an attempt at suicide that may not be intended to be successful. It is a non-fatal act in which a person deliberately causes injury to himself or herself or ingests any prescribed or generally recognised therapeutic dose in excess.

**parkinsonism:** neurologically associated movement disorders characterised by hypokinesia, **tremors** and muscle rigidity.

**partial agonist:** a pharmacological molecule that binds to a receptor and stimulates it to a lesser degree than its neurotransmitter/physiological **ligand** would, but does not have full intrinsic activity, so receptor activation can only be partial.

**passivity phenomena:** phenomena wherein people feel that some factor of themselves is under the management of other people.

**pathological gambling:** persistent and recurrent **maladaptive behaviour** characterised by an inability to control **gambling** and that leads to significant detrimental psychosocial consequences in personal, familial, financial, professional and legal matters.

**pathophysiology:** the physiology of disordered function.

**people living with HIV/Aids (PLWHA):** collective term used for people who live with HIV and Aids and who having to cope with the **stigma** and **discrimination** that accompany the **diagnosis**.

**perception:** the organisation, identification and interpretation of sensory information in order to represent and understand the environment.

**perplexity:** appearing puzzled or bewildered over what is not understood or certain.

**persecutory (delusion):** the most common type of **delusion**; it involves the theme of being followed, harassed, cheated, poisoned or drugged, conspired against, spied on, attacked or otherwise obstructed in the pursuit of one's goals.

**perseveration:** uncontrollable repetition of a particular response, such as a word, phrase, or gesture, despite the absence or cessation of the original stimulus. It is usually seen in organic disorders of the brain, delirium or **dementia** and can be seen in schizophrenia as well.

**personality:** a person's totality of innate, enduring and recognisable patterns of perceiving, relating to and thinking about themselves, others and the environment.

**person-centred psychiatry:** an initiative to place the whole person, rather than the disease, at the centre of mental health care. It is contingent on the quality of the therapeutic relationship and an integrative approach to the mind, the body and the spirit. It is described as 'a psychiatry of the person, by the person, for the person and with the person'.

**pharmacodynamics:** the **mode of action** of a drug, and thus both the therapeutic and unwanted effects of the substance on the body.

**pharmacogenetics:** the scientific study of the relationship between genetic factors and the nature of responses to drugs.

**pharmacokinetics:** the processes that determine the concentration of a substance or drug at the receptor. It encompasses all processes that the substance is subjected to in the body, and includes absorption, distribution, metabolism (biotransformation) and elimination.

**pharmacotherapy:** the treatment of disease through the administration of drugs or medication.

**phenomenology:** a term that has been and is used with many different meanings. Currently it is widely used to refer to a method for carefully describing and cataloguing particular mental states. The phenomenology of a psychiatric disorder refers to the symptoms and signs (phenomena) that characterise that disorder.

**phenotype:** the observable characteristics (e.g. appearance, physiological parameters) of an individual. The phenotype is influenced by both the **genotype** and the environment.

**phobia:** a type of anxiety disorder, it is a persistent fear of an object or situation, typically disproportional to the actual danger posed; the sufferer goes to great lengths to avoid it and often recognises it as being irrational.

**photopsia:** the presence of perceived flashes of light. It is most commonly associated with posterior vitreous detachment, migraine with **aura**, migraine aura without headache, retinal break or detachment, occipital lobe infarction and sensory deprivation (ophthalmopathic **hallucinations**).

**physical symptoms:** subjective evidence of physical disturbance (e.g. back pain, headache, bowel disturbances, dizziness, palpitations, fatigue) as observed by the patient; broadly, something that indicates the presence of a physical disorder. Physicians tend to label such symptoms as 'physical' while mental health specialists tend to use the term '**somatic**', the two adjectives are synonymous and can be used interchangeably.

**pica:** an appetite for substances that are largely non-nutritive, such as paper, clay, metal, chalk, soil, glass or sand.

**polygenic inheritance:** one characteristic that is controlled by two or more genes. Often the genes are large in quantity but small in effect. Most psychiatric disorders are thought to have a polygenic pattern of inheritance.

**polypharmacy:** the administering of many drugs together or the administering of excessive medication.

**positive health:** a definable and measurable state beyond the mere absence of disease. The focus is on well-being, with an emphasis on **recovery**, wellness and functioning. It concerns the personal experience of health, where the mind, belief system and inner attitude of the person are important. Health is seen as something that must be created; to facilitate this, the strengths of the patient must be identified.

**posturing:** bizarre poses that are maintained indefinitely.

**power of attorney:** authorisation to represent or act on another's behalf in private affairs, business or some other legal matter.

**Prader-Willi syndrome:** a rare genetic disorder with low muscle tone, short stature, incomplete sexual development, cognitive disabilities, problem behaviours and a chronic feeling of hunger that often leads to excessive eating and obesity.

**praxis (motor):** the ability of the brain to conceive, organise, and carry out a sequence of unfamiliar actions.

**prejudice:** a preconceived, usually unfavourable, opinion that results in negative attitudes and **stereotyped** beliefs about members of a specific group.

**preoccupation:** thoughts that dwell on a particular topic or theme.

**pressure of speech:** rapid and copious talk, often loud and difficult to interrupt.

**prevalence:** the number of cases of a disease that are present in a population at one point in time.

**priapism:** a painful medical condition in which the erect penis does not return to its flaccid state, often regarded as a medical emergency.

**primary psychiatric illness:** a category of mental disorder where the psychiatric symptomatology is not believed to be caused by another medical condition or by drug or **substance abuse**.

**prion:** a microscopic protein particle, apparently self-replicating despite the absence of nucleic acid, thought to be the infectious agent that causes Creutzfeld-Jakob disease and certain other neurodegenerative diseases.

**proband:** a particular subject (person or animal) being studied or reported on; the term used most often in medical genetics and other medical fields.

**problem gambler:** defining features are the emergence of negative consequences and the presence of a subjective sense of impaired control, construed as a disordered or diseased state that deviates from normal, healthy behaviour.

**prodromal:** an early symptom that indicates the onset of an attack or a disease.

**projection:** the misattribution of a person's undesired thoughts, feelings or impulses on to another person who does not have those thoughts, feelings or impulses.

**prosopagnosia:** also known as face blindness; a cognitive disorder of face **perception** where the ability to recognise faces is impaired, while other aspects of visual processing (e.g. object discrimination) and intellectual functioning (e.g. decision making) remain intact.

**protein kinase:** an enzyme that phosphorylates proteins, enzymes especially, leading to either activation or inhibition of that enzyme.

**pseudodementia:** a state of general **apathy** that resembles **dementia**, but is due to a psychiatric disorder rather than organic brain disease; it is potentially reversible (e.g. in depression).

***pseudologia phantastica*:** an elaborate, often fancifully embellished account of one's exploits, where limited factual material is effortlessly interwoven with outright fantasy. Patients appear to believe their patently fallacious stories.

**pseudoseizures:** paroxysmal events that mimic epileptic seizures and are often misdiagnosed as such; they are psychogenic in origin.

**psychoactive substance:** any chemical substance that changes brain function and results in alterations in **perception**, mood or consciousness.

**psycho-education:** education offered to individuals with a mental health condition and their families to help empower them and deal with their condition in an optimal way.

**psychological mindedness:** the ability to understand one's own and/or other people's problems in psychological terms, to self-reflect and look inwardly for possible origins of problems.

**psychological symptoms:** subjective evidence of a psychological disturbance (e.g. depressed mood, anxiety, guilt) as observed by the patient and that can affect emotions, thoughts and behaviour; they indicate the presence of a mental disorder.

**psychomimetic:** a drug or compound that engenders a psychotic-like state.

**psychomotor agitation:** a series of unintentional and purposeless motions that stem from mental tension and anxiety of an individual.

**psychomotor retardation:** a slowing down of thought processes and physical activity.

**psychoneuro-immunology:** a field that focuses on the interaction of nervous, endocrine and immune regulatory systems in the body.

**psychopathology:** the scientific study of mental disorders, including efforts to understand their genetic, biological, psychological and social causes; **nosology**; the course of mental disorders across all stages of development, their manifestations and treatment.

**psychosocial causation:** factors in the social environment (e.g. urbanicity, migration status) that play a causal role in the occurrence of mental illnesses in members of the population.

**psychosocial rehabilitation:** the process of restoring the social functioning and well-being of an individual with a psychiatric **disability**.

**psychotherapy:** the treatment of mental disorders and behavioural disturbances using such psychological techniques as support, suggestion, persuasion, re-education, reassurance and insight, in order to alter **maladaptive** patterns of coping and to encourage personality growth.

**psychotropic:** a drug or chemical substance that crosses the blood-brain barrier and affects the function of the central nervous system and mental activities like **perception**, mood, emotion, consciousness and **cognition** and that alters behaviour.

**purging:** self-induced vomiting, misuse of laxatives, diuretics or enemas to control weight or shape.

**randomised placebo-controlled trials:** the gold standard for clinical trials, used to test the **efficacy** and side-effects of a particular treatment. Study subjects, after an assessment of their eligibility and recruitment, but before the study intervention, are randomly allocated to receive one or other of the alternative treatments under study.

**rationalisation:** putting something into a different light or offering a different explanation for one's perceptions or behaviour in the face of a changing reality.

**reaction formation:** the converting of unwanted or dangerous thoughts, feelings or impulses into their opposites.

**recidivism:** the act of a person repeating an undesirable behaviour after he or she has either experienced the negative consequences of that behaviour or has been treated or trained to extinguish that behaviour.

**reductionism:** a philosophical position, which holds that a complex system is nothing but the sum of its parts, and that an account of it can be reduced to accounts of individual constituents. This can be said of objects, phenomena, explanation, theories and meanings.

**re-experience:** relive a traumatic event through spontaneous or triggered upsetting memories. Sometimes these memories feel so real it is as if the event is actually happening again. This is called a '**flashback**'. Reliving the event may cause intense feelings of fear, helplessness, and horror – similar to the feelings the person had when the event took place.

**regression:** returning to a former or less developed emotional/psychological state in the face of unacceptable thoughts or impulses.

**relapse:** a recurrence of a past (typically medical) condition.

**reliability:** the extent to which a research instrument produces consistent results.

**remission:** abatement of the symptoms of a disease and the period over which it occurs.

**repression:** the **unconscious** blocking of unacceptable thoughts, feelings and impulses.

**restricted affect:** muted emotional reactions.

**retrograde amnesia:** a loss of memory-access to events that occurred, or information that was learned, before an injury or the onset of a disease.

**ritualistic behaviour:** a repetitive behaviour systematically used by a person to neutralise or prevent anxiety, usually associated with obsessive-compulsive spectrum behaviours or autism.

**Romberg's test:** a test of the body's sense of positioning (proprioception), which requires healthy functioning of the dorsal columns of the spinal cord.

**rumination:** the compulsively focused **attention** on the symptoms of one's distress and their possible causes and consequences, as opposed to their solutions.

**saccades:** quick, simultaneous movements of both eyes in the same direction.

**salience:** the state or quality by which something stands out relative to its neighbours. Saliency detection is considered to be a key attentional mechanism that facilitates learning and survival by enabling organisms to focus their limited perceptual and cognitive resources on the most pertinent subset of the available sensory data.

**schemata:** core beliefs derived from interactions between childhood experiences and innate patterns of behaviour.

**schizotypy:** a theory that states that there is a continuum of **personality** characteristics and experiences that range from normal dissociative, imaginative states to more extreme states related to psychosis and, in particular, schizophrenia.

**secondary psychiatric illness:** a category of mental disorder where the psychiatric symptomatology is believed to be caused by another medical condition or by drug or **substance abuse**.

**second messenger:** following activation of a membrane receptor by the 'first message' (a neurotransmitter), a sequence of events follows leading to the synthesis of a second messenger molecule on the inside of the cell that ultimately determines cellular response.

**self-efficacy:** the extent or strength of one's belief in one's ability to complete tasks and reach goals.

**self-esteem:** a person's overall emotional evaluation of his or her own worth. It is a judgement of oneself as well as an attitude toward the self. Self-esteem encompasses beliefs (e.g. 'I am competent', 'I am worthy') and emotions such as triumph, despair, pride and shame.

**sensitisation:** a non-associative learning process in which the repeated administering of a stimulus results in the progressive amplification of a response.

**sensitivity:** in screening, the capacity to identify all affected people within a specific population.

**sensorium:** the sum of an organism's **perception**, the 'seat of sensation' where it experiences and interprets the environment within which it lives. It is the total character of the unique and changing sensory environments perceived by individuals. These include sensing, perceiving and interpreting information about the world around us by using the faculties of the mind such as the senses, phenomenal and psychological perception, **cognition** and **intelligence**.

**serious mental disorders:** psychiatric disorders with a lower **prevalence** (e.g. schizophrenia, bipolar mood disorder, major depressive disorder with psychotic features).

**sero-testing phenomena:** the shock, anger, anxiety, guilt and **denial** that occurs as a transition point when one has tested positive for HIV.

**sero-discordant couple:** a couple comprised of one partner who is HIV positive and the other who is HIV negative.

**sero-concordant relationship:** a relationship where both partners are either HIV positive or HIV negative.

**sexual dysfunction:** a group of disorders characterised by a disturbance in a person's ability to respond sexually or to experience sexual pleasure.

**shebeen:** in South Africa, an informal bar or pub located within the community; historically associated with unlicensed establishments.

**sleep hygiene:** recommended behavioural and environmental practices that are intended to promote better quality sleep.

***snus*:** snus is a moist powder tobacco of Scandinavian origin, from a variant of dry snuff. It is placed under the upper lip, which does not result in the need for spitting. It is known by different names in other countries like chewing tobacco in America and *makla* in Belgium and Africa. It is a precursor to snuff, which is a dry powder tobacco. Tobacco-free *snus* has been available since 2006.

**social capital:** aspects of social networks, relations, trust and power that can be studied as a property of individuals or as a property of groups (ecological). Also refers to the ability of individuals to draw on collective group level resources and that appears to be protective against mental ill-health.

**social cognition:** the evolved and normally developed ability to interact with other individuals; reading and interpreting social signals and responding appropriately to them.

**social defeat:** chronic experience of an inferior position or social exclusion, associated with the development of mental illnesses such as depression and psychosis.

**social determinants of health (SDH):** initiated by the World Health Organization, the SDH represent a focus on the economic and social conditions – and their distribution among the population – that influence individual and group differences in health status.

**social drift/selection:** the theory that people with a severe mental illness tend to drift down in social and economic class as a result of the illness, thereby explaining the increased **prevalence** of these disorders in lower socioeconomic groups.

**somatic:** of, relating to, or affecting the body, as distinguished from the mind or psyche.

**somatising:** a tendency whereby a mental event, notably a distressing one, such as anxiety, is expressed as a physical, bodily or **somatic** experience or symptom.

**somnolence:** inability to maintain alertness without constant stimulation.

**specificity:** in screening, the capacity to select 'true' cases that correspond to an established clinical concept.

**splitting:** an immature **defence mechanism** that involves a tendency to appraise others in extreme terms (i.e. as either all good or all bad). Also, a tendency to create divisions between others through one's words and behaviour.

**stereotypes:** standardised and simplified conceptions of groups based on some prior assumption that is not always factually correct.

**stereotypy:** a repetitive or **ritualistic** movement, posture or utterance; it may be simple movements, such as body rocking, or complex, such as self-caressing, crossing and uncrossing of legs and marching in place. Seen in autism, intellectual **disability**, schizophrenia, **dementia** and movement disorders.

**Stevens-Johnson syndrome:** a severe form of erythema multiforme and a variant of toxic epidermal necrolysis, causing ulceration of the skin and mucosal surfaces.

**stigma:** a mark of disgrace, infamy, stain or reproach on a person or a group.

**stupor:** extreme unresponsiveness and hypo-activitiy associated with altered arousal during which the patient fails to respond to questions or commands.

**sublimation:** the channelling of unacceptable thoughts, emotions or impulses into more acceptable ones.

**substance abuse:** a **maladaptive** pattern of substance use over a 12 month period that leads to clinically significant impairment or distress and that is manifested by one or more of the following symptoms: recurrent substance use in situations that cause physical danger to the user, recurrent substance use in the face of obvious impairment in school or work situations or recurrent substance use despite social or interpersonal problems.

**substance dependence:** a cluster of cognitive, behavioural and physiological symptoms indicating that a person continues the use of a substance despite significant substance-related problems.

**subsyndromal:** characterised by or exhibiting symptoms that are not severe enough for **diagnosis** as a clinically recognised syndrome.

**sugars:** a mixture of cannabis and cocaine. It apparently first surfaced in Chatsworth in Durban, but lost popularity when other ingredients were added to turn it into ***whoonga***.

**suicidal ideation:** thoughts of harming or killing oneself.

**suicidal intent:** the intention or considered decision to commit suicide.

**suicidality:** all suicide-related behaviours or thoughts.

**sundowning:** increased general confusion as natural light begins to fade and increased shadows appear; associated with **dementia**, especially Alzheimer's disease.

**switching (dissociative):** a sudden change or shift in executive functioning between different self-states or **alters/alter personalities**.

**switching (mood):** a shift in mood from a depressive state to an elevated state (**mania/hypomania**) related to antidepressant use (normally indicates a bipolar disorder).

**sympathomimetic:** an agent that produces effects similar to those of impulses conveyed by adrenergic postganglionic fibres of the sympathetic nervous system.

**synapse/synaptic cleft:** the fluid-filled space between the pre- and postsynaptic neuron into which transmitter is released.

**synaptic plasticity:** the ability of a synapse to change as circumstances require by altering function through increasing/decreasing sensitivity or their actual numbers.

**systematised delusion:** a fixed, false belief with a complex logical structure.

**tangentiality:** a thought disorder where there is a lack of observance to the main subject of discourse (e.g. when a person, whilst speaking on a topic, deviates from it).

**tardive dyskinesia:** a hyperkinetic movement disorder caused by long-term administration of first-generation antipsychotic medication; it manifests with quick, jerky, choreiform limb movements as well as facial and tongue movements such as chewing, tongue protrusions and facial grimacing, all of which are thought to be due to the **up-regulation** of dopamine receptors in the nigrostriatal pathway.

**teratogenicity:** the tendency to produce physical defects in embryos and foetuses.

**therapeutic index:** plasma concentration range in which a drug is effective.

**thought blocking:** complete interruption of speech before a thought or an idea has been completely expressed.

**thought content:** the ideas, beliefs and subjects of one's thoughts.

**thought flow:** the speed or rate of thoughts.

**thought form:** the structure and logical coherence of thoughts.

**thought insertion:** sensation that thoughts are being placed in one's mind.

**thought withdrawal:** sensation of having one's thoughts removed from one's mind.

**tics:** sudden, repetitive, non-rhythmic and unpredictable simple or complex movements (motor tics) and utterances (phonic tics) that involve discrete muscle groups brief movement.

**tolerance:** a phenomenon whereby an alcohol or drug user becomes physiologically accustomed to a particular dose of a substance (i.e. decreased response) and requires increasing dosages in order to obtain the same effects.

**toluene:** a clear water-insoluble liquid that smells like paint thinners. It has multiple uses, including breaking red blood cells to extract haemoglobin in biochemistry experiments, dissolving paint, rubber and silicone, acting as an octane booster in fuel, acting as a coolant because of its heat transfer properties or removing cocaine from coca leaves to make cola syrup.

**topography:** the distribution of parts or features on the surface or within an entity.

**traits:** attributes and qualities that describe the characteristic way in which a person thinks, feels and behaves in response to situations encountered in daily life.

**transcranial magnetic stimulation:** a non-invasive method to cause **depolarisation** or **hyperpolarisation** in brain neurons; sometimes used as a treatment tool for various neurological and psychiatric disorders such as Parkinson's disease, some OCDs and depression.

**transcription:** the first step of **gene expression**, in which a particular segment of DNA is copied into RNA by the enzyme RNA polymerase.

**transference:** the process whereby a patient responds and relates to the therapist in a way that mirrors his or her early relationships with caregivers.

**transgender:** the broad spectrum of individuals who transiently or persistently identify with a **gender** different from their natal gender.

**transgenerational epigenetic effects:** all processes that have evolved to achieve the non-genetic determination of **phenotype**. There has been a long-standing interest in this area from evolutionary biologists, who refer to it as non-Mendelian inheritance. Transgenerational epigenetic effects include both the physiological and behavioural transfer of information across generations. Although in most cases the underlying molecular mechanisms are not understood, modifications of the chromosomes that pass to the next generation through gametes are sometimes involved, which is called transgenerational epigenetic inheritance.

**transsexual:** an individual who seeks, or has undergone, a social transition from male to female or female to male, which in many cases also involves a **somatic** transition by cross-sex hormone treatment and sex reassignment surgery.

**transvestism:** cross-dressing behaviour used by men for the purpose of sexual excitement.

**treatment-resistant/treatment refractory depression:** cases of major depressive disorder that do not respond adequately to adequate courses of at least two antidepressants.

**tremor:** an involuntary, somewhat rhythmic, muscle contraction and relaxation involving to and from movements (oscillations or twitching) of one or more body parts.

**trichotillomania:** the compulsive urge to pull out (and in some cases, eat) one's own hair leading to noticeable hair loss, distress and social or functional impairment.

***ukuthwasa*:** a South African syndrome of ancestral calling to become a traditional healer. The individual experiences dreams of prominent ancestors and may manifest an illness including symptoms of manic states, depressive states, **hysteria** and **somatic** symptoms.

**unconscious:** the part of the mind that is inaccessible to the conscious mind but which affects behaviour and emotions.

**undoing:** an attempt to take back an **unconscious** behaviour or thought that is unacceptable or hurtful.

**up-regulation:** an increase in the number of neurotransmitter receptors at the synapse due to increased receptor synthesis.

**utilisation (stimulus-bound) behaviour:** a neurobehavioural disorder that involves the grabbing of objects in view and initiating the 'appropriate' behaviour associated with it at an 'inappropriate' time. These patients have difficulty resisting the impulse to operate or manipulate objects that are in their visual field and within reach. Characteristics include unintentional, **unconscious** actions triggered by the immediate environment. The unpreventable excessive behaviour has been linked to lesions in the frontal lobe.

**validity:** the extent to which a research instrument actually measures what it is supposed to measure.

**value judgement:** an assessment of the rightness or wrongness of something or someone, or of the usefulness of something or someone, based on a comparison or other relativity. Most commonly the term refers to one's opinion, which, of course, is formed to a degree by one's belief system and the culture to which one belongs. So a natural extension of the term *value judgement* is to include declarations seen in one way from one value system, but which may be seen differently from another.

**variable number tandem repeat (VNTR):** a location in the genome where multiple copies of short nucleotide sequences are organised as tandem repeats. These repeats vary in number.

**vegetative symptoms:** disturbances of a person's functions necessary to maintain life (vegetative functions). These include disturbances of sleep, appetite and sexual arousal and are most commonly seen in mood disorders.

**volume of distribution:** the apparent volume in which a drug is distributed; the amount of drug in a given volume of plasma.

**voluntary care, treatment and rehabilitation:** the provision of health interventions to a person who gives **consent** to such interventions.

**waxy flexibility:** also known as ***cerea flexibilitas***; a decreased response to stimuli and a tendency to remain in an immobile posture.

**whoonga:** Tanzanian in origin, it means 'the sound the brain makes'. It is a mixture of brown heroin, cut rat poison (strychrine), amnonia, tik (to make it go further) mixed with antiretrovirals (ritonavir to enhance and prolong the effects and efivarenz for colourful visions and vivid dreams.)

**withdrawal:** a substance-specific organic mental syndrome that follows the cessation of use or reduction in intake of a psycho-active substance that had been regularly used to induce a state of **intoxication**.

# Index

## A

# B

# C

# D

# E

# F

# I

# J



# K



# L



# M

# Q



# R

# T

# U